Uncommon Causes of Stroke

2nd edition

Edited by

Louis R. Caplan MD

Founding editor – Julien Bogousslavsky

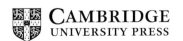

CAMBRIDGE
UNIVERSITY PRESS

CAMBRIDGE UNIVERSITY PRESS
Cambridge, New York, Melbourne, Madrid, Cape Town, Singapore, São Paulo, Delhi

Cambridge University Press
The Edinburgh Building, Cambridge CB2 8RU, UK

Published in the United States of America by Cambridge University Press, New York

www.cambridge.org
Information on this title: www.cambridge.org/9780521874373

First published 2008

First edition published 2001 © Cambridge University Press 2001

Printed in the United Kingdom at the University Press, Cambridge

A catalogue record for this publication is available from the British Library

Library of Congress Cataloguing in Publication data
Uncommon causes of stroke/edited by Louis R. Caplan; founding
editor, Julien Bogousslavsky. – 2nd ed.
    p. ; cm.
   Includes bibliographical references and index.
   ISBN 978-0-521-87437-3 (hardback)
   1. Cerebrovascular disease–Diagnosis.   2. Diagnosis, Differential.   3. Symptoms.
I. Caplan, Louis R.   II. Bogousslavsky, Julien.
   [DNLM: 1. Stroke–etiology.   2. Autoimmune Diseases–complications.
3. Genetic Diseases, Inborn–complications.   4. Infection–complications.
5. Metabolic Diseases–complications.
6. Vascular Diseases–complications. WL 355 U5414 2008]
   RC388.5.U515 2008
   616.8′1075–dc22

2008020313

ISBN 978-0-521-87437-3 hardback

CONTENTS

Contents

The color plates appear between pages 80 and 81

LIST OF CONTRIBUTORS

Harold P. Adams, Jr.
Division of Cerebrovascular Diseases
Department of Neurology
Carver College of Medicine
University of Iowa
Iowa City, Iowa, USA

Colum F. Amory
Stroke Center
Department of Neurology
The Mount Sinai School of Medicine
New York, New York, USA

Anne Angelillo-Scherrer
Service and Central Laboratory of
    Hematology
Centre Hospitalier Universitaire Vaudois
    and University of Lausanne
Lausanne, Switzerland

Irena Anselm
Department of Neurology
Children's Hospital
Boston, Massachusetts, USA

Marcel Arnold
Department of Neurology
University of Bern
Bern, Switzerland

Robert W. Baloh
Department of Neurology
UCLA School of Medicine
Los Angeles, California, USA

Ralf W. Baumgartner
Department of Neurology
University Hospital
Zürich, Switzerland

José Biller
Departments of Neurology and Neurological
    Surgery
Chairman Department of Neurology
Loyola University Chicago
Stritch School of Medicine
Maywood, Illinois, USA

Valérie Biousse
Departments of Ophthalmology and Neurology
Emory University School of Medicine
Atlanta, Georgia, USA

Matthias Bischof
Department of Neurology
University Hospital
Zürich, Switzerland

Julien Bogousslavsky
Department of Neurology
Genolier Swiss Medical Network
Valmont-Genolier, Switzerland

Natan M. Bornstein
Department of Neurology
Tel Aviv Sourasky Medical Center
Sackler Faculty of Medicine
Tel Aviv University
Tel Aviv, Israel

Marie Germaine Bousser
Department of Neurology
Hopital Lariboisière
Université Paris VII Denis Diderot
Paris, France

Robin L. Brey
Department of Neurology
University of Texas Health Science Center at San Antonio School
    of Medicine
San Antonio, Texas, USA

John C. M. Brust
Department of Neurology
Harlem Hospital Center
New York, New York, USA

Alan Bryer
Department of Neurology
University of Cape Town
South Africa

Olivier Calvetti
Departments of Ophthalmology and Neurology
Emory University School of Medicine
Atlanta, Georgia, USA

Louis R. Caplan
Department of Neurology
Beth Israel Deaconess Medical Center
Boston, Massachusetts, USA

José Castillo
Department of Neurology
Hospital Clínico Universitario
University of Santiago de Compostela
Santiago de Compostela, Spain

Hugues Chabriat
Department of Neurology
Hopital Lariboisière
Université Paris VII Denis Diderot
Paris, France

Chin-Sang Chung
Department of Neurology
Samsung Medical Center
Sungkyunkwan University School of
    Medicine
Seoul, Korea

Charlotte Cordonnier
Stroke Department
Department of Neurology
University of Lille
Roger Salengro Hospital
Lille, France

Steven C. Cramer
Department of Neurology
University of California
Irvine, California, USA

Luís Cunha
Hospitais da Universidade de Coimbra
Serviço de Neurologia
Coimbra, Portugal

Rima M. Dafer
Department of Neurology and Neurological Surgery
Loyola University Chicago
Stritch School of Medicine
Maywood, Illinois, USA

John F. Dashe
Department of Neurology
Tufts New England Medical Center
Boston, Massachusetts, USA

Cyrus K. Dastur
Department of Neurology
University of California
Irvine, California, USA

Antonio Dávalos
Department of Neurosciences
Hospital Germans Trias i Pujol
Universitat Autònoma de Barcelona, Spain

Larry E. Davis
Neurology Service
New Mexico VA Health Care System
Albuquerque, New Mexico, USA

Patricia Davis
Department of Neurology
University of Iowa Carver College of
    Medicine
Iowa City, Iowa, USA

Stephen M. Davis
Divisional Director of Neurosciences
Director of Neurology
Royal Melbourne Hospital and Professor of
    Neurology
University of Melbourne
Parkville, Victoria, Australia

Jan L. De Bleecker
Stroke Unit
Department of Neurology
University Hospital
Ghent, Belgium

Michael A. De Georgia
Neurological Intensive Care Program
The Cleveland Clinic Foundation
Cleveland, Ohio, USA

Amir R. Dehdashti
Division of Neurosurgery
Toronto Western Hospital
Toronto, Ontario, Canada

Oscar H. Del Brutto
Department of Neurological Sciences
Hospital – Clínica Kennedy
Guayaquil, Ecuador

Jacques L. De Reuck
Stroke Unit
Department of Neurology
University Hospital
Ghent, Belgium

Hans-Christoph Diener
Department of Neurology
University of Duisburg-Essen
Essen, Germany

Kathleen B. Digre
Departments of Neurology and Ophthalmology
Obstetrics and Gynecology
University of Utah
Salt Lake City, Utah, USA

Vivian U. Fritz
Department of Neurology
University of the Witwatersrand
South Africa

Nancy Futrell
Intermountain Stroke Research
Murray, Utah, USA

Bhuwan P. Garg
Department of Neurology
Indiana University School of Medicine
Indianapolis, Indiana, USA

Philip B. Gorelick
Department of Neurology and Rehabilitation
University of Illinois College of Medicine at
    Chicago, USA

Glenn D. Graham
Rehabilitation Service
New Mexico VA Health Care System
Albuquerque, New Mexico, USA

Alexander Y. Gur
Department of Neurology
Stroke Unit
Tel Aviv Sourasky Medical Center
Sackler Faculty of Medicine
Tel Aviv University
Tel Aviv, Israel

John J. Halperin
Department of Neurosciences
Atlantic Neuroscience Institute
Overlook Hospital, Summit, New Jersey
and Department of Neurology
Mount Sinai School of Medicine
New York, New York, USA

Michael Hennerici
Department of Neurology
Universitätsklinikum Mannheim
University of Heidelberg
Mannheim, Germany

Isabel Lestro Henriques
Department of Neurology
Centro Hospitalar de Lisboa and Instituto Gulbenkian de Ciência
Oeiras, Portugal

Roberto C. Heros
Department of Neurosurgery
University of Miami
Miami, Florida, USA

Daniel B. Hier
Department of Neurology and Rehabilitation
University of Illinois at Chicago
Chicago, Illinois, USA

Lorenz Hirt
Neurology Service
Centre Hospitalier Universitaire Vaudois and University of
    Lausanne
Lausanne, Switzerland

Joanna C. Jen
Department of Neurology
UCLA School of Medicine
Los Angeles, California, USA

Taro Kaibara
Department of Neurosurgery
University of Miami
Miami, Florida, USA

Sumit Kapoor
Department of Neurosurgery
Johns Hopkins Hospital
Baltimore, Maryland, USA

Sarosh M. Katrak
Department of Neurology
Grant Medical College and Sir J.J. Group of Hospitals and
    Consultant Neurologist
Jaslok Hospital and Research Centre
Mumbai, India

Siddharth Kharkar
Department of Neurosurgery
Johns Hopkins Hospital
Baltimore, Maryland, USA

Walter J. Koroshetz
National Institute of Neurological Disorders and Stroke
Bethesda, Maryland, USA

Monisha Kumar
Department of Neurology and Neurological Sciences
Stanford Stroke Center
Stanford School of Medicine
Palo Alto, California, USA

Sandeep Kumar
Department of Neurology
Beth Israel Deaconess Medical Center and Harvard Medical
    School
Boston, Massachusetts, USA

Emre Kumral
Department of Neurology
School of Medicine
Ege University
Izmir, Turkey

Tobias Kurth
Divisions of Aging and Preventive Medicine
Brigham and Women's Hospital
Harvard Medical School
Boston, Massachusetts, USA

Rogelio Leira
Department of Neurology
Hospital Clínico Universitario
University of Santiago de Compostela
Santiago de Compostela, Spain

Steven R. Levine
Stroke Center
Department of Neurology
The Mount Sinai School of Medicine
New York, New York, USA

Didier Leys
Stroke Department
Department of Neurology
University of Lille
Roger Salengro Hospital
Lille, France

Doris Lin
Division of Neuroradiology
Johns Hopkins University School of Medicine
Baltimore, Maryland, USA

Jonathan Lipton
Department of Neurology
Children's Hospital Boston and Harvard Medical School
Boston, Massachusetts, USA

Alfredo M. Lopez-Yunez
Neurohealth Ltd. of Indianapolis
Indiana, USA

Betsy B. Love
Department of Neurology
Loyola University of Chicago
Stritch School of Medicine
Maywood, Illinois, USA

Ayrton Roberto Massaro
Centro de Medicina Diagnóstica Fleury
São Paulo, Brazil

Heinrich P. Mattle
Department of Neurology
University Hospital of Bern, Switzerland

Manu Mehdiratta
Department of Neurology
Beth Israel Deaconess Medical Center
Harvard Medical School
Boston, Massachusetts, USA

John H. Menkes
Professor Emeritus of Neurology and Pediatrics
David Geffen School of Medicine at UCLA
Los Angeles, California, USA

Philippe Metellus
Department of Neurosurgery
Timone Hospital
Marseille, France

Reto Meuli
Department of Radiology
Centre Hospitalier Universitaire Vaudois and University of
    Lausanne
Lausanne, Switzerland

Patrik Michel
Neurology Service
Centre Hospitalier Universitaire Vaudois and University of
    Lausanne
Lausanne, Switzerland

Panayiotis Mitsias
Department of Neurology
Henry Ford Hospital
Detroit, Michigan, USA

Jorge Moncayo-Gaete
International University of Ecuador
Department of Neurology
Eugenio Espejo Hospital
Quito, Ecuador

Julien Morier
Neurology Service
Centre Hospitalier Universitaire Vaudois and University of
    Lausanne
Lausanne, Switzerland

Krassen Nedeltchev
Department of Neurology
University Hospital of Bern, Switzerland

Bernhard Neundörfer
Department of Neurology
University of Erlangen-Nuremberg
Erlangen, Germany

Olukemi A. Olugemo
Department of Neurology
University of Maryland
Baltimore, Maryland, USA

Nikolaos I. H. Papamitsakis
Department of Neurosciences and Director of
  Stroke Service
Department of Adult Neurology
Medical University of South Carolina
Charleston, South Carolina, USA

Stephen D. Reck
Department of Ophthalmology and Visual Sciences
University of Michigan
Ann Arbor, Michigan, USA

Luca Regli
Department of Neurosurgery
Centre Hospitalier Universitaire Vaudois and University of
  Lausanne
Lausanne, Switzerland

Marc D. Reichhart
Neurology Service
Centre Hospitalier Universitaire Vaudois and University of
  Lausanne
Lausanne, Switzerland

Daniele Rigamonti
Department of Neurosurgery
Johns Hopkins Hospital
Baltimore, Maryland, USA

Michael J. Rivkin
Harvard Medical School and Director
Stroke and Neurology In-Patient Services
Chidren's Hospital Boston
Massachusetts, USA

E. Steve Roach
Division of Child Neurology
Nationwide Children's Hospital
Ohio State College of Medicine
Columbus, Ohio, USA

Jose F. Roldan
Lupus and Vasculitis Clinic
Division of Clinical Immunology and Rheumatology
University of Texas Health Science Center at San Antonio School
  of Medicine, USA

David Z. Rose
Department of General Internal
  Medicine
Cleveland Clinic
Cleveland, Ohio, USA

Daniel M. Rosenbaum
Department of Neurology
SUNY Downstate Medical Center
Brooklyn, New York, USA

N. Paul Rosman
Department of Neurology
Floating Hospital
New England Medical Center
Boston, Massachusetts, USA

Elayna O. Rubens
Department of Neurology
Beth Israel Deaconess Medical Center
Boston, Massachusetts, USA

Sean I. Savitz
Department of Neurology
Beth Israel Deaconess Medical Center
Boston, Massachusetts, USA

Marc Schapira
Service and Central Laboratory of Hematology
Centre Hospitalier Universitaire Vaudois and University of
  Lausanne
Lausanne, Switzerland

Robert J. Schwartzman
Department of Neurology
Drexel University College of Medicine
Philadelphia, Pennsylvania, USA

Magdy Selim
Department of Neurology
Beth Israel Deaconess Medical Center
Boston, Massachusetts, USA

Yukito Shinohara
Department of Neurology
Federation of National Public Service Personnel Mutual Aid
  Associations
Tachikawa Hospital
Tachikawa, Tokyo, Japan

Aneesh B. Singhal
Department of Neurology
Massachusetts General Hospital
Harvard Medical School
Boston, Massachusetts, USA

Michael A. Sloan
Division of Neurology
Carolinas Medical Center
Charlotte, North Carolina, USA

Barney J. Stern
Department of Neurology
University of Maryland
Baltimore, Maryland, USA

Mathias Sturzenegger
Department of Neurology
Bern University Hospital
Inselspital
and University of Bern
Bern, Switzerland

Oriana Thompson
Department of Neurology
SUNY Downstate Medical Center
Brooklyn, New York, USA

A. Wesley Thevathasan
Department of Neurology
Royal Melbourne Hospital
Melbourne, Australia

Jonathan D. Trobe
Departments of Neurology and
   Ophthalmology
University of Michigan
Ann Arbor, Michigan, USA

Michael Varner
Department of Obstetrics and Gynecology
University of Utah School of Medicine
Salt Lake City, Utah, USA

Dana Védy
Service and Central Laboratory of Hematology
Centre Hospitalier Universitaire Vaudois and University of
   Lausanne
Lausanne, Switzerland

Jorge Vidaurre
Division of Child Neurology
Nationwide Children's Hospital
Ohio State College of Medicine
Columbus, Ohio, USA

Engin Y. Yilmaz
Ingalls Memorial Hospital
Neurology Associates Ltd.
Harvey, Illinois, USA

Khaled Zamel
Division of Child Neurology
Nationwide Children's Hospital
Ohio State College of Medicine
Columbus, Ohio, USA

Mathieu Zuber
Department of Neurological and Neurovascular diseases
University Paris 5 – René Descartes
Saint-Joseph Hospital
Paris, France

PREFACE

Dr. Julien Bogousslavsky and I, during a lunchtime conversation, thought of the idea of editing a book that would represent a source reference about various stroke syndromes and causes of stroke. The first publication appeared in 1995 and included: 1) patterns of symptoms and signs, 2) lesion patterns in patients with infarcts and hemorrhages in various brain locations and in various vascular territories, and 3) "patterns and syndromes that occur in unusual conditions that are known to cause stroke but that are not encountered very often." The book was conceived as a compilation of stroke syndromes and so was entitled *Stroke Syndromes*. The entire book contained 510 pages. The third section of the book entitled "particular vascular etiologic syndromes" consisted of 15 chapters covered in only 95 pages.

After the book was published and Bogousslavsky and I received considerable feedback and did our own postmortem thinking about the book, we concluded that: 1) the two main topics – *syndromes* and *uncommon causes* – were quite different, and 2) each was inadequately covered in the initial publication. We decided to edit separate greatly expanded volumes on each topic. *Stroke Syndromes, 2nd edition*, was published in 2001 and contained 54 chapters and 747 pages. A separate volume entitled *Uncommon Causes of Stroke* also appeared in 2001 and contained 48 chapters and 391 pages.

Uncommon Causes proved very successful but, as always, in carefully conducting a postmortem we found that there were many omissions and that some chapters were not optimally written. Furthermore, during the ensuing years there were important advances in diagnostic technology, more physicians and researchers became involved in cerebrovascular disease-related activities, and there were many advances in therapeutics. We decided to edit a second edition of *Uncommon Causes*.

A major change from the first edition is that I am the sole editor of this volume. Dr. Bogousslavsky and I together initially planned the outline and contributors to this second edition of *Uncommon Causes*, but he was not involved later in writing any of the chapters or in collecting or editing the chapters. The sole editorship allowed a somewhat more uniform style and language and collation of the various chapters.

In this edition, I have attempted to simplify the English to make the chapters more easily read and understood by readers. I have also expanded the number of chapters and have revised the authorship of many of the chapters. I wrote or co-authored 13 of the chapters. I have also edited each chapter in the book to ensure that it is accurate, complete, referenced sufficiently, and authoritative. I take sole responsibility for the final form of each chapter. This volume contains 71 chapters.

I owe considerable thanks to Dr. Julien Bogousslavsky, who was the progenitor of the original idea of publishing a compilation of chapters on unusual stroke-related vascular conditions. He also deserves credit for helping to plan this volume. The staff at Cambridge University Press has been involved in all of the publications in this series. Dr. Richard Barling was responsible for shepherding the first volumes in this series and was initially involved in the planning of this volume. Rachel Lazenby worked with me to ensure that the authors submitted completed chapters in the time assigned. Matthew Byrd deserves considerable credit for creating the final proofs and nursing the volume into print. Nicholas Dutton, Laura Wood, and others at Cambridge University Press were also instrumental in ensuring publication. Most of all I thank my colleagues who wrote the chapters and put up with my frequent prodding and cajoling. They have done an outstanding job.

Louis R. Caplan MD

Boston, Massachusetts

PART I: INFECTIOUS AND INFLAMMATORY CONDITIONS

ISOLATED ANGIITIS OF THE CENTRAL NERVOUS SYSTEM

Mathieu Zuber

Isolated angiitis of the central nervous system (CNS) is a rare condition with an incidence estimated at less than 1:2 000 000 (Moore, 1999). It was defined, in 1959, as an idiopathic vasculitis restricted to small leptomeningeal and parenchymal arteries and veins, without apparent systemic involvement (Cravioto and Feigin, 1959). Almost 50 years later, the affliction remains poorly recognized, and its pathogenesis mysterious, despite the growing pool of knowledge on processes responsible for CNS inflammation. The term "primary angiitis" is sometimes preferred to "isolated angiitis" because complete autopsies are rarely performed and minor abnormalities are occasionally observed in systemic organs of patients who died from so-called isolated CNS angiitis (Johnson et al., 1994). In numerous patients with no histological proof of vascular inflammation, the descriptive term "angiopathy" is more appropriate than "angiitis," but the latter term has often been overused in the recent literature.

Although stroke most often reveals the disease, it appears as the initial manifestation in only a minority of patients. Because of the protean clinical symptoms and blurred diagnostic criteria, identification is a difficult challenge for all clinicians.

Pathology and pathogenesis

Pathological picture

Isolated CNS angiitis has been referred to by several names descriptive of the pathological findings: granulomatous angiitis of the CNS, giant cell granulomatous angiitis of the CNS, and cerebral granulomatous angiitis have all been used interchangeably (Hankey, 1991; Rhodes et al., 1995). This variable terminology partly reflects the difficulty in separating isolated CNS angiitis as a pathological entity from systemic disorders, such as giant cell temporal angiitis or sarcoidosis, themselves occasionally responsible for CNS angiitis.

The nonspecific pathological pattern of isolated CNS angiitis is characterized by infiltrations of the vascular walls with mononuclear cells including lymphocytes, macrophages, and histiocytes. Fibrinoid necrosis is occasionally seen, especially in the acute phase (Craviato and Feigin, 1959; Hankey, 1991; Lie, 1992; Rhodes et al., 1995). In about 85% of patients, granulomas with epithelioid cells and giant Langerhans cells are described. The degree of this granuloma formation is variable. In early disease, granulomas are often not found. The misleading terminology "granulomatous

angiitis," should no longer be used to describe isolated CNS angiitis. The inflammatory lesions may sometimes spread to all the vascular wall layers but preservation of the media is the rule. Pure lymphocytic infiltration is rare, but it may be more frequent in childhood (Lanthier et al., 2001).

Vascular abnormalities primarily involve small- and middle-sized arteries and, less frequently, veins and venules. Arteries less than 500 μm in diameter may be solely affected. In most cases, leptomeningeal involvement is a dominating feature, with less consistent parenchymatous vascular involvement in white matter and gray matter. The segmental involvement of vessels may be responsible for false-negative histological results.

Pathogenesis

The pathogenesis of isolated CNS angiitis is unknown and progress is slow because of the rarity of tissue samples acquired from carefully documented cases. CNS inflammation activates the brainstem noradrenergic and trigeminovascular responses, contributing to reduction of regional vascular blood flow (Moore, 1998). This activation could enhance the appearance of arterial stenosis.

Isolated CNS angiitis is now regarded as an immunological, nonspecific T-cell-mediated inflammatory reaction rather than a specific entity (Calabrese et al., 1997; Ferro, 1998; Moore, 1998). This view is in accordance with:

1. the wide spectrum of diseases described in association with isolated CNS angiitis,
2. the limited known responses of the CNS blood vessels to a variety of noxious stimuli, and
3. the clinical and pathological heterogeneity of the disorder (although this may reflect individual differences in the host response).

The reason why the inflammatory response to various factors may be maladaptive and leads to disease remains mostly speculative. Chronicity of the stimuli, concurrent diseases, and genetic susceptibility are probably critical factors (Moore, 1998). According to the view that isolated CNS angiitis is probably a heterogeneous syndrome rather than a single entity, new conditions might emerge in the future that are placed in this category.

Indeed, instances of isolated CNS angiitis have been reported after various infections, such as mycoplasma, varicella zoster, or arbovirus infections (Chu et al., 1998). Both mycoplasma- and virus-like particles were identified in glial cells and cerebral blood

Uncommon Causes of Stroke, 2nd edition, ed. Louis R. Caplan. Published by Cambridge University Press. © Cambridge University Press 2008.

vessels of patients with isolated CNS angiitis (Arthur and Margolis, 1977; Linnemann and Alvira, 1980). Moreover, histological patterns very similar to isolated CNS angiitis have been reported in herpes zoster arteritis (Chu *et al.*, 1998) and a well-documented case previously published as CNS angiitis was recently shown to be in fact related to varicella zoster infection (Gilden *et al.*, 1996).

When angiitis is described in association with lymphoma, it usually remains unclear whether it is due to a malignant lymphoproliferative infiltration, the reactivation of some remote viral infection, or to nonspecific inflammatory mechanisms, such as those suspected to be responsible for isolated CNS angiitis (Greer *et al.*, 1988). Angiitis was also found to coexist with cerebral amyloid angiopathy (Fountain and Eberhard, 1996; Gray *et al.*, 1990). Angiitis is more probably an inflammatory response to β-A4-amyloid deposits than itself responsible for the amyloid deposition (Fountain and Eberhard, 1996; Yamada *et al.*, 1996). Patients with such association of both pathological lesions present with unusual clinical features (see the following Section). This so-called amyloid-related angiitis is a good example of a well-defined entity newly extracted from the wide spectrum of isolated CNS angiitis (Scolding *et al.*, 2005). More recently, a case associating isolated CNS angiitis and cerebral autosomal dominant arteriopathy with subcortical infarcts and leukoencephalopathy (CADASIL) was reported (Schmidley *et al.*, 2005).

Clinical features

The clinical presentation of CNS angiitis is highly variable because virtually any anatomic area of the CNS may be affected by the angiitis. Angiitis (whatever its cause) may thus mimic a wide range of CNS diseases. Isolated CNS angiitis has no specific symptoms that help to distinguish it from other causes of CNS vasculopathies, either infectious or noninfectious (Zuber *et al.*, 1999). A wide range of evolution has also been reported, stretching from a quasi-indolent disease to death in a few months (Calabrese and Mallek, 1988; Hankey, 1991; Johnson *et al.*, 1994). A subacute deterioration is most often observed. Relapsing symptoms are described.

Isolated CNS angiitis is twice as frequent in males as in females and onset most often occurs after 40 years of age. However, the disease can affect all age categories and cohorts of children with the condition were recently reported (Aviv *et al.*, 2006; Benseler *et al.*, 2005; Lanthier *et al.*, 2001). Conversely, mean age at presentation is unusually high (more than 65 years of age) in patients with β-amyloid-related angiitis (Scolding *et al.*, 2005).

Headache is the most common presenting symptom of isolated CNS (occurring in two-thirds of patients), and it is variable both in quality and severity (Hankey, 1991). Nonfocal symptoms, such as a fluctuating level of consciousness or a decrease in memory, associated with headaches, are typical of CNS angiitis and sometimes combine in an encephalopathic clinical pattern (Calabrese *et al.*, 1997). Abnormalities in cognition and behavior are present in most patients with β-amyloid-related angiitis (Scolding *et al.*, 2005). In some patients, headaches may suggest a chronic meningitis (Reik *et al.*, 1983).

All types of strokes have been observed in CNS angiitis including definite cerebral infarcts, transient ischemic attacks (TIAs), and

Table 1.1 Causes of cerebral angiitis *(adapted from Zuber et al., 1999)*

Infectious angiitis	Varicella zoster / Herpes zoster
	Cytomegalovirus infection
	Human immunodeficiency virus infection
	Mycotic and parasitic infections
	Syphilis
	Borrelia burgdorferi
	Tuberculosis
	Purulent bacterial meningitis
	Bacterial endocarditis
Primary systemic angiitis	Polyarteritis nodosa
Necrotizing	Churg and Strauss angiitis
Giant cell	Cogan's syndrome
– Granulomatous	Temporal angiitis
– Others	Takayasu's arteritis
	Wegener's granulomatosis
	Lymphomatoid granulomatosis
	Hypersensitivity angiitis, Kawasaki's arteritis
	Bürger's disease
	Susac's syndrome
	Kohlmeier–Degos disease
	Acute posterior multifocal placoid pigment epitheliopathy
Angiitis secondary to systemic disease	Systemic lupus erythematosus
	Sjögren's syndrome
	Behçet's disease
	Sarcoidosis
	Rheumatoid polyarthritis
	Scleroderma
	Mixed connectivitis
	Dermatomyositis
	Ulcerative colitis
	Celiac disease
Angiitis associated with neoplasia	Hodgkin's disease and non-Hodgkin's-type lymphoma
	Malignant histiocytosis
	Hairy cell leukemia
	Neoplastic meningitis
Angiitis associated with drug abuse or treatments	Illicit drugs (cocaine, crack)
	Sympathomimetic agents
	Amphetamine and relatives
	Transplantations
	Radiotherapy
Isolated angiitis of the CNS	

intraparenchymal and subarachnoid hemorrhages (Biller *et al.*, 1987; Johnson *et al.*, 1994; Koo and Massey, 1988; Kumar *et al.*, 1997; Moore, 1989). Intracranial bleedings could be more prevalent than ischemic strokes but this has not been systematically studied. These various intracranial bleedings are posited to result from vessel wall weakening resulting from transmural inflammation (Kristoferitsch *et al.*, 1984; Negishi and Sze, 1993). A multi-infarct state has been reported in some patients with CNS vasculitis (Koo and Massey, 1988).

In a critical review of isolated CNS angiitis patients, stroke was not found to be the presenting symptom in any of the histologically proven cases (Vollmer *et al.*, 1993). However, a stroke-like presentation in a patient with pre-existent diffuse cerebral symptoms should prompt a search for radiological signs in favor of angiitis. Subarachnoid hemorrhage was the presenting manifestation in several isolated CNS angiitis patients (Kumar *et al.*, 1997; Nishikawa *et al.*, 1998; Ozawa *et al.*, 1995).

Beside strokes, seizures and cranial neuropathies are other focal symptoms that occur in patients with isolated CNS angiitis (Hankey, 1991). A mass lesion presentation accounts for about 15% of patients. A necrotic unihemispheric presentation has rarely been reported (Derry *et al.*, 2002). Spinal cord involvement may be inaugural with a progressive paraparesis as the most common clinical manifestation (Bhibhatbhan *et al.*, 2006; Calabrese *et al.*, 1997). Exceptionally, the presence of spinal root pain may reveal an angiitis limited to the cauda equina (Harrison, 1976). Isolated CNS angiitis was also diagnosed in three patients with a posterior leukoencephalopathy characterized by major visual disturbances (Wijdicks *et al.*, 2003). On the whole, focal symptoms are observed in about 50% of patients (Calabrese and Mallek, 1988). However, focal symptoms nearly always occur in the setting of diffuse higher cortical impairment.

Fever is observed in 15% of patients and this confounding feature may be responsible for extensive systemic diagnostic testing (Hankey, 1991). If a patient has systemic complaints in addition to the cerebral symptoms, appropriate investigations will usually reveal some diffuse disorder responsible for multiorgan vasculitis. It is well-known that CNS angiitis, although rare, is one of the most serious complications of connective diseases and was described in most of them (Table 1.1).

Depending on the various clinical presentations, the differential diagnostic considerations are numerous. Meningoencephalitis, multiple sclerosis, abscess, and stroke of other mechanisms are the most frequently discussed in patients with acute or subacute onsets. A progressive onset may suggest neoplastic disease or dementia. Specific causes may also be discussed depending on the context, such as giant cell temporal angiitis in the elderly with headaches or Behçet's disease in a young Mediterranean patient with subacute rhombencephalitis.

Isolated CNS angiitis should also be distinguished from reversible cerebral vasoconstriction syndrome (the so-called Call–Fleming syndrome), a disease characterized by arterial vasoconstriction and much more frequent, in fact, than cerebral angiitis (Call *et al.*, 1988) (see Chapter 67). Segmental stenoses are located on medium-sized cerebral arteries and spontaneously resolve within weeks to months, although ischemic or hemorrhagic stroke may occasionally develop (Ducros *et al.*, 2007). The clinical presentation in patients with reversible angiopathy is most often different from cerebral angiitis, with an identified triggering condition for vasoconstriction, severe thunderclap headaches, and rapid improvement under nimodipine or

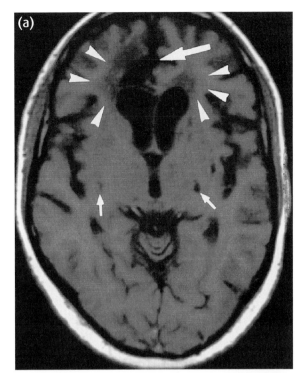

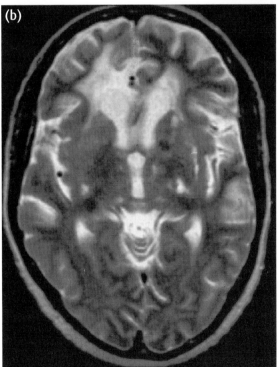

Figure 1.1 MRI abnormalities in patients with IACNS. (a) and (b) (same patient, T1- and T2-weighted sequences). Large infarction in the ACA territory (arrow) associated with deep profound infarctions (small arrows) and anterior leukoencephalopathy (arrowheads). (c) Lobar hemorrhage revealing IACNS.

other calcium channel blocker treatment (Zuber *et al.*, 2006). MR angiography shows arterial stenoses supporting the diagnosis in most cases and normalization of the vessel's caliber is observed on serial procedures, in association with clinical relief (Figure 1.1).

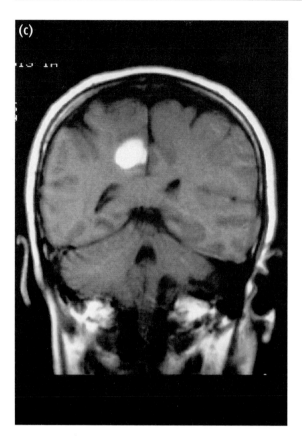

Figure 1.1 (*cont.*)

Diagnostic procedures

The cerebral arteries are separated from brain tissue by the blood–brain barrier so that biological markers supporting the diagnosis of isolated CNS angiitis are not found in most patients. The sedimentation rate is moderately increased in about 30% of biopsy-confirmed isolated CNS angiitis patients (Hankey, 1991). No immunological marker has been identified to date and antinuclear, antiphospholipid, and antineutrophil cytoplasmic antibodies are invariably normal. Cerebrospinal fluid (CSF) inflammation (moderate lymphocytic pleiocytosis, elevated protein, and normal glucose) is observed in about 90% of patients with histologically confirmed isolated CNS angiitis (Calabrese *et al.*, 1997) and is important (although highly nonspecific) for presumption of CNS vasculitis in a patient with stroke of remote origin. Oligoclonal bands are seldom reported. The CSF should always be cultured owing to possible CNS vasculitis due to viral, fungal, or indolent bacterial infections (Table 1.1).

Perivascular inflammatory lesions may be found in the retina, and fundoscopy has been reported as a valuable diagnostic tool in isolated CNS angiitis (Ohtake *et al.*, 1989). Optic fluorescein angiography could also be useful, especially in patients with normal cerebral angiography (Scolding *et al.*, 1997).

Brain imaging

Both cranial CT scans and MRIs show nonspecific abnormalities in CNS angiitis. The sensitivity of CT scan is low, at about

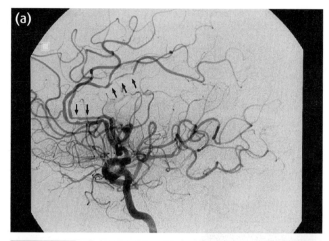

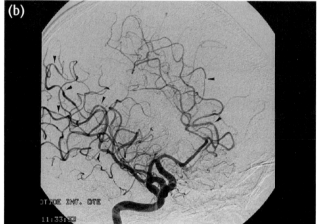

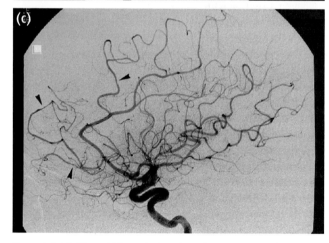

Figure 1.2 (a), (b), and (c). Cerebral angiography in patients with IACNS. Note the multiple stenoses on small- and middle-size arteries (arrows and arrowheads) delineating "sausage-like" appearances.

30%. MRI is of course more sensitive (about 80%), especially in detecting small brain lesions (Chu *et al.*, 1998) (Figure 1.2). The most common CT scan finding is focal or multifocal low density areas of varying sizes. Association with multiple parenchymal contrast enhancement and focal cerebral atrophy, or combination of both ischemic and hemorrhagic strokes, in the same patient is suggestive. Apart from signs of recent ischemic or hemorrhagic

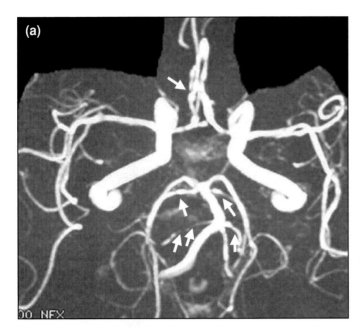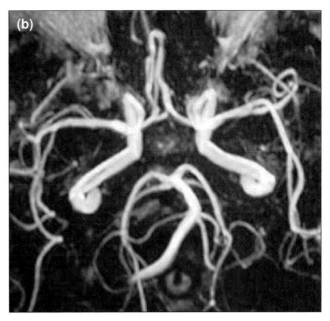

Figure 1.3 Serial MR angiography showing (a) multiple stenoses and filling defects on middle-size cerebral arteries and (b) complete resolution at one month in a reversible cerebral angiopathy. Adapted from Zuber *et al.* (2006) with kind permission of Springer Science and Business Media.

strokes, MRI frequently reveals nonspecific high intensity signals on T2-weighted sequences, sometimes responsible for leukoencephalopathy. Disseminated T2 hypersignals in white matter with no periventricular localization could indicate CNS angiitis, by contrast with the hypersignals described in multiple sclerosis (Miller *et al.*, 1987). Children with isolated CNS angiitis often have multifocal and supratentorial but unilateral lesions (Aviv *et al.*, 2006). Intracerebral hemorrhage, either in the cortex or the white matter, may occur as a result of infarction or focal necrosis of vessel walls (Hunn *et al.*, 1998). Hemorrhage is more frequent in isolated CNS angiitis than in infectious angiitis (Pierot *et al.*, 1991).

The fluid-attenuated inversion recovery (FLAIR) sequence may provide strong suspicion for distal intracranial arterial stenoses by showing several hyperintense vessel signs due to abnormal arterial blood flow kinetics (Iancu-Gontard *et al.*, 2003). Linear and punctate patterns of leptomeningeal enhancement accompanied by both hemispheric and penetrating vessels are observed in up to 60% of patients with isolated CNS angiitis, sometimes without significant parenchymal abnormalities (Chu *et al.*, 1998; Negishi and Sze, 1993). However, in my experience, visualization of leptomeningeal contrast enhancement is much less frequent. Recently, apparent diffusion coefficient mapping of the normal-appearing brain showed that abnormalities in patients with CNS angiitis are more diffuse than previously suspected (White, *et al.*, 2007).

Unusual CT scan and MRI presentations have been occasionally observed, including pseudotumoral lesions, repeated parenchymal or ventricular bleeding, multiple punctuate parenchymal contrast enhancement (milliary appearance), or diffuse white matter involvement suggesting a primary demyelinating disease (Finelli *et al.*, 1997; Hankey, 1991; Kristoferitsch *et al.*, 1984).

Angiography

The angiographic features characteristic of isolated CNS angiitis are multifocal stenoses rendering a sausage-like appearance with ectasia and occasional arterial occlusions (Figure 1.3). If the disease is restricted to arteries less than 500 μm in diameter, angiography will be reported as normal. A normal angiographical pattern is reported in up to 50% of patients, and abnormalities may only appear on repeated procedures (Kadkhodayan *et al.*, 2004; Linnemann and Alvira, 1980; Zuber *et al.*, 1999). Angiography-negative isolated CNS angiitis may be observed whatever the age, including in childhood (Benseler *et al.*, 2006). Intracerebral aneurysms and even multiple vanishing aneurysms have been seldom reported (Nishikawa *et al.*, 1998), but the pattern never mimics large ectasias of the arteries of the circle of Willis, similar to what has been typically reported in children and young adults with infections such as HIV (Kossorotoff *et al.*, 2006). Multiple microaneurysms, a very characteristic radiological pattern in peripheral tissues with vasculitis such as periarteritis nodosa, are invariably absent in isolated CNS angiitis (Chu *et al.*, 1998).

Because of the recent widespread development of the techniques, MR angiography and CT angiography are increasingly used as the first line radiological procedures for exploration of the intracerebral arteries in case of suspected CNS vasculitis. The sensitivity of both techniques for small cerebral vessel visualization has unquestionably improved over the past years. However, this sensitivity remains lower than with conventional angiography. Angiography has not been found to provide excessive risk in a large number of patients with suspected CNS vasculitis (0.8% of persistent morbidity) (Hellman *et al.*, 1992). For these different reasons, we believe that conventional angiography should still be regarded as the gold standard when CNS vasculitis is suspected.

Brain biopsy

The diagnosis of definite isolated CNS angiitis relies upon brain-leptomeningeal biopsy in all cases. The ideal diagnostic brain biopsy is a 1 cm wedge of cortex including leptomeninges and preferably containing a cortical vessel (Moore, 1989). Including leptomeninges in the biopsy is crucial because leptomeningeal involvement is a dominating pathological feature in isolated CNS angiitis (Hunn *et al.*, 1998; Zuber *et al.*, 1999). Among ten histologically confirmed isolated CNS angiitis patients, diagnostic changes were observed solely in leptomeningeal vessels in three patients (Chu *et al.*, 1998). False-negative biopsy results may be observed, particularly because of the segmental involvement of vessels, and cases with pathological features typical of isolated CNS angiitis recognized only on a recurrent biopsy have been reported. For patients without focal lesions, the preferred biopsy site is the prefrontal area or the temporal tip of the nondominant hemisphere. Nonspecific abnormalities found on brain imaging should provide useful information for selecting the biopsy site. However, mismatches between the radiological abnormalities and histological predominant lesions may explain false-negative biopsy results (Oliveira *et al.*, 1994). The use of stereotactic needle biopsies may account for a significant number of sampling errors because it lowers the sensitivity of biopsy to approximately 50% (Duna and Calabrese, 1995). This procedure should therefore be confined to cases with an isolated profound pseudotumoral lesion. Cultures of brain tissue and leptomeninges using special stains for various microorganisms should be systematically performed. The morbidity rate of brain biopsy (0.03%–2%) (Chu *et al.*, 1998; Hankey, 1991) cannot be overlooked but must be balanced against the risks of unnecessary immunosuppression.

Diagnostic strategy

Recognizing CNS angiitis is one of the most challenging neurological diagnostic problems. The reasons for this include:
1. relative rarity of the disorders,
2. lack of specificity for clinical signs and symptoms,
3. lack of efficient noninvasive diagnostic tests, and
4. inaccessibility of the end organ tissues for pathologic examination (Touzé and Méary).

The following diagnostic criteria were proposed by Moore (1989):
1. association of headaches and multiple neurological deficits that persist for at least 6 months,
2. segmental arterial stenoses on cerebral angiograms,
3. exclusion of any infectious or inflammatory cause, and
4. inflammatory lesions of the vascular wall on cerebral and/or leptomeningeal biopsy or exclusion of all other causes of cerebral angiitis.

Because of lack of specificity, there is currently no consensus regarding the appropriate use of brain imaging, angiography and brain biopsy for the diagnosis of isolated CNS angiitis (Duna and Calabrese, 1995; Harris *et al.*, 1994; Kadkhodayan *et al.*, 2004). There has been a recent trend towards diagnosing isolated CNS angiitis with angiography without tissue confirmation, at least in a subset of patients with a self-limited clinical course (Abu-Shakra

Table 1.2 Causes of segmental intracranial arterial narrowing (adapted from Zuber et al., 1999)

Cerebral angiitis, either:
– primary or secondary
– inflammatory or infectious
Intracranial dissection:
– traumatic
– spontaneous
– underlying vasculopathy (fibromuscular dysplasia)
Intracranial atherosclerosis
Recanalizing embolism
Vasospasm:
– acute hypertension
– reversible cerebral angiopathy
– migraine
Moya-moya
Cerebral radiotherapy
Tumor encasement:
– meningioma
– chordoma
– pituitary adenoma
– gliomatosis cerebri
Sickle cell anemia
Neurofibromatosis
Dysgenesis

et al., 1994). The problem is that we do not have early prognostic markers of isolated CNS angiitis and the disease may rapidly kill in the absence of appropriate treatment.

Few but important studies focused on the specificity of radiological signs suggestive for isolated CNS angiitis and asked whether these signs were predictive of a positive biopsy. Among MRI signs useful for the diagnosis of isolated CNS angiitis, leptomeningeal enhancement was found to be more sensitive than parenchymal abnormalities (Chu *et al.*, 1998; Duna and Calabrese, 1995). It should be stressed that the combination of normal MRI and CSF test results had a strong negative predictive value and allowed exclusion of CNS vasculitis in most clinical situations (Calabrese *et al.*, 1997). Whether high-resolution 3 Tesla MRI could provide more information than standard MRI for the diagnosis of isolated CNS angiitis remains to be determined.

In addition to a rather low sensitivity in showing arterial abnormalities when isolated CNS angiitis is suspected, conventional angiography has a low positive predictive value and specificity. As shown in Table 1.2, arterial stenoses in the brain may result from to various conditions, among which intracranial atherosclerosis and hypertensive vasospasms are the most frequently observed. The classical sausage-like segmental stenoses seem to be even more frequent in atherosclerosis or reversible cerebral angiopathy than in isolated CNS angiitis (Chu *et al.*, 1998). Topographical considerations may help for the differentiation: involvement of the supraclinoid carotid arteries and of the proximal MCA is usual in intracranial atherosclerosis, while more distal arteries are predominantly affected in isolated CNS angiitis. Arterial calcifications on a CT scan in the vicinity of stenoses may also be considered as indicative for intracranial atherosclerosis (Zuber *et al.*, 1999). Variations in stenoses on serial angiography are seen in CNS angiitis, but the pattern is also observed in reversible cerebral angiopathy.

Given first the lack of specific clinical and radiological features of isolated CNS angiitis, second the statistical likelihood of dealing with an alternative disorder, and third the morbidity associated with immunosuppressive regimens, we believe that early biopsy verification should be discussed in all patients with clearly suspected CNS angiitis (Calabrese *et al.*, 1997; Chu *et al.*, 1998). This assertion is reinforced by the recent publication of 25 patients with suspected primary CNS angiitis and negative brain biopsy: those who received an immunosuppressive therapy were not found to have a better outcome (Alreshaid and Powers, 2003).

The accuracy of diagnosis should be revisited periodically when the surgical procedure is delayed because of lack of evidence for CNS angiitis. Among stroke patients, the biopsy should be especially considered when headaches are prominent and associated with CSF and MRI abnormalities.

Treatment and prognosis

Reports before 1980 uniformly concluded that isolated CNS angiitis is a more or less rapidly fatal disease. This failed to account for the fact that isolated CNS angiitis was invariably diagnosed late in the evolution of the disease. In addition, no treatment regimen had been proposed in most patients.

Owing to the rarity of the disease, no controlled therapeutic trial has been conducted in isolated CNS angiitis to date, either diagnosed by leptomeningeal biopsy or by angiography. In a review of 46 patients, 19 of the 20 nontreated patients rapidly progressed either to death or to the persistence of severe sequelae, while 4 of the 13 patients treated by corticosteroids alone and 10 of the 13 treated by a combination of corticosteroids and cyclophosphamide showed favorable progression (Calabrese and Mallek, 1988). More recent analysis of isolated CNS angiitis patients suggests that the prognosis of the disease is not uniformly unfavorable. The results of a retrospective series of 105 patients showed that isolated CNS angiitis is more prone to relapse during prolonged periods when arterial abnormalities are located on small-sized arteries rather than on middle-sized arteries (MacLaren *et al.*, 2005). Combined aggressive therapy should be reserved for those patients with histologically proven isolated CNS angiitis and a deteriorating clinical status. In these patients, the combination therapy should be pursued for at least 6–12 months after the patient is in remission. According to the treatment of systemic vasculitis, cyclophosphamide is usually prescribed intravenously. Alternative treatment with azathioprine or methotrexate can be proposed when cyclophosphamide is not well-tolerated, but no valuable experience with other immunosuppressive drugs than

cyclophosphamide has yet to be published. To our knowledge, intravenous gammaglobulins, a treatment regimen occasionally proposed in cerebral angiitis with systemic diseases (Canhao *et al.*, 2000), has not been used in isolated CNS angiitis patients.

The activity of the disease under treatment is appreciated using clinical, biological, and radiological monitoring. Regression of CSF abnormalities may parallel clinical improvement (Oliveira *et al.*, 1994). The successful use of serial angiography has been reported (Alhalabi and Moore, 1994), but MR angiography or angio CT scans are also increasingly used for follow-up. Transcranial doppler occasionally reveals improvement of the cerebral circulation under treatment (Ritter *et al.*, 2002). Clinical stabilization for years with discontinuation of treatment has been described in occasional cases, as well as improvement of the MRI appearance, and the disappearance of vessel wall inflammation years after immunosuppression (Ehsan *et al.*, 1995; Johnson *et al.*, 1994; Riemer *et al.*, 1999), but a prolonged neurological supervision is necessary because relapsing episodes are possible.

In patients with a unique focal presentation such as stroke, and with isolated CNS angiitis suspected on the basis of angiography alone, a course of several-weeks of high-dose corticosteroids associated with a calcium channel blocker and no immunosuppressor has been proposed (Calabrese *et al.*, 1997). The diagnosis of reversible cerebral angiopathy should be carefully considered in these patients. Any additive vasoconstrictive stimuli including uncontrolled hypertension should be avoided.

REFERENCES

Abu-Shakra, M., Khraishi, M., Grosman, H., *et al.* 1994. Primary angiitis of the CNS diagnosed by angiography. *Q J Med*, **87**, 351–8.

Alhalabi, M., and Moore, P. M. 1994. Serial angiography in isolated angiitis of the central nervous system. *Neurology*, **44**, 1221–6.

Alreshaid, A. A., and Powers, W. J. 2003. Prognosis of patients with suspected primary CNS angiitis and negative brain biopsy. *Neurology*, **61**, 831–3.

Arthur, G., and Margolis, G. 1977. Mycoplasma-like structures in granulomatous angiitis of the central nervous system: case reports with light and electron microscope studies. *Arch Pathol Lab Med*, **101**, 382–7.

Aviv, R. I., Benseler, S. M., Silvermann, E. D., *et al.* 2006. MR imaging and angiography of primary CNS vasculitis of childhood. *Am. J Neuroradiol*, **27**, 192–9.

Benseler, S. M., de Veber, G., Hawkins, C., *et al.* 2005. Angiography-negative primary central nervous system vasculitis in children. *Arthritis Rheum*, **52**, 2159–67.

Bhibhatbhan, A., Katz, N. R., Hudon, M., *et al.* 2006. Primary angiitis of the spinal cord presenting as a conus mass: long term remission. *Surg Neurol*, **66**, 622–5.

Biller, J., Loftus, C. M., Moore, S. A., *et al.* 1987. Isolated central nervous system angiitis first presenting as spontaneous intracranial hemorrhage. *Neurosurgery*, **20**, 310–15.

Calabrese, L. H., and Mallek, J. A. 1988. Primary angiitis of the central nervous system. Report of 8 cases, review of the literature and proposal for diagnostic criteria. *Medicine*, **108**, 815–23.

Calabrese, L. H., Duna, G. F., and Lie, J. T. 1997. Vasculitis in the central nervous system. *Arthritis Rheum*, **40**, 1189–201.

Call, G. K., Fleming, M. C., Sealfon, S., *et al.* 1988. Reversible cerebral segmental vasoconstriction. *Stroke*, **19**, 1159–70.

Canhao, H., Fonseca, J. E., and Rosa, A. 2000. Intravenous gammaglobulin in the treatment of central nervous system vasculitis associated with Sjogren's syndrome. *J Rheumatol*, **27**, 1102–3.

Chu, C. T., Gray, L., Goldstein, L. B., and Hulette, C. M. 1998. Diagnosis of intracranial vasculitis: a multi-disciplinary approach. *J Neuropathol Exp Neurol*, **57**, 30–8.

Cravioto H., and Feigin I. 1959. Noninfectious granulomatous angiitis with a predilection for the nervous system. *Neurology*, **9**, 599–609.

Derry, C., Dale, R. C., Thom, M., Miller, D. H., and Giovanni, G. 2002. Unihemispheric cerebral vasculitis mimicking Rasmussen's encephalitis. *Neurology*, **58**, 327–8.

Ducros, A. Boukobza, M., Porcher, A., et al., 2007. The clinical and radiological spectrum of reversible cerebral vasoconstriction syndrome. A prospective series of 67 patients. *Brain*, **130**, 3091–101.

Duna, G., and Calabrese, L. H. 1995. Limitations of invasive modalities in the diagnosis of primary angiitis of the central nervous system. *J Rheumatol*, **22**, 662–7.

Ehsan, T., Hasan, S., Powers, J. M., and Heiserman, J. E. 1995. Serial magnetic resonance imaging in isolated angiitis of the central nervous system. *Neurology*, **45**, 1462–5.

Ferro, J. M. 1998. Vasculitis of the central nervous system. *J Neurol*, **245**, 766–76.

Finelli, P. F., Onyiuke, H. C., and Uphoff, D. F. 1997. Idiopathic granulomatous angiitis of the CNS manifesting as diffuse white matter disease. *Neurology*, **49**, 1696–9.

Fountain, N. B., and Eberhard, D. A. 1996. Primary angiitis of the central nervous system associated with cerebral amyloid angiopathy: report of two cases and review of the literature. *Neurology*, **46**, 190–7.

Gilden, D. H., Kleinschmidt-DeMasters, B. K., Wellish, M., et al. 1996. Varicella zoster virus, a cause of waxing and waning vasculitis: the *New England Journal of Medicine* case 5–1995 revisited. *Neurology*, **47**, 1441–6.

Gray, F., Viners, H. V., Le Noan, H., et al. 1990. Cerebral amyloid angiopathy and granulomatous angiitis: immunohistochemical study using antibodies to the Alzheimer A4 peptide. *Hum Pathol*, **21**, 1290–3.

Greer, J. M., Longley, S., Edwards, L., Elfenbein, G. J., and Panush, R. S. 1988. Vasculitis associated with malignancy. Experience with 13 patients and literature review. *Medicine*, **67**, 220–30.

Hankey, G. J. 1991. Isolated angiitis/angiopathy of the central nervous system. *erebrovasc Dis*, **1**, 2–15.

Harris, K. G., Tran, D. D., Sickels, W. J., Cornell, S. H., and Yuh, W. T. C. 1994. Diagnosing intracranial vasculitis: the roles of MR and angiography. *Am J Neuroradiol*, **15**, 317–30.

Harrison, P. E. 1976. Granulomatous angiitis of the central nervous system. Case report and review. *J Neurol Sci*, **29**, 335–41.

Hellmann, D. B., Roubenoff, R., Healy, R. A., and Wang, H. 1992. Central nervous system angiography: safety and predictors of a positive result in 125 consecutive patients evaluated for possible vasculitis. *J Rheumatol*, **19**, 568–72.

Hunn, M., Robinson, S., Wakefield, L., Mossman, S., and Abernethy, D. 1998. Granulomatous angiitis of the CNS causing spontaneous intracerebral haemorrhage: the importance of leptomeningeal biopsy. *J Neurol Neurosurg Psychiatry*, **65**, 956–7.

Iancu-Gontard, D., Oppenheim, C., Touzé, E., et al. 2003. Evaluation of hyperintense vessels on FLAIR MRI for the diagnosis of intracerebral arterial stenoses. *Stroke*, **34**, 1886–91.

Johnson, M. D., Maciunas, R., Creasy, J., and Collins, R. D. 1994. Indolent granulomatous angiitis. *J Neurosurg*, **81**, 472–6.

Kadkhodayan, Y., Alreshaid, A., Moran, J. C., Cross, D. T., Powers, W. J., and Derdeyn, C. P. 2004. Primary angiitis of the central nervous system at conventional angiography. *Radiology*, **233**, 878–82.

Koo, E. H., and Massey, E. W. 1988. Granulomatous angiitis of the central nervous system: protean manifestations and response to treatment. *J Neurol Neurosurg Psychiatry*, **51**, 1126–33.

Kossorotoff, M., Touz, E., Godon-Hardy, S., et al. 2006. Cerebral vasculopathy with aneurysm formation in HIV-infected young adults. *Neurology*, **66**, 1121–22.

Kristoferitsch W, Jellinger K, and Böck F. 1984. Cerebral granulomatous angiitis with atypical features. *J Neurol*, **231**, 38–42.

Kumar, R., Wijdicks, E. F. M., Brown, R. D. Jr., Parisis, J. E., and Hammond, C. A. 1997. Isolated angiitis of the CNS presenting as subarachnoid haemorrhage. *J Neurol Neurosurg Psychiatry*, **62**, 649–51.

Lanthier, S., Lortie, A., Michaud, J., Laxer, R., Jay, V., and de Veber, G. 2001. Isolated angiitis of the CNS in children. *Neurology*, **56**, 837–42.

Lie, J. T. 1992. Primary (granulomatous) angiitis of the central nervous system: a clinical pathologic analysis of 15 new cases and a review of the literature. *Hum Pathol*, **23**, 164–71.

Linnemann, C. C., and Alvira, M. M. 1980. Pathogenesis of varicella-zoster angiitis in the CNS. *Arch Neurol*, **37**, 239–40.

MacLaren, K., Gillepsie, J., Shrestha, S., Neary, D., and Ballardie, F. W. 2005. Primary angiitis of the central nervous system: emerging variants. *Q J Med*, **98**, 643–54.

Miller, D. H., Ormerod, I. E. C., Gibson, A., et al. 1987. MR brain scanning in patients with vasculitis: differentiation from multiple sclerosis. *Neuroradiology*, **29**, 226–31.

Moore, P. M. 1989. Diagnosis and management of isolated angiitis of the central nervous system. *Neurology*, **39**, 167–73.

Moore, P. M. 1998. Central nervous system vasculitis. *Curr Opin Neurol*, **11**, 241–6.

Moore, P. M. 1999. The vasculitides. *Curr Opin Neurol*, **12**, 383–8.

Negishi, C., and Sze, G. 1993. Vasculitis presenting as primary leptomeningeal enhancement with minimal parenchymal findings. *AJNR Am J Neuroradiol*, **14**, 26–8.

Nishikawa, M., Sakamoto, H., Katsuyama, J., Hakuba, A., and Nishimura, S. 1998. Multiple appearing and vanishing aneurysms: primary angiitis of the central nervous system. *J Neurosurg*, **88**, 133–7.

Ohtake, T., Yoshida, H., Hirose, K., and Tanabe, H. 1989. Diagnostic value of the optic fundus in cerebral angiitis. *J Neurol*, **236**, 490–1.

Oliveira, V. C., Povoa, P., Costa, A., and Ducla-Soares, J. 1994. Cerebrospinal fluid and therapy of isolated angiitis of the central nervous system. *Stroke*, **25**, 1693–5.

Ozawa, T., Sasaki, O., Sorimachi, T., and Tanaka, R. 1995. Primary angiitis of the central nervous system: report of two cases and review of the literature. *Neurosurgery*, **36**, 173–9.

Parisi, J. E., and Moore, P. M. 1994. The role of biopsy in vasculitis of the central nervous system. *Semin Neurol*, **14**, 341–8.

Pierot, L., Chiras, J., Debussche-Depriester, C., Dormont, D., and Bories, J. 1991. Intracerebral stenoting arteriopathies. Contribution of three radiological techniques to the diagnosis. *J Neuroradiol.*, **18**, 32–48.

Reik, L., Grunnet, M. L., Spencer, R. P., and Donaldson, J. O. 1983. Granulomatous angiitis presenting as chronic meningitis and ventriculitis. *Neurology*, **33**, 1609–12.

Rhodes, R. H., Madelaire, N. C., Petrelli, M., Cole, M., and Karaman, B. A. 1995. Primary angiitis and angiopathy of the central nervous system and their relationship to systemic giant cell arteritis. *Arch Pathol Lab Med*, **119**, 334–9.

Riemer, G., Lamszus, K., Zschaber, R., et al. 1999. Isolated angiitis of the central nervous system: lack of inflammation after long-term treatment. *Neurology*, **52**, 196–9.

Ritter, M. A., Dziewas, R., Papke, K., and Liemann, P. 2002. Follow-up examinations by transcranial doppler ultrasound in primary angiitis of the central nervous system. *Cerebrovasc Dis*, **14**, 139–42.

Schmidley, J. W., Beadle, B. A., and Trigg, L. 2005. Co-occurrence of CADASIL and isolated CNS angiitis. *Cerebrovasc Dis*, **19**, 352–4.

Scolding, N. J., Jayne, D. R., Zajicek, J. P., et al. 1997. Cerebral vasculitis – recognition, diagnosis and management. *Q J Med*, **90**, 61–73.

Scolding, N. J., Joseph, F., Kirby, P. A., et al. 2005. Aβ-related angiitis: primary angiitis of the central nervous system associated with cerebral amyloid angiopathy. *Brain*, **128**, 500–15.

Vollmer, T. L., Guarnaccia, J., Harrington, W., Pacia, S. V., and Petroff, O. A. C. 1993. Idiopathic granulomatous angiitis of the central nervous system: diagnosis challenges. *Arch Neurol*, **50**, 925–30.

White, M. L., Hadley, W. L., Zhang, Y., and Dogar, M. A. 2007. Analysis of central nervous system vasculitis with diffusion-weighted imaging and apparent diffusion coefficient mapping of the normal-appearing brain. *Am J Neuroradiol*, **28**, 933–7.

Wijdicks, E. F. M., Manno, E. M., Fulgham, J. R., and Giannini, C. 2003. Cerebral angiitis mimicking posterior leukoencephalopathy. *J Neurol*, **250**, 444–8.

Yamada, M., Itoh, Y., Shintaku, M., et al. 1996. Immune reactions associated with cerebral amyloid angiopathy. *Stroke*, **27**, 1155–62.

Zuber, M., Blustajn, J., Arquizan, C., et al. 1999. Angiitis of the central nervous system. *J Neuroradiol*, **26**, 101–17.

Zuber M, Touzé E, Domigo V, et al. 2006. Reversible cerebral angiopathy: efficacy of nimodipine. *J Neurol*, **253**, 1585–8.

2 TEMPORAL ARTERITIS

A. Wesley Thevathasan and Stephen M. Davis

Introduction

Temporal (giant cell) arteritis is a systemic disease, involving various medium-sized and larger arteries, that occurs mostly in elderly patients. In addition to the classical clinical symptoms of headache, jaw claudication, and polymyalgia rheumatica syndrome, neurological manifestations are common. Blindness due to ischemic optic neuropathy is probably the most common and most feared sinister manifestation of the disease, but stroke is the leading cause of death in patients with temporal arteritis (Caselli et al., 1988). Temporal arteritis was first described by Hutchinson (1890) and later by Horton et al. (1934). The original clinical report described an elderly man, who was unable to wear his hat because of scalp pain. He had inflamed and hardened superficial temporal arteries on examination. The disease is variously called either "temporal arteritis" or "giant cell arteritis." The term "temporal arteritis" refers to the characteristic involvement of the superficial temporal arteries, while the term "giant cell arteritis" emphasizes the systemic nature of the disease and the characteristic pathology, with giant cells being typically present in the vessel wall (Figures 2.1 and 2.2).

On a sinister historical note, it was even suggested that Adolf Hitler might have had the disease in the 1940s, with recorded symptoms of headache, impaired vision, sensitivity to pressure in the temporal regions, swollen temporal arteries, constitutional symptoms, and a raised erythrocyte sedimentation rate (Redlich, 1993). Others however, have suggested cluster headache as an alternative diagnosis (Schmidt, 1994).

Pathology

Temporal arteritis is a medium- and large-vessel vasculitis that tends to involve cranial branches of the aorta. Additionally, preference for vessels with a high elastic component means that the ophthalmic, posterior ciliary, and vertebral branches of the external carotid are most commonly affected (Goodman, 1979; Wilkinson and Russell, 1972). Intracranial involvement is very rare (Gibb et al., 1985; Mclean et al., 1993).

However, temporal arteritis is a systemic vasculitis with a well-described extracranial involvement. (Klein et al., 1975). Involvement of mesenteric vessels can cause abdominal pain. Limb claudication and Raynaud's phenomena can result from subclavian and femoral artery disease (Klein et al., 1975). Angiography is sometimes a useful procedure when used to distinguish arteritis from atherosclerotic disease in these settings (Gillanders, 1969; Klein et al., 1975;). Aortic aneurysm and dissection is now increasingly recognized as a late complication of temporal arteritis (Evans et al., 1995). One dramatic case report has even described a death resulting from an aortoduodenal fistula (Lagrand et al., 1996).

At a microscopic level, there is an inflammatory infiltrate of the vessel wall. This is usually focal and segmental, resulting in the "skip lesions" that can cause sampling error when too little of the artery is removed for a biopsy. Three histological patterns have been described (Goodman, 1979; Lie, 1990). The classical finding is granulomatous inflammation with giant cells at the junction of intima and media. (Figures 2.1 and 2.2) However, these changes are found in only about 50% of positive biopsies. Just as common is a nonspecific panarteritis without giant cells. Rarely, only a small vessel vasculitis surrounding a normal temporal artery is seen (Esteban et al., 2001).

Epidemiology and clinical features

A number of epidemiological studies have evaluated the incidence, age, and gender associations of temporal arteritis. In Olmstead County, Minnesota, the annual incidence of the disease was 17.8

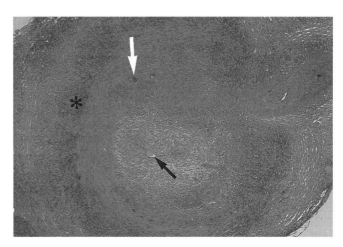

Figure 2.1 Low-powered view of the transverse section of superficial temporal artery with features of giant cell arteritis. There is a slit-like lumen (black arrow) due to intimal swelling, with disruption of the internal elastic lamina (*) and scattered, multinucleated giant cells (white arrow). See color plate.

Uncommon Causes of Stroke, 2nd edition, ed. Louis R. Caplan. Published by Cambridge University Press. © Cambridge University Press 2008.

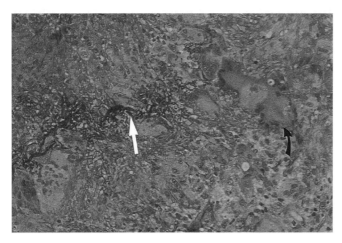

Figure 2.2 High-powered view of disrupted internal elastic lamina (white arrow), with multinucleated giant cell (black arrow). See color plate.

per 100 000 in those aged over 50 years (Machado *et al.*, 1988). Incidence increases with age and peaks between 70 and 80 years of age. Women are at least twice as often affected (Salvarani *et al.*, 2002). Prevalence is higher in those of Scandinavian and Northern European descent (Franzen *et al.*, 1992; Hunder, 2002).

Headache is the most common symptom (Goodman, 1979). Headache is often severe and associated with scalp tenderness, usually in the region of the temporal arteries. Hence the patient may have scalp pain when brushing the hair, or even resting his or her head on a pillow. However, the headache pattern is often atypical, and the diagnosis should be considered in any elderly patient presenting with headache (Huston *et al.*, 1978). Jaw claudication, meanwhile, is the most specific nonneurological feature of the condition and is due to involvement of the facial artery (Goodman, 1979; Smetana and Shmerling, 2002). Other clinical manifestations, also due to arteritis of external carotid artery branches, can include scalp, skin, and tongue necrosis (Figure 2.3; Table 2.1). Examination of the temporal arteries, typically reveals tenderness, and the temporal arteries may become firm, nodular, and pulseless (Salvarani *et al.*, 2002). The occipital arteries are also often involved and can show similar abnormalities in response to palpation.

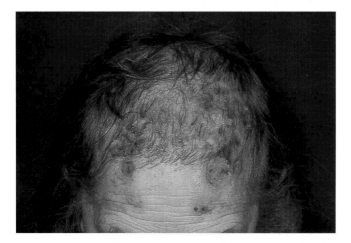

Figure 2.3 Extensive scalp necrosis in a patient with biopsy-proven temporal arteritis. See color plate.

Table 2.1 Cardinal symptoms of temporal arteritis
Headache
Polymyalgia rheumatica syndrome
Jaw claudication
Constitutional symptoms (anorexia, weight loss, malaise)
Scalp necrosis
Ischemic optic neuropathy
Stroke

Systemic symptoms can include fever, malaise, and anorexia with weight loss. These features are especially common in patients with coexisting polymyalgia rheumatica (PMR), but can be conspicuously absent. A low-grade fever can occur and may even reach 40°C. In fact, temporal arteritis is a classical cause of "pyrexia of unknown origin" in the elderly (Calamia and Hunder, 1981).

The relationship between temporal arteritis and PMR is complex. Many experts consider both to be different spectrums of the same disease (Salvarani *et al.*, 2002). About 50% of patients with temporal arteritis will also have PMR (Calamia and Hunder, 1981). Suggestive symptoms include shoulder and, less commonly, hip girdle pain. As a result, a classical complaint is difficulty hanging out the wash on a clothesline. MRI studies have implicated not only synovitis but also periarticular bursitis and tenosynovitis (Pavlica *et al.*, 2000). IT is interesting to note that only 20% of patients with PMR are said to have temporal arteritis (Franzen *et al.*, 1992; Pavlica *et al.*, 2000). However, PET studies have suggested that the rate of subclinical temporal arteritis may be significantly higher than 20% (Blockmans *et al.*, 2000). The clinical significance of these findings is yet to be determined. Currently, the usual practice is to biopsy only those patients with PMR who also have features of temporal arteritis.

Neurological and neuro-ophthalmological manifestations

Neurological complications are common in patients with temporal arteritis (Table 2.2). Caselli *et al.* (1988) reported a series of 166 consecutive patients with biopsy-proven temporal arteritis and found that approximately 30% had neurological features (Caselli *et al.*, 1988) Peripheral nervous system involvement can include mononeuropathy and peripheral polyneuropathy (Caselli *et al.*, 1984). Labyrinth dysfunction and hearing loss occur frequently (Amor-Dorado *et al.*, 2003). Numbness of the tongue can be attributed to ischemia of the lingual nerve. Neuropsychiatric manifestations, such as depression, are also well-recognized (Caselli *et al.*, 1988; Goodman, 1979). Stroke often leads to devastating consequences.

Neuro-ophthalmological manifestations are frequent. In Caselli's series, over 20% of patients with biopsy proven temporal arteritis developed ocular symptoms including amaurosis fugax, scintillating scotoma and diplopia and 8% suffered permanent visual loss (Caselli *et al.*, 1988). Other series have reported far higher rates (Reich *et al.*, 1990). The usual cause of blindness is anterior ischemic optic neuropathy (AION) (Reich *et al.*, 1990).

Table 2.2 Neurological manifestations of temporal arteritis

Neuro-ophthalmological manifestations	Ischemic optic neuropathy, central retinal artery occlusion, occipital infarction, third and sixth cranial nerve palsies
Neuropathy	Mononeuropathies and generalized peripheral neuropathy
Neuro-otological and neuropsychiatric syndromes	Particularly vertigo, depression, dementia
Tremor	
Tongue numbness	Due to lingual nerve ischemia
Myelopathy	Arteritis of spinal cord
Stroke	Most commonly due to vertebral arteritis

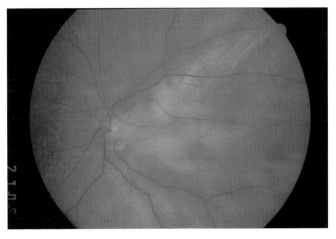

Figure 2.4 Ischemic optic neuropathy with a swollen, pale optic disc and extensive pallor of the adjacent choroid. See color plate.

Less common are retinal artery occlusion, posterior ischemic optic neuropathy, and cortical visual field defects from a posterior circulation stroke.

Transient diplopia can be the result of extraocular muscle ischemia. Pupil-sparing third nerve palsies and Horner's syndrome have been reported (Koorey, 1984; Reich *et al.*, 1990). Even an orbital inflammatory syndrome with proptosis and conjunctival injection has been described (Cockerham *et al.*, 2003; Islam *et al.*, 2003).

Ischemic optic neuropathy

Left untreated, visual symptoms in one eye will likely move on to affect the fellow eye within days or weeks (Salvarani *et al.*, 2002). Although some evidence suggests that there is potential for a limited degree of visual recovery, in fact, it is largely irreversible (Chan and O'Day, 2003; Hayreh *et al.*, 2002; Hayreh and Zimmerman, 2003a). The long-held teaching is that prompt treatment aims to protect the unaffected eye.

Transient visual loss is therefore a critically important warning symptom. Amaurosis fugax is reported to occur in 30–40% (Gonzales-Gay *et al.*, 1998; Hayreh *et al.*, 1998). Older patients with amaurosis should therefore be investigated not only for carotid and cardiac sources of emboli, but also for temporal arteritis.

The usual mechanism for blindness is arteritic AION, accounting for 80% (Hayreh and Zimmerman, 2003b). This condition is most commonly due to thrombosis, embolism, or perfusion failure of the posterior ciliary arteries, which leads to ischemia of the optic nerve head (Hayreh, 1981).Painless visual loss ensues. Typically there is chalky white-disc edema and an altitudinal visual field defect (Rucker *et al.*, 2004) (Figure. 2.4). Less commonly, central retinal artery ischemia leads to retinal infarction with cotton wool spots seen on fundoscopic examination. Pial capillary plexus ischemia can lead to posterior ischemic optic neuropathy in a patient with an initially normal fundoscopic examination (Rucker *et al.*, 2004).

A major differential diagnoses is nonarteritic AION. Arteritic AION is associated with temporal arteritis, whereas nonarteritic AION is associated with conventional atherosclerotic risk factors.

Taking the visual features in isolation, arteritic and nonarteritic AION can be indistinguishable. In the nonarteritic form, fundoscopy of the fellow eye may reveal the small-cup-disc ratio that constitutes the "disc at risk." In the arteritic form, fluorescein angiography typically demonstrates more extensive hypoperfusion involving not only the posterior ciliary vessels but also delayed filling of the choroidal circulation (Rucker *et al.*, 2004).

Optic neuritis meanwhile can also present with diminished visual acuity and optic disc edema. Usually there is pain or discomfort in the eye, particularly with eye movement. Fat-suppressed, gadolinium-enhanced MRI may show high signals in the optic nerve; however, similar findings have been reported with temporal arteritis (Morganstern *et al.*, 2003). Obviously, plaques of demyelination elsewhere may suggest an optic neuritis associated with multiple sclerosis. Visual recovery after optic neuritis is usually good, compared with the permanent deficits accompanying temporal arteritis (Beck *et al.*, 1992).

Cerebrovascular manifestations

Brain infarction is a well-recognized complication of temporal arteritis and is a leading cause of death (Table 2.3).

Stroke may be the initial presentation of temporal arteritis. Obviously, suspicion may be raised by an elderly patient with PMR who presents with stroke and elevated inflammatory markers. However, there are many reports of devastating stroke due to biopsy-proven temporal arteritis with normal ESR (Neish and Sergent, 1991). Indeed, an inverse relationship has been found

Table 2.3 Stroke in temporal arteritis

The most common cause of death in patients with temporal arteritis
Related to the degree of elastic tissue in major extracranial arteries
Usually involves extracranial vertebral artery
Intracranial arteritis is much rarer
Stroke may be a presenting manifestation of the disease (even with normal ESR)
Can produce multi-infarct dementia

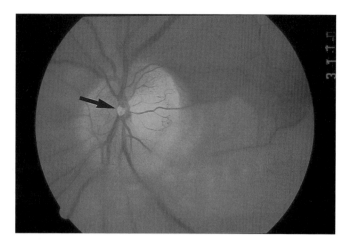

Figure 2.5 Large embolus in the central retinal artery (arrow). See color plate.

between cranial ischemic events and the presence of synovitis and "inflammatory anemia" (Peyo-Reigosa *et al.*, 2004; Smetana and Schmerling, 2002; Weyand and Goronzy, 2003).

The posterior circulation is the classical territory for strokes due to temporal arteritis. Well described are the lateral medullary syndrome, top of the basilar syndrome and occipital lobe infarction with cortical visual loss (Figure 2.5). The frequent involvement of the posterior circulation has been explained by a preference of temporal arteritis to involve vessels with significant internal elastic lamina. Hence the extracranial vertebral arteries are commonly affected but with a sharply defined upper border, typically 5mm above the point of dural perforation, correlating with the distribution of the elastic lamina (Ruegg *et al.*, 2003). However stroke in any vascular territory is possible. In fact, Caselli's series suggested that strokes due to temporal arteritis may occur at least as commonly in the carotid territories as vertebrobasilar territories (Caselli *et al.*, 1988). Intracranial vessel involvement meanwhile, is rare but has been reported. McLean et al. (1993) reported a patient who had intracranial giant cell arteritis, involving the anterior inferior cerebellar and basilar arteries. They pointed out that intracranial involvement by giant cell arteritis should be distinguished from the separate entity of primary cerebral angiitis. Even myelopathy has been reported, due to occlusion of the anterior spinal artery (Gibb *et al.*, 1985).

Caselli (1990) emphasized the unusual occurrence of dementia in patients with temporal arteritis. Such patients have multifocal cognitive impairment typical of vascular dementia, hence representing a treatable form of the disorder. Multiple cerebral infarcts, predominantly in the posterior circulation, were shown on neuroimaging. In this series, abrupt cognitive decline during periods of clinically active disease was associated with steroid reduction. The usual mechanism for stroke is an arteritis with secondary thrombosis and sometimes artery-to-artery embolization (Missen, 1972). A prothrombotic tendancy may also contribute to the pathophysiology of stroke in temporal arteritis. Studies have found associations with hyperfibrinogenaemia and thrombocytosis (Andersson *et al.*, 1986; Foroozan *et al.*, 2002; De Keyser *et al.*, 1991).

Additionally, anticardiolipin antibodies are a frequent finding in temporal arteritis patients, with titers responsive to steroid therapy (Espinosa *et al.*, 2001). However, the clinical relevance of this finding needs further examination.

Interaction with atherosclerotic risk-factors has also been found to be important. Hypertension, hyperlipidemia, diabetes mellitus, and smoking have all been found to increase stroke incidence in patients with temporal arteritis (Peyo-Reigosa, 2004; Ray *et al.*, 2005). Additionally, it has been increasingly recognized that an inflammatory milieu, as evidenced by raised CRP for instance, is a risk-factor for cardiovascular events in the general population.

Hemodynamic stroke has also been described. Bogousslavsky *et al.* (1985) reported a case with severe bilateral internal carotid artery stenosis due to temporal arteritis and progressive infarction in the vertebrobasilar territory, suggesting a "steal phenomena" from the posterior to the anterior circulations.

More proximally, another feared cardiovascular complication is aortic aneurysm formation and dissection. This is now recognized to be significantly more common in patients with giant cell arteritis (Gonzales-Gay *et al.*, 2004). Risk is estimated at seventeen times the age matched population (Evans *et al.*, 1995). As a result, a yearly chest radiograph is recommended as a screening measure (Salvarani *et al.*, 2002).

Diagnosis

The diagnosis of temporal arteritis is suggested by the presence of the cardinal clinical symptoms in an elderly patient with an elevated ESR (Table 2.4). Although patients have been reported as young as 19 years old (Thal *et al.*, 2001), it is rare under the age of 60. The clinical features found to have the greatest specificity are jaw claudication and prominent, enlarged temporal arteries (Smetana and Schmerling, 2002).

Blood tests can alter the likelihood of temporal arteritis but do not exclude the diagnosis if clinical suspicion is high. Elevated ESR is the classical finding. However temporal arteritis with normal

Table 2.4 Diagnosis and treatment of stroke due to temporal arteritis

Diagnosis and treatment	Comment
Diagnosis	
ESR	Normal in 22.5% of patients
C-reactive protein	Enhances sensitivity in combination with ESR
Temporal artery biopsy	Mandatory for all patients. Skip lesions not uncommon
Treatment	
High dose steroids as acute therapy	Controversy in literature as to initial dose
Maintenance steroids	Dose adjusted for clinical symptoms, ESR, steroid side effects
Duration of treatment	Controversial. Adverse effects of steroids balanced against risk of relapse

ESR is well-recognized. In one recent meta-analysis, 4% of biopsy-proven temporal arteritis had "normal" ESR (Smetana and Shmerling, 2002). Others report that normal ESR may occur in over 20% of patients with biopsy proven temporal arteritis (Salvarani and Hunder, 2001). C-reactive protein (CRP), a more acute marker of inflammation, significantly increases the sensitivity. In one study, the sensitivity of combined ESR and CRP was found to be 100% (Hayreh *et al.*, 1997). However, temporal arteritis with normal CRP has been reported (Weyand and Goronzy, 2003). Thrombocytosis and anemia are commonly seen on the full blood examination (Froozan *et al.*, 2002). Up to one-third of the patients are found to have abnormal liver function test results (De Keyser *et al.*, 1991).

Imaging can detect abnormalities suggestive of temporal arteritis; however, use in clinical practice is debated. Temporal artery ultrasound may reveal a characteristic hypoechoic "halo sign" indicating mural edema (Salvarani *et al.*, 2002). However the accuracy of this test is highly operator-dependant and a recent meta-analysis suggested "cautious interpretation" of results (Karassa *et al.*, 2005). Noninvasive angiography using CT or MRI may reveal sites of vascular stenoses. A typical finding is smoothly tapered stenotic lesions different from the abrupt, irregular stenoses of atherosclerotic disease (Stanson, 2000). These modalities may be helpful in assessing the extent of disease or potentially to aid diagnosis especially in biopsy negative cases. FDG-PET scanning may reveal uptake in the larger thoracic vessels including aorta, subclavian, and carotid arteries (Blockmans *et al.*, 2000). It is less useful for smaller caliber vessels, such as the temporal arteries.

Temporal artery biopsy is the gold-standard investigation. The classical finding is of granulomatous inflammation with giant cells. Complications of the procedure, such as scalp necrosis and stroke, are rare (Ghanch and Dutton, 1997). A biopsy is felt to be essential, as diagnosis of temporal arteritis commits to lengthy steroid treatment with their inherent risks. However, steroid therapy should not be delayed while awaiting biopsy if there is reasonable clinical suspicion. Blindness has been reported when this has occurred. However, a biopsy should be performed as soon as possible, as time on steroids does increase the chances of obtaining false negative or atypical histology (Guevara *et al.*, 1998; To *et al.*, 1994).

Another problem is the phenomena of "skip lesions." Normal segments of vessels may be interposed between vasculitic segments (Albert *et al.*, 1976). Various strategies are employed to optimize the chances of a positive biopsy result. First, a swollen, tender artery (if present) should be chosen. This may be the temporal artery but occipital and facial arteries are other possibilities. Second, a sufficient sample size should be obtained: a 3–5 cm sample is suggested. Some academic centers perform an intraoperative frozen section, and if it is negative, proceed to biopsy the contralateral side.

In the case of a negative unilateral temporal artery biopsy, sampling of the contralateral side will also yield a negative result 97–99% of the time (Hall *et al.*, 2003). Therefore, routine simultaneous biopsy is not recommended and when clinical suspicion is low, a unilateral biopsy is all that is needed (Hall *et al.*, 2003; Salvarani *et al.*, 2002). Importantly, even bilateral negative temporal artery biopsy does not exclude the diagnosis and a minority of patients will obtain the diagnosis of "biopsy-negative temporal arteritis" and be treated regardless.

Treatment and prognosis

The mainstay of treatment is corticosteroids, although there is much debate about the optimal dose and use of steroid sparing immunosuppressives (Table 2.4).

In the case of acute visual loss, the long held teaching is that the prognosis for the affected eye is poor and the aim of treatment is to protect the fellow eye. A study by Hayreh *et al.* (2002) supported this view. Pulsed high-dose intravenous steroids given to patients presenting with visual loss provided no significant improvement in either visual acuity or field defect. Crucially, however, in this study, patients were enrolled who had developed the visual loss many days and weeks previously. After that long, irreversible infarction would be established. In another study by Chan and O'Day, treatment with intravenous steroids was commenced within 48 hours of visual symptoms, and some improvement in visual acuity was seen after treatment (Chan and O'Day, 2003). The current practice of many neurologists is therefore to treat patients who have visual symptoms with high-dose intravenous methylprednisolone as a matter of urgency.

In the case of stroke, recognition of temporal arteritis is often made only after routine acute stroke therapy has been given. Of concern, are reports that following oral steroid initiation, new stroke, or where an extension of a stroke has occurred (Collazos *et al.*, 1994; Staunton *et al.*, 2000). Due to these concerns, authors have suggested the use of high-dose intravenous steroids and possibly anticoagulation in stroke-affected patients with temporal arteritis. In addition, there is evidence from a retrospective case-control study that the routine adjunctive use of aspirin in patients with temporal arteritis can reduce cranial ischemic events (Nesher *et al.*, 2004).

The initial corticosteroid dose in more stable settings is also controversial. It is a balance between the risks of blindness and stroke versus the need to minimize steroid complications such as vertebral fracture. Some studies suggest that starting at a low dose (e.g. 20–40 mg) may be adequate (Delecoeuillerie *et al.*, 1988; Nesher *et al.*, 1997). However, these are retrospective studies, and the usual practice of many neurologists is to start with 60–80 mg of prednisolone.

Weaning of steroids can usually begin within 4–6 weeks. This obviously needs to be tailored to the individual patient, with titration against symptoms and inflammatory markers. Unfortunately though, a rise in ESR and CRP can lag well-behind the disease process. Newer, more "upstream" markers, such as IL-6, may herald relapse more accurately and may become more widely available outside the research setting (Weyand *et al.*, 2000).

Most patients with temporal arteritis are able to be completely weaned off of steroids, but this may take years (Andersson *et al.*, 1986). Some patients may require indefinite corticosteroid treatment (Gonzalez-Gay *et al.*, 1998). Given the degree of steroid exposure, bone protection is important. Bone mineral density needs to be monitored and bisphosphonate medications considered.

For those who remain steroid dependant, the use of other immunosuppressants as "steroid sparers" has been advocated. The addition of methotrexate to steroid therapy for the treatment of temporal arteritis has been assessed in 3 randomised, double-blinded, placebo-controlled trials. In the first trial, patients had fewer relapses and required lower cumulative doses of steroids when treated with methotrexate and prednisolone compared with prednisolone alone (Jover *et al.*, 2001). However, these findings were not replicated in the 2 subsequent trials (Cantini *et al.*, 2001; Tan *et al.*, 2003). Recently, positive reports for biological agents, such as infliximab, etanercept, and rituximab have also emerged (Bhatia *et al.*, 2005; Cantini *et al.*, 2001; Tan *et al.*, 2003).

Properly treated, the prognosis for most patients with temporal arteritis is very good. Life expectancy has been found to be similar to age-matched controls (Gran *et al.*, 2001).

REFERENCES

Albert, D. M., Ruchman, M. C., and Keltner, J. L. 1976. Skip lesions in temporal arteritis. *Arch Ophthalmol*, **94**, 2072–7.

Amor-Dorado, J. C., Llarca, J., Garcia-Porrua, C. *et al.* 2003. Audiovestibular manifestations in giant cell arteritis: a prospective study. *Medicine*, **82**, 13–26.

Andersson, R., Malmvall, B. E., and Bengtsson, B. A. 1986. Acute phase reactants in the initial phase of giant cell arteritis. *Acta Med Scand*, **220**, 365–7.

Beck, R. W., Cleary, P. A., Anderson, M. M., *et al.* 1992. A randomized, controlled trial of corticosteroids in the treatment of acute optic neuritis. The Optic Neuritis Study Group. *N Engl J Med*, **326**, 581–8.

Bhatia, A., Ell, P. J., and Edwards, J. C. W. 2005. Anti CD-20 monoclonal antibody (Rituximab) as an adjunct in the treatment of giant cell arteritis. *Ann Rheumatol Dis*, **64**, 1099–100.

Blockmans, D., Stroobants, S., Maes, A. *et al.* 2000. PET in giant cell arteritis and polymyalgia rheumatica: evidence for inflammation of the aortic arch. *Am J Med*, **108**, 246–9.

Bogousslavsky, J., Deruaz, J. P., and Regli, F. 1985. Bilateral obstruction of internal carotid artery from giant cell arteritis and massive infarction limited to the vertebrobasilar area. *Eur Neurol*, **24**, 57–61.

Calamia, K. T., and Hunder, G. G. 1981. Giant cell arteritis (temporal arteritis) presenting as fever of undetermined origin. *Arthritis Rheumatol*, **24**, 1414–8.

Cantini, F., Niccoli, L., Salvarani, C., *et al.* 2001. Treatment of longstanding active giant cell arteritis with infliximab: report of 4 cases. *Arthritis Rheumatol*, **44**, 2933–5.

Caselli, R. J. 1990. Giant cell (temporal arteritis): a treatable cause of multi-infarct dementia. *Neurology*, **40**, 753–5.

Caselli, R. J., Daube, J. R., Hunder, G. G., and Whisnant, J. P. 1984. Peripheral neuropathic syndromes in giant cell arteritis. *Ann Intern Med*, **101**, 594–7.

Caselli, R. J., Hunder, G. G., and Whisnant, J. P. 1988. Neurologic disease in biopsy proven giant cell (temporal) arteritis. *Neurology*, **38**, 352–9.

Chan, C. C. K., and O'Day, J. 2003. Oral and intravenous steroids in giant cell arteritis. *Clin Exp Ophthalmol*, **31**, 179–82.

Cockerham, K. P., Cockerham, G., Brown, H., and Hidayat, A. A. 2003. Radiosensitive orbital inflammation associated with temporal arteritis. *J Neuroophthalmol*, **23**, 117–21.

Collazos, J., Garcia-Manco, C., Martin, A., Rodriguez, J., and Gomez, M. A. 1994. Multiple strokes after initiation of steroid therapy in giant cell arteritis. *Postgrad Med J*, **70**, 228–30.

De Keyser, J., De Klippel, N., and Ebinger, G. 1991. Thrombocytosis and ischaemic complications in giant cell arteritis. *BMJ*, **303**, 825.

Delecoeuillerie, G., Joly, P., Cohen de Lara A., and Paolaggi, J. B. 1988. Polymyalgia rheumatica and temporal arteritis: a retrospective analysis of prognostic features and different corticosteroid regimes (an 11-year survey of 210 patients). *Ann Rheumatol Dis*, **47**, 733–9.

Espinosa, G., Tassies, D., Font, J., *et al.* 2001. Antiphospholipid antibodies and thrombophilic factors in giant cell arteritis. *Semin Arthritis Rheumatol*, **31**, 12–20.

Esteban, M. J., Font, C., Hernandez-Rodriguez, J., *et al.* 2001. Small vessel vasculitis surrounding a spared temporal artery: clinical and pathological findings in a series of 28 patients. *Arthritis Rheumatol*, **44**, 1387–95.

Evans, J. M., O'Fallon, W. M., and Hunder, G. G. 1995. Increased incidence of aortic aneurysm and dissection in giant cell (temporal) arteritis. A population-based study. *Ann Intern Med*, **122**, 502–7.

Foroozan, R., Danesh-Meyer, H., Savino P., *et al.* 2002. Thrombocytosis in patients with biopsy proven giant cell arteritis. *Ophthalmology*, **109**, 1267–71.

Franzen, P., Sutinen, S., and von Knorring, J. 1992. Giant cell arteritis and polymyalgia rheumatica in a region of Finland: an epidemiologic, clinical and pathological study, 1984–1988. *J Rheumatol*, **19**, 273–6.

Ghanch, F. D., and Dutton, G. N. 1997. Current concepts in giant cell (temporal) arteritis. *Surv Ophthalmol*, **42**, 99–123.

Gibb, W. R., Urry, P. A., and Lees, A. J. 1985. Giant cell arteritis with spinal cord infarction and basilar artery thrombosis. *J Neurol Neurosurg Psychiatry*, **48**, 945–8.

Gillanders, L. A. 1969. Temporal arteriography. *Clin Radiol*, **20**, 149–56.

Gonzalez-Gay, M. A., Blanco, R., Rodriguez-Valverde, V., *et al.* 1998. Permanent visual loss and cerebrovascular accidents in giant cell arteritis: predictors and response to treatment. *Arthritis Rheumatol*, **41**, 1497–504.

Gonzalez-Gay, M. A., Garcia-Porrua, C., Pineiro, A., Pego-Reigosa R., Llorca J., and Hunder G. G. 2004. Aortic aneurysm and dissection in patients with biopsy proven giant cell arteritis from northwestern Spain: a population-based study. *Medicine* (Baltimore), **83**, 335–41.

Goodman, B. W. 1979. Temporal arteritis. *Am J Med*, **67**, 839–52.

Gran, J. T., Myklebust, G., Wilsgaard, T., and Jacobsen, B. K. 2001. Survival in polymyalgia rheumatica and giant cell arteritis: a study of 398 cases and matched population controls. *Rheumatology (Oxford)*, **40**, 1238–42.

Guevara, R. A., Newman, N. J., and Grossniklaus, H. E. 1998. Positive temporal artery biopsy 6 months after prednisolone treatment. *Arch Ophthalmol*, **116**, 1252–3.

Hall, J. K., Volpe, N. J., Galetta, S. L., *et al.* 2003. The role of unilateral temporal artery biopsy. *Ophthalmology*, **110**, 543–8.

Hayreh, S. S. 1981. Acute ischaemic optic neuropathy. *Arch Neurol*, **38**, 675–8.

Hayreh, S. S., Podhajsky, P. A., Raman, R., and Zimmerman, B. 1997. Giant cell arteritis: validity and reliability of various diagnostic criteria. *Am J Ophthalmol*, **123**, 285–96.

Hayreh, S. S., Podhajsky, P. A., and Zimmerman, B. 1998. Ocular manifestations of giant cell arteritis. *Am J Ophthalmol*, **125**, 509–20.

Hayreh, S. S., and Zimmerman, B. 2003a. Management of giant cell arteritis: our 27-year clinical study: New light on old controversies. *Ophthalmologica*, **217**, 239–59.

Hayreh, S. S., and Zimmerman, B. 2003b. Visual deterioration in giant cell arteritis patients while on high doses of corticosteroid therapy. *Ophthalmology*, **110**, 1204–15.

Hayreh, S. S., Zimmerman, B., and Kardon, R. H. 2002. Visual improvement with corticosteroid therapy in giant cell arteritis: report of a large study and review of literature. *Acta Ophthalmol Scand*, **80**, 355–67.

Hoffman, G. S., Cid, M. C., Hellman, D. B., *et al.* 2002. A multicenter, randomized, double-blinded, placebo controlled trial of adjuvant methotrexate treatment for giant cell arteritis. *Arthritis Rheumatol*, **46**, 1309–18.

Horton, B. T., Mastath, B., and Brown, G. E. 1934. Arteritis of the temporal vessels. A previously undescribed form. *Arch Intern Med*, **53**, 400–9.

Hunder, G. G. 2002. Epidemiology of giant cell arteritis. *Cleve Clin J Med*, **69**(**SII**), 79–82.

Huston, K. A., Hunder, G. G., Lie, J. T., Kennedy, R. H., and Elveback, L. R. 1978. Temporal arteritis. A 25-year epidemiologic, clinical, and pathological study. *Ann Intern Med*, **88**, 162–7.

Hutchinson, J. 1890. Diseases of the arteries. *Arch Surg*, **1**, 323–33.

Islam, N., Asaria, R., Plant, G. T., and Hykin, P. C. 2003. Giant cell arteritis mimicking idiopathic orbital inflammatory disease. *Eur J Ophthalmol*, **13**, 392–4.

Jover, J. A., Henandez-Garcia, C., Morado, I. C., *et al.* 2001. Combined treatment of giant cell arteritis with methotrexate and prednisolone. A randomized, double-blinded, placebo-controlled trial. *Ann Intern Med*, **134**, 106–14.

Karassa, F. B., Matsasas, M. I., Schmidt, W. A., and Ioannidis, J. P. 2005. Meta-analysis: test performance of ultrasonography for giant cell arteritis. *Ann Intern Med*, **1212**, 359–69.

Klein, R. G., Hunder, G. G., Stanson, A. W., and Sheps, S. G. 1975. Large artery involvement in giant cell (temporal) arteritis. *Ann Intern Med*, **83**, 806–12.

Koorey, D. J. 1984. Cranial arteritis. A 20-year review of cases. *Aust N Z J Med*, **14**, 143–7.

Lagrand, W. K., Hoogendoorn, M., Bakker, K., te Velde, J., and Labrie, A. 1996. Aortoduodenal fistula as an unusual and fatal manifestation of giant cell arteritis. *Eur J Vasc Endovasc Surg*, **11**, 502–3.

Lie, J. T. 1990. Illustrated histopathological classification criteria for selected vasculitis syndromes. *Arthritis Rheumatol*, **33**, 1074–87.

Machado, E. B. V., Michet, C. J., Ballard, D. J., *et al.* 1988. Trends in incidence and clinical presentation of temporal arteritis in Olmstead County, Minnesota, 1950–1985. *Arthritis Rheumatol*, **31**, 745–9.

Mclean, C. A., Gonzales, M. F., and Dowling, J. P. 1993. Systemic giant cell arteritis and cerebellar infarction. *Stroke*, **24**, 899–902.

Missen, G. A. K. 1972. Involvement of the vertebro-carotid arterial system in giant cell arteritis. *J Pathol*, **106**, 2–3.

Morganstern, K. E., Ellis, B. D., Schochet, S. S., and Linberg, J. V. 2003. Bilateral optic nerve sheath enhancement from giant cell arteritis. *J Rheumatol*, **30**, 625–7.

Neish, P. R., and Sergent, J. S. 1991. Giant cell arteritis. A case with unusual neurological manifestations and a normal sedimentation rate. *Arch Intern Med*, **151**, 378–80.

Nesher, G., Berkun, Y., Mates, M., Baras, M., Rubinow, A., and Sonnenblick, M. 2004. *Arthritis Rheumatol*, **50**, 1332–7.

Nesher, G., Rubinow, A., and Sonnenblick, M. 1997. Efficacy and adverse effects of different corticosteroid dose regimens in temporal arteritis: a retrospective study. *Clin Exp Rheumatol*, **15**, 303–6.

Pavlica, P., Barozzi, L., Salvarani, C., Cantini, F., and Olivieri, I. 2000. Magnetic resonance imaging in the diagnosis of polymyalgia rheumatica. *Clin Exp Rheumatol*, **18**, S38–9.

Peyo-Reigosa, R., Garcia-Porrua, C., Pineiro, A., *et al.* 2004. Predictors of cerebrovascular accident in giant cell arteritis in a defined population. *Clin Exp Rheumatol*, **22**, S13–7.

Ray, J. G., Mamdani, M. M., and Geerts, W. H. 2005. Giant cell arteritis and cardiovascular disease in older adults *Heart*, **91**, 324–8.

Redlich, F. C. 1993. A new medical diagnosis of Adolf Hitler. Giant cell arteritis: temporal arteritis. *Arch Intern Med*, **153**, 693–7.

Reich, K. A., Giansiracusa, D. F., and Strongwater, S. L. 1990. Neurologic manifestations of giant cell arteritis. *Am J Med*, **89**, 67–72.

Rucker, J. C., Biousse, V., and Newman, N. 2004. Ischaemic optic neuropathies. *Curr Opin Neurol*, **17**, 27–35.

Ruegg, S., Engelter, S., Jeanneret, C. *et al.* 2003. Bilateral vertebral artery occlusion resulting from giant cell arteritis. Report of 3 cases and review of literature *Medicine*, **82**, 1–12.

Salvarani, C., Cantini, F., Boiardi, L., and Hunder, G. G. 2002. Medical progress: polymyalgia rheumatica and giant cell arteritis. *N Engl J Med*, **347**, 261–71.

Salvarani, C., and Hunder, G. G. 2001. Giant cell arteritis with low ESR: frequency of occurrence in a population-based study. *Arthritis Rheumatol*, **45**, 140–5.

Salvarani, C., Silingardi, M., Ghirarduzzi, A. *et al.* 2002. Is duplex ultrasonography useful for the diagnosis of giant cell arteritis? *Ann Intern Med*, **137**, 232–8.

Schmidt, D. 1994. Giant cell arteritis and Hitler. *Arch Intern Med*, **154**, 930.

Smetana, G. W., and Shmerling, R. H. 2002. Does this patient have temporal arteritis? *JAMA*, **287**, 92–101.

Spiera, R. F., Mitnick, H. J., Kupersmith, M., *et al.* 2001. A randomized, double-blinded, placebo controlled trial of methotrexate in the treatment of giant cell arteritis. *Clin Exp Rheumatol*, **19**, 495–501.

Stanson, A. W. 2000. Imaging findings in extracranial (giant cell) temporal arteritis. *Clin Exp Rheumatol*, **18**, S43–8.

Staunton, H., Stafford, F., Leader, M., and O'Riordain, D. 2000. Deterioration of giant cell arteritis with corticosteroid therapy. *Arch Neurol*, **57**, 581–4.

Tan, A. L., Holdsworth, J., Pease, C., Emery, P., and McGonagle, D. 2003. Successful treatment of resistant giant cell arteritis with etanercept. *Ann Rheumatol Dis*, **62**, 373–4.

Thal, D. R., Barduzal, S., Franz, K., *et al.* 2001. Giant cell arteritis in a 19-year-old woman associated with vertebral artery aneurysm and subarachnoid haemorrhage. *Clin Neuropathol*, **20**, 80–6.

To, K. W., Enzer, Y. R., and Tsiaras, W. G. 1994. Temporal artery biopsy after 1 month of corticosteroid therapy. *Am J Ophthalmol*, **117**, 265–7.

Weyand, C. M., Fulbright, J. W., Hunder, G. G., Evans, J. M., and Goronzy, J. J. 2000. Treatment of giant cell arteritis: interleukin-6 as a biological marker of disease activity. *Arthritis Rheumatol*, **43**, 1041–8.

Weyand, C. M., and Goronzy, J. J. 2003. Giant cell arteritis and polymyalgia rheumatica. *Ann Intern Med*, **139**, 505–15.

Wilkinson, I. M. S., and Ross Russell, R. W. 1972. Arteries of the head and neck in giant cell arteritis. A pathological study to show the patterns of arterial involvement. *Arch Neurol*, **27**, 378–91.

3 VARICELLA ZOSTER AND OTHER VIRUS-RELATED CEREBRAL VASCULOPATHY

Matthias Bischof and Ralf W. Baumgartner

Introduction

Varicella zoster virus (VZV) is a DNA virus of the herpes family. Ten to 14 days after infection of the host, the vesicular rash characteristic of chickenpox appears (White, 1997). Subsequently, the virus migrates to the trigeminal and dorsal root including autonomic ganglia (Gilden et al., 2001), where it remains latent in neurons and satellite cells. It is assumed that waning of cellular immunity to VZV, which usually occurs decades later in life or during immunosuppression, activates the virus and causes herpes zoster (White, 1997).

Epidemiology of neurological complications related to chickenpox and herpes zoster

In temperate climates such as the United States or Europe, almost all individuals are infected by VZV as they reach adulthood, whereas in tropical countries chickenpox is often a disease of young adults (White, 1997). Neurological complications of chickenpox include cerebellar ataxia and encephalitis, which are estimated to occur in 1 per 4 000 (Guess et al., 1986) and in 1.7 per 100 000 (Preblud et al., 1984) children beyond 15 years of age, respectively. In addition, a few patients with ischemic stroke occurring after chickenpox were reported (Bodensteiner et al., 1992; Caekebeke et al., 1990; Eda et al., 1983; Gibbs and Fisher, 1986; Griffith et al., 1970; Hosseinipour et al., 1998; Hung et al., 2000; Kamholz and Tremblay, 1985; Leopold, 1993; Liu and Holmes, 1990; Shuper et al., 1990; Tsolia et al., 1995; Yilmaz et al., 1998). In a cohort study of young children (aged 6 months to 10 years) chickenpox has been identified as an independent risk factor for ischemic stroke (Askalan et al., 2001).

The risk for the development of herpes zoster is increased by age, immunosuppression, and VZV infection acquired in utero or during the first year of life, and is increased in white people compared to black people (Guess et al., 1986; Schmader et al., 1995). The estimated annual incidence rates of herpes zoster are 74 per 100 000 children younger than 10 years of age compared to 1010 per 100 000 adults aged 80–90 years (Hope-Simpson, 1965). In the immunocompetent host, complications involving the central nervous system (CNS) were 0.2% in a population-based study (Ragozzino et al., 1982). They consisted of cranial neuropathy including Ramsey-Hunt syndrome (Jemsek et al., 1983), encephalomyelitis (Rose et al., 1964), optic neuritis (Jemsek et al., 1983), and leukoencephalitis (Horton et al., 1981). In rare cases, ischemic

stroke occurs several weeks after the onset of herpes zoster. Varicella zoster virus infections of the CNS develop preferentially in immunocompromised individuals, especially those affected by HIV and cancer (Dolin et al., 1978; Gray et al., 1994; Jemsek et al., 1983). In autopsy series of immunocompromised patients, CNS affection was detected in 1.5%–4.4% (Gray et al., 1991; Gray et al., 1994; Petito et al., 1986), whereas other neuropathological series of HIV-positive individuals did not mention any case (Anders et al., 1986; Budka et al., 1987; Lang et al., 1989). In the patients with HIV infection, VZV vasculopathy of the CNS occurred often late in the course of the disease, when CD4+ cells were depleted. This was not only true in postmortem series (Baudrimont et al., 1994; Gilden et al., 1988; Gray et al., 1994; McArthur, 1987; Morgello et al., 1988; Rosenblum, 1989; Rostad et al., 1989; Ryder et al., 1986; Vinters et al., 1988), but also in clinical observations of patients whose neurological deficits improved after antiviral treatment (Rousseau et al., 1993). The introduction of highly active antiretroviral therapy (HAART) substantially decreased the morbidity and mortality due to HIV infection including HIV-associated VZV vasculopathy (Egger et al., 1997; Gulick et al., 1997; Hammer et al., 1997; Palella et al., 1998; Powderly et al., 1998).

Pathogenesis of cerebral vasculopathy related to chickenpox and herpes zoster

Chickenpox-related cerebral vasculopathy is assumed to result from hematogenous viral invasion of vessel walls by VZV as has been shown for herpes zoster (see later: cerebral vasculopathy related to herpes zoster). In addition, VZV-specific immunoglobulin G (IgG) antibodies were identified in the cerebrospinal fluid (CSF) of two patients with strokes occurring after chickenpox (Caekebeke et al., 1990; Shuper et al., 1990). However, VZV-specific IgG antibodies can still be demonstrated several months after uncomplicated herpes zoster (Haanpää et al., 1998), and do not per se provide definite evidence for active infection. In other reports, VZV-specific antibodies were either not detected (Leopold, 1993) or not mentioned (Hosseinipour et al., 1998), or the CSF/blood quotient for albumin was not given, preventing an adequate interpretation of the CSF VZV-specific antibody titers (Shuper et al., 1990). Finally, no virus particles, antigen, or DNA was demonstrated in the walls of vessels assumed to be affected by VZV after chickenpox (Bodensteiner et al., 1992; Caekebeke et al., 1990; Eda et al., 1983; Gibbs and Fisher, 1986; Griffith et al., 1970;

Uncommon Causes of Stroke, 2nd edition, ed. Louis R. Caplan. Published by Cambridge University Press. © Cambridge University Press 2008.

Hosseinipour *et al.*, 1998; Kamholz and Tremblay, 1985; Leopold, 1993; Liu and Holmes, 1990; Shuper *et al.*, 1990). Therefore, the causal relationship between chickenpox and intracranial arteriopathy is unproven and might just be a coincidence because chickenpox is a frequent disease.

Herpes zoster-related cerebral vasculopathy is well-documented as herpesvirus nucleocapsids have been detected by electron microscopy (Doyle *et al.*, 1983; Linnemann and Alvira, 1980), VZV antigen by immunocytochemistry, and VZV DNA by *in situ* hybridization or polymerase chain reaction (PCR) (Amlie-Lefond *et al.*, 1995; Eidelberg *et al.*, 1986; Gilden and Kleinschmidt-DeMasters, 1998; Gilden *et al.*, 1996; Gray *et al.*, 1994; Melanson *et al.*, 1996; Morgello *et al.*, 1988) in the walls of large and small intracranial arteries. In the pathogenesis of intracranial vasculopathy, both a VZV-induced autoimmune process and viral invasion of the vessels are proposed (Melanson *et al.*, 1996). Several possibilities for the access of VZV to the cerebral vessels have been reported.

(A) After the occurrence of herpes zoster ophthalmicus (HZO), the virus may reach the arterial wall by direct neural passage along intracranial branches of the trigeminal nerve (Eidelberg *et al.*, 1986; MacKenzie *et al.*, 1981). Trigeminovascular innervation is unilateral and more dense in the middle cerebral arteries (MCA) and anterior cerebral arteries (ACA) than in other cerebral arteries (Mayberg *et al.*, 1980; Moskowitz, 1970). This may explain why cerebral vasculopathy occurs more frequently after ophthalmic compared to segmental herpes zoster, is frequently located on the side of the skin lesion, and is often distributed in the MCA or ACA territories (Eidelberg *et al.*, 1986; MacKenzie *et al.*, 1981). (B) Hematogenous seeding of intracranial vessels. It has been shown that VZV viremia is frequent in patients with herpes zoster, and that subclinical reactivation occurs in immunocompetent and immunocompromised subjects (Mainka *et al.*, 1998). Autopsy studies suggest that, in some patients, VZV may enter the spinal cord and small vessels via axonal spread from dermatomal zoster (Amlie-Lefond *et al.*, 1995). (C) Antero- or retrograde transaxonal and trans-synaptic spread may occur within the CNS (Amlie-Lefond *et al.*, 1995; Cheatham, 1953; Gray *et al.*, 1994; Rostad *et al.*, 1989).

In a patient with chronic VZV vasculopathy, it was recently demonstrated that the oligoclonal IgG in the CSF was directed against the causative virus (Burgoon *et al.*, 2003).

Cerebral vasculopathy related to herpes zoster

The syndrome of HZO followed 2–6 weeks (range 1 week to 6 months) later by contralateral hemiplegia related to vasculopathy of large cerebral arteries was first recognized in 1896 (Brissaud, 1896). Since then, several further occurrences were reported (Doyle *et al.*, 1983; Eidelberg *et al.*, 1986; Gray *et al.*, 1994; MacKenzie *et al.*, 1981; Melanson *et al.*, 1996) suggesting that it is the most frequent zoster-related cerebral vasculopathy. In some cases zoster rash did not involve the trigeminal nerve distribution (Ahmad and Boruchoff, 2003; Hilt *et al.*, 1983; Kolodny *et al.*, 1968; Rosenblum and Hadfield, 1972), followed the CNS deficits

(Jemsek *et al.*, 1983), or was absent (Ahmad and Boruchoff, 2003; Amlie-Lefond *et al.*, 1995).

The clinical course was characterized by gradual resolution of cutaneous HZO followed by the acute onset of contralateral hemiparesis, hemisensory symptoms, or aphasia (Hilt *et al.*, 1983; Reshef *et al.*, 1985). The neurological manifestations were usually monophasic, but some patients had recurrent strokes (Hilt *et al.*, 1983; Reshef *et al.*, 1985). Transient ischemic attacks (TIAs) and amaurosis fugax were uncommon (Dalal and Dalal, 1989; Gilbert, 1974). Some patients may show symptoms and signs of optic nerve infarction or posterior ischemic optic neuropathy (Bourdette *et al.*, 1983; Gilden *et al.*, 2002; Hilt *et al.*, 1983; Lexa *et al.*, 1993; Reshef *et al.*, 1985; Terborg and Busse, 1995;). Reshef *et al.* (1985) reported diffuse CNS symptoms in 47% of 51 patients following the onset of HZO. The CNS symptoms occurred before, during, or after the appearance of contralateral hemiparesis and consisted of stupor, somnolence, confusion, delirium, memory deficits, or depression. Prognosis of stroke is guarded as mortality was 20–28% (Hilt *et al.*, 1983; Reshef *et al.*, 1985), 34% had moderate or severe neurological deficits, and 38% had slight or no neurological deficits (Hilt *et al.*, 1983). Stroke-related death usually resulted from brain edema and herniation subsequent to an acute infarction (Doyle *et al.*, 1983; Eidelberg *et al.*, 1986). Immunocompromised patients probably had a greater mortality compared to patients with cerebral infarction alone (Reshef *et al.*, 1985). This may explain that most autopsy reports of VZV vasculopathy derived from the latter group (Amlie-Lefond *et al.*, 1995; Doyle *et al.*, 1983; Eidelberg *et al.*, 1986; Gray *et al.*, 1994; Hilt *et al.*, 1983; Kolodny *et al.*, 1968; Linnemann and Alvira, 1980; Morgello *et al.*, 1988; Rosenblum, 1989; Rosenblum and Hadfield, 1972; Ryder *et al.*, 1986;) compared to the scarcity of pathological descriptions in immunocompetent patients (Bourdette *et al.*, 1983; Hilt *et al.*, 1983; Reshef *et al.*, 1985).

CSF studies were abnormal in 70% (Reshef *et al.*, 1985). Most normal CSF samples were obtained only once. The most common findings were an elevated white blood cell (WBC) count consisting of mononuclear cells (mean, 46; range, 0–1200 WBC/mm^3), elevated protein (mean, 90; range, 30–445 µg/dL), and normal levels of glucose (mean, 90; range, 30–445 µg/dL) (Reshef *et al.*, 1985). Less frequently noted abnormalities were increased polymorphonuclear leukocytes (65–100% of WBC, up to 1200/mm^3) (Doyle *et al.*, 1983; Hughes, 1951) and hypoglycorrhachia (Reshef *et al.*, 1985). Antibodies directed against VZV, VZV antigens, and DNA (PCR) can be detected in the CSF to confirm the diagnosis of VZV infection of the CNS. Definite proof of a possible causal link between vasculopathy and VZV age can only be obtained by detecting viral antigen or DNA in the wall of cerebral arteries (see above). Cerebral biopsy, however, is frequently not indicated in these patients.

Computed tomography or *MRI of the brain* showed nonspecific findings consistent with ischemic infarction. Less frequently, symptomatic hemorrhage complicating ischemic infarction (Elble, 1983), subarachnoid hemorrhage (Fukumoto *et al.*, 1986; Jain *et al.*, 2003), and basal meningitis (Gray *et al.*, 1994) were depicted. Infarcts were mainly unilateral and located in the superficial and/or deep territories of the MCA or ACA. Bilateral infarcts in the territories of the MCA or ACAs, or of the posterior cerebral (PCA) or basilar (BA) arteries, were less frequent (Baudrimont *et al.*, 1994; Eidelberg *et al.*, 1986; Linnemann and Alvira, 1980; Reshef *et al.*, 1985; Rosenblum, 1989).

Catheter or magnetic resonance angiography (MRA) showed abnormal findings in most cases. They included irregular beaded or segmental narrowing, or occlusion of one or more basal cerebral arteries and/or their main branches including the siphon and the terminal segment of the intracranial internal carotid artery (ICA), the MCA, ACA, PCA, or BA. Several authors reported obstructions of the contralateral ACA (Reshef *et al.*, 1985), both ACAs (Terborg and Busse, 1995) or both MCAs (Pratesi *et al.*, 1977), and mycotic aneurysms (Fukumoto *et al.*, 1986; Gursoy *et al.*, 1980; O'Donohue and Enzmann, 1987).

Autopsy features of VZV vasculopathy are determined by various factors, including the phase of disease at which autopsy is performed (acute vs. chronic), host immune responsiveness, the route of viral spread to the brain from latent infection, and probably treatment (Gilden and Kleinschmidt-DeMasters, 1998; Gilden *et al.*, 1996; Gray *et al.*, 1994; Schmidbauer *et al.*, 1992). Furthermore, leptomeningeal arteries showed variable abnormalities, which could be present in the same brain. On one side, thrombotic occlusion of large vessels with little or no inflammation or marked intimal proliferation producing severe luminal narrowing occasionally associated with thrombosis was detected (Eidelberg *et al.*, 1986; Gray *et al.*, 1994). On the other side, granulomatous arteritis with numerous histiocytic and fewer giant cells (Blue and Rosenblum, 1983; Fukumoto *et al.*, 1986; Gilden *et al.*, 1996; Hilt *et al.*, 1983; Rosenblum *et al.*, 1978) and rare cases with necrotizing arteritis (Doyle *et al.*, 1983; Gray *et al.*, 1994; McKelvie *et al.*, 2002) were found. One patient showed features of subarachnoid hemorrhage due to a ruptured aneurysm of the BA, which was affected by granulomatous angiitis (Fukumoto *et al.*, 1986).

There is also a more tenuous relationship between herpes zoster virus infection and primary granulomatous angiitis of the nervous system (PACNS). PACNS primarily affects small penetrating and leptomeningeal vessels in a more diffuse inflammatory process associated with giant cells and granuloma formation (Cravioto and Feigin, 1959; Kolodny *et al.*, 1968). The occasional association of PACNS with antecedent VZV infection has suggested a causal relationship (Gilbert, 1974; Rosenblum and Hadfield, 1972), and in one patient with PACNS herpesvirus nucleocapsids were detected in the wall of affected vessels (Linnemann and Alvira, 1980).

Vasculopathy of small cerebral arteries

In contrast to the abundance of reports of large vessel disease due to VZV, vasculopathy of small cerebral arteries was not appreciated until Horten *et al.* (1981) first described fatal VZV encephalitis in patients with cancer. This was later confirmed by other groups who showed that VZV-related small vessel disease occurred essentially in immunocompromised patients (Amlie-Lefond *et al.*, 1995; Baudrimont *et al.*, 1994; Blue and Rosenblum, 1983; Gilden *et al.*, 1996; Gilden and Kleinschmidt-DeMasters, 1998; Gray *et al.*, 1994; Hilt *et al.*, 1983; Kolodny *et al.*, 1968; Kronenberg *et al.*, 2002; Linnemann and Alvira, 1980; McArthur, 1987; Morgello *et al.*, 1988; Rosenblum, 1989; Rosenblum and Hadfield, 1972; Rosenblum

et al., 1978; Rostad *et al.*, 1989; Russman *et al.*, 2003; Ryder *et al.*, 1986; Vinters *et al.*, 1988). The *neurological symptoms and signs* consisted of a progressive encephalopathy with headache, cognitive and behavioral abnormalities, and focal neurological deficits. The neurological deficit was also determined by the fact that the vasculopathy affected essentially the cerebral hemispheres and, in rare cases, the brainstem (Baudrimont *et al.*, 1994; Rosenblum, 1989). In some patients, clinical features due to concomitant large cerebral artery disease, as mentioned above, were present (Amlie-Lefond *et al.*, 1995). The clinical course of small vessel disease is unknown, because no case diagnosed by brain biopsy has yet been reported.

CSF findings were similar to those observed in patients with vasculopathy of the large cerebral arteries.

CT or MRI of the brain showed multiple superficial and deep infarcts, either ischemic or hemorrhagic, with disproportionate involvement of white matter and a predilection for gray-white matter junctions (Amlie-Lefond *et al.*, 1995).

Cerebral angiography showed in some patients signs of intracranial large cerebral artery disease as described above. At *autopsy*, generally lesser degrees of blood vessel inflammation were found (Gilden and Kleinschmidt-DeMasters, 1998). Nevertheless, cases with granulomatous (Blue and Rosenblum, 1983; Gilden *et al.*, 1996; Hilt *et al.*, 1983; Kolodny *et al.*, 1968; Linnemann and Alvira, 1980; Rosenblum and Hadfield, 1972; Rosenblum *et al.*, 1978;) and necrotizing arteritis (Gilden and Kleinschmidt-DeMasters, 1998; Gray *et al.*, 1994; McKelvie *et al.*, 2002) were reported. Further findings were usually deep seated, multifocal small lesions that involved white matter more than gray matter; they were often concentrated at gray-white matter junctions. Their mixed ischemic-demyelinative composition resulted from both vasculopathy-related ischemia and from spreading of VZV into neurons, glia, and especially oligodendrocytes causing focal demyelination. Some authors appreciated the additional presence of necrotic lesions (Amlie-Lefond *et al.*, 1995; Gray *et al.*, 1994).

Concomitant parenchymal penetration by VZV

Neurological deficits in patients with VZV-related cerebral vasculopathy result from the size and location of the involved vessels as well as concomitant parenchymal penetration by VZV. Immunocompromised patients are particularly likely to develop an extension of the virus beyond the vasculature into CNS parenchyma producing combinations of large and small vessel disease, myelitis, ventriculitis, encephalitis, and leukencephalopathy (Amlie-Lefond *et al.*, 1995; Gray *et al.*, 1994). Finally, patients with HIV infection have other possible causes of CNS deficits (see "Human immunodeficiency virus-related cerebral vasculopathy").

It is unclear whether treatment of herpes zoster with antiviral agents prevents the development of subsequent cerebral vasculopathy and stroke. Case reports of cerebral vasculopathy and stroke following HZO treated by acyclovir suggest that this is not the case (Melanson *et al.*, 1996; Terborg and Busse, 1995).

No proven treatment of VZV-associated intracranial vasculopathy has been described, and in most cases, therapy did not noticeably alter the clinical course (Amlie-Lefond *et al.*, 1995; Gilden and

Kleinschmidt-DeMasters, 1998; Gray *et al.*, 1994; Hilt *et al.*, 1983; Reshef *et al.*, 1985). Nevertheless, patients with VZV-related cerebral vasculopathy have an active viral infection and should thus receive antiviral therapy. According to the guidelines of the International Herpes Management Forum (IHMF), patients with focal (large vessel) vasculopathy should be treated with intravenous acyclovir (10 mg/kg every 8 h for adults, 500 mg/m^2 body surface for children) for 7 days. Immunocompromised patients may require longer treatment (Johnson and Patrick, 2000). The role of steroid therapy (prednisone 60–80 mg daily for 3–5 days) is controversial, but should be considered to reduce inflammation (Johnson and Patrick, 2000). Although these drugs are contraindicated in patients with acute ischemic stroke (Adams *et al.*, 1994; The European Ad Hoc Consensus Group, 1997), many authors administered steroids due to the possible presence of granulomatous angiitis (Amlie-Lefond *et al.*, 1995; Doyle *et al.*, 1983; Gilbert, 1974; Hilt *et al.*, 1983; MacKenzie *et al.*, 1981; Melanson *et al.*, 1996; Pratesi *et al.*, 1977; Reshef *et al.*, 1985; Terborg and Busse, 1995). The optimal antithrombotic therapy for acute ischemic stroke and secondary prevention are unknown. Intravenous and intra-arterial thrombolysis are contraindicated (see below). Aspirin may be appropriate in the acute ischemic stroke setting due to the low hemorrhagic risk (International Stroke Trial Collaborative Group, 1997). Anticoagulation should be used with caution because of the possible presence of acute (necrotizing) vasculitis (Doyle *et al.*, 1983; Gilden and Kleinschmidt-DeMasters, 1998; Gray *et al.*, 1994) and mycotic aneurysms (Fukumoto *et al.*, 1986; Gursoy *et al.*, 1980; O'Donohue and Enzmann, 1987). Nevertheless, several patients with cerebral large artery vasculopathy were treated with anticoagulants, and there was "good recovery" in two patients (MacKenzie *et al.*, 1981) and slight (Laws, 1960) and moderate (Gilbert, 1974) disability in one patient each. Secondary prevention is probably not necessary in immunocompetent patients, because no patient with relapse of vasculopathy and stroke has been reported. Conversely, secondary prevention is justified in immunocompromised patients due to the frequently progressive course of vasculopathy.

Cerebral vasculopathy related to chickenpox

The association of chickenpox and ischemic stroke has been described in young adults (Gibbs and Fisher, 1986; Griffith *et al.*, 1970; Hosseinipour *et al.*, 1998; Leopold, 1993) and children (Bodensteiner *et al.*, 1992; Caekebeke *et al.*, 1990; Eda *et al.*, 1983; Hung *et al.*, 2000; Kamholz and Tremblay, 1985; Liu and Holmes, 1990; Shuper *et al.*, 1990; Tsolia *et al.*, 1995; Yilmaz *et al.*, 1998). A cohort study of 70 young children (aged 6 months to 10 years) showed a 3-fold increase in varicella infection in children who had an arterial ischemic stroke compared to healthy children (Askalan *et al.*, 2001). The *clinical syndrome* consisted of hemiparesis or aphasia occurring 1–3 months after the acute phase of chickenpox (Bodensteiner *et al.*, 1992; Caekebeke *et al.*, 1990; Eda *et al.*, 1983; Gibbs and Fisher, 1986; Griffith *et al.*, 1970; Hosseinipour *et al.*, 1998; Hung *et al.*, 2000; Kamholz and Tremblay, 1985; Leopold, 1993; Liu and Holmes, 1990; Shuper *et al.*, 1990; Tsolia *et al.*, 1995; Yilmaz *et al.*, 1998;). In contrast to herpes zoster–related

cerebral vasculopathy, no patient showed additional neurological and neuroradiological signs of encephalopathy. Stroke recurrence occurring 6 months later was reported in one child (Shuper *et al.*, 1990). *CSF findings* ranged from normal to a mild monocytic pleocytosis and a raised protein content (Hosseinipour *et al.*, 1998). In one patient, WBCs contained 27% segmented neutrophils (Hosseinipour *et al.*, 1998). Furthermore, VZV-specific antibodies were detected in the CSF of two patients (Caekebeke *et al.*, 1990; Shuper *et al.*, 1990). *CT or MRI of the brain* showed unilateral infarcts in the superficial or deep territories of the MCA (Hosseinipour *et al.*, 1998; Leopold, 1993; Shuper *et al.*, 1990; Yilmaz *et al.*, 1998). *Cerebral catheter or MRA* was either normal (Eda *et al.*, 1983) or showed unilateral occlusion of the supraclinoidal ICA in four patients (Bodensteiner *et al.*, 1992; Caekebeke *et al.*, 1990; Leopold, 1993; Liu and Holmes, 1990), segments of narrowing and beading or focal stenoses of the MCA and ACA, and in one patient of the PCA or the BA (Hosseinipour *et al.*, 1998; Kamholz and Tremblay, 1985; Shuper *et al.*, 1990;), sometimes associated with distal occlusions (Kamholz and Tremblay, 1985). The best treatment of ischemic stroke subsequent to chickenpox is unknown. Thrombolysis is contraindicated (see earlier). Some patients were treated without antiviral medication or steroids; other patients had intravenous acyclovir, steroids, or both (Gibbs and Fisher, 1986; Griffith *et al.*, 1970; Hosseinipour *et al.*, 1998; Leopold, 1993). Children had acyclovir, steroids, or both (Bodensteiner *et al.*, 1992; Caekebeke *et al.*, 1990; Eda *et al.*, 1983; Hung *et al.*, 2000; Kamholz and Tremblay, 1985; Liu and Holmes, 1990; Shuper *et al.*, 1990; Tsolia *et al.*, 1995; Yilmaz *et al.*, 1998). Antithrombotic therapy was either not given or consisted of aspirin (plus low-molecular-weight heparin in one case) (Bodensteiner *et al.*, 1992; Caekebeke *et al.*, 1990; Eda *et al.*, 1983; Gibbs and Fisher, 1986; Griffith *et al.*, 1970; Hosseinipour *et al.*, 1998; Hung *et al.*, 2000; Kamholz and Tremblay, 1985; Leopold, 1993; Liu and Holmes, 1990; Shuper *et al.*, 1990; Tsolia *et al.*, 1995; Yilmaz *et al.*, 1998). No antithrombotics for secondary stroke prevention were administered (Bodensteiner *et al.*, 1992; Caekebeke *et al.*, 1990; Eda *et al.*, 1983; Gibbs and Fisher, 1986; Griffith *et al.*, 1970; Hosseinipour *et al.*, 1998; Hung *et al.*, 2000; Kamholz and Tremblay, 1985; Leopold, 1993; Liu and Holmes, 1990; Shuper *et al.*, 1990; Tsolia *et al.*, 1995; Yilmaz *et al.*, 1998).

HIV-related cerebral vasculopathy

Treatment of patients infected with HIV has changed enormously in the last decade. In 1996, a combination of two nucleosides became the recommended initial regimen as several trials have shown that this therapy is superior to zidovudine alone (Carpenter *et al.*, 1996). In the following years, HAART consisting of a protease inhibitor and two non-nucleoside-analogue reverse transcriptase inhibitors, led to suppression of plasma HIV concentrations and repletion of CD4+ cell counts, translating into substantial decreases in morbidity and mortality due to AIDS (Egger *et al.*, 1997; Gulick *et al.*, 1997; Hammer *et al.*, 1997; Palella *et al.*, 1998), and reduction in the incidence of AIDS (Powderly *et al.*, 1998), including strokes associated with opportunistic infections and tumors, and advanced stages of immunosuppression. However, the use of protease inhibitors is associated with a variety of metabolic derangements that might produce accelerated atherosclerosis. The Data Collection on Adverse Events of Anti-HIV drugs (DAD) study group reported an increased incidence of myocardial infarction by an average of 26% per year of exposure to combination antiretroviral treatment in 2003 (Friis-Moller et al., 2003). In a subsequent study, an increased risk for cardio- and cerebrovascular diseases (after exclusion of secondary events from HIV CNS morbidity) was found (d'Arminio et al., 2004).

Before the introduction of HAART, CNS dysfunction frequently complicated the course of HIV infection. Involvement of the CNS occurred due to primary HIV infection or to secondary complications of immunodeficiency such as infection with opportunistic microorganisms and neoplasm. Pinto (1996) concluded that it remained unclear whether there is an association between stroke and AIDS in adults. Qureshi et al. (1997) found in a retrospective case–control study that HIV infection was associated with an increased risk of stroke. However, their patients had a mean age of 35 years, 40% used cocaine, 22% were HIV seropositive, and 9% had AIDS (Qureshi et al., 1997). Besides the possibility of cocaine-related strokes, the latter patients do not reflect the average stroke patient, and the issue of an association between HIV infection and stroke remained unanswered. A newer autopsy cohort study including 183 HIV-infected patients distinguished between cerebral infarcts associated with non-HIV CNS infection, CNS lymphoma, or cardioembolic sources and cerebral infarcts occurring in the absence of these conditions (Connor et al., 2000). Twenty-six patients without evidence of opportunistic cerebral infarction underwent a second selection process in which the presence of cerebral infarction, in the absence of the above mentioned conditions, was verified. Ten cases (5.5%) fulfilled these inclusion criteria: small vessel disease was found in all cases, vasculitis was not found. One patient had a TIA, and no patient had a stroke. It was concluded that cerebral infarcts in HIV-infected patients are not common in the absence of the above mentioned conditions.

The incidence of symptomatic cerebrovascular disease in pediatric AIDS is 1.3%, but cerebrovascular lesions were present in 25% at autopsy (Burns, 1992; Husson et al., 1992). The pathomechanisms include cardiac embolism, hypoperfusion, thrombocytopenia, and vasculopathy related to VZV, mycobacterial or fungal infections. To date, reports on 25 children (de Carvalho Neto et al., 2001; Dubrovsky et al., 1998; Fulmer et al., 1998; Husson et al., 1992; Martinez-Longoria et al., 2004; Nunes et al., 2001; Park et al., 1990; Philippet et al., 1994; Visrutaratna and Oranratanachai, 2002) and two young adults (Kossorotoff et al., 2006) document that patients with AIDS may rarely develop cerebral aneurysmal arteriopathy (CAA), which may cause ischemic and hemorrhagic stroke. Strokes in AIDS patients with VZV vasculopathy are given in Chapter 15 (see "VZV related cerebral vasculopathy").

PACNS related to HIV infection

PACNS is a disease in which CNS is the sole or dominant target organ of a vasculitic process, affecting the small and medium leptomeningeal and cortical arteries and, less frequently, the veins and venules. By definition, it is not associated with any process known to involve the CNS. An actual review of literature resulted in the detection of 22 HIV-positive patients with the histologically verified diagnosis of PACNS (Berger et al., 1990; Engstrom et al., 1989; Frank et al., 1989; Gray et al., 1992; Mizusawa et al., 1988; Nogueras et al., 2002; Rhodes, 1987; Scaravilli et al., 1989; Schwartz et al., 1986; Vinters et al., 1988; Yankner et al., 1986). The clinical features of these patients were various, consisting of both progressive encephalopathy and focal neurological deficits. *Autopsy* showed granulomatous arteritis of large and medium-sized intracerebral and leptomeningeal arteries with severe luminal narrowing and thrombosis with vessel occlusion, and infarcts located in the cortex, white matter, and basal ganglia of both cerebral hemispheres and in the pons. However, no viral material was detected in the wall of intracranial vessels, and the causal relationship between cerebral vasculopathy and HIV remains unproven. Different mechanisms – including infection of endothelial cells by HIV or other organisms, immune complex deposition, and impaired regulation of cytokines and adhesion molecules – are suggested.

CAA in childhood AIDS

Cerebral aneurysmal arteriopathy (CAA) is characterized by diffuse dilatation of the large intracranial cerebral arteries (de Carvalho Neto et al., 2001; Dubrovsky et al., 1998; Fulmer et al., 1998; Husson et al., 1992; Kossorotoff et al., 2006; Martinez-Longoria et al., 2004; Nunes et al., 2001; Park et al., 1990; Philippet et al., 1994; Visrutaratna and Oranratanachai, 2002). Dubrovsky et al. (1998) described clinical and radiological features of 13 children with CAA: cerebrovascular disease was detected 2–11 years following HIV infection, and, on average, $2^1/_2$ years after the diagnosis of AIDS. All children had a severely depressed immune system with a history of multiple opportunistic infections, and the mean CD4+ count was 23 (range, 0–107) at the time of CAA diagnosis. Ten children had strokes from ischemic infarction (eight) and fatal subarachnoid and intracerebral hemorrhage (two), the remaining three were asymptomatic. Ischemic strokes were unilateral (affecting the basal ganglia or the thalamus) in five of eight children and bihemispheric in the other three patients. A second ischemic stroke occurred in three patients. The mean survival time after diagnosis of CAA was 8 months and shortened to 5.5 months after cerebrovascular accidents.

The few performed *CSF studies* were normal. *Cerebral CT, MRI, or catheter or MRA* showed uni- or bilateral ectasia and aneurysmal dilatation of the large intracranial cerebral arteries. Three patients with ischemic stroke had catheter angiography, which showed in addition segmental stenoses (Martinez-Longoria et al., 2004; Park et al., 1990) or thrombotic occlusions (Philippet et al., 1994) of small cortical branches distal to the dilated cerebral arteries. These findings suggest that ischemic strokes may have resulted from arterioarterial thromboembolism originating in the dilated large cerebral arteries, a well-known phenomenon in cerebral aneurysms of adult patients. *Autopsy studies* were done in four children and confirmed vascular ectasia and aneurysmal dilatation limited to the large basal cerebral arteries, whereas leptomeningeal and intraparenchymal arteries and arterioles were spared. Typical findings were medial fibrosis with loss of muscularis, destruction of the internal elastic lamina, and intimal hyperplasia suggesting the prior presence of vasculitis. The very unusual presentation of the vasculopathy and the detection of HIV protein or genomic material in two autopsy cases argue in favor of HIV-related arteritis as a possible causative factor (Dubrovsky *et al.*, 1998; Kure *et al.*, 1989). Unilateral involvement of the cerebral arteries in three children and the presence of ipsilateral HZO in one of the three children suggest that also VZV may have played a pathogenetic role.

Other viruses and cerebral vasculopathy

Several observations suggest that infection with *cytomegalovirus (CMV)* or *herpes simplex virus (HSV)* plays a role in the *pathogenesis of atherosclerosis*. Clinical studies reported an increased prevalence of CMV and HSV infections among individuals with accelerated atherosclerosis in the extracranial carotid arteries (Melnick *et al.*, 1990; Nieto *et al.*, 1996; Saetta *et al.*, 2000; Sorlie *et al.*, 1994). In addition, histopathological studies have detected CMV and HSV particles within atherosclerotic vessels (Benditt *et al.*, 1983; Gyorkey *et al.*, 1984; Hendrix *et al.*, 1990; Shi and Tokunaga, 2002), and infection with HSV-induced atherosclerosis in avian models (Minick *et al.*, 1979). Furthermore, prior infection with CMV has been shown to be a strong independent risk factor for restenosis after coronary atherectomy (Zhou *et al.*, 1996). CMV was present in smooth-muscle cells from restenotic lesions of patients who had undergone coronary angioplasty, and can express immediate early gene products, which can inhibit the p53 tumor-suppressor gene product (Speir *et al.*, 1994). Conversely, two prospective studies including a nested case–control study of apparently healthy American men followed up over a 12-year period found no evidence of a positive association between baseline IgG antibodies directed against CMV or HSV and the development of future thromboembolic stroke and myocardial infarction (Fagerberg *et al.*, 1999; Ridker *et al.*, 1998). In addition, two histological studies have failed to detect CMV in the atherosclerotic tissue of coronary (Daus *et al.*, 1998) and carotid (Saetta *et al.*, 2000) arteries. In conclusion, the role of viral infection in the pathogenesis of atherosclerosis of cerebral arteries is still unclear.

Cerebral arteriitis in other viral infections

A patient treated with immunosuppressive therapy for a lymphoma developed a progressive neurological deficit characterized by decreasing alertness, epileptic seizures, blindness, deafness, and paraplegia (Koeppen *et al.*, 1981). Autopsy showed multiple infarcts in the brain and spinal cord due to occlusive arteriitis, and electron microscopy of brain and retinal tissue revealed particles compatible with *CMV*. Another patient with progressive focal neurologic deficit showed granulomatous vasculitis affecting the leptomeninx and adjacent vessels, and PCR revealed *HSV type 1* as the cause of inflammation (Schmidt *et al.*, 1992). Brain biopsy in a case with *stealth viral encephalopathy* delineated also focal perivascular lymphocytic inflammation in the leptomeninges and brain parenchyma (Martin, 1996). In all presumed viral vasculitides of the brain mentioned above, no CMV, HSV type 1, or stealth virus

material was detected in the wall of cerebral arteries. Therefore, the cause of the vasculitis remains unclear.

REFERENCES

Adams, H. P. Jr., Brott, T. G., Crowell, R. B., *et al.* 1994. Guidelines for the management of patients with acute ischemic stroke. A statement for healthcare professionals from a special writing group of the stroke council, American Heart Association. *Stroke*, **25**, 1901–14.

Ahmad, N. M., and Boruchoff, S. E. 2003. Multiple cerebral infarcts due to varicella-zoster virus large-vessel vasculopathy in an immunocompetent adult without skin involvement. *Clin Infect Dis*, **37**, 16–8.

Amlie-Lefond, C., Kleinschmidt-DeMasters, B. K., Mahalingam, R., Davis, L. E., and Gilden, D. H. 1995. The vasculopathy of varicella zoster virus encephalitis. *Ann Neurol*, **37**, 784–90.

Anders, K. H., Guerra, W. F., Tomiyasu, U., Verity, M. A., and Vinters, H.V. 1986. The neuropathology of AIDS. UCLA experience and review. *Am J Pathol*, **124**, 537–58.

Askalan, R., Laughlin, S., Mayank, S., *et al.* 2001. Chickenpox and stroke in childhood: a study of frequency and causation. *Stroke*. **32**, 1257–62.

Baudrimont, M., Moulignier, A., Huerre, M., and Dupont, B. 1994. Varicella-zoster virus (VZV) brain stem encephalitis: report of one case [abstract]. *Neuropathol Appl Neurobiol*, **20**, 313.

Benditt, E. P., Barrett, T., and McDougall, J. K. 1983. Viruses in the etiology of atherosclerosis. *Proc Natl Acad Sci USA*, **80**, 6386–9.

Berger, J. R., Harris, J. O., Gregorios, J., and Norenberg, M. 1990. Cerebrovascular disease in AIDS: a case-control study. *AIDS*, **4**, 239–44.

Blue, M. C., and Rosenblum, W. C. 1983. Granulomatous angiitis of the brain with herpes zoster and varicella encephalitis. *Arch Pathol Lab Med*, **107**, 126–8.

Bodensteiner, J. B., Hille, M. R., and Riggs, J. E. 1992. Clinical features of vascular thrombosis following varicella. *Am J Dis Child*, **146**, 100–2.

Bourdette, D. N., Rosenberg, N. L., and Yatsu, F. M. 1983. Herpes zoster ophthalmicus and delayed ipsilateral cerebral infarction. *Neurology*, **33**, 1428–32.

Brissaud, E. 1896. Du zona ophthalmique avec hémiplégie croisée. *J Med Chir*, **3**, 209–25.

Budka, H., Costanzi, G., Cristina, S., *et al.* 1987. Brain pathology induced by infection with the human immunodeficiency virus (HIV). A histological, immunocytochemical, and electron microscopical study of 100 autopsy cases. *Acta Neuropathol*, **75**, 185–98.

Burgoon, M. P., Hammack, B. N., Owens, G. P., *et al.* 2003. Oligoclonal immunoglobulins in cerebrospinal fluid during varicella zoster virus (VZV) vasculopathy are directed against VZV. *Ann Neurol*, **54**, 459–63.

Burns, D. K. 1992. The neuropathology of pediatric acquired immunodeficiency syndrome. *J Child Neurol*, **7**, 332–46.

Caekebeke, J. F. V., Boudewyn Peters, A. C., Vandvik, B., Brower, O. F., and de Bakker, H. M. 1990. Cerebral vasculopathy associated with primary varicella infection. *Arch Neurol*, **47**, 1033–5.

Carpenter, C. C. J., Fischl, M. A., Hammer, S. M., *et al.* 1996. Antiretroviral therapy for HIV infection in 1996. *JAMA*, **276**, 146–54.

Cheatham, W. J. 1953. The relation of heretofore unreported lesions to pathogenesis of herpes zoster. *Am J Pathol.*, **29**, 401–11.

Connor, M. D., Lammie, G. A., Bell, J. E., *et al.* 2000. Cerebral infarction in adult AIDS patients: observations from the Edinburgh HIV Autopsy Cohort. *Stroke*, **31**, 2117–26.

Cravioto, H., and Feigin, I. 1959. Noninfectious granulomatous angiitis with a predilection for the nervous system. *Neurology*, **9**, 599–609.

d'Arminio, A., Sabin, C. A., Phillips, A. N., *et al.* 2004. Cardio- and cerebrovascular events in HIV-infected persons. *AIDS*, **18**, 1811–7.

Dalal, P. M., and Dalal, K. P. 1989. Cerebrovascular manifestations of infectious disease. In: P. Vinken C, J F, eds., *Handbook of Clinical Neurology*. Amsterdam: Elsevier. pp. 411–41.

Daus, H., Ozbek, C., Saage, D., *et al.* 1998. Lack of evidence for a pathogenic role of Chlamydia pneumoniae and cytomegalovirus infection in coronary atheroma formation. *Cardiology*, **90**, 83–8.

de Carvalho Neto, A., Bruck, I., Coelho, L. O., *et al.* 2001. Cerebral arterial aneurysm in a child with acquired immunodeficiency syndrome: case report. *Arq Neuropsiquiatr*, **59**, 444–8.

Dolin, R., Reichman, R. C., Mazur, M. H., and Whitley, R. J. 1978. Herpes zoster-varicella infections in immunosuppressed patients. *Ann Intern Med*, **89**, 375–88.

Doyle, P. W., Gibson, G., and Dolman, C. L. 1983. Herpes zoster ophthalmicus with contralateral hemiplegia: identification of cause. *Ann Neurol*, **14**, 84–5.

Dubrovsky, T., Curless, R., Scott, G., *et al.* 1998. Cerebral aneurysmal arteriopathy in childhood AIDS. *Neurology*, **51**, 560–5.

Eda, I., Takashima, S., and Takeshia, K. 1983. Acute hemiplegia with lacunar infarct after varicella infection in childhood. *Brain Dev*, **5**, 358–60.

Egger, M., Hirschel, B., Francioli, P., *et al.* 1997. Impact of new antiretroviral combination therapies in HIV infected patients in Switzerland: prospective multicentre study. *BMJ*, **315**, 1194–9.

Eidelberg, D., Sotrel, A., Horoupian, D. S., Neumann, P. E., Pumarola-Sune, T., and Price, R. W. 1986. Thrombotic cerebral vasculopathy associated with herpes zoster. *Ann Neurol*, **19**, 7–14.

Elble, R. J. 1983. Intracerebral hemorrhage with herpes zoster ophthalmicus. *Ann Neurol*, **14**, 591–2.

Engstrom, J. W., Lowenstein, D. H., and Bredesen, D. E. 1989. Cerebral infarctions and transient neurologic deficits associated with acquired immunodeficiency syndrome. *Am J Med*, **86**, 528–32.

The European Ad Hoc Consensus Group. 1997. Optimizing intensive care in stroke: A European perspective. A report of an ad hoc consensus group meeting. *Cerebrovasc Dis*, **7**, 113–28.

Fagerberg, B., Gnarpe, J., Gnarpe, H., Agewall, S., and Wikstrand, J. 1999. Chlamydia pneumoniae but not cytomegalovirus antibodies are associated with future risk of stroke and cardiovascular disease: a prospective study in middle-aged to elderly men with treated hypertension. *Stroke*, **30**, 299–305.

Frank, Y., Lim, W., Kahn, E., *et al.* 1989. Multiple ischemic infarcts in a child with AIDS, varicella zoster infection, and cerebral vasculitis. *Pediatr Neurol*, **5**, 64–7.

Friis-Moller, N., Sabin, C. A., Weber, R., *et al.* 2003. Combination antiretroviral therapy and the risk of myocardial infarction. *N Engl J Med*, **349**, 1993–2003.

Fukumoto, S., Kinjo, M., Hokamura, K., and Tanaka, K. 1986. Subarachnoid hemorrhage and granulomatous angiitis of the basilar artery: demonstration of the varicella-zoster virus in the basilar artery lesions. *Stroke*, **17**, 1024–8.

Fulmer, B. B., Dillard, S. C., Musulman, E. M., Palmer, C. A., and Oakes, J. 1998. Two cases of cerebral aneurysms in HIV+ children. *Pediatr Neurosurg*, **28**, 31–4.

Gibbs, M.A., and Fisher, M. 1986. Cerebral infarction in an adult with disseminated varicella. *Bull Clin Neurosci 51*:65–7.

Gilbert, G. J. 1974. Herpes zoster ophthalmicus and delayed contralateral hemiparesis. *JAMA*, **229**, 302–4.

Gilden, D. H., Gesser, R., Smith, J., *et al.* 2001. Presence of VZV and HSV-1 DNA in human nodose and celiac ganglia. *Virus Genes*, **23**, 145–7.

Gilden, D.H., and Kleinschmidt-DeMasters, B.K. 1998. Reply from the authors. *Neurology*, **51**, 324–5.

Gilden, D.H., Kleinschmidt-DeMasters, B. K., Wellish, M., *et al.* 1996. Varicella zoster virus, a cause of waxing and waning vasculitis: the New England Journal of Medicine case 5–1995 revisited. *Neurology*, **47**, 1441–6.

Gilden, D. H., Lipton, H. L., Wolf, J. S., *et al.* 2002. Two patients with unusual forms of varicella-zoster virus vasculopathy. *N Engl J Med*, **347**, 1500–3.

Gilden, D. H., Murray, R. S., Wellish, M., Kleinschmidt-DeMasters, B. K., and Vafai, A. 1988. Chronic progressive varicella-zoster virus encephalitis in an AIDS patient. *Neurology*, **38**, 1150–3.

Gray, F., Bélec, L., Lescs, M. C., *et al.* 1994. Varicella-zoster virus infection of the central nervous system in the acquired immune deficiency syndrome. *Brain*, **117**, 987–99.

Gray, F., Geny, C., Lionnet, F., *et al.* 1991. Etude neuropathologique de 135 cas adultes de syndrome d'immuno-déficience acquise (SIDA). *Ann Pathol*, **11**, 236–47.

Gray, F., Lescs, M. C., Keohane, C., *et al.* 1992. Early brain changes in HIV infection: neuropathological study of 11 HIV seropositive, non-AIDS cases. *J Neuropathol Exp Neurol*, **51**, 177–85.

Griffith, J. F., Salam, M.V., and Adams, R.D. 1970. The nervous system diseases associated with varicella. *Acta Neurol Scand*, **46**, 279–300.

Guess, H. A., Broughton, D. D., Melton, L. J. III, Kurland, L. D. 1986. Population-based studies of varicella complications. *Pediatrics*, **78**(**suppl**), 723–7.

Gulick, R. M., Mellor, J. W., Havlir, D., *et al.* 1997. A controlled trial of two nucleoside analogues plus indinavir in persons with human immunodeficiency virus infection and prior antiretroviral therapy. *N Engl J Med*, **33**, 734–9.

Gursoy, G., Aktin, E., Bahar, S., Tolun, R., Ozden, B. 1980. Postherpetic aneurysm in the intrapetrosal portion of the internal carotid artery. *Neuroradiology*, **19**, 279–82.

Gyorkey, F., Melnick, J. L., Guinn, G. A., Gyuorkey, P., DeBakey, M. E. 1984. Herpes viridiae in the endothelial and smooth muscle cells of the proximal aorta of atherosclerotic patients. *Exp Mol Pathol*, **40**, 328–39.

Haanpää, M., Dastidar, P., Weinberg, A., *et al.* 1998. CSF and MRI findings in patients with acute herpes zoster. *Neurology*, **51**, 1405–11.

Hammer, S. M., Squires, K. E., Hughes, M. D., *et al.* 1997. A controlled trial of two nucleoside analogues plus indinavir in persons with human immunodeficiency virus and CD4 cell counts of 200 per cubic millimeter or less. *N Engl J Med*, **337**, 725–33.

Hendrix, M. G., Salimans, M. M., van Boven, C. P., and Bruggemann, C. A. 1990. High prevalence of latently present cytomegalovirus in arterial walls of patients suffering from grade III atherosclerosis. *Am J Pathol*, **136**, 23–8.

Hilt, D. C., Buchholz, D., and Krumholz, A. 1983. Herpes zoster ophthalmicus and delayed contralateral hemiparesis caused by cerebral angiitis: diagnosis and management approaches. *Ann Neurol*, **14**, 543–53.

Hope-Simpson, R. E. 1965. The nature of herpes zoster: a long-term study and a new hypothesis. *Proc Roy Soc Med*, **58**, 9–20.

Horton, B., Price, R. W., and Jimenez, D. 1981. Multifocal varicella-zoster virus leukoencephalitis temporally remote from herpes zoster. *Ann Neurol*, **9**, 151–266.

Hosseinipour, M. C., Smith, N. H., Simpson, E. P., Greenberg, S. B., Armstrong, R. M., and White, A. C. Jr. 1998. Middle cerebral artery vasculitis and stroke after varicella in a young adult. *South Med J*, **91**, 1070–2.

Hughes, W. N. 1951. Herpes zoster of the right trigeminal nerve with left hemiplegia. *Neurology*, **1**, 167–9.

Hung, P. Y., Lee, W. T., and Shen, Y. Z. 2000. Acute hemiplegia associated with herpes zoster infection in children: report of one case. *Pediatr Neurol*, **23**, 345–8.

Husson, R. N., Salni, R., Lewis, L. L., Butler, K. M., Patronas, N., and Pizzo, P. A. 1992. Cerebral artery aneurysms in children infected with human immunodeficiency virus. *J Pediatr*, **121**, 927–30.

International Stroke Trial Collaborative Group. 1997. The International Stroke Trial (IST): a randomised trial of aspirin, subcutaneous heparin, both, or neither among 19435 patients with acute ischemic stroke. *Lancet*, **349**, 1569–81.

Jain, R., Deveikis, J., Hickenbottom, S., and Mukherji, S. K. 2003. Varicella-zoster vasculitis presenting with intracranial hemorrhage. *AJNR Am J Neuroradiol*, **24**, 971–4.

Jemsek, J., Greenberg, S. B., Taber, L., Harvey, D., Gershon, A., and Couch, R. B. 1983. Herpes zoster-associated encephalitis: clinicopathologic report of 12 cases and review of the literature. *Medicine*, **62**, 81–97.

Johnson, R., and Patrick, D. 2000. *Improving the Management of Varicella, Herpes Zoster and Zoster-Associated Pain*. Worthing: PAREXEL MMS Europe Ltd.

Kamholz, J., and Tremblay, G. 1985. Chickenpox with delayed contralateral hemiparesis caused by cerebral angiitis. *Ann Neurol*, **18**, 358–60.

Koeppen, A. H., Lansing, L. S., Peng, S. K., and Smith, R. S. 1981. Central nervous system vasculitis in cytomegalovirus infection. *J Neurol Sci*, **51**, 395–401.

Kolodny, K. H., Rebeiz, J. J., Caviness, V. S., and Richardson, E. P. 1968. Granulomatous angiitis of the central nervous system. *Arch Neurol.* **19**, 510–24.

Kossorotoff, M., Touze, E., Godon-Hardy, S., *et al.* 2006. Cerebral vasculopathy with aneurysm formation in HIV-infected young adults. *Neurology*, **66**, 1121–2.

Kronenberg, A., Schupbach, R., Schuknecht, B., *et al.* 2002. Multifocal vasculopathy due to Varicella-Zoster Virus (VZV): serial analysis of VZV DNA and intrathecal synthesis of VZV antibody in cerebrospinal fluid. *Clin Infect Dis*, **35**, 330–3.

Kure, K., Park, Y. D., Kim, T. S., *et al.* 1989. Immunohistochemical localization of an HIV epitope in cerebral aneurysmal arteriopathy in pediatric acquired immunodeficiency syndrome (AIDS). *Pediatr Pathol*, *9*, 655–67.

Lang, W., Miklossy, J., Deruaz, J. P., *et al.* 1989. Neuropathology of the acquired immune deficiency syndrome (AIDS): a report of 135 consecutive autopsy cases from Switzerland. *Acta Neuropathol*, **77**, 379–90.

Laws, H. W. 1960. Herpes zoster ophthalmicus complicated by contralateral hemiplegia. *Arch Ophthalmol*, **63**, 273–80.

Leopold, N. A. 1993. Chickenpox stroke in an adult. *Neurology*, **43**, 1852–3.

Lexa, F., Galetta, S. L., Yousem, D. M., *et al.* 1993. Herpes zoster ophthalmicus with orbital pseudotumor syndrome complicated by optic nerve infarction and cerebral granulomatous angiitis: MR-pathologic correlation. *AJNR Am J Neuroradiol*, **14**, 185–90.

Linnemann, C. C., and Alvira, M. 1980. Pathogenesis of the varicella-zoster angiitis in the CNS. *Arch Neurol*, **37**, 239–40.

Liu, G. T., and Holmes, G. L. 1990. Varicella with delayed contralateral hemiparesis detected by MRI. *Pediatr Neurol*, **6**, 131–4.

MacKenzie, R. A., Forbes, G. S., and Karnes, W. E. 1981. Angiographic findings in herpes zoster arteritis. *Ann Neurol*, **10**, 458–64.

Mainka, C., Fuss, B., Geiger, H., Hofelmayr, H., and Wolff, M. H. 1998. Characterization of viremia at different stages of varicella-zoster virus infection. *J Med Virol*, **56**, 91–8.

Martin, W. J. 1996. Stealth viral encephalopathy: report of a fatal case complicated by cerebral vasculitis. *Pathobiology*, **64**, 59–63.

Martinez-Longoria, C. A., Morales-Aguirre, J. J., Villalobos-Acosta, C. P., Gomez-Barreto, D., and Cashat-Cruz, M. 2004. Occurrence of intracerebral aneurysm in an HIV-infected child: a case report. *Pediatr Neurol*, **31**, 130–2.

Mayberg, M., Langer, R., and Moskowitz, M. A. 1980. Perivascular connections from the trigeminal ganglia of the cat: a possible neuroanatomical substrate for vascular headaches in humans. *Ann Neurol*, **8**, 120.

McArthur, J. C. 1987. Neurologic manifestations of AIDS. *Medicine*, **66**, 407–37.

McKelvie, P. A, Collins, S., Thyagarajan, D., *et al.* 2002. Meningoencephalomyelitis with vasculitis due to varicella zoster virus: a case report and review of the literature. *Pathology*, **34**, 88–93.

Melanson, M., Chalk, C., Georgevich, L., *et al.* 1996. Varicella-zoster virus DNA in CSF and arteries in delayed contralateral hemiplegia: evidence for viral invasion of cerebral arteries. *Neurology*, **47**, 569–70.

Melnick, J. L., Adam, E., and DeBakey, M. E. 1990. Possible role of cytomegalovirus in atherogenesis. *JAMA*, **263**, 2204–7.

Minick, C. R., Fabricant, C. R., Fabricant, J., and Litrenta, M. M. 1979. Atherosclerosis induced by infection with herpes virus. *Am J Pathol*, **96**, 673–706.

Mizusawa, H., Hirano, A., Llena, J. F., Shintaku, M. 1988. Cerebrovascular lesions in acquired immune deficiency syndrome (AIDS). *Acta Neuropathol (Berl)*, **76**, 451–7.

Morgello, S., Block, G. A., Price, R. W., and Petito, C. K. 1988. Varicella-zoster virus leukoencephalitis and cerebral vasculopathy. *Arch Pathol Lab Med*, **112**, 173–7.

Moskowitz, M. A. 1970. The neurobiology of vascular head pain. *Ann Neurol*, **16**, 157–68.

Nieto, F. J., Adam, E., Sorlie, P., *et al.* 1996. Cohort study of cytomegalovirus infection as a risk factor for carotid intimal-medial thickening, a measure of subclinical atherosclerosis. *Circulation*, **94**, 922–7.

Nogueras, C., Sala, M., Sasal, M., *et al.* 2002. Recurrent stroke as a manifestation of primary angiitis of the central nervous system in a patient infected with human immunodeficiency virus. *Arch Neurol*, **59**, 468–73.

Nunes, M. L., Pinho, A. P., and Sfoggia, A. 2001. Cerebral aneurysmal dilatation in an infant with perinatally acquired HIV infection and HSV encephalitis. *Arq Neuropsiquiatr*, **59**, 116–8.

O'Donohue, J. M., and Enzmann, D. R. 1987. Mycotic aneurysm in angiitis associated with herpes zoster ophthalmicus. *AJNR Am J Neuroradiol*, **8**, 615–9.

Palella, F. J. Jr., Delaney, K. M., Moorman, A. C., *et al.* 1998. Declining morbidity and mortality among patients with advanced human immunodeficiency virus infection. *N Engl J Med*, **338**, 853–60.

Park, Y. D., Belman, A. L., Kim, T. S., *et al.* 1990. Stroke in pediatric acquired immunodeficiency syndrome. *Ann Neurol*, **28**, 303–11.

Petito, C. K., Cho, E. S., Lemann, W., Navia, B. A., and Price, R. W. 1986. Neuropathology of acquired immunodeficiency syndrome (AIDS): an autopsy review. *J Neuropathol Exp Neurol*, **45**, 635–46.

Philippet, P., Blanche, S., Sebag, G., Rodesch, G., Griscelli, C., and Tardieu, M. 1994. Stroke and cerebral infarcts in children infected with human immunodeficiency virus. *Arch Pediatr Adolesc Med*, **148**, 965–70.

Pinto, A. N. 1996. AIDS and cerebrovascular disease. *Stroke*, **27**, 538–43.

Powderly, W. G., Landay, A., and Lederman, M. M. 1998. Recovery of the immune system with antiretroviral therapy. *JAMA*, **280**, 72–7.

Pratesi, R., Freemon, F. R., and Lowry, J. L. 1977. Herpes zoster ophthalmicus with contralateral hemiplegia. *Arch Neurol*, **34**, 640–1.

Preblud, S. R., Orenstein, W. A., and Bart, K. J. 1984. Varicella: clinical manifestations, epidemiology and health impact in children. *Pediatr Infect Dis*, **3**, 505–9.

Qureshi, A. I., Janssen, R. S., Karon, J. M., *et al.* 1997. Human immunodeficiency virus infection and stroke in young patients. *Arch Neurol*, **54**, 1150–3.

Ragozzino, M. W., Melton, L. J., Kurland, L. T., Chu, C. P., and Perry, H. O. 1982. Population-based study on herpes zoster and its sequelae. *Medicine*, **61**, 310–6.

Reshef, E., Greenberg, S. B., and Jankovic, J. 1985. Herpes zoster ophthalmicus followed by contralateral hemiparesis: report of two cases and review of the literature. *J Neurol Neurosurg Psychiatry*, **48**, 122–7.

Rhodes, R. H. 1987. Histopathology of the central nervous system in the acquired immunodeficiency syndrome. *Hum Pathol*, **18**, 636–43.

Ridker, P. M., Hennekens, C. H., Stampfer, M. J., and Wang, F. 1998. Prospective study of herpes simplex virus, cytomegalovirus, and the risk of future myocardial infarction and stroke. *Circulation*, **98**, 2796–9.

Rose, F. C., Brett, E. M., and Burston, J. 1964. Zoster encephalomyelitis. *Arch Neurol*, **11**, 155–72.

Rosenblum, M. K. 1989. Bulbar encephalitis complicating trigeminal zoster in the acquired immune deficiency syndrome. *Hum Pathol*, **20**, 292–5.

Rosenblum, W. I., and Hadfield, M. G. 1972. Granulomatous angiitis of nervous system in cases of herpes zoster and lymphosarcoma. *Neurology*, **22**, 348–54.

Rosenblum, W. I., Hadfield, M. G., Young, H. F. 1978. Granulomatous angiitis of the brain with herpes zoster and varicella encephalitis. *Ann Neurol*, **3**, 374–5.

Rostad, S. W., Olson, K., McDougall, J., Shaw, C. M., and Alvord, E. C. J. 1989. Transsynaptic spread of varicella zoster virus through the visual system: a mechanism of viral dissemination in the central nervous system. *Hum Pathol*, **20**, 174–9.

Rousseau, F., Perronne, C., Rauguin, G., Thouvenot, D., Vidal, A., and Leport, C. 1993. Necrotizing retinitis and cerebral vasculitis due to varicella-zoster virus in patients infected with the human immunodeficiency virus [letter]. *Clin Infect Dis*, **17**, 943–4.

Russman, A. N., Lederman, R. J., Calabrese, L. H., *et al.* 2003. Multifocal varicella-zoster virus vasculopathy without rash. *Arch Neurol*, **60**, 1607–9.

Ryder, J. W., Croen, K., Kleinschmidt-DeMasters, B. K., *et al.* 1986. Progressive encephalitis three months after resolution of cutaneous zoster in patients with AIDS. *Ann Neurol*, **19**, 182–8.

Saetta, A., Fanourakis, G., Agapitos, E., and Davaris, P. S. 2000. Atherosclerosis of the carotid artery: absence of evidence for CMV involvement in atheroma formation. *Cardiovasc Pathol*, **9**, 181–3.

Scaravilli, F., Daniel, S. E., Harcourt-Webster, N., and Guiloff, R. J. 1989. Chronic basal meningitis and vasculitis in acquired immunodeficiency syndrome. A possible role for human immunodeficiency virus. *Arch Pathol Lab Med*, **113**, 192–5.

Schmader, K., George, L. K., Burchett, B. M., Pieper, C. F., and Hamilton, J. D. 1995. Racial differences in the occurrence of herpes zoster. *J Infect Dis*, **171**, 701–4.

Schmidbauer, M., Budka, H., Pilz, P., Kurata, T., and Hondo, R. 1992. Presence, distribution and spread of productive varicella zoster virus infection in nervous tissues. *Brain*, **115**, 383–98.

Schmidt, J. A., Dietzmann, K., Müller, U., and Krause, P. 1992. Granulomatous vasculitis – an uncommon manifestation of herpes simplex infection of the central nervous system. *Zentralbl Allg Pathol*, **138**, 298–302.

Schwartz, N. D., So, Y. T., Hollander, H., Allen, S., and Fye, K. H. 1986. Eosinophilic vasculitis leading to amaurosis fugax in a patient with acquired immunodeficiency syndrome. *Arch Intern Med*, **146**, 2059–60.

Shi, Y., and Tokunaga, O.. 2002. Herpesvirus (HSV-1, EBV and CMV) infections in atherosclerotic compared with non-atherosclerotic aortic tissue. *Pathol Int*, **52**, 31–9.

Shuper, A., Vining, E. P., and Freeman, J. M. 1990. Central nervous system vasculitis after chickenpox – cause or coincidence? *Arch Dis Child*, **65**, 1245–8.

Sorlie, P. D., Adam, E., Melnick, S. L., *et al.* 1994. Cytomegalovirus/herpesvirus and carotid atherosclerosis: the ARIC study. *J Med Virol* **42**:33–7.

Speir, E., Modali, R., Huang, E. S., *et al.* 1994. Potential role of human cytomegalovirus and p53 interaction in coronary restenosis. *Science*, **265**, 391–4.

Terborg, C., and Busse, O. 1995. Granulomatous vasculitis of the CNS as a complication of herpes zoster ophthalmicus. *Fortschr Neurol Psychiatr*, **63**, 383–7.

Tsolia, M., Skardoutsou, A., Tsolas, G., et al. 1995. Pre-eruptive neurologic manifestations associated with multiple cerebral infarcts in varicella. *Pediatr Neurol*, **12**, 165–8.

Vinters, H. V., Guerra, W. F., Eppolito, L., and Keith, P. E. 3rd. 1988. Necrotizing vasculitis of the nervous system in a patient with AIDS-related complex. *Neuropathol Appl Neurobiol*, **14**, 417–24.

Visrutaratna, P., and Oranratanachai, K. 2002. Clinics in diagnostic imaging: HIV encephalopathy and cerebral aneurysmal arteriopathy. *Singapore Med J*, **43**, 377–80.

White, C. J. 1997. Varicella-zoster virus vaccine. *Clin Infect Dis*, **24**, 753–64.

Yankner, B. A., Skolnik, P. R., Shoukimas, G. M., *et al.* 1986. Cerebral granulomatous angiitis associated with isolation of human T-lymphotropic virus type III from the central nervous system. *Ann Neurol*, **20**, 362–4.

Yilmaz, K., Caliskan, M., Akdeniz, C., *et al.* 1998. Acute childhood hemiplegia associated with chickenpox. *Pediatr Neurol*, **18**, 256–61.

Zhou, Y. F., Leon, M. B., Waclawiw, M. A., *et al.* 1996. Association between prior cytomegalovirus infection and the risk of restenosis after coronary atherectomy. *N Engl J Med*, **335**, 624–30.

4 TAKAYASU DISEASE

Yukito Shinohara

Introduction

The clinical signs and symptoms caused by stenosing and obstructing processes in the aortic arch and the origin of its major branches, the innominate arteries, the carotid arteries, and the subclavian arteries, have an enormous variety of nomenclatures. These include Takayasu disease (Pahwa *et al.*, 1959), Takayasu's syndrome (Ask-Upmark and Fajers, 1956), Takayasu's arteritis (Hirsch *et al.*, 1964), Takayasu–Ohnishi's disease (Hirose and Baba, 1963), aortic arch syndrome (Frövig, 1946), aortic arch arteritis (Koszewski, 1958), aortitis syndrome, pulseless disease (Shimizu and Sano, 1951), pulseless syndrome (Lessoff and Glynn, 1959), reversed coarctation (Giffin, 1939), carotid-subclavian arteritis, brachiocephalic arteritis, chronic subclavian-carotid obstruction syndrome (Bustamante *et al.*, 1954), chronic subclaviocarotid syndrome, syndrome of obliteration of supra-aortic branches (Martorell and Fabbé Tersol, 1944), obliterative brachiocephalic arteritis (Gibbons and King, 1957), thromboarteritis obliterans subclaviocarotica, thromboangiitis obliterans of the branches of the aortic arch (Kalmanson and Kalmansohn, 1957), panarteritis branchiocephalica (Gilmour, 1941), idiopathic medial aortopathy and arteriopathy (Marquis *et al.*, 1968), Martorell syndrome, and so on. Among them, aortic arch syndrome and Takayasu disease or Takayasu's arteritis are most often used to describe the overall clinical picture of this syndrome or disease. However, the term "aortic arch syndrome" can be used to describe many conditions including arteriosclerosis, syphilitic aortitis, young female arteritis of unknown etiology, and other pathological conditions (traumatic, congenital, thrombotic, neoplastic, embolic, and so on) (Judge *et al.*, 1962; Ross and McKusick, 1953; Thurlbeck and Currens, 1959). In contrast, Takayasu disease usually means an arteritis of unknown origin, involving the aortic arch, with inflammatory narrowing or obstruction of the proximal portion of the major branches, and occurring predominantly in young women. Therefore, Takayasu disease is one of the causes of aortic arch syndrome and should be defined separately from other types of aortic arch syndrome.

Historical review

At the Annual Meeting of the Japanese Ophthalmological Society in 1905, Takayasu, a Japanese ophthalmologist, presented a 21-year-old woman with peculiar eye ground findings in both eyes (1908). She had a wreath-like anastomosis surrounding the optic disc at a distance of 2 or 3 mm, and surrounding this was another circular anastomosis. There were anastomotic shunts of arterioles and venules. Both the surrounding vessels and their branches had lumps that were seen to move from day to day. Although Takayasu did not understand the etiology of the disease, this was the first description of the so-called Takayasu retinopathy (Ito, 1995). At the same meeting, Ohnishi mentioned a similar patient who had circular anastomosis and aneurysm-like lumps in the optic fundi, with no palpable radial pulses. Immediately afterwards, Kagoshima also mentioned a similar pulseless patient with cataracts. Those presentations and discussions were the origin of the term Takayasu disease or Takayasu–Ohnishi's disease. However, according to Judge *et al.* (1962), Pokrovsky *et al.* (1980), and Bleck (1989), the first description of this kind of disorder, i.e. Takayasu disease, observed usually in young women, was not by Takayasu and Ohnishi, but by Davy (1839), and somewhat later it was also noted independently by Savory (1856) and by Kussmaul (1873). Because the term Takayasu disease is now most commonly used, we have adopted it in this chapter.

Epidemiology

Koide and his colleagues (1992) performed epidemiological studies in Japan from 1973 to 1991. The age distribution of the aortic arch syndrome, mainly Takayasu disease, is shown in Table 4.1. The female-to-male ratio was 11 to 1, and the great majority of patients developed their initial symptoms in their third or fourth decade; more recent results delineate slightly different manifestations in an older population, probably due to the upward shift of the average age of the female population in Japan. As shown on the right of Table 4.1, the estimated age of onset was rather similar in all the studies. Children and teenagers may be affected, and it is also seen, although rarely, in infants (Stanley *et al.*, 2003).

In China, Deyu *et al.* (1992) reported 530 cases of Takayasu disease. The age distribution was quite similar to that in Japan, but the female-to-male ratio was 2.9 to 1, which is very different from that in Japan. Hall *et al.* (1985) suggested that the North American incidence of this disease was 2.6 per million per year.

These results suggest that, while this disease has an unexplained predilection for Asians, it occurs in all racial groups.

Uncommon Causes of Stroke, 2nd edition, ed. Louis R. Caplan. Published by Cambridge University Press. © Cambridge University Press 2008.

Table 4.1 Age distribution and estimated age of onset of Takayasu disease in Japan

Age distribution Year examined:	Estimated age of onset 1973–5	1982–4	1991	1973–5	1982–4	1991
Age						
<9	22	3	2	11	19	10
10 < 19	180	128	47	285	333	182
20 < 29	637	397	168	453	625	342
30 < 39	527	714	213	253	408	281
40 < 49	448	601	387	96	233	187
50 < 59	218	512	357	39	138	100
60 < 69	84	203	228	13	22	35
70 < 79	20	46	72	3	10	10
Unknown	12	2	1	233	818	328
Total number of patients	2148	2606	1475	1386	2606	1475

Pathogenesis

The etiology of this disease is unknown. An autoimmune pathogenesis is often suggested, but so far there is no direct evidence for this. Coexistent tuberculosis was also suspected to be one of the causes, but no direct evidence has been found, including the case of Takayasu (1908).

Because Takayasu disease seems to occur predominantly in Asian countries and twin patients with this disease are sometimes observed, there is a possibility that hereditary factors may participate in its pathophysiology. Dong *et al.* (1992) examined HLA-DP antigen in 64 patients with Takayasu disease and in 317 healthy individuals in the Japanese population, and found that the combination or haplotype of HLA–Bw52-DRB1*1502-DRB5*0102-DQA1*0103-DQB1*0601-DPA1*02-DPB1*0901 may confer susceptibility to this disorder, whereas another combination or haplotype of HLA–Bw54- DRB1*0405-DRB4*0101-DQA1*0301-DQB1*0401 may confer resistance to the disease.

Pathology and hemodynamics

In Takayasu disease, the aortic arch, with its main arterial trunks and the descending aorta, as well as renal arteries, is the main site of inflammation. The lymphoplasmacytic inflammation affects primarily the tuna media, causing destruction of the elastic lamellae (acute phase). In the intermediate stage, the inflammatory infiltrate subsides, and the partially necrotic media is revascularized by new branches of the vasa vasorum. Secondary fibrosis of all layers causes thickening and loss of compliance of the vessel walls. The involved arteries are finally transformed into rigid, thick-walled tubes with severe narrowing or occlusion by superimposed thrombosis. Saccular aneurysms may also arise during this phase (sclerosing stage).

Cerebral blood flow (CBF) studies were done in some patients by using single photon emission computed tomography (SPECT) (Grosset *et al.*, 1992) and positron emission tomography (PET) (Takano *et al.*, 1993). However, the results were different depending on the patients and on their stages. In some patients, CBF was reduced in the watershed territories of the brain (Grosset *et al.*, 1992). In others, CBF and cerebral oxygen extraction fraction were well maintained (Takano *et al.*, 1993), but the hemodynamic reserve and oxygen metabolism were impaired in patients with cerebral infarction (Takano *et al.*, 1993).

Classification of Takayasu disease

Four types of aortic arch involvements in Takayasu disease had been proposed (Lupi-Herrera *et al.*, 1979; Nakao *et al.*, 1967). However, the most recently devised classification was suggested in 1996, and this divided the disease into six types (Hata *et al.*, 1996; Moriwaki *et al.*, 1997), as follows:

1. Type I involves only the branches of the aortic arch.
2. Type IIa involves the aorta only at its ascending portion and/or at the aortic arch. The branches of the aortic arch may be involved as well. The rest of the aorta is not affected.
3. Type IIb affects the descending thoracic aorta with or without involvement of the ascending aorta or the aortic arch with its branches. The abdominal aorta is not involved.
4. Type III is concomitant involvement of the descending thoracic aorta, the abdominal aorta, and/or the renal arteries. The ascending aorta and the aortic arch and its branches are not involved.
5. Type IV involves only the abdominal aorta and/or the renal arteries.
6. Type V is a generalized type, with combined features of the other types.

Note: Involvement of the coronary and pulmonary arteries should be indicated as C(+) or P(+), respectively.

Clinical manifestations and prognosis

Initial manifestations

Takayasu disease is thought to begin clinically with symptoms of systemic inflammation (Bleck, 1989) or with eye symptoms (Takayasu, 1908). Bleck (1989) described myalgias, arthralgias, fatigue, fever, and weight loss as prominent early symptoms. He also mentioned that the occurrence of neurological symptoms such as claudication, transient ischemic attack, and stroke-like symptoms can seldom be categorized into early or late phenomena. However, Kerr *et al.* (1994) mentioned that only 33% of their patients had systemic symptoms. In a large study of more than 1000 patients in Japan (Koide, 1992), the most frequent chief complaints at the first visit in patients with Takayasu disease were symptoms related to ischemia of the extremities, such as paresthesia, cold sensation, pulselessness, claudication, and so on (72.3%, 969/1341), followed by systemic symptoms such as fever, easy fatigability, or lassitude (66.8%, 885/1324) and symptoms related to cerebral ischemia such as dizziness, headache, syncope, and so on (64.6%, 837/1351 patients), although some headaches may not have been related to cerebral ischemia.

Neurological symptoms related to stroke

It is known that serious illness and death in younger patients with Takayasu disease is often due to central nervous system involvement. Cerebral vascular disease is usually a consequence of severe hypertension, or carotid or brachiocephalic obstruction. Among his 81 patients with Takayasu disease, Ishikawa (1981) reported that 5 of 16 deaths resulted from stroke. These 16 patients also had serious morbidity, including two subarachnoid hemorrhages, one intracerebral hemorrhage, two cases of acute unilateral blindness, and two cases of bilateral blindness.

In contrast, Rose and Sinclair-Smith (1980) reported that 3 of 16 deaths (mean age 20 years) were due to hypertensive intracerebral hemorrhages. In a large study in Japan (Koide, 1992), 8 of 69 deaths were due to stroke in 1972 to 1975, and 5 of 59 deaths were due to stroke in a study that was done in 1991. In the latter study, only 3 of 5 stroke deaths were from intracerebral hemorrhage. Among the more than 59 deaths, 21 were from cardiac disorders and 12 were from rupture of aortic aneurysms. However, in a Chinese study (Deyu *et al.*, 1992), cerebral hemorrhage was the most common cause of death; 23.6% of deaths (13 of 55 among 530 patients) were from cerebral hemorrhage, and 3.6% (2 of 55 among 530) from cerebral infarction (Deyu *et al.*, 1992).

Because the subclavian artery proximal to the origin of the vertebral artery is often involved earlier, diversion of blood from the vertebrobasilar territory into the subclavian artery via retrograde flow through the ipsilateral vertebral artery may occur. This steal phenomenon of the blood from the posterior circulation of the brain, if symptomatic, is called the "subclavian steal syndrome" (Reivich *et al.*, 1961).

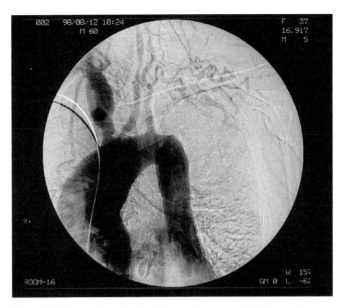

Figure 4.1 X-ray angiography of a 57-year-old woman with Takayasu disease (estimated age of onset 23 years). Note occlusion of the left subclavian artery and collateral circulation through the left vertebral artery, although this patient did not show symptomatic subclavian steal syndrome.

Diagnosis and laboratory data

It is well known that the erythrocyte sedimentation rate (ESR) is elevated in most patients, particularly in the stage of exacerbation. At the first visit to the hospital, the laboratory abnormalities usually found were elevation of ESR, positive C-reactive protein (CRP), anemia, elevated serum gamma globulin, leukocytosis, and so on, in that order.

Usually, physical examinations reveal weakness or right-to-left difference of radial pulsation, weakness of femoral arterial pulsation, asymmetry of blood pressure, hypertension, cardiac murmur, bruit (especially in the neck, supraclavicular region, anterior chest), abnormal ocular findings, and so on.

If such physical abnormalities and abnormal laboratory data are found, especially in young women, angiography should be performed to confirm the diagnosis. Angiography still remains the cornerstone of diagnosis (Figure 4.1). Magnetic resonance angiography (MRA) is also a useful tool for diagnosing Takayasu disease (Figure 4.2), because it avoids the risks of arterial puncture, iodinated contrast load, and radiation exposure.

Recently, it has been emphasized that use of Doppler ultrasound, computed tomography angiography, and PET (Kissin and Merkel, 2004, as well as MRI and MRA (Nastri *et al.*, 2004), in combination, may facilitate the detection of Takayasu disease activity at a more treatable stage.

Differential diagnosis

Disorders that should be differentiated from Takayasu disease include arteriosclerosis, Bürger's disease, congenital vessel anomalies, coarctation of the aorta, dissecting aneurysm, collagen disease, and Behçet's disease.

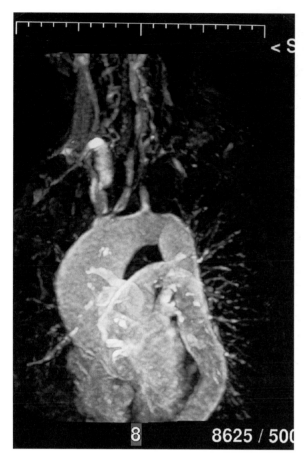

Figure 4.2 Magnetic resonance angiography of the same patient as in Figure 4.1.

Complications

Major complications of this disease include aortic regurgitation (33%), dilatation of aortic arch (27%), and renovascular hypertension (21%) (Koide, 1992). Others include coarctation of the aorta, pulmonary infarction, myocardial infarction, and so on.

As regards stroke, 16 patients with intracranial aneurysms were reported, and among them 13 were ruptured and 3 were unruptured (Asaoka *et al.*, 1998). Intracranial aneurysms arose predominantly along the course of collateral flow, especially in the vertebrobasilar system, and a high incidence of multiple aneurysms has been reported. In contrast, although extracranial carotid aneurysm caused by Takayasu disease is said to be extremely rare, 6 among 106 cases have been reported by Tabata *et al.* (2001).

Therapy

Concerning the treatment and management of Takayasu disease patients with stroke, one has to consider the treatment of Takayasu disease and stroke separately. Intracerebral hemorrhage in Takayasu disease can be managed in the same way as usual hypertensive intracerebral hemorrhage. Because the patients may have aortic regurgitation, aortic arch dilation, or intracranial aneurysms, the control of high blood pressure is essential, especially in patients with hemorrhagic stroke. In patients with

subarachnoid hemorrhage, immediate detection of the site of the ruptured aneurysm is necessary, and immediate surgery should be performed. In patients with ischemic stroke, systemic blood pressure should not be reduced abruptly, but attention must always be paid to the control of extremely high blood pressure in order to prevent the development of cardiac failure. The use of antiplatelet drugs such as aspirin (81–350 mg/day) is recommended in ischemic stroke if blood pressure is not too high. In cerebral thrombosis, a thromboxane A2 inhibitor may be used in the acute stage.

Together with the management of stroke, treatment for Takayasu disease itself is also necessary in the active stage of the disease. Although there has been no randomized controlled study regarding the efficacy of medical and surgical treatments of Takayasu disease, it is generally believed that corticosteroids are effective in controlling the inflammatory symptoms. The dose of steroid is initially in the 0.5–1.5 mg/kg/day or 20–75 mg/day predonisolone-equivalent range. Usually, the dose of steroid should be reduced by 5–10 mg every 2–3 weeks. Five to 10 mg should be continued until the ESR drops below 20 mm/h or CRP becomes negative. During the acute stage, surgical procedures, angiography with contrast media, or percutaneous angioplasty should be avoided. In this connection, MRA (Figure 4.2) is a useful noninvasive method to diagnose this disease atraumatically. Immunosuppressants such as cyclophosphamide, methotrexate, mycophenolate mofetil, azathioprine, or 6-mercaptopurine added to corticosteroids may induce remission. Anticoagulants such as heparin or warfarin have been used in the hope of preventing thrombosis distal to the stenosis or occlusions, but so far no data concerning efficacy are available.

A better understanding of the pathogenesis has led to trials with anti–tumor necrosis factor-β in patients with refractory disease, and preliminary results are encouraging (Hoffman *et al.*, 2004: Liang and Hoffman, 2004).

Surgical procedures, including intravascular techniques, are necessary in some cases with severe aortic regurgitation, aortic coarctation, or renovascular hypertension. However, these procedures should not be undertaken in the acute stage of inflammation or stroke. Aneurysms or aneurysm-like dilation may be observed in the territories of the brachiocephalic artery, subclavian arteries, descending aorta, or the carotid arteries as well as cerebral arteries. If the aneurysm increases in size during observation, surgical treatment should be done before rupture. Subclavian steal syndrome or moderate carotid stenosis, as well as renal artery stenosis (Sharma *et al.*, 1992), may be an indication for angioplasty and/or stenting.

REFERENCES

Asaoka, K., Houkin, K., Fujimoto, S., Ishikwa, T., and Abe, H. 1998. Intracranial aneurysms associated with aortitis syndrome: case report and review of the literature. *Neurosurgery*, **42**, 157.

Ask-Upmark, E., and Fajers, C. M. 1956. Further observations on Takayasu's syndrome. *Acta Med Scand*, **155**, 275.

Bleck, T. P. 1989. Takayasu's disease. In *Handbook of Clinical Neurology*, ed. J. F. Toole. Vol. 11: Part III chap. 20pp. p. 335. Elsevier Science, pp. 335.

Bustamante, R. A., Milanes, B., Casas, M., and De-La Torre, A. 1954. The chronic subclavian-carotid obstruction syndrome (pulseless disease). *Angiology*, **5**, 479.

Davy, J. 1839. Researches, Physiological and Anatosiscal. Vol. 1, London: Smith Elder and Co., pp. 426 (quoted from Judge *et al.*, 1962).

Deyu, Z., Dijun, F., and Lisheng, L. 1992. Takayasu arteritis in China: a report of 530 cases. *Heart Vessels*, Suppl **7**, 32.

Dong, R. P., Kimura, A., Numano, F., *et al.* 1992. HLA-DP antigen and Takayasu arteritis. *Tissue Antigens*, **39**, 106.

Frøvig, A. G. 1946. Bilateral obliteration of the common carotid artery. Thrombangitis obliterans? *Acta Psychiatr Neurol Scand*, Suppl, **39**.

Gibbons, T. B., and King, R. L. 1957. Obliterative brachiocephalic arteritis: pulseless disease of Takayasu. *Circulation*, **15**, 845.

Giffin, H. M. 1939. Reversed coarctation and vasomotor gradient: report of a cardiovascular anomaly with symptoms of brain tumor. *Proc Mayo Clin*, **14**, 561.

Gilmour, J. R. 1941. Giant-cell arteritis. *J Pathol Bacteriol*, **53**, 263.

Grosset, D. G., Patterson, J., and Bone, I. 1992. Intracranial haemodynamics in Takayasu's arteritis. *Acta Neurochir (Wien)*, **119**, 161.

Hall, S., Barr, W., Lie, J. T., *et al.* 1985. Takayasu arteritis. *Medicine*, **94**, 89.

Hata, A., Noda, M., Moriwaki, R., and Numano, F. 1996. Angiographic findings of Takayasu arteritis: new classification. *Int J Cardiol*, **54 (Suppl)**, s155.

Hirose, K., and Baba, K. 1963. A study of fundus changes in the early stages of Takayasu–Ohnishi (pulseless) disease. *Am J Ophthalmol*, **55**, 293.

Hirsch, M. S., Aikat, B. K., and Basu, A. K. 1964. Takayasu arteritis. *Bull Johns Hopkins Hosp*, **115**, 29.

Hoffman, G. S., Merkel, P. A., Brasington, R. D., Lenschow D. J., and Liang, P. 2004. Anti-tumor necrosis factor therapy in patients with difficult to treat Takayasu arteritis. *Arthritis Rheum*, **50**, 2296.

Ishikawa, K. 1981. Survival and morbidity after diagnosis of occlusive thromboaortopathy (Takayasu's disease). *Am J Cardiol*, **47**, 1026.

Ito, I. 1995. Aortitis syndrome (Takayasu's arteritis). A historical perspective. *Jpn Heart J*, **36**, 273.

Judge, R. D., Currier, R. D., Gracie, W. A., and Figley, M. M. 1962. Takayasu's arteritis and the aortic arch syndrome. *Am J Med*, **32**, 379.

Kalmanson, R. B., and Kalmansohn, R. W. 1957. Thrombotic obliteration of the branches of the aortic arch. *Circulation*, **15**, 237.

Kerr, G. S., Hallahan, C. W., Gierdant, J., *et al.* 1994. Takayasu arteritis. *Ann Intern Med*, **120**, 919.

Kissin, E. Y., and Merkel, P. A. 2004. Diagnostic imaging in Takayasu arteritis. *Curr Opin Rheumatol*, **16**, 31.

Koide, K. 1992. Aortitis syndrome. *Nihon Rinsho*, **50**, 343 (in Japanese).

Koszewski, B. J. 1958. Branchial arteritis or aortic arch arteritis. A new inflammatory arterial disease (pulseless disease). *Angiology*, **9**, 180.

Kussmaul, A. 1873. Zwei Falle von spontaner allmaliger Verschliessung grosser Halsarterienstamme. *Deutsche Klinik*, **24**, 461.

Lessoff, M. H., and Glynn, L. E. 1959. Pulseless syndrome. *Lancet*, 799.

Liang, P., and Hoffman, G. S. 2004. Advances in the medical and surgical treatment of Takayasu arteritis. *Curr Opin Rheumatol*, **17**, 16.

Lupi-Herrera, E., Sanchez-Torres, G., Marcushamer, J., *et al.* 1979. Takayasu's arteritis. Clinical study of 107 cases. *Am Heart J*, **73**, 94.

Marquis, J., Richardson, J. B., Ritchie, A. C., and Wigle, E. D. 1968. Idiopathic medial aortopathy and arteriopathy. *Am J Med*, **44**, 939.

Martorell, F., and Fabbé Tersol, J. 1944. El síndrome de obliteración de los troncos supraaorticos. *Medicina Clínica (Barcelona)*, **2**, 26.

Moriwaki, R., Noda, M., Yjima, M., Sharma, B. K., and Numano, F. 1997. Clinical manifestations of Takayasu arteritis in India and Japan: new classification of angiographic findings. *Angiology*, **48**, 369.

Nakao, K., Ikeda, M., Kimata, S. *et al.* 1967. Takayasu's arteritis. Clinical report of eighty-four cases and immunological studies of seven cases. *Circulation*, **35**, 1141.

Nastri, M. V., Baptista, L. P. S., Baroni, R. H., *et al.* 2004. Gadolinium-enhanced three-dimensional MR angiography of Takayasu arteritis. *Radio Graphics*, **24**, 773.

Pahwa, J. M., Pandey, M. P., and Gypha, D. P. 1959. Pulseless disease, or Takayasu's disease. *Br Med J*, **2**, 1439.

Pokrovsky, A. V., Tsereshkin, D. M., and Golossovskaya, M. A. 1980. Pathology of non-specific aortoarteritis. *Angiology*, **31**, 549.

Reivich, M., Holling, H. E., Roberts, B., and Toole, J. F. 1961. Reversal of blood flow through the vertebral artery and its effects on cerebral circulation. *N Engl J Med*, **265**, 878.

Rose, A. G., and Sinclair-Smith, C. C. 1980. Takayasu's arteritis; a study of 16 autopsy cases. *Arch Pathol Lab Med*, **104**, 231.

Ross, R. S., and McKusick, V. A. 1953. Aortic arch syndromes. Diminished or absent pulses in arteries arising from arch of aorta. *Arch Intern Med*, **92**, 701.

Savory, W. S. 1856. Case of a young woman in whom the main arteries of both upper extremities and of the left side of the neck were throughout completely obliterated. *Transactions Medical-Chirurgical Society (London)*, **39**, 205, (quoted from Judge *et al.*, 1962).

Sharma, S., Saxena, A., Talwar, K. K., *et al.* 1992. Renal artery stenosis caused by nonspecific arteritis (Takayasu disease): results of treatment with percutaneous transluminal angioplasty. *Am J Radiol*, **158**, 417.

Shimizu, K., and Sano, K. 1951. Pulseless disease. *J Neuropathol Exp Neurol*, **1**, 37.

Stanley, P., Roebuck, D., and Barboza, A. 2003. Takayasu's arteritis in children. *Tech Vasc Interv Radiol*, **6**, 158.

Tabata, M., Kitagawa, T., Saito, T., et al. 2001. Extracranial carotid aneurysm in Takayasu's arteritis. *J Vasc Surg*, **34**, 739.

Takano, K., Sadoshima, S., Ibayashi, S., Ichiya, Y., and Fujishima, M. 1993. Altered cerebral hemodynamics and metabolism in Takayasu's arteritis with neurological deficits. *Stroke*, **24**, 1501.

Takayasu, M. 1908. A case with peculiar changes of the central retinal vessels. *Acta Societatis Ophthalmologicae Japonicae*, **12**, 554, (in Japanese).

Thurlbeck, W. M., and Currens, J. H. (1959). The aortic arch syndrome (pulseless disease): a report of ten cases with three autopsies. *Circulation*, **19**, 499.

5 BÜRGER'S DISEASE (THROMBOANGIITIS OBLITERANS)

Hans-Christoph Diener and Tobias Kurth

Introduction

Bürger's disease or thromboangiitis obliterans (TAO) is a nonatherosclerotic segmental inflammatory obliterative vascular disease that affects medium- and small-sized arteries as well as superficial veins. Distal vessels of the legs and arms are mainly involved. Affected patients are mostly young male smokers, who can develop ulcers and gangrene of the toes and fingers as a result of the vascular ischemia, often requiring minor and sometimes major limb amputation. TAO rarely affects cerebral and visceral vessels and even more rarely deep veins. It was first described by von Winiwarter in 1879 and later by Bürger in 1908. The pathological examination may show two phases of the disease. In the acute phase, arteries or veins are occluded by a fresh thrombus (Crawford, 1977) and the intima is inflamed. Endothelial cells proliferate, and lymphocytes can be observed in the intima, which, in addition can show fibrinoid necrosis (Leu, 1969; Leu and Brunner, 1973). In the chronic phase, pathological changes are nonspecific and include recanalization of the organized thrombus and perivascular fibrosis.

According to Zülch and Pilz (1989), Bürger's disease manifested in the brain has the following morphologic characteristics:

1. arterial occlusions caused by thrombosis in small arteries without arteriosclerosis,
2. spatial predilection for the cerebral surface in the watershed region between the middle cerebral, anterior, and posterior cerebral arteries.

Lindenberg and Spatz (1940) described two neuropathologically distinct forms of cerebral TAO:

1. one form with changes of the arteries with a diameter less than 1 mm; and
2. another form with thrombosis of the large basal arteries (internal carotid artery or middle cerebral artery) in combination with involvement of distal small arteries (Briebach et al., 1991).

The cerebral form of TAO was criticized by Fisher (1957), who doubted that a cerebral form of TAO existed. Others contended that the vascular changes could be caused by pial artery occlusion in the presence of systemic arterial hypotension (Romanuel and Abramowitz, 1964).

Epidemiology

The incidence of TAO strongly varies by gender. A male-to-female ratio variation between 8:1 and 3.3:1 has been reported (Mills and Porter, 1991; Olin et al., 1990). Recent studies have shown a ratio as large as 14:1 or even greater (Jimenez-Paredes et al., 1998; Puchmayer, 1996). In white men younger than 45 years, the incidence is estimated between 8 and 12 per 100 000 per year (DeBakey and Cohen, 1963; Lie, 1989). It is more common in Eastern Europe, the Middle East, and Asia than in Western countries, most likely due to heavy smoking habits in these countries (Reny and Cabane, 1998). During the last decade, a decrease of the prevalence of TAO has been reported (Matsushita et al., 1998). The median age at the time of diagnosis is between 35 and 45 years. The cerebral form of TAO accounts for about 2% of all cases of TAO (Lippmann, 1952; Zülch and Pilz, 1989). Inzelberg et al. (1989) evaluated 46 TAO patients during 833 patient-years. Only one patient with no other risk factor for stroke developed a transient aphasia and right hemiparesis (Inzelberg et al., 1989). The result of this study suggests that the rarity of the cerebral manifestation makes it difficult to conclude that cerebrovascular manifestations are part of this disease.

Pathogenesis

The pathogenesis of TAO is still poorly understood, and there is no specific marker of the disease. TAO in the limbs is seen almost exclusively in smokers. Cessation of smoking leads to regression of the vessel lesions and finally to remission. Several studies indicate that autoimmune mechanisms act via a cell-mediated immune response to human artery type-specific collagens (Adar et al., 1983; Papa et al., 1992). A tobacco antigen has been suggested as a cause of vascular reactivity in cigarette smokers. A study by Papa et al. (1992) of 13 patients with TAO, 16 healthy smokers, and 12 nonsmokers found identical cellular responses to tobacco glycoprotein in smokers and patients with TAO. Patients with TAO had a significantly higher frequency of HLA-DR4 and a lower frequency of HLA-DRW6 antigens. Other studies report a significant increase in other HLA antibodies (HLA-B40, HLA-B35, and HLA-DR2) and anticollagen antibodies in patients with TAO (Fernandez-Miranda et al., 1993; Jaini et al., 1998). These results indicate that an autoimmune mechanism may be involved. Pietraszek et al. (1993) found an increased blood level of free serotonin and a decreased maximal platelet serotonin uptake velocity. This may lead to platelet activation via 5–HT2 receptors (Pietraszek et al., 1993). Another possible association is between Bürger's disease and hyperhomocysteinemia (Calgüneri et al., 2004).

Uncommon Causes of Stroke, 2nd edition, ed. Louis R. Caplan. Published by Cambridge University Press. © Cambridge University Press 2008.

Table 5.1 *Diagnostic criteria*

A. Onset of distal extremity ischemic symptoms before 45 years of age

B. Normal arteries proximal to the popliteal or distal brachial level

C. Distal occlusive disease documented by distinctive plethysmographic, arteriographic, or pathological findings

D. Absence of any of the following conditions:

    1. proximal embolic source

    2. trauma

    3. autoimmune disease

    4. diabetes

    5. hyperlipidemia

Source: From Mills and Porter (1991)

Clinical features

TAO is characterized by claudication or ischemia of both legs and less so of the arms. The disease begins distally and progresses more proximally. With disease progression, Raynaud's phenomenon (34%), involvement of the upper extremities (34%), and superficial phlebitis (37%) occur (Mills and Porter, 1991). Two limbs are affected in 16%, three in 41%, and all limbs in 43% (Shionoya, 1989). Later during the disease, gangrene, ulcerations, and rest pain are the leading symptoms. Leg amputation is required in 5–15% and finger amputations in 15–20% of patients (Joyce, 1990). Diagnostic criteria are shown in Table 5.1.

The clinical picture of neurological disturbances is nonspecific; monoparesis, hemiparesis, visual field defects, aphasia, dysarthria, and cerebellar symptoms may occur (Harten *et al.*, 1996; Zülch and Pilz, 1989). One patient with involvement of the external carotid artery showing vascular lesions in the oral cavity was described by Farish *et al.* (1990).

The diagnosis of TAO requires the exclusion of an embolic source, autoimmune disease, diabetes, and hyperlipidemia. Arteriography should show the distal involvement with normal arterial lumen proximal to the popliteal or distal brachial level and the absence of atheromatous changes in the large vessels.

Therapy

Abstinence from tobacco will likely halt disease progression and sometimes result in regression of vascular changes. Among TAO patients, ex-smokers have a significantly lower frequency of amputations than smokers do. It is not known whether immunosuppressive therapy with azathioprine is helpful. Corticosteroids, reserpine, calcium channel blockers, alpha-blockers, antiplatelet drugs, and anticoagulants are not effective (Olin *et al.*, 1990). There are no reports of a specific therapy for the cerebral form of TAO.

REFERENCES

Adar, R., Papa, M. Z., Halpern, Z., *et al.* 1983. Cellular sensitivity of collagen in thrombangiitis obliterans. *N Engl J Med*, **308**, 1113–6.

Briebach, T., Gräfin Vitzthum, H., Hahn, J., Schlote, W., and Fischer, P. A. 1991. Ein Fall von zerebraler Thrombangiitis obliterans. Klinische und autoptische Befunde beim verlaustyp I nach Spatz und Lindenberg. *Nervenarzt*, **62**, 247–51.

Bürger, L. 1908. Thrombo-angiitis obliterans: a study of the vascular lesion leading to pre-senile spontaneous gangrene. *Am J Med Sci*, **136**, 567–80.

Calgüneri, M., Öztürk, M. A., Ay H., *et al.* 2004. Buerger's disease with multisystem involvement. A case report and review of the literature. *Angiology*, **55**, 325–8.

Crawford, T. 1977. Blood and lymphatic vessels, thrombangiitis obliterans (Buerger's disease). In *Pathology* Vol. 1, ed. W. A. D. Anderson and J. M. Kissane. St. Louis: Mosby, pp. 897–927.

DeBakey, M. E., and Cohen, B. 1963. *Buerger's Disease: Follow-up Study of World War II Army Cases.* Springfield, IL: Charles C. Thomas Publishing.

Farish, S. E., el Mofty, S. K. and Colm, S. J. 1990. Intraoral manifestation of thromboangiitis obliterans (Buerger's disease). *Oral Surg Oral Med Oral Pathol*, **69**, 223–6.

Fernandez-Miranda, C., Rubio, R., Vicario, J. L., *et al.* 1993 [Thromboangiitis obliterans (Buerger's disease). Study of 41 cases]. *Med Clin (Barc)*, **101**, 321–6.

Fisher, M. C. 1957. Cerebral thromboangiitis obliterans (including a critical review of the literature). *Medicine*, **36**, 169–209.

Harten, P., Müller-Huelsbeck, S., Regensburger, D., and Loeffler, H. 1996 Multiple organ manifestations in thromboangiitis obliterans (Buerger's disease). *Angiology*, **47**, 419–25.

Inzelberg, R., Bornstein, N. M., and Korczyn, A. D. 1989. Cerebrovascular symptoms in thromboangiitis obliterans. *Acta Neurol Scand*, **80**, 347–50.

Jaini, R., Mandal, S., Khazanchi, R. K., and Mehra, N. K. 1998. Immunogenetic analysis of Buerger's disease in India. *Int J Cardiol*, **66 Suppl. 1**, S283–5.

Jimenez-Paredes, C. A., Canas-Davila, C. A., Sanchez, A., *et al.* 1998. Buerger's disease at the 'San Juan De Dios' Hospital, Santa Fe De Bogota, Colombia. *Int J Cardiol*, **66 Suppl 1**, S267–72.

Joyce, J. W. 1990. Buerger's disease (thromboangiitis obliterans). *Rheum Dis Clin North Am*, **16**, 463–70.

Leu, H. J. 1969. Die entzündlichen Arterien- und Venenerkrankungen. *Zentralblatt für Phlebologie*, **8**, 164–4.

Leu, H. J., and Brunner, U. 1973. Zur pathologisch-anatomischen Abgrenzung der Thrombangiitis obliterans von der Arteriosklerose. *Deutsche Medizinische Wochenschrift*, **98**, 158–61.

Lie, J. T. 1989. The rise and fall of resurgence of thromboangiitis obliterans (Buerger's disease). *Acta Pathol Jpn*, **39**, 153.

Lindenberg, R., and Spatz, H. 1940. Über die Thrombendarteriitis obliterans der Hirngefäße (cerebrale Form der Winiwarter-Buergerschen Krankheit). *Virchows Arch A Pathol Pathol Anat*, **305**, 531–57.

Lippmann, H. I. 1952. Cerebrovascular thrombosis in patients with Buerger's disease. *Circulation*, **5**, 680–92.

Matsushita, M., Nishikimi, N., Sakurai, T., and Nimura, Y. 1998. Decrease in prevalence of Buerger's disease in Japan. *Surgery*, **124**, 498–502.

Mills, J. L., and Porter, J. M. 1991. Buerger's disease (Thrombangiitis obliterans). *Ann Vasc Surg*, **5**, 570–2.

Olin, J. W., Young, J. R., Graor, R. A., Ruschhaupt, W. F., and Bartholomew, J. R. 1990. The changing clinical spectrum of thromboangiitis obliterans (Buerger's disease). *Circulation*, **82 Suppl. IV**, IV3–8.

Papa, M., Bass, A., Adar, R., *et al.* 1992. Autoimmune mechanisms in thromboangiitis obliterans (Buerger's disease): the role of tobacco antigen and the major histocompatibility complex. *Surgery*, **111**, 527–31.

Pietraszek, M. H., Choudhury, N. A., Baba, S., *et al.* 1993. Serotonin as a factor involved in pathophysiology of thromboangiitis obliterans. *Int J Angiol*, **12**, 9–12.

Puchmayer, V. 1996. [Clinical diagnosis, special characteristics and therapy of Buerger's disease]. *Bratislava Lek Listy*, **97**, 224–9.

Reny, J. L., and Cabane, J. 1998. [Buerger's disease or thromboangiitis obliterans]. *Rev Med Interne*, **19**, 34–43.

Romanuel, F. C. A., and Abramowitz, A. 1964. Changes in brain and pial vessels in arterial boundary zones. *Arch Neurol*, **11**, 40–65.

Shionoya, S. 1989. Buerger's disease (thromboangiitis obliterans). In *Vascular Surgery*, ed. R. B. Rutherford. Philadelphia: W.B. Saunders, pp. 207–17.

von Winiwarter, F. 1879. Über eine eigentümliche Form von Endarteritis und Endophlebitis mit Gangrän des Fußes. *Archiv für Klinische Chirurgie*, **23**, 202–26.

Zülch, K. J., and Pilz, P. 1989. Thrombangitis obliterans (von Winiwarter-Buerger). In *Handbook of Clinical Neurology*, ed. J. F. Toole. Amsterdam: Elsevier Science Publishers, pp. 307–16.

6 NEUROSYPHILIS AND STROKE

Larry E. Davis and Glenn D. Graham

Treponema pallidum

Treponema pallidum spirochetes are slender, tightly coiled, unicellular, helical bacteria 5–15 nm in length and 0.09–0.18 nm wide (Tramont, 2005). The genome is a single, circular chromosome of about 1 138 000 base pairs, which places it in the lowest range for all bacteria. In addition, unlike most other pathogenic bacteria, the genome lacks apparent transposable elements. These observations may explain why *T. pallidum* has remained sensitive to penicillin for more than 60 years and is so difficult to cultivate. *T. pallidum* has not been successfully cultured in vitro although the spirochete will infect experimental animals such as rabbits and monkeys. The width of *T. pallidum* is so narrow that the spirochetes are not visualized by light microscopic examination of fixed cerebrospinal fluid (CSF) sediment or brain tissues using Gram or hematoxylin and eosin stains. However, spirochetes may be detected by light microscopy when silver stains or immunohistochemistry stains are used.

In nature, the only host for *T. pallidum* is man. The organism is transmitted from person to person, mainly through sexual intercourse, when the spirochete penetrates intact mucosal membranes. However, occasional transmission has followed kissing or close contact with an infected primary lesion, via infected fresh blood transfusion, from accidental inoculation, or by spread across the placenta from an infected mother to her fetus (congenital syphilis). The number of spirochetes required to infect a human is unknown but rabbits can be infected with as few as four organisms.

History and epidemiology of neurosyphilis

The origin of syphilis remains unknown. However, by the sixteenth century it had rapidly spread throughout Europe, reportedly causing high morbidity and mortality. Unfortunately, little is known about what syphilis did to the central nervous system (CNS) and the types of vascular disease it may have caused in past centuries. By the twentieth century, but before the advent of penicillin, syphilis had become less virulent. It was estimated that approximately 10% of adults living in New York, Paris, or Berlin had a positive Wasserman blood test (nontreponemal antibody test similar to the rapid plasma reagin [RPR] or Venereal Disease Research Laboratory [VDRL] assay). In spite of the high prevalence of syphilis, relatively few patients developed severe disease. In one study of 473 patients with untreated early syphilis, two-thirds never developed clinical symptoms and only 9.5% developed neurosyphilis (Moore, 1941). A separate study estimated that only 6.5% of infected individuals subsequently developed symptomatic neurosyphilis, with 2.3% developing meningovascular syphilis (Clark and Danbolt, 1955). The change in disease severity might reflect a spontaneous decrease in the organism's virulence or adaptation to the host.

With the discovery of penicillin, the prevalence of syphilis in the United States rapidly fell from about 400 cases/100,000 population in the 1940s to less than 100 cases/100,000 in the late 1950s and to less than 30 cases/100,000 by 1990 (Peterman *et al.*, 2005). However, the prevalence of primary and secondary syphilis rose again in early 2000, particularly in young men (Peterman *et al.*, 2005; San Francisco Department of Public Health, 2005). In San Francisco, the incidence of neurosyphilis has risen sixfold since 2000 (San Francisco Department of Public Health, 2005). Fortunately, syphilis still remains uncommon in developed countries. Unfortunately, worldwide syphilis remains a serious disease with an estimated 12 million new cases occurring each year (Hook and Peeling, 2004).

Pathogenesis of early neurosyphilis

Neurosyphilis begins with invasion of the CNS by spirochetes during the period of spirochete dissemination from the primary lesion (called "secondary syphilis"). The term "early neurosyphilis" refers to meningitis associated with secondary syphilis, asymptomatic neurosyphilis, and meningovascular syphilis and lasts up to two decades (Merritt *et al.*, 1946; Simon, 1985). Late neurosyphilis involves general paresis and tabes dorsalis, develops from spirochete invasion of the brain or spinal cord parenchyma, and typically develops decades after the initial infection (Marra, 2004; Simon, 1985).

Secondary syphilis begins 2–12 weeks (mean 6 weeks) after the primary infection (Marra, 2004). In 40% of these patients, there is dissemination to the CNS. Cerebrospinal fluid findings include a mononuclear cell pleocytosis, slightly elevated protein, normal glucose, reactive CSF-VDRL test, and identification of spirochetes by animal inoculation, polymerase chain reaction, or histologic staining (Davis and Sperry, 1978; Lukehart *et al.*, 1988; Merritt and Moore, 1935; Noordhoek *et al.*, 1991).

While most patients with secondary syphilis do not develop signs of meningitis, occasionally patients develop aseptic

Uncommon Causes of Stroke, 2nd edition, ed. Louis R. Caplan. Published by Cambridge University Press.   © Cambridge University Press 2008.

meningitis with headaches, nausea, stiff neck, and low-grade fever (Merritt and Moore, 1935). A few patients will also develop unilateral or bilateral cranial nerve palsies, especially peripheral facial palsy, deafness and/or vertigo, diplopia, or difficulty in swallowing or protruding the tongue (Alpers, 1954). A few patients with secondary syphilis also develop strokes (Merritt and Moore, 1935).

In most patients with CNS involvement during secondary syphilis, the spirochetes disappear from the CSF and the meningitis spontaneously terminates. In some patients the CNS infection persists and a stage of asymptomatic neurosyphilis begins. Five to 10 years later, growth of spirochetes in the meninges may result in meningovascular syphilis (Simon, 1985).

Meningovascular syphilis

The incidence of strokes from meningovascular syphilis in the prepenicillin era had been estimated to range from 2.3% to 20% of all neurosyphilis cases (Clark and Danbolt, 1955; Kierland et al., 1942; Merritt et al., 1946; Moore, 1941). In the postantibiotic era, the reported incidence of strokes from meningovascular syphilis ranges from 7% to 23% of all patients with neurosyphilis (Aho et al., 1969; Burke and Schaberg, 1985; Danielsen et al., 2004; Hooshmand et al., 1972; Hotson, 1981; Nordenbo and Sorensen, 1981; Perdrup et al., 1981; Timmermans and Carr, 2004). Some of these reports gave data only on meningovascular syphilis and did not distinguish between those patients with strokes and those with only cranial nerve palsies.

The percentage of strokes due to neurosyphilis fell because of a dramatic reduction in syphilis in developed countries. A study of 218 consecutive patients with a transient ischemic attack (TIA) or stroke concluded that meningovascular syphilis is an uncommon cause for strokes, accounting for only 0.4% of stroke patients (Kelley et al., 1989). Another Australian study of 700 stroke patients (14 of whom were young) failed to find syphilis as the cause in any (Chambers et al., 1981).

The pathology of meningovascular syphilis has two major components. The cause of most cerebrovascular disease is syphilitic endarteritis, usually involving medium-to-large meningeal arteries, called Heubner's endarteritis (Gray and Alonso, 2002). These arteries have concentric collagenous thickening of the intima (endarteritis obliterans) and corresponding thinning of the media. The elastic lamina remains intact, but there may be splitting. Lymphocytes and plasma cells infiltrate the thickened adventitia and penetrate the media. Lumen constriction occurs from endothelial proliferation and thickening that can be sufficient to produce ischemic lesions of the brain and spinal cord. The middle cerebral artery is the most commonly involved vessel leading to a stroke, but occasionally the anterior cerebral, posterior cerebral, or basilar artery branches are involved (Merritt et al., 1946). The pathology of the cerebral infarction does not differ from that of other ischemic strokes.

The meninges primarily along the base of the brain have a diffuse or localized chronic inflammation, and some arteries within the meninges are affected by Huebner's endarteritis (Gray and Alonso, 2002). Lymphocytes and some plasma cells combine with fibrous tissue to form perivascular infiltrates around blood vessels along the brainstem in the thickened meninges. The periarteritis may produce cranial nerve palsies and occasionally brainstem ischemic strokes from thrombosis of small penetrating arteries from the vertebral or basilar artery (Brightbill et al., 1995; Johns et al., 1987; Tyler et al., 1994; Umashankar et al., 2004).

The clinical features of brain ischemia from meningovascular syphilis differ from those usually seen in other causes of ischemic strokes. The patient's age at stroke onset is much younger than the typical patient age seen in the more common causes of ischemic stroke. Ninety percent of neurosyphilis strokes are in patients between 30 and 50 years of age (Merritt et al., 1946). The stroke incidence is higher in men than women.

About 25% of patients develop a prodrome of headaches, dizziness, and/or emotional disturbances days to weeks prior to the stroke (Merritt et al., 1946). Signs and symptoms of cerebral vascular syphilis vary by site of the infarction. Overall, about 80% develop a hemiparesis, 30% aphasia, 15% hemihypesthesia, 7% hemianopia, and 15% seizures (Alpers, 1954; Merritt et al., 1946; Perdrup et al., 1981). Because the patient may have coexistent chronic basilar meningitis, about 10% will also have cranial nerve palsies, and 30% will have abnormal pupils. Of note, 25% of patients with stroke will have their symptoms evolve over several days instead of the typical sudden onset (Merritt et al., 1946). Because T. pallidum can simultaneously infect the meninges and brain parenchyma, some patients also may have cognitive decline or frank dementia from general paresis.

Brain CT or MRI of patients with meningovascular syphilis and stroke typically show abnormalities consistent with ischemic lesions, which may be multiple (Brightbill et al., 1995; Holland et al., 1986). Conventional angiography or magnetic resonance angiography typically shows evidence of arteritis with concentric narrowing of large vessels and often focal narrowing and occasionally dilatation of smaller arteries (Brightbill et al., 1995; Flint et al., 2005; Gaa et al., 2004; Gallego et al., 1994; Peters et al., 1993; Vatz et al., 1974). The findings are not specific and are compatible with other types of CNS vasculitis and with vasoconstriction unrelated to vasculitis. In a few patients with a stroke and CSF evidence of meningovascular syphilis, arterial imaging may show another cause for the stroke, such as atherosclerosis. At other times, atherosclerosis may be present along with arteritis (Landi et al., 1990). MRI with gadolinium often shows enhancement and thickening of the meninges around the cisterns and brainstem and, occasionally, over the cerebral cortex (Brightbill et al., 1995; Good and Jager, 2000). Nontreponemal extracranial vascular disease may also be present (Aldrich et al., 1983).

The CSF should always be abnormal. The opening pressure in a lumbar puncture may be normal to slightly elevated. The CSF typically has a mononuclear cell pleocytosis of 20 to several hundred cells per microliter, normal glucose levels, and protein levels range from normal to 250 mg/dL. Oligoclonal bands and elevated CSF immunoglobulin G (IgG) levels are often present (Vartdal et al., 1982). In meningovascular syphilis, the ability to isolate spirochetes by animal inoculation of CSF is very difficult in contrast to secondary syphilis, in which spirochetes can be isolated in up to 30% (Lukehart et al., 1988).

Syphilitic myelitis and spinal cord stroke

Syphilis of the spinal cord is a clinical rarity and usually accompanies other forms of cerebral syphilitic involvement. In the classic preantibiotic series at Boston City Hospital, only 31 (1%) of the 2263 patients with syphilis had nontabetic spinal cord damage (Merritt *et al.*, 1946). Only one-third of those with spinal cord disease had spinal vascular syphilis. Patients could present with an insidious onset or suddenly develop an acute transverse myelitis syndrome. The principal symptoms include paraparesis or paraplegia, urinary and fecal incontinence, and sensory abnormalities with paresthesias, pain, or sensory loss in the lower back and legs. Available pathology shows that the patients had a chronic spinal meningitis with some larger vessels showing typical Heubner's endarteritis. The thoracic spinal cord is the most commonly affected, and patients may present like an acute transverse myelitis. Spinal syphilis is only rarely seen today (Fisher and Poser, 1977; Harrigan *et al.*, 1984; Lowenstein *et al.*, 1987; Silber, 1989). The MRI typically shows short segment, high signal intensity in the thoracic cord on T2-weighted images and abnormal enhancement, predominately in the superficial parts of the spinal cord, on gadolinium-enhanced images (Lowenstein *et al.*, 1987; Nabatame *et al.*, 1992).

Involvement of the cervical spinal cord with quadriplegia is extraordinarily rare but has developed following a syphilitic gumma necrosing the cervical cord or from development of a firm fibrous sheath surrounding the cervical cord (syphilitic hypertrophic pachymeningitis) (Merritt *et al.*, 1946; Silber, 1989).

HIV and neurosyphilis

Considerable evidence shows that immunodeficiency impairs the clearance of *T. pallidum* from the CNS and may accelerate the course of neurosyphilis (Funnye and Akhtar, 2003; Marra, 2004). Individuals with *T. pallidum* are at higher risk of concurrent HIV infection. The dual infection results in a higher HIV load (Buchacz *et al.*, 2004). Accordingly, HIV tests are recommended in every patient with neurosyphilis (Golden *et al.*, 2003). In addition, HIV patients with untreated syphilis have an increased risk (24%) of neurosyphilis (Bordon *et al.*, 1995). Thus, a CSF-VDRL test is needed in every HIV patient who develops cerebrovascular disease, especially if the serum Fluorescent Treponemal Antibody Absorption Assay (FTA-ABS) or RPR test is reactive.

Currently, in the HIV patient both the CSF-VDRL and CSF-FTA-ABS tests appear adequate for diagnosis of meningovascular syphilis, but slightly more false-positive serum RPR tests are encountered. Treating the patient infected with both *T. pallidum* and HIV may be difficult. There is evidence that penicillin treatment for a duration longer than 14 days is required for meningovascular syphilis in the HIV patient (Marra *et al.*, 2004).

Diagnostic evaluation for syphilis in a patient with cerebrovascular disease

Although cerebrovascular disease from neurosyphilis is uncommon in developed countries, there are several risk factors that increase the probability (Table 6.1).

Table 6.1 Diagnostic work-up for syphilis in patients with cerebrovascular disease

Risk factors that increase the probability of neurosyphilis

1)	Patient is 25–50 years old (younger than expected age in most causes of strokes or TIAs).
2)	Patient has a history of syphilis (treated or unknown treatment) or other sexually transmitted diseases.
3)	Patient is infected with HIV.
4)	Patient immigrated to the United States as an adult from a high-syphilis-risk country such as sub-Saharan Africa, south or southeast Asia, Latin America, or the Caribbean.
5)	Patient has stroke symptoms progressing over 24 hours.
6)	Patient is young adult with stroke plus history of progressive cognitive impairment or prior cranial nerve palsies.
7)	Patient has neuroimaging suggestive of arteritis.

Recommended laboratory tests*

Serum:
    RPR
    FTA-ABS or other treponemal-specific antibody test

CSF
    Cell count
    Glucose
    Protein
    IgG level or IgG index
    Oligoclonal bands
    CSF-VDRL
    CSF-FTA-ABS test under specific conditions

Neuroimaging*
    MR angiography or conventional arteriography

*See text for details of interpretation of results

The following laboratory tests help to establish the diagnosis. More than 95% of patients with early neurosyphilis have a positive serum RPR test with titers ranging from 1:2 to >1:128. The RPR and VDRL tests are nontreponemal tests and measure IgG and immunoglobulin M (IgM) antibodies to a cardiolipin–lecithin–cholesterol antigen. The reactivity of these tests generally reflects the activity of disease, and titers decline often to zero following effective antibiotic treatment. A reactive serum RPR test must be confirmed with a positive serum FTA-ABS or *T. pallidum* particle agglutination (TPPA) test to insure that the RPR reactivity is specific for syphilis. These treponemal tests measure IgG and IgM antibodies to *T. pallidum*. Most patients who have reactive specific treponemal tests will have reactive tests for the remainder of their lives, regardless of treatment or disease activity. A reactive serum RPR or FTA-ABS test confirms that the patient has active syphilis but does not signify that the patient has neurosyphilis.

The diagnosis of neurosyphilis requires a lumbar puncture and CSF examination. The CSF should always have a pleocytosis of 10 to several hundred white blood cells (predominately lymphocytes and plasma cells) per microliter. The CSF glucose is normal. The CSF protein is typically elevated in the range of 60–250 mg/dL and usually contains an elevated IgG index and the presence of several oligoclonal bands (Vartdal *et al.*, 1982). The oligoclonal bands are directed against *T. pallidum* antigens when tested in a research laboratory.

The CSF-VDRL test is highly specific, but is relatively insensitive. The test is reactive only in about 75% of patients with syphilis (Centers for Disease Control and Prevention [CDC], 2002). A reactive CSF-VDRL test is diagnostic for neurosyphilis because factors that cause false-positive serum RPR titers are only rarely present in CSF (CDC, 2002).

The difficulty comes when the patient lacks a positive CSF-VDRL test but has clinical, arteriographic, and CSF findings that are suspicious for neurosyphilis. This occasionally develops in patients who have vascular disease from secondary syphilitic meningitis or from meningovascular syphilis (CDC, 2002; Marra, 2004). If the clinical picture and the rest of the CSF are suspicious for meningovascular syphilis, a reactive CSF-FTA-ABS (without blood contamination in the CSF) is usually considered diagnostic (CDC, 2002). Conversely, a negative CSF-FTA-ABS test excludes neurosyphilis (CDC, 2002; Davis and Schmitt, 1989)

Treatment

Penicillin is the main treatment for neurosyphilis, but penicillin must achieve sustained treponemicidal CSF levels for a prolonged period to cure. The long treatment period is necessary because penicillin kills only during bacterial cell division and *T. pallidum* has a slow replication rate of 30 hours. Aqueous crystalline penicillin G in adults is administered as 3–4 million units intravenously every 4 hours or by continuous infusion for 10–14 days (CDC, 2002). Following the end of the intravenous treatment, the patient often is given intramuscular benzathine penicillin (2.4 million units) at 1-week intervals for 3 weeks, especially if there is also HIV infection (Jay, 2006). The major adverse effects of penicillin include anaphylaxis, rash, Stevens–Johnson syndrome, drug-induced eosinophilia, hemolytic anemia, thrombocytopenia, neutropenia, seizures, interstitial nephritis, and pseudomembranous enterocolitis. Because each million units of penicillin contain 1.7 meQ of potassium, serum potassium levels should be carefully followed in patients with renal insufficiency (Jay, 2006).

If the patient is allergic to penicillin, desensitization to penicillin should be considered (see CDC, 2002, for method). The CDC syphilis treatment guidelines are published about every 4 years, so one should always consult the latest version. Ceftriaxone (in adults, 2 g intravenously once daily for 14 days) is currently the alternative treatment of choice in the few patients who cannot be desensitized to penicillin (Marra, 2004). Of note, azithromycin as an alternative antibiotic should seldom be used because macrolide-resistant mutations of *T. pallidum* are being detected (Lukehart *et al.*, 2004).

Stroke rehabilitation

No studies have been specifically conducted regarding the rehabilitation of patients following stroke related to syphilis. However, individual case reports describe clinical improvement in syphilitic stroke patients with rehabilitation (Umashankar *et al.*, 2004). We recommend that current guidelines for provision of rehabilitation services following stroke be followed (Bates *et al.*, 2005; Duncan *et al.*, 2005). Patients diagnosed with meningovascular or other forms of syphilis following presentation for acute stroke will typically spend several weeks as hospital inpatients to receive intravenous penicillin therapy. This treatment period provides a natural time frame within which to initiate inpatient rehabilitation, either in an acute neurological/medical or rehabilitation ward setting.

Follow-up

Even though the peak infectious period for syphilis transmission occurs many years before a stroke, it is still important to urge the patient to notify all sexual partners (even if the relationship was years ago) to have serum RPR and FTA-ABS tests.

Every patient with neurosyphilis requires clinical and serological follow-up at 3, 6, and possibly 12 months (CDC, 2002; Golden *et al.*, 2003; Marra, 2004). The first repeat CSF examination is best at 3 months after treatment to decrease patient loss in follow-up. One prospective study found that the median time for normalization of CSF, including the white blood cell count, CSF-VDRL, and serum RPR, was 3–4 months (Marra *et al.*, 2004). CSF protein resolves slower. If the CSF is normal at 3 months, then further lumbar punctures are not needed. CDC guidelines recommend that, if the CSF cell count has not markedly decreased by 6 months or the CSF is not normal after 2 years, retreatment should be considered (CDC, 2002). Other experts recommend retreatment when there is failure of the serum RPR and CSF-VDRL to decline fourfold or to negative by 1 year (Marra, 2004). Remember that syphilitic re-infections do occur, so recurrence may not indicate treatment failure.

What happens to the cerebral arteritis and arterial stenosis following penicillin therapy is unclear, as limited follow-up imaging studies have been performed (Kelley *et al.*, 2003). Because of this, patients should also receive daily aspirin, or another antiplatelet agent, to minimize further strokes.

REFERENCES

Aho, K., Sievers, K., and Salo, O. P. 1969. Late complications of syphilis: a comparative epidemiological and serological study of cardiovascular syphilis and various forms of neurosyphilis. *Acta Derm Venereol*, **49**, 336–42.

Aldrich, M. S., Burke, J. M., and Gulati, S. M. 1983. Angiographic findings in a young man with recurrent stroke and positive fluorescent treponemal antibody (FTA). *Stroke*, **14**, 1001–4.

Alpers, B. J. 1954. *Clinical Neurology*, 3rd edn. Philadelphia: FA Davis.

Bates, B., Choi, J. Y., Duncan, P. W., *et al.* 2005. Veterans Affairs/Department of Defense Clinical Practice Guideline for the Management of Adult Stroke Rehabilitation Care: executive summary. *Stroke*, **36**, 2049–56.

Bordon, J., Martinez-Vazquez, C., Alvarez, M., *et al.* 1995. Neurosyphilis in HIV-infected patients. *Eur J Clin Microbiol Infect Dis*, **14**, 864–9.

Brightbill, T. C., Ihmeidan, I. H., Post, M. J., Berger, J. R., and Katz, D. A. 1995. Neurosyphilis in HIV-positive and HIV-negative patients: neuroimaging findings. *Am J Neuroradiol*, **16**, 703–11.

Buchacz, K., Patel, P., Taylor, M., *et al.* 2004. Syphilis increases HIV viral load and decreases CD4cell counts in HIV-infected patients with new syphilis infections. *AIDS*, **18**, 2075–9.

Burke, J. M., and Schaberg, D. R. 1985. Neurosyphilis in the antibiotic era. *Neurology*, **35**, 1368–71.

Centers for Disease Control and Prevention (CDC). 2002. *Sexually Transmitted Diseases Treatment Guidelines 2002*. Atlanta, GA: CDC, 51 (RR06).

Chambers, B. R., Bladin, P. F., McGrath, K., and Goble, A. J. 1981. Stroke syndromes in young people. *Clin Exp Neurol*, **18**, 132–44.

Clark, E. G., and Danbolt, N. 1955. The Oslo study of the natural history of untreated syphilis; an epidemiologic investigation based on a restudy of the Boeck-Bruusgaard material; a review and appraisal. *J Chronic Dis*, **2**, 311–44.

Danielsen, A. G., Weismann, K., Jorgensen, B. B., Heidenheim, M., and Fugleholm, A. M. 2004. Incidence, clinical presentation and treatment of neurosyphilis in Denmark 1980–1997. *Acta Derm Venereol*, **84**, 459–62.

Davis, L., and Schmitt, J. 1989. Clinical significance of cerebrospinal fluid tests for neurosyphilis. *Ann Neurol*, **25**, 50–5.

Davis, L., and Sperry, S. 1978. Bell's palsy and secondary syphilis: CSF spirochetes detected by immunofluorescence. *Ann Neurol*, **4**, 378–80.

Duncan, P. W., Zorowitz, R., Bates, B., *et al.* 2005. Management of adult stroke rehabilitation care: a clinical practice guideline. *Stroke*, **36**, e100–43.

Fisher, M., and Poser, C. M. 1977. Syphilitic meningomyelitis: a case report. *Arch Neurol*, **34**, 785.

Flint, A. C., Liberato, B. B., Anziska, Y., Schantz-Dunn, J., and Wright, C. B. 2005. Meningovascular syphilis as a cause of basilar artery stenosis. *Neurology*, **64**, 391–2.

Funnye, A. S., and Akhtar, A. J. 2003. Syphilis and human immunodeficiency virus co-infection. *J Natl Med Assoc*, **95**, 363–82.

Gaa, J., Weidauer, S., Sitzer, M., Lanfermann, H., and Zanella, F. E. 2004. Cerebral vasculitis due to Treponema pallidum infection: MRI and MRA findings. *Eur Radiol*, **14**, 746–7.

Gallego, J., Soriano, G., Zubieta, J. L., Delgado, G., and Villanueva, J. A. 1994. Magnetic resonance angiography in meningovascular syphilis. *Neuroradiology*, **36**, 208–9.

Golden, M. R., Marra, C. M., and Holmes, K. K. 2003. Update on syphilis: resurgence of an old problem. *JAMA*, **290**, 1510–4.

Good, C. D., and Jager, H. R. 2000. Contrast enhancement of the cerebrospinal fluid on MRI in two cases of spirochaetal meningitis. *Neuroradiology*, **42**, 448–50.

Gray, F., and Alonso, J. M. 2002. Bacterial infections of the central nervous system. In *Greenfield's Neuropathology*, 7th edn. D. I. Graham and P. L. Lantos, eds. London: Arnold, pp. II:178–II:184.

Harrigan, E. P., McLaughlin, T. J., and Feldman, R. G. 1984. Transverse myelitis due to meningovascular syphilis. *Arch Neurol*, **41**, 337–8.

Holland, B. A., Perrett, L. V., and Mills, C. M. 1986. Meningovascular syphilis: CT and MRI findings. *Radiology*, **158**, 439–42.

Hook, E. W. III, and Peeling, R. W. 2004. Syphilis control – a continuing challenge. *N Engl J Med*, **351**, 122–4.

Hooshmand, H., Escobar, M. R., and Kopf, S. W. 1972. Neurosyphilis. A study of 241 patients. *JAMA*, **219**, 726–9.

Hotson, J. R. 1981. Modern neurosyphilis: a partially treated chronic meningitis. *West J Med*, **135**, 191–200.

Jay, C. A. 2006. Treatment of neurosyphilis. *Curr Treat Options Neurol*, **8**, 185–92.

Johns, D. R., Tierney, M., and Parker, S. W. 1987. Pure motor hemiplegia due to meningovascular neurosyphilis. *Arch Neurol*, **44**, 1062–5.

Kelley, R. E., Bell, L., Kelley, S. E., and Lee, S. C. 1989. Syphilis detection in cerebrovascular disease. *Stroke*, **20**, 230–4.

Kelley, R. E., Minagar, A., Kelley, B. J., and Brunson, R. 2003. Transcranial Doppler monitoring of response to therapy for meningovascular syphilis. *J Neuroimaging*, **13**, 85–7.

Kierland, R. R., O'Leary, P. A., and Vandoren, E. 1942. Symptomatic neurosyphilis. *J Vener Dis Inf*, **22**, 360–77.

Landi, G., Villani, F., and Anzalone, N. 1990. Variable angiographic findings in patients with stroke and neurosyphilis. *Stroke*, **21**, 333–8.

Lowenstein, D. H., Mills, C., and Simon, R. P. 1987. Acute syphilitic transverse myelitis: unusual presentation of meningovascular syphilis. *Genitourin Med*, **63**, 333–8.

Lukehart, S. A., Godornes, C., Molini, B. J., *et al.* 2004. Macrolide resistance in Treponema pallidum in the United States and Ireland. *N Engl J Med*, **351**, 154–8.

Lukehart, S. A., Hook, E. W. III, Baker-Zander, S. A., *et al.* 1988. Invasion of the central nervous system by Treponema pallidum: implications for diagnosis and treatment. *Ann Intern Med*, **109**, 855–62.

Marra, C. M. 2004. Neurosyphilis. In *Infections of the Central Nervous System*, 3rd edn. Philadelphia: Lippincott, Williams & Wilkins, pp. 649–57.

Marra, C. M., Maxwell, C. L., Tantalo, L., *et al.* 2004. Normalization of cerebrospinal fluid abnormalities after neurosyphilis therapy: does HIV status matter? *Clin Infect Dis*, **38**, 1001–6.

Merritt, H. H., Adams, R. D., and Solomon, H. C. 1946. *Neurosyphilis*. New York: Oxford University Press, pp. 83–174.

Merritt, H. H., and Moore, M. 1935. Acute syphilitic meningitis. *Medicine*, **14**, 119–83.

Moore, J. 1941. *The Modern Treatment of Syphilis*, 2nd edn., Springfield: CC Thomas.

Nabatame, H., Nakamura, K., Matuda, M., *et al.* 1992. MRI of syphilitic myelitis. *Neuroradiology*, **34**, 105–6.

Noordhoek, G. T., Engelkens, H. J., Judanarso, J., *et al.* 1991. Yaws in West Sumatra, Indonesia: clinical manifestations, serological findings and characterization of new Treponema isolates by DNA probes. *Eur J Clin Microbiol Infect Dis*, **10**, 12–9.

Nordenbo, A. M., and Sorensen, P. S. 1981. The incidence and clinical presentation of neurosyphilis in Greater Copenhagen, 1974 through 1978. *Acta Neurol Scand*, **63**, 237–46.

Perdrup, A., Jorgensen, B. B., and Pedersen, N. S. 1981. The profile of neurosyphilis in Denmark. A clinical and serological study of all patients in Denmark with neurosyphilis disclosed in the years 1971–1979 incl. by Wassermann reaction (CWRM) in the cerebrospinal fluid. *Acta Derm Venereol Suppl (Stockh)*, **96**, 1–14.

Peterman, T., Heffelfinger, J., Swint, E., and Groseclose, S. 2005. The changing epidemiology of syphilis. *Sex Transm Dis*, **32**, S4–S10.

Peters, K. M., Adam, G., Biedermann, M., Zilkens, K. W., and Gunther, R. 1993. [Osteomyelitis today – diagnostic imaging and therapy]. *Zentralbl Chir*, **118**, 637–45.

San Francisco Department of Public Health. 2005. San Francisco Sexually Transmitted Disease Annual Summary, 2004.

Silber, M. H. 1989. Syphilitic myelopathy. *Genitourin Med*, **65**, 338–41.

Simon, R. P. 1985. Neurosyphilis. *Arch Neurol*, **42**, 606–13.

Timmermans, M., and Carr, J. 2004. Neurosyphilis in the modern era. *J Neurol Neurosurg Psychiatry*, **75**, 1727–30.

Tramont, E. C. 2005. Treponema pallidum (syphilis). In *Principles and Practices of Infectious Diseases*, 6th edn., eds. G. L. Mandell, J. Bennett, and R. Dolin. Philadelphia: Elsevier, Churchill, Livingstone, pp. 2768–85.

Tyler, K. L., Sandberg, E., and Baum, K. F. 1994. Medical medullary syndrome and meningovascular syphilis: a case report in an HIV-infected man and a review of the literature. *Neurology*, **44**, 2231–5.

Umashankar, G., Gupta, V., and Harik, S. I. 2004. Acute bilateral inferior cerebellar infarction in a patient with neurosyphilis. *Arch Neurol*, **61**, 953–6.

Vartdal, F., Vandvik, B., Michaelsen, T. E., Loe, K., and Norrby, E. 1982. Neurosyphilis: intrathecal synthesis of oligoclonal antibodies to Treponema pallidum. *Ann Neurol*, **11**, 35–40.

Vatz, K. A., Scheibel, R. L., Keiffer, S. A., and Ansari, K. A. 1974. Neurosyphilis and diffuse cerebral angiopathy: a case report. *Neurology*, **24**, 472–6.

7 VASCULITIS AND STROKE DUE TO TUBERCULOSIS

Sarosh M. Katrak

Tuberculosis (TB) is considered one of the oldest diseases known to man. A human skeleton with evidence of spinal TB from a neolithic cemetery was found near Heidelberg in 1904. This is considered to be the first documented record of human TB (Morse, 1961). It is unfortunate that, despite advances in prophylactic and therapeutic measures, this disease still remains a scourge in large parts of the world. To make matters worse, the HIV pandemic has brought about a resurgence of this dreaded disease in many developed countries (Berenguer et al., 1992; Dube et al., 1992) and an explosion of all forms of TB in developing countries, some of which are the poorest in the world.

Tuberculous meningitis (TBM) is the most common form of neurotuberculosis, accounting for 70–80% of the cases (Udani et al., 1971). TBM is still a crippling disease with a high degree of morbidity and mortality. One of the most severe complications of TBM is stroke resulting from vascular involvement. Although the first clinical description of arteritis in TBM in the indexed literature was by Collomb et al. (1967), Baumgarten (1881) is believed to be the first to describe these changes in autopsy specimens. Since the early 1970s, considerable work has been published from the Indian subcontinent on the clinical, pathological, and angiographic studies of vasculitis and strokes in TBM. The newer techniques of neuroimaging – CT scans, MRI, and digital subtraction angiography (DSA) – have added to our understanding of this dreaded complication of TBM.

TBM is invariably secondary to a primary involvement of some extracranial organ, very often pulmonary TB (Vashishta and Banerjee, 1999). Our understanding of the pathogenesis of TBM begins with comprehensive and meticulous studies by Rich and McCordock (1933). They showed that there was a subcortical or meningeal focus, later called the "Rich focus," from which bacilli gained access to the subarachnoid space. Once it gains entry, there are many factors that determine the type of lesions seen in the central nervous system (CNS). The time lapse between onset of infection and institution of therapy, the age of the patient, the immune status of the patient, and the virulence and drug sensitivity of the bacillus are important determinants modifying the pathology of neurotuberculosis. Gross examination of the brain at autopsy showed that a thick exudate was most frequently present on the basal aspect (Dastur and Lalitha, 1973; Thomas et al., 1997), where the structures are obscured. Coronal slices of the brain reveal thick organized exudates all around the optic chiasm, extending into the Sylvian fissures entrapping the middle cerebral arteries and its branches.

Askanazy (1910) first described the triad of vascular changes in TBM: panarteritis involving all three coats in a tuberculous process, caseation of the vessel wall, and fibrinoid swelling. Since then, changes involving the vessels in the brain are the most intensively studied and one of the landmark histopathological features of TBM. Macroscopically, the basal arteries, particularly the MCA and its branches are maximally involved. Microscopically, the vascular changes include endoarteritis, periarteritis, vascular edema, fibrinoid necrosis, and thrombosis (Dastur and Lalitha, 1973; Deshpande et al., 1969; Shankar, 1989; Vashishta and Banerjee, 1999). However, the pathogenesis of the infarcts found predominantly in the MCA territory is controversial. Based on angiographic and pathological studies, some believe that the MCA and its perforating branches are preferentially involved in the copious exudates with "throttling and occlusion" of the larger arteries (Dastur et al., 1970; Rojas-Echeverri et al., 1996; Vashishta and Banerjee, 1999; Wadia and Singhal, 1967), producing infarcts in the basal ganglia. However, "there was an absence of thrombosis" in the occluded vessels (Dastur and Lalitha, 1973). In a prospective study, Dalal (1979) noted that softening of the brain often occurred in areas where the degree of luminal stenosis was not pronounced and, conversely, significant reduction in the vascular lumen was found in patients with no neurological deficit. Others have had similar experiences (Deshpande et al., 1969; Rojas-Echeverri et al., 1996; Shankar, 1989). This implies that throttling and occlusion is but one of the pathogenic mechanisms producing infarcts, preferentially in the basal ganglia region, and that a true arteritis with no relation to the basal exudates also occurs. It would be logical to presume that other pathogenetic factors – such as changes in microvascular reactivity to neurochemicals, cytokines, and the state of cell-mediated immunity (CMI) of the patient at that particular time – play an important role in the genesis of these lesions.

In a review of pathological data, Shankar found intracytoplasmic vacuolations of the muscular coat of the vessels. He felt that these changes were nonspecific as they were noted in blood vessels even in subarachnoid hemorrhage but pointed to a common pathogenic mechanism – vasospasm – and that the latter explained the "reversible" stenotic segment described by Dalal (1979). The vasospasm in turn could be chemically mediated by vasoactive eicosanoids or cytokines. Dastur and Dave (1977) postulated that the basement membrane proliferation seen around small arterioles played a role in initiating an immunologic reaction. Shankar, in contrast, showed that various components of the tuberculoprotein are antigenic and selectively bind to various components of

Uncommon Causes of Stroke, 2nd edition, ed. Louis R. Caplan. Published by Cambridge University Press. © Cambridge University Press 2008.

the vessel wall, thus initiating and maintaining an immunological injury (Shankar, 1989). However, neither of them showed the presence of *Mycobacterium tuberculosis* in the vicinity of these blood vessels.

In HIV-infected individuals with TBM, the immune response to the tuberculous bacilli is altered; therefore, pathological features are very different from those seen in patients with relatively normal CMI. The brains of such individuals showed minimal inflammatory response with parenchymal infarcts and vasculitis, not only in the basal ganglia but in the cortical parenchyma as well (Katrak *et al.*, 2000). The exact reason for this extensive vasculopathy was not clear. It is known that polyclonal B-cell activation occurs in HIV-infected patients with resultant hypergammaglobulinemia and circulating immune complexes (Cotran *et al.*, 1999). However, it remains speculative that such B-cell activation occurred due to mycobacteria in these patients (Katrak *et al.*, 2000).

The controversy over the pathogenesis of vasculitis, therefore, is far from resolved. Whether morphological changes, chemically mediated vasospasm, or an immunologic attack of the vessel wall by various components of the tuberculoprotein, with or without impaired CMI, plays a major role, is undetermined as adequate systematic immunopathological studies of this entity are lacking. The truth may lie in a combination of these factors.

The clinical features are usually preceded by a prodromal phase of fatigue, malaise, low-grade fever, and loss of appetite. The further temporal evolution depends on the rapidity with which the disease and complications associated with the involvement of basal structures (namely, cranial nerve palsies, paraplegia, strokes, hydrocephalus, and loss of consciousness) progress. Traditionally, the severity of the disease is grouped into three stages: mild (stage 1), moderate (stage 2), and severe (stage 3), with a good correlation with the final outcome (Singhal *et al.*, 1975; Streptomycin in Tuberculosis Trial Committee, 1948). Strokes usually occur in patients in stages 2 or 3. Hence, this dreaded complication is associated with a high mortality and morbidity (Katrak *et al.*, 2000; Misra *et al.*, 2000).

Focal neurological deficits occur in 10–47% of patients with TBM in different series (Chan *et al.*, 2005; Deshpande *et al.*, 1969; Osuntokun *et al.*, 1971; Paul, 1967; Thomas *et al.*, 1977). In one series, 8% of strokes in the young were due to tuberculous vasculitis (Dalal and Dalal, 1989). The highest incidence (47%) has been reported from Taiwan (Lan *et al.*, 2001). Focal neurological deficits usually occur acutely and involve the basal ganglia and subcortical structures. Thus aphasia, apraxia, and agnosia are uncommon. However, when these occur insidiously, they should arouse suspicion of an evolving tuberculoma in the appropriate area. Infarcts in the vertebrobasilar territory are uncommon, and intracerebral or intraventricular hemorrhages are rare (Dalal and Dalal, 1989). Convulsions may present at any stage of TBM. They are more common in children. They occurred in 37.5% of patients with vascular involvement as compared to only 20% of those without strokes in a case study (Thomas *et al.*, 1997). Convulsions may also occur due to associated tuberculomas, hydrocephalus, or tuberculous meningoencephalitis. Clinically, strokes in individuals co-infected

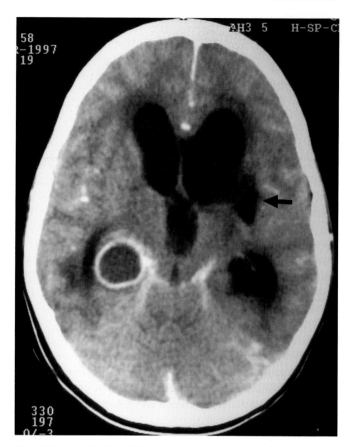

Figure 7.1 Postcontrast axial CT scan showing dense basal exudates around the quadrigeminal cistern, hydrocephalus, right parahippocampal tuberculous abscess, and left basal ganglia infarct (*arrow*).

with HIV are no different than those in persons without HIV infection, as reported by several case series (Berenguer *et al.*, 1992; Dube *et al.*, 1992; Katrak *et al.*, 2000; Porkert *et al.*, 1997; Yechoor *et al.*, 1990).

The diagnosis of TBM is usually established by the demonstration of acid-fast bacilli, by direct smear or culture in the cerebrospinal fluid, brain parenchyma, tuberculomas, or meninges in biopsy or autopsy material. Newer techniques, particularly polymerase chain reaction, have increased the diagnostic yield (Takahashi *et al.*, 2005). Neuroimaging techniques and procedures are not diagnostic for TBM but have become the standard for its complications.

CT or MRI of the head may reveal intense basal enhancement after intravenous contrast administration, communicating or noncommunicating hydrocephalus, cerebral infarcts, parenchymatous tuberculomas, or a combination of two or more of these features (Figure 7.1). Basal enhancement and tuberculomas are direct signs of TBM, whereas ischemic infarcts and hydrocephalus are signs of its complications. Although the CT scan lacks the sensitivity of the MRI, especially for infarcts, it is readily available in most centers, particularly in developing countries. It is cost effective and obviates the need for sedation in an acutely ill patient as the duration of the study is short.

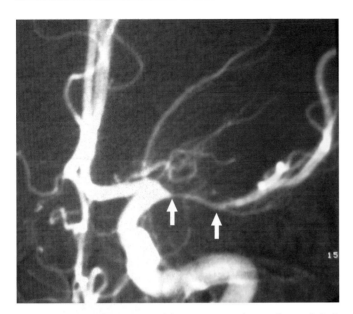

Figure 7.2 Left carotid angiogram of the same patient showing "strangulation" of the M1 segment of the middle cerebral artery (*between arrows*).

Neuroimaging findings usually are in tandem with the pathological data, especially in immunocompetent individuals. In the western literature, neuroimaging findings were no different in HIV-infected individuals when compared to noninfected cases (Berenguer *et al.*, 1992; Villora *et al.*, 1995; Yechoor *et al.*, 1990). In contrast to the above findings, we found distinct differences. The basal exudates were sparse and infrequent, tending to occur only after initiation of antituberculous therapy. Ventricular dilatation occurred secondary to atrophy. Granulomatous lesions included tuberculomas as well as toxoplasma granulomas. An interesting observation was that of the occurrence of cortical infarcts in these patients with angiographic evidence of arteritis (Katrak *et al.*, 2000). Similar findings have been described from other centers in India and abroad (Karve *et al.*, 2001; Sze and Zimmerman, 1988). Infarcts are more common in children than in adults (Kingsley *et al.*, 1987; Mishra and Goyal, 1999), and the incidence is significantly higher on MRI as compared to CT scans (Chan *et al.*, 2005; Mishra and Goyal, 1999).

The role of cerebral angiography is limited in TBM. It is usually necessary in patients with focal neurological deficits and in those with altered mentation. Lehrer described an angiographic triad of a sweeping pericallosal artery, narrowing of the supraclinoid portion of the internal carotid artery, and narrowed or occluded small or medium-sized intracranial arteries with scanty collaterals (Lehrer, 1966). This was later subsequently confirmed in many studies (Dalal, 1979; Mishra and Goyal, 1999; Rojas-Echeverri *et al.*, 1996; Wadia and Singhal, 1967). The clinico-angiographic analysis correlation is not good. Normal angiograms have been found in patients with clinical or MRI evidence of infarcts in 42–57% of cases (Dalal, 1979; Rojas-Echeverri *et al.*, 1996; Wadia and Singhal, 1967). Conversely, a significant reduction in the vascular lumen has been found in patients with no neurological deficit (Dalal, 1979; Deshpande *et al.*, 1969; Rojas-Echeverri *et al.*, 1996) or neuropathological changes (Dalal, 1979). Even the mechanism for the

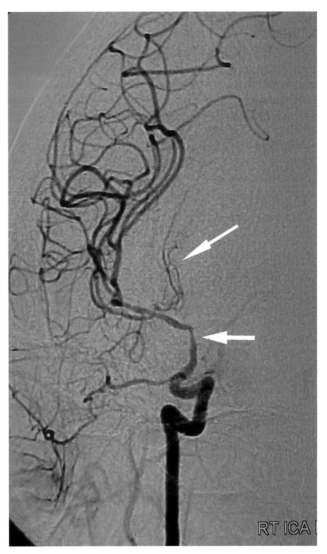

Figure 7.3 Right carotid angiogram showing marked narrowing of the supraclinoid internal carotid artery with segmental narrowing of M1 segments of the middle cerebral artery (*between thick arrows*). Note: only the lateral lenticulostriate perforators are seen (*thin arrow*).

angiographic changes is debated, as mentioned earlier in the discussion of pathogenesis. It could be due to morphological changes in the vessel due to thick basal exudates (Figure 7.2) (Dastur *et al.*, 1970; Vashishta and Banerjee, 1999; Wadia and Singhal, 1967) or due to arteritis (Figure 7.3) (Dalal, 1979; Rojas-Echeverri *et al.*, 1996). In our cases of TBM with HIV infection and cortical infarcts, we had angiographic and pathological evidence of widespread arteritis (Figure 7.4) (unpublished data). However, there is agreement that the majority of infarcts are in the area supplied by the lenticulostriate and thalamoperforating branches of the MCA, the so-called "TB zone" described by Hsieh *et al.* (1992). In conclusion, angiography is not routinely indicated in TBM and should be performed only in cases with focal neurological deficit and altered sensorium.

Despite the availability of antimicrobial agents in various combinations, the morbidity and mortality of TBM remains high,

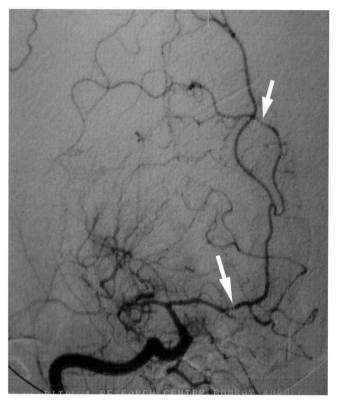

Figure 7.4 Right carotid angiogram, oblique view of a patient with tuberculous meningitis and HIV infection. Total block of the right middle cerebral artery and areas of segmental narrowing – arteritis – along the right anterior cerebral artery (*arrows*).

especially in patients who seek treatment late. Besides chemotherapy, patients of TBM with vasculitis and infarcts should be given corticosteroids in a dose of 1 mg/kg/day, tapering this over 4–6 weeks (Thwaites *et al.*, 2004).

REFERENCES

Askanazy, M. 1910. (Quoted by Winkleman, N. W., and Moore, T. 1940). Meningeal blood vessels in tuberculous meningitis. *Am Rev Tuberc*, **42**, 315–33.

Baumgarten, P. 1881. Gammose arteritis und entsprechende tuberculöse veränderungen. *Virchows Arch Pathol Anat Physiol Klin Med*. **179**, 86.

Berenguer, J., Moreno, S., Laguna, F. *et al.* 1992. Tuberculous meningitis in patients infected with the human immunodeficiency virus infection. *N Engl J Med*, **326**, 668–72.

Chan, K. H., Cheung, R. T., Lee, R., Mak, W., and Ho, S. L. 2005. Cerebral infarcts complicating tuberculous meningitis. *Cerebrovasc Dis*, **19**, 391–5.

Collomb, H., Lemercier, G., Virieu, R., and Dumas, M. 1967. Multiple cerebral vascular thrombosis due to arteritis associated with tuberculous meningitis. *Bulletin Societè Medècin Africa Noire Langue Français*, **12**, 813–22.

Cotran, R. S., Kumar, V., and Collins, T. 1999. Diseases of immunity. In *Robbins Pathological Basis of Disease*, eds. R. S. Cotran, V. Kumar, and T. Collins Philadelphia: W. B. Saunders, pp.188–259.

Dalal, P. M. 1979. Observations on the involvement of cerebral vessels in tuberculous meningitis in adults. In *Advances in Neurology*, ed. M. Goldstein, L. Bolis, C. Fieschi, S. Gorini, and C. H. Millikan. New York: Raven Press, **25**, pp. 149–59.

Dalal, P. M., and Dalal, K. P. 1989. Cerebrovascular manifestations of infectious disease. In *Handbook of Clinical Neurology*, Vol 11: Vascular diseases, Part III, ed. J. F. Toole. Amsterdam: Elsevier, pp. 411–41.

Dastur, D. K., and Dave, U. P. 1977. Ultrastructural basis of the vasculopathy in and around brain tuberculomas. *Am J Pathol*, **89**, 35–50.

Dastur, D. K., and Lalitha, V. S. 1973. The Many Facets of Neurotuberculosis: An Epitome of Neuropathology. In *Progress in Neuropathology*, ed. H. Zimmerman. New York: Grune and Stratton, pp. 351–408.

Dastur, D. K., Lalitha, V. S., Udani, P. M., and Parekh, U. 1970. The brain and meninges in TBM. Gross pathology and pathogenesis in 100 cases. *Neurol India*, **18**, 86–100.

Deshpande, D. H., Bharucha, E. P., and Mondkar, V. P. 1969. Tuberculous meningitis in adults. *Neurol India*, **17**, 28–35.

Dube, M. P., Holton, P. D., and Larsen, R. A. 1992. Tuberculous meningitis in patients with and without human immunodeficiency virus infection. *Am J Med*, **93**, 520–4.

Hsieh, F., Chia, L., and Shen, W. 1992. Location of cerebral infarctions in tuberculous meningitis. *Neuroradiology*, **34**, 197–9.

Karve, K. K., Satishchandra, P., Shankar, S. K., *et al.* 2001. Tuberculous meningitis with and without HIV infection. *Abstracts of Annual Conference of Neurological Society of India, A225*, 311–2.

Katrak, S. M., Shembalkar, P. K., Bijwe, S. R., and Bhandarkar, L. D. 2000. The clinical, radiological and pathological profile of tuberculous meningitis in patients with and without human immunodeficiency virus infection. *J Neurol Sci*, **181**, 118–26.

Kingsley, D. P. E., Hendrickse, W. A., Kendall, B. E., Swash, M., and Singh, V. 1987. Tuberculous meningitis: role of CT in management and prognosis. *J Neurol Neurosurg Psychiatry*, **50**, 30–6.

Lan, S. H., Chang, W. N., Lu. C. H., Lui, C. C., and Chang, H. W. 2001. Cerebral infarction in chronic meningitis: a comparison of tuberculous meningitis and cryptococcal meningitis. *Q J Med*, **94**, 247–53.

Lehrer, H. 1966. The angiographic triad in tuberculous meningitis. *Radiology*, **87**, 829.

Mishra, N. K., Goyal, M. 1999. *Imaging of CNS Tuberculosis*. In: *Neurology in Tropics*, eds. J. S. Chopra, and I. M. S. Sawhney. New Delhi: BI Churchill Livingstone Pvt. Ltd, pp. 370–90.

Misra, U. K., Kalita, J., Roy, A. K., Mandal, S. K., and Srivastava, M. 2000. Role of clinical, radiological and neurophysiological changes in predicting the outcome of tuberculous meningitis: a multivariate analysis. *J Neurol Neurosurg Psychiatry*, **68**, 300–3.

Morse, D. 1961. Prehistoric TB in America. *Am Rev Respir Dis*, **83**, 489.

Osuntokun, B. O., Adeuja, A. O. G., Familusi, J. B. 1971. Tuberculous meningitis in Nigerians: a review of 194 patients. *Trop Geogr Med*, **23**, 225–31.

Paul, F. M. 1967. Tuberculous meningitis in children in the department of paediatrics over a 10 year period. *Singapore Med J*, **8**, 102–4.

Porkert, M. T., Sotir, M., Parrott-Moore, P., Blumberg, H. M. 1997. Tuberculous meningitis at a large inner city medical centre. *Am J Med Sci*, **313**, 325–31.

Rich, A. R., McCordock, H. A. 1933. The pathogenesis of tuberculous meningitis. *Bull John Hopkins Hosp*, **53**, 5–37.

Rojas-Echeverri, L. A., Soto-Hernandez, J. L., Garza, S., *et al.* 1996. Predictive value of digital subtraction angiography in patient with tuberculous meningitis. *Neuroradiology*, **38**, 20–4.

Shankar, S. K. 1989. CNS vasculopathy–revisited. In *Progress in Clinical Neurosciences 5*, eds. K. K. Sinha, and P. Chandra. Ranchi, India: Neurological Society of India, Catholic Press, pp. 93–101.

Singhal, B. S., Bhagwati, S. N., Sayed, A. H., Laud, G. W. 1975. Raised intracranial pressure in tuberculous meningitis. *Neurol India*, **23**, 32–9.

Streptomycin in Tuberculosis Trial Committee. 1948. Medical Research Council Streptomycin treatment of tuberculous meningitis. *Lancet*, **i**, 582–96.

Sze, G., Zimmerman, R. D. 1988. The magnetic resonance imaging of infections and inflammatory diseases. *Radiol Clin North Am*, **26**, 839–59.

Takahashi, T., Nakayama, T., Tamura, M., *et al.* 2005. Nested polymerase chain reaction for assessing the clinical cause of tuberculous meningitis. *Neurology*, **64**, 1789–93.

Thomas, M. D., Chopra, J. S., Banerjee, A. K., and Singh, M. S. 1997. Tuberculous meningitis: a clinicopathological study. *Neurol India*, **25**, 26–34.

Thwaites, G. E., Bang, N. D., Dung, N. H., *et al.* 2004. Dexamethasone for the treatment of tuberculous meningitis in adolescents and adults. *N Engl J Med*, **351**, 1741–51.

Udani, P. M., Parekh, U. C., and Dastur, D. K. 1971. Neurological and related syndromes in CNS tuberculosis: clinical features and pathogenesis. *J Neurol Sci*, **14**, 341–57.

Vashishta, R. K., and Banerjee, A. K. 1999. CNS Tuberculosis–Pathology. In *Neurology in Tropics*, eds. J. S. Chopra, and I. M. S. Sawhney. New Delhi: BI Churchill Livingstone Pvt. Ltd, pp. 391–8.

Villora, M. F., Fortea, F., Moreno, S., Munoz, L., Manero, M., and Benito, C. 1995. MR imaging and CT of central nervous system tuberculosis in patients with AIDS. *Radiol Clin North Am*, **33**, 805–20.

Wadia, N. H., Singhal, B. S. 1967. Cerebral arteriography in tuberculous meningitis. *Neurol India*, **15**, 127–32.

Yechoor, V. K., Shandera, W. X., Rodriguez, P., Cate, T. R. 1990. Tuberculous meningitis among adults with or without HIV infection. *Arch Intern Med*, **156**, 1710–6.

8 STROKE DUE TO FUNGAL INFECTIONS

Daniel B. Hier and Louis R. Caplan

Stroke due to fungal infection is rare. Walshe *et al.* (1985b) reviewed the 1953–1978 autopsy records of the Johns Hopkins Hospital. There were 60 autopsied cases with central nervous system (CNS) involvement by fungus. The most common pathogens were aspergillus (16), candida (27), and cryptococcus (14). In addition, there were two cases of mucor and one case of histoplasmosis. Meningeal signs were common with cryptococcus (86%) but uncommon with either aspergillus or candida (less than 10%). Focal neurological signs, focal seizures, hemiplegia, and cranial nerve deficits occurred in 50% of the patients with aspergillus, 21% of those with cryptococcus, and 4% of those with candida. Pathological examination showed meningeal inflammation in the cases of cryptococcus. Angioinvasion occurred in all cases of aspergillus, 7% of the cases of candida, and none of the cryptococcal cases. Of the three most common fungal pathogens, stroke and stroke-like syndromes are most likely to occur with aspergillus, unlikely to occur with candida, and are unreported with cryptococcus.

Not all patients with invasive fungal infection will have CNS involvement. Schwesinger *et al.* (2005) reviewed 2027 autopsies at Greifswald University Institute of Pathology between 1994 and 2003. They found 137 cases of invasive candidiasis (6.7%) and 31 cases of invasive aspergillosis (1.5%). In only five cases of candidiasis and two cases of aspergillosis was there CNS involvement. Liu *et al.* (2003) examined 149 cases of nosocomial fungal infections over a 20-year period at Peking Union Medical College Hospital. The most common pathogens were *Candida albicans*, *Candida tropicalis*, *Candida parapsilosis*, *Cryptococcus neoformans*, and various aspergillus species. The most common risk factors for nosocomial infection included steroids, cytotoxic therapy, prolonged use of broad-spectrum antibiotics, immunosuppression, and intravenous lines. Baddley *et al.* (2002) reviewed their experience with 1620 transplant patients over a 3-year period including 230 hematopoietic stem cell transplants and 1390 organ transplants. Fungal brain abscesses were diagnosed in 17 patients (1.05%). None of the 17 cases presented as strokes although 35% had hemiplegia. Sixty-five percent of the infections were due to aspergillus species.

Coplin *et al.* (2001) identified 36 patients with stroke among 1245 bone marrow transplant cases over a 3-year period. Infarction or hemorrhage was caused by fungus in 30.6% of the bone marrow transplant patients with a stroke during that period. Nine of the 12 strokes from infection were caused by aspergillus, predominantly the angioinvasive form of infection. Mortality in the series of Coplin *et al.* (2001) was 89%. Stroke due to infection can complicate cancer. In an autopsy study of 3426 patients at the Memorial Sloan-Kettering Cancer Center, 500 patients were found to have sustained a stroke. In 33 cases, the stroke was attributed to a septic embolism. The most common pathogens were aspergillus and candida, with aspergillus more likely to present with focal signs and seizures and candida more likely to present with encephalopathy (Rogers, 2003).

Aspergillus

Among fungal pathogens, aspergillus is most likely to present as a stroke or stroke-like syndrome (Walshe *et al.*, 1985a). The most common pathogen is *Aspergillus fumigatus*, but infections may also occur with *A. flavus*, *A. niger*, *A. terreus*, and other species (Lass-Flörl *et al.*, 2005). Invasive fungal infection with aspergillus is a major problem in immunocompromised patients including those with malignancy and those undergoing organ transplantation. Aspergillus spores are ubiquitous. They are often found in hospital ventilation systems and throughout the community environment. The mode of infection is usually by inhalation with the upper respiratory tract the most common initial site of infection. Occasionally airborne spores may infect an open wound or surgical drain (Fungal Infections, 2004). Pulmonary infections with aspergillus may lead to hematogenous spread of the organism to the brain.

Kleinschmidt-DeMasters (2002) found invasive Aspergillus in 71 patients (1.8%) in 3897 autopsies over a 20-year period. There was CNS involvement in 42 of 71. Pathological changes ranged from subtle abscesses to massive areas of hemorrhagic infarction. Other pathological changes in other cases included cerebral hemorrhage, bland cerebral infarction, and purulent meningitis. Beal *et al.* (1982) reported 12 patients with CNS aspergillosis in immunosuppressed patients or patients on high dose corticosteroids. Pulmonary infiltrates were present in all patients. Sudden onset of neurological deficits that were stroke-like in onset occurred in nine patients. Pathologically there were multiple abscesses with prominent arterial invasion by the fungus. Boes *et al.* (1994) reported on 26 patients with autopsy-proven CNS aspergillosis. Most presented with fever and a stroke-like syndrome. Pathologically there were multiple areas of cerebral infarction with thrombosis due to Aspergillus invasion of arteries. Underlying illnesses included bone marrow transplant, liver transplant, AIDS, and other immune compromised conditions.

Uncommon Causes of Stroke, 2nd edition, ed. Louis R. Caplan. Published by Cambridge University Press. © Cambridge University Press 2008.

Aspergillus may produce intracerebral or subarachnoid hemorrhage. Hemorrhage may occur due to direct invasion of the artery by aspergillus or rupture of a mycotic aneurysm. Cleri *et al.* (2003) reported a fatal case of intracerebral hemorrhage in a patient with hemolytic anemia treated with corticosteroids complicated by pulmonary aspergillus and candida. Asari *et al.* (1988) reported an unusual case of death due to a mycotic aneurysm at the site of surgery for an anterior communicating artery aneurysm treated by clipping. Corvisier *et al.* (1987) reported a 54-year-old woman with Hodgkin's disease treated with cytotoxic drugs and steroids with invasion of the carotid artery by aspergillus leading to a fatal rupture of the right carotid artery. Takahashi *et al.* (1998) reported Aspergillus infection of the orbit and ethmoid sinus that extended posteriorly into the brain and involved the cavernous sinus and internal carotid artery. Pathological examination of the internal carotid artery showed chronic inflammatory cells and hyphae. *Aspergillus fumigatus* was cultured from the brain. Terminally there was rupture of the internal carotid artery with subarachnoid and intracerebral hemorrhage. Davutgolu *et al.* (2004) reported a 36-year-old man with aspergillus vegetations in the left ventricle. The patient died of a massive intracerebral hemorrhage due to a mycotic aneurysm. Embolic material from the heart likely lodged in the middle cerebral artery branches leading to mycotic aneurysm formation and fatal intracerebral hemorrhage. Endo *et al.* (2002) reported a 50-year-old woman who underwent successful surgery for an anterior communicating artery aneurysm. She sustained a second subarachnoid hemorrhage on the 26th postoperative day. The patient died on the 40th postoperative day with evidence of bilateral cerebellar hemisphere infarcts. Postmortem examination of the brain showed fusiform dilation of the basilar artery with Aspergillus invasion of the basilar artery and vertebral arteries. Microscopically there were branching hyphae of aspergillus with vascular wall necrosis. Thrombotic occlusion of the basilar artery was caused by aspergillus hyphae. Breadmore *et al.* (1994) reported a case of invasive aspergillus of the cavernous sinus with rupture of the internal carotid artery. Haran and Chandy (1993) reported 13 patients with intracranial Aspergillus in Vellore, India. One of the 13 patients presented with a stroke-like syndrome.

Aspergillus has been reported to produce a septic thrombosis of the cavernous sinuses (Ebright *et al.*, 2001). Matsumura *et al.* (1988) reported two cases of intracerebral hemorrhage due to cerebral Aspergillosis. Lau *et al.* (1991) reported a case of fatal subarachnoid hemorrhage due to mycotic aneurysm of the carotid artery due to Aspergillus. Ihara *et al.* (1990) reported a fatal subarachnoid hemorrhage from a mycotic aneurysm of the basilar artery. Murthy *et al.* (2000) reported on 21 patients with CNS involvement with Aspergillus. In 16, aspergillus spread to the brain from sinus infections. Skull-based syndromes were found in 16; 6 presented as a brain abscess and 2 had stroke-like onsets. Pagano *et al.* (1996) reported on 100 patients with leukemia and aspergillosis. Fourteen had CNS involvement. Autopsies showed invasive Aspergillus; clinical presentation was generally as a brain abscess with hemiparesis and seizures. The primary focus was generally in the lungs. Suzuki *et al.* (1995) reported a case of fatal subarachnoid hemorrhage due to a mycotic aneurysm of the middle cerebral artery. Piotrowski and Pilz (1994) reported aspergillus arteritis after aneurysm clipping that mimicked vasospasm.

Clues to the presence of CNS aspergillosis include the gradual extension of infarction during a few days and spread of involvement across arterial territories. The spinal fluid usually does not show a major pleocytosis because cerebral involvement is due to a necrotizing arteritis and not meningitis. Other fungi (except Mucor) and the tubercle bacillus are organisms that almost invariably cause meningitis.

Mucor

Mucorales are filamentous fungi that are ubiquitous. Like Aspergillus, Mucor species are angioinvasive and can cause stroke through hemorrhagic infarction, bland infarction, and vascular thrombosis (Fungal Infections, 2004). They are found in soil, manure, plants, and decaying materials. They are airborne pathogens that commonly infect immunocompromised patients through the lungs and nasal passages (Eucker *et al.*, 2001). Mucormycosis is the third leading invasive fungal infection after aspergillus and candida. Mortality with disseminated forms of the disease is in excess of 95% (Eucker *et al.*, 2001). Fungi of the order Mucorales include rhizopus, absidia, and rhizomucor. Less common pathogens include cunninghamella, mortierella, saksenaea, and apophysomyces (Eucker *et al.*, 2001). Prognosis in mucormycosis with cerebral involvement is almost uniformly poor with most series showing 100% fatality rates when the brain is involved.

Rangel-Guerra *et al.* (1996) reviewed their experience with 36 cases of mucormycosis over a 15-year period. Rhinocerebral mucormycosis was diagnosed in 22 patients. The underlying disorder was diabetes in 20 cases, renal failure in 1, and myelodysplastic syndrome in 1. Among the 22 patients with rhinocerebral mucormycosis, 4 presented with a cavernous sinus syndrome, 4 with an orbital apex syndrome, and 5 with thrombosis of the internal carotid artery (with hemiparesis). Hall and Nussbaum (1995) reviewed their experience with 11 cases of mucormycosis at the University of Minnesota over a 13-year period. In four cases the mucor spread to the brain hematogenously from a pulmonary focus, and in three a nasal infection spread to the brain. Risk factors in their patients included immunosuppression (7), leukemia (4), diabetes mellitus (3), organ transplant (1), and hematological disorders (2). All seven with brain involvement died. They reported no stroke-like symptoms in their series.

The most common presentation is so-called rhinocerebral mucormycosis in which the fungus enters the brain from the nasal passages through the sinuses and orbit into the brain. Rhino-orbital Mucormycosis has been reported to extend into the cavernous sinus and produce carotid artery thrombosis (Dooley *et al.*, 1992). De Medeiros *et al.* (2001) reported another case of mucormycosis with invasion of the cavernous sinus and thrombosis after bone marrow transplantation. Mucormycosis has been reported to produce a septic thrombosis of the cavernous sinuses (Ebright *et al.*, 2001).

Sundaram *et al.* (2005) reported experience with 56 patients with mucormycosis (zygomycosis) seen between 1971 and 2001. Forty-six patients had the rhinocerebral form with infection in the nasal sinuses leading to brain involvement. Twelve patients had isolated mucormycosis of the brain without evidence of nasal sinus involvement. Patients with the isolated form of mucormycosis had a variety of comorbidities including diabetes mellitus, renal transplantation, renal failure, and steroid use. Six of the patients presented with a stroke-like syndrome: two with meningitis, and four with a brain abscess. Pathologically, patients with a stroke-like syndrome had areas of hemorrhagic infarction with evidence of arteritis with branching aseptate hyphae invading the vessel wall. Gollard *et al.* (1994) reported a case of isolated cerebral mucormycosis without evidence of pulmonary or nasal involvement in a young intravenous drug abuser without HIV. MRI of the brain showed a mass in the left basal ganglia. Biopsy showed epithelioid granulomas and nonseptate hyphae typical of mucor. He recovered with intravenous amphotericin treatment.

Mucor may also enter the brain hematogenously after pulmonary infection. A few patients with cerebral mucormycosis have been reported without nasal or pulmonary infection after intravenous drug abuse. Verma *et al.* (2005) reported a case of primary cerebral mucormycosis without evidence of pulmonary or nasal infection and without a history of intravenous drug abuse. Autopsy showed infarction and hemorrhage in the brain with extensive vascular necrosis related to branching hyphae consistent with mucormycosis. Mathur *et al.* (1999) reported a single case of massive cerebral infarction in a patient with acute myelogenous leukemia that occurred on day 2 of induction chemotherapy. Mucormycosis was found in both the lung and the brain. The fungus presumably spread from the lung to the brain by a hematogenous route. The brain at autopsy showed a hemorrhagic infarction in the right frontal and temporal lobes with cerebral edema and uncal herniation and brainstem compression with Duret hemorrhages. Fungi consistent with mucormycosis were found in the brain infarct. No source of the infection was identified.

Kameh and Gonzalez (1997) report a fatal case of mucormycosis with fungal cerebritis due to Rhizopus species and multiple cerebral infarctions and cerebral edema. Zhang *et al.* (2002) reported a rare case of *Cunninghamella bertholletiae* infection in a renal transplant patient. *Cunninghamella bertholletiae* is a saprophytic soil fungus that rarely infects humans. It is of the class Zygomycetes and order Mucorales. The patient died with a lung abscess containing *C. bertholletiae*. Autopsy showed fungal endocarditis as well as diffuse hemorrhagic vasculitis affecting the brainstem, cerebrum, and cerebellum.

Candida

Candida is not an angioinvasive pathogen, and reports of stroke after candida infection are distinctly uncommon. In our autopsy series of 27 cases, there were no strokes and no stroke-like syndromes (Walshe *et al.*, 1985b). Candida generally produces oral thrush or Candida esophagitis. Enterocolitis with candida is less common. Candida frequently colonizes the gastrointestinal tract, especially in hospitalized patients receiving broad-spectrum antibiotics. Candida may also colonize the urinary tract of patients with indwelling Foley catheters and the female genital tract. Candida is the fifth most common organism isolated from blood

cultures (Girishkumar *et al.*, 1999). In immunocompromised patients, candida may spread hematogenously from the gastrointestinal tract; in immunocompetent patients, candida may reach the blood through indwelling venous catheters. Mucosal injury and surgical manipulation of the gastrointestinal tract may predispose to dissemination and fungemia (Fungal Infections, 2004). In 43 patients at Bronx-Lebanon Hospital with positive blood cultures for candida, Girishkumar *et al.* (1999) reported none with a stroke. CNS involvement with candidiasis was about 10% of cases and was more common when endocarditis was present. Disseminated candidiasis requires disruption of normal epithelial barrier in intestines, antibiotic use that permits colonization of gastrointestinal tract with yeast, and decreased host defenses that allow disseminated spread of the yeast. The yeast usually spreads hematogenously to the brain. Unlike aspergillus, candida is not angioinvasive. Stroke is uncommon even with CNS involvement. The usual manifestation in the CNS is meningitis, but rarely the candida may produce a cerebritis and stroke-like syndrome.

Cimbaluk *et al.* (2005) describe a 43-year-old immunosuppressed man with systemic lupus erythematosus and lupus nephritis who had an infiltrating candida enterocolitis. He developed leg weakness after hemicolectomy. Blood cultures were positive for *Candida albicans*. CT showed hemorrhagic infarction in the brain due to hematogenous spread of *C. albicans*. Cerebritis, cerebral infarction, and cerebral hemorrhage were confirmed at autopsy. Cimbaluk *et al.* (2005) describe a second patient with candida enterocolitis in an immunosuppressed 50-year-old woman with lymphocytic leukemia. After colectomy she developed a hemorrhagic stroke in the frontal and parietal regions bilaterally complicated by subarachnoid hemorrhage. Kieburtz *et al.* (1993) reported a single case of cerebral infarction in an HIV patient with an opportunistic infection with *C. albicans*. The infarction was attributed to vasculopathy due to Candida. Terol *et al.* (1994) reported 10 cases with sepsis due to *Candida tropicalis*. All were granulocytopenic, had intravenous catheters, had positive blood cultures for *C. tropicalis*, and were on broad-spectrum antibiotics. Two died from intracerebral hemorrhage.

A separate entity is chronic mucocutaneous candidiasis. This is an immunodeficiency disorder that has been poorly characterized and is associated with persistent or recurrent infections of the mucous membranes with *C. albicans*. Grouhi *et al.* (1998) reported two patients with chronic mucocutaneous candidiasis associated with cerebral vasculitis, multiple intracranial arterial occlusions, and cerebral hemorrhage.

Cryptococcus

Like candida species, cryptococcus is not angioinvasive. *Cryptococcus neoformans* is an encapsulated yeast. It is a ubiquitous fungus with a worldwide distribution (Vilchez *et al.*, 2002). None of the 14 cases in our autopsy series presented as a stroke (Walshe *et al.*, 1985). Infection is usually by inhalation in an immunocompromised host (HIV or transplant). Cryptococcus may spread from the lungs to the nervous system hematogenously. Twenty to sixty percent of cases of cryptococcosis in HIV-negative patients occur in transplant patients. Cryptococcosis of the nervous system usually presents as meningitis with headache, decreased alertness, and fever (de Pauw and Meunier, 1999; Walshe *et al.*, 1985). Nuchal rigidity, visual loss, and seizures are frequent (Vilchez *et al.*, 2002). Stroke has not been reported as a complication of cryptococcal infections (Doi *et al.*, 1998; Vilchez *et al.*, 2002).

As in tuberculous meningitis, the origins and first few millimeters of the penetrating arteries at the base of the brain may show thickening of the medial coats, usually referred to as Huebner's arteritis. Infarction may occur in the territories of those arteries that penetrate from the anterior and posterior perforated substance of the brain, regions that are bathed in fungal infected cerebrospinal fluid at the base of the brain.

Other fungi

Coccidioidomycosis is endemic in the San Joaquin Valley in the USA. The clinical findings are identical to cryptococcus infection. A variety of less common fungi that can rarely infect immuno-compromised patients include fusarium (a septate mold), Trichosporon (a pathogenic yeast), paecilomyces, pseudallescheria, Scopulariopsis, and the endemic fungi (coccidioides immitis, histoplasma capsulatum). Reports of CNS involvement or stroke-like syndromes are limited with these less common fungi (Fungal Infections, 2004). de Almeida *et al.* (2004) reviewed 24 patients with CNS involvement by the fungus Paracoccidioides brasiliensis endemic in subtropical areas of Central and South America. The most common presentation was as seizures or meningitis. Kleinschmidt-DeMasters (2002) reported single cases of cerebritis with fungi Pseudallescheria boydii and Scedosporium inflatum that resembled the pathological changes found with aspergillus.

REFERENCES

Asari, S., Nishimoto, A., and Murakami, M. 1988. A rare case of cerebral Aspergillus aneurysm at the site of the temporary clip application. *No Shinkie Geka*, **16**, 1079–82.

Baddley, J. W., Salzman, D., and Pappas, P. G. 2002. Fungal brain abscess in transplant recipients: epidemiologic, microbiologic, and clinical features. *Clin Transplant*, **16**, 419–24.

Beal, M. F., O'Carroll, C. P., Kleinman, G. M., and Grossman, R. I. 1982. Aspergillosis of the central nervous system. *Neurology*, **32**, 473–9.

Boes, B., Bashir, R., Boes, C., Hahn, F., McConnell, J. R., and McComb, R. 1994. Central nervous system aspergillosis: Analysis of 26 cases. *J Neuroimaging*, **4**, 123–9.

Breadmore, R., Desmond, P., and Opeskin, K. 1994. Intracranial aspergillosis producing cavernous sinus syndrome and rupture of internal carotid artery. *Australas Radiol*, **38**, 72–5.

Cimbaluk, D., Scudiere, J., Butsch, J., and Jakate, S. 2005. Invasive candidal enterocolitis followed shortly by fatal cerebral hemorrhage in immunocompromised patients. *J Clin Gastroenterol*, **39**, 795–7.

Cleri, D. J., Moser, R. L., Villota, F. J., *et al.* 2003. Pulmonary aspergillosis and central nervous system hemorrhage as complications of hemolytic anemia treated with corticosteroids. *South Med J*, **96**, 592–5.

Coplin, W. M., Cochran, M. S., Levine, S. R., and Crawford, S. W. 2001. Stroke after bone marrow transplantation: frequency, aetiology and outcome. *Brain*, **124**, 1043–51.

Corvisier, N., Gray, F., Cherardi, R., *et al.* 1987. Aspergillosis of ethmoid sinus and optic nerve, with arteritis and rupture of the internal carotid artery. *Surg Neurol*, **28**, 311–5.

Davutoglu, V., Soydine, S., Aydin, A., and Karakok, M. 2005. Rapidly advancing invasive endomyocardial aspergillosis. *J Am Soc Echocardiogr*, **18**, 185–7.

de Almeida, S. M., Querioz-Telles, F., Tieve, H. A., Ribeiro, C. E., and Wernek, L. C. 2004. Central nervous system paracoccidioidmycosis: clinical features and laboratorial findings. *J Infect*, **48**, 193–8.

de Medeiros, C. R., Bleggi-Torres, L. F., Faoro, L. N., *et al.* 2001. Cavernous sinus thrombosis caused by zygomycosis after unrelated bone marrow transplantation. *Transplant Infectious Diseases*, **3**, 231–4.

de Pauw, B. D. E., and Meunier, F. 1999. The challenge of invasive fungal infections. *Chemotherapy*, **45**(**suppl**), 1–14.

Doi, S. A., Tan, C. T., Liam, C. K., and Naganathan, K. 1998. Cryptococcosis at the University Hospital, Kuala Lampur. *Trop Doct*, **28**, 34–9.

Dooley, D. P., Hollsten, D. A., Grimes, S. R., and Moss, J. Jr. 1992. Indolent orbital apex syndrome caused by occult mucormycosis. *J Clin Neuroophthalmol*, **12**, 245–9.

Ebright, J. R., Pace, M. T., and Niazi, A. F. 2001. Septic thrombosis of the cavernous sinuses. *Arch Intern Med*, **161**, 2671–6.

Endo, T., Tominaga, T., Konno, H., and Yoshimoto, T. 2002. Fatal subarachnoid hemorrhage, brainstem and cerebellar infarction, caused by aspergillus infection after cerebral aneurysm surgery: case report. *Neurosurgery*, **50**, 1147–51.

Eucker, J., Sezer, O., Graf, B., and Possinger, K. 2001. Mucormycoses. *Mycoses*, **44**, 253–60.

Fungal infections. 2004. *Am J Transplant*, **4** (**supplement 10**), 110–34. doi:10.1111/j.1600–6135.2004.00735.xa

Girishkumar, H., Yousuf, A. M., Chivate, J., and Geisler, E. 1999. Experience with invasive candida infections. *Postgrad Med J*, **75**, 151–2.

Gollard, R., Rabb, C., Larsen, R., and Chandrasoma, P. 1994. Isolated cerebral Mucormycosis: case report and therapeutic considerations. *Neurosurgery*, **34**, 174–7.

Grouhi, M., Ilan, D., Misbet-Brown, E., and Roifman, C. M. 1998. Cerebral vasculitis associated with chronic mucocutaneous candidiasis. *J Pediatrics*, **133**, 571–4.

Hall, W. A., and Nussbaum, E. S. 1995. Isolated cerebral mucormycosis: case report and therapeutic considerations [correspondence]. *Neurosurgery*, **36**, 623.

Haran, R. P., Chandy, M. J. 1993. Intracranial aspergillus granuloma. *Br J Neurosurg*, **7**, 383–88.

Kameh, D. S., and Gonzalez, O. R. 1997. Fatal rhino-orbital-cerebral zygomycosis. *South Med J*, **90**, 1133–7.

Kieburtz, K. D., Eskin, T. A., Ketonen, T. A., and Tuite, M. J. 1993. Opportunistic cerebral vasculopathy and stroke in patients with acquired immunodeficiency syndrome. *Arch Neurol*, **50**, 430–2.

Kleinschmidt-DeMasters, B. K. 2002. Central nervous system aspergillosis: a 20-year retrospective series. *Hum Pathol*, **33**, 116–24.

Ihara, K., Makita, Y., Nabeshima, S., Tei, T., Keyaki, A., and Nioka, H. 1990. Aspergillosis of the central nervous system causing subarachnoid hemorrhage from mycotic aneurysm of the basilar artery: case report. *Neurol Med Chir*, **30**, 618–23.

Lass-Flörl, C. X., Griff, K., Mayr, A., *et al.* 2005. Epidemiology and outcome of infections due to aspergillus terries: 10-year single centre experience. *Br J Haematol*, **312**, 201–7.

Lau, A. H., Takeshita, M., and Ishii, N. 1991. Mycotic (aspergillus) arteritis resulting in fatal subarachnoid hemorrhage: a case report. *Angiology*, **42**, 251–5.

Liu, Z. Y., Sheng, R. Y., Li, X. L., Li, T. S., and Wang, A. X. 2003. Nocosomial fungal infections, analysis of 149 cases. *Zhonghua Yi Xue Za Zhi*, **83**, 399–403.

Mathur, S. C., Friedman, H. D., Kende, A. J., Davis, R. L., and Graziano, S. L. 1999. Cryptic mucor infection leading to massive cerebral infarction at initiation of antileukemic chemotherapy. *Ann Hematol*, **78**, 241–5.

Matsumura, S., Sato, S., Fujiwara, H., *et al.* 1988. Cerebral aspergillosis as a cerebral vascular accident. *Brain Nerve*, **40**, 225–32.

Murthy, J. M., Sundaram, C., Prasad, V. S., Purohit, A. K., Rammurti, S., and Laxmi, V. 2000. Aspergillosis of the central nervous system: a study of 21 patients seen in a university hospital in south India. *J Assoc Physicians India*, **48**, 677–81.

Pagano, L., Ricci, P., Montillo, M., *et al.* 1996. Localization of aspergillosis to the central nervous system among patients with acute leukemia: a report of 14 cases. Gruppo Italiano Malattie Ematologiche dell'Audulto Infection Program. *Clin Infect Dis*, **23**, 628–30.

Piotrowski, W. P., and Pilz, P. 1994. Postoperative fungal arteritis mimicking vasospasm: case report. *Neurol Medic Chir*, **34**, 315–8.

Rangel-Guerra, R., Martínez, H. R., Sáenz, C., Bosques-Padilla, F., and Estrada-Bellman, I. 1996. Rhinocerebral and system mucormycosis. Clinical experience with 36 cases. *J Neurol Sci*, **143**, 19–30.

Rogers, L. R. 2003. Cerebrovascular complications in cancer patients. *Neurol Clin*, **21**, 167–92.

Schwesinger, G., Junghans, D., Schröder, G., Bernhardt, H. and Knoke, M. 2005. Candidosis and aspergillosis as autopsy findings from 1994 to 2003. *Mycoses*, **48**, 176–80.

Sundaram, C., Mahadevan, A., Laxmi, V., *et al.* 2005. Cerebral zygomycosis. *Mycoses*, **48**, 396–407.

Suzuki, K., Iwabuchi, N., Kuramochi, S., *et al.* 1995. Aspergillus aneurysm of the middle cerebral artery causing a fatal subarachnoid hemorrhage. *Intern Med*, **34**, 550–3.

Takahashi, Y., Sugita, Y., Maruiwa, H., *et al.* 1998. Fatal hemorrhage from rupture of the intracranial internal carotid artery caused by Aspergillus arteritis. *Neurosurg Rev*, **21**, 198–201.

Terol, M. J., Tassies, D., Lopez-Guillermon, A., *et al.* 1994. Sepsis by Candida tropicalis in patients with granulocytopenia: a study of 10 cases. *Med Clin (Barc)*, **103**, 579–82.

Verma, A., Brozman, B., and Petito, C. K. 2005. Isolated cerebral mucormycosis: report of a case and review of the literature. *J Neurol Sci*, **240**, 65–9.

Vilchez, R. A., Fung, J., and Kusne, S. 2002. Cryptococcosis in organ transplant recipients: an overview. *Am J Transplant*, **2**, 576–80.

Walshe, T. J., Hier, D. B., and Caplan, L. R. 1985a. Aspergillosis of the central nervous system: clinicopathological analysis of 17 patients. *Ann Neurol*, **18**, 574–82.

Walshe, T. J., Hier, D. B., and Caplan, L. R. 1985b. Fungal infections of the central nervous system: comparative analysis of risk factors and clinical signs. *Neurology*, **35**, 1654–7.

Zhang, R., Zhang, J. W., and Szerlip, H. M. 2002. Endocarditis and hemorrhagic stroke caused by Cunninghamella bertholletiae infection after kidney transplantation. *Am J Kidney Dis*, **40**, 842–6.

9 STROKE AND VASCULITIS IN PATIENTS WITH CYSTICERCOSIS

Oscar H. Del Brutto

Cysticercosis is caused by infection with the larval stage of *Taenia solium*, the pork tapeworm. This cestode has a complex life cycle involving both pigs and humans. In the usual cycle of transmission, humans are definitive hosts and carry the adult parasite in the small intestine. Eggs detached from the distal end of *T. solium* are passed with feces to contaminate – in places where open-air defecation is common – soil and vegetation. Free-roaming pigs eat human feces and get infected with hundreds of eggs. After ingestion, eggs hatch into oncospheres in the intestine of pigs (the natural intermediate hosts). Then, oncospheres cross the intestinal wall, enter the bloodstream, and are carried into the tissues of the pig where larvae (cysticercus) develop. When humans ingest improperly cooked pork infected with cysticerci, larvae evaginate in the small intestine, get attached to the intestinal wall, and begin forming proglottides, thus completing the life cycle of *T. solium*. Humans also become intermediate hosts of this parasite by ingesting its eggs from the soil or from contaminated food handled by a taenia carrier, or directly by the fecal–oral route in individuals harboring the adult parasite. In these cases, human cysticercosis develops (García *et al.*, 2003).

Cysticerci usually invade the central nervous system (CNS) and its coverings, causing neurocysticercosis (NCC), a severe disease that constitutes a threat to millions of people living in developing countries in Latin America, Africa, and Asia. In these areas, NCC accounts for up to 10% of all admissions to neurological hospitals and is a leading cause of acquired epilepsy and other neurological conditions (Del Brutto *et al.*, 1998; Murrell, 2005). Increased traveling and migratory movements of people from endemic to nonendemic areas has produced a recent increase in the prevalence of NCC in North America and some European countries, where this condition was considered rare (Wallin and Kurtzke, 2004). More than 50 000 new deaths due to NCC occur every year, and many more patients survive but are left with irreversible brain damage. This makes NCC an important public health problem because most affected people are at productive ages.

Cerebrovascular disease is one of the most feared complications of NCC and represents an important cause of death and disability in these patients. Cysticercotic angiitis was probably first recognized in the nineteenth century by the German pathologist Askanazy, who described inflammatory changes in the arteries at the base of the brain in a patient with meningeal NCC (Henneberg, 1912). Thereafter, Moniz *et al.* (1932) suggested that angiographic changes in NCC may resemble those seen in tuberculosis, syphilis, or other infections that cause angiitis of intracranial

vessels. During the first half of the twentieth century, many neuropathologists described in detail the changes that may occur in the intracranial arteries in association with cysticerci infection of basal leptomeninges (Asenjo, 1950; Dolpogol and Neustaedter, 1935; Trelles and Ravens, 1953). Despite this, angiitis remained an under-recognized complication of NCC for many years, until the introduction of modern neuroimaging techniques that allowed a better recognition of cysticercosis angiitis and NCC-related stroke (Del Brutto, 1992).

Neuropathology

A brief description of the many changes that cysticerci induce in the CNS is necessary to understand the pathogenesis of NCC-related stroke. Cysticerci are vesicles consisting of two main parts, the vesicular wall and the invaginated scolex. Their appearance varies according to their location within the CNS. Parenchymal brain cysticerci measure less than 10 mm and tend to lodge in the cerebral cortex or the basal ganglia due to the high vascular supply of these areas. Subarachnoid cysticerci may be located within cortical sulci or in the cisterns at the base of the brain. The latter may attain a size of 50 mm or more as their growth is not limited by the pressure effects from the brain parenchyma. In some of these parasites, the scolex can not be identified as they are composed of only several membranes attached to each other (racemose form of cysticerci). Ventricular cysticerci have a variable size and may or may not have a scolex; these cysts may be attached to the choroid plexus or may be freely floating within the ventricular cavities. Other locations of cysticerci within the CNS include the subdural space, the sellar region, and the spinal cord (Pittella, 1997).

After entering the CNS, cysticerci elicit little inflammatory changes in the surrounding tissues. In this stage, called the vesicular stage, viable parasites have a thin membrane, a clear vesicular fluid, and a normal scolex. Cysticerci may remain for decades in this stage or, as the result of a complex immunological attack from the host, enter in a process of degeneration. The first stage of involution of cysticerci is the colloidal stage, in which the transparent vesicular fluid is replaced by a viscous and turbid fluid, and the scolex shows signs of hyaline degeneration. Colloidal cysticerci are surrounded by a thick collagen capsule, and the surrounding brain parenchyma shows astrocytic gliosis associated with microglial proliferation, diffuse edema, neuronal degenerative changes, and perivascular cuffing of lymphocytes. Thereafter, the wall of the cyst thickens, and the scolex is transformed into

Uncommon Causes of Stroke, 2nd edition, ed. Louis R. Caplan. Published by Cambridge University Press. © Cambridge University Press 2008.

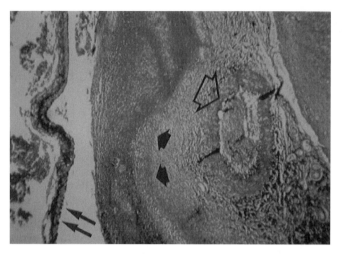

Figure 9.1 Section of occluded small leptomeningeal vessel (*open arrow*) affected by endarteritis. Collagen capsule surrounds the vessel (*arrowheads*) and parasite membranes (*solid arrows*). (Reproduced from: Rodriguez-Carbajal *et al.*, 1989, with permission.)

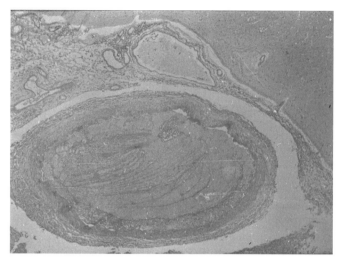

Figure 9.2 Atheroma-like deposit occluding major branch of middle cerebral artery in patient with cysticercotic angiitis. (Reproduced from: Rodriguez-Carbajal *et al.*, 1989, with permission.)

mineralized granules; this stage, in which the cysticercus is no longer viable, is called the granular nodular stage. Finally, in the calcified stage parasite remnants appear as mineralized (calcified) nodules (Escobar and Weidenheim, 2002). When parasites enter into the granular and calcified stages, the edema subsides, but astrocytic changes in the vicinity of the lesions become more intense than in the preceding stages. The duration of each of these stages varies considerably among individuals.

Meningeal cysticerci elicit a severe inflammatory reaction in the subarachnoid space with formation of an exudate composed of collagen fibers, lymphocytes, multinucleated giant cells, eosinophils, and hyalinized parasitic membranes leading to abnormal thickening of the leptomeninges (Pittella, 1997). Cranial nerves located at the base of the brain are often encased in this leptomeningeal thickening. The foramina of Luschka and Magendie may be occluded, with the subsequent development of obstructive hydrocephalus. Small and medium-sized arteries arising from the circle of Willis are frequently affected by this inflammatory reaction, providing a substrate for the occurrence of NCC-related stroke. The walls of penetrating arteries are invaded by inflammatory cells, leading to endarteritis with thickening of the adventitia, fibrosis of the media, and endothelial hyperplasia (Figure 9.1). This hyperplasia reduces or occludes the lumen of the vessel. Besides endarteritis, the lumen of major intracranial arteries may be occluded by atheroma-like deposits resulting from disruption of the endothelium (Figure 9.2). Finally, adherence of cysticerci to subarachnoid blood vessels may weaken the vessel wall with the subsequent development of a mycotic aneurysm.

Stroke syndromes

NCC may cause ischemic or hemorrhagic strokes. As expected, different stroke subtypes are related to different pathogenetic mechanisms and produce varied clinical manifestations (Table 9.1). Transient ischemic attacks have been described in some patients with NCC, and are most often caused by intermittent stenoses of major intracranial arteries secondary to meningeal cysticerci engulfing such vessels. Many of the patients eventually develop a cerebral infarction when the inflammatory process occludes the affected artery (Aditya *et al.*, 2004; Lee and Chang, 1998; McCormick *et al.*, 1983).

Lacunar infarctions occur as the result of inflammatory occlusion of small penetrating branches of the middle cerebral artery (MCA). These infarctions are usually located in the posterior limb of the internal capsule or the subcortical white matter, and produce lacunar syndromes (ataxic hemiparesis, pure motor hemiparesis, sensorimotor stroke) indistinguishable from those caused by atherosclerosis (Barinagarrementeria and Del Brutto, 1988a, 1989; Barinagarrementeria *et al.*, 1988; Gauthier *et al.*, 1995). Large cerebral infarctions, related to the occlusion of the internal carotid artery, or the anterior or MCA, also occur in patients with NCC. Such infarctions cause profound neurological deficits, signs of cortical dysfunction, or cognitive decline when both anterior cerebral arteries are affected (Arteaga-Rodriguz *et al.*, 2004; Jha and Kumar, 2000; Kohli *et al.*, 1997; Monteiro *et al.*, 1994; Rocha *et al.*, 2001; Rodriguez-Carbajal *et al.*, 1989; terPenning *et al.*, 1992). Subarachnoid cysticerci located at the base of the brain may cause inflammatory occlusion of small branches of the basilar artery with the subsequent development of brainstem infarctions. In these cases, clinical manifestations include somnolence, pupillary abnormalities, impaired vertical gaze, paraparesis, and urinary incontinence (Del Brutto, 1992).

Another cerebrovascular complication of NCC is hemorrhagic stroke. Most of these cases have been related to the formation and subsequent rupture of a mycotic aneurysm located in the vicinity of subarachnoid cysticerci engulfing an intracranial artery (Guevara-Dondé *et al.*, 1987; Huang *et al.*, 2000; Kim *et al.*, 2005; Soto-Hernández *et al.*, 1996). Parenchymal brain hemorrhages have occasionally been reported as secondary to the damage of a small artery in the vicinity of a parenchymal brain cyst (Alarcón *et al.*, 1992; Tellez-Zenteno *et al.*, 2003).

Table 9.1 Stroke syndromes due to NCC.

Clinical manifestations	Stroke subtype	Pathogenetic mechanism
Transient ischemic attacks	– – –	Narrowing of the intracranial internal carotid or basilar artery
Lacunar syndromes: ataxic hemiparesis, pure motor hemiparesis	Lacunar infarct in the internal capsule or the corona radiata	Inflammatory occlusion of small penetrating branches arising from the circle of Willis
Sensorimotor deficit, aphasia, signs of cortical dysfunction, coma	Large cerebral infarction involving the entire territory of the anterior or middle cerebral artery	Occlusion of major cerebral arteries due to atheroma-like deposits
Cognitive decline	Infarction in both frontal lobes	Occlusion of both anterior cerebral arteries
Top of the basilar syndrome, Parinaud's syndrome	Infarction involving the brainstem and thalamus	Inflammatory occlusion of penetrating branches of the basilar artery
Headache, vomiting, neck stiffness, coma	Subarachnoid hemorrhage	Rupture of a mycotic aneurysm
Headache, vomiting, focal neurological deficits	Parenchymal brain hemorrhage	Rupture of a small artery in the vicinity of a parenchymal brain cyst

Relationship between NCC and stroke

Stroke is common among patients with subarachnoid NCC, but it is seldom observed in other forms of the disease. Some patients with parenchymal NCC present with acute stroke-like episodes that are not related to a cerebral infarction or a hemorrhage, but to a strategically located cyst (Barinagarrementeria and Del Brutto, 1988b; Catapano and Marx, 1986; Wraige et al., 2003). The actual prevalence of stroke among patients with NCC, as well as the impact of NCC as a cause of stroke in endemic areas, has been a subject of debate (Alarcón et al., 1992; Barinagarrementeria and Cantú, 1992). In a preliminary series of 403 patients with ischemic stroke from Mexico, NCC accounted for 2.5% of cases, and was the second most prevalent cause of nonatherosclerotic cerebral infarction (Barinagarrementeria, 1989).

Two recent studies have improved our knowledge of the relationship between NCC and stroke (Barinagarrementeria and Cantú, 1998; Cantú and Barinagarrementeria, 1996). One of them evaluated 65 patients with NCC-related stroke who were classified in two groups according to whether NCC was focal or diffuse, and settled the wide clinical and neuroimaging spectrum of this association (Cantú and Barinagarrementeria, 1996). Thirty-five of these patients had focal cysticercotic lesions in the subarachnoid space, and 30 patients had diffuse arachnoiditis. Among the 35 patients with focal cysticercosis, only 13 had small-vessel disease and the remaining 22 had evidence of large-vessel disease. In contrast, most patients with diffuse arachnoiditis had evidence of both small- and large-vessel involvement. Clinical manifestations also differed among the two groups. Whereas a stroke syndrome was the most common form of presentation of patients with focal disease, intracranial hypertension and subacute meningitis were the most common manifestations of patients with diffuse arachnoiditis.

A second study settled the prevalence of angiitis in patients with subarachnoid cysticercosis (Barinagarrementeria and Cantú, 1998). The authors found that 15 of 28 patients (53%) with subarachnoid cysticercosis had angiographic evidence of angiitis. Of the 15 patients with angiitis, 8 had a cerebral infarction, 3 had transient ischemic attacks, and 1 had an intracranial hemorrhage. In contrast, only 1 of the 13 patients without angiographic evidence of angiitis had a cerebral infarction. The middle and posterior cerebral arteries were the most frequently affected vessels. In most cases, only one or two vessels were affected. Results from this study confirmed that angiitis is most often a focal process associated with the presence of a parasite in the vicinity of a blood vessel.

Diagnosis

In endemic areas, a patient may have NCC and a stroke from unrelated reasons. Therefore, the cause-and-effect relationship between NCC and stroke must be supported by CT or MRI evidence of meningeal cysts or arachnoiditis adjacent to the infarction, or by cerebrospinal fluid (CSF) findings suggesting arachnoiditis (Del Brutto, 1992). In a preliminary report, five of seven patients with a lacunar syndrome related to cysticercotic angiitis had a suprasellar cysticercus located near the origin of penetrating branches of the MCA (Barinagarrementeria and Del Brutto, 1989). This finding has been confirmed in a number of case reports in which neuroimaging studies have shown, besides the infarction, subarachnoid cysticerci located in the vicinity of affected vessels (Aditya et al., 2004; Jha and Kumar, 2000; Monteiro et al., 1994; Rocha et al., 2001; Rodriguez-Carbajal et al., 1989; terPenning et al., 1992).

Diagnosis of NCC-related stroke is possible in most cases after proper interpretation of data provided by neuroimaging studies

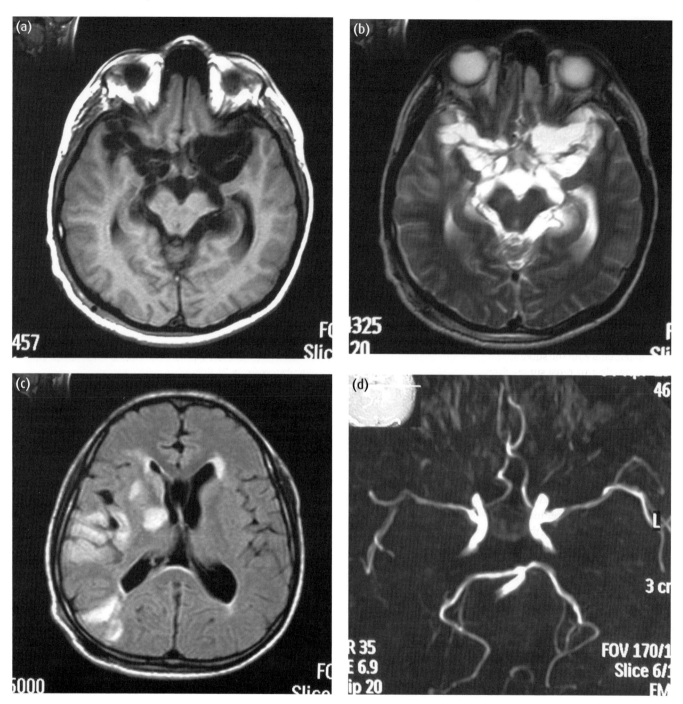

Figure 9.3 Cerebral infarction in patient with cysticercotic angiitis. T1- (**a**) and T2-weighted (**b**) MRI show huge subarachnoid racemose cysts in sylvian fissures engulfing both MCAs, fluid-attenuated inversion recovery (FLAIR) sequences (**c**) shows fresh infarction in entire territory of right MCA, and MRA (**d**) shows stenosis of major branches arising from circle of Willis. (Courtesy of Dr. Julio Lama, Guayaquil, Ecuador.)

and results of immunologic tests (García *et al.*, 2005). CT and MRI show the infarction as well as the characteristic findings of subarachnoid NCC, including abnormal enhancement of leptomeninges, hydrocephalus, and cystic lesions located at the sylvian fissure or basal cisterns (Figure 9.3). Angiography or magnetic resonance angiography (MRA) may show segmental narrowing or occlusion of intracranial arteries (Monteiro *et al.*, 1994;

Rodriguez-Carbajal *et al.*, 1989; terPenning *et al.*, 1992). CSF analysis shows lymphocytic pleocytosis and increased protein contents. Immune diagnostic tests are a valuable complement to neuroimaging, but they should never be used alone to exclude or confirm the diagnosis (Del Brutto, 2005).

A recent study evaluated the role of transcranial Doppler in the diagnosis and follow-up of patients with cysticercotic angiitis

(Cantú *et al.*, 1998). The authors studied nine patients with cysticercosis-related stroke, and found a good correlation between arterial lesions seen with both angiography and transcranial Doppler. Abnormalities in transcranial Doppler were evidenced by a high systolic blood-flow velocity in patients with angiographic evidence of arterial narrowing and by absence of blood-flow velocity in patients with arterial occlusion. Transcranial Doppler also allowed a noninvasive follow-up of stenotic lesions. Therefore, transcranial Doppler appears as a bedside, noninvasive test that allows the detection of arterial lesions in patients with subarachnoid cysticercosis, and may be useful for the follow-up of patients with cysticercotic angiitis.

Treatment

In general terms, therapy of NCC depends on the location of parasites and the degree of disease activity (García and Del Brutto, 2005). Introduction of cysticidal drugs (albendazole and praziquantel) have greatly improved the prognosis of NCC by destroying intracranial cysts and improving the neurological manifestations in most patients with parenchymal NCC. The scenario is totally different in patients with the subarachnoid form of the disease. Cysticidal drugs destroy most subarachnoid cysts (Del Brutto, 1997). However, owing to the proximity of these cysts to intracranial blood vessels, the inflammatory reaction that occurs during cyst destruction may enhance the process of endarteritis and may precipitate the occurrence of a cerebral infarction (Bang *et al.*, 1997; Levy *et al.*, 1995; Woo *et al.*, 1988). Dexamethasone must be given simultaneously to reduce the risk of this complication (Del Brutto *et al.*, 1992). For patients with associated hydrocephalus, shunt placement must be contemplated before medical therapy. Actually, little is known about the proper management of cerebrovascular complications of NCC because there are no published trials on this subject. Current practice is to give corticosteroids to reduce the inflammatory reaction in the subarachnoid space (García *et al.*, 2002). Long-term follow-up with repeated CSF examinations and transcranial Doppler may be of value to determine the length of corticosteroid therapy. The role of neuroprotective drugs is still unknown (Del Brutto, 1997).

REFERENCES

Aditya, G. S., Mahadevan, A., Santosh, V., *et al.* 2004. Cysticercal chronic basal arachnoiditis with infarcts, mimicking tuberculous pathology in endemic areas. *Neuropathology*, **24**, 320–5.

Alarcón, F., Hidalgo, F., Moncayo, J., Viñán, I., and Dueñas, G. 1992. Cerebral cysticercosis and stroke. *Stroke*, **23**, 224–8.

Alarcón, F., Vanormelingen, K., Moncayo, J., and Viñán, I. 1992. Cerebral cysticercosis as a risk factor for stroke in young and middle-aged people. *Stroke*, **23**, 1563–5.

Arteaga-Rodríguez, C., Naréssi-Munhoz, A. H., and Hernández-Fustes, O. J. 2004. Infarto cerebral extenso y neurocisticercosis. *Rev Neurol*, **39**, 583.

Asenjo, A. 1950. Setenta y dos casos de cisticercosis en el instituto de neurocirugía. *Revista de Neuro-Psiquiatría*, **13**, 337–53.

Bang, O. Y., Heo, J. H., Choi, S. A., and Kim, D. I. 1997. Large cerebral infarction during praziquantel therapy in neurocysticercosis. *Stroke*, **28**, 211–3.

Barinagarrementería, F. 1989. Causas no aterosclerosas de isquemia cerebral. *Archivos del Instituto Nacional de Neurología y Neurocirugía de México*, **4(suppl)**, 33.

Barinagarrementería, F., and Cantú, C. 1992. Neurocysticercosis as a cause of stroke. *Stroke*, **23**, 1180–1.

Barinagarrementería, F., and Cantú, C. 1998. Frequency of cerebral arteritis in subarachnoid cysticercosis. An angiographic study. *Stroke*, **29**, 123–5.

Barinagarrementería, F., and Del Brutto, O. H. 1988a. Neurocysticercosis and pure motor hemiparesis. *Stroke*, **19**, 1156–8.

Barinagarrementería, F., and Del Brutto, O. H. 1988b. Ataxic hemiparesis from parenchymal brain cysticercosis. *J Neurol*, **235**, 325.

Barinagarrementería, F., and Del Brutto, O. H. 1989. Lacunar syndrome due to neurocysticercosis. *Arch Neurol*, **46**, 415–7.

Barinagarrementería, F., Del Brutto, O. H., and Otero, E. 1988. Ataxic hemiparesis from cysticercosis. *Arch Neurol*, **45**, 246.

Cantú, C., and Barinagarrementería, F. 1996. Cerebrovascular complications of neurocysticercosis. Clinical and neuroimaging spectrum. *Arch Neurol*, **53**, 233–9.

Cantú, C., Villarreal, J., and J. L., and Barinagarrementeria, F. 1998. Cerebral cysticercotic arteritis: detection and follow-up by transcranial doppler. *Cerebrovasc Dis*, **8**, 2–7.

Catapano, M. S., and Marx, J. A. 1986. Central nervous system cysticercosis simulating an acute cerebellar hemorrhage. *Ann Emerg Med*, **15**, 847–9.

Del Brutto, O. H. 1992. Cysticercosis and cerebrovascular disease: a review. *J Neurol Neurosurg Psychiatry*, **55**, 252–4.

Del Brutto, O. H. 1997a. Albendazole therapy for subarachnoid cysticerci: clinical and neuroimaging analysis of 17 patients. *J Neurol Neurosurg Psychiatry*, **62**, 659–61.

Del Brutto, O. H. 1997b. Clues to prevent cerebrovascular hazards of cysticidal drug therapy. *Stroke*, **28**, 1088.

Del Brutto, O. H. 2005. Neurocysticercosis. *Semin Neurol*, **25**, 243–51.

Del Brutto, O. H., Sotelo, J., Aguirre, R., Diaz-Calderon, E., and Alarcón, T. A. 1992. Albendazole therapy for giant subarachnoid cysticerci. *Arch Neurol*, **49**, 535–8.

Del Brutto, O. H, Sotelo, J., and Román, G. C. 1998. *Neurocysticercosis: A Clinical Handbook*. Lisse, The Netherlands: Swets & Zeitlinger.

Dolpogol, V. B., and Neustaedter, M. 1935. Meningo-encephalitis caused by *Cysticercus cellulosae*. *Arch Neurol Psychiatry*, **33**, 132–47.

Escobar, A., and Weidenheim, K. M. 2002. The pathology of neurocysticercosis. In *Taenia solium cysticercosis. From basic to clinical science.* eds. G. Singh, and S. Prabhakar. Oxon, UK: CAB International, pp. 289–305.

García, H. H., and Del Brutto, O. H. 2005. Neurocysticercosis: updated concepts about an old disease. *Lancet Neurol*, **4**, 653–61.

García, H. H., Del Brutto, O. H., Nash, T. E., White, C. A. Jr., Tsang, V. C. W., and Gilman, R. H. 2005. New concepts in the diagnosis and management of neurocysticercosis (Taenia solium). *Am J Trop Med Hyg*, **72**, 3–9.

García, H. H., Evans, C. A. W., Nash, T. E., *et al.* 2002. Current consensus guidelines for treatment of neurocysticercosis. *Clin Microbiol Rev*, **15**, 747–56.

García, H. H., Gonzalez, A. E., Evans, C. A. W., and Gilman, R. H. 2003. *Taenia solium* cysticercosis. *Lancet*, **361**, 547–56.

Gauthier, N., Sangla, S., Stroh-Marcy, A., and Payen, L. 1995. Neurocysticercose révélée par un accident vasculaire cérébral. *J Radiol*, **76**, 119–23.

Guevara-Dondé, J. E., Gadea-Nieto, M. S., and Gómez-Llata, A. S. 1987. Cisticerco recubriendo un aneurisma de la arteria basilar. *Archivos del Instituto Nacional de Neurología y Neurocirugía de México*, **2**, 41–2.

Henneberg, R. 1912. Die tierischen parasiten des zentralnervensystems. I. Des Cysticercus cellulosae. In *Handbuch der Neurologie, Vol III*, Spezielle Neurologie II, ed. M. Lewandowsky. Berlin: Verlag von Julius Springer, 642–83.

Huang, P. P., Choudhri, H. F., Jallo, G., and Miller, D. C. 2000. Inflammatory aneurysm and neurocysticercosis: further evidence for a causal relationship? Case report. *Neurosurgery*, **47**, 466–7.

Jha, S., and Kumar, V. 2000. Neurocysticercosis presenting as stroke. *Neurol India*, **48**, 391–4.

Kim, I. Y., Kim, T. S., Lee, J. H., *et al.* 2005. Inflammatory aneurysm due to neurocysticercosis. *J Clin Neurosci*, **12**, 585–8.

Kohli, A., Gupta, R., and Kishore, J. 1997. Anterior cerebral artery infarction in neurocysticercosis: evaluation by MR angiography and in vivo proton MR spectroscopy. *Pediatr Neurosurg*, **26**, 93–6.

Lee, S. I., and Chang, G. Y. 1998. Recurrent brainstem transient ischemic attacks due to neurocysticercosis: a treatable cause. *Eur Neurol*, **40**, 174–5.

Levy, A. S., Lillehei, K. O., Rubinstein, D., and Stears, J. C. 1995. Subarachnoid neurocysticercosis with occlusion of the major intracranial arteries: case report. *Neurosurgery*, **36**, 183–8.

McCormick, G. F., Giannotta, S., Zee, C. S., and Fisher, M. 1983. Carotid occlusion in cysticercosis. *Neurology*, **33**, 1078–80.

Moniz, E., Loff, R., and Pacheco, L. 1932. Sur le diagnostic de la cysticercose cérébrale. *L'Encephale*, **27**, 42–53.

Monteiro, L., Almeida-Pinto, J., Leite, I., Xavier, J., and Correia, M. 1994. Cerebral cysticercus arteritis: five angiographic cases. *Cerebrovasc Dis*, **4**, 125–33.

Murrell, K. D. 2005. WHO/FAO/OIE guidelines for the surveillance, prevention and control of taeniosis/cysticercosis. Paris, France: Office International des Epizooties.

Pittella, J. E. H. 1997. Neurocysticercosis. *Brain Pathol*, **7**, 681–93.

Rocha, M. S. G., Brucki, S. M. D., Ferraz, A. C., and Piccolo, A. C. 2001. Doença cerebrovascular e neurocisticercose. *Arq Neuropsiquiatr*, **59**, 778–83.

Rodriguez-Carbajal, J., Del Brutto, O. H., Penagos, P., Huebe, J., and Escobar, A. 1989. Occlusion of the middle cerebral artery due to cysticercotic angiitis. *Stroke*, **20**, 1095–9.

Soto-Hernández, J. L., Gomez-Llata, S. A., Rojas-Echeverri, L. A., *et al.* 1996. Subarachnoid hemorrhage secondary to a ruptured inflammatory aneurysm: a possible complication of neurocysticercosis: case report. *Neurosurgery*, **38**, 197–9.

Tellez-Zenteno, J. F., Negrete-Pulido, O. R., Cantú, C., *et al.* 2003. Hemorrhagic stroke associated to neurocysticercosis. *Neurología*, **18**, 272–5.

terPenning, B., Litchman, C. D., and Heier, L. 1992. Bilateral middle cerebral artery occlusions in neurocysticercosis. *Stroke*, **23**, 280–3.

Trelles, J. O., and Ravens, R. 1953. Estudios sobre neurocisticercosis. II. Lesiones vasculares, meníngeas, ependimarias y neuróglicas. *Revista de Neuro-Psiquiatría*, **16**, 241–70.

Wallin, M. T., and Kurtzke, J. F. 2004. Neurocysticercosis in the United States. Review of an important emerging infection. *Neurology*, **63**, 1559–64.

Woo, E., Yu, Y. L., and Huang, C. Y. 1988. Cerebral infarct precipitated by praziquantel in neurocysticercosis – a cautionary note. *Trop Geogr Neurol*, **40**, 143–6.

Wraige, E., Graham, J., Robb, S. A., and Jan, W. 2003. Neurocysticercosis masquerading as a cerebral infarct. *J Child Neurol*, **18**, 298–300.

STROKE IN PATIENTS WITH LYME DISEASE

John J. Halperin

Introduction

Lyme disease, the multisystem infectious disease caused by the tick-borne spirochete *Borrelia burgdorferi*, readily invades the central nervous system (CNS) and, in up to 15% of patients, causes symptomatic meningitis or involvement of the cranial or spinal nerves. Parenchymal CNS disease is far less common; its pathophysiologic basis remains poorly understood. Proposed mechanisms range from direct infection, to vasculitis, to demyelination. Because it has not yet been reported in animal models, and because clinical data are extremely limited, it is necessary to try to deduce mechanisms by analogy to involvement in the peripheral nervous system and elsewhere, and to other related diseases. In particular, many have compared nervous system Lyme disease (neuroborreliosis) to neurosyphilis – a comparison that immediately raises the specter of meningovascular involvement. Several dozen case reports describing *B. burgdorferi* infection–associated strokes have been published; whether a specific causal relationship exists is unclear.

To understand the complexities of proving this association, it is important to appreciate some of the difficulties inherent in proving the diagnosis of Lyme disease in general, and nervous system infection in particular.

Diagnosis of Lyme disease

The biology of pathogenic spirochetes imposes several inherent limitations on diagnostic strategies. Unlike most bacterial infections, culturing these organisms is challenging – to this day the only (marginally) practical way to culture *Treponema pallidum* remains a cumbersome animal inoculation technique. Although it is possible to grow *B. burgdorferi* in vitro, this requires specialized medium (BSK II) not normally available in commercial diagnostic laboratories, incubation at 33°C, then maintaining the culture for weeks. Moreover, much like in syphilis, although the primary cutaneous lesion (the chancre in syphilis, erythema migrans in Lyme disease) contains huge numbers of readily demonstrable spirochetes, once the organism has disseminated, the bacterial load in obtainable specimens (such as cerebrospinal fluid [CSF]) is so low that even polymerase chain reaction (PCR)-based strategies for organism detection are of very low sensitivity. In Lyme meningitis, which clearly is caused by CNS invasion by spirochetes, sensitivity of culture is about 10%, and is improved minimally with PCR.

Because of this, diagnosis in both diseases rests heavily on demonstration of the host's immune response to the organism. All serodiagnostic approaches share several inherent limitations. Because it takes time for the immune system to produce detectable levels of antibody after exposure to new antigens, serologic tests are often negative very early in infection. In most diseases, this is addressed by obtaining acute and convalescent sera – a practice that, for unclear reasons, has not been adopted in Lyme disease. (This may relate to overanalogizing to syphilis, in which one-time detection of nonspecific reaginic antibodies – the fairly high titer anti-cardiolipin antibodies that are detected by all screening blood tests for syphilis – is considered diagnostic.)

However, fully adopting a syphilis analogy would have led logically to an immediate appreciation of the importance of addressing other disorders that cause false positives in the screening test – something done routinely with positive syphilis screening tests, but inconsistently in Lyme disease. This raises the second limitation of Lyme serodiagnosis shared with other serologies – because many epitopes are not unique to specific organisms, there can be important cross-reactivities among assays. The most commonly used serodiagnostic tool for screening for Lyme disease is an enzyme-linked immunosorbent assay (ELISA) – a technique that measures immunoreactivity to a combination of *B. burgdorferi*'s antigens. Many of these antigens are shared by other borrelia – such as those that cause relapsing fever, as well as the treponemata responsible for syphilis (*T. pallidum*) and even periodontal disease (*T. denticola*). Differentiating between Lyme and relapsing fever is usually straightforward based on symptoms and epidemiology – there is little geographic overlap between the two disorders. Differentiating from syphilis, particularly in a suspected meningovascular case, is best done by checking a reaginic test such as the Venereal Disease Research Laboratory (VDRL) or Rapid plasma reagin (RPR), because these are rarely if ever positive in Lyme disease.

A related challenge in serodiagnosis is that many inflammatory disorders can induce a broad range of nonspecific seropositivity. Patients with vasculitis, endocarditis, or other hyperimmune states can overproduce all immunoglobulins, giving rise to nonspecific false positives – a particularly important issue in many of the reported patients with stroke. This is addressed technically by doing Western blots on samples that are positive or borderline in the ELISA (but *not* in negative ELISAs, as Western blot criteria are not defined in this population). Western blots identify the specific bacterial antigens to which patients have developed an

Uncommon Causes of Stroke, 2nd edition, ed. Louis R. Caplan. Published by Cambridge University Press. © Cambridge University Press 2008.

Table 10.1 Western blot criteria

	IgM (2/3 Required)	IgG (5/10 Required)
	(acute disease)	(established disease)
Bands	23, 39, 41	18, 23, 28, 30, 39, 41, 45, 58, 66, 93
Sensitivity	32%	83%

antibody response. Criteria for positive blots do not rely on identification of responses to unique antigens present only in patients with Lyme disease, but rather on identification of combinations of immunoreactivities that are statistically known to indicate a very high probability of exposure to this organism. The Western blot criteria were developed for very high specificity; as in any such approach, there is a concomitant loss of sensitivity (Table 10.1). However this approach is very useful in identifying false positives due to nonspecific B-cell proliferation, seen in many inflammatory states. Notably, Western blot criteria developed to improve specificity in North American patients are not helpful in Europe, where greater strain variability makes it more difficult to identify specific bands that differentiate between true infection and cross-reactive immunoreactivity.

The third problem inherent in all serologic techniques relates to the inherent memory function of the immune system – when exposed to an organism, the immune response tends to persist, to provide future immunity. Even though this response does not provide effective immunity in syphilis or Lyme disease, in both, the specific antibody response typically remains detectable for many years. Consequently, identifying a patient as having a positive Lyme ELISA and Western blot merely proves exposure – without establishing that current signs and symptoms are caused by this infection.

Because of these issues, the concepts of positive and negative predictive value become particularly important when attempting serodiagnosis in Lyme disease. Lyme occurs in very specific geographically defined endemic areas – in suburban and rural regions of the Northeast, the upper Midwest, and northern California. In patients who have never left urban centers, or who spend all their time in places where Lyme is not endemic, obtaining a serology is counterproductive. Because, as in many such tests, positive cutoffs are statistically defined, and are calculated based on the mean plus 3 standard deviations in an uninfected population, about 1 sample per 1000 will be a false positive. Because nationwide in the United States the incidence is about 1/10 000, in a population not at risk, false positives will outnumber true positives by at least 10 to 1.

Identifying neurologic disorders as causally related to this infection poses additional challenges. However, several basic principles, analogous to lessons learned from neurosyphilis, can be helpful. First, because this constitutes a chronic bacterial infection of the CNS, there should usually be a CSF pleocytosis and elevated protein. Effective treatment is typically accompanied by these values returning towards normal. In longstanding infection, there often is enough B-cell proliferation within the CNS that immunoglobulin (Ig) measures (such as the IgG index) are increased; oligoclonal bands may be present (reported more often in Europe than in the United States). Specific antibody measures can also be helpful. As in many other chronic infections, the prolonged presence of organisms in the CNS leads to production of specifically targeted antibodies within the CNS. Thus demonstrating intrathecally produced antibodies (ITAb) can be diagnostic of CNS infection. This must be done correctly, measuring specific antibody in CSF and serum, and normalizing for blood–brain barrier disruption or nonspecific immune stimulation within the CNS, but when done (and after neurosyphilis is eliminated) this provides a very specific indicator of CNS infection. Estimates of the technique's sensitivity vary – in Europe, demonstration of ITAb is required for the diagnosis of CNS Lyme. In the United States, sensitivity estimates in different patient populations range from 90% to 50%. Most agree that, in patients with obvious immune stimulation in the CNS (increased overall IgG synthesis, oligoclonal bands, etc.) caused by *B. burgdorferi* infection, the demonstrated antibody excess should be targeted against *B. burgdorferi* – i.e. there should be specific ITAb production.

This technique has two major limitations. When established, the relative excess production of antibody in the CNS can persist for many years, despite effective treatment. An elevated CSF/serum antibody index indicates that there has been active CNS infection in the past, not necessarily currently. In contrast, combining this value with measures of CSF cell count and protein can provide valuable insights into the etiology and activity of a particular disorder.

The other limitation is technical. If the Lyme-specific antibody values are not appropriately corrected for the total concentration of Ig in the CSF relative to blood (and many labs do not do this), results can be meaningless. Particularly problematic are patients who have had a CNS bleed, have blood–brain barrier disruption for other reasons, or who have other causes of CNS inflammation (for example, multiple sclerosis). All of these circumstances will raise total CSF Ig concentrations, spuriously elevating CSF concentration of antibodies that react in the Lyme assay. If not adjusted appropriately, all will result in false positives.

Stroke in Lyme disease

The first reports suggesting that neuroborreliosis, like neurosyphilis, might cause a meningovascular process, appeared almost two decades ago (Hanny and Hauselmann, 1987; Midgard and Hofstad, 1987; Uldry *et al.*, 1987). Since then, reports of at least another 32 patients with purported meningovascular neuroborreliosis (Table 10.2) have appeared. However the relationship between *B. burgdorferi* infection and vascular disease remains unclear, reflected in the fact that none of the three sets of published practice guidelines that address diagnosis of nervous system Lyme disease (Brouqui *et al.*, 2004; Halperin *et al.*, 1996; Wormser *et al.*, 2000) would permit diagnosis of a stroke or cerebral vasculitis as a manifestation of Lyme disease. Therefore, a critical analysis of these case reports is needed.

The presumed mechanism has been a vasculitis, by analogy to meningovascular syphilis. Interestingly, although different vasculitides generally preferentially affect specific classes of blood

Table 10.2 Summary of published reports describing apparent cerebrovascular disorders in patients thought to have Lyme disease.

Author	Serology		MRI	Angiogram	CSF				ITAb Index	VDRL	Rx
	ELISA	Western blot			WBC	Protein	IgG Index	OCB			
Series											
Corral et al., 1997	+				nl	nl			neg		
105 sero+; 9 CVA											
Hammers-Berggren et al., 1993	1075				74	190			66; index+	neg	Dox->improved
281 CVA; 1 CSF+ w/HA, transient neuro											
Hanny and Hauselmann 1987	+	n/d	stroke	n/d	+				n/d	n/d	
45 sero+; 6 CVA											
Lyme, not vascular											
Cox et al., 2005			"infarct"	MCA sten	13	72	2.8	+	IgG 12.9 (?corr)	≠reported	CFTX->CSF Nl
9 F; awoke hemiparesis, dysphasia											
Deloizy et al., 2000	180 (n<6)	3 IgG	lesion, edema	n/d	140	220			5.6	neg	CFTX
27M, awoke hemi											
Henriksen, 1997	+				incr	185			+		PCN->resolved
66 F, Bannwarth											
Kohler et al., 1988	+				30	66	1.59	+	c 128; s 16		
#3: 20 M, bilat hemi 2 m apart, HA											
#4: 36 M HA, 2 L hemisphere attacks, HA					550	299	2.2	+	c 256:s 64		PCN->Clin improved
Laroche et al., 1999	3.21		whole putamen		65	nl			(<3.49)	n/d	CFTX 3 W->improved
9 M, L hemi											
May and Jabbari, 1990	1.016 (.106)	+	l thal		770	210			1.12	neg	CFTX 2 w->improved
20 M; HA × 2 mo, bilat thalamic											
Olsson and Zbornikova, 1990	3800		CT nl		30		2.97	+	1300/3800		PCN->improved
55 M, L hemi evolve over days											
Reik, 1993	+	+	Mult		238	174			6.17; +wb	neg	CFTX 30 d->stable
56 F; EM, HA, VII, Rx doxy, pred->evolving deficit											
Romi et al., 2004	+		"vasculitic foci"	n/d	250	180		+	2.5		PCN,CFTX
56 M, fever, HA, VII, evolving hemi											
Schmiedel et al., 2004	+		R BG, temp Cx	L ICA sten	298	746	8.6			n/d	CFTX->improved
38 F; 4 mo HA, N, V, wk->hemi, encephalopathic											

(cont.)

Table 10.2 (*cont.*)

Author	Serology		MRI	Angiogram	CSF					VDRL	Rx
	ELISA	Western blot			WBC	Protein	IgG Index	OCB	ITAb Index		
Wilke *et al.*, 2000	?		L BG/IC		65	113			g 14.7 m 4.2	n/d	PCN × 14 d, CFTX × 14 d->CSF improved
	#3: 15 F, 5 wk HA, Rt hemi over 1 wk										
Zhang *et al.*, 2000	IgM only	IgG & M	R BG	R MCA sl	5	67			neg	n/d rpr	CFTX
	+	+	Old biparietal							neg	CFTX ->improved
	#4: episodes L hemi — 74 M, 1 wk progressive L hemi, neuropathy										
Vascular, Lyme unclear											
Brogan *et al.*, 1990	.200/.091	n/d	CT R thal	Irreg aa	1	178			0.84	neg	Pred, Cfrx->Agram better
	37 F, 10 d postpartum; HA, seizure									rpr	
Heinrich *et al.*, 2003	???		Lesion	R MCA sten	72				+	neg	CFTX, methylpred->improved
	17 F, EM, HA										
Jacobi *et al.*, 2006	+	+	Neg	Irreg R P1	1067				15.6 (?corr)	n/d	Cefuroxime, methylpred->improved
	58 F, EM, acute HA										
Scheid *et al.*, 2003	1000		Bleed residua	Neg	–				2.3 (93u)	n/d	
	56 F, R VII'72, tick '93, Jt pain '95, HA5/98, +1 wk = hem										
Schmitt *et al.*, 1999	+	IgM, C, & S		Vasculitis	9	280		+	0.3972	neg	No response pred, CFTX->CTX
	50, multi infarcts										
Seijo Martinez, *et al.*, 2001	3.37 (1.2)	34, 57, 59, 62		R MCA spasm	10	592			1.17	neg	CFTX × 4 w
	48 M, evolving paraparesis mos, acute HA										
Klingebiel, *et al.*, 2002	"strongly +"		Multi MCA, ACA	Mult stenoses	45	750	7.43	+	–	n/d	CFTX, Cefotaxime × 3 w->resolved
	12 F, 3 mo prodrome->acute R hemi										
Misc, Lyme unlikely											
Chehrenama *et al.*, 1997	1.17/1	CSF 5 IgG	Pial enhance	Neg	86	300			2.36 (≠corr)	≠reported	Dox->improved
	25 F, 2 mos HA, jt pain, wk; demyelinating EMG										

Oksi et al., 1996	#1: 51 F multisystem disease	–	n/d	atrophy	n/d	–				–	neg	
	#2: 40 M, seizures	+	n/d	3 sm fr lesions	n/d						neg	
	#3: 11 F RLE weakness	+	n/d	Periventric	n/d						n/d	
Oksi et al., 1998	#1: 43 F, L ICA aneurysm, SAH	–			L ICA aneur	nl	nl	nl		–	–	CFTX
	#2: 18 M, HA, R VI	–			R ICA aneur	nl	nl	nl		–	–	CFTX
	#3: 42 F 5 mo "EM", polyradic; 13 mo p Rx- SAH	+			Bas aneur	5	62	nl		1.5 (Dako)	neg	CFTX improved
Lyme & Vascular												
Keil et al., 1997	20 M, R Thal acute event		+	Thal	R Thal sten	1550	297		+	13	n/d	cftx->resolved sx
Midgard and Hofstad, 1987	#1: 49 M, Bannwarth-like, then bilat wkness	+		L capsule	Mult sten	54	94	0.77	+	"20" not defined	neg	vasc, cva, prob lyme dexa & pcn
Uldry et al., 1987	40 F, EM, 1 y later HA, multifocal sx BP 170/120	M 1:32;G 1:256		CT bilat Thal	A/MCA sten	28	267	2.13	+	IgM 1':4; g 1:128		pcn × 10 d, pred × 8 w->CSF better
Veenendaal-Hilbers et al., 1988	#1: 27 F, 3 mo HA, 2 episodes, 1 min ea L wk	0.375		CT nl	Bas occlud	250	200	1.19	+		tpha-	
	#2: evolving paraparesis				Bas occlud	33	142	1.56		c 1:32	tpha -; fta+	pcn × 10 d; CSF better

vessels (e.g. small arteries vs. large), these reports describe everything from lacunar-size strokes to internal carotid artery (ICA) and basilar artery disease. Similarly, although the pathologic diagnosis of a vasculitis typically requires evidence of damage to the blood vessel walls (Schoen, 2005), the little histopathologic material available at best shows perivascular inflammatory infiltrates, a rather nonspecific finding.

To assess the validity of the published literature, the following would seem a rigorous and appropriate approach for each case:

1. Did the patient have a stroke? Was the clinical event stroke-like in onset and evolution, and did imaging studies show characteristic findings, including damage in a vascular distribution and, if available, appropriate changes on diffusion-weighted MRI and angiography?

2. Was there compelling evidence for Lyme disease? Although published guidelines for the diagnosis of nervous system Lyme disease explicitly exclude strokes, were other criteria met (possible exposure, positive serology)? If serology was negative, was there otherwise truly compelling evidence – a classic erythema migrans; positive culture in a reliable reference laboratory; PCR positivity using at least two distinct primers, performed in a reliable laboratory known not to have difficulties with false positives? (Brouqui et al., 2004; Wormser et al., 2000)

3. Was there compelling evidence of CNS Lyme disease? If the assumption is that this is analogous to meningovascular syphilis, did the CSF show a meningeal inflammatory process, with a lymphocytic pleocytosis, increased protein, and increased immunoglobulin? If there was felt to be an inflammatory process due to B. burgdorferi infection, was there evidence of intrathecal production of anti–B. burgdorferi antibodies, including demonstration that the inflammatory process was not due to neurosyphilis?

Case reviews

Three papers have looked systematically at series of patients from Lyme-endemic areas with this issue in mind. The first, from Switzerland (Hanny and Hauselmann, 1987), identified 45 patients with suspected neuroborreliosis. Six were felt to have stroke-like presentations. Although all had a CSF pleocytosis, none had angiography, none were tested for intrathecal production of anti–B. burgdorferi antibody (ITAb), and none were screened for neurosyphilis. Autopsy in one case showed perivascular inflammatory infiltrates but no vessel wall damage. The authors concluded that this infection did not cause cerebrovascular disease.

A similar study from Spain (Corral et al., 1997) identified 105 seropositive patients seen over 8 years. Forty-one had typical neuroborreliosis; nine others had strokes, but on careful review in none was this considered causally related to B. burgdorferi infection. The third study, from Sweden (Hammers-Berggren et al., 1993) tested sera from all patients presenting with stroke or transient ischemic attacks (TIAs) over the course of 1 year. Of 495 patients screened, 24 had positive serologies for B. burgdorferi exposure. One of these, a 66-year-old woman with a several-hour episode of dysphasia, had a CSF pleocytosis and ITAb, in the context of a several-month systemic illness. No other patient had

anything to suggest that his or her symptoms were related to B. burgdorferi infection.

Fourteen patients (Table 10.2) were described as having Lyme-associated cerebrovascular disease (Cox et al., 2005; Deloizy et al., 2000; Henriksen, 1997; Kohler et al., 1988; Laroche et al., 1999; May and Jabbari, 1990; Olsson and Zbornikova, 1990; Reik, 1993; Romi et al., 2004; Schmiedel et al., 2004; Wilke et al., 2000), and the reason for labeling it cerebrovascular disease is unclear. Only two had angiography; in both this demonstrated unifocal arterial stenosis – involving the MCA in one (Cox et al., 2005) and the ICA in another (Schmiedel et al., 2004; Zhang et al., 2000). In one other (Wilke et al., 2000), a magnetic resonance angiography showed slight narrowing of the MCA. In all, clinical presentations and imaging studies could be more readily explained by a multifocal inflammatory than vascular process. In most, syphilis testing was not described.

Seven reported patients (Chehrenama et al., 1997; Oksi et al., 1996, 1998) have had little to suggest that they had neuroborreliosis. One, with a spinal subarachnoid hemorrhage (Chehrenama et al., 1997) had a minimally positive peripheral blood serology without Western blot confirmation and a positive CSF serology and ITAb index but with grossly bloody CSF, a common source of false positives. This patient had prominent peripheral nerve demyelination, a process rarely if ever seen in Lyme disease (Halperin, 2003) and had negative cerebral angiography. Syphilis serology was not described. In the other two papers, only 3 of 6 patients had positive blood serologies, none with Western blot confirmation. None had a CSF pleocytosis. One was said to have ITAb, but the reported index (1.5) did not meet the usual cutoff recommended (2.0) for the kit used. Three were diagnosed based on positive PCR results (two in plasma), a procedure that the authors performed only with a single primer, to flagellin. Pathology was reported in two patients; in both there were perivascular inflammatory infiltrates without vessel wall damage. None of these seven patients would meet standard diagnostic criteria for neuroborreliosis.

In seven reported patients with vascular processes, the diagnosis of B. burgdorferi infection was unclear. One (Brogan et al., 1990), a 10-day postpartum woman, had angiographic findings of multifocal vasospasm or vasculitis, only one white cell in her CSF, a marginally positive serum Lyme ELISA without Western blot confirmation, and no ITAb. Whether she had a postpartum vasculopathy or a vasculitis is unclear; however, the evidence for neuroborreliosis was tenuous at best. A second (Scheid et al., 2003) patient who almost certainly had had B. burgdorferi infection developed a temporoparietal hemorrhage. One week prior to the hemorrhage, CSF (obtained because of severe headaches) had been completely normal. Cerebral angiography showed no bleeding source or vasculitis. On evaluation a year later, she was found to have positive blood and CSF Lyme serologies, with a positive ITAb index; there was no CSF pleocytosis. In this patient, the relationship between prior neuroborreliosis and a cerebral hemorrhage is unclear.

In the other five patients, a link between Lyme and the cerebrovascular process is possible but not entirely compelling. The first report of a Lyme-associated cerebral hemorrhage (Seijo Martinez et al., 2001) described a 48-year-old man evaluated for 4 months of progressive paraparesis, in retrospect presumably

Bannwarth's syndrome. He presented a month after this initial assessment with a right temporal lobe hemorrhage with subarachnoid extension. Angiography demonstrated only some vasospasm in the right MCA; follow-up angiography 17 days later was normal. Serum and CSF Lyme ELISAs were elevated with an ITAb index of 1.17 (borderline); there was a mild CSF pleocytosis, and syphilis testing was negative. He was treated with ceftriaxone, and the CSF improved. Like the previous patient, this man may have had prior neuroborreliosis and, for unrelated reasons, developed a cerebral hemorrhage. Because both had angiograms with no evidence of vasculitis or aneurysms, it is difficult to postulate a mechanism inter-relating the infection and the hemorrhage.

Three other case reports are of interest. A 58-year-old woman developed an occipital subarachnoid hemorrhage while being evaluated for apparent Lyme-associated thoracic radiculopathy (Bannwarth's syndrome) (Jacobi et al., 2006). Cerebral angiography did not show a bleeding source or vasculitis. CSF showed a pleocytosis and ITAb (although technical details regarding correction for subarachnoid blood were not provided). Peripheral blood Lyme serology and Western blot were positive.

A 17-year-old woman (Heinrich et al., 2003) with acute left arm and face weakness, and prior events thought to be focal seizures or TIAs, had angiographically demonstrated right MCA stenosis and stenotic segments in the right anterior cerebral artery (ACA) and posterior cerebral artery (PCA), a CSF pleocytosis, and ITAb. Results of peripheral blood serology were not reported, although CSF results were said to be confirmed by immunoblot. She was treated with 14 days of ceftriaxone and 6 months of methylprednisolone, with improvement in her CSF, vascular studies, and clinical status. Similarly (Schmitt et al., 1999), a 50-year-old patient with "cerebral vasculitis" on angiography and multiple infarcts had a CSF pleocytosis, positive Lyme serologies in CSF and serum, and evidence of ITAb. This patient did not respond to ceftriaxone and prednisolone but did to cyclophosphamide. In these two, the treatment response seems to suggest an immune-mediated rather than infectious process, but by conventional criteria it is possible that B. burgdorferi was responsible for their vasculitis.

Finally, a 12-year-old developed multifocal brain disease with angiographic demonstration of multiple stenotic areas around the circle of Willis, the left ICA, and the left ACA and MCA. Peripheral blood serologies demonstrated strongly positive IgG but weakly positive IgM antibodies to B. burgdorferi. She had a mild CSF pleocytosis but did not have ITAb. She was treated with ceftriaxone and cefotaxime, and largely recovered.

In the final group, consisting of just three patients, the relationship appears more plausible. The two earliest reports (Midgard and Hofstad, 1987; Uldry et al., 1987) described patients with multifocal brain disease, angiographically demonstrated vasculitis, CSF pleocytosis, and positive serologies in serum and CSF whose CSF improved after high dose penicillin treatment. In one patient (Midgard and Hofstad, 1987), the cerebral event was preceded by a month of thoracic pain (presumably Bannwarth's syndrome). The other had a prolonged, waxing and waning course spanning 3 years. Both cases predated current Western blot and ITAb criteria and, as such, the validity of the diagnoses can be questioned on

technical grounds, although, at least the first patient probably did have B. burgdorferi infection.

The next year, two patients with basilar artery occlusion and a CSF pleocytosis were reported (Veenendaal-Hilbers et al., 1988). In both, blood and CSF Lyme serologies were slightly positive (one patient also had a positive fluorescent treponemal antibody (FTA) but negative treponemal pallidum hemagglutination (TPHA), a known cross-reactivity); in both, CSF improved significantly following high dose penicillin. A decade later, Keil et al. (1997) reported a 20-year-old man with an apparent thalamocapsular infarct, stenosis of the feeding arteries, a CSF pleocytosis, ITAb, and positive Western blots (though values of quantitative serologic tests were not provided). He was treated with 14 days of ceftriaxone; his CSF improved significantly.

The clinical evidence supporting an association between B. burgdorferi infection and cerebral vasculitis or stroke is tenuous at best. In light of this, it is worthwhile to ask if any other data support such an association. Unfortunately, parenchymal brain disease has not been reported in any animal model. Peripheral nerve disease occurs fairly commonly both in infected patients (Halperin, 2003) and in experimentally infected rhesus macaque monkeys (Roberts et al., 1998). Although in both humans and monkeys this is a patchy multifocal disease (mononeuritis multiplex), with perivascular inflammatory infiltrates evident in biopsied nerves, in neither has there ever been evidence of a true vasculitis or significant vasculopathy. Thus, although neurosyphilis has been known for many years to cause vascular inflammation and damage, to date there is little proof that this occurs in Lyme disease.

Should one consider screening for Lyme disease in patients with stroke? Unless in an endemic area, clearly not. In endemic areas it may be worth testing individuals who have had other systemic or neurologic symptoms prior to the acute event – virtually all the patients in the literature in whom there is a possible association had a significant prodrome. If the diagnosis is considered, CSF examination is mandatory, as is a careful consideration of other potential causes of cerebral vasculitis or vasculopathy.

REFERENCES

Brogan, G. X., Homan, C. S., and Viccellio, P. 1990. The enlarging clinical spectrum of Lyme disease: Lyme cerebral vasculitis, a new disease entity. *Ann Emerg Med*, **19**(5), 572–6.

Brouqui, P., Bacellar, F., Baranton, G., et al.. 2004. Guidelines for the diagnosis of tick-borne bacterial diseases in Europe. *Clin Microbiol Infect*, **10**(12), 1108–32.

Chehrenama, M., Zagardo, M., and Koski, C. 1997. Subarachnoid hemorrhage in a patient with Lyme disease. *Neurology*, **48**(2), 520–3.

Corral, I., Quereda, C., Guerrero, A., Escudero, R., and Marti-Belda, P. 1997. [Neurological manifestations in patients with sera positive for Borrelia burgdorferi]. *Neurologia*, **12**(1), 2–8.

Cox, M. G., Wolfs, T. F., Lo, T. H., Kapelle, L. J., and Braun, K. P. 2005. Neuroborreliosis causing focal cerebral arteriopathy in a child. *Neuropediatrics*, **36**(2), 104–7.

Deloizy, M., Devos, P., Stekelorom, T., Testard, D., and Belhadia, A. 2000. [Left sided sudden hemiparesis linked to a central form of Lyme disease]. *Rev Neurol (Paris)*, **156**(12), 1154–6.

Halperin, J. J. 2003. Lyme disease and the peripheral nervous system. *Muscle Nerve*, **28**(2), 133–43.

Halperin, J. J., Logigian, E., Finkel, M., and Pearl, R. 1996. Practice parameters for the diagnosis of patients with nervous system Lyme borreliosis (Lyme disease). *Neurology*, **46**, 619–27.

Hammers-Berggren, S., Grondahl, A., Karlsson, M. *et al.* 1993. Screening for neuroborreliosis in patients with stroke. *Stroke*, **24**(**9**), 1393–6.

Hanny, P. E., and Hauselmann, H. J. 1987. Die Lyme-krankheit aus der sicht des neurologen. *Schwiez med Wsch*, **117**, 901–15.

Heinrich, A., Khaw, A. V., Ahrens, N., Kirsch, M., and Dressel, A. 2003. Cerebral vasculitis as the only manifestation of Borrelia burgdorferi infection in a 17-year-old patient with basal ganglia infarction. *Eur Neurol*, **50**(**2**), 109–12.

Henriksen, T. B. 1997. [Lyme neuro-borreliosis in a 66-year old women. Differential diagnosis of cerebral metastases and cerebral infarction]. *Ugeskr Laeger*, **159**(**21**), 3175–7.

Jacobi, C., Schwark, C., Kress, B., *et al.* 2006. Subarachnoid hemorrhage due to Borrelia burgdorferi-assiciated vasculitis. *Eur J Neurol*, **13**, 536.

Keil, R., Baron, R., Kaiser, R., and Deuschl, G. 1997. [Vasculitis course of neuroborreliosis with thalamic infarct]. *Nervenarzt*, **68**(**4**), 339–41.

Klingebiel, R. G., Benndorf, M., Schmitt, A., von Moers and Lehmann, R. 2002. Large cerebral vessel occlusive disease in Lyme neuroborreliosis. *Neuropediatrics* **33**(**1**), 37–40.

Kohler, J., Kern, U., Kasper, J., Rhese-Kupper, B., and Thoden, U. 1988. Chronic central nervous system involvement in Lyme borreliosis. *Neurology*, **38**(**6**), 863–7.

Laroche, C., Lienhardt, A., and Boulesteix, J. 1999. [Ischemic stroke caused by neuroborreliosis]. *Arch Pediatr*, **6**(**12**), 1302–5.

May, E. F., and Jabbari, B. 1990. Stroke in neuroborreliosis. *Stroke*, **21**(**8**), 1232–5.

Midgard, R., and Hofstad, H. 1987. Unusual manifestations of nervous system Borrelia burgdorferi infection. *Arch Neurol*, **44**(**7**), 781–3.

Oksi, J., Kalimo, H., Marttila, J., *et al.* 1996. Inflammatory brain changes in Lyme borreliosis. A report on three patients and review of literature. *Brain*, **119**(**Pt 6**), 2143–54.

Oksi, J., Kalimo, H., Marttila, J., *et al.* 1998. Intracranial aneurysms in three patients with disseminated Lyme borreliosis: cause or chance association? *J Neurol Neurosurg Psychiatry*, **64**(**5**), 636–42.

Olsson, J. E., and Zbornikova, V. 1990. Neuroborreliosis simulating a progressive stroke. *Acta Neurol Scand*, **81**(**5**), 471–4.

Reik, L. Jr. 1993. Stroke due to Lyme disease. *Neurology*, **43**(**12**), 2705–7.

Roberts, E. D., Bohm, R. P. Jr., Lowrie, R. C. Jr., *et al.* 1998. Pathogenesis of Lyme neuroborreliosis in the rhesus monkey: the early disseminated and chronic phases of disease in the peripheral nervous system. *J Infect Dis*, **178**(**3**), 722–32.

Romi, F., Krakenes, J., Aarli, J. A., and Tysnes, O. B. 2004. Neuroborreliosis with vasculitis causing stroke-like manifestations. *Eur Neurol*, **51**(**1**), 49–50.

Scheid, R., Hund-Georgiadis, M., and von Cramon, D. Y. 2003. Intracerebral haemorrhage as a manifestation of Lyme neuroborreliosis? *Eur J Neurol*, **10**(**1**), 99–101.

Schmiedel, J., Gahn, G., von Kummer, R., and Reichmann, H. 2004. Cerebral vasculitis with multiple infarcts caused by lyme disease. *Cerebrovasc Dis*, **17**(**1**), 79–81.

Schmitt, A. B., Kuker, W., and Nacimiento, W. 1999. [Neuroborreliosis with extensive cerebral vasculitis and multiple cerebral infarcts]. *Nervenarzt*, **70**(**2**), 167–71.

Schoen, F. J. 2005. Blood vessels. In *Robbins and Cotran, Pathologic Basis of Disease*, eds. V. Kumar, A. K. Abbas, and N. Fausto. Elsevier Saunders, 511–37.

Seijo Martinez, M., Grandes Ibanez, J., Sanchez Herrero, J., and Garcia-Monco, J. C. 2001. Spontaneous brain hemorrhage associated with Lyme neuroborreliosis. *Neurologia*, **16**(**1**), 43–5.

Uldry, P. A., Regli, F., and Bogousslavsky, J. 1987. Cerebral angiopathy and recurrent strokes following Borrelia burgdorferi infection. *J Neurol Neurosurg Psychiatry*, **50**, 1703–4.

Veenendaal-Hilbers, J. A., Perquin, W. V., Hoogland, P. H., and Doornbos, L. 1988. Basal meningovasculitis and occlusion of the basilar artery in two cases of Borrelia burgdorferi infection. *Neurology*, **38**(**8**), 1317–9.

Wilke, M., Eiffert, H., Christen, H. J., and Hanefeld, F. 2000. Primarily chronic and cerebrovascular course of Lyme neuroborreliosis: case reports and literature review. *Arch Dis Child*, **83**(**1**), 67–71.

Wormser, G., Nadelman, R., Dattwyler, R., *et al.* 2000. Practice guidelines for the treatment of Lyme disease. *Clin Infect Dis*, **31**(**Suppl 1**), S1–S14.

Zhang, Y., Lafontant, G., and Bonner, F. J. Jr., 2000. Lyme neuroborreliosis mimics stroke: a case report. *Arch Phys Med Rehabil*, **81**(**4**), 519–21.

11 BEHÇET'S DISEASE

Emre Kumral

Introduction

Behçet's disease (BD) is a multisystemic inflammatory disorder of unknown etiology, and neurologic involvement is one of the major clinical features (International Study Group for Behçet's Disease, 1990; Yazici, 2002). The most known triad of the disease, described as the components of this disease entity in 1937 by Behçet, includes recurrent oral and genital ulcerations and hypopyon iritis (Behçet, 1937). Since then, many other organ system involvements have been described such as mucocutaneous, ocular, articular, vascular, pulmonary, gastrointestinal, renal, and nervous, extending the borders of BD to a multisystem disorder (Serdaroglu, 1998). Knapp (1941) described the first clinical report of neurological involvement in BD. Cavara and D'Ermo (1954) introduced the term "neuro-Behçet's disease" (n-BD) to describe a patient with meningoencephalitis. It is well known that other neurological manifestations such as aseptic meningitis, myelitis, optic neuritis, peripheral neuritis, myositis, cerebral venous thrombosis, and arterial stroke may occur in n-BD (Kawakita *et al.*, 1967; O'Duffy *et al.*, 1971; O'Duffy and Goldstein, 1976; Rougemont *et al.*, 1982; Serdaroglu, 1998; Serdaroglu *et al.*, 1989; Wolf *et al.*, 1965).

Authors whose patient populations were sufficiently high have suggested a prevalence of 5.3% in Istanbul (Serdaroglu *et al.*, 1989), 16% in Casablanca (Benamour *et al.*, 1990), 25% in Alexandria (Assaad-Khalil *et al.*, 1993), and 3.3% in a nationwide survey in Iran (Davitchi *et al.*, 1997). In an autopsy series, 20% of 170 cases of patients with Behçet's syndrome showed pathological evidence for neurological involvement (Lakhanpal *et al.*, 1985). Male gender frequency and the association with human leukocyte antigen (HLA)-B51 split of HLA-5 were more frequent in western than eastern countries (Yazici and Moutsopoulos, 1985). In Turkey and Japan, skin pathergy reaction is correlated with the presence of the disease, whereas no association between them could be found in Western countries (O'Duffy, 1990).

Etiology

The central pathological process in BD is vasculitis. There is evidence suggesting a role of immunological mechanisms in this vasculitis. The clinical picture may be the consequence of the interaction of intrinsic (i.e. genetic) and extrinsic (i.e. some microorganisms) factors (Emmi *et al.*, 1995; Mizuki and Ohno, 1996). Neutrophil hyperfunction and an increase in the CD8+/CD4+ cell ratio occur. There is an increase in circulating T cells bearing receptors; indeed, peptides derived from the 65-kd heat shock proteins (hsp) have been shown to stimulate T cells specifically from patients with the disease (Lehner, 1997; Suzuki *et al.*, 1992). Such cells have been shown to be uveitogenic to Lewis rats (Stanford *et al.*, 1994). Occurrence of familial cases and association of the disease with HLA-B51, at least in some populations, have accelerated genetic studies. The suspected region of susceptibility gene(s) for the disease is between the tumor necrosis factor (TNF) and HLA-B or HLA-C genes (Mizuki and Ohno, 1996). Moreover, some pathogenetic microorganisms such as some streptococcal strains, herpes simplex virus type 1, or hsp 65 may induce specific immunopathological responses in genetically predisposed individuals. However, there is no evidence of a direct infectious cause. Antigenic cross-reactivity seems to be a better explanation, because antigens such as hsp have been shown to be shared between microorganisms and samples from patients with BD (Lehner *et al.*, 1991; Stanford *et al.*, 1994; Tasçi *et al.*, 1998), suggesting that BD has an autoimmune nature (Sakane, 1997). However, there is opposition to this autoimmune theory based on facts such as its male predominance, the lack of concurrent autoimmune diseases, the lack of any specific antigen or antibody, and the lack of any relationship with HLA class II antigens (Yazici, 1997). Genetic susceptibility to BD has been noted in certain populations. In the Mediterranean region and the Middle East, HLA-B51 is significantly more common among BD patients. For example, up to 84% of patients with BD in Turkey are positive for HLA-B51 (Yazici *et al.*, 1980), a marker that is not found in other populations, such as British and North American patients (O'Duffy, 1994).

Pathology

When the clinicopathological and neuroradiological findings are combined, two different patterns of central nervous system (CNS) involvement in BD can be established: parenchymal (82% of cases) and neurovascular (18% of cases). The pathological process within the nervous parenchyma occurs mainly in the brainstem, basal ganglia, diencephalic structures (Figure 11.1), and internal capsules, and is also disseminated throughout the CNS as a low-grade inflammation. Neuropathological examination shows small foci of softening, lymphocytic perivascular infiltration, diffuse microglial activity, and small areas of demyelination (Shimizu, 1962; Totsuka and Midorikawa, 1972; Totsuka *et al.*, 1979). Other pathological processes in the vascular system of the CNS are cerebral venous thrombosis, large-artery occlusion, aneurysm, and hemorrhage. The visible lesions of parenchyma usually correspond

Uncommon Causes of Stroke, 2nd edition, ed. Louis R. Caplan. Published by Cambridge University Press.   © Cambridge University Press 2008.

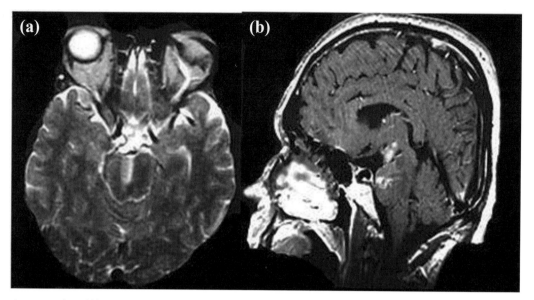

Figure 11.1 (a and b). Axial and sagittal T2-weighted MRI of a 40-year-old man with BD who presented with an acute brainstem syndrome showing very pronounced high-signal-intensity abnormalities throughout the brainstem.

well to a main vascular territory in this type of involvement. This type of vascular involvement should be called vasculo-BD (Akman-Demir *et al.*, 1996; Wechsler *et al.*, 1992). The large arterial lesion in vasculo-BD represents inflammation occurring in the media and adventitia. In the affected arteries, vasculitis is usually considered to be the central pathological feature (Ehrlich, 1997; O'Duffy, 1990). However, a vasculitic process is usually not evident in the CNS (Hadfield *et al.*, 1997). Studies on the pathology of the CNS involvement have shown that both a low-grade chronic lymphocytic or neutrophilic infiltration and multifocal necrotic foci, predominantly in the brainstem and basal ganglion region, are seen (Rubinstein and Urich, 1963; Sugihara *et al.*, 1969). Saccular aneurysms are probably produced by severe destruction of the media due to intense active inflammation (Matsumoto *et al.*, 1991).

Neuro-Behçet's disease

Neurologic involvement is one of the most devastating manifestations of BD. This involvement may occur primarily within the nervous parenchyma (n-BD) or secondarily in the cerebral vascular system (vasculo[angio]-BD) (Serdaroglu, 1998). Meningoencephalitis of n-BD begins months or years after the mucocutaneous manifestations and often develops with exacerbations of the non-neurological symptoms. Neurologic deficits may be seen acutely or by gradual onset and usually progress in a halting manner with periods of acceleration and incomplete remission. The meningoencephalitis predominates in the brainstem and is characterized by a variety of symptoms that have fluctuating courses and include headache, pyramidal tract signs, cerebellar incoordination, pseudobulbar palsy, seizures, and stupor (Kawakita *et al.*, 1967; O'Duffy and Goldstein, 1976; Rougemont *et al.*, 1982; Tsutsui *et al.*, 1998; Wolf *et al.*, 1965). Examination of the spinal fluid may reveal a slight pleocytosis with a preponderance of lymphocytes,

a moderate increase in total protein, and an elevation of gamma globulins. CT scans may show focal areas of decreased density that may be enhanced after contrast injection (Herskovitz *et al.*, 1988; Patel *et al.*, 1989) MRI may show focal regions of increased signal on T2-weighted images, mainly in the brainstem, basal ganglia, and hypothalamus. These lesions do not conform to arterial territories, are often larger than those encountered in arteritis, and have a tendency to resolve over time (following treatment), although in chronic cases they are particularly associated with brainstem atrophy (Banna and El Ramahi, 1991; Montalban *et al.*, 1990; Wechsler *et al.*, 1993).

In contrast, symptoms that are considered typical of multiple sclerosis, such as paroxysmal attacks, can occasionally be observed in n-BD cases. MRI findings are discriminative in most of the cases where the major lesion is located in the brainstem–diencephalon– basal ganglion region (Akman-Demir *et al.*, 1998; Gerber *et al.*, 1996; Wechsler *et al.*, 1993). However, the predominant lesion may be in the periventricular white matter (Miller *et al.*, 1987; Morissey *et al.*, 1993), in which case it will be difficult to discriminate from multiple sclerosis (Çoban *et al.*, 1999). In such cases, cerebrospinal fluid (CSF) pleocytosis with polymorphonuclear predominance, and the absence of more than two oligoclonal immunoglobulin G (IgG) bands may indicate n-BD (Saruhan-Direskeneli *et al.*, 1996). Other than multiple sclerosis, in certain cases of CNS infection – especially when there is CSF pleocytosis and fever – cerebrovascular disease, brain tumors, and compressive myelopathy should be considered in the differential diagnosis of n-BD.

In patients with vasculo-BD, neurologic abnormalities may develop due to cerebral venous or large- or small-artery involvement, and a variety of clinical features such as pseudotumor cerebri, cerebral venous thrombosis, transient ischemic attacks (TIAs), stroke, and bulbar and pseudobulbar palsy may be seen (Bousser *et al.*, 1980; Iragui and Maravi, 1986; Shimizu *et al.*, 1979; Uruyama *et al.*, 1979). The pathophysiology of vasculo-BD is not clear, and our knowledge is limited with the data derived from pathological and angiographic studies.

Vasculo-Behçet's disease

CNS vasculature involvement is rare in BD. The main vascular pathological process in the CNS is thrombosis of large sinuses and veins, which has a special place and importance in BD and may be considered as vasculo-BD. Arterial involvement is extremely rare, but does occur and can have a wide range of manifestations such as arterial malformations, intracranial hemorrhages, and occlusive arterial disease.

Cerebral sinus and venous thrombosis

Thrombosis of cerebral large veins and sinuses is the most common feature of vasculo-BD, although thrombosis of the vena cava and portal vein may also occur in one third of these patients. It is well known that papilledema and pseudotumor cerebri or benign intracranial hypertension are reported frequently as a manifestation of cerebral sinus and venous thrombosis (CSVT) in patients with BD (Ben-Itzhak *et al.*, 1985; Bousser *et al.*, 1980, 1985; Imaizumi *et al.*, 1980; Kawakita *et al.*, 1967; Masheter, 1959; Pamir *et al.*, 1981; Serdaroglu *et al.*, 1989; Shakir *et al.*, 1990; Wechsler *et al.*, 1986 Wilkins *et al.*, 1986). CT and MRI and/or magnetic resonance angiography (MRA) are important investigations to either disclose or exclude dural sinus thrombosis in patients with benign intracranial hypertension, particularly in the context of BD (Ameri and Bousser, 1992; Bousser *et al.*, 1985; Harper *et al.*, 1985).

Isolated intracranial hypertension is not the only manifestation of CSVT in BD. Most of the patients develop focal signs such as focal seizures or focal deficits that can have highly variable patterns of onset: acute, mimicking an arterial stroke, or subacute, during days and sometimes weeks, mimicking meningoencephalitis (Ameri and Bousser, 1992; Bousser *et al.*, 1985; Medejel *et al.*, 1986). Such patients are often misdiagnosed as n-BD, whereas the association of CSVT with n-BD is rare (Serdaroglu *et al.*, 1989). The signs and symptoms of CSVT in BD are similar to the mode of onset in patients with CSVT due to other causes. It most frequently affects, in order of decreasing frequency, the superior sagittal sinus (SSS), lateral sinuses, cortical veins, veins of the galenic system, and cavernous sinuses (Figure 11.2). In most patients, thrombosis affects several sinuses, or sinuses together with cerebral veins, which explains the frequent association between signs of intracranial hypertension and focal signs (Ameri and Bousser, 1992; Bousser *et al.*, 1985). Isolated cortical and deep vein thrombosis may be seen in BD with seizures, concurrent meningitis, and intracranial hypertension (Kidd *et al.*, 1999; Sagduyu *et al.*, 2006) (Figure 11.3).

Although CT is normal in 20% of patients with isolated intracranial hypertension, CT scan may show direct signs of SSS thrombosis in the majority of cases such as empty-delta signs; dense-triangle, localized, or diffuse swelling; intense contrast enhancement of the falx and tentorium; or a spontaneous hyperdensity or hypodensity, more or less suggestive of a venous infarct (Ameri and Bousser, 1992; Bousser *et al.*, 1985). Digital subtraction angiography (DSA) is the gold method to reveal the thrombosis itself, but it

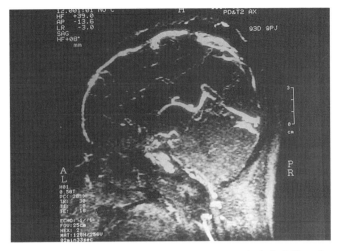

Figure 11.2 MRA of a 25-year-old man with n-BD. Notice the lack of filling of the superior sagittal and transverse sinuses.

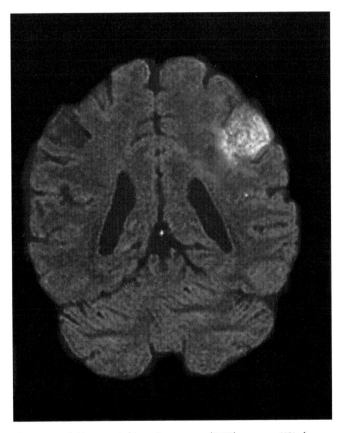

Figure 11.3 Fluid-attenuated inversion recovery (FLAIR) sequence MRI of a patient who presented with headache and hemiparesis due to cortical vein thrombosis with infarction.

seems to have been replaced by MRI and MRA, the major advantage of which was noninvasiveness with higher sensitivity to show CSVT (Ameri and Bousser, 1992; Macchi *et al.*, 1986; Montalban *et al.*, 1990; Wechsler *et al.*, 1992).

The neuro-BD form frequently occurs with exacerbations of the extraneurological and inflammatory signs, whereas CSVT seems to

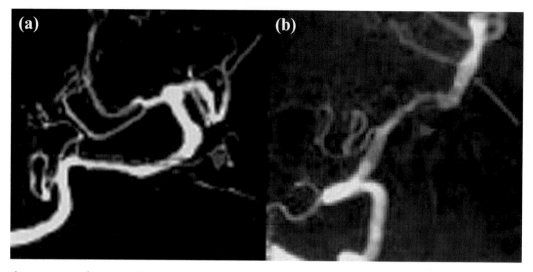

Figure 11.4 DSA of a patient with vasculitis. (**a**) Slight stenosis of distal part of the V4 segment of right VA and irregularities of the basilar artery (BA). (**b**) Ectasic appearance of proximal segment of BA and beading of P1 and P2 segment of left posterior cerebral artery (PCA).

belong to the vasculo-BD subgroup. The prognosis of patients with CSVT is usually good; in this respect it again differs from neuro-BD meningoencephalitis. The treatment of choice is heparin or low-molecular-weight heparin followed by long-term oral anticoagulants that can be combined with corticosteroid treatment for long-term suppression of the immunopathological status (Ameri and Bousser, 1992; Bousser *et al.*, 1985). In a previous series, worsening of a patient under anticoagulation was not related to treatment itself (Wechsler *et al.*, 1992).

Ischemic stroke

Ischemic cerebrovascular manifestations are less frequent in patients with BD than in those with aseptic meningitis or meningoencephalitis. During the course of BD, arterial involvement is rare (1–5%), and peripheral arteries are most often involved with aneurysm and pseudo-aneurysm formation or occlusion (Dilsen, 2000). Occlusions of the large cerebral arteries have been uncommonly reported, both clinically (Bienenstock and Murray, 1961; Iragui and Maravi, 1986; Shimizu *et al.*, 1979; Uruyama *et al.*, 1979) and pathologically (Totsuka *et al*, 1979). In Japanese series, the incidence of intracerebral large-artery occlusive disease was around 0.15% (Shimizu *et al.*, 1979; Uruyama *et al.*, 1979), which is lower than the 2.3% incidence for extracerebral large-artery involvement (Shimizu *et al.*, 1979). In a series of 868 BD patients, only 2 had cerebral artery occlusion (Uruyama *et al.*, 1979). Shimizu *et al.* (1979) reported 2 patients with common carotid artery occlusion among 81 cases of vasculo-BD investigated from a series of 1731 patients with BD. In a study of 323 patients with BD, 2 patients had supratentorial infarct in the centrum semiovale and internal capsule, and the other 3 patients had brainstem involvement with Wallenberg's syndrome, pseudobulbar signs, and brief loss of consciousness. One case had a cerebral angiogram with normal carotid and vertebral arteries (Serdaroglu *et al.*, 1989). In another case report, the patient presented TIAs that preceded the mucocutaneous symptoms of the disease by several years. Angiography

showed a high-grade stenosis of the left middle cerebral artery (MCA) that became occluded during the procedure. In a few years, the patient developed almost total blindness in the left eye with fundoscopic signs of ischemic retinopathy due to an occlusion of the left internal carotid artery (Iragui and Maravi, 1986). An autopsied patient was reported who had MCA occlusion on angiography that appeared after mucocutaneous lesions (Suga *et al.*, 1990), and another autopsy study of a BD patient clearly showed neuropathological findings consistent with panarteritis of branches of the MCA causing occlusion and infarction in its territories (Nishimura *et al.*, 1991).

BD is usually included among the systemic vasculitides (Allen, 1993) but documented cerebral arteritis is extremely rare and even a debatable mechanism for CNS involvement. However, some patients have been reported as having a typical appearance of arteritis with multiple segments of stenosis, dilatations, or occlusion of proximal segments of medium-sized intracranial vessels, usually of the MCA, which were sometimes associated with more peripheral small-vessel involvement (Bienenstock and Murray, 1961; Buge *et al.*, 1987; Nishimura *et al.*, 1991; Zelenski *et al.*, 1989). In all patients, there was convincing evidence that a vasculitic process underlined the arterial changes. High protein content and/or pleocytosis of CSF were seen in all the patients. In two patients there was vasculitis elsewhere; pulmonary in one case (Buge *et al.*, 1987), and retinal in two cases (Buge *et al.*, 1987; Zelenski *et al.*, 1989). Spontaneous progression (Buge *et al.*, 1987) or regression of the arterial changes under immunosuppressive therapy (Iragui and Maravi, 1986; Zelenski *et al.*, 1989) pleaded also in favor of vasculitis in three patients (Iragui and Maravi, 1986; Zelenski *et al.*, 1989). In a large registry, including 200 n-BD patients, cerebral vasculitis and brain infarction was present in only one patient (Krespi *et al.*, 2001). In this series, another patient reported with right brainstem infarction had right extracranial vertebral artery (VA) dissection due to vasculitis (Bahar et al., 1993) (Figure 11.4). Histological studies show a nonspecific vasculitis with mononuclear cells or neutrophilic infiltration, endothelial cell proliferation, destruction of internal elastic lamina, fibrinoid necrosis, and thrombus formation. Vasculitis of vasa vasorum is usually considered to be responsible for aneurysm or pseudoaneurysm formation (Matsumoto *et al.*, 1991; Totsuka and Midorikawa, 1972).

Some patients with CT signs of hemispheric infarction have been reported. In these reports, the patients have had arterial strokes, but no angiographic or pathological details concerning the underlying arterial lesions (Shakir *et al.*, 1990). Zelenski *et al.* (1989) reported a single patient with dramatic improvement of arterial lesions after 8 months of aggressive treatment with an initial course of intravenous nitrogen mustard and a long-term administration of chlorambucil and prednisolone.

Our recent study showed that one third of the 55 patients with BD had microembolic signals (MES) on transcranial Doppler examination, especially with a preponderance in the frequency of MES in patients with neurological involvement (Kumral *et al.*, 1999). It is notable that MES were present in all patients with neurological involvement, including basal ganglia (4 patients) and upper brainstem (1 patient) involvement and cerebral venous thrombosis (1 patient). The high prevalence of MES in the patient with cerebral venous thrombosis may be explained by generalized activation of thrombotic system due to an immunopathologic process in the blood. It is probable that, in some patients with BD, immunological mechanisms promote the formation of microthrombi, and thereafter yield to embolization of the distal vascular system. Previous studies showed an activation of blood coagulation such as shortening of prothrombin time, decreases in concentrations and activities of plasma antithrombin III, and elevated levels of the plasma thrombin–antithrombin-III complex. Moreover, increased plasma levels of protein C and total protein S levels, plasminogen activator activity, and decreased levels of alpha 2-plasmin inhibitor also indicated an activation of fibrinolysis in these patients (Fusegawa *et al.*, 1991; Hampton *et al.*, 1991).

Hemorrhagic stroke

In BD, subarachnoid and intracerebral hemorrhages are uncommon. A patient with three recurrent massive intracranial hemorrhages had severe hypertension (Nagata, 1985). Postmortem examination showed the usual features of n-BD and concomitant hypertensive changes in the cerebral small penetrating arteries. The author accepted that the recurrent hemorrhages were more likely due to the hypertension than to the perivascular lesions of BD.

A rare instance of a spinal subarachnoid hemorrhage due to a dissection of the extracranial VA in its V2 segment and an aneurysmal dilatation of a radiculomedullary branch in its intradural portion at the C5 level was reported (Bahar *et al.*, 1993). A spinal subarachnoid hematoma was also found in another man with BD. The hematoma was completely evacuated, but there was no description of histological examination (Arias *et al.*, 1987). In BD, aneurysm (either saccular or dissecting type) formation occurs most commonly in the aorta (Matsumoto *et al.*, 1991). In the affected arteries, active arteritis occurs initially, followed by destruction of the media and fibrosis. Saccular aneurysms were

probably produced by severe destruction of the media by active inflammation.

A few patients with single or multiple cerebral aneurysms have been reported (Bartlett *et al.*, 1988; Buge *et al.*, 1987; Godeau *et al.*, 1980; Shakir *et al.*, 1990; Shimizu *et al.*, 1979). They are less frequent than systemic aneurysms with which they are frequently associated. They can be asymptomatic, or can yield to subarachnoid or intracerebral hemorrhage or to ischemic stroke (Buge *et al.*, 1987). A unique patient was reported with multiple systemic arterial lesions and right leg weakness of sudden onset. On angiography, she was found to have both an aneurysm of the left anterior communicating artery and a large arteriovenous malformation (Hassen Khoda *et al.*, 1991). Another patient with arteriovenous malformation was reported, but it was a dural malformation draining into the right transverse sinus in this patient, who had bilateral occlusion of the lateral sinuses (Imaizumi *et al.*, 1980).

Treatment of vascular manifestations

Certain factors influence the course and prognosis of n-BD cases. According to recent findings, the most important of these is the correlation between the acute-stage CSF findings and the clinical course. Normal CSF at the acute stage is associated with a better prognosis, i.e. a stable course and less disability, whereas high cellular and/or protein content is significantly associated with a worse prognosis. This should be kept in mind when initiating treatment at the acute stage and making a decision about the addition of immunosuppressants to corticosteroid treatment. Other associations with a poor prognosis, such as "brainstem +" type involvement and a progressive course, are less surprising. The long-term prognosis in n-BD may not be as favorable as that observed in short-term follow-up. On 7-year follow-up of 42 patients with n-BD, 2 had had dural sinus thrombosis and the other 2 had gone through a Wallenberg-like brainstem syndrome, which could be attributable to the vascular events (Akman-Demir *et al.*, 1996). The overall prognosis for patients with arterial involvement in BD is far worse than that for patients with venous manifestations, because of aneurysm relapse, recurrence after vascular surgery, and rupture of the vascular wall. In a series of 24 patients with extracerebral arterial involvement, death occurred in 6 cases, mostly because of aneurysm rupture (Huong du *et al.*, 1993).

There has been no controlled trial of therapy on cerebral ischemic events, although immunosuppressive agents are the main choice of drugs as well as in many immunopathological states. Corticosteroids control many symptoms, although they do not prevent end points such as blindness, recurrent CNS vasculature involvement, or death (Yazici, 2002). Corticosteroids can be applied in oral or pulsed regimens especially in the acute phase. Some groups recommend chlorambucil, but it is not widely utilized because of the side effects (O'Duffy, 1990). Intravenous immunoglobulin, plasma exchange, tacrolimus, cyclosporin, interferon-2a, total nodal lymphoid irradiation, and transfer factor are not widely used (O'Duffy *et al.*, 1996; Sakane, 1997). For long-term suppression of the disease, steroids can be combined with azathioprine, colchicine, and cyclophosphamide. Treatment for dural sinus venous thrombosis involves anticoagulation; some authors advocate the concurrent use of corticosteroids for large-artery involvement (Wechsler *et al.*, 1992; Yazici *et al.*, 1996), although again this has not been established by means of a prospective clinical trial.

Conclusion

Cerebrovascular complications of BD are rarer than parenchymal involvement of the CNS and aseptic meningitis. The most common vascular manifestation is CSVT, which accounts for about 11–35% of the neurological manifestations of BD. It usually entails a good prognosis but requires early and prolonged anticoagulation together with corticosteroid treatment. Cerebral arterial manifestations such as aneurysms, arteriovenous malformations, intracranial or spinal hemorrhages, arterial dissections, large-artery occlusions, and arteritis are extremely rare. They are usually associated with systemic arterial lesions and entail a severe prognosis. Abnormal CSF and parenchymal involvement, especially of the "brainstem +" type, justify more aggressive treatment. A combination of steroids, immunosuppressants, and anticoagulants is required in occlusive cases. No formal trial of treatment for this disorder has been published, so there is now an urgent need to do so through multicenter clinical trials.

REFERENCES

Akman-Demir, G., Bahar, S., Çoban, O., *et al.* 1998. Cranial MRI findings in Behçet's disease: a study of 134 MRI of 98 cases. *J Neurol*, **245**, 362.

Akman-Demir, G., Baykan-Kurt, B., Serdaroglu, P., *et al.* 1996. Seven-year follow-up of neurologic involvement in Behçet's syndrome. *Arch Neurol*, **53**, 691–4.

Ameri, A., and Bousser, M. G. 1992. Cerebral venous thrombosis. *Neurol Clin*, **10**, 87–111.

Arias, M. J., Calero, E., Gil, J. F., and Paz, J. 1987. Spinal subarachnoid hematoma in Behçet's disease. *Neurosurgery*, **20**, 62–3.

Assaad-Khalil, S., Abou-Seif, M., Abou-Seif, S., El-Sewy, F., and El-Sewy, M. 1993. Neurologic involvement in Behçet's disease: clinical, genetic and computed tomographic study. In B. Wechsler and P. Godeau, eds., *Behçet's Disease*. Amsterdam: Excerpta Medica International Congress Series, 1037, pp. 409–14.

Bahar, S., Çoban, O., Gürvit, I. H., Akman-Demir, G., and Gökyiğit, A. 1993. Spontaneous dissection of the extracranial vertebral artery with spinal subarachnoid haemorrhage in a patient with Behçet's disease. *Neuroradiology*, **35**, 352–4.

Banna, M., and El Ramahi, K. 1991. Neurologic involvement in Behçet's disease: imaging findings in 16 patients. *Am J Neuroradiol*, **12**, 791–6.

Bartlett, S. T., McCarthy, W. J. III, Palmer, A. S., *et al.* 1988. Multiple aneurysms in Behçet's disease. *Arch Surg*, **123**, 1004–8.

Behçet, H. 1937. Ueber rezidivierende Aphtöse durch ein Virus verursachte Geschwüre am Mund am Auge und an den Genitalen. *Dermatologische Wochenschrift*, **36**, 1152–7.

Ben-Itzhak, J., Keren, S., and Simon, J. 1985. Intracranial venous thrombosis in Behçet's syndrome. *Neuroradiology*, **27**, 450–1.

Benamour, S., Zeroual, B., Bennis, R., Amraoui, A., and Bettal, S. 1990. Maladie de Behçet: 316 cas. *Presse Medicine*, **19**, 1485–9.

Bienenstock, H., and Murray, E. M. 1961. Behçet's syndrome: report of a case with extensive neurologic manifestations. *N Engl J Med*, **264**, 1342–5.

Bousser, M. G., Bletry, O., Launay, M., *et al.* 1980. Thromboses veineuses cérébrales au cours de la maladie de Behçet. *Revue Neurologique*, **136**, 753–62.

Bousser, M. G., Chiars, J., and Bories, J. 1985. Cerebral venous thrombosis: a review of 38 cases. *Stroke*, **16**, 199–211.

Buge, A., Vincent, D., Rancurel, G., Dechy, H., Dorra, M., and Betourne, C. 1987. Maladie de Behçet avec anévrysmes artériels multiples intracraniens. *Revue Neurologique*, **143**, 832–5.

Cavara, V., and D'Ermo, F. 1954. A case of Behçet's syndrome. XVII Concilium. *Acta Ophthalmol (Copenh)*, **3**, 1489–505.

Çoban, O., Bahar, S., Akman-Demir, G., *et al.* 1999. Masked assessment of MRI findings: is it possible to differentiate neuro-Behçet's disease from other central nervous system diseases? *Neuroradiology*, **41**, 255–60.

Davitchi, F., Shavran, F, Akbarin, M., *et al.* 1997. Behçet's disease: analysis of 3443 cases. *APLAR Journal of Rheumatology*, **1**, 2–5.

Dilsen, N. 2000. About diagnostic criteria for Behçet's disease: our new proposal. In: D. Bang, E. S. Lee, S. Lee, eds., *Behcet's Disease*. Seoul, South Korea: Design Mecca Publishing Co., pp. 101–4.

Dilsen, N., Konice, M., Aral, O., and Aykut, S. 1986. Standardization and evaluation of the skin pathergy test in Behçet's disease and controls. In T. Lehner and C. G. Barnes, eds., *Recent Advances in Behçet's Disease*. London, UK: London Royal Society of Medicine Services, pp. 169–72.

Ehrlich, G. E. 1997. Vasculitis in Behçet's disease. *Int Rev Immunol*, **14**, 81–8.

Emmi, L., Salvati, G., Brugnolo, F., and Morchione, T. 1995. Immunopathological aspects of Behçet's disease. *Clin Exp Rheumatol*, **13**, 687–91.

Fusegawa, H., Ichikawa, Y., Tanaka, Y., *et al.* 1991. Blood coagulation and fibrinolysis in patients with Behçet's disease. *Rinsho Byori*, **39**, 509–16.

Gerber, S., Biondi, A., Dormont, D., Wechsler, B., and Marsault, C. 1996. Long-term MR follow-up of cerebral lesions in neuro-Behçet's disease. *Neuroradiology*, **38**, 761–8.

Godeau, P., Wechsler, B., Maaouni, A., Fagard, M., and Herreman, G. 1980. Manifestations cardiovasculaires de la maladie de Behçet. *Annales de Dermatologie et de Vénéréologie*, **167**, 741–7.

Hadfield, M. G., Aydin, F., Lippman, H. R., and Sanders, K. M. 1997. Neuro-Behçet's disease. [Review]. *Clin Neuropathol*, **16**, 55–60.

Hampton, K. K., Chamberlain, M. A., Menon, D. K., and Davies, J. A. 1991. Coagulation and fibrinolytic activity in Behçet's disease. *Thromb Haemost*, **66**, 292–4.

Harper, M. C., O'Neill, B. P., O'Duffy, J. D., and Forbes, G. S. 1985. Intracranial hypertension in Behçet's disease: demonstration of sinus occlusion with use of digital substraction angiography. *Mayo Clin Proc*, **60**, 419–22.

Hassen Khoda, R., Declemy, S., Batt, M., *et al.* 1991. Maladie de Behçet avec atteinte artérielle multiple et volumineux angiome intra-cérébrale. *Journal des Maladies Vasculaires*, **16**, 383–6.

Herskovitz, S., Lipton, R. B., and Lantos, G. 1988. Neuro-Behçet's disease. CT and clinical correlates. *Neurology*, **38**, 1714–20.

Huong du, L. T., Wechsler, B., Piette, J. C., *et al.*, 1993. Long term prognosis of arterial lesions in Behçet's disease. In B. Wechsler and P. Godeau, eds., *Behçet's Disease*. Amsterdam: Excerpta Medica, pp. 557–62.

Imaizumi, M., Nukada, T., Toneda, S., and Abe, H. 1980. Behçet's disease with sinus thrombosis and arteriovenous malformation in brain. *J Neurol*, **222**, 215–8.

International Study Group for Behçet's Disease. 1990. Criteria for Behçet's disease. *Lancet*, **335**, 1078–80.

Iragui, V. J., and Maravi, E. 1986. Behçet's syndrome presenting as cerebrovascular disease. *J Neurol Neurosurg Psychiatr*, **49**, 838–40.

Kawakita, H., Nishimura, N., Satoh, Y., and Shibata, N. 1967. Neurological aspects of Behçet's disease. *J Neurol Sci*, **5**, 417–39.

Kidd, D., Steuer, A., Denman, M., and Rudge, P. 1999. Neurological complications in Behçet's syndrome. *Brain*, **122**, 2183–94.

Knapp, P. 1941. Beitrag zur Symptomatologie und Therapie der rezidivierenden Hypopyoniritis und der begleitenden aphtözen Schleimhauterkrankungen. *Schweizerische Medizinische Wochenschrift*, **71**, 1288–90.

Krespi, Y., Akman-Demir, G., Poyraz, M., *et al.* 2001. Cerebral vasculitis and ischaemic stroke in Behçet's disease: report of one case and review of the literature. *Eur J Neurol*, **8**, 719–22.

Kumral, E., Evyapan, D., Oksel, F., Keser, G., and Bereketoglu, M. A. 1999. Transcranial Doppler detection of MES in patients with Behçet's disease. *J Neurol*, **246**, 592–5.

Lakhanpal, S., Tani, K., Lie, J. T., *et al.* 1985. Pathologic features of Behçet's syndrome: a review of Japanese autopsy registry data. *Hum Pathol*, **16**, 790–5.

Lehner, T. 1997. The role of heat shock protein, microbial and autoimmune agents with the aetiology of Behçet's disease. *Int Rev Immunol,* **14,** 21–32.

Lehner, T., Lavery, R., Smith, R., *et al.* 1991. Association between the 65-kilodalton heat shock protein, Streptococcus sanguis, and the corresponding antibodies in Behçet's syndrome. *Infect Immun,* **59,** 1434–41.

Macchi, P., Grossman, R. I., Gomori, J. M., *et al.* 1986. High field MR imaging of cerebral venous thrombosis. *J Comput Assist Tomogr,* **10,** 10–5.

Masheter, H. C. 1959. Behçet's syndrome complicated by intracranial thrombophlebitis. *Proc R Soc Med,* **52,** 1039–40.

Matsumoto, T., Uekusa, T., and Fukuda, Y. 1991. Vasculo-Behçet's disease: a pathologic study of eight cases. *Hum Pathol,* **22,** 45–51.

Medejel, A., El Alaoui Faris, M., Al-Zemmouri, K., *et al.* 1986. Les manifestations neurologiques de la maladie de Behçet. *Semaine des Hôpitaux,* **62,** 1325–8.

Miller, D. H., Ormerod, I. E., Gibson, A., *et al.* 1987. MR brain scanning in patients with vasculitis: differentiation from multiple sclerosis. *Neuroradiology,* **29,** 226–31.

Mizuki, N., and Ohno, S. 1996. Immuno-genetic studies of Behçet's disease. *Revue de Rhumatologie (English Edition),* **63,** 520–7.

Montalban, J., Codina, A., Alijotas, J., Ordi, J., and Khamashta, M. 1990. Magnetic resonance imaging in Behçet's disease. *J Neurol Neurosurg Psychiatr,* **53,** 442.

Morissey, S. P., Miller, D. H., Hermaszewski, R., *et al.* 1993. Magnetic resonance imaging of the central nervous system in Behçet's disease. *Eur Neurol,* **33,** 287–93.

Nagata, K. 1985. Recurrent intracranial hemorrhage in Behçet's disease. *J Neurol Neurosurg Psychiatr,* **48,** 190–1.

Nishimura, M., Satoh, K., Suga, M., and Oda, M. 1991. Cerebral angio- and neuro-Behçet's syndrome: neuroradiological and pathological study of one case. *J Neurol Sci,* **106,** 19–24.

O'Duffy, J. D. 1990. Behçet's syndrome. *N Engl J Med,* **322,** 326–7.

O'Duffy, J. D., Carney, J. A., and Deodhar, S. 1971. Behçet's disease. Report of 10 cases, 3 with new manifestations. *Ann Intern Med,* **75,** 561–9.

O'Duffy, J. D. 1994. Behçet's disease. [Review]. *Curr Opin Rheumatol,* **6,** 39–43.

O'Duffy, J. D., Cohen, S., Jorizzo, J., *et al.* 1996. Alpha-interferon (IFN-a) treatment in Behçet's disease. *Revue Rhumatologie (English Edition),* **63,** 560.

O'Duffy, J. D., and Goldstein, N. P. 1976. Neurological involvement in seven patients with Behçet's disease. *Am J Med,* **61,** 170–8.

Pamir, M. N., Kansu, T., Erbengi, A., and Zileli, T. 1981. Papilledema in Behçet's syndrome. *Arch Neurol,* **38,** 643–5.

Patel, D. V., Neuman, M. J., and Hier, D. B. 1989. Reversibility of CT and MR findings in neuro-Behçet's disease. *J Comput Assist Tomogr,* **13,** 669–73.

Rougemont, D., Bousser, M. G., Wechsler, B., Bletry, O., Castaigne, P., and Godeau, P. 1982. Manifestations neurologiques de la maladie de Behçet. *Revue Neurologique,* **138,** 493–505.

Rubinstein, L. J., and Urich, H. 1963. Meningo-encephalitis of Behçet's disease: case report with pathological findings. *Brain,* **86,** 151–60.

Sagduyu, A., Sirin, H., Mulayim, S., *et al.* 2006. Cerebral cortical and deep venous thrombosis without sinus thrombosis: clinical-MRI correlates. *Acta Neurol Scand,* **114,** 254–60.

Sakane, T. 1997. New perspective on Behçet's disease [Review]. *Int Rev Immunol,* **14,** 89–96.

Saruhan-Direskeneli, G., Akman-Demir, G., Tasçi, B., Serdaroglu P, and Eraksoy, M. 1996. Local synthesis of oligoclonal IgG is infrequent in Behçet's disease. *Rev Rheumatol,* **63 Suppl,** 552.

Serdaroglu, P., Yazici, H., Özdemir, Ç., *et al.* 1989. Neurologic involvement in Behçet's syndrome. A prospective study. *Arch Neurol,* **46,** 265–9.

Serdaroglu, P. 1998. Behçet's disease and the nervous system. *J Neurol,* **245,** 197–205.

Shakir, R. A., Sulaiman, K., Kahn, R. A., and Rudwan, M. 1990. Neurological presentation of neuro-Behçet's syndrome: clinical categories. *Eur Neurol,* **30,** 249–53.

Shimizu, T. 1962. Epidemiological and clinico-pathological studies on neuro-Behçet's syndrome. *Adv Neurol Sci (Tokyo),* **16,** 167–78.

Shimizu, T., Ehrlich, G. E., Inaba, G., and Hayashi, K. 1979. Behçet's disease. *Semin Arthritis Rheum,* **8,** 223–60.

Stanford, M. R., Kasp, E., Whiston, R., *et al.* 1994. Heat shock protein peptides reactive in Behçet's disease are uveitogenic in Lewis rats. *Clin Exp Immunol,* **97,** 226–31.

Suga, M., Sato K., Nishimura, M., and Oda, M. 1990. An autopsy case of neuro-Behçet's disease with the middle cerebral artery occlusion on cerebral angiogram. *Rinsho Shinkeigaku,* **30,** 1005–9.

Sugihara, H., Muto, Y., and Tsuchiyama, H. 1969. Neuro-Behçet's syndrome: report of two autopsy cases. *Acta Pathology (Japan),* **19,** 95–101.

Suzuki, Y., Hoshi, K., Matsuda, T., and Mizushima, Y. 1992. Increased peripheral blood T cells and natural killer cells in Behçet's disease. *J Rheumatol,* **19,** 588–92.

Tasçi, B., Direskeneli, H., Serdaroglu, P., Akman-Demir, G., Eraksoy, M., and Saruhan-Direskeneli, G. 1998. Humoral immune response to mycobacterial heat shock protein (hsp) 65 in the cerebrospinal fluid of neuro-Behçet patients. *Clin Exp Immunol,* **113,** 100–4.

Totsuka, S., Hattori, T., and Yazari, M. 1979. Clinico-pathology of neuro-Behçet's syndrome. In T. Kehner and C. G. Barnes, eds., *Behçet's Disease. Clinical and Immunological Features.* London: Academic Press, pp. 133–96.

Totsuka, S., and Midorikawa, T. 1972. Some clinical and pathological problems in neuro-Behçet's syndrome. *Folia Psychiatrica et Neurologica (Japan),* **28,** 275–84.

Tsutsui, K., Hasegawa, M., Takata, M., and Takehara, K. 1998. Behçet's disease. *J Rheumatol,* **25,** 326–8.

Uruyama, A., Sakuragi, S., and Sakai, F. 1979. Angio-Behçet syndrome. In T. Lehner and C. G. Barnes, eds., Behçet's Syndrome. Clinical and Immunological Features. London: Academic Press, pp. 176–6.

Wechsler, B., Dell'Isola, B., Vidailhet, M., *et al.* 1993. Magnetic resonance imaging in 31 patients with Behçet disease and neurological involvement: prospective study with clinical correlation. *J Neurol Neurosurg Psychiatr,* **56,** 793–8.

Wechsler, B., Vidailhet, M., Piette, J. C., *et al.* 1992. Cerebral venous thrombosis in Behçet's disease-clinical study and long term follow-up of 25 cases. *Neurology,* **42,** 614–8.

Wilkins, M. R., Gove, R. I., Roberts, S. D., and Kendall, M. J. 1986. Behçet's disease presenting as benign intracranial hypertension. *Postgrad Med J,* **62,** 36–41.

Wolf, S. M., Scrotland, D. L., and Phillips, L. L. 1965. Involvement of nervous system in Behçet's syndrome. *Arch Neurol,* **12,** 315–25.

Yazici, H. 2002. Behçet's syndrome: where do we stand? *Am J Med,* **112,** 75–6.

Yazici, H. 1997. The place of Behçet's syndrome among the autoimmune diseases. *Int Rev Immunol,* **14,** 1–10.

Yazici, H., Basaran, E. G., Hamuryudan, V., *et al.* 1996. The ten-year mortality in Behçet's syndrome. *Br J Rheumatol,* **35,** 139–41.

Yazici, H., and Moutsopoulos, H. H. 1985. Behçet's disease. In L. M. Lichenstein and A. S. Fauci, eds., *Current Therapy in Allergy, Immunology and Rheumatology.* Philadelphia: Decker, pp. 194–7.

Yazici, H., Tüzün, Y., Pazarlı, H., Yalçın, B., Yurdakul, S., and Müftüoglu, A. 1980. The combined use of HLA-B5 and the pathergy test as diagnostic markers of Behçet's disease in Turkey. *J Rheumatol,* **7,** 206–10.

Zelenski, J. D., Caparo, J. A., Holden, D., and Calabrese, L. H. 1989. Central nervous system vasculitis in Behçet's syndrome: angiographic improvement after therapy with cytotoxic agents. *Arthritis Rheum,* **32,** 217–20.

Olukemi A. Olugemo and Barney J. Stern

Introduction

Stroke is the third leading cause of death in the United States, and the leading cause of disability in the adult population. Most of the well-known risk factors for hemorrhagic and ischemic stroke can be controlled to some extent with medications and lifestyle and dietary modifications. In contrast, the contribution to stroke risk from disease entities such as inflammatory and infectious disorders may be less readily managed. One of the exceptional causes of stroke is granulomatous inflammation of primarily small and medium-sized blood vessels in patients with neurosarcoidosis.

Sarcoidosis is often referred to as a "disease of exclusion" (Gullapalli and Phillips, 2002). The definitive diagnosis of sarcoidosis requires histopathologic demonstration of noncaseating epithelioid granulomas that are not due to infection or malignancy.

Epidemiology of sarcoidosis

The term "sarkoid" was first coined in 1899 by Boeck, a Norwegian dermatologist, to describe a skin lesion that he thought resembled a sarcoma histologically. The disorder is now known to be a multisystem granulomatous disease of unknown etiology that primarily affects the lungs and the lymphatic system. Other typical organs affected include the skin, liver, eyes, heart, and the musculoskeletal system. Central nervous system (CNS) involvement occurs in approximately 5% of patients with sarcoidosis (Stern, 2004), although there have been reports of incidence as high as 26% (Allen *et al.*, 2003). Approximately 50% of patients with neurosarcoidosis present with neurologic disease at the time sarcoidosis is first diagnosed.

The incidence of sarcoidosis is approximately 40 per 100 000 persons. African Americans, Swedes, and Danes have the highest prevalence rates in the world (Burns, 2003). The disease affects both sexes almost equally. Young adults in the third to fourth decade of life are most likely to develop this disease, although sarcoidosis has been diagnosed in patients as young as 3 months and as old as 78 years. Both familial clustering of cases and the racial variation in epidemiology argue for the role of genetics in the pathogenesis of sarcoidosis.

Immunopathogenesis of sarcoidosis

Non-necrotizing granulomas in sarcoidosis comprise epithelioid cells, macrophages, lymphocytes, monocytes, and fibroblasts (Stern, 2004; Van Gundy and Sharma, 1987). The precise etiology of granuloma formation is unknown; however, it is widely accepted that sarcoidosis is caused by exaggerated immune responses. There has been speculation about various organisms such as mycobacteria, propionibacterium, borrelia, or viruses being potential triggers for the inflammatory response. Additionally, noninfectious agents such as beryllium, zirconium, and aluminum have also been implicated because of their ability to induce a granulomatous response (Moller and Chen, 2002b).

Much of the information now known about the immunopathogenesis of granuloma formation in sarcoidosis is gleaned from studies of patients with lung involvement, primarily through bronchoalveolar lavage specimens. The cascade of events begins with the deposition of a poorly soluble antigen that becomes the core of granuloma formation (Moller and Chen, 2002). Shortly after this step, there is an accumulation of T lymphocytes and mononuclear cells at the site of inflammation. These lymphocytes and other inflammatory cells secrete cytokines such as interleukin-2 (IL-2), interleukin-1 (IL-1), interferon-γ, and tumor necrosis factor (TNF-α). IL-2 promotes lymphocyte proliferation, and interferon-γ activates macrophages. TNF-α steers the inflammatory process towards fibrosis and granuloma formation. Cytokines lead to the differentiation of B cells, which further contributes to the inflammatory process. If these processes remain exuberant, obliterative fibrosis eventually develops. This is one potential mechanism that might be responsible for occlusion of vessels and subsequent cerebral infarction in patients with neurosarcoidosis.

Clinical manifestations of neurosarcoidosis

Patients can be classified as having possible, probable, or definite neurosarcoidosis based on the certainty of the diagnosis of multisystem sarcoidosis, the pattern of neurological disease, and the response to therapy. The following is adapted from Zajicek *et al.* (1999):

1. Possible: the clinical syndrome and neurodiagnostic evaluation are suggestive of neurosarcoidosis. Infection and malignancy have not been rigorously excluded, or there is no pathologic confirmation of systemic sarcoidosis.
2. Probable: the clinical syndrome and neurodiagnostic evaluation are suggestive of neurosarcoidosis, and alternative diagnoses have been excluded, especially infection and malignancy. There is pathologic evidence of systemic sarcoidosis.
3. Definite: (a) the clinical presentation is suggestive of neurosarcoidosis, other possible diagnoses are excluded, and there is the presence of supportive nervous system pathology; or (b) the

Uncommon Causes of Stroke, 2nd edition, ed. Louis R. Caplan. Published by Cambridge University Press.   © Cambridge University Press 2008.

criteria for a "probable" diagnosis are met, and the patient has had a beneficial response to therapy for neurosarcoidosis over a 1- to 2-year observation period.

As reviewed by Stern in 2004, the neurologic manifestations of sarcoidosis and their approximate frequencies are cranial neuropathies (overall 50–75%; facial palsy 25–50%); meningeal disease, including aseptic meningitis and mass lesion (10–25%); hydrocephalus (10%); parenchymal disease (overall 50%), including endocrinopathy, encephalopathy, vasculopathy (5–10%), seizures (5–10%), vegetative dysfunction, extramedullary or intramedullary spinal canal disease, and cauda equina syndrome; neuropathy (15%), including demyelinating, axonal, sensory, motor, sensorimotor, mononeuropathy multiplex, and Gullain–Barré syndrome; and lastly myopathy including nodule(s), polymyositis, and atrophy.

The entire CNS axis is vulnerable to granulomatous infiltration from neurosarcoidosis. Stroke is, however, an exceedingly rare complication of neurosarcoidosis, with very few case reports in the literature.

Pathophysiology and clinical presentations of stroke in sarcoidosis

One or more mechanisms may be responsible for the development of stroke in patients with neurosarcoidosis. These include small-vessel disease with *in situ* thrombosis from perivascular granulomatous inflammation, cardiogenic emboli caused by either restrictive or dilated cardiomyopathy and associated arrhythmias or conduction disturbances, large artery compression from adjacent granulomatous mass lesions, large artery inflammation with *in situ* thrombosis, and, possibly, artery-to-artery emboli.

Cytokines have been found to influence both procoagulant and anticoagulant pathways. Previous studies identified TNF-α, IL-1, IL-6, IL-12, and IL-2 as cytokines that can induce thrombin generation in human subjects. Van der Poll *et al.* (1990) discovered that TNF activates the common pathway of coagulation, probably induced through the extrinsic route. Paleolog *et al.* (1994) reported that "stimulation of endothelial cells in vitro by TNF-α increases the surface expression of leukocyte adhesion molecules, enhances cytokine production, and induces tissue factor procoagulant activity." They studied the actions of two surface receptors for TNF-α (p55 and p75) on endothelial cells, and found that "endothelial cell responses to TNF-α, such as expression of tissue factor and adhesion molecules for mononuclear cells, may be important in the pathogenesis of atherosclerosis, and are mediated predominantly, but not exclusively, by the p55 TNF receptor."

Other authors have reported abnormalities in fibrinolysis and coagulation in patients with sarcoidosis (Hasday *et al.*, 1988). These include increased tissue thromboplastin activity, decreased plasminogen activator activity, decreased protein C activity, increased factor VII activity, and increased thrombin-activatable fibrinolysis inhibitor. These observations provide additional explanations for the development of cerebral infarction in patients with neurosarcoidosis.

Although transient ischemic attacks (TIAs) and stroke rarely develop in patients with neurosarcoidosis, pathologic studies often show evidence of vascular involvement. Parenchymal granulomas can abut or encase arteries or veins. According to Brown *et al.*, (1989), numerous studies have shown "granulomatous invasion of the blood vessel walls, with vasculitic disruption of the media and the internal elastic lamina." Other reports have shown granulomatous vessel stenosis or occlusion, sometimes clearly associated with small brain infarcts. Rather than presenting with signs or symptoms of acute stroke, these patients had "a slowly progressive encephalopathy characterized by headache, seizures, confusion, dementia or coma" (Brown *et al.*, 1989). The discrepancy between the frequent neuropathological findings of vasculopathy and the rarity of clinical stroke in neurosarcoidosis may reflect the chronic nature of the inflammation.

Caplan *et al.* (1983) described pertinent neuro-ophthalmologic findings in two patients with postmortem granulomatous angiitis. The first patient was a 21-year-old man with biopsy-proven sarcoidosis involving the lymphatic system, lungs, eyes, and CNS. His initial presentation was the development of fever, cough, night sweats, and headache. He also had right eye uveitis. He responded to treatment with corticosteroids, but 6 months after his corticosteroids had been tapered, he had a relapse of headache, right eye pain, and blurry vision. Fundoscopic examination at that time revealed "bilateral optic disc edema, periphlebitis with sheathing, scattered peripheral exudates, and cells in the vitreous." Treatment with corticosteroids was re-initiated, but after a subsequent taper, the patient had a decline in gait and mental status, and died shortly after a diagnostic lumbar puncture was performed. Pathologic examination of the brain showed extensive herniation of the cerebellar tonsils; a swollen left hemisphere with several areas of discrete hemorrhage in the left cerebellar hemisphere, vermis, and pons; and multiple epithelioid granulomas throughout the meninges. These granulomatous changes affected the entire wall of veins and the adventitia of the arteries.

The second patient presented with hypopituitarism and transient episodes of slurred speech, right face and arm numbness, and trouble controlling the right arm. The spells lasted approximately 10–20 minutes. They were often preceded by an odd taste in the mouth. Electroencephalogram showed diffuse slowing. CT scan of the brain and bilateral carotid angiography showed no abnormalities. Multiple lumbar punctures revealed increased cerebrospinal fluid (CSF) protein and pleocytosis. The patient later developed acute shock and respiratory distress, and died approximately 18 months after his initial presentation. Pathologic studies revealed evidence of severe granulomatous meningitis. There were tiny white plaques on the surface of the brain, "milky perivenous exudates," "arterial cuffing by lymphocytes," and multiple infarcts of various ages in the anterior pituitary gland. Cultures for fungi, bacteria, tuberculosis, and viruses were all negative; hence the presumed diagnosis was neurosarcoidosis.

Other authors have reported the occurrence of angiitis in patients with sarcoidosis (Caplan *et al.*, 1983). The granulomas tend to involve the Virchow–Robin perivascular spaces and adventitia, sometimes extending into the media and intima of arteries. Panarteritis often leads to thrombosis. Veins can also become infiltrated with epithelioid cells, lymphocytes, and plasma cells (see Figures 12.1–12.3 for representative biopsy specimens).

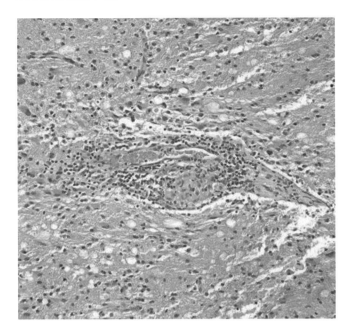

Figure 12.1 Photomicrograph of a frontal lobe biopsy specimen at 200 magnification showing perivascular lymphocytes and a collection of epithelioid histiocytes (i.e. granuloma). See color plate. (Courtesy of Dr. Rudy Castellani, Dept. of Pathology at University of Maryland School of Medicine.)

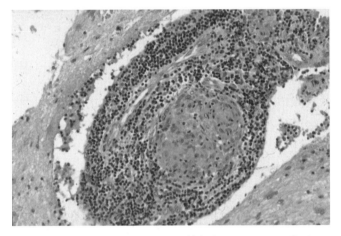

Figure 12.2 Photomicrograph of a temporal lobe biopsy at 60 magnification showing perivascular Virchow–Robin space infiltration by lymphocytes and one well-formed granuloma. See color plate. (Courtesy of Dr. Rudy Castellani, Dept. of Pathology at University of Maryland School of Medicine.)

Corse and Stern (1989) presented the case of a 38-year-old patient with biopsy-proven sarcoidosis involving the lungs, eyes, skin, and lymph nodes. The patient developed acute left hemiparesis after 2 weeks of transient neurologic deficits. Physical examination revealed a pure motor hemiparesis without any cortical signs. Brain CT and MRI showed an enhancing suprasellar mass adjacent to the internal carotid artery (ICA) and anterior cerebral artery (ACA). There was also an area of increased signal intensity in the posterior limb of the internal capsule on the T2-weighted MRI images. A transthoracic echocardiogram showed moderate concentric left ventricular hypertrophy and apical hypokinesis.

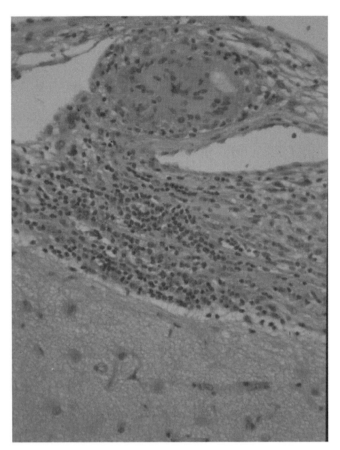

Figure 12.3 Photomicrograph at 60 magnification showing leptomeningeal, perivascular lymphocytic, and granulomatous infiltration, with gliosis of the molecular layer of the neocortex. See color plate. (Courtesy of Dr. Rudy Castellani, Dept. of Pathology at University of Maryland School of Medicine.)

Angiography demonstrated "a tapering stenosis of the right anterior cerebral artery." The patient's total cholesterol was slightly elevated at 240 mg/dL. Westergren sedimentation rate was also elevated at 37 mm/h (normal 0–8 mm/h). Examination of the CSF was consistent with inflammation. The total protein was 89 mg/dL, glucose 60 mg/dL, and white blood cell count 118 per mm^3 with 36% mononuclear cells and 64% polymorphonuclear cells. Immunoglobulin G (IgG) index was elevated at 0.79 (normal 0.34–0.66).

The patient was treated with oral prednisone for several months, and follow-up imaging showed a progressive decrease in the size of the suprasellar mass. The conclusion was drawn that the capsular infarct that this patient sustained was due to neurosarcoidosis.

A handful of other investigators have reported similar patients with focal recurrent neurological deficits attributable to neurosarcoidosis. Nakagaki *et al.* (2004) reported a 75-year-old woman with sarcoidosis who developed sudden weakness of the left arm and leg. Diffusion-weighted MRI showed an acute right parieto-occipital infarct, and a biopsy specimen from the occipital cortex revealed epithelioid granulomas without caseous necrosis. Dakdouki *et al.* (2005) reported a case of intracerebral bleeding in a patient with neurosarcoidosis while on corticosteroid therapy. This was the third of such known cases in the literature of intracerebral hemorrhage attributed to sarcoidosis. The authors propose an increase in vascular permeability as a potential mechanism of intracerebral hemorrhage in neurosarcoidosis.

Dural sinus thrombosis has also been reported in patients with neurosarcoidosis, presumably due to either an acquired coagulopathy or direct infiltration of the sinovenous system. Akova *et al.* (1993) reported a 35-year-old man with "pseudotumor cerebri" and meningeal sarcoidosis as the presenting feature of neurosarcoidosis. The patient initially presented with diabetes insipidus (polyuria and polydipsia), followed by horizontal diplopia and left gaze palsy within 1 month. Of note, there was a 6-year history of severe occipital headaches and convulsions without any identified etiology. A lumbar puncture performed approximately 3 months after diabetes insipidus ensued was notable for an opening pressure of 340 mm H_2O, protein of 62 mg/dL, glucose of 41 mg/dL, and elevation of IgG levels in the serum and CSF. Chest radiography was normal, but a gallium scan revealed bilateral perihilar involvement. CT showed a left occipital infarct, and MRI revealed diffuse leptomeningeal enhancement, pituitary gland enlargement, left occipital and subtemporal infarcts, and sagittal sinus thrombosis (confirmed by digital subtraction angiography). The patient's symptoms improved rapidly after treatment with 80 mg of prednisone per day. Table 12.1 shows selected cases of TIA or clinical stroke in patients with neurosarcoidosis. Additionally, a representative brain MRI and magnetic resonance angiography (MRA) of a patient with neurosarcoidosis and stroke involving the anterior circulation is illustrated in Figure 12.4.

Treatment

Corticosteroids are the mainstay of treatment for patients with symptomatic neurosarcoidosis; however, the severity and chronicity of this disease in some patients often leads to reluctance in subjecting patients to the long-term sequelae of corticosteroid treatment. Furthermore, corticosteroid therapy can lead to diabetes mellitus, which can lead to atherosclerosis and endothelial dysfunction (Iuchi *et al.*, 2003; Molnar *et al.*, 2002).

There is a body of evidence, mostly gathered from case series and expert opinions, that treatment with other forms of immune-modulating drugs can shorten exacerbations and alleviate symptoms. Examples of such adjunct or alternative drugs include methotrexate, cyclophosphamide, azathioprine, cyclosporine, mycophenolate mofetil, and chlorambucil (Stern, 2004). Pentoxifylline (Trental) inhibits TNF-α production from macrophages in patients with sarcoidosis (Baughman and Lower, 1997). Other agents that antagonize TNF-α include thalidomide and infliximab (Remicade). None of these drugs have been subjected to controlled clinical trials, largely because of the low prevalence of patients with the relapsing or chronic form of sarcoidosis and, from the perspective of this chapter, the rarity of sarcoidosis-associated stroke syndromes. Nonetheless, it is reasonable to decrease sarcoidosis-associated inflammation to decrease stroke risk. What represents the best strategy is unknown, but anecdotal evidence suggests that concurrent use of corticosteroids and adjunctive agents is a reasonable approach (Stern,

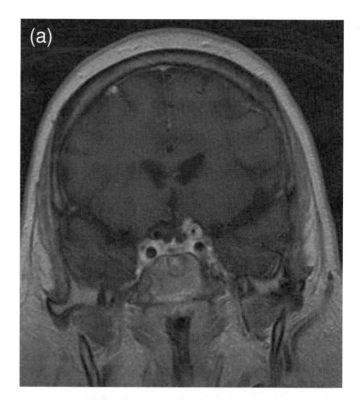

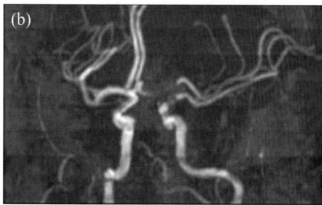

Figure 12.4 a and **b**. CNS sarcoidosis. Stroke developed on prednisone 10 mg/day. Note encasement of left ICA on MRI and abnormal ICA and ACA on MRA.

2004). Because TNF-α plays a central role in both sarcoidosis-associated inflammation and inflammation-associated thrombogenicity, it may be reasonable to consider agents that specifically decrease TNF-α activity.

In those patients who have had an ischemic infarct that can be directly attributed to neurosarcoidosis, the question of acute treatment strategies and additional preventative regimens will arise. Are acute therapies such as intravenous thrombolytics using tissue plasminogen activator or intra-arterial lysis of fresh clot contraindicated, given the underlying inflammatory process? What role do antiplatelet medications such as aspirin or clopidogrel play in these patients, if any? Should patients receive warfarin due to the association of exaggerated coagulation with cytokine production in sarcoidosis? Lastly, will the rapidly growing trend of stenting

Table 12.1 Selected cases of stroke or TIAs in neurosarcoidosis

Etiology of stroke	Age at onset of sarcoidosis	Age at onset of first stroke or TIA	Race/Sex	Systemic disease	Neurologic manifestation	Relevant diagnostic tests	Treatment and outcome
Large Artery							
Nakagaki *et al.*, 2004	Unknown	75	Asian/F	Lymphatic system	Hemiparesis, hyperreflexia hypesthesia disorientation psychosis	+MRI +EEG +CSF +Biopsy of lymph node and brain	Prednisone Improved psychosis and encephalopathy
Small Artery							
Corse and Stern, 1989	25	38	White/M	Lungs, eyes, skin, lymph nodes	Hemiparesis, hyperreflexia	−ACE +MRI brain +angiography	Prednisone Resolution of symptoms at 4 weeks
Brown *et al.*, 1989	6	25	Black/M	Lungs	Recurrent CN VII palsy, numbness, hemiparesis, hyperreflexia	+Kveim +ACE +PFTs +bronchoscopy −Lung biopsy −CSF	None Resolution of weakness at 4 weeks
Sinovenous disease							
Akova *et al.*, 1993	29	35	Asian/M	Lungs, eyes	Vision loss, gaze palsy, headache, convulsions polydipsia, polyuria	+CSF +CT +MRI	Steroids Ocular and systemic recovery
Sethi *et al.*, 1986	40	43	U/M	None	Aphasia, weakness, numbness, incontinence, headache	+CSF +CT +cerebral angiography +Brain biopsy −EEG, CXR	Steroids Resolution of intracerebral mass; cessation of TIA symptoms
Intracranial hemorrhage							
Dakdouki *et al.*, 2005	25	25	Asian/M	Lung, liver	CN III, X palsies, headache, diplopia, gait disturbance	+ACE +CXR +BAL and bronchial biopsy +MRI brain	Prednisone and methotrexate Remission in 12 months
Berek *et al.*, 1993	35	35	U/M	None	Blurred vision, bitemporal hemianopia	+ACE in CSF +Visual evoked potentials +CT +MRI	Steroids. Complete recovery

Key: ACE, angiotensin-converting enzyme; BAL, bronchoalveolar lavage; CXR, chest x-ray; EEG, electroencephalogram; PFTs, pulmonary function tests; U, unknown.

intra- or extracranial stenotic lesions benefit patients with large-artery granulomatous angiitis or cause more harm in patients who are already susceptible to vascular injury and may have compromised vascular integrity?

These questions, although currently unanswered, will likely be the subject of further investigations, as more progress is being made in understanding the pathogenesis of neurosarcoidosis and stroke. The authors have used antiplatelet agents as a stroke-preventive strategy but have avoided thrombolytic interventions. It is prudent to address all other applicable stroke risk factors to treat these patients.

Prognosis

There is significant variation in the morbidity and mortality of those persons affected with sarcoidosis. African Americans tend to be younger at the time of diagnosis, have increased rates of pulmonary involvement, and present with more severe disease. Children with sarcoidosis have the same organ involvement as adults but a more favorable prognosis. Spontaneous remission occurs in approximately two thirds of patients. Others have either a relapsing remitting course or a chronic progressive course, especially patients with parenchymal brain and spinal cord disease and optic nerve involvement. Personal observations suggest that patients with large and small artery and sinovenous compromise have a guarded prognosis.

REFERENCES

Akova, Y. A., Kansu, T., and Duman, S. 1993. Pseudotumor cerebri secondary to dural sinus thrombosis in neurosarcoidosis. *J Clin Neuroophthalmol*, **13**, 188–9.

Allen, R. K. A., Sellars, R. E., and Sandstrom, P. A. 2003. A prospective study of 32 patients with neurosarcoidosis. *Sarcoidosis Vasc Diffuse Lung Dis*, **20**, 118–25.

Baughman, R. P., and Lower, E. E. 1997. Steroid-sparing alternative treatments for sarcoidosis. *Clin Chest Med*, **18**, 853–64.

Berek, K., Kiechl, S., Willeit, J., *et al*. 1993. Subarachnoid hemorrhage as presenting feature of isolated neurosarcoidosis. *Clin Investig*, **71**, 54–6.

Boeck, C. 1899. Multiple benign sarkoid of the skin. *J Cutan Dis*, **17**, 543–50.

Brown, M. M., Thompson, A. J., Wedzicha, J. A., and Swash, M. 1989. Sarcoidosis presenting with stroke. *Stroke*, **20**, 400–5.

Burns, T. M. 2003. Neurosarcoidosis. *Arch Neurol*, **60**, 1166–8.

Caplan, L., Corbett, J., Goodwin, J., *et al*. 1983. Neuro-ophthalmologic signs in the angiitic form of neurosarcoidosis. *Neurology*, **33**, 1130–5.

Corse, A. M., and Stern, B. J. 1989. Neurosarcoidosis and stroke. *Stroke*, **20**, 152–3.

Dakdouki, G. K., Kanafani, Z. A., Ishak, G., Hourani, M., and Kanj, S. S. 2005. Intracerebral bleeding in a patient with neurosarcoidosis while on corticosteroid therapy. *South Med J*, **98**, 492–4.

Gullapalli, D., and Phillips, L. H. 2002. Neurologic manifestations of sarcoidosis. *Neurol Clin*, **20**, 59–83.

Hasday, J. D., Bachwich, P. R., Lynch, J. P., *et al*. 1988. Procoagulant and plasminogen activator activities of bronchoalveolar fluid in patients with pulmonary sarcoidosis. *Exp Lung Res*, **14**, 261–78.

Iuchi, T., Akaike, M., Mitsui, T., *et al*. 2003. Glucocorticoid excess induces superoxide production in vascular endothelial cells and elicits vascular endothelial dysfunction. *Circ Res*, **92**, 81–7.

Matsumoto, K., Awata, S., Matsuoka, H., Nakamura, S., and Sato, M. 1998. Chronological changes in brain MRI, SPECT, and EEG in neurosarcoidosis with stroke-like episodes. *Psychiatry Clin Neurosci*, **52**, 629–33.

Moller, D. R., and Chen, E. C. 2002a. Genetic basis of remitting sarcoidosis: triumph of the trimolecular complex? *Am J Respir Cell Mol Biol*, **27**, 391–5.

Moller, D. R., and Chen, E. C. 2002b. What causes sarcoidosis? *Curr Opin Pulm Med*, **8**, 429–34.

Molnar, J., Nijland, M. J., Howe, D., and Nathanielsz, P. W. 2002. Evidence for microvascular dysfunction after prenatal dexamethasone at 0.7, 0.75, and 0.8 gestation in sheep. *Am J Physiol Regul Integr Comp Physiol*, **283**, R561–7.

Nakagaki, H., Furuya, J., Nagata T., *et al*. 2004. An elder case of neurosarcoidosis associated with brain infarction. *Rinsho Shinkeigaku*, **44**, 81–5.

Paleolog, E. M., Delasalle, S. A., Buurman, W. A., Feldmann, M. 1994. Functional activities of receptors for tumor necrosis factor-alpha on human vascular endothelial cells. *Blood*, **84**, 2578–90.

Russegger, L., Weiser, G., Twerdy, K., and Grunert, V. 1986. Neurosarcoid reaction in association with a ruptured ACA aneurysm. *Neurochirurgia*, **29**, 42–4.

Sethi, K. D., el Gammal, T., Patel, B. R., and Swift, T. R. 1986. Dural sarcoidosis presenting with transient neurologic symptoms. *Arch Neurol*, **43**, 595–7.

Sharma, O. P. 2001. Tumor necrosis factor polymorphism in sarcoidosis. *Chest*, **119**, 678–9.

Stern, B. J. 2004. Neurological complications of sarcoidosis. *Curr Opin Neurol*, **17**, 311–6.

Van der Poll T., Büller, H. R., ten Cate, H., *et al*. 1990. Activation of coagulation after administration of tumor necrosis factor to normal subjects. *N Engl J Med*, **322**, 1622–7.

Van Gundy, K., and Sharma, O. P. 1987. Pathogenesis of sarcoidosis. *West J Med*, **147**, 168–74.

Zajicek, J. P., Scolding, N. J., Foster, O., *et al*. 1999. Central nervous system sarcoidosis: diagnosis and management. *Q J Med*, **92**, 103–17.

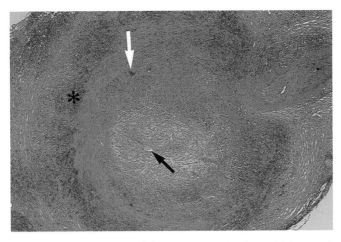

Figure 2.1 Low-powered view of the transverse section of superficial temporal artery with features of giant cell arteritis. There is a slit-like lumen (*black arrow*) due to intimal swelling, with disruption of the internal elastic lamina (*) and scattered, multinucleated giant cells (*white arrow*).

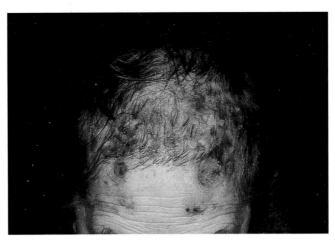

Figure 2.3 Extensive scalp necrosis in a patient with biopsy-proven temporal arteritis.

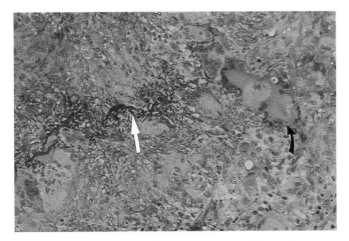

Figure 2.2 High-powered view of disrupted internal elastic lamina (*white arrow*), with multinucleated giant cell (*black arrow*).

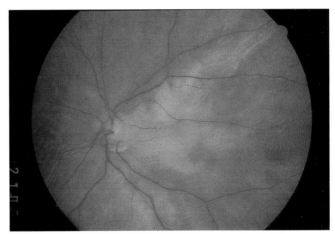

Figure 2.4 Ischemic optic neuropathy with a swollen, pale optic disc and extensive pallor of the adjacent choroid.

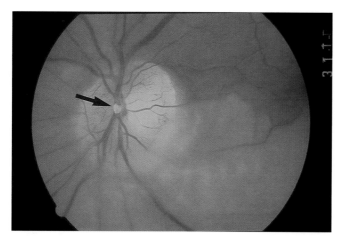

Figure 2.5 Large embolus in the central retinal artery (*arrow*).

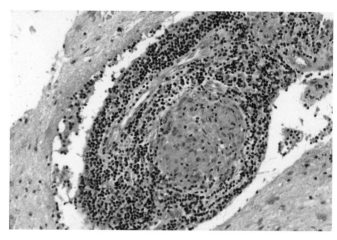

Figure 12.2 Photomicrograph of a temporal lobe biopsy at 60 magnification showing perivascular Virchow–Robin space infiltration by lymphocytes and one well-formed granuloma. [Courtesy of Dr. Rudy Castellani, Dept. of Pathology at University of Maryland School of Medicine.]

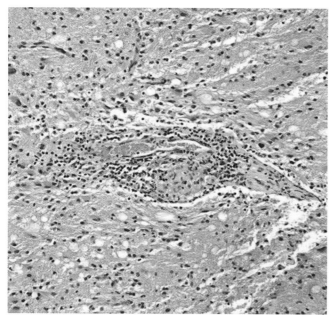

Figure 12.1 Photomicrograph of a frontal lobe biopsy specimen at 200 magnification showing perivascular lymphocytes and a collection of epithelioid histiocytes (i.e. granuloma). [Courtesy of Dr. Rudy Castellani, Dept. of Pathology at University of Maryland School of Medicine.]

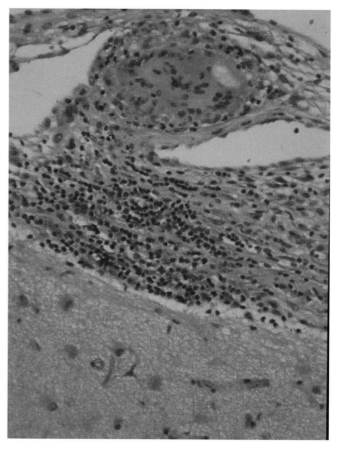

Figure 12.3 Photomicrograph at 60 magnification showing leptomeningeal, perivascular lymphocytic, and granulomatous infiltration, with gliosis of the molecular layer of the neocortex. [Courtesy of Dr. Rudy Castellani, Dept. of Pathology at University of Maryland School of Medicine.]

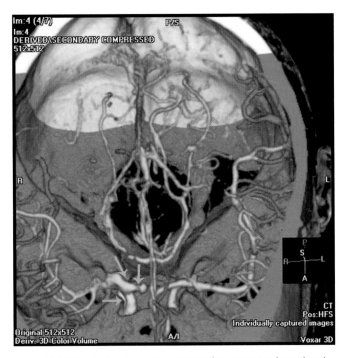

Figure 15.2 CT cerebral angiogram in patient with HIV-associated vasculopathy with fusiform dilatation of the right distal supraclinoid internal carotid (*bottom arrow*) and proximal M1 and A1 segments of the right middle and anterior cerebral artery (*top left arrow*). There is a postdilatation stenosis and occlusion of the right anterior cerebral artery (*top right arrow*).

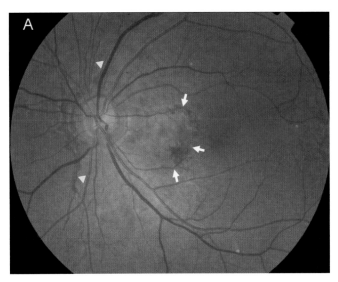

Figure 21.3 Funduscopic findings of a patient with PXE. Angioid streaks (*arrow heads*) radiating from the optic disk and mottling of the temporal retina are conspicuous. Angioid streak represents the rupture of Bruch's membrane. Notice the development of choroidal neovascular membrane (*arrows*) secondary to angioid streak. (Image courtesy of Professor Se Woong Kang, MD, Sungkyunkwan University School of Medicine, Seoul, Korea.)

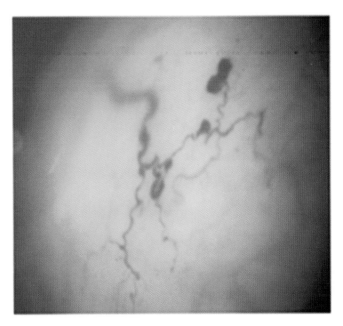

Figure 19.1 Abnormal conjunctival vessels in a man with Fabry's disease. (Courtesy of Dr. Alan H. Friedman, M. D., Department of Ophthalmology, The Mount Sinai School of Medicine).

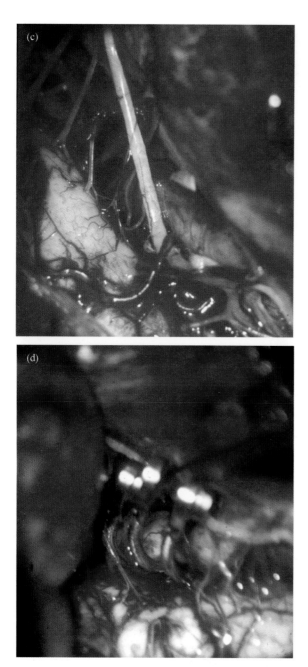

Figure 27.2 A 53-year-old man presenting with posterior inferior cerebellar artery infarct related to vertebral artery fusiform aneurysm: vertebral arteriogram and intraoperative photograph demonstrating obliteration of aneurysm and preservation of vertebral artery lumen with three fenestrated clips placed in a "picket-fence" fashion.

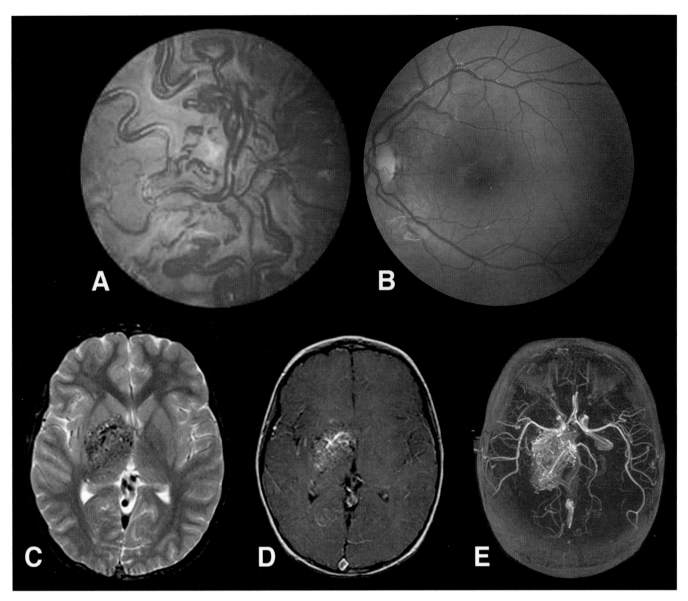

Figure 32.1 WMS. **A**. Fundus photograph of the right eye shows tortuous arteriovenous anastomoses centered over the optic disc and extending to the equator of the eye. **B**. Fundus photograph of the left eye is normal. **C**. T2-weighted axial MRI with fat suppression shows flow voids in the right basal ganglia and thalamus, consistent with a large AVM. **D**. Enhanced T1-weighted axial MRI shows high signal in areas of anomalous vessels. **E**. Three-dimensional reformatted magnetic resonance angiogram, viewed from above, shows an AVM. (Reprinted with permission from Reck, S. D., Zacks, D. N., and Eibschitz-Tsimhoni, M. 2005. Retinal and intracranial arteriovenous malformations: Wyburn-Mason syndrome. *J Neuro-Ophthalmol*, **25**, 205–8.)

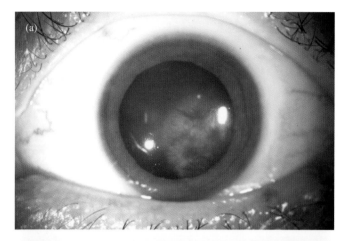

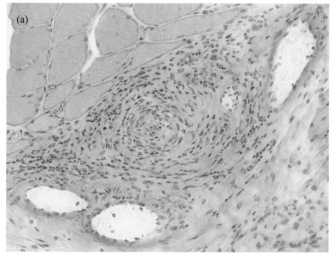

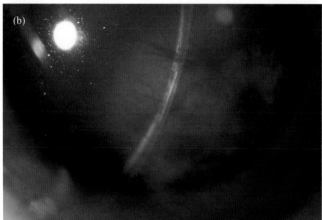

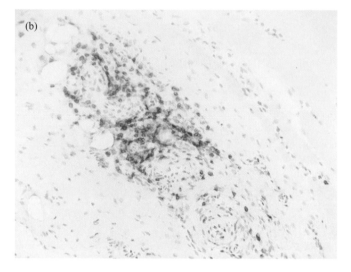

Figure 37.1 a and **b**. Interstitial keratitis in Cogan's syndrome. Slit-lamp examination showing corneal stromal opacities.

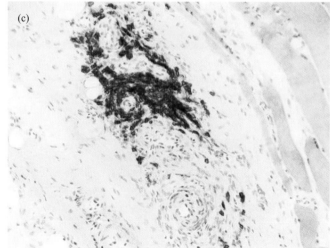

Figure 43.3 Muscular biopsy of Patient 6, 2004, Lausanne. Hematoxylin and eosin staining shows typical inflammation of a small-sized artery, with perivascular inflammation (**A**). Staining for CD3 confirms T lymphocytes infiltration (**B**). Staining for CD20 shows B lymphocyte infiltration (**C**). Figures courtesy of Prof. R. Janzer, Department of Pathology, Lausanne.

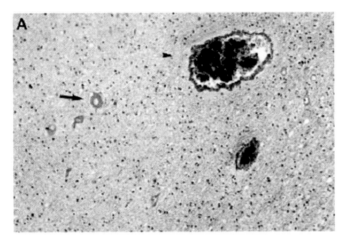

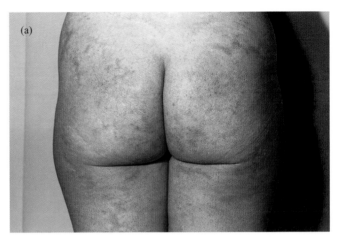

Figure 43.4 Microscopic examination of cerebral arteries of Patient 1, 1982, Lausanne (Van Gieson-Luxol), showing arterial wall fibrosis (*purple-red*) of arterioles and small arteries with fibrosis of the media and adventitia (*full arrow*). Two small venules (*arrowhead*) are normal. (Reichhart *et al.*, 2000).

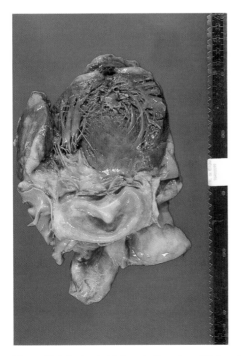

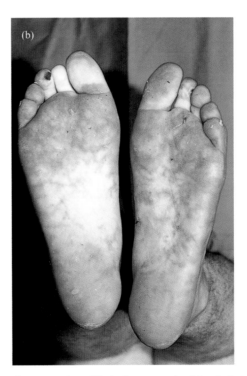

Figure 56.1 (a and **b)** Livedo racemosa involving the buttocks, feet, and lower legs in two SS patients. (Courtesy of Prof. J.-M. Naeyaert, Ghent University Hospital.)

Figure 50.1 Nonbacterial thrombotic endocarditis in patients with adenocarcinoma of the lung.

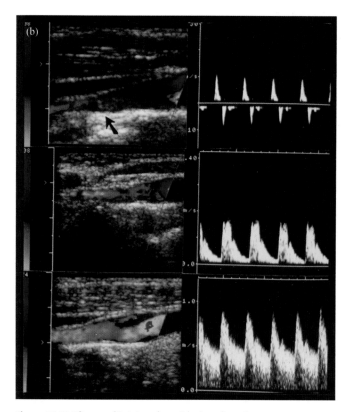

Figure 60.15 Ultrasound in internal carotid artery dissection.

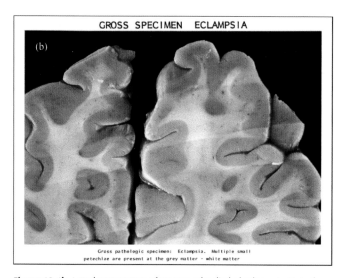

Figure 68.6b Actual postmortem of woman who died of eclampsia. Note the small petechial hemorrhages at the gray-white junction. From Digre *et al.*, 1993 with permission. Copyright © 1993, American Medical Association. All rights reserved.

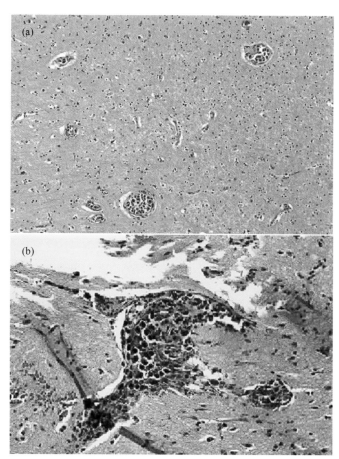

Figure 70.1 (**a**) Hematoxylin and eosin staining showing lymphocyte accumulation in small to medium-sized vessels in the brain. (**b**) Higher power hematoxylin and eosin staining showing lymphocyte accumulation in small to medium-sized vessels in the brain.

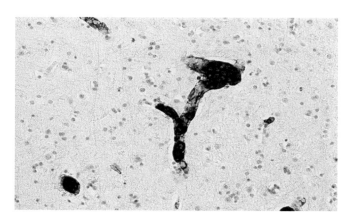

Figure 70.2 The tumor cells within the vessels stain with B-cell marker CD20.

13 KAWASAKI DISEASE: CEREBROVASCULAR AND NEUROLOGIC COMPLICATIONS

Jonathan Lipton and Michael J. Rivkin

Introduction

Kawasaki (1967) first described the "mucocutaneous lymph node syndrome" that now bears his name. Kawasaki disease comprises a usually self-limited, necrotizing, panvasculitis that affects vessels of the entire body, most notably, the coronary arteries. Vessels of the nervous system can also be affected, although the aneurysms that ravage the coronary vessels have only rarely been described in the brain (Amano and Hazama, 1980; Amano *et al.*, 1979b; Bell *et al.*, 1983; Ferro, 1998; Morens and O'Brien, 1978). The diagnosis and treatment of Kawasaki disease has advanced with concomitant improvement in prognosis. However, the cause of the disease remains unknown. Neurological signs and symptoms are common in Kawasaki disease and most often include aseptic meningitis, encephalopathy, and sensorineural hearing loss. Stroke has been described but is extremely rare. The long-term neurological sequelae of Kawasaki disease have not been fully determined.

Etiology

The etiology of Kawasaki disease is unknown although an infectious agent has long been suspected based on available epidemiologic evidence (Burns *et al.*, 2000; Shulman and Rowley, 1997; Yanagawa *et al.*, 2001, 2006). The disease tends to occur in localized epidemics, and the incidence of disease among family members significantly surpasses that of the general population. Further support for the infectious hypothesis derives from the observation that the disease has not been observed in neonates and only rarely in adults, thus, suggesting universally acquired immunity and the passive transfer of protective maternal antibodies against a ubiquitous transmissible agent. Finally, recurrence is unusual, arguing against an autoimmune process.

Kawasaki disease occurs in all races, but individuals of Asian descent have repeatedly been shown to be more susceptible, irrespective of either their geographic origin or location. As a result, many have considered that this suggests a genetic predisposition to Kawasaki disease in this population (Bell *et al.*, 1983; Kawasaki, 1967; Kawasaki *et al.*, 1974; Morens and O'Brien, 1978; Newburger *et al.*, 2004b; Shulman and Rowley, 1997; Yanagawa *et al.*, 2006).

Epidemiology

About 80% of instances of Kawasaki disease occur in children younger than 5 years, and most affected children are younger than 2 years at time of diagnosis. Rare occurrences of Kawasaki disease have been reported in adolescents and adults (Jackson *et al.*, 1994; Rauch, 1989). Boys are affected 1.5 times more often than are girls; this sexually dimorphic pattern of disease prevalence further suggests an underlying genetic influence on disease susceptibility.

Death due to Kawasaki disease occurs as a result of myocardial infarction or sudden unexplained cardiac death. The estimated in-hospital case fatality rate in the United States is 0.17%, virtually all the result of cardiac disease (Chang, 2002). Sudden death has been reported even years after disease remission in children who had a significant burden of coronary disease or myocardial infarction prior to symptom resolution (Newburger *et al.*, 2004b).

Pathogenesis

Kawasaki disease is classified as a systemic panvasculitis of medium-sized vessels (Dillon and Ozen, 2006). The observed necrotizing endarteritis in Kawasaki disease has often been compared to the infantile form of polyarteritis nodosa. Kawasaki disease and infantile polyarteritis nodosa are pathologically and clinically similar. Polyarteritis nodosa is characterized by skin biopsy–proven endarteritis, and at least two of the following: myalgia, systemic hypertension, testicular pain or tenderness, livedo reticularis, or subcutaneous nodules (Dillon and Ozen, 2006; Ozen *et al.*, 2006). Peripheral nervous system involvement in polyarteritis nodosa is present in about 70% of patients. In contrast to that in Kawasaki disease, the clinical course in polyarteritis nodosa tends to be chronic.

Although involvement of the intracranial vasculature has been shown in Kawasaki disease, it is infrequently described in the literature due to the low mortality rate of this disorder. The most complete neuropathological evaluations were performed on autopsy specimens of patients severely affected with coronary disease, all of whom died from cardiac death (Amano and Hazama, 1980; Amano *et al.*, 1979b). In these patients, carotid disease was observed in 79%, and involvement of the aorta was seen in 75%.

Several stages of vascular involvement have been described. First, the arterial lesions are characterized by endothelial cell degeneration and hyperplasia with fibrin mass, platelet deposition, and swelling of the internal elastic lamina. Necrotizing panarteritis develops next, characterized by predominant lymphocytic infiltration with desquamation and degeneration of the endothelium. Eventually, granulation and scar formation develop in the vessel wall. These developments are the hypothesized harbingers of vascular aneurysm development. When these aneurysms develop, they are located in the coronary arteries, most often in the main coronary artery (Amano *et al.*, 1979a).

Neuropathology from children with prominent CNS involvement demonstrates swollen, edematous brain with dilation of subarachnoid vessels and thickening of the leptomeninges. The meninges were infiltrated with lymphocytes and mononuclear cells. Necrosis within the brain parenchyma with a "spongy" quality has been described (Amano *et al.*, 1980). Infiltration of the parasympathetic ganglion with atrophy, inflammation, and degeneration has also been described (Amano and Hazama, 1980).

Clinical manifestations and diagnosis

Patients are almost always children younger than five years who present with unexplained sustained high fever, polymorphous rash, mucous membrane inflammation, conjunctivitis, acral extremity changes (particularly of the fingers), and cervical adenopathy. Fully, 15–20% of untreated patients develop aneurysms of the coronary vessels (Amano *et al.*, 1979a, 1979b; Newburger *et al.*, 2004b). These complications of Kawasaki disease constitute one of the most intensively studied aspects of the disorder and remain a leading cause of cardiac death in children (Newburger *et al.*, 2004b).

There is no definitive diagnostic test for Kawasaki disease. Diagnosis is clinically based on evolving diagnostic criteria (Newburger *et al.*, 2004b). Four of the following five criteria must be met after establishing the persistence of fever for 5 consecutive days: bilateral conjunctivitis, changes in mucous membranes, peripheral edema and/or erythema and/or periungual desquamation, polymorphous rash, and cervical adenopathy (Burns *et al.*, 2000; Dajani *et al.*, 1993; Dillon and Ozen, 2006; Mason and Burns, 1997; Morens and O'Brien, 1978; Newburger *et al.*, 2004b; Ozen *et al.*, 2006).

Natural history

The acute phase of illness is heralded by an erratic, high fever that may be prolonged (up to 3 or 4 weeks) while remaining unresponsive to antipyretics or antibiotics (Kawasaki, 1967; Kawasaki *et al.*, 1974; Newburger *et al.*, 2004a, 2004b). A non-exudative conjunctivitis appears within the first 48 hours of fever. Erythema of the oral mucosa with cracking of the labial, buccal, and pharyngeal mucosa is frequent. Prominent involvement of the vallate papillae of the tongue creates the classically described "strawberry tongue," also seen with scarlet fever. Confluent, erythematous lesions of the palms and soles, perineal area, and prominent, painful swelling of the hands and feet are common. Finally, cervical adenopathy featuring nodes 1.5 cm or larger can be found, often in a unilateral array. Acute cervical lymphadenopathy occurs in 50–75% of patients. Because these symptoms are shared by other viral exanthems of childhood, diagnosis can be challenging, especially in the youngest children in whom viral syndromes or meningitis is often suspected at presentation.

Other manifestations of Kawasaki disease appear later. Coronary artery aneurysms are usually detected days to weeks after symptom onset but may also be present during the acute phase. Most patients have some degree of left ventricular dysfunction

(Mason, 1997). Later in the convalescent period, subungual membranous desquamation occurs. Transverse grooves in the fingernails, known as "Beau's lines," can be seen 1–2 weeks after fever initiation and are thought to be the manifestation of arrested nail growth during the acute phase of disease.

Many laboratory abnormalities have been reported in Kawasaki disease including thrombocytosis, elevation in liver enzymes, and alteration in lipid profile. Specifically, there is a depression in plasma total cholesterol and high-density lipoprotein (HDL) cholesterol with a concomitant elevation in triglycerides (Newburger *et al.*, 1991a). The relevance of these findings to the incidence of neurological sequelae and stroke in Kawasaki disease patients is unknown.

Neurology of Kawasaki disease

Although neurological symptoms at presentation are varied, a mild encephalopathy in young children with fever and irritability sometimes occurs and may mimic viral meningitis (Newburger *et al.*, 2004b). Aseptic meningitis is estimated to occur in 30–50% of Kawasaki disease patients, most often during the first 30 days of illness (Amano and Hazama, 1980; Amano *et al.*, 1980; Kawasaki, 1967; Kawasaki *et al.*, 1974). One retrospective study found cerebrospinal fluid (CSF) pleocytosis in 39% of patients with a median white blood cell count of $22.5/mm^3$, featuring a monocytosis. CSF glucose was less than 45 mg/dL in 2.2%, and CSF protein was "elevated" in 17.4% (Dengler *et al.*, 1998). We could find only one reported case of focal neurological symptoms described as the presenting feature of Kawasaki disease (Table 13.1). Tabarki *et al.* (2001) reported a 4-year-old child who had a febrile illness with coronary aneurysms who developed hemiparesis and at subsequent follow-up had persistent myoclonic seizures and autistic features. The etiological relationship between the patient's Kawasaki disease and the neuropsychiatric morbidity is unclear in this patient.

Other neurological complications of Kawasaki disease include myositis, peripheral facial palsy, hearing loss, subdural hemorrhage, ischemic stroke, moyamoya disease, and seizures (Amano and Hazama, 1980; Bailie *et al.*, 2001; Fujiwara *et al.*, 1992; Knott *et al.*, 2001; Koutras, 1982; Lapointe *et al.*, 1984; Laxer *et al.*, 1984; Suda *et al.*, 2003; Tabarki *et al.*, 2001; Tanaka *et al.*, 2007; Templeton and Dunne, 1987; Terasawa *et al.*, 1983; Wada *et al.*, 2006). Overall, neurological symptoms other than mild encephalopathy are uncommon and their long-term sequelae poorly understood. There have been few systematic studies concerning nervous system involvement in Kawasaki disease. The largest of these is a Japanese study in which focal neurological deficits were reported in 6 of 540 (1.1%) patients. Two of these children had hemiplegia, and four had lower motor neuron facial palsy. In the two former cases, hemiplegia developed in a distribution consistent with stroke; however, no evidence of infarction was disclosed on neuroimaging in either case. One patient showed only mild ventriculomegaly and enlargement of the extra-axial spaces; arteriography did not show aneurysms in either the carotid or vertebral arterial systems. The hemiparesis completely resolved in both patients when seen at follow-up 2 months later (Table 13.1) (Terasawa *et al.*, 1983).

Table 13.1 Case reports of hemiparesis or stroke in children with Kawasaki disease

Reference	Age/Sex (in months)	Symptoms	Imaging Findings	CAA Present	Outcome
Hosaki et al., 1978	4/M	HP	Occlusion of MCA	Yes	Myoclonic seizures
Lauret et al., 1979	60/F	HP, hemianopsia	Right ICA occlusion	NA	NA
Terasawa et al., 1983	24/F	HP	Extra-axial space and ventricular enlargement	Yes	HP resolved at 2 mo
Terasawa et al., 1983	5/M	HP	Increased extra-axial spaces	Yes	HP resolved at 1 mo
Boespflug et al., 1984	9/F	HP	NA	Yes, MI	NA
Lapointe et al., 1984	4/M	Seizure, HP	MCA branch occlusion.	Yes	11-mo follow-up angio recanalization of occluded MCA branches Mild left HP at age 5 y
Laxer et al., 1984	26/F	Seizure, HP, hemianopsia	MCA branch, low flow	Yes	Choreo-athetosis of right arm, mild spastic HP at 5 y of age
Laxer et al., 1984	5	HP, seizure	Right MCA branch occlusion	Yes	Left HP at 5 y, cognitive delay
Templeton and Dunne, 1987	6/NA	HP	MCA infarction (total)	Yes, with mural aneurysm	Sudden death 1 d post presentation
Fujiwara et al., 1992	22/M	Asymptomatic	Right caudate, putamen infarction	Yes, giant	NA
Tabarki et al., 2001	48/F	Seizure, HP	Normal MRI at presentation Diffuse atrophy at 12 mo	Yes	Hemiparesis resolved by 3 mo. At 12 mo, autistic features noted; seizures, bilateral sensorineural hearing loss
Suda et al., 2003	8/M	HP	CT / NA	Yes	NA
Wada et al., 2006	36/M	HP, "motor aphasia"	MRI:T2 hyperintensity in area of posterior branch left MCA No vessel imaging reported	No	Complete recovery at 12 mo
Muneuchi et al., 2006	48/M	Asymptomatic	Likely cerebellar hemispheric infarct with absence of PICA flow void on MRA	Yes	NA

Key: HP, hemiparesis; MCA, middle cerebral artery; ICA, internal carotid artery; CAA, coronary artery aneurysm; MI, myocardial infarction; NA, not available; PICA; MRA, magnetic resonance angiography.

Stroke

Although stroke in patients with Kawasaki disease has not been methodically studied, several reports exist of hemiparesis in children diagnosed with Kawasaki disease, some of which include angiographically diagnosed vascular lesion(s) (see Table 13.1) (Beiser et al., 1998; Boespflug et al., 1984; Fujiwara et al., 1992; Hosaki et al., 1978; Lapointe et al., 1984; Laxer et al., 1984; Lauret et al., 1979; Muneuchi et al., 2006; Suda et al., 2003; Tabarki et al., 2001; Templeton and Dunne, 1987; Terasawa et al., 1983). In virtually all patients, coronary aneurysms were present. Importantly,

cerebral aneurysms have not been detected despite the occurrence of coronary aneurysms and, in some patients, aneurysms elsewhere in the vascular tree (Lapointe et al., 1984). The reason for the apparent sparing of the cerebral vasculature from aneurysm formation in Kawasaki disease is unknown. One isolated report describes a child with a history of Kawasaki disease who developed a noncongenital posterior cerebral artery aneurysm with subsequent postoperative stroke. However, it is uncertain whether the occurrence of Kawasaki disease contributed to the aneurysm discovered years later (Tanaka et al., 2007).

One group posits that changes in cerebral perfusion may exist in patients without signs, symptoms, or neuroradiological evidence of infarction (Ichiyama *et al.*, 1998). This limited prospective study of brain perfusion characteristics in acute Kawasaki disease using single photon emission computed tomography showed localized hypoperfusion in 6 of 21 (28.6%) neurologically asymptomatic children (Ichiyama *et al.*, 1998). One patient had transient mitral regurgitation on echocardiography, whereas the remainder of the group had neither cardiac lesion nor dysfunction. Despite the finding of diffuse hypoperfusion, no angiographic data that support an underlying vascular etiology could be found. Our review of the literature reveals no report of stroke in Kawasaki disease patients in whom MRA or conventional angiogram showed vascular lesions typical of a diffuse CNS vasculopathy such as primary CNS angiitis (Benseler *et al.*, 2006). Further investigation is needed.

There are two case reports of asymptomatic brain infarction in children with Kawasaki disease (Fujiwara *et al.*, 1992; Muneuchi *et al.*, 2006). Coronary artery aneurysms were identified in both patients. These reports raise the important possibility that neurologic sequelae (stroke specifically) may be underestimated in Kawasaki disease. Most Kawasaki disease patients with hemiparesis also developed coronary aneurysms regardless of the presence of documented brain infarction. This association suggests that the mechanism of stroke in these patients may be related to the concomitant presence of heart disease. Thus, thorough clinical neurological investigation of all patients with coronary involvement is recommended. Whether coronary involvement might *predict* cerebrovascular involvement has not been formally studied.

The long-term neurological outcome of most patients with Kawasaki disease and hemiparesis and/or stroke has been favorable. Few of the patients in the available literature had neurological and/or developmental symptoms at follow-up visits. This has not been formally studied, however, and the true developmental prognosis of children with Kawasaki disease (with or without neurological symptoms) is unknown.

Treatment

Early attempts to treat Kawasaki disease focused on the use of aspirin, glucocorticoids, and immune modulators such as azathioprine. The demonstration by one study of increased cardiac morbidity associated with the use of steroids has led to the discontinuation of use of this agent in routine management (Kato *et al.*, 1979). Furthermore, a trial of pulsed methylprednisolone in addition to intravenous gamma globulin demonstrated no additional benefit to intravenous gamma globulin alone (Newburger *et al.*, 2007).

Currently, high-dose intravenous gamma globulin, given as a single dose (2 g/kg), has had the greatest impact on the treatment of Kawasaki disease (Newburger *et al.*, 1986, 1991b). This regimen replaced 0.4 g/kg for four consecutive days (Furusho *et al.*, 1984; Newburger *et al.*, 1986). High-dose intravenous gamma globulin reduces the incidence of coronary artery aneurysms by more than 75%, including a reduction in the incidence of giant aneurysms (those > 8 mm in diameter) (Sundel and Newburger, 1997). High-dose intravenous gamma globulin with aspirin (see below) reduces the incidence of coronary aneurysms to about 5%.

There is a single case report of brain infarction attributed to high-dose intravenous gamma globulin therapy in a patient with Kawasaki disease, but no angiography was performed to confirm vascular occlusion (Table 13.1) (Wada *et al.*, 2006). The authors hypothesized that high-dose intravenous gamma globulin resulted in increased blood viscosity, increased thrombin production due to contamination by factor XI, or direct toxicity to the vascular endothelium. The case was potentially confounded by a history of *Varicella* infection – a well-documented cause of cerebral arteriopathy in children (Alehan *et al.*, 2002; deVeber *et al.*, 2000; Takeoka and Takahashi, 2002).

Aspirin (3–5 mg/kg/day) is still a mainstay of therapy in the acute phase of illness for its anti-inflammatory effects, but it has no effect on incidence of coronary artery aneurysm (Israels and Michelson, 2006; Sundel and Newburger, 1997). After 6–8 weeks, if no coronary abnormality is evident, aspirin is discontinued. When coronary artery aneurysm is found, aspirin treatment is continued although the duration of therapy has not been determined with certainty. When giant aneurysms are present, aspirin is often accompanied by an anticoagulant. Increased awareness of Kawasaki disease and early use of high-dose intravenous gamma globulin have reduced the frequency with which the full spectrum of disease is seen. Often the presence of persistent fever combined with appearance of coronary aneurysms is sufficient to diagnose Kawasaki disease for implementation of therapy (Newburger *et al.*, 2004b).

Conclusion

Kawasaki disease remains one of the most important causes of vasculitis and cardiac death in children. Its cause has eluded identification, and there is still no definitive diagnostic test. Clinical acumen remains the main diagnostic tool. Serious neurological complications are rare but do occur. Our review of the current literature suggests that stroke, and specifically asymptomatic brain infarction, may be more common than now recognized, especially in patients with coronary artery abnormalities. Thorough clinical, neuroradiological, and neuropsychological assessments of these patients are indicated to gain a full appreciation of the nervous system involvement and the long-term neurodevelopmental sequelae resulting from this disease.

REFERENCES

Alehan, F. K., Boyvat, F., Baskin, E., Derbent, M., and Ozbek, N. 2002. Focal cerebral vasculitis and stroke after chickenpox. *Eur J Paediatr Neurol*, **6**, 331–3.

Amano, S., and Hazama, F. 1980. Neural involvement in Kawasaki disease. *Acta Pathol Jpn*, **30**, 365–73.

Amano, S., Hazama, F., and Hamashima, Y. 1979a. Pathology of Kawasaki disease: I. Pathology and morphogenesis of the vascular changes. *Jpn Circ J*, **43**, 633–43.

Amano, S., Hazama, F., and Hamashima, Y. 1979b. Pathology of Kawasaki disease: II. Distribution and incidence of the vascular lesions. *Jpn Circ J*, **43**, 741–8.

Amano, S., Hazama, F., Kubagawa, H., *et al.* 1980. General pathology of Kawasaki disease. On the morphological alterations corresponding to the clinical manifestations. *Acta Pathol Jpn*, **30**, 681–94.

Bailie, N. M., Hensey, O. J., Ryan, S., Allcut, D., and King, M. D. 2001. Bilateral subdural collections–an unusual feature of possible Kawasaki disease. *Eur J Paediatr Neurol*, **5**, 79–81.

Beiser, A. S., Takahashi, M., Baker, A. L., Sundel, R. P., and Newburger, J. W. 1998. A predictive instrument for coronary artery aneurysms in Kawasaki disease. US Multicenter Kawasaki Disease Study Group. *Am J Cardiol*, **81**, 1116–20.

Bell, D. M., Morens, D. M., Holman, R. C., Hurwitz, E. S., and Hunter, M. K. 1983. Kawasaki syndrome in the United States 1976 to 1980. *Am J Dis Child*, **137**, 211–4.

Benseler, S. M., Silverman, E., Aviv, R. I., et al. 2006. Primary central nervous system vasculitis in children. *Arthritis Rheum*, **54**, 1291–7.

Boespflug, O., Tardieu, M., Losay, J., and Leroy, D. 1984. [Acute hemiplegia complicating Kawasaki disease]. *Rev Neurol (Paris)*, **140**, 507–9.

Burns, J. C., Kushner, H. I., Bastian, J. F., et al. 2000. Kawasaki disease: a brief history. *Pediatrics*, **106**, E27.

Chang, R. K. 2002. Hospitalizations for Kawasaki disease among children in the United States, 1988–1997. *Pediatrics*, **109**, e87.

Dajani, A. S., Taubert, K. A., Gerber, M. A., et al. 1993. Diagnosis and therapy of Kawasaki disease in children. *Circulation*, **87**, 1776–80.

Dengler, L. D., Capparelli, E. V., Bastian, J. F., et al. 1998. Cerebrospinal fluid profile in patients with acute Kawasaki disease. *Pediatr Infect Dis J*, **17**, 478–81.

deVeber, G., Roach, E. S., Riela, A. R., and Wiznitzer, M. 2000. Stroke in children: recognition, treatment, and future directions. *Semin Pediatr Neurol*, **7**, 309–17.

Dillon, M. J., and Ozen, S. 2006. A new international classification of childhood vasculitis. *Pediatr Nephrol*, **21**, 1219–22.

Ferro, J. M. 1998. Vasculitis of the central nervous system. *J Neurol*, **245**, 766–76.

Fujiwara, S., Yamano, T., Hattori, M., Fujiseki, Y., and Shimada, M. 1992. Asymptomatic cerebral infarction in Kawasaki disease. *Pediatr Neurol*, **8**, 235–6.

Furusho, K., Kamiya, T., Nakano, H., et al. 1984. High-dose intravenous gamma-globulin for Kawasaki disease. *Lancet*, **2**, 1055–8.

Hosaki, J., Abe, S., Shoback, B. R., Yoshimatu, A., and Migita, T. 1978. Mucocutaneous lymph node syndrome with various arterial lesions. *Helv Paediatr Acta*, **33**, 127–33.

Ichiyama, T., Nishikawa, M., Hayashi, T., et al. 1998. Cerebral hypoperfusion during acute Kawasaki disease. *Stroke*, **29**, 1320–1.

Israels, S. J., and Michelson, A. D. 2006. Antiplatelet therapy in children. *Thromb Res*, **118**, 75–83.

Jackson, J. L., Kunkel, M. R., Libow, L., Gates, R. H. 1994. Adult Kawasaki disease. Report of two cases treated with intravenous gamma globulin. *Arch Intern Med*, **154**, 1398–405.

Kato, H., Koike, S., and Yokoyama, T. 1979. Kawasaki disease: effect of treatment on coronary artery involvement. *Pediatrics*, **63**, 175–9.

Kawasaki, T. 1967. [Acute febrile mucocutaneous syndrome with lymphoid involvement with specific desquamation of the fingers and toes in children]. *Arerugi*, **16**, 178–222.

Kawasaki, T., Kosaki, F., Okawa, S., Shigematsu, I., and Yanagawa, H. 1974. A new infantile acute febrile mucocutaneous lymph node syndrome (MLNS) prevailing in Japan. *Pediatrics*, **54**, 271–6.

Knott, P. D., Orloff, L. A., Harris, J. P., Novak, R. E., and Burns, J. C. 2001. Sensorineural hearing loss and Kawasaki disease: a prospective study. *Am J Otolaryngol*, **22**, 343–8.

Koutras, A. 1982. Myositis with Kawasaki's disease. *Am J Dis Child*, **136**, 78–9.

Lapointe, J. S., Nugent, R. A., Graeb, D. A., and Robertson, W. D. 1984. Cerebral infarction and regression of widespread aneurysms in Kawasaki's disease: case report. *Pediatr Radiol*, **14**, 1–5.

Lauret, P., Lecointre, C., and Billard, J. L. 1979. [Kawasaki disease complicated by thrombosis of the internal carotid artery]. *Ann Dermatol Venereol*, **106**, 901–5.

Laxer, R. M., Dunn, H. G., and Flodmark, O. 1984. Acute hemiplegia in Kawasaki disease and infantile polyarteritis nodosa. *Dev Med Child Neurol*, **26**, 814–8.

Mason, W. H., and Burns, J. C. 1997. Clinical presentation of Kawasaki disease. *Prog Pediatr Cardiol*, **6**, 193–201.

Morens, D. M., O'Brien, R. J. 1978. Kawasaki disease in the United States. *J Infect Dis*, **137**, 91–3.

Muneuchi, J., Kusuhara, K., Kanaya, Y., et al. 2006. Magnetic resonance studies of brain lesions in patients with Kawasaki disease. *Brain Dev*, **28**, 30–3.

Newburger, J. W., Burns, J. C., Beiser, A. S., and Loscalzo, J. 1991a. Altered lipid profile after Kawasaki syndrome. *Circulation*, **84**, 625–31.

Newburger, J. W., Sleeper, L. A., McCrindle, B. W., et al. 2007. Randomized trial of pulsed corticosteroid therapy for primary treatment of Kawasaki disease. *N Engl J Med*, **356**, 663–75.

Newburger, J. W., Takahashi, M., Beiser, A. S., et al. 1991b. A single intravenous infusion of gamma globulin as compared with four infusions in the treatment of acute Kawasaki syndrome. *N Engl J Med*, **324**, 1633–9.

Newburger, J. W., Takahashi, M., Burns, J. C., et al. 1986. The treatment of Kawasaki syndrome with intravenous gamma globulin. *N Engl J Med*, **315**, 341–7.

Newburger, J. W., Takahashi, M., Gerber, M. A., et al. 2004a. Diagnosis, treatment, and long-term management of Kawasaki disease: a statement for health professionals from the Committee on Rheumatic Fever, Endocarditis and Kawasaki Disease, Council on Cardiovascular Disease in the Young, American Heart Association. *Circulation*, **110**, 2747–71.

Newburger, J. W., Takahashi, M., Gerber, M. A., et al. 2004b. Diagnosis, treatment, and long-term management of Kawasaki disease: a statement for health professionals from the Committee on Rheumatic Fever, Endocarditis, and Kawasaki Disease, Council on Cardiovascular Disease in the Young, American Heart Association. *Pediatrics*, **114**, 1708–33.

Ozen, S., Ruperto, N., Dillon, M. J., et al. 2006. EULAR/PReS endorsed consensus criteria for the classification of childhood vasculitides. *Ann Rheum Dis*, **65**, 936–41.

Rauch, A. M. 1989. Kawasaki syndrome: issues in etiology and treatment. *Adv Pediatr Infect Dis*, **4**, 163–82.

Shulman, S. T., and Rowley, A. H. 1997. Etiology and pathogenesis of Kawasaki disease. *Prog Pediatr Cardiol*, **6**, 187–92.

Suda, K., Matsumura, M., and Ohta, S. 2003. Kawasaki disease complicated by cerebral infarction. *Cardiol Young*, **13**, 103–5.

Sundel, R., and Newburger, J. W. 1997. Management of acute Kawasaki disease. *Prog Pediatr Cardiol*, **6**, 203–9.

Tabarki, B., Mahdhaoui, A., Selmi, H., Yacoub, M., and Essoussi, A. S. 2001. Kawasaki disease with predominant central nervous system involvement. *Pediatr Neurol*, **25**, 239–41.

Takeoka, M., and Takahashi, T. 2002. Infectious and inflammatory disorders of the circulatory system and stroke in childhood. *Curr Opin Neurol*, **15**, 159–64.

Tanaka, S., Sagiuchi, T., and Kobayashi, I. 2007. Ruptured pediatric posterior cerebral artery aneurysm 9 years after the onset of Kawasaki disease: a case report. *Childs Nerv Syst*, **23**, 701–6.

Templeton, P. A., and Dunne, M. G. 1987. Kawasaki syndrome: cerebral and cardiovascular complications. *J Clin Ultrasound*, **15**, 483–5.

Terasawa, K., Ichinose, E., Matsuishi, T., and Kato, H. 1983. Neurological complications in Kawasaki disease. *Brain Dev*, **5**, 371–4.

Wada, Y., Kamei, A., Fujii, Y., Ishikawa, K., and Chida, S. 2006. Cerebral infarction after high-dose intravenous immunoglobulin therapy for Kawasaki disease. *J Pediatr*, **148**, 399–400.

Yanagawa, H., Nakamura, Y., Yashiro, M., et al. 2001. Incidence survey of Kawasaki disease in 1997 and 1998 in Japan. *Pediatrics*, **107**, E33.

Yanagawa, H., Nakamura, Y., Yashiro, M., et al. 2006. Incidence of Kawasaki disease in Japan: the nationwide surveys of 1999–2002. *Pediatr Int*, **48**, 356–61.

14 CEREBROVASCULAR PROBLEMS IN CHAGAS' DISEASE

Ayrton Roberto Massaro

It is clear that the basic epidemiological fact of the disease is constituted by an insect, a constant companion of men in their houses, and thus easily vulnerable to destruction. . . . Sanitary measures in this sense, especially improvement of the living conditions, would certainly represent an administrative act of major importance.

Carlos Chagas

Introduction

American trypanosomiasis or Chagas' disease was discovered in 1909 and gradually revealed to be widespread throughout Latin America, affecting millions of people with a high impact on morbidity and mortality (Schofield *et al.*, 2006). By 1960, the first World Health Organization (WHO) Expert Committee meeting on Chagas' disease estimated global prevalence of the infection to be seven million people. By the end of the 1980s, data from serological surveys showed that there were 16–18 million people infected with Chagas' disease. After the Southern Cone Initiative (the Disease Control Priorities Project of the National Institutes of Health and the World Bank), the prevalence was estimated at 9.8 million people (Schofield *et al.*, 2006).

Chagas' disease is caused by *Trypanosoma cruzi*, a parasite that shares some epidemiological features with other pathogens that cause latent illness. Geographical strain differences result in distinct tissue tropism virulence and clinical manifestation. From an epidemiological classification, *T. cruzi* II is the agent of Chagas' disease in the southern cone countries of South America, whereas *T. cruzi* I is endemic in northern South America and Central America, where chronic Chagas' disease is said to be more benign (Miles *et al.*, 2003).

Historical background

The use of a DNA probe targeting a segment of *T. cruzi* DNA extracted from nearly 300 Andean mummified human soft tissues has reconstructed the action of Chagas' disease among entire ancient populations in the Andean area (Aufderheide *et al.*, 2004), but the breakthrough regarding this disease started when the Brazilian Government tried to connect Belém (city in the extreme north of the country) to Rio de Janeiro, and the construction was stopped in the state of Minas Gerais due to a malaria epidemic that occurred among the railroad workers. Then, Carlos Chagas was sent to a city called Lassance and noticed the existence of hematophagus insects that, because of their typical behavior of biting persons on the face during the night, were known as "barbeiros" ("barbers") or "kissing bugs" (Morel, 1999). In 1909, he discovered the acute disease in a young girl, Berenice.

Unfortunately after the first published report in 1909, there was an extensive dispute about whether the discovery was important or even true. The arguments at that time contributed to the successive denial of a well-deserved Nobel Prize in recognition of Carlos Chagas' outstanding and remarkable studies (Coutinho *et al.*, 1999).

Transmission of *Trypanosoma cruzi*

Trypanosoma cruzi is transmitted to humans by triatomine bugs, large bedbugs that deposit feces on the mucous membranes or scraped skin while they bite. These triatomine insects are known popularly in the different countries as "vinchuca," "barbeiro," and "chipo" (Miles *et al.*, 2003). When people rub the bite wound and, subsequently, their eyes or mouth, the feces, which contain the parasite, enter the bloodstream (Miles *et al.*, 2003). Chagas' disease can also be transmitted during pregnancy and via infected blood transfusions or organ transplants (Pirard *et al.*, 2005). Occasionally, adult triatomine bugs contaminate palm juice presses or other foods, causing orally transmitted outbreaks (Cardoso *et al.*, 2006).

The transmission cycles of *T. cruzi* by vectors are complex. More than 130 species of triatomine insect are known, most of them confined to the Americas. A few triatomine species have adapted to colonize and thrive in houses, where they transmit *T. cruzi* to humans and domestic animals, such as dogs or cats (Miles *et al.*, 2003). *Triatoma infestans*, which is found in South American countries, has spread far beyond its initial silvatic habitats, and is exclusively domestic or peridomestic throughout most of its geographic range. Domestic and silvatic transmission cycles in a given locality can be considered as separate or overlapping based on the degree of interaction between them.

Owing to a huge migratory movement inside some endemic countries (like Brazil), mortality from Chagas' disease occurs even in regions classified as free of vector transmission. The emigration of Latin Americans to more developed countries has also raised concerns regarding a possible increased risk of transfusion-transmitted *T. cruzi* in the developed world. It may account for the estimated 100 000 or more chronically infected persons now living in the United States (Kirkchoff, 1993) and more than a dozen

Uncommon Causes of Stroke, 2nd edition, ed. Louis R. Caplan. Published by Cambridge University Press. © Cambridge University Press 2008.

transfusion- and transplantation-associated cases in the United States, Canada, and countries in Europe, which do not screen donors serologically for Chagas' disease (Maguire, 2006).

Epidemiological strategies to control Chagas' disease

Chagas' disease is a disease of poverty and international neglect. Efforts to eradicate triatomines persist, but pesticide administration appears to be largely ineffective. Treatment is toxic and resource-intensive and people can be re-infected.

The main control strategy relies on prevention of transmission by eliminating the domestic insect vectors and controlling transmission by blood transfusion. A national control program only began to be implemented after the 1970s, when technical questions were overcome and the scientific demonstration of the high social impact of Chagas' disease was used to encourage national campaigns (Dias *et al.*, 2002). Recently, the Intergovernment Commission of the Southern Cone Initiative against Chagas' disease declared Brazil to be free of Chagas' disease transmission due to *T. infestans* (Schofield *et al.*, 2006). Because the rate of new infection has declined over such substantial areas, the prevalence has been progressively reduced to a current 9.8 million people infected. However, it is less clear whether interventions should also be considered against silvatic populations (Pinto *et al.*, 2004).

General clinical features of Chagas' disease

Chagas' disease progresses in stages, most patients being infected during childhood (Punukollu *et al.*, 2007). In the acute phase, following the infection, there are no helpful signs and symptoms other than fever, myalgias, sweating, hepatosplenomegaly, and swollen lymph glands. At the site of exposure to infected bug feces an initial lesion may occur, and *T. cruzi* may multiply locally, giving rise to unilateral conjunctivitis and edema (Romaña's sign) or to a cutaneous chagoma (Punukollu *et al.*, 2007). However, the initial acute phase of infection is usually asymptomatic and unrecognized, although trypanosomes may be detectable in blood by microscopy. There is intense parasitism noted on microscopic examination in most of the organs. Cardiac involvement is present in more than 90% of cases, although diagnosis is established in less than 10% of cases, due to mild symptoms. Laboratory findings are nonspecific and include leukocytosis with an absolute increase of lymphocyte count. Electrocardiography may show low voltage, diffuse ST-T changes, and various conduction abnormalities. Serologic tests for *T. cruzi* infection are usually negative during the first weeks, but the circulating parasite can be detected by xenodiagnosis, an early stage diagnostic tool achieved by exposing a presumably infected individual or tissue to a clean, laboratory-bred bug and then examining the vector for the presence of *T. cruzi*. A reactivated acute phase can occur in immunocompromised patients. Both immunocompromised and congenital cases may be associated with meningoencephalitis, which has a poor prognosis (Sartori *et al.*, 2007).

After initial infection, the transient parasitemia resolves and the asymptomatic indeterminate stage begins, which may last for many years. During this phase, the patient remains asymptomatic with positive serology and no physical signs or clinical evidence of organ involvement. Much later, in a proportion of infected people, the disease manifests with cardiac (cardiac dilatations, arrhythmias, and conduction abnormalities) and/or intestinal (megaesophagus, megacolon) involvement.

Chagas' cardiomyopathy

Despite the effective public health measures in combating vectorial and blood transfusion transmission, there is still a significant number of people in Latin America with Chagas' cardiomyopathy; therefore, it should remain one of the leading causes of heart failure for the next few years. Patients with Chagas' cardiomyopathy have usually had a lower level of education than have persons with other cardiomyopathies (Braga *et al.*, 2006). In addition, a higher frequency of family history of Chagas' disease links this disease to the socioeconomic status of the population affected.

Chagas' cardiomyopathy has been considered a type of dilated cardiomyopathy (Braga *et al.*, 2006). Involvement of the autonomic nerves that supply the heart is considered the major cause of the myocardiopathy rather than direct infection of the heart muscle by parasites. Symptoms and physical signs of Chagas' cardiomyopathy arise from heart failure, cardiac arrhythmias, and arterial thromboembolism. Atypical chest pain is common in patients with Chagas' cardiomyopathy. Heart failure caused by Chagas' cardiomyopathy is the most frequent and severe clinical manifestation of chronic Chagas' disease, and is associated with poor prognosis and high mortality rate. Cardiac arrhythmias may cause palpitations, lightheadedness, dizziness, and syncope. Autonomic dysfunction results in marked heart rate abnormalities, especially bradycardia. Sudden death is an occasional complication that may be precipitated by exercise and can be explained by ventricular tachycardia or fibrillation or complete heart block. Mural thrombi form in cardiac chambers and may result in systemic emboli. Stroke is the most important complication of embolism in Chagas' cardiomyopathy and may be found in 19% of those patients (Braga *et al.*, 2006).

Diagnostic tests for Chagas' disease

There is no straightforward diagnostic test for Chagas' disease. In the acute phase, diagnosis is established by demonstration of the parasite in the blood, by direct examination, or after hemoconcentration or xenodiagnosis. The diagnosis of chronic Chagas' disease is routinely achieved with methods that detect circulating antibodies that bind to *T. cruzi* antigens. The most commonly used test is based on complement fixation, immunofluorescence, or enzyme-linked immunofluorescence assays. Chagas' disease can be diagnosed with greater sensitivity by the detection of *T. cruzi*–specific sequence of DNA.

Specific treatment options for Chagas' disease

Nifurtimox and benznidazole are specific therapy to treat Chagas' disease during the acute phase, irrespective of the mechanism of transmission and when reactivation of chronic disease occurs during immunosuppressive conditions. Neither drug is effective after the disease has progressed to the chronic stage. There is no definitive evidence that these drugs cure the cardiac disease. A systematic review from the Cochrane database detected only a few trials that allocated patients with chronic Chagas' disease without symptomatic cardiac Chagas' to trypanocidal treatments given for at least 30 days at any dose. Parasite-related outcome was improved, but no hard clinical outcome changes were reported in any of these trials (Villar *et al.*, 2002). New target interventions may develop after the recent genome sequence of *T. cruzi* (El-Sayed *et al.*, 2005).

Prognosis of Chagas' disease

Death in Chagas' disease is predominantly cardiovascular. The mechanism of cardiovascular death is either an arrhythmic event (often ventricular fibrillation), a nonarrhythmic episode such as severe congestive heart failure, or an embolic episode. Noncardiovascular causes consist of complications of megaesophagus and megacolon. Sudden death in Chagas' disease occurs mainly between 30 and 50 years of age, being uncommon after the sixth decade of life, and predominates in men (Bestetti *et al.*, 1993).

Prognosis of Chagas' cardiomyopathy

In a longitudinal, case–control follow-up study carried out in endemic areas over a period of 10 years, more than one third of patients with chronic Chagas' disease developed clinical or electrocardiographic deterioration (Coura *et al.*, 1985). Some epidemiological studies showed that male gender was associated with a poorer prognosis of Chagas' cardiomyopathy and a more severe progression (Basquiera *et al.*, 2003). The ejection fraction has been shown to be an effective predictor of survival in patients with Chagas' cardiomyopathy (Mady *et al.*, 1994). In addition, the prognosis of patients with heart failure due to Chagas' cardiomyopathy in functional class III and IV is worse than that of patients with functional class III and IV with idiopathic, ischemic, or hypertensive heart disease (Freitas *et al.*, 2005).

Rassi *et al.* (2006) reported their evaluation of 424 patients with known Chagas' cardiomyopathy in an attempt to devise a risk score to predict the likelihood of death. In descending order of importance, these features are New York Heart Association class III or IV, cardiomegaly on chest radiography, segmental or global wall-motion abnormalities on echocardiography, nonsustained ventricular tachycardia on Holter monitoring, low QRS voltage on electrocardiography, and male sex. A risk score derived by combining points for each of these features accurately classified patients into subgroups at low, medium, and high risk for death.

Among patients in the high-risk category, the 10-year mortality was 84%. Mortality was considerably lower among those classified as low risk (10%) or intermediate risk (44%), but the long-term outcome for many of these patients is not promising, given the progressive nature of the disease.

Stroke and Chagas' disease

Chagas' disease is a risk factor for stroke in endemic areas, independent of the severity of cardiac failure (Oliveira-Filho *et al.*, 2005). Stroke in Chagas' disease has been described in several autopsy reports of individuals, but the stroke mechanism was not defined.

Brain infarction has been reported in 5–15% of the autopsies of chagasic persons in an endemic area in the northeastern region of Brazil (Braga *et al.*, 1995). Samuel *et al.* (1983) reported 39 individuals with brain infarction, 28% of whom had infarction characterized as the cause of death. Usually the autopsy series suggest that chagasic patients with older age (>40 years), advanced heart failure, thrombosis in the left cardiac chambers, atrial fibrillation, ventricular arrhythmias, previous embolism, and ventricular aneurysm have a high risk of ischemic stroke (Aras *et al.*, 2003). However, despite the high frequency of embolic events in autopsy cases with Chagas' disease, most of them were not diagnosed during life (Aras *et al.*, 2003).

Demographic features and stroke risk factors

Stroke occurs in Chagas' disease patients at least 50 years of age, after the period of a higher risk of cardiac death (Oliveira-Filho *et al.*, 2005). A survival advantage for women with Chagas' disease may be one clarification for the observed higher frequency of Chagas' disease with stroke in women. Although most Chagas' disease patients with stroke had at least one associated risk factor, the most frequent being hypertension (Carod-Artal *et al.*, 2005), the frequency of stroke risk factors in Chagas' disease patients is lower than that found in other stroke causes.

Ischemic stroke subtypes

Chagas' cardiomyopathy increases the risk occurrence of embolic ischemic stroke, and its treatment is one of the most important strategies for stroke prevention in Chagas' disease patients. The most common stroke syndrome in Chagas' disease patients is a partial anterior circulation infarct, with the middle cerebral artery being the most often affected vascular territory (Carod-Artal *et al.*, 2005).

Serological Chagas' disease results in endemic areas can show that up to 25% of patients have positive chagasic serology. Although there is an association between *T. cruzi* infection and stroke (regardless of cardiac abnormalities), in endemic areas (Leon-Sarmiento *et al.*, 2004), socioeconomic disparities in multiple associated stroke risk factors may predispose Chagas' disease patients to other ischemic stroke subtypes, such as atherosclerosis. A 13% frequency of carotid occlusion or at least a moderate to severe carotid stenosis (>50%) has been found in a series of patients with stroke and Chagas' disease who were studied using carotid ultrasound (Carod-Artal *et al.*, 2003).

Using the Trial of Org 10172 in Acute Stroke Treatment (TOAST) criteria, Carod-Artal *et al.* (2003) classified the strokes of 37% of Chagas' disease stroke patients as having an unknown cause. Some of those patients probably also had the indeterminate form of Chagas' disease that may require further cardiac investigation. Thrombophilia states such as protein C or S deficiency, antithrombin III deficiency, factor V Leiden, and anticardiolipin antibodies were not associated with Chagas' disease and stroke (Carod-Artal *et al.*, 2005).

Cardiac investigation in patients with Chagas' disease and stroke

Almost 70% of patients with Chagas' disease and stroke have shown some electrocardiogram (ECG) alterations. The common changes on ECG are ventricular premature beats, right bundle branch block, left anterior hemiblock, diffuse repolarization abnormality, runs of nonsustained ventricular tachycardia, heart block, and abnormal Q waves. In advanced stages of Chagas' disease, atrial fibrillation, and low QRS voltage may occur.

Radiological study of the thorax is a routine investigation in patients with Chagas' disease to detect cardiac impairment and to evaluate the degree of ventricular dysfunction.

Usually, in the early stages of cardiac involvement, echocardiography may reveal one or more areas of abnormal wall motion. More advanced cardiac disease is characterized by global cardiac dilatation and diffuse hypokinesis, often associated with mitral and tricuspid regurgitation. Left ventricular aneurysms may develop at the cardiac apex, a hallmark morphological sign of Chagas' disease. Apical aneurysms may occur in 16% of Chagas' disease patients with stroke. These patients often have associated ECG abnormalities (Carod-Artal *et al.*, 2005).

Other techniques may provide novel approaches to identifying cardiac lesions, particularly in the indeterminate phase of Chagas' disease. Regional myocardial perfusion disturbances may occur early in the course of Chagas' cardiomyopathy even before wall-motion abnormalities develop (Simões *et al.*, 2000). Myocardial delayed enhancement by MRI is a noninvasive diagnosis to evaluate myocardial fibrosis in Chagas' disease patients (Rochitte *et al.*, 2005). MRI can also show that the degree of myocardial fibrosis may increase progressively from mild to the most severe Chagas' disease stages, and may be a marker of disease severity.

Brain imaging and transcranial Doppler in Chagas' disease patients with stroke

Usually patients with Chagas' disease and stroke have embolic infarcts detected by early CT or MRI. In addition, cerebral blood flow impairment can also be found in Chagas' disease patients with refractory congestive heart failure (Massaro *et al.*, 2006).

Treatment of Chagas' disease patients with stroke

Chagas' disease patients with acute ischemic stroke may also benefit from recombinant tissue plasminogen activator (rtPA), as do patients with other causes of acute ischemic stroke who arrive at the emergency service within the therapeutic window (Trabuco *et al.*, 2005).

There is a higher frequency of Chagas' cardiomyopathy in stroke patients; therefore, prevention of subsequent stroke by long-term anticoagulation with warfarin should be indicated. Heart failure is treated in a manner similar to other causes. The maximal tolerated dose of angiotensin-converting enzyme inhibitors is usually lower in heart failure patients with Chagas' cardiomyopathy and may be a marker of pump failure death (Bestetti and Muccillo, 1997). Patients with Chagas' cardiomyopathy more often need an artificial permanent pacemaker than do patients with other causes of cardiomyopathies. Cardiac transplantation has been successful in selected patients with refractory congestive heart failure. Despite the risk of immunosuppression, only a few patients developed cutaneous or myocardial reactivation (Malheiros *et al.*, 1997). In addition, Chagas' disease patients with Chagas' cardiomyopathy seem to have lower stroke rates during heart transplantation compared to patients with ischemic cardiomyopathy, suggesting that stroke is mainly associated with previous atherosclerotic cardiovascular disease rather than with the surgical procedure (Malheiros *et al.*, 2002).

REFERENCES

Aras, R., da Matta, J. A., Mota, G., Gomes, I., and Melo, A. 2003. Cerebral infarction in autopsies of Chagasic patients with heart failure. *Arq Bras Cardiol*, **81**, 414–6.

Aufderheide, A. C., Salo, W., Madden, M., *et al.* 2004. A 9,000-year record of Chagas' disease. *Proc Natl Acad Sci U S A*, **101**, 2034–9.

Basquiera, A. L., Sembaj, A., Aguerri, A. M., *et al.* 2003. Risk progression to chronic Chagas cardiomyopathy: influence of male sex and of parasitaemia detected by polymerase chain reaction. *Heart*, **89**, 1186–90.

Bestetti, R. B., Freitas, O. C., Muccillo, G., and Oliveira, J. S. 1993. Clinical and morphological characteristics associated with sudden cardiac death in patients with Chagas' disease. *Eur Heart J*, **14**, 1610–4.

Bestetti, R. B., and Muccillo, G. 1997. Clinical course of Chagas' heart disease: a comparison with dilated cardiomyopathy. *Int J Cardiol*, **60**, 187–93.

Braga, J. C., Labrunie, A., Villaca, F., do Nascimento, E., and Quijada, L. 1995. Thromboembolism in chronic Chagas' heart disease. *São Paulo Med J*, **113**, 862–6.

Braga, J. C., Reis, F., Aras, R., *et al.* 2006. Clinical and therapeutics aspects of heart failure due to Chagas disease. *Arq Bras Cardiol*, **86**, 297–302.

Cardoso, A. V. N., Lescano, S. A. Z., Amato Neto, V., Gakiya, E., and Santos, S. V. 2006. Survival of *Trypanosoma cruzi* in sugar cane used to prepare juice. *Rev Inst Med Trop S Paulo*, **48**, 287–9.

Carod-Artal, F. J., Vargas, A. P., Horan, T. A., and Nunes, L. G. 2005. Chagasic cardiomyopathy is independently associated with ischemic stroke in Chagas disease. *Stroke*, **36**, 965–70.

Carod-Artal, F. J., Vargas, A. P., Melo, M., and Horan, T. A. 2003. American trypanosomiasis (Chagas' disease): an unrecognised cause of stroke. *J Neurol Neurosurg Psychiatry*, **74**, 516–8.

Coura, J. R., de Abreu, L. L., Pereira, J. B., and Willcox, H. P. 1985. Morbidity in Chagas' disease. IV. Longitudinal study of 10 years in Pains and Iguatama, Minas Gerais, Brazil. *Mem Inst Oswaldo Cruz*, **80**, 73–80.

Coutinho, M., Freire, O. Jr, and Dias, J. C. 1999. The noble enigma: Chagas' nominations for the Nobel prize. *Mem Inst Oswaldo Cruz*, **94 Suppl 1**, 123–9.

Dias, J. C., Silveira, A. C., and Schofield, C. J. 2002. The impact of Chagas disease control in Latin America: a review. *Mem Inst Oswaldo Cruz*, **97**, 603–12.

El-Sayed, N. M., Myler, P. J., Bartholomeu, D. C., *et al.* 2005. The genome sequence of *Trypanosoma cruzi*, etiologic agent of Chagas disease. *Science*, **309**, 409–15.

Freitas, H. F., Chizzola, P. R., Paes, A. T., Lima, A. C., and Mansur, A. J. 2005. Risk stratification in a Brazilian hospital-based cohort of 1220 outpatients with heart failure: role of Chagas' heart disease. *Int J Cardiol,* **102**, 239–47.

Kirchhoff, L. V. 1993. American trypanosomiasis (Chagas' disease): a tropical disease now in the United States. *N Engl J Med,* **329**, 639–44.

Leon-Sarmiento, F. E., Mendoza, E., Torres-Hillera, M., *et al.* 2004. Trypanosoma cruzi-associated cerebrovascular disease: a case-control study in Eastern Colombia. *J Neurol Sci,* **217**, 61–4.

Mady, C., Cardoso, R. H. A., Barretto, A. C. P., *et al.* 1994. Survival and predictors of survival in patients with congestive heart failure due to Chagas' cardiomyopathy. *Circulation,* **90**, 3098–102.

Maguire, J. R. 2006. Chagas' disease – can we stop the deaths? *N Engl J Med,* **355**, 760–1.

Malheiros, S. M. F., Almeida, D. R., Massaro, A. R., *et al.* 2002. Neurologic complications after heart transplantation. *Arq Neuropsiquiatr,* **60(2-A)**, 192–7.

Malheiros, S. M. F., Gabbai, A. A., Brucki, S. M. D, *et al.* 1997. Neurologic outcome after heart transplantation in Chagas' disease. Preliminary results. *Acta Neurol Scand,* **96**, 252–5.

Massaro, A. R., Dutra, A. P., Almeida, D. R., Diniz, R. V. Z., and Malheiros, S. M. F. 2006. Transcranial Doppler assessment of cerebral blood flow: effect of cardiac transplantation. *Neurology,* **66**, 124–6.

Miles, M. A., Feliciangeli, M. D., and de Arias, A. R. 2003. American trypanosomiasis (Chagas' disease) and the role of molecular epidemiology in guiding control strategies. *BMJ,* **326**, 1444–8.

Morel, C. M. 1999. Chagas disease, from discovery to control – and beyond: history, myths and lessons to take home. *Mem Inst Oswaldo Cruz,* **94 Suppl 1**, 3–16.

Oliveira-Filho, J., Viana, L. C., Vieira de Melo, R. M., *et al.* 2005. Chagas disease is an independent risk factor for stroke: baseline characteristics of a Chagas disease cohort. *Stroke,* **36**, 2015–17.

Pinto, A. Y. N., Valente, S. A. S., Valente V da C. 2004. Emerging acute Chagas disease in Amazonian Brazil: case reports with serious cardiac involvement. *Braz J Infect Dis,* **8**, 454–60.

Pirard, M., Iihoshi, N., Boelaert, M., Basanta, P., Lopez, F., and Van der Stuyft, P. 2005. The validity of serologic tests for *Trypanosoma cruzi* and the effectiveness of transfusional screening strategies in a hyperendemic region. *Transfusion,* **45**, 554–61.

Punukollu, G., Gowda, R. M., Khan, I. A., Navarro, V. S., and Vasavada, B. C. 2007. Clinical aspects of the Chagas' heart disease. *Int J Cardiol,* **115**, 279–83.

Rassi, A. Jr, Rassi, A., Little, W. C., *et al.* 2006. Development and validation of a risk score for predicting death in Chagas' heart disease. *N Engl J Med,* **355**, 799–808.

Rochitte, C. E., Oliveira, P. F., Andrade, J. M., *et al.* 2005. Myocardial delayed enhancement by magnetic resonance imaging in patients with Chagas' disease: a marker of disease severity. *J Am Coll Cardiol.* **46**, 1553–8.

Samuel, J., Oliveira, M., Correa de Araújo, R. R., Navarro, M. A., and Muccillo, G. 1983. Cardiac thrombosis and thromboembolism in chronic Chagas' heart disease. *Am J Cardiol,* **52**, 147–51.

Sartori, A. M., Ibrahim, K. Y., Nunes Westophalen, E. V., *et al.* 2007. Manifestations of Chagas disease (American trypanosomiasis) in patients with HIV/AIDS. *Ann Trop Med Parasitol,* **101**, 31–50.

Schofield, C. J., Jannin, J., and Salvatella, R. 2006. The future of Chagas disease control. *Trends Parasitol,* **22**, 583–8.

Simões, M. V., Pintya, A. O., Bromberg-Marin, G., *et al.* 2000. Relation of regional sympathetic denervation and myocardial perfusion disturbance to wall motion impairment in Chagas' cardiomyopathy. *Am J Cardiol,* **86**, 975–81.

Trabuco, C. C., Pereira de Jesus, P. A., Bacellar, A., and Oliveira-Filho, J. 2005. Successful thrombolysis in cardioembolic stroke from Chagas disease. *Neurology,* **64**, 170–1.

Villar, J. C., Marin-Neto, J. A., Ebrahim, S., and Yusuf, S. 2002. Trypanocidal drugs for chronic asymptomatic *Trypanosoma cruzi* infection. *Cochrane Database Syst Rev,* **1**, CD003463.

STROKE IN PERSONS INFECTED WITH HIV

Vivian U. Fritz and Alan Bryer

Introduction

Stroke is uncommon in HIV-positive individuals. The question arises as to whether stroke is incidental to the HIV status of the individual or whether HIV infection confers increased risk of stroke. Most studies do not distinguish between stroke due to medical conditions and stroke due to an HIV-associated vasculopathy. Sub-Saharan Africa has one of the most rapidly expanding HIV epidemics in the world. The nature of the virus with delayed onset of manifestations of infection makes it very difficult to track the progress of the epidemic. In this region, most available data concerning the scale of the epidemic are from South Africa. This country's population has grown to approximately 48 million people and, of these, 5.4 million were estimated to be infected with HIV (11% of the total population) by the middle of 2006 (Dorrington et al., 2006). Nineteen percent of the working age population (ages 20–64) was HIV positive. The HIV prevalence rate in women was highest between ages 25 and 29 (33%), and in men prevalence was highest between ages 30 and 34 (27%). In South Africa, 1.8 million AIDS deaths had occurred since the start of the epidemic. South Africa is uniquely positioned to study the association between HIV infection and stroke in a region with a high seropositive prevalence in the general population. A number of studies concerning this issue have been published from this region in the past 7 years (Chetty, 2005; Connor et al., 2000; Hoffman et al., 2000; Kumwenda et al., 2005; Mochan et al., 2003, 2005; Patel et al., 2005; Tipping et al., 2007).

Is there an increased risk of stroke in patients infected with HIV?

Controversy exists as to whether HIV infection confers an increased risk of stroke, and there are few data to quantify any such HIV-associated stroke risk.

In 1989, Engstroom et al. undertook a retrospective study in which 1600 AIDS patients were analyzed. They found 12 strokes over a 5-year period. This group was compared with age-matched controls in the age range of 35–45 years. The conclusion reached was that stroke was more common in the group with AIDS than in the age-matched control group.

A case-controlled study (Berger et al., 1990) in the late 1980s compared the prevalence of cerebrovascular disease in autopsied patients between the ages of 20 and 50 years with and without AIDS. Thirteen of 154 patients (8%) had strokes. There was no statistically significant difference between the prevalence of stroke in

dying patients with AIDS and that in dying patients matched for age and sex who did not have AIDS. In contrast, a retrospective, case–control, hospital-based study suggested that HIV infection was associated with an increased stroke risk, particularly cerebral infarction, in young people (Qureshi et al., 1997). Data from a cohort study on 772 consecutive HIV-infected patients that evaluated the rate of transient ischemic attack (TIA) and stroke suggest that ischemic cerebrovascular events were more common in the HIV-infected patients than in the general population (Evers et al., 2003).

Another retrospective, case–control study was carried out on patients registered in the South African Durban stroke data bank (Hoffmann et al., 2000). Sixteen percent of all strokes in young (<50 years old) black Africans living in KwaZulu-Natal province recorded on this register occurred in association with HIV infection. The area is estimated to have the highest estimated incidence of HIV seropositivity in Sub-Saharan Africa, reported as 36% in the South African Department of Health national HIV and syphilis seroprevalence study of women attending public health clinics in South Africa (2000). The incidence rate of HIV in this population paralleled that of the young black population at large, suggesting no overall increased rate of stroke in association with HIV. However, when compared to strokes occurring in an age- and sex-matched HIV-seronegative control population, large-vessel cryptogenic stroke was more common in the HIV-infected population.

A subsequent hospital-based study was undertaken in KwaZulu-Natal province in order to determine whether HIV infection confers a predisposition to stroke in young adults (Patel et al., 2005). Patients who were HIV-positive with no other identifiable etiology were compared to age- and race-matched HIV-negative patients. The HIV-positive and -negative groups did not differ in angiographic, cardiac, or serologic tests, and a positive HIV test did not provide causal information or diagnosis. However, there was a trend towards more frequent internal carotid artery/common carotid artery occlusions in the HIV-positive group when compared with the HIV-negative group.

In a short review on AIDS and stroke risk, Berger (2004) noted that an increased risk of stroke in people with AIDS has been suggested by clinical (Evers et al., 2003), radiographic (Gillams et al., 1997), and pathological series (Anders et al., 1986; Budka et al., 1987; Connor et al., 2000; Kuwe et al., 1991; Lang et al., 1989; Mizusawa et al., 1988; Petito et al., 1986; Rhodes, 1987).

In the first ever population-based study to quantify AIDS-associated stroke risk, Cole et al. (2004) found that AIDS was strongly associated with ischemic stroke and intracranial hemorrhage. They identified all incident ischemic stroke and intracranial hemorrhage cases in young adults (15–44 years old) in central Maryland and Washington DC over a 4-year period and were able to determine the number of AIDS cases in the area during this period. After exclusion of cases in AIDS patients in whom other potential causes were identified, AIDS patients continued to have an increased risk of stroke (adjusted relative risk 9.1; 95% confidence interval [CI]: 3.4–24 for ischemic stroke and 12.7; 95% CI, 4.0–40.0 for intracranial hemorrhage). Although the study concluded that AIDS is strongly associated with both ischemic stroke and intracerebral hemorrhage, it was limited by the small number of AIDS cases, particularly women (2 of the 12 AIDS patients were female). Other limiting factors were that there may have been underreporting of AIDS patients in the cohort studied and that only inpatients were reported. This study was conducted in the pre-HAART therapy era (Highly Active Antiretroviral Therapy), and most patients were only treated with zidovudine (AZT) or not treated at all. No histopathology was carried out in this study.

In a setting of high HIV seropositive prevalence in the general population, cerebral infection is an important consideration in the differential diagnosis of stroke (Kumwenda *et al.*, 2005).

Possible mechanisms of the increased stroke risk

The information obtained above has suggested that there is a risk of stroke in AIDS patients that is higher than that in age-matched controls. The reason that there is an increased risk of stroke in AIDS patients has been the source of many investigations. The most common mechanisms cited for stroke development in AIDS patients are:

- Hypercoagulable or prothrombotic states
- Other secondary causes such as brain embolism and cerebral infections
- Direct primary HIV-associated vasculopathies

Prothrombotic states

The suggestion that there was a prothrombotic state in AIDS patients has been made by several authors. In a retrospective case–control study comparing stroke etiologies in young, predominantly African American subjects with and without HIV infection, the investigators found protein S deficiency in 20% and meningitis in 25% of the HIV-positive cohort. They concluded that meningitis and protein S deficiency were significantly associated with stroke (Qureshi *et al.*, 1997). However, the relationship between the protein S deficiency and the occurrence of cerebral infarction was not clearly defined.

In a subsequent hospital-based series, 35 HIV-infected heterosexual adult patients presenting with stroke to a large South African public hospital were investigated for stroke cause (Mochan *et al.*, 2003). They did not abuse intravenous drugs, and the strokes were prospectively studied. Smoking, oral contraceptive use, and dyslipidemia were not risk factors in this cohort, and none of them had been treated with antiretroviral therapy. Their mean age was

32.1 years, and there were more women (21) than men (14). Ninety-four percent (33 patients) had cerebral infarctions, 6% (2 patients) had intracerebral hemorrhages, and there were no venous strokes in this series. There was no control group. A possible cause of the cerebral infarction was found in 22 of the 33 patients, and coagulopathy was the most common. Seventeen patients (49%) had a coagulopathy, and of these latter patients protein S deficiency occurred in 11 of the patients, protein C deficiency in 1 patient, and anti-phospholipid antibody syndrome in 5. This study precluded other epidemiological observations because there was no stroke registry in the hospital and hospital admission statistics were not available. The authors also noted that they had no data available on the prevalence of protein S deficiency and anti-phospholipid antibodies in the HIV-positive and HIV-negative populations.

There was a low incidence of intracerebral hemorrhages in this study and also a higher number of women with stroke and HIV. Patients with intracerebral space-occupying lesions were excluded. Five patients had elevated anti-phospholipids and immunoglobulin G (IgG) antibody titers; these antibodies are known to occur frequently in patients with HIV infection and AIDS (Abuaf *et al.*, 1997; Casado Naranjo *et al.*, 1992; Hassell *et al.*, 1994; Rubbert *et al.*, 1994), but the clinical relevance of elevated anti-phospholipid IgG antibody titers in patients who are HIV-positive remains uncertain.

In 2005, Mochan *et al.* undertook a study to determine the relevance of protein S deficiency in HIV-infected patients with ischemic stroke. Thirty-three HIV-positive patients with ischemic stroke who were previously described were prospectively compared with control groups for occurrence of protein S deficiency. The control groups comprised an equal number of consecutive, matched HIV-positive and -negative patients with and without stroke, respectively. Protein S deficiency was found to occur significantly more frequently in HIV-positive patients compared with HIV-negative stroke patients. A second set of controls of HIV-positive patients with other medical conditions (pulmonary tuberculosis, pneumonia, Guillain–Barré syndrome, bilateral Bell's palsy) but without stroke was then included as a control group, and this group was compared with the HIV-positive stroke group. When these patients were compared with the previously reported group of HIV-positive stroke patients (Mochan *et al.*, 2003), a significant association was found between HIV infection and protein S deficiency but not between stroke and protein S deficiency. The observation that HIV infection is associated with protein S deficiency had been made by a number of previous authors (Bissuel *et al.*, 1992; Erbe *et al.*, 2003; Hassell *et al.*, 1994; Sorice *et al.*, 1994; Stahl *et al.*, 1993; Sugerman *et al.*, 1996). However, the inclusion of HIV-positive patients without stroke as a control group indicated that protein S deficiency is related to HIV infection rather than stroke occurrence. In terms of HIV infection, the data supported the concept that the occurrence of protein S deficiency is an epiphenomenon of HIV infection and not a likely cause of stroke. The study was limited by relatively small numbers of patients, but the patients were all from the same region and hospital, and the control groups were appropriately matched. An editorial comment following the article acknowledged that protein S deficiency is probably not related to the increased risk of stroke in HIV (Qureshi, 2005). Other potential mechanisms for the increased stroke risk have been proposed.

Secondary causes of stroke

Traditionally, stroke occurrence with HIV infection has been associated with opportunistic infection, malignancy, and cardioembolic causes of stroke. These are discussed briefly below.

1. Cardiac sources of emboli have been well described. These include HIV-associated cardiomyopathy, infective endocarditis, and nonbacterial thrombotic endocarditis (Anders *et al.*, 1986; Berger *et al.*, 1990).
2. Cerebral opportunistic infections are important causes of secondary infective vasculitis and cause both cerebral infarcts and hemorrhages. These include fungal and tuberculous meningitis. Intracerebral hemorrhage was documented in patients who had infectious or neoplastic intracerebral space-occupying lesions such as primary central nervous system (CNS) lymphoma, metastatic Kaposi's sarcoma, and cerebral toxoplasmosis (Pinto, 1996), and can mimic stroke. Cerebral infections that have been associated with stroke and vasculitis are listed in Table 15.1.
3. Hypercoagulable states. Apart from the questionable role of protein S deficiency and the presence of anti-phospholipid antibodies as a previously mentioned risk for stroke, infrequent reports of other prothrombotic states have been described to cause stroke in the HIV-positive patient. These include disseminated intravascular coagulation (Berger *et al.*, 1990), hyperviscosity syndrome (Martin *et al.*, 1989), and cerebral venous thrombosis with cachexia and dehydration (Berger *et al.*, 1990). Unrecognized prothrombotic states have been suspected of being responsible for cryptogenic stroke in HIV-positive individuals (Hoffmann *et al.*, 2000) but no proof has been offered to support this hypothesis.
4. Malignancy. Lymphoma can invade the vessel wall resulting in thrombosis with subsequent infarction, but this is a very uncommon cause of stroke in the HIV-positive patient.
5. Substance abuse. Patients may be predisposed to developing stroke by virtue of falling into a specific risk group for HIV. In particular, this category includes all patients who misuse drugs intravenously and use substances that are known to cause stroke such as cocaine, heroin, and amphetamines.
6. Accelerated atherosclerosis with use of protease inhibitors. The spectrum of the HIV epidemic is changing. The use of HAART has resulted in a clear reduction in the incidence of comorbid conditions and premature mortality, and this could account for a growing prevalence of atherosclerosis in HIV-infected persons as they get older (Rabinstein, 2003). There is anecdotal evidence that treatment with protease inhibitors is associated with severe premature atherosclerotic vascular disease (Henry *et al.*, 1998; Behrens *et al.*, 1998; Vittecoq *et al.*, 1998). Protease inhibitors can induce a variety of metabolic abnormalities including hypercholesterolemia, hypertriglyceridemia, increased serum insulin and peptide C levels with insulin resistance, and lipodys-

Table 15.1 Infections associated with cerebral vasculitis

Varicella zoster virus
Herpes simplex virus
Cytomegalovirus
Cryptococcus
Aspergillosis
Candida albicans
Coccidioidomycosis
Syphilis
Tuberculosis
Mucormycosis
Toxoplasmosis
Trypanosomiasis

trophy (Sklar and Masur, 2003). These lipid and other abnormalities have been extensively reviewed by Rabinstein (2003).

HIV-associated vasculopathy and vasculitis

The association of systemic vasculitis syndromes with infectious disease is a well-described phenomenon. The co-occurrence of systemic vasculitis and infection with HIV was the subject of an early review (Calabrese, 1991). At that time, efforts were made to determine whether the coexisting diseases were causally or merely coincidentally associated and were limited by the absence of controlled epidemiological investigations, leaving only clinical descriptions and pathophysiologic studies to address the issue (which to this day has not been adequately resolved). The issue is compounded by the fact that HIV infection is frequently associated with coexisting infections – such as Epstein–Barr virus (EBV), varicella zoster virus (VZV), cytomegalovirus (CMV), hepatitis B virus, and others – all of which have been linked causally to various vasculitic syndromes. The author described a spectrum of systemic vasculitic syndromes reported in the literature in association with HIV infection including polyarteritis (Gherardi *et al.*, 1993; Gisselbrecht *et al.*, 1998; Libman *et al.*, 1995; Valeriano-Marcet *et al.*, 1990), Churg–Strauss, hypersensitivity vasculitis, lymphomatoid granulomatosis, and primary angiitis of the central nervous system (PACNS). Apart from PACNS, these conditions manifested with systemic pathology not confined to the CNS. PACNS is a rare condition, and only six case reports in association with HIV are cited in this review. It was not possible to determine whether these cases represent the same disease described in the pre-HIV era or whether they represent some new nosologic entity.

Calabrese (1991) cited a number of tentative mechanisms for an HIV-associated vasculitis, including the possibilities that HIV may be invading the vascular endothelium directly and that the expression of adhesion molecules on the surface of endothelial cells causes lymphocyte trafficking. In addition, the possibility was proposed that virally stimulated immune-competent cells interact with endothelial cells causing the cells to release chemotactic factors or inducing endothelial cells to serve as the focus of altered self-antigenic presentation with a subsequent autoimmune response.

Subsequent to this review, HIV-related cerebral vasculitis is often cited as a cause of stroke. This may be the result of the misinterpretation of perivascular inflammatory cells, which are common in the HIV setting, and the inclusion of cases in which either potential or more likely causes of vasculitis have not been excluded. The pathological diagnosis of a vasculitis should be reserved for cases in which there is infiltration of the vessel wall by inflammatory cells with subsequent vessel wall damage.

The primary vasculopathies of the CNS described in association with HIV include:
1. Small-vessel vasculopathy
2. Large- and medium-vessel vasculopathy

Small-vessel HIV-associated vasculopathy

Mounting evidence supports the occurrence of a disease involving small vessels in the CNS (Rabinstein, 2003). An autopsy study revealed the presence of an asymptomatic vasculopathy in 10 patients characterized by hyaline small-vessel wall thickening, perivascular space dilatation, rarefaction and pigment deposition with vessel wall mineralization, and occasional perivascular inflammatory cell infiltrates (Connor et al., 2000). This study sought to determine whether cerebral infarcts occur in the Edinburgh autopsy cohort in the absence of causes other than HIV infection. The pathologic findings were detected in all patients with hypoxic/ischemic pathologic lesions who had no intercurrent CNS opportunistic infections or embolic sources. These lesions (that were found in 5.5% of this large 183-case autopsy series) were typically multiple, small, and composed of palely stained and rarefied brain tissue with loss of neurons and variable numbers of associated reactive astrocytes and microglial cells with varying degrees of cavitation. Infection of endothelial cells with consequent breakdown of the blood–brain barrier has been advanced as at least a theoretical possible mechanism of HIV entry into the CNS (Budka 1989; Ho et al., 1987; Rhodes and Ward, 1991). Vasculitis was not found in any of the 10 patients, and although 1 patient had had a TIA, no patients had had a stroke. These vascular changes were similar to those found in cases of cerebral arteriosclerosis seen in elderly, hypertensive, and diabetic patients. They were also similar to the changes seen in AIDS-related leukoencephalopathy. However, these patients were young (range 22–47 years) and mostly free of the traditional vascular risk factors (although 5 of the 10 patients with vasculopathy were previously intravenous drug users). Most of the patients had not been on modern antiretroviral drugs when the study was done; therefore, microinfarcts seen were not drug induced. Neither the degree of vasculopathy nor the extent of cerebral microinfarcts was associated with viral load, although all were severely immunodepressed.

The study confirmed the presence of an HIV-associated small-vessel vasculopathy although the associated cerebral microinfarcts are not common (5.5% of cases that went to autopsy) in the absence of cerebral opportunistic infection, lymphoma, non-HIV infection, or embolic sources.

Large- and medium-vessel HIV-associated vasculopathy

Cerebral aneurysmal arteriopathy in childhood AIDS

A cerebral vasculopathy with aneurysms is a rare HIV-specific condition leading to stroke that was previously reported only in children with AIDS. Typically the arteriopathy developed in children between 2 and 12 years of age, was characterized by fusiform dilatation of the arteries of the Circle of Willis with sparing of the leptomeningeal and intraparenchymal arteries and arterioles, and presented with ischemic stroke or intracranial hemorrhage (Dubrovsky et al., 1998). The vascular pathology (in four patients who had postmortem examinations) showed medial fibrosis with loss of the muscularis, destruction of the internal elastic lamina, and intimal hyperplasia. In those patients tested, immunostains for HSV, VZV, and CMV were negative. All these patients had a severely depressed immune system with a history of multiple opportunistic infections preceding the diagnosis of aneurysmal arteriopathy. Although vascular inflammation was sparse or absent in the few autopsy cases, the pathology was considered consistent with a prior vasculitis, and the clinical histories clearly indicated an acquired lesion of subacute onset. The pathogenesis of this vasculopathy was unclear, but the authors suggested a role for VZV or a vasculitis due to HIV itself. Evidence for HIV was the detection of HIV protein or genomic material in two of the four autopsy cases. Other case reports have confirmed the presence of this distinct entity with single but typically multiple fusiform or saccular aneurysms located near or in the Circle of Willis in children with AIDS (Martinez-Longoria et al., 2004; Mazzoni et al., 2000; Nunes et al., 2001; Patsalides et al., 2002)

Large- and medium-vessel HIV-associated vasculopathy in adults

As early as 1996, case reports of saccular cerebral aneurysms in adult patients with full blown AIDS presenting with subarachnoid hemorrhage appeared in the literature (Maniker and Hunt, 1996). Histopathology was not available, and the authors had no reason to suggest that HIV was a causal agent in the formation of cerebral aneurysms. They cited the pediatric literature (Joshi et al., 1987) as evidence that HIV is implicated in cerebral vascular disease by virtue of a vasculitis shown at autopsy. Subsequently, a large to medium-sized extra- and intracranial vasculopathy peculiar to HIV was reported. In 2000, Chetty et al. reported a series of 16 HIV-positive adult patients (age range 18–38 years) with large-vessel disease consisting of either aneurysms (usually multiple) or occlusive disease. These patients presented with rupture of aneurysm, TIA, hypertension, ischemia to the lower extremity, or a mass at the site of the aneurysm. Arteries commonly affected were the common carotid, abdominal aorta, common iliac, femoral, and popliteal.

Pathological specimens from these 16 patients were sent for histological assessment of aneurysmal and nonaneurysmal vessel wall. Special stains for acid-fast bacilli, fungi, spirochetes, and bacteria were performed on all specimens. Patients had the relevant serologic tests for syphilis, typhoid, anti-nuclear factor, and anticardiolipin antibodies, but viral cultures were not performed.

None of the patients had any obvious infective vascular lesion, and none were treated for HIV/AIDS. Histopathology of the vessel wall revealed that the key features were within the adventitia – showing a leukocytoclastic vasculitis of the vasa vasorum and periadventitial vessels, proliferation of slit-like vascular channels, chronic inflammation, and fibrosis. There was associated medial fibrosis with loss and fragmentation of muscle and elastic tissue. Intimal changes were slight and consisted of duplication and fragmentation of the internal elastic lamina with calcification. Atheroma and marked intimal thickening were not evident.

The authors suggested that the occurrence of this large-vessel vasculopathy (mainly aneurysmal), often with multiple lesions in young HIV-positive patients, was characteristic of possible infective or immune complex origin, with leukocytoclastic vasculitis of vasa vasorum and periadventitial vessels being pivotal in many cases. The histological changes described in this study suggest that two patterns are present:

1. An acute or active phase that shows leukocytoclastic vasculitis of the vasa vasorum with resultant ischemia of the media
2. A chronic healed/healing phase with less obvious leukocytoclastic vasculitis, and fibrosis in the media ultimately leading to weakening of the vessel and aneurysm formation. Occlusive disease or aneurysm formation is most likely secondary to vessel wall damage after leukocytoclastic vasculitis.

The authors made a cogent argument that the clinicopathological changes described in their study are characteristic and consistent enough to suggest that this large-vessel disease represents a distinct subset of vasculopathy in HIV-positive patients.

In a subsequent report, the same group reported a spontaneous arteriovenous fistula of the superficial femoral artery in an HIV-infected person (Nair *et al.*, 2001). Histological examination of the artery showed similar features to those seen in HIV-related aneurysm (Chetty *et al.*, 2000). In an ongoing clinical survey to determine the spectrum of vascular disease in HIV/AIDS patients conducted at the University of Pretoria Academic Hospital in South Africa a similar spectrum of clinical vascular pathology was reported. This involved occlusive disease of large arteries (including the extracranial carotid arteries) as well as striking aneurysms of large vessels, but histology was not provided.

Subsequently isolated case reports of intracranial cerebral vasculopathy have been reported by a few authors. Kossorotoff *et al.* (2006) described two adult patients with this characteristic angiographic appearance: a 23-year-old infected with HIV presenting with recurrent large vessel ischemic stroke as well as interhemispheric meningeal hemorrhage in which angiography revealed a vasculopathy characterized by multiple ectasias and stenotic lesions of medium-sized arteries and aneurysmal dilatation of the terminal internal carotid artery, and a 32-year-old HIV-positive patient with ischemic stroke in the right middle cerebral artery territory who had angiography that showed multiple ectasias and focal stenoses of medium- and small-sized cerebral arteries. Serology for a variety of infective causes (including CMV, EBV, VZV, and HSV) were all negative. In another report (Ake, 2006) a 29-year-old African American with AIDS is described who presented with an acute intracranial hemorrhage and was shown to have many

fusiform aneurysms and stenoses involving the anterior and posterior circulations. Extensive evaluations for infectious, autoimmune, or metabolic causes were all negative.

Tipping *et al.* (2006) described a 27-year-old HIV-infected South African woman who presented with ischemic stroke and was shown to have an intracranial vasculopathy on angiography characterized by fusiform dilatation of the arteries of the Circle of Willis. Subsequent autopsy and histological examination of the internal carotid and middle cerebral arteries showed luminal thrombosis, concentric intimal fibrosis with hyalinization, and thinning of the elastic lamina. Neutrophils were present on the luminal surface related to the thrombus. Arteries on the nonaneurysmal side had thickened internal elastic lamina with fragmentation and focal intimal proliferation with calcification. The media was preserved. There was deposition of mucopolysaccharides in the intima and media of the arteries with splaying of the myocytes. No microorganisms or cytopathic changes were observed, and immunoperoxidase stains showed moderate numbers of CD68 macrophages and some CD3 lymphocytes. HIV p24 antigen staining of the vessel sections was negative. As there was no evidence of active vasculitis, the authors suggest that the pathology of intracranial HIV-associated vasculopathy may be different from the extracranial aneurysms in HIV-positive patients because of a vasculitis involving the vasa vasorum, which is absent in the intracranial vessels.

In a subsequent study (Tipping *et al.*, 2007), 67 patients with confirmed first stroke, infected with HIV, and prospectively included in the University of Cape Town/Groote Schuur Hospital stroke register between September 2000 and July 2006 were identified and reviewed. Patients with nonstroke intracranial lesions were excluded. Mean age was 33.4 years with 90% of these patients younger than 45 years. Cerebral infarction occurred in 64 patients (96%) and intracerebral hemorrhage in 3 (4%). The etiology of the intracerebral hemorrhages was hypertension in all three patients. Underlying causes of cerebral infarction were identified in the majority of patients. However, seven patients (10%) were identified with an extracranial vasculopathy for which no obvious cause could be found. This manifested clinically as either a total or significant occlusion of the carotid bifurcation. Seven patients (10%) had radiological evidence of an intracranial vasculopathy for which no cause could be found and which was not seen without cause in the HIV-negative group of stroke patients in our register of 1087 South African stroke patients. Intracranial vasculopathy is characterized as medium-vessel occlusion with or without fusiform dilatation, stenosis, and vessel caliber variation by angiography (Figures 15.1, 15.2, 15.3, and 15.4).

The study also emphasized the approach that, in HIV-positive patients presenting with a stroke or TIA, potentially treatable causes such as cerebral coinfection or tumor should be excluded before assuming that the cause is related to HIV infection itself as a result of a vasculopathy or some as yet unrecognized pathogenetic mechanism.

In HIV-infected patients with stroke, underlying intra- and extracranial vasculopathy is being increasingly recognized after infective vasculitides have been excluded. The precise mechanisms of this vasculopathy, the role of the HIV, and the potential influence of HAART remain to be determined.

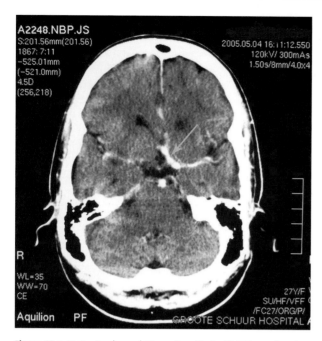

Figure 15.1 Contrast-enhanced CT scan in patient with HIV vasculopathy showing fusiform dilatation of the A1 segment of the anterior cerebral artery.

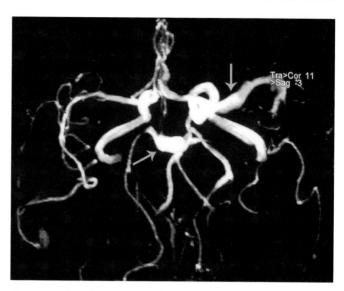

Figure 15.3 Three-dimensional time-of-flight magnetic resonance angiography (MRA) of Circle of Willis: fusiform dilatation of the left M1 segment (*top arrow*) with attenuation of the left M2 and M3 vessels; fusiform dilatation of the terminal basilar artery and right P1 segment of the posterior cerebral artery (*bottom arrow*).

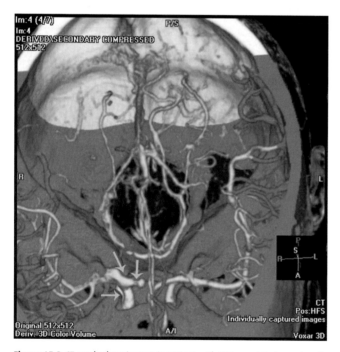

Figure 15.2 CT cerebral angiogram in patient with HIV-associated vasculopathy with fusiform dilatation of the right distal supraclinoid internal carotid (*bottom arrow*) and proximal M1 and A1 segments of the right middle and anterior cerebral artery (*top left arrow*). There is a postdilatation stenosis and occlusion of the right anterior cerebral artery (*top right arrow*). See color plate.

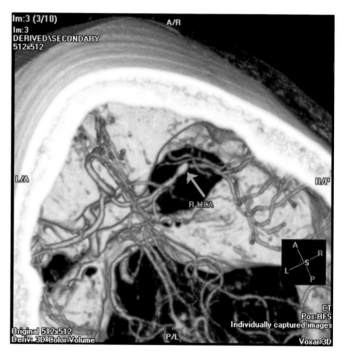

Figure 15.4 CT angiogram: fusiform segmental dilatation of the right middle cerebral artery (distal M1).

Approach to stroke therapy in a patient that is found to be HIV positive or has AIDS

The management of the HIV-infected patient presenting with a stroke should be directed primarily towards determining the underlying cause of the stroke.

The occurrence of stroke in the younger patient who is HIV positive should not preclude comprehensive evaluation, as HIV status may be incidental particularly in a population with a high HIV seropositive prevalence in the general population. A thorough history and clinical examination frequently reveal a likely cause for stroke. This should include enquiry concerning drug misuse and symptoms and signs of opportunistic infection such as tuberculosis and prior VZV.

A coagulation abnormality is often found associated with HIV and stroke. As discussed above, protein S deficiency has been associated with HIV and stroke and is probably an epiphenomenon, and the role of elevated anti-phospholipid antibodies is uncertain.

AIDS is frequently found in developing countries and in medical environments in which a rational and cost-effective approach is recommended. A CT scan is essential in any young patient with a stroke that is HIV positive in order to establish whether there has been a hemorrhage or an infarct and to exclude other conditions that often mimic stroke in the HIV-positive patient such as toxoplasmosis, tuberculoma, or lymphoma. If the CT scan does not reveal evidence of a space-occupying lesion, a lumbar puncture is usually indicated in order to exclude chronic meningitis (tuberculosis, syphilis, fungal infection, zoster). Given the high prevalence of cardioembolic causes of stroke in this group, careful cardiac examination, electrocardiogram, and often echocardiography is required. Although full blood count, serology for syphilis, and chest x-ray is routinely done, a CD4 count is not essential but does provide information about the degree of immunosuppression in the HIV-infected person.

Other investigations including angiography should be individualized and should follow routine stroke management guidelines. Regardless of angiographic appearance, stroke should not be attributed to an HIV-associated vasculopathy unless thorough evaluation has excluded infective and other causes.

The patient should ideally be treated in a stroke unit, and long-term care plans would need to be tailored to the patient's specific needs. The severity of the primary disease and the association of secondary opportunistic infections are of major importance in the management of these patients. The rehabilitation of the HIV-infected patient, particularly with a stroke, should not be neglected. With the predicted future increased use of HAART in patients diagnosed with AIDS, attention will need to be directed to the potential metabolic abnormalities (including the lipid abnormalities with atherogenic potential due to the protease inhibitors) that may develop on treatment.

Conclusions

There is mounting evidence to indicate that HIV infection is associated with an increased risk for both ischemic and hemorrhagic stroke. A number of mechanisms, discussed in detail in this chapter, have been proposed for this increased risk including prothrombotic states, other secondary causes such as cerebral infections and cardioembolic causes, as well as a primary HIV-associated vasculopathy. Two forms of vasculopathy have been described that have been considered to be HIV-specific:

Small vessel HIV-associated vasculopathy

This is largely an asymptomatic vasculopathy that has been described in patients that have died with AIDS and is characterized by hyaline small-vessel wall thickening, perivascular space dilatation, rarefaction and pigment deposition with vessel wall mineralization, and occasional perivascular inflammatory cell infiltrates, and is associated with microinfarcts.

Large- and medium-vessel HIV-associated vasculopathy

This was first described in children and then later in adults. The vasculopathy involves both extracranial arteries (including the carotids but also other large arteries) as well as medium-sized intracranial vessels, particularly those near or part of the Circle of Willis. The extracranial vasculopathy presents with occlusive disease or aneurysm formation and is most likely secondary to vessel wall damage after leukocytoclastic vasculitis. The intracranial vasculopathy is characterized as medium-vessel occlusion with or without fusiform dilatation, stenosis, and vessel caliber variation by angiography and can present as either ischemic stroke or intracranial hemorrhage.

A number of possible mechanisms have been proposed to be implicated in the pathogenesis of this condition, but the exact role of HIV in the etiology of the condition remains uncertain.

REFERENCES

Abuaf, N., Laperche, S., Rajoely, B., et al. 1997. Auto antibodies to phospholipid and to the coagulation proteins in AIDS. Thromb Haemost, 77, 856–61.

Ake, J. A., 2006. Cerebral aneurysmal arteriopathy associated with HIV infection in an adult. Clin Infect Dis, 43, e46–50.

Anders, K. H., Guerra, W. F., Tomiyasu, U., Verity, M. A., and Vinters, H. V. 1986. The neuropathology of AIDS: UCLA experience and review. Am J Pathol, 124, 537–58.

Behrens, G., Schmidt, H., Meyer, D., Stoll, M., and Schmidt, R. E. 1998. Vascular complications associated with the use of HIV protease inhibitors. Lancet, 351, 1958.

Berger, J. R., 2004. AIDS and stroke risk. Lancet Neurol, 3, 206–7.

Berger, J. R., Harris, J. O., Gregarios, J., and Norenberg, M. 1990. Cerebrovascular disease in AIDS: a case control study. AIDS, 4, 239–44.

Bissuel, F., Berruyer, M., and Causse, X. 1992. Acquired protein S deficiency: correlation with advanced disease in HIV-1 infected patients. J Acquir Immune Defic Syndr, 5, 484–9.

Budka, H. 1989. Human immunodeficiency virus (HIV)–induced disease of the central nervous system: pathology and implications for pathogenesis. Acta Neuropathol, 77, 225–36.

Budka, H., Costanzi, G., and Cristina, S. 1987. Brain pathology induced by infection with the human immunodeficiency virus (HIV): a histological, immunocytochemical and electron microscopical study of 100 autopsy cases. Acta Neuropathol (Berlin), 75, 185–98.

Calabrese, L. H. 1991. Vasculitis and infection with the human immunodeficiency virus. Rheum Dis Clin North Am, 17, 131–47.

Casado Naranjo, I., Toledo Santos, J. A., and Antolin Rodriguez, M. A. 1992. Ischemic stroke as the sole manifestation of human immunodeficiency virus infection. Stroke, 23, 117–8.

Chetty, R. 2005. Vasculitides associated with HIV infection. J Clin Pathol, 54, 275–8.

Chetty, R., Batitang, S., and Nair, R. 2000. Large artery vasculopathy in HIV positive patients. Another vasculitic enigma. Hum Pathol, 31, 374–9.

Cole, J. W., Pinto, A. N., Hebel, J. R., et al. 2004. Acquired immunodeficiency syndrome and the risk of stroke. Stroke, 35, 51–6.

Connor, M. D., Lammie, G. A., Bell, J. A., Warlow, C. P., Simmonds, P., and Brettle, R. D. 2000. Cerebral infarction in adult AIDS patients. Observations from the Edinburgh HIV autopsy cohort. Stroke, 31, 2117–26.

Dorrington, R. E., Johnson, L. F., Bradshaw, D., and Daniel, T. 2006. The demographic impact of HIV/AIDS in South Africa. National and Provincial Indicators for 2006. Cape Town: Centre for Actuarial Research, South African Medical Research Council and Actuarial Society of South Africa. Available at: http://www.assa.org.za/aids or http://www.mrc.ac.za.

Dubrovsky, T., Curless, R., Scott, G., et al. 1998. Cerebral aneurysmal arteriopathy in childhood AIDS. Neurology, 51, 560–5.

Engstroom, J. W., Lowenstein, D. H., and Bredesen, D. E. 1989. Cerebral infarction and transient neurological deficits associated with acquired immune deficiency syndrome. *Am J Med*, **86**, 528–32.

Erbe, M., Rickerts, V., and Bauersachs, R. M. 2003. Acquired protein C and protein S deficiency in HIV infected patients. *Clin Appl Thromb Haemost*, **9**, 325–31.

Evers, S., Nabavi, D., Ratiman, A., *et al.* 2003. Ischemic cerebrovascular events in HIV infection, a cohort study. *Cerebrovasc Dis*, **15**, 199–205.

Gherardi, R., Belec, L., and Mhin, C. 1993. The spectrum of vasculitis in human immunodeficiency virus–infected patients. *Arthritis Rheum*, **36**, 1164–74.

Gillams, A. R., Allen, E., Hrieb, K., *et al.* 1997. Cerebral infarction in patients with AIDS. *AJNR Am J Neuroradiol*, **18**, 1581–5.

Gisselbrecht, M., Cohen, P., and Lortholary, D. 1998. Human immunodeficiency virus–related vasculitis. Clinical presentation of and therapeutic approach to eight cases. *Ann Med Interne (Paris)*, **149**, 398–405.

Hassell, K. L., Kressin, D. C., Neumann, A., Ellison, R., and Marlar, R. A. 1994. Correlation of antiphospholipid antibodies and protein S deficiency with thrombosis in HIV infected men. *Blood Coagul Fibrinolysis*, **5**, 455–62.

Henry, K., Melroe, H., Heubesch, J., *et al.* 1998. Severe premature coronary artery disease with protease inhibitors. *Lancet*, **351**, 1328.

Ho, D. D., Pomerantz, R. J., and Kaplan, J. C. 1987. Pathogenesis of infection with human immunodeficiency virus. *N Engl J Med*, **317**, 278–86.

Hoffman, M., Berger, J. R., Nath, A., and Rayens, M. 2000. Cerebrovascular disease in young HIV infected black Africans in the Kwa-Zulu Natal Province of South Africa. *J Neurovirol*, **6**, 229–36.

Joshi, V. V., Pawel, B., Connor, E., *et al.* 1987. Arteriopathy in children with acquired immune deficiency syndrome. *Pediatr Pathol*, **7**, 261–75.

Kossorotoff, M., Touzé, E., Godon-Hardy, S., *et al.* 2006. Cerebral vasculopathy with aneurysm formation in HIV-infected young adults. *Neurology*, **66**, 1121–2.

Kumwenda, J. J., Mateyu, G., Kampondeni, S., *et al.* 2005. Differential diagnosis of stroke in a setting of high HIV prevalence in Blantyre, Malawi. *Stroke*, **36**, 960–4.

Kuwe, K., Llena, J. F., and Lyman, W. D. 1991. Human immunodeficiency virus–1 infection of the nervous system: an autopsy study of 268 adult, paediatric and foetal brains. *Hum Pathol*, **22**, 700–10.

Lang, W., Miklossy, J., Deruaz, J. P., *et al.* 1989. Neuropathology of the acquired immune deficiency syndrome (AIDS): a report of 135 consecutive autopsy cases from Switzerland. *Acta Neuropathol (Berlin)*, **77**, 379–90.

Libman, B. S., Quismorio, F. P. Jr, and Stimmler, M. M. 1995 Polyarteritis nodosa like vasculitis in human deficiency virus infection. *J Rheumatol*, **22**, 351–5.

Maniker, A. L., and Hunt, C. D. 1996. Cerebral aneurysm in the HIV patient: a report of six cases. *Surg Neurol*, **46**, 49–54.

Martin, C. M., Matlow, A. G., Chew, E., Sutton, D., and Pruzanski, W. 1989. Hyperviscosity syndrome in a patient with acquired immunodeficiency syndrome. *Arch Intern Med*, **149**, 1435–6.

Martinez-Longoria, C. A., Morales-Aguirre, J. J., Villalobos-Acosta, C. P., Gomez-Barreto, D., and Cashat-Cruz, M. 2004. Occurrence of intracerebral aneurysm in an HIV-infected child: a case report. *Pediatr Neurol*, **31**, 130–2.

Mazzoni, P., Chiriboga, C. A., Millar, W. S., and Rogers, A. 2000. Intracerebral aneurysms in human immunodeficiency virus infection: case report and literature review. *Pediatr Neurol*, **23**, 252–5.

Mizusawa, H., Hirano, A., Llena, J. F., and Shintaku, M. 1988. Cerebrovascular lesions in acquired immune deficiency syndrome (AIDS). *Acta Neuropathol*, **76**, 451–7.

Mochan, A., Modi, M., and Modi, G. 2003. Stroke in black South African HIV positive patients, a prospective analysis. *Stroke*, **34**, 10–5.

Mochan, A., Modi, M., and Modi, G. 2005. Protein S deficiency in HIV associated ischemic stroke: an epiphenomenon of HIV infection. *J Neurol Neurosurg Psychiatry*, **76**, 1455–6.

Nair, R., Chetty, R., Woolgar, J., Naidoo, N. G., and Robbs, J. V. 2001. Spontaneous arteriovenous fistula resulting from HIV arteritis. *J Vasc Surg*, **33**, 186–7.

The National HIV and syphilis seroprevalence study of women attending public health clinics in SA. 2000. South Africa: Department of Health. www.doh.gov.za/docs/reports/2000/hivreport.html

Nunes, M. L., Pinho, A. P., and Sfoggia, A. 2001. Cerebral aneurysmal dilatation in an infant with perinatally acquired HIV infection and HSV encephalitis. *Arq Neuropsiquiatr*, **59**(3-B), 830.

Patel, V. B., Sacoor, Z., Francis, P., *et al.* 2005. Ischemic stroke in young HIV positive patients in Kwa-Zulu Natal, South Africa. *Neurology*, **65**, 759–61.

Patsalides, A. D., Wood, L. V., Atac, G. K., Sandifer, E., Butman, J. A., and Patronas, N. J. 2002. Cerebrovascular disease in HIV-infected pediatric patients. *AJR Am J Roentgenol*, **179**, 999–1003.

Petito, C. K., Cho, E. S., Lemann, W., Naria, B. A., and Price, R. W. 1986. Neuropathology of Acquired Immunodeficiency Syndrome (AIDS): an autopsy review. *J Neuropathol Exp Neurol*, **45**, 635–646.

Pinto, A. N. 1996. AIDS and cerebrovascular disease. *Stroke*, **27**, 538–43.

Qureshi, A. I. 2005. HIV infection and stroke: if not protein S deficiency then what explains the relationship. *J Neurol Neurosurg Psychiatry*, **76**, 1331.

Qureshi, A. I., Janssen, R. S., Karon, J. M., *et al.* 1997. Human immunodeficiency virus infection and stroke in young patients. *Arch Neurol*, **54**, 1150–3.

Rabinstein, A. A. 2003. Stroke In HIV-infected patients: a clinical perspective. *Cerebrovasc Dis*, **15**, 37–44.

Rhodes, R. H. 1987. Histopathology of the central nervous system in the acquired immunodeficiency syndrome. *Hum Pathol*, **18**, 636–43.

Rhodes, R. H., and Ward, J. M. 1991. AIDS meningoencephalomyelitis: pathogenesis and changing neuropathological findings. *Pathol Annu*, **26**, 247–76.

Rubbert, A., Bock, E., Schwab, J., *et al.* 1994. Anticardiolipin antibodies in HIV infection: association with cerebral perfusion defects as detected by 99 mTc–HMPAO SPECT. *Clin Exp Immunol*, **98**, 361–8.

Sklar, P., and Masur, H. 2003. HIV infection and cardiovascular disease–is there really a link? *N Engl J Med*, **349**, 2065–7.

Sorice, M., Griggi, T., and Arceria, P. 1994. Protein S and HIV infection. The role of anticardiolysis and antiprotein S. *Thromb Res*, **73**, 65–175.

Stahl, C. P., Wideman, C. S., and Spira, T. J. 1993. Protein S deficiency in men with long term human immunodeficiency virus infection. *Blood*, **81**, 1801–7.

Sugerman, R. W., Church, J. A., and Goldsmith, J. C. 1996. Acquired protein S deficiency in children infected with human immunodeficiency virus. *Pediatr Infect Dis J*, **15**, 106–11.

Tipping, B., de Villiers, L., Candy, S., and Wainwright, H. 2006. Stroke caused by human immunodeficiency virus-associated intracranial large-vessel aneurysmal vasculopathy. *Arch Neurol*, **63**, 1640–2.

Tipping, B., de Villiers, L., Wainright, H., Candy, S., and Bryer, A. 2007. Stroke in human immunodeficiency virus infections. *J Neurol, Neurosurg, and Psychiatry*, **78**, 1320–4.

Valeriano-Marcet, J., Ravichandran, L., and Kerr, L. D. 1990. HIV associated systemic necrotising vasculitis. *J Rheumatol*, **17**, 1091–3.

Vittecoq, D., Escaut, L., and Monsuez, J. J. 1998. Vascular complications associated with the use of HIV protease inhibitors. *Lancet*, **351**, 1958–9.

PART II: HEREDITARY AND GENETIC CONDITIONS AND MALFORMATIONS

16 PULMONARY ARTERIOVENOUS MALFORMATIONS

Julien Morier and Patrik Michel

Introduction

Pulmonary arteriovenous malformations (PAVMs) are rare occurrences among the population. With patent foramen ovale (PFO), congenital cardiac defects, and patent ductus arteriosus, they belong to the group of pathological arteriovenous communications that increase the risk of paradoxical embolism. Since their first description in 1897 (Churton, 1897), they have been called hemangiomas of the lung, pulmonary telangiectasias, cavernous angiomas of the lung, pulmonary arteriovenous aneurysms, or pulmonary arteriovenous fistulae. Although uncommon, their detection is of the utmost importance as they are a treatable cause of potentially devastating conditions. Complications such as hemothorax or a massive hemoptysis may occur. Their presence is associated with neurological complications such as acute ischemic stroke, transient ischemic attack (TIA), intracerebral hemorrhage, seizure, migraine, and cerebral abscess in 30–45% of patients. This incidence may reach 70% in case of a diffuse disease (Faughnan et al., 2000).

These malformations can be acquired in various clinical settings or be congenital. Indeed most of them (~70%) are associated with Hereditary hemorrhagic telangiectasia (HHT), also known as Osler–Weber–Rendu disease (see Chapter 17), which is an inherited autosomal dominant disorder characterized by recurrent epistaxis, mucocutaneous telangiectases, and visceral involvement. Older reports assert that PAVM patients with HHT tend to have a more pronounced symptomatology, a more rapid disease progression, a higher frequency of multiple arteriovenous malformations, and more complications (Dines et al., 1974, 1983; Monsour et al., 1970). Given this poorer prognosis, the use of the diagnostic criteria of HHT, also known as the Curaçao criteria (positive family history for HHT, visceral lesion, telangiectasia, recurrent and spontaneous epistaxis), is encouraged (Shovlin et al., 2000).

The clinical course of pulmonary malformations is usually slowly progressive, although a more rapid growth has been described during pregnancy and adolescence. If the symptoms are left untreated, morbidity and mortality can rise significantly. Fortunately, thanks to recent advances in genetics, radiological imaging, and interventional radiology, this disease is better understood and is treated earlier and more efficiently.

Pathology

Congenital PAVMs consist of direct arteriovenous connections without any intervening capillary bed. They are usually made of two parts: a thin-wall part corresponding to the endothelium, and a surrounding connective tissue stroma in a variable amount. Precise distinction between venous and arterial components is usually not possible. They are classified as either simple PAVMs (2/3 of patients), when their feeding arteries arise from a single subsegmental artery, or as complex (1/3), when they are perfused by more than one artery. Based on embryological development, an anatomical classification of PAVMs has been proposed that divides these lesions into five groups according to their size and the presence of an aneurysm or a fistula (Anabtawi et al., 1965).

A thorough review of the pathologic characteristics of patients with PAVMs showed that 36% had multiple lesions, whereas 8–25% had bilateral disease (Bosher et al., 1959). Thirty to 70% of solitary PAVMs are located in the lower lobes (Swanson et al., 1999; White et al., 1988), more frequently in the left lower lobe. Their size is usually 1–5 cm, but some can be bigger than 10 cm. About 7–11% of patients have diffuse microvascular PAVMs that might occur in association with larger arteriovenous malformations, leading to a higher risk of developing cerebral complications. It is widely accepted that PAVMs with a diameter >2 cm and/or a feeding artery >3 mm are associated with an increased risk of developing neurological complications and therefore must be treated even in asymptomatic patients (White et al., 1988). The natural history of smaller PAVMs remains unclear, and it is unproved whether vessels smaller than 1 mm in diameter could allow emboli to enter the systemic circulation. If untreated, about half of the PAVMs gradually enlarge at an approximate rate of 0.3–2 mm per year (Mager et al., 2004; Vase et al., 1985).

Epidemiology

About 45–90% of the cases of PAVM are linked to HHT, whereas 15–50% of patients with HHT have a PAVM (Gallitelli et al., 2005; Gossage and Kanj, 1998; Hinterseer et al., 2006; Moussouttas et al., 2000). The prevalence of HHT is 2–3 per 100 000 population, but it might be higher than 1 in 10 000 in certain areas like the Danish island of Fyn (Vase et al., 1985), the Dutch Antilles (Jessurun et al., 1993), and even some Northern regions of France (Plauchu et al., 1989). A positive family history is found in 70–94% of patients studied. There is a female predominance of 1.5–2:1.

Symptoms related to PAVM, especially when they are congenital, will develop between the third and sixth decades. More than two thirds of neurological manifestations of HHT are related to PAVMs (Guttmacher et al., 1995). In the remaining third, cerebral

Uncommon Causes of Stroke, 2nd edition, ed. Louis R. Caplan. Published by Cambridge University Press. © Cambridge University Press 2008.

or spinal arteriovenous malformations may cause subarachnoid hemorrhage, seizures, or (in very rare cases) paraparesis (Roman *et al.*, 1978). The complications of PAVM involve the central nervous system in about 30–70%.

Pathogenesis and etiology

The etiology of PAVMs remains unexplained. Several mechanisms have been proposed on the basis of histology. It is believed that a defect in the terminal arterial loop could induce a dilation of capillary sacs, and that an incomplete resorption of the vascular septae between the arterial and venous plexuses during fetal development could lead to the formation of these defects (Gossage and Kanj, 1998). In patients with HHT, two disease-causing gene mutations on chromosomes 9 (locus 9q34) and 12 (locus 12q1) have been identified as HHT type 1 and HHT type 2, respectively. A third uncommon subtype is associated with juvenile polyposis coli, which is due to a mutation of SMAD-4 (Gallione *et al.*, 2004). The gene on chromosome 9 encodes for endoglin (CD105), which is a cell-surface component of the transforming growth factor-alpha (TGF-alpha) receptor complex, whereas activin receptor-like kinase 1 (ALK-1) encoded on chromosome 12 belongs to the TGF-alpha superfamily type I receptor. Both are implicated in controlling migration, proliferation, adhesion, and extracellular matrix composition of the endothelial cells (Marchuk, 1997). A molecular diagnostic test (quantitative multiplex polymerase chain reaction [PCR], sequence analysis, reverse-transcriptase PCR) has been available since late 2003. It may help to identify patients with HHT and to classify families. However, the heterogeneity of the mutations (deletions, insertions, missense, and point mutations) emphasizes the difficulties of the task. Even if PAVMs are 10 times more likely in families with HHT 1 than with HHT 2 (Berg *et al.*, 1996), the phenotype of endoglin families can be mild for successive generations before an individual presents with a symptomatic PAVMs. These families could also be more prone to develop cerebral arteriovenous malformations, but this has not been shown unambiguously so far. Despite the description of several endoglin mutations, no differences have been observed with respect to the clinical presentation (Shovlin and Letarte, 1999). The pathophysiological mechanism responsible for neurological complications such as strokes and brain abscesses is probably paradoxical embolism across the PAVMs. The malformation eliminates the physiological filter of the lungs, so that shunt flow is able to cross through the PAVMs. In contrast to the intermittent passage of emboli through PFOs that occurs during increased pressure in the right atrium, materials can pass through PAVMs continuously. In this aspect, PAVM patients are considered at a higher risk of paradoxical embolism. The total surface area of all the arteriovenous channels should be considered when evaluating the risk of embolism, although others have opined that shunt size is not correlated with the risk of brain abscesses, for instance (Gallitelli *et al.*, 2006). It remains debatable whether embolism originates from the peripheral venous circulation or directly from a local thrombosis within the PAVM.

Other than paradoxical embolism, thrombotic events because of polycythemia, hypoxia, or even air embolism from a defect in the wall of the PAVM could promote brain ischemia. Polycythemia or anemia during pregnancy might worsen hemodynamics within the arteriovenous malformation. Brain abscesses occur in 50% of the cases after a recent visit to the dentist. Less frequently, PAVMs are found in other medical conditions such as hepatopulmonary syndrome or in mitral stenosis, trauma, actinomycosis, schistosomiasis, metastatic thyroid cancer, or Fanconi's syndrome. Other causes of pulmonary shunt must be considered in case of surgery for congenital cardiac disease, moderate-to-severe bronchiectasis, or as a result of venous atresia. To our knowledge, only one case has been described in association with Adams–Oliver syndrome, which is a rare entity characterized by terminal transverse limb malformation of variable severity and congenital scalp defects (Maniscalco *et al.*, 2005). In contrast to PFO (where it is a real concern), only one case of dysbaric air embolism associated with HHT has been reported (Hsu *et al.*, 2004). The concomitant presence of PFO and PAVM in a right-to-left shunt should not be overlooked (Peters *et al.*, 2005).

Clinical features

The clinical manifestations of PAVMs in patients with HHT as well as those without HHT are quite variable, as is the phenotype of HHT. Asymptomatic patients account for up to 50% of patients, making this diagnosis moderately related to the clinical status. PAVMs may manifest themselves early in life with congestive heart failure, cyanosis, or severe respiratory failure, but symptoms usually develop between the third and the sixth decade. Single PAVMs <2 cm in diameter may be asymptomatic. The severity of symptoms is believed to be proportionally related to the size (diameter) of the PAVMs.

Epistaxis resulting from PAVM is the most common complaint, noted in 50% of patients by the age of 20 and 90% by the age of 45 (Plauchu *et al.*, 1989), but usually the bleeding is not severe enough to cause anemia. Epistaxis precedes the development of cutaneous telangiectases by 10–30 years. Dyspnea is the second most common symptom in about 55% of all patients, especially in those with large or multiple PAVMs. Cyanosis and clubbing are not directly related to the size of the PAVMs or to the intensity of the dyspnea. Some patients have platypnea-orthodeoxia (improvement in breathing on reclining and hypoxemia in the sitting or upright position). Hemoptysis is the third symptom in terms of frequency (8–15%). Life-threatening hemoptysis may occur as the initial symptom, although nowadays the mortality from such an event is moderate. Gastrointestinal bleeding from telangiectases develops after the age of 58 in half of the patients. Hemothorax occurs less often, but the risk seems higher during the second half of pregnancy. Other less specific symptoms such as chest pain, cough, and syncope have also been mentioned in patients with PAVMs (Gossage and Kanj, 1998).

Neurological symptoms are present in about half of the patients (43–67%). Confusion, syncope, paresthesias, paresis, headache, and vertigo represent the major symptoms. Tinnitus, dizziness, dysarthria, and diplopia are more likely due to cerebrovascular complications. Age increases the risk of neurological complications; they occur in 10% of PAVM patients younger than

30 years and in 45% of patients older than 30 years (Maher *et al.*, 2001; Moussouttas *et al.*, 2000). The following incidence of neurological complications from single PAVM has been observed in the studies by White *et al.* (1988, 1996): TIA in 37%, acute ischemic stroke in 18%, brain abscess in 9%, seizure in 8%, and migraine in 43%. In the study by Cottin *et al.* (2007) that included single and multiple PAVMs with HHT, slightly different figures were found: TIA (6.3%), acute ischemic stroke (9.5%), brain abscess (19%), migraine (16%), and cerebral hemorrhage (2.4%). Only four cases of paradoxical brain embolism related to an isolated PAVM without HHT have been reported so far (Kimura *et al.*, 2004).

The prevalence of cerebral vascular malformation in patients with HHT is about 10–15% (Haitjema *et al.*, 1995; Willinsky *et al.*, 1990), with one study reporting up to 36% (Roman *et al.*, 1978). It comprises arteriovenous malformations (mostly low-grade Spetzler I or II), cavernous malformations, dural arteriovenous fistulae, and aneurysms. Very few studies about intracranial hemorrhage in relation to HHT are available, and the bleeding risk is supposedly low, between 2 and 4% (Ondra *et al.*, 1990; Willemse *et al.*, 2000). It is unknown whether the risk of bleeding in HHT patients is greater than that in non-HHT patients (Haitjema *et al.*, 1995).

The overall risk of developing central nervous system complications, especially of stroke or abscess, increases according to the number of PAVMs. The prevalence of infarction in a single PAVM is 32% and increases to 60% in multiple PAVMs (Moussouttas *et al.*, 2000). Brain abscess in a patient with a single PAVM occurs in 8% and in 16% of patients who have multiple PAVMs.

Few cases of infections in the meninges, spine (Blanco *et al.*, 1998; David *et al.*, 1997), joints (mainly knees; Desproges-Gotteron *et al.*, 1973), kidney (Edigo *et al.*, 1991), and liver have been described. About 5% of patients have a more diffuse and multifocal pattern of PAVMs that conveys a poorer prognosis. In this particular group, neurological complications can occur in up to 70% of the patients with a much higher prevalence of brain abscess and stroke (Faughnan *et al.*, 2000). Lung transplantation is sometimes considered in these patients; however, the 2-year survival rate is much better in those treated with embolotherapy (91%) than with transplantation (63%) (Trulock, 1997).

After PAVMs are treated, 2% of patients develop strokes or brain abscesses during 5 years, and about 10–15% of treated PAVMs show recanalization. The development of new PAVMs, the growth of new feeding arteries to a previously occluded PAVM, and the appearance of pleurisy late after embolotherapy have been observed in a few patients (Lee *et al.*, 1997; Mager *et al.*, 2004).

The prevalence of migraine is also increased in PAVM patients (21–59% vs. 10–12% in the general population), with a predominance of migraine with aura (81%) (Thenganatt *et al.*, 2006). In patients with HHT, this prevalence is elevated as well (38%). The causal relation between a right-to-left shunt and migraine is debated, especially as PFO has been related to a higher migraine prevalence as well (Post *et al.*, 2004; Schwerzmann *et al.*, 2004; Wilmshurst *et al.*, 2000). So far, the pathogenesis of migraine in patients with PAVMs is unexplained (Post *et al.*, 2005). One hypothesis is a genetic substrate that might lead to both the formation of a right-to-left shunt and the development of migraine. Another explanation may be the more likely passage of vasoactive migraine trigger substances through the pulmonary shunt (Steele *et al.*, 1993).

On clinical examination, telangiectases are the most frequent clinical signs of the disease (66%). They are 1- to 2-mm-diameter, papular, well-demarcated lesions that blanch partially with pressure, are located preferentially on nasal mucosa (68–100%), but are often seen on oral mucosa (58–79%), on the face (30–63%), chest or trunk (13–85%), upper extremities (25–67%), conjunctiva or retina (45%), and digestive tract (unknown percentage). They must be differentiated from the spider nevi in liver disease, senile angiomas, or venectasia. Pulmonary auscultation is helpful in localizing a murmur over the site of the PAVMs, which can be heard in 46% of patients. It usually increases in a standing position or any position that would bring some pressure on the malformation due to gravitation. Digital clubbing and cyanosis are seen in 39% and 34% of patients, respectively. The classical triad of PAVMs – dyspnea, cyanosis, and clubbing – is present in only 10% of patients (Puskas *et al.*, 1993).

The early recognition of symptoms and signs of PAVMs is mandatory as the mortality rate in patients with brain abscesses can be as high as 41%. Recurrent stroke may occur in patients with HHT patients until the correct diagnosis is made (Cohen *et al.*, 2006). Untreated PAVMs have a propensity to provoke stroke and brain abscess, and are associated with a mortality of 4–22% (Dines *et al.*, 1974, 1983; Swanson *et al.*, 1999). Besides, an increase in existing PAVMs or the development of new malformations in pregnant patients with HHT represents a particularly high risk for hemorrhage in the chest (hemoptysis or hemothorax). In these circumstances, treatment must not be postponed.

Diagnosis

No international consensus has been reached on the best diagnostic tool for PAVMs. Until recently, patients suspected of harboring a PAVM usually had a measurement of the shunt fraction by the 100% oxygen method. Then another examination, such as contrast echocardiography or pulmonary angiography, was requested. Since the publication of more recent studies (Cottin *et al.*, 2004; Lee *et al.*, 2003) contrast echocardiography is the first recommended test in suspected patients to screen for PAVMs and to check for recanalization after treatment. The combination of an anteroposterior chest radiograph and contrast echocardiography has the best diagnostic values as a screening test with a sensitivity of 100%, a negative predictive value of 100%, and a negative likelihood ratio of 0.04 (Cottin *et al.*, 2004). The specific anatomy of the vascular malformation must then be analyzed either with helical CT or magnetic resonance angiography (MRA). Digital subtraction angiography is eventually performed.

Shunt fraction measurement

The abnormal communication between pulmonary arteries and veins results in a right-to-left shunt that reduces SaO_2. The fraction of cardiac output that is shunted can be measured. The normal value should be $\leq 5\%$. The shunt fraction is high in most

PAVM patients (88–100%). The best method to assess shunt fraction, using the 100% oxygen method, is described by Gossage and Kanj (1998). Its sensitivity for detecting clinically relevant PAVMs is estimated to be 97%. As a screening test, its specificity is insufficient, however. Pulse oximetry is also believed to be an inaccurate screening method, and its use is not recommended in this setting, whereas pulmonary function testing could be useful in assessing suspected cases of PAVMs. One study noted the presence of platypnea-orthodeoxia in selected patients (Dutton *et al.*, 1995).

Chest radiography

The chest radiograph shows some abnormality in 98% of patients with PAVMs. In patients with HHT, chest radiography has been helpful in only 45% of patients (Cottin *et al.*, 2007). Chest radiographs can be normal in patients with microvascular telangiectases. PAVMs appear as round or oval masses of uniform density, frequently lobulated but sharply defined, more commonly located in the lower lobes, and ranging from 1 to 5 cm in diameter. Only a minority of feeding vessels can be spotted on this examination. Their size ranges from 4 to 7 mm and very rarely exceed 20 mm.

CT, MRI

Three-dimensional helical CT yields an accurate analysis of the presence or absence of a PAVM and of the anatomical structure of the vascular malformation (Remy *et al.*, 1994), and so provides a useful tool to decide on the most appropriate treatment.

MRI can help to differentiate between an aneurysm within the PAVMs with a rapid blood flow resulting in low-intensity signals and other low signal intensity such as hematoma, cystic lesion, air cyst, or calcified lesion. Unfortunately, most PAVMs consist of a low-blood-flow lesion leading to a poor sensitivity of MRI (Gossage and Kanj, 1998). MRA is more sensitive and can detect quite reliably PAVMs >5 mm and feeding arteries >3 mm. Both examinations can be used in the follow-up to detect recurrences.

In order to exclude cerebral arteriovenous malformations, patients with PAVMs should undergo a MRI with and without gadolinium. In case of a negative result, this examination does not need to be repeated, as most of these lesions are congenital.

Pulmonary angiography

Digital subtraction angiography (or conventional pulmonary angiography) remains the gold standard in the diagnosis of PAVMs. It is used after non-invasive diagnostic tools have indicated a high suspicion of PAVMs in a patient. It will give more information about the architecture of the lesion and will usually identify malformations that may benefit from embolotherapy.

Contrast echocardiography

Contrast echocardiography is probably the most accurate method for identifying clinically relevant PAVMs. It has a sensitivity between 94% and 100% (Barzilai *et al.*, 1999), a specificity of 80% (Nanthakumar *et al.*, 2001), and a negative predictive value of 93%

(Cottin *et al.*, 2004). Technically, a delay of 3–8 cardiac cycles is expected before contrast (produced by injection of 10 mL of agitated saline) is visualised in the left atrium. It is easily differentiated from intracardiac shunts in which the contrast reaches the left side of the heart within the first cardiac cycle. A new grading system has been proposed to predict the probability of a PAVM that would allow this examination to be used in a screening algorithm (Zukotynski *et al.*, 2007). One problem might be that it may also detect clinically nonrelevant PAVMs (Lee *et al.*, 2003). This is exemplified by examinations that remain positive after embolization therapy in quite a large number of patients (Lee *et al.*, 2003), indicating that many patients have additional small PAVMs that are not detected by standard screening methods.

Radionuclide perfusion lung scanning

This technique has a few disadvantages as a screening test because of its cost and limited availability. Nevertheless, it shows a sensitivity of 71–87% and a specificity of 61% for the uncovering of residual PAVM after embolotherapy (Thompson *et al.*, 1999). As opposed to other means of investigation, one notes that arterial blood sampling is not necessary and that shunt measurement during exercise is possible. These potential advantages may be applied to specific clinical situations.

Transcranial Doppler ultrasonography

The sensitivity of transcranial Doppler ultrasonography has been estimated to be 100% for PFO, whereas for intrapulmonary shunt it is 50%. Although reliable in demonstrating a right-to-left shunt in patients who have a PFO (Devuyst, 1999), saline contrast transcranial Doppler has not yet been used in a comparative study addressing the screening methods to distinguish a pulmonary from an intracardiac shunt. It remains a useful procedure to assess the result of embolotherapy and follow up in patients at risk of recurrence (Del Sette *et al.*, 1998; Todo *et al.*, 2004; Yeung *et al.*, 1995).

Transpleural Doppler ultrasound

The demonstration of blood within the thoracic cavity and blood flow anomalies can be studied directly with Doppler ultrasound (Groves *et al.*, 2004; Hsu *et al.*, 2004). Although it is not a recommended screening test, it may contribute to the diagnosis in some cases.

Treatment

The aims of treatment are to prevent neurological complications and pulmonary hemorrhage and to improve hypoxemia. It is recommended that PAVMs that are symptomatic, progressively enlarging, or >2 cm in diameter should be treated. Medical therapy may be challenging in cases of neurological manifestations or concomitant prothrombotic disorders, as antiaggregants should be avoided in all individuals with HHT. There are no randomized data of medication for PAVMs. Hormones, danazol, octreotide, desmopressin, and aminocaproic acid have been used without relevant success in epistaxis and gastrointestinal bleeding in patients with HHT.

Surgery

Surgery was the method of choice before any other treatment was available. Since the first embolotherapy in 1977, lobectomy or pneumonectomy is performed only in rare situations, such as in patients in whom the feeding artery is so short that there is a risk of coil migration. Thoracoscopic procedures render this approach less stressful and reduce the morbidity risk (Watanabe *et al.*, 1995). Major complications following surgery include recurrence of PAVMs, enlargement of undetected malformation, stroke, and increase of pulmonary hypertension (Puskas *et al.*, 1993).

In cases where there are cerebral arteriovenous malformations larger than 1 cm in diameter, neurovascular surgery is preferred. It can be combined with stereotactic surgery or embolotherapy according to the size, location, or structure of the lesion.

Embolization therapy

Embolization therapy is applied for PAVMs with a feeding artery of at least 3 mm in diameter. This technique is carried out by transcatheter embolotherapy, which consists in obliterating the feeding artery. Several devices have been used to achieve this maneuver: metal coils (Lee *et al.*, 1997; White *et al.*, 1988), Guglielmi detachable coils (Dinkel and Triller, 2002), the Amplatzer duct occluder (Ayed *et al.*, 2005; Beck *et al.*, 2006; Hinterseer *et al.*, 2006), vascular plug (Beck *et al.*, 2006; Cil *et al.*, 2006; Rossi *et al.*, 2006), or detachable balloons (Barth *et al.*, 1982; Saluja *et al.*, 1999). Contrary to surgery, selective closure of the PAVMs preserves the unaffected branching vessels and lung parenchyma. The average success rate of immediate occlusion of PAVMs (98.7%) as well as the rate of persistent occlusion at 1 year (>85%) render this therapy quite attractive (Coley and Jackson, 1998; Dinkel and Triller, 2002; Haitjema *et al.*, 1995). About 70% of the cases benefit from this treatment, whereas the others undergo surgery (Cottin *et al.*, 2007).

Major complications occur in about 2% and include stroke, brain abscesses, systemic embolization (limb ischemia, bowel infarction), infection, or recanalization of occluded vessels (Mager *et al.*, 2001). The most frequent minor complications (14%) are short time pleurisy and angina caused by air embolism, segmental or subsegmental lung infarction, or superficial femoral thrombosis. During the procedure, the reported risk of paradoxical embolization of coils or balloons is about 2–4% (White *et al.*, 1988). Long-term results concerning new devices are not yet available. All in all, due to the low morbidity and mortality, this method has become the first line of treatment for PAVM and may even be used in the later stage of pregnancy. In case of recanalization, the procedure should be repeated as long as the PAVMs remain detectable by radiography.

Embolotherapy of PAVMs seems to decrease significantly the overall prevalence of migraine (Post *et al.*, 2006), but further data are needed before such a treatment can be recommended for patients with migraine as the only indication for treatment of PAVMs.

Prevention

Due to the potential severity of infectious complications, antibiotic prophylaxis before any dental or surgical procedure is recommended despite the lack of direct evidence. Although the penetrance of the disease may vary, the risk of developing disabling complications in an affected member of a known HHT family is sizeable, with an incidence of PAVMs of approximately 35%. Therefore, international associations for PAVMs advocate that all children of a parent with HHT should undergo screening tests. Pulse oximetry is recommended for babies every 1–2 years in both lying and sitting positions, followed by contrast echocardiography if oximetry is <97% or if classical symptoms are present and for every child (12 years old or older) of HHT patients. Any abnormal contrast echocardiography will require a chest CT scan.

For patients with a known and untreated PAVM, physical examination and measurement of the artery blood gases is a yearly requisite, and unenhanced CT is recommended every 2–3 years in order to detect growth. Specific conditions such as pregnancy or puberty require stricter controls. The same examinations are performed annually after embolotherapy to detect recanalization.

Dedication

This chapter is dedicated to Dr Gerald Devuyst, who wrote this chapter in the first edition of this book. We hope that our work is up to his high scientific standards and that he would have appreciated this update.

REFERENCES

Anabtawi, I. N., Ellison, R. G., and Ellison, L. T. 1965. Pulmonary arteriovenous aneurysms and fistulas. Anatomical variations, embryology, and classification. *Ann Thorac Surg,* **122,** 277–85.

Ayed, K. A., Bazerbashi, S., and Uthaman, B. 2005. Pulmonary arteriovenous malformation presenting with severe hypoxemia. *Med Princ Pract,* **14,** 430–3.

Barth, K. H., White, R. I., Kaufman, S. L., *et al.* 1982. Embolotherapy pulmonary arteriovenous malformations with detachable balloons. *Radiology,* **142,** 599–606.

Barzilai, B., Waggoner, A. D., Spessert, C., Picus, E., and Goodenberger D. 1999. Two-dimensional contrast echocardiography in the detection and follow-up of congenital pulmonary arteriovenous malformations. *Am J Cardiol,* **68,** 1507–10.

Beck, A., Dagan, T., Matitiau, A., *et al.* 2006. Transcatheter closure of pulmonary arteriovenous malformation with Amplatzer devices. *Catheter Cardiovasc Interv,* **67,** 932–7.

Berg, J. N., Guttmacher, A. E., Marchuk, D. A., *et al.* 1996. Clinical heterogeneity in hereditary haemorrhagic telangiectasia: are pulmonary arteriovenous malformations more common in families linked to endoglin? *J Med Genet,* **33,** 256–7.

Blanco, P., Schaeverbeke, T., Baillet, L., *et al.* 1998. Rendu-Osler familial telangiectasia angiomatosis and bacterial spondylodiscitis [in French]. *Rev Med Interne,* **19,** 938–9.

Bosher, L. H., Blake, D. A., and Byrd, B. R. 1959. Analysis of the pathologic anatomy of pulmonary arteriovenous aneurysms with particular reference to the applicability of local excision. *Surgery,* **45,** 91–104.

Churton, T. 1897. Multiple aneurysms of the pulmonary artery. *Br Med J*, **1**, 1223–5.

Cil, B., Canyigit, M., Ozkan, O. S., *et al.* 2006. Bilateral multiple pulmonary arteriovenous malformations: endovascular treatment with the Amplatzer vascular plug. *J Vasc Interv Radiol*, **17**, 141–5.

Cohen, R., Cabanes, L., Burckel, C., *et al.* 2006. Pulmonary arteriovenous fistulae recurrent stroke. *J Neurol Neurosurg Psychiatry*, **77**, 707–8.

Coley, S. C., and Jackson, J. E. 1998. Endovascular occlusion with a new mechanical detachable coil. *AJR Am J Roentgenol*, **171**, 1075–9.

Cottin, V., Chinet, T., Lavole, A., *et al.* 2007. Pulmonary arteriovenous malformations in hemorrhagic hereditary telangiectasia: a series of 126 patients. *Medicine (Baltimore)*, **86**, 1–17.

Cottin, V., Plauchu, H., Bayle, J. Y., *et al.* 2004. Pulmonary arteriovenous malformations in patients with hereditary hemorrhagic telangiectasia. *Am J Respir Crit Care Med*, **169**, 994.

David, C., Brasme, L., Peruzzi, P., *et al.* 1997. Intramedullary abscess of the spinal cord in a patient with a right-to-left shunt: case report. *Clin Infect Dis*, **24**, 89–90.

Del Sette, M., Angeli, S., Leandri, M., *et al.* 1998. Migraine with aura and right to-left shunt on transcranial Doppler: a case-control study. *Cerebrovasc Dis*, **8**, 327–30.

Desproges-Gotteron, R., Francon, F., and Diaz, R. 1973. Un cas d'arthrite purulente au cours d'une angiomatose de Rendu-Osler (telangiectasia hereditaria hemorrhagica). *Vie Méd Can F*, **2**, 223–5.

Devuyst, G. 1999. New trends in neurosonology. In M. Fisher and J. Bogouslavsky, eds., *Current Review of Cerebrovascular Disease*. Philadelphia: Current Medicine, Inc., pp. 65–76.

Dines, D. E., Arms, R. A., Bernatz, P. E., *et al.* 1974. Pulmonary arteriovenous fistulas. *Mayo Clin Proc*, **49**, 460–5.

Dines, D. E., Seward, J. B., Bernatz, P. E., *et al.* 1983. Pulmonary arteriovenous fistulas. *Mayo Clin Proc*, **58**, 176–81.

Dinkel, H. P., and Triller, J. 2002. Pulmonary arteriovenous malformations: embolotherapy with the superselective coaxial catheter placement and filling of venous sac with Guglielmi detachable coils. *Radiology*, **223**, 709–14.

Dutton, J. A. E., Jackson, J. E., Hughes, J. M. B., *et al.* 1995. Pulmonary arteriovenous malformations: results of treatment with coil embolization in 53 patients. *AJR Am J Roentgenol*, **165**, 1119–25.

Edigo, R., Panades, M. J., Ramos, J., Guajardo, J., and Parra, R. 1991. Renal actinomycosis: presentation of a case. *Acta Urol Esp*, **15**, 580–2.

Faughnan, M. E., Lui, Y. W., Wirth, J. A., *et al.* 2000. Diffuse pulmonary arteriovenous malformations: characteristics and prognosis. *Chest*, **117**, 31–8.

Gallione, C. J., Repetto, G. M., Legius, E., *et al.* 2004. A combined syndrome of juvenile polyposis and hereditary haemorrhagic telangiectasia associated with mutations in MADH4(SMAD4). *Lancet*, **363**, 852–9.

Gallitelli, M., Guastamacchia, E., Resta, F., *et al.* 2006. Pulmonary arteriovenous malformations, hereditary haemorrhagic telangiectasia coma and brain abscess. *Respiration*, **73**, 553–7.

Gallitelli, M., Lepore, V., Pasculli, G., *et al.* 2005. Brain abscess: a need to screen for pulmonary arteriovenous malformations. *Neuroepidemiology*, **24**, 76–8.

Gossage, J. R., Kanj, G. 1998. Pulmonary arteriovenous malformations. A state of the art review. *Am J Respir Crit Care Med*, **158**, 643–61.

Groves, A. M., See, T. C., Appleton, D. S., *et al.* 2004. Transpleural ultrasound diagnosis of pulmonary arteriovenous malformation. *Br J Radiol*, **77**, 620–32.

Guttmacher, A. E., Marchuk, D. A., and White, R. I. Jr. 1995. Hereditary hemorrhagic telangiectasia. *N Engl J Med*, **333**, 918–24.

Haitjema, T., Westermann, C. J., Overtoom, T. T., *et al.* 1996. Hereditary hemorrhagic telangiectasia (Osler-Weber-Rendu disease): new insights in pathogenesis, complications, and treatment. *Arch Intern Med*, **156**, 714–9.

Haitjema, T. J., Disch, F., Overtoom, T. T. C., *et al.* 1995. Screening family members of patients with hereditary haemorrhagic telangiectasia. *Am J Med*, **99**, 519–24.

Haitjema, T. J., Overtoom, T. T. C., Westermann, C. J. J., *et al.* 1995. Embolization of pulmonary arteriovenous malformation: results and follow up in 32 patients. *Thorax*, **15**, 719–23.

Hinterseer, M., Becker, A., Barth, A. S., *et al.* 2006. Interventional embolization of a giant pulmonary arteriovenous malformation with right-left-shunt

associated with hereditary hemorrhagic telangiectasia. *Clin Res Cardiol*, **95**, 174–8

Hsu, Y. L., Wang, H. C., and Yang, P. C. 2004. Desbaric air embolism during diving: an unusual complication of Osler-Weber-Rendu disease. *Br J Sports Med*, **38**, e6

Jessurun, G. A., Kamphuis, D. J., van der Zande, E. H., *et al.* 1993. Cerebral arteriovenous malformations in the Netherlands Antilles: high prevalence of hereditary haemorrhagic telangiectasia-related single and multiple cerebral arteriovenous malformations. *Clin Neurol Neurosurg*, **95**, 193–8.

Kimura, K., Minematsu, K., Nakajima, M. 2004. Isolated primary arteriovenous fistula without Rendu-Osler-Weber disease as a cause of cryptogenic stroke. *J Neurol Neurosurg Psychiatry*, **75**, 311–3.

Lee, D. W., White, R. I., Egglin, T. K., *et al.* 1997. Embolotherapy of large pulmonary arteriovenous malformations: long-term results. *Ann Thorac Surg*, **64**, 930–40.

Lee, W. L., Graham, A. F., Pugash, R. A., *et al.* 2003. Contrast echocardiography remains positive after treatment of pulmonary arteriovenous malformations. *Chest*, **123**, 351–8.

Mager, J. J., Overtoom, T. T., Blauw, H., Lammers, J. W., and Westermann, C. J. 2004. Embolotherapy of pulmonary arteriovenous malformations: long-term results in 112 patients. *J Vasc Interv Radiol*, **15**, 451–6.

Mager, J. J., Overtoom, T. T., Mauser, H. W., *et al.* 2001. Early cerebral infarction after embolotherapy of pulmonary arteriovenous malformation. *J Vasc Interv Radiol*, **12**, 122–3.

Maher, C. O., Piepgras, D. G., Brown, R. D., *et al.* 2001. Cerebrovascular manifestations in 321 cases of hereditary hemorrhagic telangiectasia. *Stroke*, **32**, 877–82.

Maniscalco, M., Zedda, A., Faraone, S., *et al.* 2005. Association of Adams-Oliver syndrome with pulmonary arterio-venous malformation in the same family. *Am J Med Genet*, **136**, 269–74.

Marchuk, D. A. 1997. The molecular genetics of hereditary haemorrhagic telangiectasia. *Chest*, **111 (Suppl)**, 79s–82s.

Monsour, K. A., Hatcher, C. R. Jr, Logan, W. D., *et al.* 1970. Pulmonary arteriovenous fistula. *Am Surg*, **37**, 203–8.

Moussouttas, M., Fayad, P., Rosenblatt, M., *et al.* 2000. Pulmonary arteriovenous malformations: cerebral ischemia and neurologic manifestations. *Neurology*, **55**, 959–64.

Nanthakumar, K., Graham, A. T., Robinson, T. I., *et al.* 2001. Contrast echocardiography for detection of pulmonary arteriovenous malformations. *Am Heart J*, **141**, 243–6.

Ondra, S. L., Troupp, H., George, E. D., and Schwab, K. 1990. The natural history of symptomatic arteriovenous malformations of the brain: a 24-year follow-up assessment. *J Neurosurg*, **73**, 387–91.

Peters, B., Ewert, P., Schubert, S., *et al.* 2005. Rare case of pulmonary arteriovenous fistula simulating residual defect after transcatheter closure of patent foramen ovale for recurrent paradoxical embolism. *Catheter Cardiovasc Interv*, **64**, 348–51.

Plauchu, H., de Chadarevian, J. P., Bideau, A., *et al.* 1989. Age-related clinical profile of hereditary haemorrhagic telangiectasia in an epidemiologically recruited population. *Am J Med Genet*, **32**, 291–7.

Post, M. C., Letteboer, T. G. W., Mager, J. J., *et al.* 2005. A pulmonary right to left shunt in patients with hereditary haemorrhagic telangiectasia is associated with an increased prevalence of migraine. *Chest*, **128**, 2485–9.

Post, M. C., Thijs, V., Herroelen, L., *et al.* 2004. Closure of a patent foramen ovale is associated with a decrease in prevalence of migraine. *Neurology*, **62**, 1439–40.

Post, M. C., Thijs, V., Schonewille, W. J., *et al.* 2006. Embolization of pulmonary arteriovenous malformations and decrease in prevalence of migraine. *Neurology*, **66**, 202–5.

Puskas, J. D., Allen, M. S., Moncure, A. C., *et al.* 1993. Pulmonary arteriovenous malformations: therapeutic options. *Ann Thorac Surg*, **56**, 253–8.

Remy, J., Remy-Jardin, M., Giraud, F., *et al.* 1994. Angioarchitecture of pulmonary arteriovenous malformations: clinical utility of three-dimensional helical CT. *Radiology*, **191**, 657–64.

Roman, G., Fisher, M., Perl, D. P., *et al.* 1978. Neurological manifestations of hereditary haemorrhagic telangiectasia (Rendu-Osler-Weber disease): report of 2 cases and review of the literature. *Ann Neurol*, **4**, 130–44.

Rossi, M., Rebonato, A, Greco L, *et al.* 2006. A new device for vascular embolization: report on case of two pulmonary arteriovenous fistulas embolization using the amplatzer vascular plug. *Cardiovasc Intervent Radiol,* **29,** 902–6.

Saluja, S., Sitko, L., Lee, R. W., *et al.* 1999. Embolotherapy of pulmonary AVM with detachable balloons: long-term durability and efficiency. *J Vasc Interv Radiol,* **10,** 883–9.

Schwerzmann, M., Wiher, S., Nedeltchev, K., *et al.* 2004. Percutaneous closure of patent foramen ovale reduces the frequency of migraine attacks. *Neurology,* **62,** 1399–401.

Shovlin, C. L., Guttmacher, A. E., Buscarini, E., *et al.* 2000. Diagnostic criteria for hereditary hemorrhagic telangiectasia (Rendu-Osler-Weber syndrome). *Am J Med Genet,* **91,** 66–7.

Shovlin, C. L., and Letarte, M. 1999. Hereditary haemorrhagic telangiectasia and pulmonary arteriovenous malformations: issues in clinical management and review of pathogenic mechanisms. *Thorax,* **54,** 714–29.

Steele, J. G., Nath, P. U., Burn, J., *et al.* 1993. An association between migrainous aura and hereditary haemorrhagic telangiectasia. *Headache,* **33,** 145–8.

Swanson, K. L., Prakash, U. B., and Stanson, A. W. 1999. Pulmonary arteriovenous fistulas: Mayo Clinic experience, 1982–1997. *Mayo Clin Proc,* **74,** 671–80.

Thenganatt, J., Schneiderman, J., Hyland, R. H., *et al.* 2006. Migraines linked to intrapulmonary right-to-left shunt. *Headache,* **46,** 439–43.

Thompson, R. D., Jackson, J., Peters, A. M., *et al.* 1999. Sensitivity and specificity of radioisotope right-left shunt measurement and pulse oximetry for the early detection of pulmonary arteriovenous malformations. *Chest,* **115,** 109–13.

Todo, K., Moriwaki, H., Higashi, M., *et al.* 2004. A smell pulmonary arteriovenous malformation as a cause of recurrent brain embolism. *AJNR Am J Neuroradiol,* **25,** 428–30.

Trulock, E. P. 1997. Lung transplantation. *Am J Respir Crit Care Med,* **155,** 789–818.

Vase, P., Holm, M., and Arendrup, H. 1985. Pulmonary arteriovenous fistulas in hereditary haemorrhagic telangiectasia. *Acta Med Scand,* **218,** 105–9.

Watanabe, N., Munakata, Y., Ogiwara, M., *et al.* 1995. A case of pulmonary arteriovenous malformation in a patient with brain abscess successfully treated with video-assisted thoracoscopic resection. *Chest,* **108,** 1724–7.

White, R. I. Jr, Lunch-Nyhan, A., Terry, P., *et al.* 1988. Pulmonary arteriovenous malformations: techniques and long-term outcome of embolotherapy. *Radiology,* **169,** 663–9.

White, R. I. Jr, Pollak, J. S., and Wirth, J. A. 1996. Pulmonary arteriovenous malformations: diagnosis and transcatheter embolotherapy. *J Vasc Interv Radiol,* **7,** 787–804.

Willemse, R. B., Mager, J. J., Westermann, C. J., *et al.* 2000. Bleeding risk of cerebrovascular malformations in hereditary hemorrhagic telangiectasia. *J Neurosurg,* **92,** 779–84.

Willinsky, R. A., Lasjaunias, P., Terbrugge, K., *et al.* 1990. Multiple cerebral arteriovenous malformation: review of our experience from 203 patients with cerebral vascular lesions. *Neuroradiology,* **32,** 207–10.

Wilmshurst, PT, Nightingale S, Walsh KP, *et al.* 2000. Effect on migraine of closure of cardiac right-to-left shunts to prevent recurrence of decompression illness or stroke or for haemodynamic reasons. *Lancet,* **356,** 1648–51.

Yeung, M., Khan, K. A., Antecol, D. H., *et al.* 1995. Transcranial Doppler ultrasonography and transesophageal echocardiography in the investigation of pulmonary arteriovenous and formation in a patient with hereditary haemorrhagic telangiectasia presenting with stroke. *Stroke,* **26,** 1941–4.

Zukotynski, K., Chan, R. P., Chow, C. M., *et al.* 2007. Contrast echocardiography grading predicts pulmonary arteriovenous malformations on CT. *Chest,* **132,** 18–23.

17 HEREDITARY HEMORRHAGIC TELANGIECTASIA (OSLER–WEBER–RENDU DISEASE)

Mathieu Zuber

Hereditary hemorrhagic telangiectasia (HHT, also known as Osler–Weber–Rendu syndrome) is one of the most common autosomal dominant disorders. It is characterized by epistaxis, cutaneous telangiectasia, and visceral vascular malformations.

The disease has been subject to under-reporting for many years. Careful epidemiological studies recently revealed an incidence of 1 in 5000–8000 (Begbie *et al.*, 2003). The degree of penetrance is high, but clinical manifestations are usually not present at birth and develop with increasing age: epistaxis, the earliest sign of disease in most individuals, often occurs during childhood, pulmonary arteriovenous malformations (PAVMs) becoming apparent from puberty, with mucocutaneous and gastrointestinal telangiectasia developing with age. It is considered that more than two thirds of patients will have developed some sign of HHT by the age of 16 years, rising to more than 90% by the age of 40 years (Porteous *et al.*, 1992). Neurological symptoms occur in 10–20% of HHT patients (Adams *et al.*, 1977; Begbie *et al.*, 2003; Peery, 1987) and include infectious and vascular involvement of the central nervous system (CNS).

Pathology

Telangiectasia, the most prominent lesion of HHT, is defined by focal dilatations of postcapillary venules and some degree of perivascular lymphocytic infiltrate (Peery, 1987). As the telangiectasia develops, venules become more markedly dilated and convoluted, with excessive layers of smooth muscle without elastic fibers. The connecting arterioles also become dilated and communicate directly with the venules without intervening capillaries (Braverman *et al.*, 1990). In addition to the telangiectases, HHT patients also present with arteriovenous malformations (AVMs) and arteriovenous fistulae (AVFs), which account for the most devastating clinical complications of the disease. The largest AVMs (up to several centimeters in diameter) occur in the lungs, liver, and CNS. Intracranial arterial aneurysms are exceptionally reported (Roman *et al.*, 1978). The various vascular malformations may combine in the same patient.

Three different phenotypes of vascular malformations have been differentiated in the CNS, including large fistulae characterized by a direct arteriovenous shunt without nidus but with an an ectatic draining vein, small AVMs with a nidal size between 1 and 3 centimeters, and micro-AVMs with a nidus smaller than 1 centimeter (Krings *et al.*, 2005; Matsubara *et al.*, 2000). There is no argument supporting a possible evolution of one type of CNS vascular malformation to another, but serial radiological studies are lacking. CNS malformations in HHT do not differ from those observed in non-HHT patients, both from the histological and angiographical points of view (Guttmacher *et al.*, 1995; Krings *et al.*, 2005). One single vein draining the lesion is the rule. Location of the malformation is almost exclusively near the surface of the CNS. Pial AVFs are also reported (Garcia-Monaco *et al.*, 1995). More than three cerebral AVMs in a single patient are rarely reported (Putman *et al.*, 1996). Recent studies highlight the age dependence of the different forms of phenotypical HHT appearances in the CNS. AVFs are most frequently discovered on angiography in children younger than 5 years, whereas small AVMs predominantly reveal in adolescents and micro-AVMs in young adults (Krings *et al.*, 2005). Accordingly, it was suggested that maturity of the vessel is a determining factor of the disease manifestations, in addition to the presence of genetic mutations. Venules seem to be the initial target of the pathological process in all cases.

Pathogenesis

Important advances were made during the last decade in understanding the molecular basis of HHT, which appears as a genetically heterogeneous group of disorders.

Since 1994 (McAllister *et al.*, 1994), HHT was found to be related to mutations in at least two genes, endoglin and activin receptor-like kinase 1 (ALK1), that both encode proteins expressed predominantly on vascular endothelial cells. The two genes are localized on chromosomes 9 and 12, respectively, and mutations are responsible for the so-called HHT1 and HHT2 subgroups of the disease, respectively. Numerous distinctive mutations of each of the two genes may be responsible for the HHT phenotype. In a recent French series of 160 unrelated HHT patients, 100 different mutations (36 in the endoglin and 64 in ALK1) were observed (Lesca *et al.*, 2004). There seems to be no definite relationship between the type of mutation and the phenotype of the disease (Begbie *et al.*, 2003). Transgenic models have been generated (murine and mice), confirming that the mutations are causative for the disease (Bourdeau *et al.*, 1999). Levels of proteins expressed in endothelial cells from the two genes are about half of the normal levels in HHT patients, supporting the view that the disease results from haplo-insufficiency (Begbie *et al.*, 2003).

Both endoglin and ALK1 play distinct roles in the transforming growth factor-beta signaling pathway. Transforming growth factor-beta is a complex of polypeptides that regulates several

Uncommon Causes of Stroke, 2nd edition, ed. Louis R. Caplan. Published by Cambridge University Press. © Cambridge University Press 2008.

fundamental pathways in cell development and takes part in vascular remodeling by controlling the extracellular matrix production (Marchuk *et al.*, 2003). Physiologically, endoglin and ALK1 bind to the transforming growth factor-beta proteins and therefore influence angiogenesis. Alterations in the process lead to abnormal vessels and abnormal connections between vessels (Krings *et al.*, 2005).

Despite the recent advances in understanding the molecular basis of HHT, several issues remain. First, endoglin and ALK1 genes mutations are not responsible for all HHT cases. Some patients are known to suffer from an HHT–juvenile polyposis overlap syndrome due to specific mutations (Gallione *et al.*, 2004). Recently, a new locus for HHT was mapped to chromosome 5 (Cole *et al.*, 2005). Pulmonary involvement could be prominent in this so-called HHT3 subgroup of the disease. Second, the presentation of HHT may vary considerably from one patient to another, even in the same family (Begbie *et al.*, 2003 Guttmacher *et al.*, 1995). This suggests that genetic influences other than gene mutations or environmental factors play some important role in the manifestations of the disease. Depending on the timing of these triggers, one or the other of the vascular manifestations could dominate (Krings *et al.*, 2005).

Extraneurological features

Nasal and mucocutaneous telangiectases

Epistaxis caused by spontaneous bleeding from telangiectases of the nasal mucosa appears to be the first complaint in 50% of affected patients and is often present in childhood. Recurrent epistaxis (sometimes on a daily basis) is the most common symptom of HHT and present in 50–80% of affected patients (Begbie *et al.*, 2003; Haitjema *et al.*, 1996). It can be severe, but most patients require no treatment other than iron supplementation, in order to avoid chronic anemia.

Telangiectases of the skin and buccal mucosa occur in about 75% of individuals and are typically present later in life than epistaxis (Plauchu *et al.*, 1989). They occur on the face, lips, tongue, palate, and fingertips. Telangiectasias of the tongue and of the lips should systematically be chased when HHT is suspected, because they can easily be overlooked or misinterpreted. The size and number of telangiectases progressively increase with patient age and become constant after the age of 60 years. The risk of hemorrhages parallels the anatomical progression (Peery, 1987; Plauchu *et al.*, 1989).

Gastrointestinal involvement

Recurrent gastrointestinal hemorrhages occur in up to 30% of patients with HHT (Kjeldsen and Kjeldsen, 2000). They do not usually start until the fifth or sixth decade, and are related to mucosal telangiectases that are more common in the stomach and duodenum than in the colon. In a minority of patients, gastrointestinal angiography may find AVMs or aneurysms. Blood transfusions are seldom required.

Liver involvement often remains asymptomatic (Garcia-Tsao *et al.*, 2000). When multiple hepatic AVMs are present, portal hypertension and biliary disease may develop. Because of left-to-right shunting, high cardiac output leading to heart failure has been occasionally observed. Portosystemic encephalopathy is reported, particularly in cases of gastrointestinal tract bleeding (Roman *et al.*, 1978).

Pulmonary manifestations

The prevalence of PAVM in series of HHT patients ranges from 5% to 20% (Guttmacher *et al.*, 1995; White *et al.*, 1988). It could be more frequent in the HHT3 subgroup of patients (Cole *et al.*, 2005). Conversely, about 70% of all PAVMs occur in HHT patients (Begbie *et al.*, 2003).

PAVMs predominate in the lower lobes, enlarge with increasing age, and often become symptomatic during the third or the fourth decade. Because of the direct right-to-left shunt and the consecutive arterial oxygen saturation decrease with hypoxemia, fatigue, dyspnea, cyanosis, or polycythemia may then occur. A wide range of hemorrhagic manifestations have been documented, from mild hemoptysis to catastrophic hemothorax (Hodgson *et al.*, 1959; White *et al.*, 1988).

Non-invasive procedures such as finger oximetry and chest radiography are important tools for screening PAVMs in patients with HHT (Begbie *et al.*, 2003; Haitjema *et al.*, 1996). Because of the recent widespread development of helical CT, the technique is now routinely used to analyze architecture of the vessels, and has simplified the diagnostic approach (Love *et al.*, 1992).

The most frequent and frightful complications of PAVMs are not local hemorrhages but CNS complications, in relation to paradoxical embolism. Clearly, neurological complications are more frequent (about 40%) among HHT patients with PAVM than among those without PAVM (Fulbright *et al.*, 1998; Roman *et al.*, 1978). Embolic cerebral events can occur regardless of the degree of respiratory symptoms, and can be the revealing manifestation of a PAVM (Begbie *et al.*, 2003).

Neurological features

Neurological complications in HHT are reported at all ages, with peak incidence in the third to fourth decades, and result from PAVMs (60%), vascular malformations from the brain (28%) and spinal cord (8%), and portosystemic encephalopathy (3%) (Roman *et al.*, 1978). Depending on the mechanism and the location of the CNS involvement, numerous neurological symptoms are reported in HHT patients, including headache, syncope, focal deficits, focal and generalized seizures, vertigo, and diplopia.

Neurological complications due to PAVMs

Right-to-left shuntings due to PAVMs facilitate the crossing of septic and bland emboli into the cerebral circulation. A CNS complication may reveal not only a previously unknown PAVM but even the disease itself (Guttmacher *et al.*, 1995; Hewes *et al.*, 1985).

When septic paradoxical emboli lodge within the CNS vasculature, bacterial encephalitis, meningitis, abscess, or mycotic aneurysm may occur (Peery, 1987). Cerebral abscess is the most

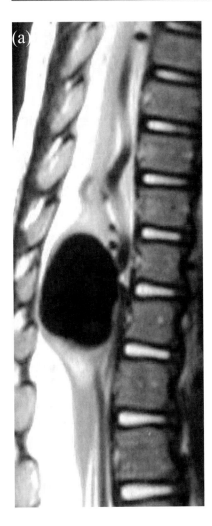
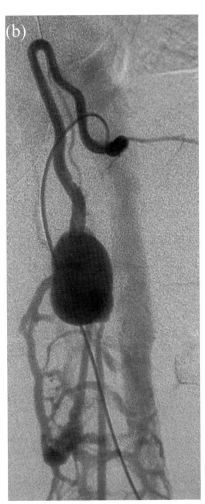

Figure 17.1 MRI (**a**) and conventional angiography (**b**) showing a large spinal AVF in a 2-year-old boy with HHT. (Courtesy of Professor P. Lasjaunias.)

frequent septic complication in HHT. The abscess is usually a solitary and supratentorial lesion (Dong *et al.*, 2001; Thompson *et al.*, 1977). In a patient with recurrent cerebral abscesses, screening for HHT should be systematically performed (Wilkins *et al.*, 1983). The incidence of cerebral abscess in patients with PAVMs is estimated at 5% to 6% (Adams *et al.*, 1977; Wilkins *et al.*, 1983).

Cerebral ischemic manifestations are severe complications of the paradoxical embolism in patients with HHT. Emboli most often provide from peripheral sites but may also, in case of large ectatic PAVM, develop locally on the walls of the malformation (Krings *et al.*, 2005). Both transient ischemic attacks and strokes are reported (Albucher *et al.*, 1996; Love *et al.*, 1992; Neau *et al.*, 1987; Sisel *et al.*, 1970). The middle cerebral artery seems to be the most frequent site of embolism. In a minority of patients, ischemic stroke is the initial manifestation of HHT (Albucher *et al.*, 1996; Fressinaud *et al.*, 2000; Love *et al.*, 1992). Nevertheless, screening for HHT in a patient with a PAVM revealed by stroke may also be negative (Kimura *et al.*, 2004).

Apart from paradoxical embolism, two other mechanisms could favor cerebral ischemic manifestations in HHT patients, including blood hyperviscosity related to polycythemia and air embolism from the lung to the brain (Peery, 1987). The latter probably results from air seepage into the arterial circulation through the AVM wall during cough, and is associated with hemoptysis (Neau *et al.*, 1987). Exceptionally, embolism from an associated intracranial carotid aneurysm is also suspected in a patient with HHT (Fisher and Zito, 1983).

Hemorrhagic neurological complications

Approximately one third of the neurological complications in patients with HHT are consecutive to hemorrhages from cerebral or spinal vascular malformations, meaning that about 5% of all HHT patients are concerned. Prevalence of cerebrovascular malformations in HHT is estimated at 5% using only CT (White *et al.*, 1988), but it increases up to approximately 20% when MRI is performed (Fulbright *et al.*, 1998). Nevertheless, false-negatives are reported with MRI as well (Willemse *et al.*, 2000). Malformations that are not detected by MRI are thought to be from the micro-AVM type and bear a small, if any, risk of hemorrhage (Krings *et al.*, 2005). Larger cerebrovascular malformations are associated with a 1.4–2.0% risk of hemorrhage per year, a rate similar to the one observed in non-HHT patients (Ondra *et al.*, 1990). Occasionally, symptoms due to a CNS malformation may be linked to thrombosis of the venous pouch or to venous congestion with venous ischemia rather than vessel rupture (Yoshida *et al.*, 2004). Subarachnoid hemorrhages induced by AVFs or arterial aneurysms are scarce (Garcia-Monaco *et al.*, 1995).

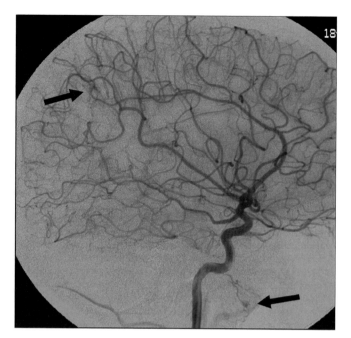

Figure 17.2 Supra- and infratentorial micro-AVMs in a patient with HHT. (Courtesy of Professor P. Lasjaunias.)

Table 17.1 International diagnostic criteria of HHT (Shovlin *et al.*, 2000)

1–	Epistaxis: spontaneous, recurrent nose bleeds
2–	Telangiectases, multiple and at characteristic sites:
	– lips
	– oral cavity
	– fingers
	– nose
3–	Visceral lesions such as:
	– gastrointestinal telangiectasia (with or without bleeding)
	– PAVM
	– hepatic AVM
	– cerebral AVM
	– spinal AVM
4–	Family history of first-degree relative with HHT according to these criteria

HHT is:

"definite" if three criteria are present

"possible" or "suspected" if two criteria are present

"unlikely" if fewer than two criteria are present

In a large, recent series of 50 consecutive HHT patients with CNS malformations explored by conventional angiography, a total of 75 vascular malformations was found, including 7 spinal cord AVFs, 34 cerebral AVFs, 16 small AVMs, and 18 micro-AVMs (Figures 17.1, 17.2, and 17.3) (Krings *et al.*, 2005). Mean age at diagnosis was 2.2, years, 3.0 years, 23.1 years, and 31.8 years, respectively. Epilepsy (21%) and headache (12%) were the prominent initial symptoms. Bleeding was observed in only 11% of patients (Krings *et al.*, 2005). Cerebral malformations were supratentorial in most of the cases. Spinal arteriovenous fistula (AVFs) are often large and associated with a high risk of hemorrhage. Rapidly progressive para- or tetraplegia is the usual presentation, with hematomyelia visualized on MRI.

Diagnosis criteria

In the nineteenth century, the medical entity combining nose and gastrointestinal bleeding with mucocutaneous telangiectasia had been well recognized through the eponym Osler–Weber–Rendu syndrome or HHT. During the first part of the twentieth century, visceral AVMs were described and appeared as a cornerstone of the syndrome (Fuchizaki *et al.*, 2003; Osler, 1901; Rendu, 1896). Recently, international consensus diagnostic criteria (the so-called Curaçao criteria) were proposed (Shovlin *et al.*, 2000), including personal and familial information (Table 17.1). Such criteria are likely to be further refined as molecular diagnostic tests become available. It should be stressed that, considering the progressive apparition of symptoms during life, no child of a patient with HHT can be informed he has no disease on clinical grounds only.

Treatment of neurological complications and practical considerations

Acute treatments for infectious or vascular CNS manifestations do not differ from those used in non-HHT patients. Complications of a PAVM can be limited if the condition is recognized and treated. In addition, treatment of the malformation with transcatheter embolotherapy has now proved to be safe. Accordingly, in order to prevent abscesses and ischemia, the tendency is now to screen putative HHT patients for PAVM (Begbie *et al.*, 2003). When a specific treatment is not decided, follow-up with helical CT should be regularly performed in order to detect any enlargement of the malformation (Guttmacher *et al.*, 1995). Prophylactic antibiotics are recommended at the time of dental or surgical procedures.

Various therapies for CNS AVMs have been proposed including surgical resection, stereotactic radiosurgery, embolization, or a combination of these treatments (Krings *et al.*, 2005). The optimal treatment remains to be agreed upon, and probably has to be discussed for each individual patient. Uncertainties are similar to those in non-HHT patients with AVM (Stapf *et al.*, 2006). There is complete paucity of data about the risk/benefit ratio for presymptomatic intervention in CNS neurovascular malformations in HHT. Indeed, the management approaches markedly differ across countries. Agreement is roughly obtained on the one hand for micro-AVMs that do not tend to bleed, and on the other hand for large spinal fistulae that bear a high risk of hemorrhagic complications (Krings *et al.*, 2005). However, the question of whether HHT patients with no neurological symptoms should be systematically screened for cerebral AVMs remains hotly debated, remembering the potential risks and interventional modalities (Begbie *et al.*, 2003). To sum up, screening is performed in most North American centers (Morgan *et al.*, 2002) but not in European centers (Krings *et al.*, 2005).

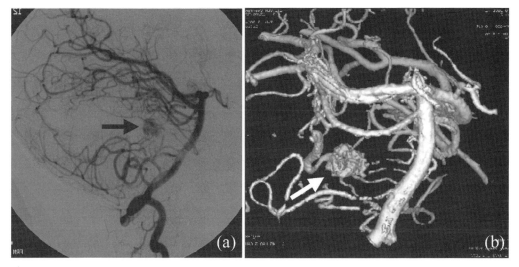

Figure 17.3 Conventional angiography (**a**) and CT angiography (**b**) showing the AVM nidus in the posterior cranial fossa of a patient with HHT. (Courtesy of Professor P. Lasjaunias.)

During pregnancy, PAVMs may enlarge with an increased risk of hemorrhage (White *et al.*, 1988), and the presence of a spinal AVM leads to contraindication of epidural analgesia. For these reasons, women with known HHT should be screened for PAVM and spinal AVF before conception, and optimal treatments decided on time.

Finally, practitioners in charge of HHT patients should be convinced that the disease and its potential complications have to be carefully explained. The use of educational materials is recommended (Guttmacher *et al.*, 1995).

REFERENCES

Adams, H. P., Subbiah, B., and Bosch, E. P. 1977. Neurologic aspects of hereditary haemorrhagic telangiectasia. *Arch Neurol*, **34**, 101–4.

Albucher, J. F., Carles, P., Giron, P., Guiraud-Chaumeil, B., and Chollet, F. 1996. Accident vasculaire cérébral ischémique au cours de la maladie de Rendu Osler: à propos d'un cas. *Rev Neurol (Paris)*, **152**, 283–7.

Begbie, M. E., Wallace, G. M., and Shovlin, C. L. 2003. Hereditary haemorrhagic telangiectasia (Osler-Weber-Rendu syndrome): a view from the 21st century. *Postgrad Med J*, **79**, 18–24.

Bourdeau, A., Dumont, D. J., and Letarte, M. 1999. A murine model of hereditary haemorrhagic telangiectasia. *J Clin Invest*, **104**, 1343–51.

Braverman, I. M., Keh, A., and Jacobson, B. S. 1990. Ultrastructure and three-dimensional organization of the telangiectases of hereditary haemorrhagic telangiectasia. *J Invest Dermatol*, **95**, 422–7.

Cole, S. G., Begbie, M. E., Wallace, G. M. F., and Shovlin, C. L. 2005. A new locus for hereditary hemorrhagic telangiectasia (HHT3) maps to chromosome 5. *J Med Genet*, **42**, 577–82.

Dong, S. L., Reynolds, S. F., and Steiner, I. P. 2001. Brain abscess in patients with hereditary hemorrhagic telangiectasia: case report and literature review. *J Emerg Med*, **20**, 247–51.

Fisher, M., and Zito, J. L. 1983. Focal cerebral ischemia distal to a cerebral aneurysm in hereditary hemorrhagic telangiectasia. *Stroke*, **14**, 419–21.

Fressinaud, C., Pasco-Papon, A., Brugeilles-Baguelin, H., and Emile, J. 2000. Complication inhabituelle de la maladie de Rendu-Osler-Weber: le syndrome bulbaire paramédian. *Rev Neurol (Paris)*, **156**, 388–91.

Fuchizaki, U., Miyamori, H., Kitagawa, S., *et al.* 2003. Hereditary haemorrhagic telangiectasia (Rendu-Osler-Weber disease). *Lancet*, **362**, 1490–4.

Fulbright, R., Chaloupka, J., Putman, C., *et al.* 1998. MR of hereditary haemorrhagic telangiectasia: prevalence and spectrum of cerebrovascular malformations. *Am J Neuroradiol*, **19**, 477–84.

Gallione, C., Repetto, G. M., Leguis, E., *et al.* 2004. A combined syndrome of juvenile polyposis and hereditary haemorrhagic telangiectasia is associated with mutations in MADH4 (SMAD4). *Lancet*, **363**, 852–9.

Garcia-Monaco, R., Taylor, W., Rodesch, G., *et al.* 1995. Pial arteriovenous fistula in children as presenting manifestation of Rendu-Osler-Weber disease. *Neuroradiology*, **37**, 60–4.

Garcia-Tsao, G., Korzenik, J. R., Young, L., *et al.* 2000. Liver disease in patients with hereditary haemorrhagic telangiectasia. *N Engl J Med*, **343**, 931–6.

Guttmacher, A. E., Marchuk, D. A., and White, R. I. 1995. Hereditary hemorrhagic telangiectasia. *N Engl J Med*, **333**, 918–24.

Haitjema, T., Westerman, C. J. J., Overtoom, T. T. C., *et al.* 1996. Hereditary haemorrhagic telangiectasia (Osler-Weber- Rendu disease). New insights in pathogenesis complications and treatment. *Arch Intern Med*, **156**, 714–19.

Hewes, R. C., Auster, M., and White, R. I. 1985. Cerebral embolism – first manifestation of pulmonary arteriovenous malformation in patients with hereditary haemorrhagic telangiectasia. *Cardiovasc Intervent Radiol*, **8**, 151–5.

Hodgson, C. H., Burchell, H. B., Good, G. A., and Clagett, O. T. 1959. Hereditary haemorrhagic telangiectasia and pulmonary arteriovenous fistula. Survey of a large family. *N Engl J Med*, **261**, 625–36.

Kimura, K., Minematsu, K., and Nakajima, M. 2004. Isolated pulmonary arteriovenous fistula without Rendu-Osler-Weber disease as a cause of cryptogenic stroke. *J Neurol Neurosurg Psychiatr*, **75**, 311–3.

Kjeldsen, A., and Kjeldsen, J. 2000. Gastrointestinal bleeding in patients with hereditary haemorrhagic telangiectasia. *Am J Gastroenterol*, **95**, 415–8.

Krings, T., Chng, S. M., Ozanne, A., *et al.* 2005. Hereditary haemorrhagic telangiectasia in children: endovascular treatment of neurovascular malformations. *Neuroradiology*, **47**, 946–54.

Krings, T., Ozanne, A., Chng, S. M., *et al.* 2005. Neurovascular phenotypes in hereditary haemorrhagic telangiectasia patients according to age. Review of 50 consecutive patients aged 1 day–60 years. *Neuroradiology*, **47**, 711–20.

Lesca, G., Plauchu, H., Coulet, F., *et al.* 2004. Molecular screening of ALK1/ACVRL1 and ENG genes in hereditary haemorrhagic telangiectasia in France. *Hum Mutat*, **23**, 289–99.

Love, B. B., Biller, J., Landas, S. K., and Hoover, W. W. 1992. Diagnosis of pulmonary arteriovenous malformation by ultrafast chest computed tomography in Rendu-Osler-Weber syndrome with cerebral ischemia: a case report. *Angiology*, **43**, 552–8.

Marchuk, D. A., Srinivasan, S., Squire, T. L., and Zawitowski, J. S. 2003. Vascular morphogenesis: tales of two syndromes. *Hum Mol Genet*, **12**, R97–112.

Matsubara, S., Mandzia, J. L., ter Brugge K., Willinsky, R. A., and Faughnan, N. E. 2000. Angiographic and clinical characteristics of patients with cerebral arteriovenous malformations associated with hereditary haemorrhagic telangiectasia. *AJNR Am J Neuroradiol*, **21**, 1016–20.

McAllister, K. A., Grogg, K. M.,Gallione, C. J., *et al*. 1994. Endoglin, a TGF-β binding protein of endothelial cells, is the gene for haemorrhagic telangiectasia type 1. *Nat Genet*, **8**, 345–51.

Morgan, T., McDonald, J., Anderson, C., *et al*. 2002. Intracranial hemorrhage in infants and children with hereditary haemorrhagic telangiectasia (Osler-Weber-Rendu syndrome). *Pediatrics*, **109**, E12.

Neau, J. P., Boissonnot, L., Boutaud, P., *et al*. 1987. Manifestations neurologiques de la maladie de Rendu-Osler-Weber. A propos de 4 observations. *Rev Méd Interne*, **8**, 75–8.

Ondra, S. L., Troupp, H., George, E. D., and Schwab, K. 1990. The natural history of symptomatic arteriovenous malformations of the brain: a 24-year follow-up assessment. *J Neurosurg*, **73**, 331–7.

Osler, W. 1901. On a family form of recurring epistaxis, associated with multiple telangiectases of the skin and mucous membranes. *John Hopkins Hospital Bulletin*, **12**, 333–7.

Peery, W. H. 1987. Clinical spectrum of hereditary haemorrhagic telangiectasia (Osler-Weber-Rendu disease). *Am J Med*, **82**, 989–97.

Plauchu, H., de Chadarévian, J. P., Bideau, A., and Robert, J. M. 1989. Age-related clinical profile of hereditary haemorrhagic telangiectasia in an epidemiologically recruited population. *Am J Med Genet*, **32**, 291–7.

Porteous, M. E. M., Burn, J., and Proctor, S. J. 1992. Hereditary haemorrhagic telangiectasia: a clinical analysis. *J Med Genet*, **29**, 527–30.

Putman, C. M., Chaloupka J. C., Fulbright, R. K., *et al*. 1996. Exceptional multiplicity of cerebral arteriovenous malformations associated with hereditary haemorrhagic telangiectasia (Osler-Weber-Rendu syndrome). *Am J Neuroradiol*, **17**, 1733–42.

Rendu, H. 1896. Epistaxis répétées chez un sujet porteur de petits angiomes cutanés et muqueux. *Bulletin des Membres de la Société de Médecine Hospitalière de Paris*, **13**, 731–3.

Roman, G., Fisher, M., Perl, D. P., and Poser, C. M. 1978. Neurological manifestations of hereditary haemorrhagic telangiectasia (Rendu-Osler-Weber disease): report of two cases and review of the literature. *Ann Neurol*, **4**, 130–44.

Shovlin, C. L., Guttmacher, A. E., Buscarini, E., *et al*. 2000. Diagnostic criteria for hereditary haemorrhagic telangiectasia (Rendu-Osler-Weber disease). *Am J Med Genet*, **91**, 66–7.

Sisel, R. J., Parker, B. M., and Bahl, O. P. 1970. Cerebral symptoms in pulmonary arteriovenous fistula. A result of paradoxical emboli? *Circulation*, **46**, 123–8.

Stapf, C., Mast, H., Sciacca, R. R., *et al*. 2006. Predictors of hemorrhage in patients with untreated brain arteriovenous malformation. *Neurology*, **66**, 1350–5.

Thompson, R. L., Cattaneo, S. M., and Barnes, J. 1977. Recurrent brain abscess: manifestation of pulmonary arteriovenous fistula and hereditary haemorrhagic telangiectasia. *Chest*, **72**, 654–5.

White, R. I., Lynch-Nyhan, A., Terry, P., *et al*. 1988. Pulmonary arteriovenous malformations: techniques and long-term outcome of embolotherapy. *Radiology*, **169**, 663–9.

Wilkins, E. G. L., O'Feaeghail, M., and Carroll, J. D. 1983. Recurrent cerebral abscess in hereditary haemorrhagic telangiectasia. *J Neurol Neurosurg Psychiatr*. **46**, 963–5.

Willemse, R. B., Mager, J. J., Westermann, C. J., *et al*. 2000. Bleeding risk of cerebrovascular malformations in hereditary haemorrhagic telangiectasia. *J Neurosurg*, **92**, 779–84.

Yoshida, Y., Weon, Y. C., Sachet, M., *et al*. 2004. Posterior cranial fossa single-hole arteriovenous fistulae in children: 14 consecutive cases. *Neuroradiology*, **46**, 474–81.

18 CEREBRAL AUTOSOMAL DOMINANT ARTERIOPATHY WITH SUBCORTICAL INFARCTS AND LEUKOENCEPHALOPATHY (CADASIL)

Hugues Chabriat and Marie Germaine Bousser

Introduction

Cerebral autosomal dominant arteriopathy with subcortical infarcts and leukoencephalopathy (CADASIL) (Tournier-Lasserve et al., 1993) is an inherited small artery disease of mid-adulthood caused by mutations of the NOCTH3 gene on chromosome 19 (Joutel et al., 1996).

The exact frequency of CADASIL remains unknown. The disease is not limited to white families and has been reported worldwide. In a consecutive series of 212 patients with lacunar stroke, the screening of mutations in exons 3, 4, 5, and 6 of the NOCTH3 gene revealed only one affected patient. For patients with onset of lacunar stroke younger than 65 years with leukoaraiosis, the yield was estimated at 2%. The screening of mutations in exons 3 and 4 was negative in limited samples of subjects with stroke or dementia in the absence of selective criteria (Wang et al., 2000). Finally, based on a register for the disease in western Scotland, Ravzi et al. (2005) estimated that the prevalence in 2004 of NOCTH3 gene mutation is about 4.14 per 100 000 adults in this population. This frequency is possibly largely underestimated.

Clinical manifestations

The first clinical manifestations in CADASIL are attacks of migraine with aura occurring between age 20 and 40 years (Chabriat et al., 1997; Desmond et al., 1999; Dichgans et al., 1998). They are observed in 20–30% of patients. Ischemic manifestations are reported in 60–80% of patients, usually during the fourth and fifth decade. They can be associated with severe mood disturbances or seizures, most often in association with various degrees of cognitive impairment. Dementia is usually detected between 50 and 60 years and is found nearly constant at the end stage of the disorder (Chabriat et al., 1997; Desmond et al., 1999; Dichgans et al., 1998).

In contrast to migraine without aura, the frequency of which is identical to that estimated in the general population, migraine with aura is reported in 20–40% of CADASIL patients, a frequency four- to fivefold higher than in the general population. Migraine with aura is the predominating clinical feature in some families (Chabriat, Tournier-Lasserve et al., 1995) but is absent in others (Lv et al., 2004). The mean age at onset is between 28 and 30 years (Desmond et al., 1999; Vahedi et al., 2004), with a large range from 6 to 48 years. Thus, attacks of migraine with aura may occur in some patients before the appearance of MRI signal abnormalities.

In the largest series of Vahedi et al. (2004), the frequency of attacks appeared extremely variable among affected individuals, from two per week to one every 3–4 years. Triggering factors of migraine with aura are similar to those of migraine in the general population. The most frequent symptoms are visual, sensory, or aphasic. Motor symptoms are reported in one fifth of CADASIL patients who have attacks of migraine with aura. In contrast with the aura symptoms reported in the general population, more than half of patients have a history of atypical aura such as basilar, hemiplegic, or prolonged aura (Headache Classification Committee of the International Headache Society, 1988). A few patients have severe attacks with unusual symptoms such as confusion, fever, meningitis, or coma (Feuerhake et al., 2002; Le Ber et al., 2002; Schon et al., 2003). Acetazolamide was found to reduce the frequency of attacks of migraine with aura in anecdotal cases (Forteza et al., 2001; Weller et al., 1998). The pathophysiology of migraine with aura in CADASIL is still unknown.

Ischemic manifestations are the most frequent clinical events in CADASIL: 60–85% of patients have had transient ischemic attacks (TIAs) or complete strokes (Bousser and Tournier-Lasserve, 1994; Chabriat, Vahedi et al., 1995; Dichgans et al., 1998; Singhal et al., 2004). They occur at a mean age of 45–50 years (extreme limits from 20 to 70 years) (Chabriat, Vahedi et al., 1995, 1997; Desmond et al., 1998; Dichgans et al., 1998). Age at onset does not differ between men and women. In a recent follow-up study, Peters et al. (2004) estimated the incidence rate of stroke at 10.4 per 100 person-years. Two thirds of them are classical lacunar syndromes: pure motor stroke, ataxic hemiparesis, pure sensory stroke, sensory motor stroke (Chabriat, Vahedi et al., 1995). Other focal neurologic deficits of abrupt onset are less frequent: dysarthria (either isolated or associated with motor or sensory deficit), monoparesis, paresthesia of one limb, isolated ataxia, nonfluent aphasia, hemianopia (Chabriat, Vahedi et al., 1995). The onset of the neurological deficit can progress for several hours (Chabriat, Vahedi et al., 1995; Dichgans et al., 1998). Some neurological deficits occur suddenly and are associated with headache. When they are transient, they can mimick attacks of migraine with aura. Vahedi et al. (2004) reported that 4/41 CADASIL migraine sufferers had attacks with sudden aura difficult to differentiate from ischemic events. TIAs and stroke may be observed in the absence of vascular risk factors (Chabriat, Tournier-Lasserve et al., 1995). However, in the largest and most recent series, one fifth of patients are hypertensive, 20–50% are current smokers or have an increased serum level of cholesterol (Peters et al., 2004; Singhal et al., 2004).

Higher median plasma homocysteine levels are also detected in CADASIL patients (Flemming *et al.*, 2001). Singhal *et al.* (2004) recently reported 9% of 127 patients having hyperhomocysteinemia and 4% with diabetes. Only current smoking at the time of the event was found to be associated with earlier onset of ischemic manifestations (Singhal *et al.*, 2004). In contrast, the mutation site within the *NOCTH3* gene does not seem to influence the age of onset or risk of ischemic events. In addition, the homozygous status for the mutation in the *NOCTH3* gene does not seem to influence the clinical presentation (Tuominen *et al.*, 2001).

Five to 10% of CADASIL patients have seizures, either focal or generalized (Desmond *et al.*, 1998; Dichgans *et al.*, 1998; Malandrini *et al.*, 1997). They are usually reported in patients with a positive history of stroke. Epilepsy is usually well-controlled by current antiepileptic drugs.

About one fifth of CADASIL patients have severe episodes of mood disturbances. Their frequency is widely variable between families (Chabriat, Vahedi *et al.*, 1995, 2000). These episodes can be inaugural and lead to misdiagnosis (Chabriat, Vahedi *et al.*, 1995, 2000). Few patients have severe depression of the melancholic type sometimes alternating with typical manic episodes suggesting bipolar mood disorder (Kumar and Mahr, 1997), although the *NOCTH3* gene is not involved in familial forms of this disease (Ahearn *et al.*, 2002). The location of ischemic lesions in the basal ganglia and the frontal location of white-matter lesions may play a key role in the occurrence of mood disturbances observed in affected individuals (Aylward *et al.*, 1994; Bhatia and Marsden, 1994).

Cognitive impairment and dementia represent the second most frequent clinical manifestation in CADASIL. At the onset of the disease, the cognitive profile is most often heterogeneous and usually involves very few cognitive domains. The alteration of executive functions is the most frequent deficit observed even in young patients and several decades before dementia. Executive dysfunction was detected in all individuals between 35 and 50 years old in a recent series of 42 symptomatic patients (Buffon *et al.*, 2006). These cognitive changes are insidious at onset and may also appear a long time before TIAs or stroke (Lesnik Oberstein *et al.*, 2003). The Wisconsin Card Sorting Test or the Trail Making Test is particularly sensitive to detect early changes in executive performance (Taillia *et al.*, 1998). With aging, cognitive decline becomes more homogenous with significant changes in all cognitive domains. Dementia is reported in one third of symptomatic patients at the late phase of the disorder. The frequency of dementia increases considerably with age. Thus, about 60% of patients older than 60 years are demented, and more than 80% of deceased subjects were reported to be demented before death. When dementia is present, the neuropsychological deficit is usually extensive involving not only executive functions, attention and memory, but also reasoning and language performances (Buffon *et al.*, 2006). Dementia is often associated with apathy. Conversely, severe aphasia, apraxia, or agnosia is rare (Buffon *et al.*, 2006; Peters *et al.*, 2005). Dementia is observed in the absence of any other clinical manifestations in 10% of cases (Buffon *et al.*, 2006).

Dementia is always associated with pyramidal signs. Gait difficulties are present in 90%, urinary incontinence in 80–90%, and pseudobulbar palsy in 50% of demented individuals. At the end stage of the disorder, CADASIL patients become bedridden. In a large retrospective study of 411 patients, Opherk *et al.* (2004) found that the median age at onset for inability to walk without assistance was 59 years in men and 62 years in women, and for becoming bedridden, 62 years in men and 66.5 years in women.

CADASIL patients usually die after they develop the pulmonary complications of dysphagia (Chabriat *et al.*, 1997; Opherk *et al.*, 2004). Age at death was found significantly lower in men than in women (median age 64.6 years vs 70.7 years) (Opherk *et al.*, 2004). In contrast to the normal median survival time observed in women, affected men may have a mean decrease of 5 years of their life expectancy (Opherk *et al.*, 2004).

Imaging investigations

MRI shows on T2-weighted images widespread areas of increased signal in the white matter associated with focal hyperintensities in the basal ganglia, thalamus, and brainstem (Chabriat *et al.*, 1998;

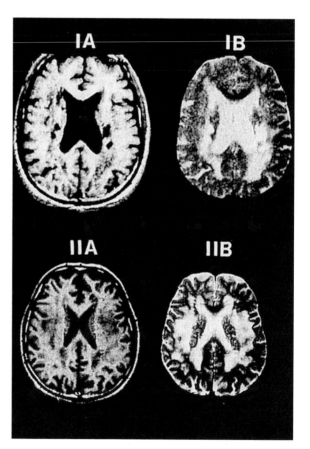

Figure 18.1 (IA) T1-weighted MRI from a patient, showing numerous low-signal subcortical lesions (left and right thalami, posterior limb of left internal capsule, right external capsule, and left temporo-occipital white matter). **(IB)** T2-weighted MRI showing corresponding areas of high signal, with a more diffuse increased signal in white matter. **(IIA)** T1-weighted MRI from an asymptomatic subject, showing that the signal returned from white matter is abnormal, but no focal areas are seen. **(IIB)** T2-weighted MRI showing diffuse high signal intensity of the subcortical white matter. (From Tournier-Lasserve *et al.*, 1993, with permission. Copyright American Heart Association.)

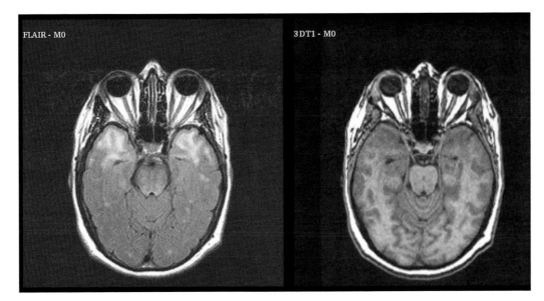

Figure 18.2 MRI (Fluid-Attenuated Inversion Recovery [FLAIR] images), and three-dimensional T1 showing the characteristic bilateral signal changes in the subcortical white matter of CADASIL patients within the anterior part of temporal lobes.

Dichgans *et al.*, 1999). The extent of white-matter signal abnormalities is highly variable. It increases dramatically with age. In subjects younger than 40 years, T2 hypersignals are usually punctate or nodular with a symmetrical distribution, and predominate in periventricular areas and within the centrum semiovale. Later in life, white-matter lesions are diffuse (Figure 18.1) and can involve the whole of white matter, including the U fibers under the cortex (Chabriat *et al.*, 1998, 1999; Coulthard *et al.*, 2000; Dichgans *et al.*, 1999). The frequency of signal abnormalities in the external capsule (2/3 of patients) and in the anterior part of the temporal lobes (60%) is noteworthy (Figure 18.2) and particularly useful for differential diagnosis with other small-vessel diseases (Auer *et al.*, 2001; Markus *et al.*, 2002; O'Sullivan *et al.*, 2001). T2 hyperintensities also can be detected in the corpus callosum (Coulthard *et al.*, 2000; Iwatsuki *et al.*, 2001). Brainstem lesions predominate in the pons in areas irrigated by perforating arteries and can involve the mesencephalon (Chabriat *et al.*, 1999). In contrast, the medulla is usually spared.

On T1-weighted images, punctiform or larger focal hypointensities are frequent in the same areas and are detected in about two thirds of individuals with T2 hyperintensities (Chabriat *et al.*, 1998). They are observed both in the white matter and basal ganglia, but also in the brainstem, and correspond mostly to lacunar infarcts. The total load of such lesions appears significantly related to different scores of clinical severity (Chabriat *et al.*, 1998). Numerous hypointensities on T1-weighted images may also correspond to Virchow–Robin spaces, which are more frequent and extensive in CADASIL than in healthy subjects (Cumurciuc *et al.*, 2006). Such MRI signal abnormalities within the temporal white matter in CADASIL and particularly within the subcortical white matter are considered as a characteristic feature of the disease (van Den Boom *et al.*, 2002). Cortical or cerebellar lesions are exceptional. They have been observed in only two cases older than 60 years (unpublished data) and may be related

to the involvement of medium-sized or large arteries (Choi *et al.*, 2005).

On gradient-echo images or T2*-weighted images, microbleeds are easily detected in 30–50% of patients (Dichgans *et al.*, 2002; Lesnik Oberstein *et al.*, 2001; van den Boom *et al.*, 2003). Only age was found to influence the occurrence of microhemorrhage in these small series of patients.

Cerebral angiography obtained in 14 patients belonging to the first large series was found normal except in one patient who had several narrowings of medium-sized arteries (Chabriat, Vahedi *et al.*, 1995). Since that date, isolated CADASIL patients with lumen irregularities mimicking angiitis have been detected (Engelter *et al.*, 2002; Schmidley *et al.*, 2005; Williamson *et al.*, 1999). However, a high frequency of neurological worsening after angiography has been reported in large series of patients (Dichgans and Petersen, 1997).

Pathology

Macroscopic examination of the brain shows a diffuse myelin pallor and rarefaction of the hemispheric white matter sparing the U fibers (Baudrimont *et al.*, 1993). Lesions predominate in the periventricular areas and centrum semiovale. They are associated with lacunar infarcts located in the white matter and basal ganglia (lentiform nucleus, thalamus, caudate) (Ruchoux *et al.*, 2002; Ruchoux and Maurage, 1997). The most severe hemispheric lesions are the most profound (Baudrimont *et al.*, 1993; Davous and Fallet-Bianco, 1991; Ruchoux *et al.*, 1995). In the brainstem, the lesions are more marked in the pons and are similar to the pontine ischemic rarefaction of myelin described by Pullicino *et al.* (1995). Small deep infarcts and dilated Virchow–Robin spaces are also associated with the white-matter lesions. The vessels close to these lesions do not appear occluded (Santa *et al.*, 2003).

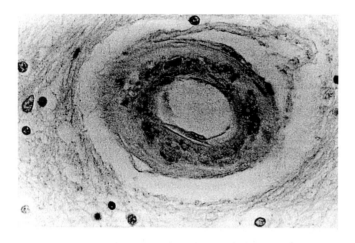

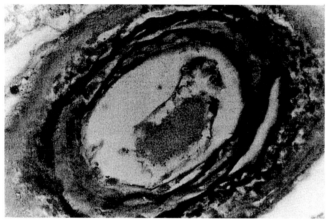

Figure 18.3 Vascular changes in small arteries of the white matter. *Top*: Granular eosinophilic material in the media (hematoxylin and eosin stain × 284). *Bottom*: Thickening and reduplication of the internal elastic lamellae (orcein stain × 284). (From Baudrimont *et al.*, 1993, with permission. Copyright American Heart Association.)

Microscopic investigations show that the wall of cerebral and leptomeningeal arterioles is thickened with a significant reduction of the lumen (Baudrimont *et al.*, 1993), so penetrating arteries in the cortex and white matter appear stenosed (Miao *et al.*, 2004; Okeda *et al.*, 2002). A distinctive feature is the presence of a granular material within the media (Figure 18.3) extending into the adventitia (Baudrimont *et al.*, 1993; Bergmann *et al.*, 1996; Desmond *et al.*, 1998; Filley *et al.*, 1999; Gray *et al.*, 1994; Mikol *et al.*, 2001; Ruchoux *et al.*, 1995). The periodic acid–Schiff (PAS)-positive staining suggested the presence of glycoproteins; the staining for amyloid substance and elastin is negative (Ruchoux *et al.*, 1995; Ruchoux and Maurage, 1997). By contrast, the endothelium of the vessels is usually spared. Sometimes, the smooth muscle cells are not detectable and are replaced by collagen fibers (Zhang *et al.*, 1994). On electron microscopy, the smooth muscle cells appear swollen and often degenerated, some of them with multiple nuclei. There is a granular, electron-dense, osmiophilic material (GOM) within the media (Gutierrez-Molina *et al.*, 1994). This material consists of granules of about 10–15 nm in diameter. It is localized close to the cell membrane of the smooth muscle cells, where it appears very dense. The smooth muscle cells are separated by large amounts of this

unidentified material. These vascular abnormalities observed in the brain are also detectable in other organs or territories (Ruchoux *et al.*, 1995; Ruchoux and Maurage, 1997). The GOM surrounding the smooth muscle cells as seen with electron microscopy is also present in the media of arteries located in the spleen, liver, kidneys, muscle, and skin and also in the wall of carotid arteries and the aorta (Robinson *et al.*, 2001; Ruchoux *et al.*, 1995; Ruchoux and Maurage, 1997). These vascular lesions can be detected by nerve or muscle biopsy (Goebel *et al.*, 1997; Schroder *et al.*, 1995). The presence of the GOM in the skin vessels now allows confirmation of the diagnosis of CADASIL using punch skin biopsies (Chabriat *et al.*, 1997; Ebke *et al.*, 1997; Jen *et al.*, 1997; Ruchoux *et al.*, 1994, 1995), although the sensitivity and specificity of this method have not yet been completely established. Joutel *et al.* (2001) proposed to use anti-*NOCTH3* antibodies to reveal the accumulation of *NOCTH3* products within the vessel wall in CADASIL patients as an alternative diagnostic method.

Genetics

CADASIL is caused by stereotyped mutations of the *NOCTH3* gene (Joutel *et al.*, 1996). The *NOCTH3* gene is expressed only in vascular smooth mucle cells (Joutel, Andreux *et al.*, 2000) of arterial vessels (Villa *et al.*, 2001). It encodes a single-pass transmembrane receptor of a 2321-amino-acid protein, with an extracellular domain containing 34 epidermal growth factor (EGF) repeats (including 6 cystein residues) and 3 Lin repeats associated with intracellular and transmembrane domains (Joutel *et al.*, 1996, 1997). Domenga *et al.* (2004) recently showed that *NOCTH3* is required specifically to generate functional arteries in mice by regulating arterial differentiation and maturation of vascular smooth muscle cells.

The stereotyped missense mutations (Joutel *et al.*, 1996) or deletions (Joutel, Chabriat *et al.*, 2000) responsible for CADASIL are within EGF-like repeats and are located only in the extracellular domain of the *NOCTH3* protein (Dotti *et al.*, 2005; Peters *et al.*, 2005). In 70% of cases, they are located within exons 3 and 4, which encode the first five EGF domains (Joutel *et al.*, 1997). All mutations responsible for the disease lead to an uneven number of cystein residues.

The *NOCTH3* protein usually undergoes complex proteolytic cleavages leading to an extracellular and a transmembrane fragment (Blaumueller *et al.*, 1997). After cleavage, these two fragments form a heterodimer at the cell surface of smooth muscle cells. In CADASIL, the ectodomain of the *NOCTH3* receptor accumulates within the vessel wall of affected subjects (Joutel, Andreux *et al.*, 2000). This accumulation is found near but not within the characteristic GOM seen on electron microscopy. It is observed in all vascular smooth mucle cells and in pericytes within all organs (brain, heart, muscles, lungs, skin). An abnormal clearance of the *NOCTH3* ectodomain from the smooth muscle cell surface is presumed to cause this accumulation (Joutel, Andreux *et al.*, 2000; Joutel, Francois *et al.*, 2000c; Joutel and Tournier-Lasserve, 2002). The exact mechanisms underlying this phenomenon are not elucidated yet.

Diagnosis and treatment

The diagnosis is confirmed by genetic testing or skin biopsy. Genetic tests are initially focused on exons where the mutations are most frequent (Joutel *et al.*, 1997). Peters *et al.* (2005) found 90% of mutations within exons 2–6. Diagnostic testing with immunostaining using anti-*NOCTH3* antibodies is an alternative method that seems easier than electron microscopy and particularly useful before initiating a complete screening of the gene in difficult cases (Joutel *et al.*, 2001). As previously detailed, angiography with contrast agents should be avoided because of possible neurological complications (Dichgans and Petersen, 1997).

No treatment has been evaluated for CADASIL. Because CADASIL is a vascular disorder responsible for cerebral ischemic events, different authors prescribe aspirin for secondary prevention, but its benefit in the disease has not been shown. The occurrence of intracerebral hemorrhage in two anecdotal cases (Maclean *et al.*, 2005; Ragoschke-Schumm *et al.*, 2005) and in one patient, at the time of death (Baudrimont *et al.*, 1993), suggests that anticoagulant therapy may be dangerous in CADASIL. Whether this risk is related to the number of silent microbleeds is still unknown. For migraine, all vasoconstrictive drugs such as ergot derivatives and triptans are not recommended during the course of the disease. Treatment of migraine should be restricted to analgesic agents and nonsteroidal anti-inflammatory drugs. As reported for other ischemic diseases, rehabilitation procedures are crucial, particularly when a new ischemic event occurs. If stroke occurs at an early stage of the disease, recovery is often complete. Psychological support for the patient and family is crucial in this disorder, and genetic counseling and testing should be performed only at specialized centers that have the necessary experience.

REFERENCES

Ahearn, E. P., Speer, M. C., Chen, Y. T., *et al.* 2002. Investigation of Notch3 as a candidate gene for bipolar disorder using brain hyperintensities as an endophenotype. *Am J Med Genet*, **114**, 652–8.

Auer, D. P., Putz, B., Gossl, C., *et al.* 2001. Differential lesion patterns in CADASIL and sporadic subcortical arteriosclerotic encephalopathy: MR imaging study with statistical parametric group comparison. *Radiology*, **218**, 443–51.

Aylward, E. D., Roberts-Willie, J. V., Barta, P. E., *et al.* 1994. Basal ganglia volume and white matter hyperintensities in patients with bipolar disorder. *Am J Psychiatry*, **5**, 687–93.

Baudrimont, M., Dubas, F., Joutel, A., Tournier-Lasserve, E., and Bousser, M. G. 1993. Autosomal dominant leukoencephalopathy and subcortical ischemic stroke. A clinicopathological study. *Stroke*, **24**, 122–5.

Bergmann, M., Ebke, M., Yuan, Y., *et al.* 1996. Cerebral autosomal dominant arteriopathy with subcortical infarcts and leukoencephalopathy (CADASIL): a morphological study of a German family. *Acta Neuropathol (Berl)*, **92**, 341–50.

Bhatia, K., and Marsden, C. 1994. The behavioural and motor consequences of focal lesions of the basal ganglia in man. *Brain*, **117**, 859–76.

Blaumueller, C. M., Qi, H., Zagouras, P., and Artavanis-Tsakonas, S. 1997. Intracellular cleavage of Notch leads to a heterodimeric receptor on the plasma membrane. *Cell*, **90**, 281–91.

Bousser, M. G., and Tournier-Lasserve, E. 1994. Summary of the proceedings of the First International Workshop on CADASIL. Paris, May 19–21, 1993. *Stroke*, **25**, 704–7.

Buffon, F., Porcher, R., Hernandez, K., *et al.* 2006. Cognitive profile in CADASIL. *J Neurol Neurosurg Psychiatr*, (in press).

Chabriat, H., Joutel, A., Vahedi, K., *et al.* 1997. [CADASIL. Cerebral Autosomal Dominant Arteriopathy with Subcortical Infarcts and Leukoencephalophathy]. *Rev Neurol (Paris)*, **153**, 376–85.

Chabriat, H., Joutel, A., Vahedi, K., *et al.* 2000. [CADASIL (cerebral autosomal dominant arteriopathy with subcortical infarcts and leukoencephalopathy): clinical features and neuroimaging]. *Bull Acad Natl Med*, **184**, 1523–31; discussion 1531–3.

Chabriat, H., Levy, C., Taillia, H., *et al.* 1998. Patterns of MRI lesions in CADASIL. *Neurology*, **51**, 452–7.

Chabriat, H., Mrissa, R., Levy, C., *et al.* 1999. Brain stem MRI signal abnormalities in CADASIL. *Stroke*, **30**, 457–9.

Chabriat, H., Tournier-Lasserve, E., Vahedi, K., *et al.* 1995. Autosomal dominant migraine with MRI white-matter abnormalities mapping to the CADASIL locus. *Neurology*, **45**, 1086–91.

Chabriat, H., Vahedi, K., Iba-Zizen, M. T., *et al.* 1995. Clinical spectrum of CADASIL: a study of 7 families. Cerebral autosomal dominant arteriopathy with subcortical infarcts and leukoencephalopathy. *Lancet*, **346**, 934–9.

Choi, E. J., Choi, C. G., and Kim, J. S. 2005. Large cerebral artery involvement in CADASIL. *Neurology*, **65**, 1322–4.

Coulthard, A., Blank, S. C., Bushby, K., Kalaria, R. N., and Burn, D. J. 2000. Distribution of cranial MRI abnormalities in patients with symptomatic and subclinical CADASIL. *Br J Radiol*, **73**, 256–65.

Cumurciuc, R., Guichard, J. P., Reizine, D., *et al.* 2006. Dilation of Virchow-Robin spaces in CADASIL. *Eur Neurol*, in press.

Davous, P., and Fallet-Bianco, C. 1991. [Familial subcortical dementia with arteriopathic leukoencephalopathy. A clinico-pathological case]. *Rev Neurol (Paris)*, **147**(5), 376–84.

Desmond, D. W., Moroney, J. T., Lynch, T., Chan, S., Chin, S. S., and Mohr, J. P. 1999. The natural history of CADASIL: a pooled analysis of previously published cases. *Stroke*, **30**, 1230–3.

Desmond, D. W., Moroney, J. T., Lynch, T., *et al.* 1998. CADASIL in a North American family: clinical, pathologic, and radiologic findings. *Neurology*, **51**, 844–9.

Dichgans, M., Filippi, M., Bruning, R., *et al.* 1999. Quantitative MRI in CADASIL: correlation with disability and cognitive performance. *Neurology*, **52**, 1361–7.

Dichgans, M., Holtmannspotter, M., Herzog, J., *et al.* 2002. Cerebral microbleeds in CADASIL: a gradient-echo magnetic resonance imaging and autopsy study. *Stroke*, **33**, 67–71.

Dichgans, M., Mayer, M., Uttner, I., *et al.* 1998. The phenotypic spectrum of CADASIL: clinical findings in 102 cases. *Ann Neurol*, **44**, 731–9.

Dichgans, M., and Petersen, D. 1997. Angiographic complications in CADASIL. *Lancet*, **349**, 776–7.

Domenga, V., Fardoux, P., Lacombe, P., *et al.* 2004. Notch3 is required for arterial identity and maturation of vascular smooth muscle cells. *Genes Dev*, **18**, 2730–5.

Dotti, M. T., Federico, A., Mazzei, R., *et al.* 2005. The spectrum of Notch3 mutations in 28 Italian CADASIL families. *J Neurol Neurosurg Psychiatr*, **76**, 736–8.

Ebke, M., Dichgans, M., Bergmann, M., *et al.* 1997. CADASIL: skin biopsy allows diagnosis in early stages. *Acta Neurol Scand*, **95**, 351–7.

Engelter, S. T., Rueegg, S., Kirsch, E. C., *et al.* 2002. CADASIL mimicking primary angiitis of the central nervous system. *Arch Neurol*, **59**, 1480–3.

Feuerhake, F., Volk, B., Ostertag, C. B., *et al.* 2002. Reversible coma with raised intracranial pressure: an unusual clinical manifestation of CADASIL. *Acta Neuropathol (Berl)*, **103**, 188–92.

Filley, C. M., Thompson, L. L., Sze, C. I., *et al.* 1999. White matter dementia in CADASIL. *J Neurol Sci*, **163**, 163–7.

Flemming, K. D., Nguyen, T. T., Abu-Lebdeh, H. S., *et al.* 2001. Hyperhomocysteinemia in patients with cerebral autosomal dominant arteriopathy with subcortical infarcts and leukoencephalopathy (CADASIL). *Mayo Clin Proc*, **76**, 1213–8.

Forteza, A. M., Brozman, B., Rabinstein, A. A., Romano, J. G., and Bradley, W. G. 2001. Acetazolamide for the treatment of migraine with aura in CADASIL. *Neurology*, **57**, 2144–5.

Goebel, H. H., Meyermann, R., Rosin, R., and Schlote, W. 1997. Characteristic morphologic manifestation of CADASIL, cerebral autosomal-dominant arteriopathy with subcortical infarcts and leukoencephalopathy, in skeletal muscle and skin. *Muscle Nerve*, **20**, 625–7.

Gray, F., Robert, F., Labrecque, R., *et al.* 1994. Autosomal dominant arteriopathic leuko-encephalopathy and Alzheimer's disease. *Neuropathol Appl Neurobiol*, **20**, 22–30.

Gutierrez-Molina, M., Caminero Rodriguez, A., Martinez Garcia, C., *et al.* 1994. Small arterial granular degeneration in familial Binswanger's syndrome. *Acta Neuropathol (Berl)*, **87**, 98–105.

Headache Classification Committee of the International Headache Society. 1988. Classification and diagnostic criteria for headache disorders, cranial neuralgias and facial pain. *Cephalalgia*, **8 Suppl 7**, 1–96.

Iwatsuki, K., Murakami, T., Manabe, Y., *et al.* 2001. Two cases of Japanese CADASIL with corpus callosum lesion. *Tohoku J Exp Med*, **195**, 135–40.

Jen, J., Cohen, A. H., Yue, Q., *et al.* 1997. Hereditary endotheliopathy with retinopathy, nephropathy, and stroke (HERNS). *Neurology*, **49**, 1322–30.

Joutel, A., Andreux, F., Gaulis, S., *et al.* 2000. The ectodomain of the Notch3 receptor accumulates within the cerebrovasculature of CADASIL patients. *J Clin Invest*, **105**, 597–605.

Joutel, A., Chabriat, H., Vahedi, K., *et al.* 2000. Splice site mutation causing a seven amino acid Notch3 in-frame deletion in CADASIL. *Neurology*, **54**, 1874–5.

Joutel, A., Corpechot, C., Ducros, A., *et al.* 1996. Notch3 mutations in CADASIL, a hereditary adult-onset condition causing stroke and dementia. *Nature*, **383**, 707–10.

Joutel, A., Corpechot, C., Ducros, A., *et al.* 1997. Notch3 mutations in cerebral autosomal dominant arteriopathy with subcortical infarcts and leukoencephalopathy (CADASIL), a Mendelian condition causing stroke and vascular dementia. *Ann N Y Acad Sci*, **826**, 213–7.

Joutel, A., Favrole, P., Labauge, P., *et al.* 2001. Skin biopsy immunostaining with a Notch3 monoclonal antibody for CADASIL diagnosis. *Lancet*, **358**, 2049–51.

Joutel, A., Francois, A., Chabriat, H., *et al.* 2000. [CADASIL: genetics and physiopathology]. *Bull Acad Natl Med*, **184**, 1535–42; discussion 1542–4.

Joutel, A., and Tournier-Lasserve, E. 2002. [Molecular basis and physiopathogenic mechanisms of CADASIL: a model of small vessel diseases of the brain]. *J Soc Biol*, **196**, 109–15.

Joutel, A., Vahedi, K., Corpechot, C., *et al.* 1997. Strong clustering and stereotyped nature of Notch3 mutations in CADASIL patients. *Lancet*, **350**, 1511–5.

Kumar, S. K., and Mahr, G. 1997. CADASIL presenting as bipolar disorder. *Psychosomatics*, **38**, 397–8.

Le Ber, I., Carluer, L., Derache, N., *et al.* 2002. Unusual presentation of CADASIL with reversible coma and confusion. *Neurology*, **59**, 1115–6.

Lesnik Oberstein, S. A., van den Boom, R., Middelkoop, H. A., *et al.* 2003. Incipient CADASIL. *Arch Neurol*, **60**, 707–12.

Lesnik Oberstein, S. A., van den Boom, R., van Buchem, M. A., *et al.* 2001. Cerebral microbleeds in CADASIL. *Neurology*, **57**, 1066–70.

Lv, H., Yao, S., Zhang, W., *et al.* 2004. [Clinical features in 4 Chinese families with cerebral autosomal dominant arteriopathy with subcortical infarcts and leukoencephalopathy (CADASIL).]. *Beijing Da Xue Xue Bao*, **36**, 496–500.

Maclean, A. V., Woods, R., Alderson, L. M., *et al.* 2005. Spontaneous lobar haemorrhage in CADASIL. *J Neurol Neurosurg Psychiatr*, **76**, 456–7.

Malandrini, A., Carrera, P., Ciacci, G., *et al.* 1997. Unusual clinical features and early brain MRI lesions in a family with cerebral autosomal dominant arteriopathy. *Neurology*, **48**, 1200–3.

Markus, H. S., Martin, R. J., Simpson, M. A., *et al.* 2002. Diagnostic strategies in CADASIL. *Neurology*, **59**, 1134–8.

Miao, Q., Paloneva, T., Tuominen, S., *et al.* 2004. Fibrosis and stenosis of the long penetrating cerebral arteries: the cause of the white matter pathology in cerebral autosomal dominant arteriopathy with subcortical infarcts and leukoencephalopathy. *Brain Pathol*, **14**, 358–64.

Mikol, J., Henin, D., Baudrimont, M., *et al.* 2001. [Atypical CADASIL phenotypes and pathological findings in two new French families]. *Rev Neurol (Paris)*, **157**, 655–67.

Okeda, R., Arima, K., and Kawai, M. 2002. Arterial changes in cerebral autosomal dominant arteriopathy with subcortical infarcts and leukoencephalopathy (CADASIL) in relation to pathogenesis of diffuse myelin loss of cerebral white matter: examination of cerebral medullary arteries by reconstruction of serial sections of an autopsy case. *Stroke*, **33**, 2565–9.

Opherk, C., Peters, N., Herzog, J., Luedtke, R., and Dichgans, M. 2004. Long-term prognosis and causes of death in CADASIL: a retrospective study in 411 patients. *Brain*, **127(Pt 11)**, 2533–9.

O'Sullivan, M., Jarosz, J. M., Martin, R. J., *et al.* 2001. MRI hyperintensities of the temporal lobe and external capsule in patients with CADASIL. *Neurology*, **56**, 628–34.

Peters, N., Herzog, J., Opherk, C., and Dichgans, M. 2004. A two-year clinical follow-up study in 80 CADASIL subjects: progression patterns and implications for clinical trials. *Stroke*, **35**, 1603–8.

Peters, N., Opherk, C., Bergmann, T., *et al.* 2005. Spectrum of mutations in biopsy-proven CADASIL: implications for diagnostic strategies. *Arch Neurol*, **62**, 1091–4.

Peters, N., Opherk, C., Danek, A., *et al.* 2005. The pattern of cognitive performance in CADASIL: a monogenic condition leading to subcortical ischemic vascular dementia. *Am J Psychiatry*, **162**, 2078–85.

Pullicino, P., Ostow, P., Miller, L., Snyder, W., and Muschauer, F. 1995. Pontine ischemic rarefaction. *Ann Neurol*, **37**, 460–6.

Ragoschke-Schumm, A., Axer, H., Witte, O. W., *et al.* 2005. Intracerebral haemorrhage in CADASIL. *J Neurol Neurosurg Psychiatr*, **76**, 1606–7.

Razvi, S. S., Davidson, R., Bone, I., and Muir, K. W. (2005). The prevalence of cerebral autosomal dominant arteriopathy with subcortical infarcts and leucoencephalopathy (CADASIL) in the west of Scotland. *J Neurol Neurosurg Psychiatr*, **76**, 739–41.

Robinson, W., Galetta, S. L., McCluskey, L., Forman, M. S., and Balcer, L. J. 2001. Retinal findings in cerebral autosomal dominant arteriopathy with subcortical infarcts and leukoencephalopathy (CADASIL). *Surv Ophthalmol*, **45**, 445–8.

Ruchoux, M. M., Brulin, P., Brillault, J., *et al.* 2002. Lessons from CADASIL. *Ann N Y Acad Sci*, **977**, 224–31.

Ruchoux, M. M., Chabriat, H., Bousser, M. G., Baudrimont, M., and Tournier-Lasserve, E. 1994. Presence of ultrastructural arterial lesions in muscle and skin vessels of patients with CADASIL. *Stroke*, **25**, 2291–2.

Ruchoux, M. M., Guerouaou, D., Vandenhaute, B., *et al.* 1995. Systemic vascular smooth muscle cell impairment in cerebral autosomal dominant arteriopathy with subcortical infarcts and leukoencephalopathy. *Acta Neuropathol (Berl)*, **89**, 500–12.

Ruchoux, M. M., and Maurage, C. A. 1997. CADASIL: cerebral autosomal dominant arteriopathy with subcortical infarcts and leukoencephalopathy. *J Neuropathol Exp Neurol*, **56**, 947–64.

Santa, Y., Uyama, E., Chui D, H., *et al.* 2003. Genetic, clinical and pathological studies of CADASIL in Japan: a partial contribution of Notch3 mutations and implications of smooth muscle cell degeneration for the pathogenesis. *J Neurol Sci*, **212**, 79–84.

Schmidley, J. W., Beadle, B. A., and Trigg, L. 2005. Co-occurrence of CADASIL and isolated CNS angiitis. *Cerebrovasc Dis*, **19**, 352–4.

Schon, F., Martin, R. J., Prevett, M., *et al.* 2003. "CADASIL coma": an underdiagnosed acute encephalopathy. *J Neurol Neurosurg Psychiatr*, **74**, 249–52.

Schroder, J. M., Sellhaus, B., and Jorg, J. 1995. Identification of the characteristic vascular changes in a sural nerve biopsy of a case with cerebral autosomal dominant arteriopathy with subcortical infarcts and leukoencephalopathy (CADASIL). *Acta Neuropathol (Berl)*, **89**, 116–21.

Singhal, S., Bevan, S., Barrick, T., Rich, P., and Markus, H. S. 2004. The influence of genetic and cardiovascular risk factors on the CADASIL phenotype. *Brain*, **127(Pt 9)**, 2031–8.

Taillia, H., Chabriat, H., Kurtz, A., *et al.* 1998. Cognitive alterations in non-demented CADASIL patients. *Cerebrovasc Dis*, **8**, 97–101.

Tournier-Lasserve, E., Joutel, A., Melki, J., *et al.* 1993. Cerebral autosomal dominant arteriopathy with subcortical infarcts and leukoencephalopathy maps to chromosome 19q12. *Nat Genet*, **3**, 256–9.

Tuominen, S., Juvonen, V., Amberla, K., *et al.* 2001. Phenotype of a homozygous CADASIL patient in comparison to 9 age-matched heterozygous patients with the same R133 C Notch3 mutation. *Stroke*, **32**, 1767–74.

Vahedi, K., Chabriat, H., Levy, C., *et al.* 2004. Migraine with aura and brain magnetic resonance imaging abnormalities in patients with CADASIL. *Arch Neurol*, **61**, 1237–40.

van den Boom, R., Lesnik Oberstein, S. A., Ferrari, M. D., Haan, J., and van Buchem, M. A. 2003. Cerebral autosomal dominant arteriopathy with subcortical infarcts and leukoencephalopathy: MR imaging findings at different ages–3rd-6th decades. *Radiology*, **229**, 683–90.

van Den Boom, R., Lesnik Oberstein, S. A., van Duinen, S. G., *et al.* 2002. Subcortical lacunar lesions: an MR imaging finding in patients with cerebral autosomal dominant arteriopathy with subcortical infarcts and leukoencephalopathy. *Radiology*, **224**, 791–6.

Villa, N., Walker, L., Lindsell, C. E., Gasson, J., Iruela-Arispe, M. L., and Weinmaster, G. 2001. Vascular expression of Notch pathway receptors and ligands is restricted to arterial vessels. *Mech Dev*, **108**, 161–4.

Wang, T., Sharma, S. D., Fox, N., *et al.* 2000. Description of a simple test for CADASIL disease and determination of mutation frequencies in sporadic ischaemic stroke and dementia patients. *J Neurol Neurosurg Psychiatr*, **69**, 652–4.

Weller, M., Dichgans, J., and Klockgether, T. 1998. Acetazolamide-responsive migraine in CADASIL. *Neurology*, **50**, 1505.

Williamson, E. E., Chukwudelunzu, F. E., Meschia, J. F., *et al.* 1999. Distinguishing primary angiitis of the central nervous system from cerebral autosomal dominant arteriopathy with subcortical infarcts and leukoencephalopathy: the importance of family history. *Arthritis Rheum*, **42**, 2243–8.

Zhang, W. W., Ma, K. C., Andersen, O., *et al.* 1994. The microvascular changes in cases of hereditary multi-infarct disease of the brain. *Acta Neuropathol (Berl)*, **87**, 317–24.

19 CEREBROVASCULAR COMPLICATIONS OF FABRY'S DISEASE

Panayiotis Mitsias, Nikolaos I. H. Papamitsakis, Colum F. Amory, and Steven R. Levine

Introduction

Fabry's disease (FD), or angiokeratoma corporis diffusum, is a rare X-linked inherited disorder of glycosphingolipid metabolism (Desnick *et al.*, 2001). Deficiency of a lysosomal hydrolase, *a*-galactosidase, leads to progressive accumulation of glycosphingolipids (mainly ceramide trihexoside) in most visceral tissues and primarily in the lysosomes of the vascular endothelium. Progressive endothelial glycosphingolipid accumulation results in tissue ischemia and infarction, and leads to the major clinical manifestations of the disease (Desnick *et al.*, 2001). The disease is genetically heterogeneous, as it has been linked to multiple mutations in the *a*-galactosidase gene (Chen *et al.*, 1998; Takenaka *et al.*, 1996; Topaloglou *et al.*, 1999).

While the prevalence of FD has been estimated to be around 1 in 40 000 males (Desnick *et al.*, 2001), a recent study (Spada *et al.*, 2006) found 12 of 37 104 consecutive male neonates with specific mutations in the *a*-galactosidase gene. This prevalence of 1 in 3 100 males suggests a vast underdiagnosis of FD.

Hemizygote males usually have characteristic skin lesions and angiokeratomas, and often have unexplained fever, acroparesthesias, episodic crises of excruciating pain, corneal and lenticular opacities, hypohidrosis, and cardiac and renal dysfunction (Desnick *et al.*, 2001). Tinnitus and hearing loss are also very common. Death usually occurs in adult life from renal, cardiac, and/or cerebral complications of their vascular disease (Desnick *et al.*, 2001).

Heterozygote females either are asymptomatic or exhibit fewer signs and symptoms of the disease, although occasional females have been described with symptoms similar to males (Bird and Lagunoff, 1978).

The neurological complications of FD include peripheral neuropathy, autonomic neuropathy, and cerebrovascular disease (Desnick *et al.*, 2001). Heterozygotes usually present either with no symptoms (Desnick *et al.*, 2001) or with milder manifestations of FD as compared to hemizygotes (Bird and Lagunoff, 1978). However, cerebrovascular manifestations are common in both the hemizygote and the symptomatic heterozygote groups. Furthermore, these manifestations may be the first indication of the disease: in a prospective study, 4% of patients (both hemizygotes and heterozygotes) with cryptogenic strokes had mutations in the *a*-galactosidase gene (Rolfs *et al.*, 2005).

In this chapter, we analyze the clinical, radiologic, and pathologic features of hemizygote and heterozygote FD patients and cerebrovascular involvement based on our experience and a comprehensive review of the literature (Archer, 1927; Bass, 1958; Becker *et al.*, 1975; Bethune *et al.*, 1961; Bird and Lagunoff, 1978; Brown, 1952; Cable *et al.*, 1982; Colley *et al.*, 1958; Curry *et al.*, 1961; De Groot, 1964; DiLorenzo *et al.*, 1969; Grewal and Barton, 1992; Grewal and McLatchey, 1992; Guin and Saini, 1976; Hasholt *et al.*, 1990; Ho and Feman, 1981; Jensen, 1966; Kahn, 1973; Kaye *et al.*, 1988; Lou and Reske-Nielsen, 1971; Maisey and Cosh, 1980; Menzies *et al.*, 1988; Mitsias and Levine, 1996; Morgan *et al.*, 1990; Moumdjian *et al.*, 1989; Mutoh *et al.*, 1988; Petersen *et al.*, 1989; Pompen *et al.*, 1947; Roach, 1989; Schatzki *et al.*, 1979; Scully *et al.*, 1984; Sher *et al.*, 1978; Steward and Hitchcock, 1968; Stoughton and Clendenning, 1959; Tagliavini *et al.*, 1982; Wallace and Cooper, 1965; Wise *et al.*, 1962; Zeluff *et al.*, 1978).

Early diagnostic features

The most consistent early symptoms of FD are episodic crises of pain, lasting for minutes to hours, mostly affecting the feet or the hands, usually precipitated by exercise, fever, or hot weather, and modified by acetophenacetin. The mechanisms responsible for production of the pain crises are not well known, but it is possible that storage of glycophospholipids within the endothelial cells of the vasa nervorum, the perineural cells, or the dorsal root and autonomic ganglia can cause altered vasomotor reactivity, resulting in a hypoxic state (Desnick *et al.*, 2001).

Anhidrosis, due to infiltration of lipids into the sweat glands and loss of unmyelinated nerve fibers innervating the sweat glands, usually complicates the problem of heat intolerance.

The most often observed sign is the angiokeratoma, appearing in clusters within the superficial layers of the skin. They are usually first noted in the periumbilical area, the extensor surfaces of the elbows and knees, and the hip and genital areas (Desnick *et al.*, 2001).

Ophthalmological examination typically reveals whirl-like, corneal opacities, dilatation and tortuosity of the conjunctival vessels, and abnormalities of retinal vessels (Desnick *et al.*, 2001). These changes do not usually impair vision. (Figure 19.1).

Clinical manifestations of cerebrovascular disease

Male hemizygotes develop symptomatic cerebrovascular disease at a young age for stroke, usually in the fourth decade (mean age 32) (Mitsias and Levine, 1996). Hemiparesis, vertigo, dysarthria, diplopia, ataxia, hemisensory symptoms, nystagmus, and nausea and/or vomiting are the most common symptoms and

Uncommon Causes of Stroke, 2nd edition, ed. Louis R. Caplan. Published by Cambridge University Press. © Cambridge University Press 2008.

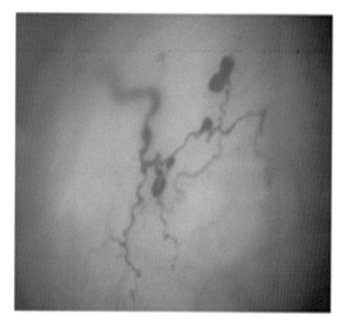

Figure 19.1 Abnormal conjunctival vessels in a man with Fabry's disease. See color plate. (Courtesy of Dr. Alan H. Friedman, MD., Department of Ophthalmology, The Mount Sinai School of Medicine).

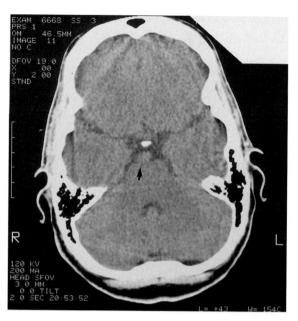

Figure 19.2 Unenhanced head CT from a heterozygote patient, demonstrating basilar artery dilatation and compression of the right side of the ventral pons.

signs (Mitsias and Levine, 1996). Headache is rather infrequent, reported by 20% of patients (Mitsias and Levine, 1996). In the majority (58%) of patients, the presentation was consistent with vertebrobasilar territory ischemia, whereas the anterior circulation was definitely symptomatic in approximately 20% of the patients (Mitsias and Levine, 1996).

Vascular dementia from penetrating small-vessel disease has also been described in patients with FD and should be a consideration in the evaluation of otherwise unexplained dementia, particularly in men younger than 65 years (Mendez et al., 1997).

Heterozygote women develop symptomatic cerebrovascular disease usually a decade later than the hemizygotes (Mitsias and Levine, 1996). Memory loss, vertigo, ataxia, hemiparesis, depressed level of consciousness, hemisensory symptoms, and headache are the predominant symptoms and signs (Mitsias and Levine, 1996). In half of the patients, the clinical presentation was consistent with involvement within the vertebrobasilar territory, whereas in only 10% the carotid territory was definitely involved (Mitsias and Levine, 1996). Central retinal artery occlusion (Utsumi et al., 1997) and central retinal vein occlusion (Oto et al., 1998) have also been reported.

Neuroradiologic findings

A multitude of findings on head CT scans has been reported, ranging from completely normal results, to the presence of large superficial territorial infarctions, to multiple small deep infarcts in the cerebral hemispheres, brainstem, or cerebellum (Mitsias and Levine, 1996). In addition, dilatation and ectasia of the basilar or vertebral arteries are often seen in both hemizygotes and heterozygotes (Mitsias and Levine, 1996) (Figure 19.2).

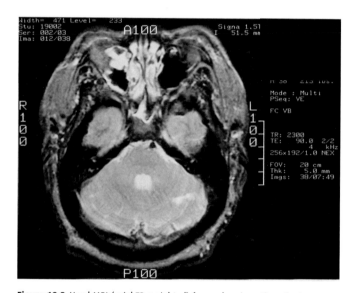

Figure 19.3 Head MRI (axial T2-weighted) from a hemizygotic patient, revealing ectasia of the basilar artery and a left cerebellar infarct.

In a large series of patients with FD evaluated with serial head MRI scans, it was observed that patients younger than 26 years did not have visible lesions, whereas all patients older than 54 years had MRI-visible hyperintense lesions, typical for small-vessel disease. Of all patients evaluated, 32% had no lesions (mean age 36 years), 26% had white-matter lesions (mean age 43 years), and 26% had lesions in both white and gray matter (mean age 47 years). Approximately one third of the patients with lesions on MRI had neurological symptoms (Crutchfield et al., 1998). In addition, other MRI reports indicated that prominent, ectatic, intracranial basal vessels may be found (Mitsias and Levine, 1996) (Figure 19.3).

Cerebral angiography could be normal. However, often dolichoectatic intracranial vessels, especially basilar or vertebral

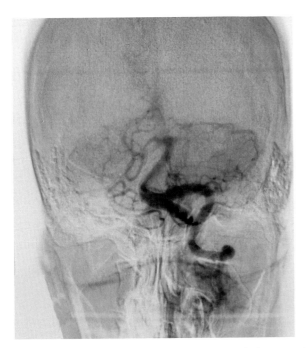

Figure 19.4 Selective right vertebral artery catheter cerebral angiography from a heterozygous patient demonstrating an ectatic, tortuous vertebrobasilar system.

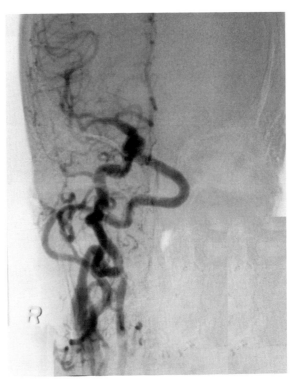

Figure 19.5 Conventional right carotid angiography from a hemizygotic patient, revealing tortuous and ectatic external and internal carotid arteries.

arteries, and occasionally the internal carotid artery are seen in hemizygotic and heterozygotic patients (Mitsias and Levine, 1996) (Figures 19.4 and 19.5).

In one study (Tedeschi *et al.*, 1999), proton magnetic resonance spectroscopy (MRS) imaging revealed that the ratios of *N*-acetylaspartate (NAA) to creatine (Cr)-phosphocreatine and NAA to choline were significantly decreased compared to controls, whereas the choline/Cr ratio was not different between FD patients and controls. These findings led to the conclusion that there is decreased NAA in FD patients, possibly due to either direct metabolic neuronal dysfunction or to diffuse subclinical ischemia leading to neuronal loss. This neuronal involvement extended beyond the areas of MRI-visible abnormalities. In another study (Marino *et al.*, 2006), changes in NAA/Cr ratios were correlated with clinical measures of disability. This information could be of help in the assessment of potential therapeutic interventions.

Diffusion tensor imaging (DTI), which measures the random translational motion of water molecules, can be used to evaluate the relative restriction of that movement in certain tissues (such as along axons) as well as to measure the general structural integrity of brain parenchyma. In one study (Fellgiebel *et al.*, 2006), DTI demonstrated increased mean diffusivity even in normal-appearing areas of the brain in patients with FD. It is possible that DTI could be used for early evaluation of cerebral pathology, although it is not yet clear what clinical significance can be attached to these findings.

Positron emission tomography (PET) scanning has demonstrated increased resting cerebral blood flow distributed fairly evenly throughout gray and white matter (Moore *et al.*, 2001). Despite the increase in blood flow, however, regional cerebral glucose metabolism is significantly decreased in the white matter of

FD patients (Moore *et al.*, 2003). These findings suggest an underlying local metabolic insufficiency stimulating global increased blood flow.

Cerebrovascular pathology

Neuropathologic autopsy findings are consistent with prior events of cerebral ischemia and, rarely, hemorrhage. Large, superficial cerebral hemispheric infarcts; multiple small, deep infarcts; and brainstem and/or cerebellar infarcts are often seen in hemizygotes and symptomatic heterozygotes (Mitsias and Levine, 1996). Intracerebral hemorrhage is rarely observed (Mitsias and Levine, 1996).

The vessels of the Circle of Willis often appear thickened. Narrowing of the lumina and intracellular deposits in arteries and arterioles are additional findings. Dolichoectasia of the basilar and vertebral arteries, and less often of the carotid arteries, is a frequent finding in both hemizygotes and symptomatic heterozygotes (Mitsias and Levine, 1996).

Ischemic cerebrovascular disease

The majority of patients (male hemizygotes and symptomatic female heterozygotes) present with symptoms and signs related to vertebrobasilar ischemia, whereas symptoms due to anterior circulation involvement are relatively uncommon. This is in contrast with the general frequency of anterior versus posterior circulation cerebrovascular disease (Bamford *et al.*, 1991; Bogousslavsky *et al.*, 1988), and suggests a general predilection for involvement of the arteries of the posterior circulation in FD. The combination of large intracranial artery dolichoectasia, especially in the vertebrobasilar system (Colley *et al.*, 1958; Mitsias and Levine, 1996; Petersen *et al.*, 1989; Wallace and Cooper, 1965; Wise *et al.*, 1962), and marked thickening and luminal compromise of the medium- and small-sized arteries (Jensen, 1966; Kahn, 1973; Lou and Reske-Nielsen, 1971; Scully *et al.*, 1984; Tagliavini *et al.*, 1982) may cause reduction of blood flow and also stretching, distortion, and obstruction of the already stenotic basilar tributaries, thus resulting in brainstem or cerebellar ischemia (Nishizaki *et al.*, 1986). Complete or partial thrombosis resulting in unilateral restricted pontine infarct in the territory of a penetrating artery, large bilateral pontine infarcts from basilar artery occlusion, cerebellar infarcts, or embolic infarction of the occipital lobe or the thalamus have been observed in several patients with FD (Mitsias and Levine, 1996).

Deep small cerebral infarcts, usually multiple, are also a frequent finding (Mitsias and Levine, 1996). The most likely underlying mechanism is progressive occlusion of the small intracranial arteries or arterioles, secondary to deposition of the glycosphingolipid in the vessel wall, as shown pathologically in several patients (Jensen, 1966; Lou and Reske-Nielsen, 1971; Schatzki *et al.*, 1979; Tagliavini *et al.*, 1982). Other risk factors (hypertension secondary to renal involvement, diabetes mellitus, etc.) may also play a role, but the extent to which each of these factors contributes is unclear. However, uncontrolled hypertension is widely prevalent in patients with FD (Kleinert *et al.*, 2006).

Cardiac abnormalities are frequently encountered, and they can potentially lead to cardiogenic embolism. Coronary artery disease, due to deposition of the glycosphingolipid, resulting in premature myocardial infarction (Scully *et al.*, 1984; Wise *et al.*, 1962; Zeluff *et al.*, 1978), can cause left ventricular wall-motion abnormalities, mural thrombus formation, and subsequent cardiogenic embolism. Valvular heart disease, especially of the mitral valve, is frequently encountered. Mitral valve prolapse is found in 54–56% of hemizygotes and 39–58% of heterozygotes (Goldman *et al.*, 1986; Sakuraba *et al.*, 1986). The presence of glycolipid deposits in all the structures of the heart is one of the reasons for the increased incidence of mitral valve prolapse in FD (Becker *et al.*, 1975). Mitral valve prolapse has a role in cerebral ischemia (Avierinos *et al.*, 2003; Barnett *et al.*, 1980).

Hypertrophic cardiomyopathy is known to complicate FD (Cohen *et al.*, 1983; Yokoyama *et al.*, 1987), especially in heterozygote women who exhibit a more severe form of cardiac disease (Goldman *et al.*, 1986; Sakuraba *et al.*, 1986). Hypertrophic obstructive cardiomyopathy is associated with increased risk for stroke (Russel *et al.*, 1991), especially when associated with atrial fibrillation (Furlan *et al.*, 1984; Nishide *et al.*, 1983).

Carotid artery atherosclerotic plaque appears to be less prevalent in patients with FD when compared with controls. However, the intima-media thickness (IMT) is diffusely greater in patients with FD. Although increased IMT has been shown to be independently related to risk of ischemic stroke and coronary artery disease, it is not clear what clinical significance this finding of increased nonatherosclerotic carotid IMT has in patients with FD (Barbey *et al.*, 2006).

Impaired autonomic function in male (Cable *et al.*, 1982) and female (Mutoh *et al.*, 1988) patients with FD, presumably related

Table 19.1 Mechanisms of brain ischemia in patients with FD

1. Intracranial arterial dolichoectasia
   a. Complete or partial thrombosis of main arterial trunk
   b. Stretching, distortion, and obstruction of tributary vessels
   c. Artery-to-artery embolism
2. Progressive occlusion of small arteries or arterioles secondary to deposition of glycosphingolipid in the vessel wall
3. Cardiogenic embolism
   a. Wall-motion abnormalities secondary to ischemic heart disease
   b. Valvular heart disease, especially mitral valve prolapse
   c. Hypertrophic cardiomyopathy
4. Impaired autonomic function
   a. Hypertension
   b. Hypotension
5. Prothrombotic states
   a. Platelet activation
   b. Activation of endothelial factors

to glycolipid deposition in the peripheral nervous system and vascular beds, is known to occur. The resulting severe orthostatic hypotension could lead to transient or permanent cerebral ischemia, especially in the presence of cerebral vessel occlusive disease (Dobkin, 1989).

Prothrombotic states are not uncommon in patients with FD. Widespread endothelial abnormalities (Desnick *et al.*, 2001) – related to tissue deposits of glycophospholipids, predominantly ceramide trihexoside, and to a lesser extent ceramide digalactoside and the tissue blood type B substance – can lead to platelet activation. This has been demonstrated even in patients without a prior history of thrombotic episodes (Igarashi *et al.*, 1986). In addition, analysis of plasma from FD patients for multiple endothelial factors reveals elevated concentrations of soluble intercellular adhesion molecule-1, vascular cell adhesion molecule-1, P-selectin, and plasminogen activator inhibitor; lower levels of thrombomodulin; and elevated levels of integrin CDIIb, compared to normal controls (DeGraba *et al.*, 2000). Furthermore, up to 35% of all patients with FD have been discovered to have the Factor V Leiden mutation (Hughes and Mehta, 2005), and patients with FD with deep white-matter lesions on MRI are far more likely to have the same mutation (Altarescu *et al.*, 2005). These findings are consistent with a prothrombotic state in FD patients, and could also provide markers of efficacy for therapeutic interventions in the disease (see Table 19.1).

The vasculature itself is also abnormal in patients with FD. The nitric oxide pathway for regulation of vascular reactivity appears to be down-regulated, and the non-nitric oxide pathways emerge as the main regulators of endothelial reactivity (Altarescu *et al.*, 2005). Enhanced nitrotyrosine immunohistochemical staining in the cerebral and dermal vascular beds is consistent with increased oxidative stress (Moore *et al.*, 2001), which may lead to continued vasodilation as well as accelerated atherosclerosis. Decreased levels of vitamin C and increased levels of myeloperoxidase in patients with FD also contribute to an inability to handle oxidative stress (Moore *et al.*, 2004).

Intracranial arterial dolichoectasia

In FD, in addition to cerebral ischemia, dolichoectatic intracranial arteries may also cause neurovascular compression syndromes. Triventricular hydrocephalus related to dolichoectatic basilar artery has been reported in hemizygotic (Kahn, 1973) and heterozygotic (Colley et al., 1958; Maisey and Cosh, 1980; Wise et al., 1962) patients. Other presentations, including isolated third nerve palsy (De Groot, 1964), trigeminal neuralgia (Morgan et al., 1990), isolated eighth nerve dysfunction (De Groot, 1964; Prüss et al., 2006; Wallace and Cooper, 1965; Wise et al., 1962), and dysfunction of the hypoglossal nerve (Maisey and Cosh, 1980) can also be attributed to compression of the individual nerves by dolichoectatic basilar or vertebral arteries. Optic atrophy, observed in three patients (Steward and Hitchcock, 1968; Wallace and Cooper, 1965; Wise et al., 1962), also can be attributed to compression of the optic nerve by a dolichoectatic supraclinoid segment of the internal carotid artery (Schwartz et al., 1993).

The deposition of the glycosphingolipid occurs in all areas of the body, but predominantly in the lysosomes of endothelial, perithelial, and smooth-muscle cells of blood vessels (Desnick et al., 2001), resulting thus in extensive vascular smooth muscle involvement and loss of structural integrity of the arterial wall, eventually leading to the development of intracranial artery dolichoectasia.

Intracerebral hemorrhage

There are rare reports of intracerebral hemorrhage in hemizygotes (Bass, 1958; Wise et al., 1962) and heterozygotes (Steward and Hitchcock, 1968). Despite incomplete descriptions, it appears likely that this was a consequence of malignant hypertension secondary to uremia. It is possible, however, that the degeneration of the cerebral vessels due to deposition of glycosphingolipid in the vessel wall strongly contributes to the development of this process.

Outcome

The majority (75%) of hemizygotic males presenting with cerebral ischemia will eventually develop recurrent cerebrovascular events, and most of them more than one event (Mitsias and Levine, 1996). In three quarters of patients, the recurrence will be in the vertebrobasilar territory (Mitsias and Levine, 1996). Intracerebral hemorrhage is rare as a recurrent event (Mitsias and Levine, 1996). The mean interval between the first cerebrovascular event and the first recurrence is 6.4 years (range 0–19 years) (Mitsias and Levine, 1996). During follow-up time, approximately 50% of patients die within a mean interval of 8.2 years (67.4, range 0–20). In the majority of patients, death is directly linked to the cerebrovascular event, whereas others die of consequences of renal failure.

The prognosis of symptomatic heterozygotes is also quite poor. One third die as a direct consequence of the initial cerebrovascular event, usually within 1 year of presentation with cerebrovascular disease (Mitsias and Levine, 1996). Reported causes of death are progressively deepening coma and pontine hemorrhage. Of the survivors, the vast majority (85%) develop recurrent cerebrovascular disease (Mitsias and Levine, 1996), almost always in the posterior circulation, and usually within 1–4 years (Mitsias and Levine, 1996).

Management

Treatment is far from satisfactory as no specific therapy for the cerebrovascular complications of FD is available. Administration of antiplatelet agents may help to prevent the atherosclerotic and thromboembolic effects of damage to the vascular endothelium, but experience with this approach is limited. In one study, administration of ticlopidine significantly modified platelet aggregation in patients with FD (Sakuraba et al., 1987), but whether this is of value in a clinical setting remains to be shown. Management of underlying cardiac dysfunction, and the use of oral anticoagulant agents (if there are conditions predisposing to cardiogenic embolism) should also be considered.

In addition to correcting renal function, renal transplantation may also prevent the further development of vascular lesions, thus preventing cerebrovascular manifestations, by providing a source of normal enzyme for release into the circulation, although a report of progressive cardiac involvement despite successful renal allotransplantation (Kramer et al., 1985) emphasizes the importance of long-term follow-up studies. Genetic counseling and prenatal diagnosis based on enzyme assay in amniocytes and chorionic villi (Kleijer et al., 1987) should be offered.

Enzyme replacement therapy (ERT) with recombinant human a-galactosidase A clears endovascular deposits of globotriaosylceramide from the kidneys, heart, and skin of patients with FD with return to normal or near-normal histology on biopsy from each site (Eng et al., 2001). Renal function is also improved with ERT (Schiffman et al., 2001). Furthermore, uncontrolled hypertension is reduced with ongoing ERT (Kleinert et al., 2006), although this result may be secondary to the improvement in renal function. Current recommendations are that all patients diagnosed with FD should be treated with ERT as soon as clinical signs are observed (Desnick et al., 2003).

The response to ERT in patients with cerebrovascular pathology is not well studied. The increase in nitrotyrosine staining seen in the cerebral vasculature is reversible with infusion of recombinant human a-galactosidase A (Moore et al., 2001), as is global cerebral hyperperfusion (Moore et al., 2002). In addition, ERT decreases regional cerebral blood flow (Moore et al., 2002). Vitamin C infusion also reduces cerebral blood flow in both control subjects and patients treated with ERT (Moore et al., 2004). However, these changes have not yet been shown to translate into clinical reductions in cerebrovascular pathology. MRI studies show progression of white-matter lesion load despite ERT, although these patients did not show clinical neurologic progression (Ginsberg et al., 2006).

The Mainz Severity Score Index (MSSI) is a scoring system developed in order to describe the severity of disease in patients with FD as well as to monitor the response to treatment. It covers the general, neurologic, cardiologic, and renal manifestations of the disease. The MSSI has been validated in that patients with FD have significantly higher scores than do patients presenting with similar symptoms who were later demonstrated not to have FD. In addition, MSSI scores go down in patients who have been treated and who have shown clinical improvement (Beck, 2006).

Future directions

A virus-producing cell line, producing high-titer recombinant retrovirus constructed to transduce and correct target cells, has been developed; skin fibroblasts from FD patients were infected with the recombinant virus, and secreted enzyme was observed to be taken up by uncorrected cells. Similar endogenous enzyme correction and a small amount of secretion, as well as uptake by uncorrected cells, were demonstrated in transduced immortalized B-cell lines from FD patients. These observations lead to the possibility that corrected stem cells (and their progeny) from FD patients, after ex vivo transduction and reimplantation, may become a continuous source of secreted a-galactosidase A activity in vitro. This then could be delivered and taken up by various target cell and tissue types (metabolic cooperativity) (Medin *et al.*, 1996).

In a further move towards clinical utility of a therapeutic approach, cells originating from the bone marrow of FD patients and also healthy volunteers (isolated CD34+-enriched cells and long-term bone marrow culture cells, including non-adherent hematopoietic cells and adherent stromal cells) could be effectively transduced, demonstrating metabolic cooperativity. Increased intracellular a-galactosidase A enzyme activity was demonstrated, as well as functional correction of lipid accumulation. These results demonstrate that a gene transfer approach to bone marrow cells could be of therapeutic benefit for FD patients (Ohsugi *et al.*, 2000; Takenaka *et al.*, 1999). It certainly remains to be shown whether the above-mentioned approaches could eventually become useful in the daily practice of etiologic treatment of FD and, therefore, primary prevention of cerebrovascular complications.

The use of a knockout mouse model for reproducing the pathology of FD holds promise for understanding the vascular and cerebral disturbances of FD. By using gene expression analysis, it is possible to gather information on the actual genetic environment in the FD cells, as well as on the genetic responses following treatment. Furthermore, each individual tissue may be separately examined in this fashion. Although it remains to be seen exactly how this will affect clinical practice, our understanding of the complex consequences of single gene disorders will be enhanced (Moore *et al.*, 2006).

Low-density lipoprotein apheresis was used in one 39-year-old patient with FD who had had three prior ischemic cerebrovascular events. Not only were lipid levels reduced, levels of adhesion molecules, particularly p-selectin, were reduced, leading to a potentially less thrombotic state (Utsumi *et al.*, 2006). This treatment, in addition to ERT, may reduce ischemic events, and needs to be studied in a controlled fashion.

Acknowledgment

Supported in part by National Institutes of Health grants NS23393 and NS43992.

REFERENCES

Altarescu, G., Moore, D. F., Pursley, R., *et al.* 2001. Enhanced endothelium-dependent vasodilation in Fabry disease. *Stroke*, **32**, 1559–62.

Altarescu, G., Moore, D. F., and Schiffmann, R. 2005. Effect of genetic modifiers on cerebral lesions in Fabry disease. *Neurology*, **64**, 2148–50.

Archer, B. W. C. 1927. Multiple cavernous angiomata of the sweat glands associated with hemiplegia. *Lancet*, **ii**, 595–6.

Avierinos, J-F., Brown, R. D., Foley, D. A., *et al.* 2003. Cerebral ischemic events after diagnosis of mitral valve prolapse. *Stroke*, **34**, 1339–44.

Bamford, J., Sandercock, P., Dennis, M., *et al.* 1991. Classification and natural history of clinically identifiable subtypes of cerebral infarction. *Lancet*, **337**, 1521–6.

Barbey, F., Brakch, N., Linhart, A., *et al.* 2006. Increased carotid intima-media thickness in the absence of atherosclerotic plaques in an adult population with Fabry disease. *Acta Paediatr*, **95(Suppl 451)**, 63–8.

Barnett, H. J. M., Boughner, D. R., Taylor, D. W. *et al.* 1980. Further evidence relating mitral-valve prolapse to cerebral ischemic events. *N Engl J Med*, **302**, 139–44.

Bass, B. H. 1958. Angiokeratoma corporis diffusum. *Br Med J*, **1**, 1418.

Beck, M. 2006. The Mainz Severity Score Index (MSSI): development and validation of a system for scoring the signs and symptoms of Fabry disease. *Acta Paediatr*, **95(Suppl 451)**, 43–6.

Becker, A. E., Schoorl, R., Balk, A. G. and van der Heide, R. M. 1975. Cardiac manifestations of Fabry's disease. *Am J Cardiol*, **36**, 829–35.

Bethune, J. E., Landrigan, P. L. and Chipman, C. D. 1961. Angiokeratoma corporis diffusum universale (Fabry's disease) in two brothers. *N Engl J Med*, **264**, 1280–5.

Bird, T. D. and Lagunoff, D. 1978. Neurological manifestations of Fabry disease in female carriers. *Ann Neurol*, **4**, 537–40.

Bogousslavsky, J., Van Melle, G., and Regli, F. 1988. The Lausanne Stroke Registry: analysis of 1,000 consecutive patients with first stroke. *Stroke*, **19**, 1083–92.

Brown, A. 1952. Diffuse angiokeratoma: report of two cases with diffuse skin changes, one with neurological symptoms and splenomegaly. *Glasgow Med J*, **33**, 361–8.

Cable, W. J. L., Kolodny, E. H., and Adams, R. D. 1982. Fabry disease: impaired autonomic function. *Neurology*, **32**, 498–502.

Chen, C. H., Shyu, P. W., Wu, S. J., *et al.* 1998. Identification of a novel point mutation (S65T) in alpha-galactosidase A gene in Chinese patients with Fabry disease. Mutations in brief no. 169. Online. *Hum Mutat*, **11**, 328–30.

Cohen, I. S., Fluri-Lundeen, J., and Wharton, T. P. 1983. Two dimensional echocardiographic similarity of Fabry's disease to cardiac amyloidosis: a function of ultrastructural analogy? *J Clin Ultrasound*, **11**, 437–41.

Colley, J. R., Miller, D. L., Hutt, M. S. R., and Wallace, H. J. 1958. The renal lesion in angiokeratoma corporis diffusum. *Br Med J*, **1**, 1266–8.

Crutchfield, K. E., Patronas, N. J., Dambrosia, J. M., *et al.* 1998. Quantitative analysis of cerebral vasculopathy in patients with Fabry disease. *Neurology*, **50**, 1746–9.

Curry, H. B., Fleisher, T. L., and Howard, F. 1961. Angiokeratoma corporis diffusum–a case report. *JAMA*, **175**, 864–8.

DeGraba, T., Azhar, S., Dignat-George, F., *et al.* 2000. Profile of endothelial and leukocyte activation in Fabry patients. *Ann Neurol*, **47**, 229–33.

De Groot, W. P. 1964. Angiokeratoma corporis diffusum Fabry. *Dermatologica*, **128**, 321–49.

Desnick, R. J., Brady, R., Barranger, J., *et al.* 2003. Fabry disease, an under-recognized multi-systemic disorder: expert recommendations for diagnosis, management, and enzyme replacement therapy. *Ann Intern Med*, **138**, 338–46.

Desnick, R. S., Ioannou, Y. A., and Eng, C. M. 2001. a-Galactosidase A deficiency: Fabry disease. In C. R. Scriver, A. L. Beaudet, W. S. Sly, and D. Valle, eds., *The Metabolic Basis of Inherited Disease*, 8th edn. New York: McGraw Hill; pp. 3733–74.

DiLorenzo, P. A., Kleinfeld, J., Tellman, W., and Nay, L. 1969. Angiokeratoma corporis diffusum (Fabry's disese). *Acta Derm Venereol*, **49**, 319–25.

Dobkin, B. H. 1989. Orthostatic hypotension as a risk factor for symptomatic occlusive cerebrovascular disease. *Neurology*, **39**, 30–4.

Eng, C. M., Guffon, N., Wilcox, W. R., et al. 2001. Safety and efficacy of recombinant human α-galactosidase A replacement therapy in Fabry's disease. N Engl J Med, 345, 9–16.

Fellgiebel, A., Mazanek, M., Whybra, C., et al. 2006. Pattern of microstructural brain tissue alterations in Fabry disease. J Neurol, 253, 780–7.

Furlan, A. J., Craciun, A. R., Raju, N. R., and Hart, N. 1984. Cerebrovascular complications associated with idiopathic hypertrophic subaortic stenosis. Stroke, 15, 282–4.

Ginsberg, L., Manara, R., Valentine, A. R., et al. 2006. Magnetic resonance imaging changes in Fabry disease. Acta Paediatr, 95(Suppl 451), 57–62.

Goldman, M. E., Cantor, R., Schwartz, M. F., et al. 1986. Echocardiographic abnormalities and disease severity in Fabry's disease. J Am Coll Cardiol, 7, 1157–61.

Grewal, R. P., and Barton, N. W. 1992. Fabry's disease presenting with stroke. Clin Neurol Neurosurg, 94, 177–9.

Grewal, R. P., and McLatchey, S. K. 1992. Cerebrovascular manifestations in a female carrier of Fabry's disease. Acta Neurol Belg, 92, 36–40.

Guin, G. H., and Saini, N. 1976. Diffuse angiokeratoma (Fabry's disease): case report. Mil Med, 141, 259–63.

Hasholt, L., Sorensen, S. A., Wandall, A., et al. 1990. A Fabry's disease heterozygote with a new mutation: biochemical, ultrastructural, and clinical investigations. J Med Genet, 27, 303–6.

Ho, P. C. and Feman, S. S. 1981. Internuclear ophthalmoplegia in Fabry's disease. Ann Ophthalmol, 13, 949–51.

Hughes, D. A., and Mehta, A. B. 2005. Vascular complications of Fabry disease: enzyme replacement and other therapies. Acta Paediatr, 94(Suppl 447), 23–33.

Igarashi, T., Sakuraba, H., and Suzuki, Y. 1986. Activation of platelet function in Fabry's disease. Am J Hematol, 22, 63–7.

Jensen, E. 1966. On the pathology of angiokeratoma corporis diffusum (Fabry). Acta Pathol Microbiol Scand, 68, 313–31.

Kahn, P. 1973. Anderson–Fabry disease: a histopathological study of three cases with observations on the mechanism of production of pain. J Neurol Neurosurg Psychiatr, 36, 1053–62.

Kaye, E. M., Kolodny, E. H., Logigian, E. L., and Ullman, M. D. 1988. Nervous system involvement in Fabry's disease: clinicopathological and biochemical correlation. Ann Neurol, 23, 505–9.

Kleijer, W. J., Hussaarts-Odijk, L. M., Sachs, E. S., et al. 1987. Prenatal diagnosis of Fabry's disease by direct analysis of chorionic villi. Prenat Diagn, 7, 283–7.

Kleinert, J., Dehout, F., Schwarting, A., et al. 2006. Prevalence of uncontrolled hypertension in patients with Fabry disease. Am J Hypertens, 19, 782–7.

Kramer, W. J., Thormann, J., Mueller, K., and Frenzel, H. 1985. Progressive cardiac involvement by Fabry's disease despite successful renal allotransplantation. Int J Cardiol, 7, 72–5.

Lou, H. O. C., and Reske-Nielsen, E. 1971. The central nervous system in Fabry's disease. Arch Neurol, 25, 351–9.

Maisey, D. N., and Cosh, J. A. 1980. Basilar artery aneurysm and Anderson–Fabry disease. J Neurol Neurosurg Psychiatr, 43, 85–7.

Marino, S., Borsini, W., Buchner, S., et al. 2006. Diffuse structural and metabolic brain changes in Fabry disease. J Neurol, 253, 434–40.

Medin, J. A., Tudor, M., Simonovitch, R., et al. 1996. Correction in trans for Fabry disease: expression, secretion and uptake of alpha-galactosidase A in patient-derived cells driven by a high-titer recombinant retroviral vector. Proc Natl Acad Sci USA, 93, 7917–22.

Mendez, M. F., Stanley, T. M., Medel, N. M., Li, Z., and Tedesco, D. T. 1997. The vascular dementia of Fabry's disease. Dement Geriatr Cogn Disord, 8, 252–7.

Menzies, D. G., Campbell, I. W., and Kean, D. M. 1988. Magnetic resonance imaging in Fabry's disease. J Neurol Neurosurg Psychiatr, 51, 1240–1.

Mitsias, P., and Levine, S. R. 1996. Cerebrovascular complications of Fabry's disease. Ann Neurol, 40, 8–17.

Moore, D. F., Altarescu, G., Barker, W. C., et al. 2003. White matter regions in Fabry disease occur in 'prior' selectively hypometabolic and hyperperfused brain regions. Brain Res Bull, 62, 231–40.

Moore, D. F., Altarescu, G., Herscovitch, P., and Schiffmann, R. 2002. Enzyme replacement reverses abnormal cerebrovascular responses in Fabry disease. BMC Neurol, 2, 4.

Moore, D. F., Gelderman, M. P., Fuhrmann, S. R., et al. 2006. Fabry disease and vascular risk factors: future strategies for patient-based studies and the knockout murine model. Acta Paediatr, 95(Suppl 451), 69–71.

Moore, D. F., Scott, T. C. S., Gladwin, M. T., et al. 2001. Regional cerebral hyperperfusion and nitric oxide pathway dysregulation in Fabry disease. Circulation, 104, 1506–12.

Moore, D. F., Ye, F., Brennan, M., et al. 2004. Ascorbate decreases Fabry cerebral hyperperfusion suggesting a reactive oxygen species abnormality: an arterial spin tagging study. J Magn Reson Imaging, 20, 674–83.

Morgan, S. H., Rudge, P., Smith, S. J. M., et al. 1990. The neurological complications of Anderson–Fabry disease (a-galactosidase A deficiency). Investigation of symptomatic and presymptomatic patients. Q J Med, 75, 491–504.

Moumdjian, R., Tampieri, D., Melanson, D., and Ethier, R. 1989. Anderson–Fabry disease: a case report with MR, CT, and cerebral angiography. Am J Neuroradiol, 10, S69–70.

Mutoh, T., Senda, Y., Sugimura, K., et al. 1988. Severe orthostatic hypotension in a female carrier of Fabry's disease. Arch Neurol, 45, 468–72.

Nishide, M., Irino, T., Gotoh, M., et al. 1983. Cardiac abnormalities in ischemic cerebrovascular disease studied in two-dimensional echocardiography. Stroke, 14, 541–5.

Nishizaki, T., Tamaki, N., Takeda, N., et al. 1986. Dolichoectatic basilar artery: a review of 23 cases. Stroke, 17, 1277–81.

Ohsugi, K., Kobayashi, K., Itoh, K., Sakuraba, H., and Sakuragawa, N. 2000. Enzymatic corrections for cells derived from Fabry disease patients by a recombinant adenovirus vector. J Hum Genet, 45, 1–5.

Oto, S., Kart, H., Kadayifcilar, S., Ozdemir, N., and Aydin, P. 1998. Retinal vein occlusion in a woman with heterozygous Fabry's disease. Eur J Ophthalmol, 8, 265–7.

Petersen, R. C., Garrity, J. A., Houser, O. W. 1989. Fabry's disease: an unusual cause of stroke with unique angiographic findings. Neurology, 39(Suppl. 1), 123.

Pompen, A. W. M., Ruiter, M., and Wyers, H. J. G. 1947. Angiokeratoma corporis diffusum (universale) Fabry, as a sign of an unknown internal disease; two autopsy reports. Acta Med Scand, 128, 234–55.

Prüss, H., Bohner, G., and Zschenderlein, R. 2006. Paroxysmal vertigo as the presenting symptom of Fabry disease. Neurology, 66, 249.

Roach, E. S. 1989. Congenital cutaneouvascular syndromes. In J. F. Toole, ed., Handbook of Clinical Neurology, vol. II (55): Vascular Diseases, Part III. Amsterdam–New York: Elsevier Science Publishers B.V., pp. 443–62.

Rolfs, A., Böttcher, T., Zschiesche, M., et al. 2005. Prevalence of Fabry disease in patients with cryptogenic stroke: a prospective study. Lancet, 366, 1794–6.

Russel, J. W., Biller, J., Hajduczok, Z. D., et al. 1991. Ischemic cerebrovascular complications and risk factors in idiopathic hypertrophic subaortic stenosis. Stroke, 22, 1143–7.

Sakuraba, H., Igarashi, T., Shibata, T., and Suzuki, Y. 1987. Effect of vitamin E and ticlopidine on platelet aggregation in Fabry's disease. Clin Genet, 31, 349–54.

Sakuraba, H., Yanagawa, Y., Igarashi, T., et al. 1986. Cardiovascular manifestations in Fabry's disease. A high incidence of mitral valve prolapse in hemizygotes and heterozygotes. Clin Genet, 29, 276–83.

Schatzki, P. F., Kipreos, B., and Payne, J. 1979. Fabry's disease. Primary diagnosis by electron microscopy. Am J Surg Pathol, 3, 211–9.

Schiffman, R., Koff, J. B., Austin, H. A., et al. 2001. Enzyme replacement therapy in Fabry disease. JAMA, 285, 2743–9.

Schwartz, A., Rautenberg, W., and Hennerici, M. 1993. Dolichoectatic intracranial arteries: review of selected aspects. Cerebrovasc Dis, 3, 273–9.

Scully, R. E., Mark, E. J., and McNeely, B. U. 1984. Case records of Massachusetts General Hospital: case 2, 1984. N Engl J Med, 310, 106–14.

Sher, N. A., Reiff, W., Letson, R. D., and Desnick, R. J. 1978. Central retinal artery occlusion complicating Fabry's disease. Arch Ophthalmol, 96, 815–7.

Spada, M., Pagliardini, S., Yasuda, M., et al. 2006. High incidence of later-onset Fabry disease revealed by newborn screening. Am J Med Genet, 79, 31–40.

Steward, V. W., and Hitchcock, C. 1968. Fabry's disease (Angiokeratoma corporis diffusum). Pathol Eur, 3, 377–88.

Stoughton, R. B., and Clendenning, W. E. 1959. Angiokeratoma corporis diffusum (Fabry). Arch Dermatol, 79, 601–2.

Tagliavini, F., Pietrini, V., Gemignani, F., et al. 1982. Anderson–Fabry's disease: neuropathological and neurochemical investigation. Acta Neuropathol (Berlin), 56, 93–8.

Takenaka, T., Hendrickson, C. S., Tworeck, D. M., *et al.* 1999. Enzymatic and functional correction along with long-term enzyme secretion from transduced bone marrow hematopoietic stem/progenitor and stromal cells derived from patients with Fabry disease. *Exp Hematol*, **27**, 1149–59.

Takenaka, T., Sakuraba, H., Hashimoto, K., *et al.* 1996. Coexistence of gene mutations causing Fabry disease and Duchenne muscular dystrophy in a Japanese boy. *Clin Genet*, **49**, 255–60.

Tedeschi, G., Bonavita, S., Banerjee, T. K., Virta, A., and Schiffmann, R. 1999. Diffuse central neuronal involvement in Fabry disease. A proton MRS imaging study. *Neurology*, **52**, 1663–7.

Topaloglou, A. K., Ashley, G. A., Tong, B., *et al.* 1999. Twenty novel mutations in the alpha-galactosidase A gene causing Fabry disease. *Mol Med*, **5**, 806–11.

Utsumi, K., Seta, T., Katsumata, T., *et al.* 2006. Effect of selective LDL-apheresis in a Fabry patient with recurrent strokes. *European Journal of Neurology*, **13**, 429–30.

Utsumi, K., Yamamoto, N., Kase, R., *et al.* 1997. High incidence of thrombosis in Fabry's disease. *Intern Med*, **36**, 327–9.

Wallace, R. D., and Cooper, W. J. 1965. Angiokeratoma corporis diffusum universale (Fabry's disease). *Am J Med*, **39**, 656–61.

Wise, D., Wallace, H. J., and Jellinek, E. H. 1962. Angiokeratoma corporis diffusum. *Q J Med*, **122**, 177–206.

Yokoyama, A., Yamazoe, M., and Shibata, A. 1987. A case of heterozygous Fabry's disease with a short PR interval and giant T waves. *Br Heart J*, **57**, 296–9.

Zeluff, G. W., Caskey, C. T., and Jackson, D. 1978. Heart attack or stroke in a young man? Think Fabry's disease. *Heart Lung*, **7**, 1056–61.

20 MARFAN'S SYNDROME

Luís Cunha

Bernard Marfan described the disease that still bears his name at a meeting of the Medical Society of Paris in 1896. He presented the case of a 5-year-old girl called Gabrielle, pointing out what is still considered to be one of the hallmarks of the disease, her disproportionately long limbs. Further elucidation of the clinical features of the disease would be aggregated in the following decades. The more complex discussion on its causes and treatment still continues today.

Marfan's syndrome is a connective tissue disorder responsible for an extensive and generalized malformation of organs and systems (Pyeritz, 2000). The skeleton is disproportionately arranged and unstable, the eyes often have lens dislocations and are myopic, and a cystic disease of the lungs can be present. All the organic departments can be affected in different degrees, leading to multiple medical problems. Nevertheless, defective formation of cardiac valves and blood vessels are the origin of the more serious occurrences in Marfan's syndrome.

Marfan's syndrome is present in 1 in 5 000–10 000 people, and both men and women of any ethnic group can be affected. The disease is an inherited disorder transmitted as a dominant trait, being sporadic in less than one fourth of the cases. A gene defect is located in the long arm of chromosome 15, in which a mutation in the FBN1 gene that encodes fibrillin-1 was first reported in 1991 (Kainulainen *et al.*, 1990, 1991; Magenis *et al.*, 1991). Since then, more than 600 mutations have been identified, most of them causing marfanoid phenotypes or fragments of the Marfan's syndrome phenotype. The FBN1 mutations include missense and nonsense mutations, exon-splicing errors, and small genomic deletions. Only 12% of the mutations related to Marfan's disease have been reported more than once in unrelated individuals.

Other mutations, not related to fibrillin-1, have recently been described in Marfan patients (Mizuguchi *et al.*, 2004). The so-called second locus for Marfan's syndrome was mapped to 3p24–25, and mutations of indefinite significance in transforming growth factor-alphaβ (TGF-alphaβ) are currently under investigation.

Fibrillin-1 is a major component of the extracellular matrix and seems to offer the fibrillar structure for elastin deposition. Studies of patients with Marfan's syndrome show a decreased content of fibrillin in microfibrillar fibers of skin and cultured fibroblasts (Hollister *et al.*, 1990). Some clinical features, such as the ectopic lens and the cardiovascular malformations, are accepted as obvious consequences of the defective support tissue. Others, like bone overgrowth, are not so clearly explained by that model.

Basic investigations and experimental models are still being pursued to better understand the pathology of Marfan's disease and related disorders.

Clinical features

The clinical spectrum of Marfan's syndrome is large and its complete extent has gradually been clarified. That was the origin of distinct denominations during the last century (dolichostenomelia, arachnodactyly [long fingers], etc.) and, almost certainly, of the inclusion in clinical series of patients who had different diseases. Genetic definition of the Marfan's entity allows a more precise identification of the cases, but is not a definite criterion for diagnosis. Actually, the better studied FBN1 mutations can lead to several conditions related to Marfan's syndrome, including myopia, mitral valve prolapse, aortic dilatation, and skin and skeletal anomalies (MASS), familial ectopia lentis, familial aortic aneurysms and dissections, familial Marfan-like habitus, and so forth. So, Marfan's syndrome diagnosis remains based on a careful clinical assessment of patients (American Academy of Pediatrics Committee on Genetics, 1996). A methodical exploration of the organic departments and the hierarchic organization of the findings in *major* and *minor* criteria were proposed and are currently adopted.

Skeletal system

The skeletal peculiarities, particularly the long and thin extremities, were first recognized by Marfan and were the core of his original description. An excessive length of the long bones, usually (but not always) resulting in tall stature, is one the most striking features of the Marfan's patient. Pectus carinatum and pectus excavatum, the consequence of an excessive growth of ribs, are other *major* signals. Pes planus, arachnodactyly, scoliosis, and other vertebral deformities, are very often present. Joint laxity is common.

Ocular system

The eye abnormalities were described by Boerger only two decades after the Marfan communication. Ectopia lentis, provoked by the lassitude or rupture of the suspensory ligaments of the lens, is one of the cardinal manifestations of the syndrome, present in nearly half of the cases and the single *major* ocular criterion. Increased axial length of the globe with myopia and a tendency to detachment of the retina are also common.

Uncommon Causes of Stroke, 2nd edition, ed. Louis R. Caplan. Published by Cambridge University Press. © Cambridge University Press 2008.

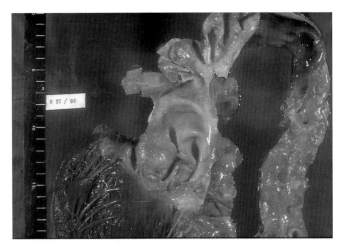

Figure 20.1 Aorta rupture and dissection in a Marfan's patient.

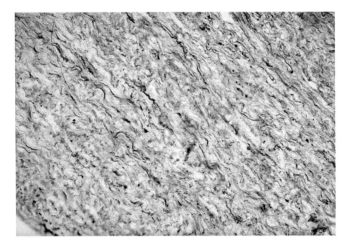

Figure 20.2 Shortened and thickened elastic fibers (elastin and Alcian Blue 200 × 2.5).

Cardiovascular system

Cardiovascular abnormalities, the other *major* component of Marfan's syndrome, are the cause of the most damaging or even fatal complications of the disease. More than 90% of Marfan patients die from a cardiovascular complication. Surprisingly, these abnormalities were first described only in 1943, despite the fact that a dissecting aneurysm of the aorta was reported in association with a left recurrent laryngeal nerve palsy as early as 1909.

Dilatation of the ascending aorta with or without aortic regurgitation, and involving at least the sinuses of Valsalva or dissection of the ascending aorta, is the *major* criterion. Aortic root dilatation is present in 80% of cases (Hwa *et al.*, 1993). The first identifiable enlargement can be seen as early as 10 years of age or as late as the sixth decade. Aorta and large arteries are unusually wide and fragile, even in very young patients, and can rapidly progress to aneurysms and aneurysm dissection. The main histologic abnormality affects the aortic media, which presents with a severe loss of elastic fibers in advanced forms (Figures 20.1 and 20.2).

Mitral valve prolapse affects two thirds of the patients, and mitral regurgitation and cardiac rhythm abnormalities are very often associated. Mitral valve lesions, as well as the more rare dilatation of the pulmonary artery and dilatation or dissection of the descending aorta, are *minor* criteria of the disease.

Other findings

Lumbosacral dural ectasia is present in 60% of the patients having back pain, and is a *major* criterion when confirmed by CT or MRI. Emphysema and pneumothoraces, related to the fragility of support tissues, are common. Also frequent are recurrent hernias, striae atrophicae, and other skin signs. All the pulmonary and skin manifestations are considered *minor* criteria. Other *major* criteria are a positive family and genetic history.

The final diagnosis of Marfan's syndrome requires a minimal cluster of the signals mentioned. In the absence of family history, final diagnosis requires the presence of *major* criteria in two organ systems and involvement of a third organ system. No cerebrovascular manifestation is considered to contribute to the diagnosis. Nevertheless, the occurrence of a cerebrovascular event during the natural course of Marfans syndrome is possible. Secondary placement of neurological manifestations relates to their lower frequency, because the most dramatic consequences of cardiovascular anomalies are not expressed primarily by neurological syndromes.

The cerebral complications of Marfan's syndrome

An estimate of the risk of developing a cerebrovascular event in Marfan's syndrome is entirely elusive, both in general and for a particular patient. Severity of the vascular malformations differs from patient to patient and, in the worst cases, the chance of a disastrous event is largely related to other than neurological causes. Two main causes underlie the neurological complications of Marfan's syndrome.

Dissection of the ascending aorta, and the carotid and vertebral arteries

The first reference to a neurological complication in a Marfan's patient was in 1909 and consisted of a recurrent laryngeal paralysis. It was not a stroke or other vascular occurrence, but its cause was a dissecting aneurysm of the aorta. Since then, most references to cerebrovascular events relate to the presence of an arterial malformation: dilatation, aneurysm, or dissection, extending from the aorta (Schievink *et al.*, 1994b) or occurring independently in the internal carotid (Schievink *et al.*, 1994a) or vertebral arteries (Youl *et al.*, 1990).

Embolic mechanisms

Valvular dysfunction and disturbances of cardiac rhythm can produce embolic strokes basically no different from any other embolic stroke. Intracerebral aneurysms and aneurysmal rupture have for a long time been considered frequent complications of Marfan's syndrome. The controversy has not been resolved but has come closer to a conclusion: there is an excess of aneurysms in Marfan's syndrome (Schievink *et al.*, 1997) but not an excess of subarachnoid hemorrhages (van den Berg *et al.*, 1996).

Other neurological complications of Marfan's syndrome

Other neurological complications have been described in Marfan's syndrome. Particular attention must be given to spinal defects, particularly at the craniospinal junction. As many as 54% of patients with Marfan's syndrome have increased atlantoaxial translation, and a radiographic prevalence of 36% for basilar impression was described in the same population (Hobbs *et al.*, 1997). Distinct varieties of headaches (Fukutake *et al.*, 1997; Zambrino *et al.*, 1999) and other craniofacial manifestations (Nagatani *et al.*, 1998) have been related to spinal and vascular anomalies.

Diagnostic considerations

Despite the advances in the genetics of Marfan's syndrome, a simple diagnostic test does not exist. Diagnosis of Marfan's syndrome is difficult and remains based on clinical criteria (De Paepe *et al.*, 1996). Unfortunately, clinical appearance varies greatly among affected people, and, in the absence of familial history (15–20% of the cases) and congenital ectopia lentis (perhaps the most specific trait of the syndrome), considerable risk of misdiagnosis exists.

Homocystinuria is the main condition to be distinguished from Marfan's syndrome. Both diseases can present with skeletal deformities, eye defects, and vascular disease. However, patients with homocystinuria have a high frequency of mental retardation; homocystinuria is transmitted as a recessive trait and can be identified by specific tests.

Congenital contractural arachnodactyly, like Marfan's syndrome, is a dominant inherited disorder. The habitus is marfanoid, and cardiovascular defects, although somewhat different, may be also present. Ocular anomalies may be present (Huggon *et al.*, 1990) or not (Ramos Arroyo *et al.*, 1985) but, if present, are not as serious.

Prognosis and treatment

A complete physical examination, focusing on the systems affected by the disorder, is crucial for diagnosis, but equally is the most effective way to follow the progress of the malformations. In the absence of corrective treatment for the basic defect of Marfan's syndrome, the malformations tend to progress continuously, so the principal concerns in the management of these patients are the early identification of functional and structural defects and implementation of corrective measures. Some basic protective procedures and careful medical management that can greatly improve the prognosis and lengthen the life span, are listed below.

1. Lifestyle adaptations, such as the avoidance of strenuous exercise
2. Monitoring of the skeletal system, especially during childhood and adolescence
3. Annual echocardiogram to monitor the size and function of the heart and aorta
4. Regular ophthalmologic evaluation, including slit-lamp eye examination

Early manifestations are associated with the worst prognosis (Gray *et al.*, 1998). In particular, cardiac valvular defects present at birth bear a severe prognosis. Nevertheless, life expectancy was estimated to have increased from 37 to 61 years between 1972 and 1995, largely because of advances in medical and surgical treatment. Beta-blockers to reduce aortic stress, and cardiovascular surgery, are specifically directed to patients with aortic dilatation. There is some evidence that beta-blockers slow aortic root growth, decrease rates of cardiac events, and improve survival. An aortic diameter greater than 50–60 mm (or, in children, doubling its normal dimension) is critical and makes a decision on the surgical repair of the vessel urgent. Concerning when to perform elective surgery on Marfan's syndrome patients who have dilatation of their ascending aortas, a number of factors should be considered, including the diameter of the aortic root (Kim *et al.*, 2005).

The approach to valvular dysfunctions is basically analogous to that to similar conditions in non-Marfan patients, including reconstructive surgery and valvular replacement. Heart transplantation, with or without replacement of aortic and pulmonary vessels, is proposed in the neonatal period.

Anticoagulation is indicated for patients who have graft surgery. Antibiotics are recommended before dental or genitourinary treatment in patients who have mitral valve prolapse or artificial heart valves or in those who have had aortic surgery.

The future

The main defective component of connective tissue, the fibrilllin, and the functional and structural modifications with which it operates, have been investigated for the last decades. Some hundred mutations in the critical gene for fibrillin have been discovered. Other abnormalities in the structural or functional components of cells and organic systems have been identified and scrutinized. Prenatal diagnosis is now available for some families, at least for those families in which a mutation in the fibrillin gene has been shown. Experimental models have been delineated and are now available (Pereira *et al.*, 1997).

However, there are currently no prophylactic or curative medical treatments for the crucial Marfan's anomalies. The optimistic idea that the comprehension of genetic determinants of a disease would be the last step for a logical and easy treatment lacks confirmation in Marfan's syndrome, and we are probably far from the possibility of genetic intervention. This makes the managment of the disease largely based on early diagnosis of complications and correction, chemical or surgical, of the functional and structural defects.

Additional progress in understanding genetics and biochemical defects and in the elucidation of the ultimate mechanisms related to malformations in Marfan's syndrome are expected in the near future. Then, perspectives will be no different than usual: an easy and effective test for prenatal and presymptomatic diagnosis and a treatment effective in the prevention or eradication of the disease by acting on the genes responsible (Gott, 1998).

REFERENCES

American Academy of Pediatrics Committee on Genetics. 1996. Health supervision for children with Marfan syndrome. *Pediatrics*, **98**, 978–82.

De Paepe, A., Devereux, R. B., Dietz, H. C., Hennekam, R. C., and Pyeritz, R. E. 1996. Revised diagnostic criteria for the Marfan syndrome. *Am J Med Genet*, **62**, 417–26.

Fukutake, T., Sakakibara, R., Mori, M., Araki, M., and Hattori, T. 1997. Chronic intractable headache in a patient with Marfan's syndrome. *Headache*, **37**, 291–5.

Gott, V. L. 1998. Antoine Marfan and his syndrome: one hundred years later. *Md Med J*, **47**, 247–52.

Gray, J. R., Bridges, A. B., West, R. R., *et al.* 1998. Life expectancy in British Marfan syndrome populations. *Clin Genet*, **54**, 124–8.

Hobbs, W. R., Sponseller, P. D., Weiss, A. P., and Pyeritz, R. E. 1997. The cervical spine in Marfan syndrome. *Spine*, **22**, 983–9.

Hollister, D. W., Godfrey, M., Sakai, L. Y., and Pyeritz, R. E. 1990. Immunohistologic abnormalities of the microfibrillar-fiber system in the Marfan syndrome. *N Engl J Med*, **323**, 152–9.

Huggon, I. C., Burke, J. P., and Talbot, J. F. 1990. Contractural arachnodactyly with mitral regurgitation and iridodonesis. *Arch Dis Child*, **65**, 317–9.

Hwa, J., Richards, J. G., Huang, H., *et al.* 1993. The natural history of aortic dilatation in Marfan syndrome. *Med J Aust*, **158**, 558–62.

Kainulainen, K., Pulkkinen, L., Savolainen, A., Kaitila, I., and Peltonen, L. 1990. Location on chromosome 15 of the gene defect causing Marfan syndrome. *N Engl J Med*, **323**, 935–9.

Kainulainen, K., Steinmann, B., Collins, F., *et al.* 1991. Marfan syndrome: no evidence for heterogeneity in different populations, and more precise mapping of the gene. *Am J Hum Genet*, **49**, 662–7.

Kim, S. Y., Martin, N., Hsia, E., Pyeritz, R. E., and Albert, D. A. 2005. Management of aortic disease in Marfan Syndrome: a decision analysis. *Arch Intern Med*, **165**, 749–55.

Magenis, R. E., Maslen, C. L., Smith, L., Allen, L., and Sakai, L. Y. 1991. Localization of the fibrillin (FBN) gene to chromosome 15, band q21.1. *Genomics*, **11**, 346–51.

Mizuguchi, T., Collod-Beroud, G., Akyiama, T., *et al.* 2004. Heterozigous TGFBR2 mutations in Marfan syndrome. *Nat Genet*, **36**, 855–60.

Nagatani, T., Inao, S., and Yoshida, J. 1998. Hemifacial spasm associated with Marfan's syndrome: a case report. *Neurosurg Rev*, **21**, 152–4.

Pereira, L., Andrikopoulos, K., Tian, J., *et al.* 1997. Targetting of the gene encoding fibrillin-1 recapitulates the vascular aspect of Marfan syndrome. *Nat Genet*, **17**, 218–22.

Pyeritz, R. E. 2000. The Marfan syndrome. *Annu Rev Med*, **51**, 481–510.

Ramos Arroyo, M. A., Weaver, D. D., and Beals, R. K. 1985. Congenital contractural arachnodactyly. Report of four additional families and review of literature. *Clin Genet*, **27**, 570–81.

Schievink, W. I., Björnsson, J., and Piepgras, D. G. 1994a. Coexistence of fibromuscular dysplasia and cystic medial necrosis in a patient with Marfan's syndrome and bilateral carotid artery dissections. *Stroke*, **25**, 2492–6.

Schievink, W. I., Michels, V. V., and Piepgras, D. G. 1994b. Neurovascular manifestations of heritable connective tissue disorders. A review. *Stroke*, **25**, 889–903.

Schievink, W. I., Parisi, J. E., Piepgras, D. G., and Michels, V. V. 1997. Intracranial aneurysms in Marfan's syndrome: an autopsy study. *Neurosurgery*, **41**, 866–70.

The FBN1 mutations database. http://www.umd.be

van den Berg, J. S., Limburg, M., Hennekam, R. C. 1996. Is Marfan syndrome associated with symptomatic intracranial aneurysms? *Stroke*, **27**, 10–2.

Youl, B. D., Coutellier, A., Dubois, B., Leger, J. M., and Bousser, M. G. 1990. Three cases of spontaneous extracranial vertebral artery dissection. *Stroke*, **21**, 618–25.

Zambrino, C. A., Berardinelli, A., Martelli, A., Vercelli, P., Termine, C., and Lanzi, G. 1999. Dolicho-vertebrobasilar abnormality and migraine-like attacks. *Eur Neurol*, **41**, 10–4.

21 PSEUDOXANTHOMA ELASTICUM

Louis R. Caplan and Chin-Sang Chung

Introduction

Pseudoxanthoma elasticum (PXE) is an inherited connective tissue disorder, characterized predominantly by skin, eye, cardiac, and vascular abnormalities. Hypertension is common, and elevated blood pressure and vascular lesions often lead to strokes and damage to many body organs.

The skin manifestations were first described by the French dermatologist Rigal in 1881. Two Swedish physicians, Grönblad (an ophthalmologist) and Strandberg (a dermatologist), in 1929 recognized that the skin findings were accompanied by angioid streaks in the retina. PXE is often referred to as Grönblad-Strandberg disease after these two physicians.

Prevalence and inheritance

About 1 in 25 000–100 000 individuals have PXE (Laube and Moss, 2005; Neldner, 1993; Schievink *et al.*, 1994; Viljoen, 1993). There is an approximately 2:1 female preponderance (Laube and Moss, 2005). The genetics are complex: two autosomal recessive and two autosomal dominant forms have been described (Schievink *et al.*, 1994). Most patients probably have the autosomal recessive form (Neldner, 1993). Patients with the autosomal dominant form may develop more severe vascular disease.

The genetic defect has now been mapped to the ABCC6 gene on chromosome 16p13.1 (Bergen *et al.*, 2000; Laube and Moss, 2005; Ringpfeil *et al.*, 2000). The ABCC6 gene encodes multidrug resistance associated protein 6 that belongs to the ABC (ATP binding cassette) transmembrane transporter family of proteins (Laube and Moss, 2005). Genetic studies have identified about 60 mutations as well as large deletions in the gene (Laube and Moss, 2005). The biological effect of this genetic defect is still not known. Curiously, patients with B-thalassemia seem to have an unexpectedly high frequency of PXE (Aessopos *et al.*, 1989, 1997).

Clinical findings and organ involvement

Skin

The characteristic skin lesions are linear, round, or oval yellow-orange elevated skin lesions that resemble xanthomas (Viljoen, 1993). The flexor surfaces are most often involved. The face, neck, axilla, and the antecubital, inguinal, and periumbilical regions contain the most frequent skin lesions (Neldner, 1988, 1993; Strole

and Margolis, 1983). The skin in affected regions can become thickened and grooved resembling course-grained leather. Later the skin becomes lax and redundant (Lebwohl, 1993). Figure 21.1 shows an example of very abnormal redundant lax skin within the upper arm of a patient with PXE (Mayer *et al.*, 1994).

The lips show similar lesions. The mucosa of the palate, buccal region, vagina, and rectum may also show typical xanthomas. In some patients the skin abnormalities are very subtle, and abnormalities can only be definitively shown by biopsy (Lebwohl *et al.*, 1993). The same process that affects mucocutaneous surfaces can also affect other regions that contain elastic fibers. Endoscopy sometimes shows similar lesions in the gastric mucosa and within the gastrointestinal tract (Strole and Margolis, 1983); the process also may involve the endocardium and the heart valves (Lebwohl *et al.*, 1982).

The skin and mucosal abnormality consists of very abnormal elastic tissue. Biopsy early in the course of illness shows irregularity, fragmentation, and clumping of elastic fibers in the skin. Calcification of the abnormal mucocutaneous regions develops later. Penicillamine treatment can produce skin abnormalities

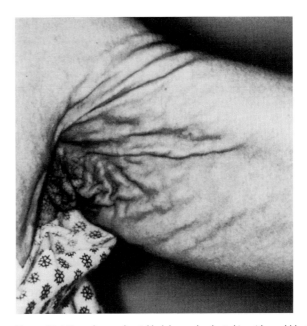

Figure 21.1 Very abnormal wrinkled, lax, redundant skin with a cobblestone appearance in the upper arm of a patient with PXE. (From Mayer *et al.*, 1994 with permission.)

Uncommon Causes of Stroke, 2nd edition, ed. Louis R. Caplan. Published by Cambridge University Press. © Cambridge University Press 2008.

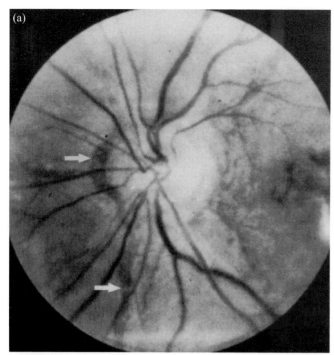

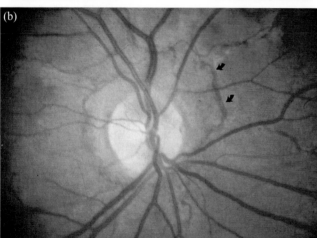

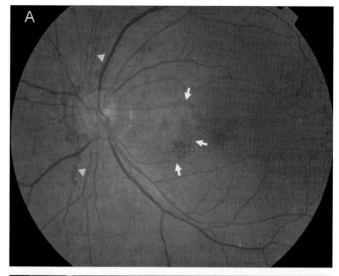

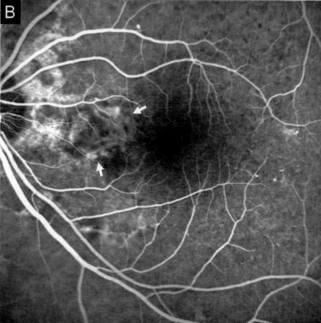

Figure 21.2 Fundus photographs of angioid streaks in patients with PXE. (**a**) Large angioid streak (*white arrows*) in the patient whose skin is shown in Figure 21.1. A macular scar is also present. (From Mayer *et al.*, 1994 with permission.) (**b**) Large tortuous angioid streak (*curved black arrows*) in a patient with PXE.

Figure 21.3 Funduscopic (**a**) and fluorescein angiographic (**b**) findings of a patient with PXE. Angioid streaks (*arrow heads*, **a**) radiating from the optic disk and mottling of the temporal retina are conspicuous. Angioid streak represents the rupture of Bruch's membrane. Notice the development of choroidal neovascular membrane (*arrows*, **a** and **b**) secondary to angioid streak. See color plate. (Image courtesy of Professor Se Woong Kang, MD, Sungkyunkwan University School of Medicine, Seoul, Korea.)

indistinguishable from those found in PXE (Bolognia and Braverman, 1992).

Eye

The most characteristic and diagnostic feature of PXE is the angioid streaks found in the retina. The streaks are red-brown or gray, are usually wider than veins, and radiate from the optic disc (Strole and Margolis, 1983). The retinal streaks are thought to be the result of cracks or ruptures in Bruch's membrane, which has been weakened by disruption of elastic fibers. Figure 21.2 shows two examples of angioid streaks. Figure 21.3 shows a fundus photograph

after a fluorescein angiogram that shows the cracking well. The angioid streaks radiate outward from the disc like spokes on a tire. Autofluorescence photography of the fundus shows the angioid streaks quite well (Sawa *et al.*, 2006).

Another fundoscopic finding seen in some patients with PXE is a speckled, yellowish mottling of the posterior pole of the retina temporal to the macula. This appearance has been dubbed "peau d'orange" because it resembles the skin of an orange. This finding is attributed to changes in the retinal pigmented epithelium overlying a calcified and degenerating Bruch's membrane. This finding may be present even before the appearance of angioid streaks (Gomolin, 1992).

Chorioretinal scarring, hemorrhages, pigmentary deposits, and macular degeneration also occur, and many patients with PXE have diminished visual acuity. PXE may also cause infarction of the optic nerve related to abnormalities in its posterior ciliary artery blood supply (Murthy and Prasad, 2004). About 85% of patients with PXE have angioid streaks (Pessin and Chung, 1995).

Angioid streaks also occur in other conditions. Patients with sickle cell anemia and Paget's disease of bone often have angioid streaks when ophthalmoscopy is thoroughly performed (Clarkson and Altman, 1982; Lebwohl et al., 1993; Neldner, 1988). Angioid streaks have occasionally been described in patients with hyperphosphatemia, Ehlers-Danlos syndrome, lead poisoning, trauma, idiopathic thrombocytopenic purpura, and pituitary diseases (Lebwohl et al., 1993).

Heart

Cardiac abnormalities are common and may dominate the clinical presentation. Cardiac manifestations relate to premature coronary artery disease and to endocardial abnormalities. Coronary artery disease with resulting angina pectoris, myocardial infarction, and sudden death are common and may occur at quite a young age (Lebwohl et al., 1993). Some patients have an ischemic cardiomyopathy. Histological examination of coronary artery specimens in patients with PXE shows loss of elastic tissue, fragmentation of the internal elastic membrane, and calcifications between the intima and media (Wiemer et al., 2003).

Abnormalities in the elastic tissue of the endocardium can produce dramatic cardiac findings. Huang et al. (1967) described thickened mitral valves, mitral annular calcification, and mitral stenosis in patients with PXE. The abnormal mitral valve can show fragmentation, coiling, and disruption of collagen bundles (Davies et al., 1978). Lebwohl et al. (1982) reported a high frequency of mitral valve prolapse in patients with PXE who had echocardiography.

The elastic tissue abnormalities also can cause dramatic calcification of the endocardium and a restrictive cardiomyopathy (Navarro-Lopez et al., 1980; Rosenzweig et al., 1993). Echocardiography may show diastolic dysfunction in patients with PXE (Nguyen et al., 2006). Rosenzweig et al. (1993) described a woman with PXE who had extensive mitral annulus calcification. The calcification extended from the mitral valve into the left ventricular endocardium. The entire left atrium was encircled with calcific endocardial plaques. A 5-mm mobile calcific lesion was attached to the junction of the left atrial appendage and the left atrium (Rosenzweig et al., 1993).

Gastrointestinal tract

Gastrointestinal hemorrhages are quite common in patients with PXE (Laube and Moss, 2005), and are often the presenting symptom. Superficial mucosal and intestinal erosions and a diffuse gastritis are the result of vascular lesions. Gastroscopic examination may show yellow cobblestone-like changes in the gastric mucosa. Examination of gastric tissue removed at surgery and autopsy show mucosal and submucosal capillaries, and veins may be dilated. Small and medium-sized arteries show degenerative abnormalities that predominantly involve the internal elastic lamina (Kaplan and Hartman, 1954; Strole and Margolis, 1983). Angiography of abdominal arteries may show tortuosity with narrowing and occlusions. Microaneurysms and angiomatous malformations also occur (Strole and Margolis, 1983). Abdominal angina and ischemic bowel disease occasionally develop.

Aorta and peripheral blood vessels

The aorta may be involved and show aneurysmal dilatation. Peripheral limb arteries are often calcified. Intermittent claudication is common. Extremity arteries may become firm on palpation, and plain x-rays may show calcification. Hypertension is also very common in patients with PXE and often contributes to the cardiac and cerebrovascular pathology.

Cerebrovascular disease

Premature occlusive cervicocranial disease and aneurysmal subarachnoid hemorrhage are the two cerebrovascular problems directly attributable to PXE. The carotid arteries are thicker and more elastic in patients with PXE than in controls as judged by ultrasound analysis (Kornet et al., 2004). Intimal-medial thickness is increased, as are distensibility and compliance. These abnormalities are posited to be related to fragmentation of elastic fibers and accumulation of proteoglycans in the vessel wall (Kornet et al., 2004).

Rios-Montenegro et al. (1972) described a patient with PXE who had a moyamoya-like syndrome of bilateral, internal carotid artery occlusion at the skull base associated with a "rete-mirabile" of abnormal small vessels. Their patient also had a carotid-cavernous fistula. Koo and Newton (1972) also reported a patient with PXE and a carotid 'rete mirabile.' Internal carotid artery and basilar artery occlusive disease has also been reported (Goto, 1975; Iqbal et al., 1978; Sharma et al., 1974; Tay, 1970). The occlusive lesions can be extracranial or intracranial (Schievink et al., 1994). Brain ischemic symptoms most often develop in the fifth or sixth decade of life, but occasional patients develop cervicocranial occlusive disease in their twenties. Some patients with PXE show tortuosity and ectasia of the neck arteries on angiography (Schievink et al., 1994).

Some patients with PXE show the common complications of hypertension – intracerebral hemorrhages, multiple lacunar infarcts, and microvascular disease of the Binswanger type (Mayer et al., 1994). Cerrato et al. (2005) described a patient with multiple white matter lesions of the Binswanger type who had no recognized neurological symptoms or signs.

Mayer et al. (1994) reported two women with PXE who had multiple strokes and extensive white matter abnormalities on MRI. Both of these patients had longstanding hypertension. Pavlovic et al. (2005) reported three patients with lacunes and extensive white matter abnormalities; two of the three had slight hypertension. I have cared for a patient with angioid retinal streaks, blindness, pseudobulbar palsy, gait abnormalities, dementia, and Binswanger-like abnormalities on MRI who had PXE and hypertension. Hypertension is common in patients with PXE. It is difficult in patients with Binswanger-like abnormalities, PXE, and hypertension to know how much of the abnormalities, if any, relate directly to PXE and how much are attributable to the hypertension.

Aneurysm formation and subarachnoid hemorrhage (SAH) have also been reported in patients with PXE. Some of the aneurysms are located within the cavernous sinus, and patients have presented with cranial nerve palsies rather than SAH. Kito *et al.* (1983) reported a 37-year-old woman with PXE who ruptured an aneurysm that arose from the thoracic portion of the anterior spinal artery.

Dissections have occasionally also been reported in patients with PXE, but it is not certain if the association is a chance one. The frequency of dissection in patients with PXE does not approach that known for Ehlers-Danlos syndrome and Marfan's syndrome. Josien (1992) described a 17-year-old boy who had PXE and a cervical vertebral artery dissection. One patient of Mokri *et al.* (1979), with a spontaneous cervical, internal carotid artery dissection, had an angioid retinal streak.

REFERENCES

Aessopos, A., Farmakis, D., Karagiorga, M., Rombos, I. and Loucopoulos, D. 1997. Pseudoxanthoma elasticum lesions and cardiac complications as contributing factors for strokes in B-thalassemia patients. *Stroke*, **28**, 2421–4.

Aessopos, A., Stamatelos, G., Savvides, P., *et al.* 1989. Angioid streaks in homozygous B thalassemia. *Am J Ophthalmol*, **108**, 356–9.

Bergen, A. A., Plomp, A. S., Schuurman, E. J., *et al.* 2000. Mutations in ABCC6 cause pseudoxanthoma elasticum. *Nat Genet*, **25**, 228–31.

Bolognia, J. L., and Braverman, I. 1992. Pseudoxanthoma-elasticum-like skin changes induced by penicillamine. *Dermatology*, **184**, 12–8.

Cerrato, P., Giraudo, M., Baima, C., *et al.* 2005. Asymptomatic white matter ischemic lesions in a patient with pseudoxanthoma elasticum. *J Neurol*, **252**, 848–9.

Clarkson, J. G., and Altman, R. D. 1982. Angioid streaks. *Surv Ophthalmol*, **26**, 235–46.

Davies, M. J., Moore, B. P., and Brainbridge, M. V. 1978. The floppy mitral valve: study of incidence, pathology, and complications in surgical, necropsy, and forensic material. *Br Heart J*, **40**, 468–81.

Gomolin, J. E. 1992. Development of angioid streaks in association with pseudoxanthoma elasticum. *Can J Ophthalmol*, **27**, 30–1

Goto, K. 1975. Involvement of central nervous system in pseudoxanthoma elasticum. *Folia Psychiatr Neurol Jpn*, **29**, 263–77.

Grönblad, E. 1929. Angioid streaks: pseudoxanthoma elasticum. *Acta Opthalmol*, **7**, 329–33.

Huang, S., Kumar, G., Steele, H. D., and Parker, J. O. 1967. Cardiac involvement in pseudoxanthoma elasticum: report of a case. *Am Heart J*, **74**, 680–6.

Iqbal, A., Alter, M., and Lee, S. H. 1978. Pseudoxanthoma elasticum: a review of neurological complication. *Ann Neurol*, **4**, 18–20.

Josien, E. 1992. Extracranial vertebral artery dissection: nine cases. *J Neurol*, **239**, 327–30

Kaplan, L., and Hartman, S. W. 1954. Elastica disease: case of Gronblad-Strandberg syndrome with gastrointestinal hemorrhage. *Arch Intern Med*, **94**, 489–92.

Kito, K., Kobayashi, N., Mori, N., and Kohno, H. 1983. Ruptured aneurysm of the anterior spinal artery associated with pseudoxanthoma elasticum: case report. *J Neurosurg*, **58**, 126–8.

Koo, A. H., Newton, T. H. 1972. Pseudoxanthoma elasticum associated with carotid rete mirabile: a case report. *AJR Am J Roentgenol*, **116**, 16–22.

Kornet, L., Bergen, A. A., Hoeks, A. P., *et al.* 2004. In patients with pseudoxanthoma elasticum a thicker and more elastic carotid artery is associated with elastin fragmentation and proteoglycan accumulation. *Ultrasound Med Biol*, **30**, 1041–8.

Lebwohl, M. 1993. Pseudoxanthoma elasticum. *N Engl J Med*, **329**, 1240.

Laube, S., and Moss, C. 2005. Pseudoxanthoma elasticum. *Arch Dis Child*, **90**, 754–6.

Lebwohl, M., Halperin, J., and Phelps, R. G. 1993. Brief report: occult pseudoxanthoma elasticum in patients with premature cardiovascular disease. *N Engl J Med*, **329**, 1237–9.

Lebwohl, M. G., Distefano, D., Prioleau, P. G., Uram, M., Yannuzzi, L. A., and Fleischmajer, R. 1982. Pseudoxanthoma elasticum and mitral-valve prolapse. *N Engl J Med*, **307**, 228–31.

Mayer, S., Tatemichi, T. K., Spitz, J., *et al.* 1994. Recurrent ischemic events and diffuse white matter disease in patients with pseudoxanthoma elasticum. *Cerebrovasc Dis*, **4**, 294–7.

Mokri, B., Sundt, T. M. Jr., and Houser, O. W. 1979. Spontaneous internal carotid artery dissection, hemicrania, and Horner's syndrome. *Arch Neurol*, **36**, 677–80.

Murthy, S., and Prasad, S. 2004. Pseudoxanthoma elasticum and nonarteritic anterior ischaemic optic neuropathy. *Eye*, **18**, 201–2.

Navarro-Lopez, F., Liorian, A., Ferrer-Roca, O., Betriu, A., and Sans, G. 1980. Restrictive cardiomyopathy in pseudoxanthoma elasticum. *Chest*, **78**, 113–15.

Neldner, K. H. 1988. Pseudoxanthoma elasticum. *Clin Dermatol*, **6**, 1–159.

Neldner, K. H. 1993. Pseudoxanthoma elasticum. In *Connective Tissue and its Heritable Disorders: Molecular, Genetic, and Medical Aspects*, ed. P. M. Royce and B. Steinman. New York: Wiley-Liss, pp. 425–36.

Nguyen, L. D., Terbah, M., Daudon, P., and Martin, L. 2006. Left ventricular systolic and diastolic function by echocardiogram in pseudoxanthoma elasticum. *Am J Cardiol*, **97**, 1535–7.

Pavlovic, A. M., Zidverc-Trajkovic, J., Milovic, M. M., *et al.* 2005. Cerebral small vessel disease in pseudoxanthoma elasticum: three cases. *Can J Neurol Sci*, **32**, 115–8.

Pessin, M. S., and Chung, C. S. 1995. Eales's disease and Gronenblad-Strandberg disease (pseudoxanthoma elasticum). In *Stroke Syndromes*, 1st edn, eds. J. Bogousslavsky and L. R. Caplan. Cambridge, UK: Cambridge University Press, pp. 443–7.

Rigal, D. 1881. Observation pour servir a l'histoire de la cheloide diffuse xanthelasmique. *Arch Derm Syphilol*, **2**, 491–501.

Ringpfeil, F., Lebwohl, M. G., Christiano, A. M., *et al.* 2000. Pseudoxanthoma elasticum mutations in the gene encoding a transmembrane ATP binding cassette (ABC) transporter. *Proc Natl Acad Sci U S A*, **97**, 6001–6.

Rios-Montenegro, E. N., Behrens, M. M., and Hoyt, W. F. 1972. Pseudoxanthoma elasticum. Association with bilateral carotid rete mirabile and unilateral carotid-cavernous sinus fistula. *Arch Neurol*, **26**, 151–5.

Rosenzweig, B. P., Guarneri, E., and Kronzon, I. 1993. Echocardiographic manifestations in a patient with pseudoxanthoma elasticum. *Ann Intern Med*, **119**, 487–90.

Sawa, M., Ober, M. D., Freund, K. B., and Spaide, R. F. 2006. Fundus autofluorescence in patients with pseudoxanthoma elasticum. *Opthalmology*, **113**, 820.e1–2.

Schievink, W. I., Michels, V. V., and Piepgras, D. G. 1994. Neurovascular manifestations of heritable connective tissue disorders: a review. *Stroke*, **25**, 889–903.

Sharma, N. G. K., Beohar, P. C., Ghosh, S. K., and Gupta, P. S. 1974. Subarachnoid hemorrhage in pseudoxanthoma elasticum. *Postgrad Med J*, **50**, 774–6.

Strandberg, J. V. 1929. Pseudoxanthoma elasticum. *Zentralbl Haut Und Geschlechtskr*, **31**, 689–93.

Strole, W. E., and Margolis, R. 1983. Case records of the Massachusetts General Hospital: case 10–1983. *N Engl J Med*, **308**, 579–85.

Tay, C. H. 1970. Pseudoxanthoma elasticum. *Postgrad Med J*, **46**, 97–108.

Viljoen, D. 1993. Pseudoxanthoma elasticum. In *McKusick's Heritable Disorders of Connective Tissue*, 5th edn, ed. P. Beighton. St. Louis, MO: Mosby Co., pp. 335–365.

Wiemer, M., Muller, W., Heintzen, M., and Horstkotte, D. 2003. Pseudoxanthoma elasticum. Coronary vascular specimen from atherectomy. *Circulation*, **108**, e19–20.

22 EHLERS-DANLOS SYNDROME

E. Steve Roach

The Ehlers-Danlos syndromes (EDS) are a group of connective tissue diseases classically characterized by fragile or hyperelastic skin, hyperextensible joints, vascular lesions, and easy bruising and excessive scarring after an injury (Beighton, 1993). Based on the clinical manifestations, inheritance pattern, and (in some cases) specific collagen defects, there are at least 10 subtypes of EDS (Byers, 1994). Exact categorization is not always possible because of overlapping clinical features and because there is substantial phenotypic variability even among patients with the same subtype (Byers *et al.*, 1979). More than 80% of EDS patients have types I, II, or III. Most individuals with cerebrovascular complications, however, have type IV EDS, which occurs in 1 in 50 000–500 000 individuals (Byers, 1995).

All confirmed cases of type IV EDS have shown autosomal dominance (Beighton, 1993; Germain and Herrera-Guzman, 2004). Earlier reports of autosomal recessive transmission may be due to parental mosaicism (Byers, 1994). Affected patients have abnormal production of type III procollagen, which is the major collagen type in blood vessels, bowel, and uterus (Germain and Herrera-Guzman, 2004; Gilchrist *et al.*, 1999; North *et al.*, 1995). Numerous mutations of the COL3A1 gene on chromosome 2, including point mutations, exon skipping mutations, and multi-exon deletions, have been described. All result in abnormal type III procollagen that causes tissue to be thin and friable (Byers, 1994; Cikrit *et al.*, 2002; Pepin *et al.*, 2000). Characteristic facial features and/or easy bruising are described in some individuals (Schievink, 1997), but neither hyperelastic skin (Figure 22.1) nor hyperextensible joints are prominent features of type IV EDS, and diagnosis is often delayed in these patients until major vascular complications occur.

Intracranial aneurysm, carotid-cavernous fistula, and arterial dissection result from EDS type IV, and the likelihood of these complications increases steadily with increasing age. (Oderich *et al.*, 2005). Summarizing 220 individuals with EDS type IV, Pepin *et al.* (2000) noted that 25% of the patients developed one or more vascular complications by age 25 years and that 80% had a vascular complication by age 40 years. This complication rate was higher than that reported by North *et al.* (1995), who identified 20 cerebrovascular complications in 19 of 202 individuals with type IV EDS from 121 families in which the diagnosis was confirmed by molecular or biochemical studies. Outside the central nervous system, spontaneous hemorrhage, aneurysms, arterial dissection, bowel perforation, and uterine rupture are major causes of morbidity and mortality in patients with type IV EDS (Bergqvist, 1996; Freeman *et al.*, 1996; Peaceman and Cruikshank, 1987).

The diagnosis depends on recognition of the typical clinical findings and, for type IV, demonstration of defective synthesis of type III collagen. A family history of sudden unexplained death (especially during childbirth) or of spontaneous hemorrhage, major hemorrhage from relatively minor trauma, hemorrhagic complications during surgery, or bowel rupture may be important clues to the diagnosis in individuals with subtle findings.

Aneurysms

Rubinstein and Cohen (1964) first reported the occurrence of intracranial aneurysms due to EDS in a 47-year-old woman with aneurysms of both the internal carotid and vertebral arteries. Numerous patients with extracranial and intracranial aneurysms have since been reported, including several individuals with multiple intracranial aneurysms (Krog *et al.*, 1983; Mirza *et al.*, 1979; North *et al.*, 1995; Schievink *et al.*, 1990). The internal carotid artery is the most likely site of aneurysm formation, typically in the cavernous sinus or just as it emerges from the sinus (Figures 22.2 and 22.3). Aneurysms occur in most of the other intracranial arteries as well (Imahori *et al.*, 1969). Rupture of an intracavernous carotid aneurysm to create a carotid-cavernous fistula or rupture with subarachnoid hemorrhage is the most common presentation. Rupture of the aneurysm can occur spontaneously or during vigorous activity (McKusick, 1972; North *et al.*, 1995; Rubinstein and Cohen, 1964; Schievink *et al.*, 1990).

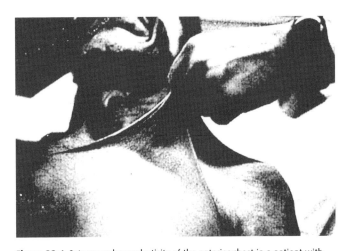

Figure 22.1 Cutaneous hyperelasticity of the anterior chest in a patient with EDS. Reproduced from Roach (1989) with permission.

Uncommon Causes of Stroke, 2nd edition, ed. Louis R. Caplan. Published by Cambridge University Press.   © Cambridge University Press 2008.

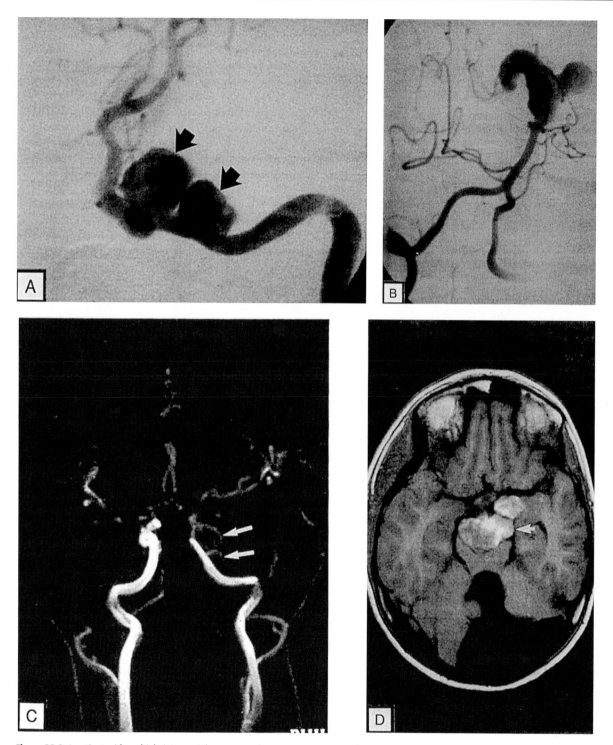

Figure 22.2 A patient with multiple intracranial aneurysms due to type IV EDS. **A.** Left internal carotid angiogram shows two adjacent aneurysms (*arrows*). **B.** Right vertebral angiogram demonstrates another large fusiform aneurysm with saccular component at the tip of the basilar artery. **C.** Magnetic resonance angiogram, frontal projection, reveals two aneurysms (*arrows*) of the left internal carotid artery. **D.** The T1-weighted magnetic resonance scan with gadolinium showed the vertebral artery aneurysm (*arrows*) plus incidental cerebellar hypoplasia.

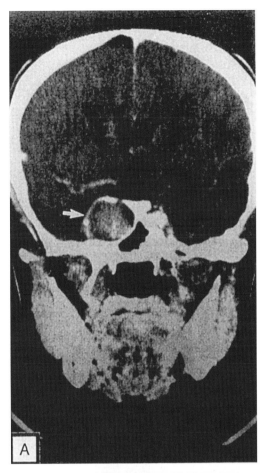

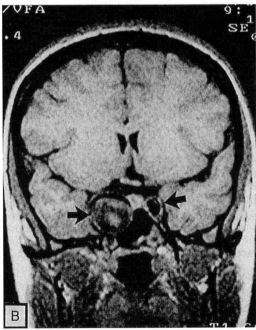

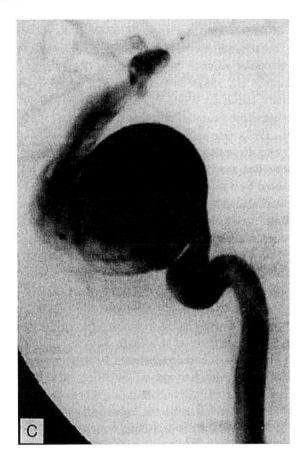

Figure 22.3 (*cont.*)

Figure 22.3 An 18-year-old with a family history of EDS type IV presented with headache. **A.** Coronal CT with contrast reveals a giant aneurysm (*arrow*) of the right intracavernous carotid artery. **B.** Coronal T1-weighted magnetic resonance scan shows bilateral intracavernous carotid aneurysms (*arrows*). **C.** Right internal carotid angiogram shows the giant aneurysm of the intracavernous carotid artery.

Although aneurysms are common in individuals with EDS type IV, relatively few patients with intracranial aneurysms have hereditary connective tissue disorders (Grond-Ginsbach *et al.*, 2002). Mutations of the COL3A1 gene are rare in unselected patients with cerebral aneurysms (Hamano *et al.*, 1998; Kuivaniemi *et al.*, 1993). Aneurysms occasionally occur in people with EDS type I (Krog *et al.*, 1983) or with Marfan's syndrome (Hainsworth and Mendelow, 1991; Stehbens *et al.*, 1989). Giant aneurysms have been reported in Marfan patients (Finney *et al.*, 1976; Hainsworth and Mendelow, 1991; Matsuda *et al.*, 1979), and, as with EDS type IV, these lesions tend to affect the intracranial portion of the internal carotid artery. Occasional reports of berry aneurysms in Marfan patients (Stehbens *et al.*, 1989) could be coincidental.

Carotid-Cavernous Fistulas

Graf (1965) described two EDS patients with a spontaneous carotid-cavernous fistula, and numerous patients have subsequently been reported (Chuman *et al.*, 2002; Debrun *et al.*, 1996; Pollock *et al.*, 1997; Schievink *et al.*, 1991; Zimmerman *et al.*, 1994). Symptoms sometimes develop after minor head trauma (Krog *et al.*, 1983), but most occur spontaneously. The patient may report periorbital swelling, blurred or double vision, pain, and pulsatile tinnitus. Clinical findings include proptosis, chemosis, abnormal ocular motility, tortuous episcleral vessels (from arterialized blood flow), elevated intraocular pressure, and retinal venous engorgement. Vision may be lost if the fistula is not treated.

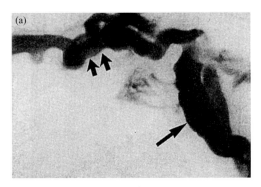

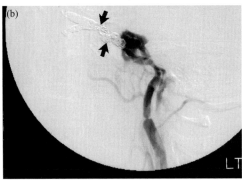

Figure 22.4 A 28-year-old woman with EDS type IV. **A**. Her left internal carotid angiogram revealed a carotid-cavernous fistula and an enlarged, tortuous internal carotid artery (*single arrow*). The superior orbital vein (*double arrows*) is markedly dilated. **B**. The fistula has been occluded with platinum coils.

Most carotid-cavernous fistulae in EDS patients result from rupture of an internal carotid artery aneurysm within the cavernous sinus (direct fistula) (Fox *et al.*, 1988; Graf, 1965; Schievink *et al.*, 1991). Schoolman and Kepes (1967) describe bilateral carotid-cavernous fistulae in a 39-year-old woman with EDS. At autopsy she had fragmentation of the internal elastic membrane and fibrosis of portions of the carotid wall. Similar fragmentation of the internal elastic membrane was recorded by Krog and colleagues (1983) along with several arteries with microscopic ruptures between the media and adventitia.

The fistula is most reliably demonstrated by catheter angiography (Figure 22.4). However, the vascular fragility of type IV EDS makes both standard angiography and intravascular occlusion of the fistula difficult (Beighton and Thomas, 1969). Driscoll and colleagues (1984) reported the perforation of the superior vena cava during intravenous digital angiography, and other patients have developed localized hematomas or cutaneous tears at the site of catheter insertion. Complications of diagnostic angiography may be as high as 67%, and 6–17% of patients die from the procedure (Cikrit *et al.*, 1987; Freeman *et al.*, 1996; Schievink *et al.*, 1991). Consequently, Magnetic resonance angiography or computed tomographic angiography are generally preferable to catheter angiography for initial diagnosis.

Endovascular embolization (Figure 22.4) is the procedure of choice for treating carotid-cavernous fistulae, and this procedure has also been successful in some EDS patients (Desal *et al.*, 2005; Forlodou *et al.*, 1996; Halbach *et al.*, 1990; Kanner *et al.*, 2000; Schievink *et al.*, 1991; Zimmerman *et al.*, 1994). Others have reported death as a direct complication of the embolization procedure or occurring in the days to months following a successful procedure, due to complications of the disease (Halbach *et al.*, 1990; Horowitz *et al.*, 2000; Pollock *et al.*, 1997; Schievink *et al.*, 1991). Although vascular complications are common in individuals with EDS type IV who undergo angiography or surgery, these procedures can be done successfully (Mirza *et al.*, 1979; Oderich *et al.*, 2005). In some individuals, transvenous access to occlude the cavernous sinus and superior ophthalmic vein may be safer than transarterial balloon occlusion (Zimmerman *et al.*, 1994). Still others may require "trapping" of the fistula by occlusion of the carotid artery proximal and distal to the fistula.

Arterial Dissections

It is not surprising that EDS patients develop arterial dissections. Surgeons have likened the tissue of these patients to wet blotting paper (Schievink *et al.*, 1990). During surgery, the arteries fail to hold sutures, and handling the tissue leads to tears of the artery or separation of the arterial layers (Sheiner *et al.*, 1985). Dissection has been documented in most of the intracranial and extracranial arteries, and the clinical presentation depends primarily on which artery is affected. Carotid dissection may cause ipsilateral oculosympathetic paresis and headache. One patient with a vertebral artery dissection developed a painful, pulsatile mass in the neck (Edwards and Taylor, 1969). Dissection of an intrathoracic artery can secondarily occlude cervical vessels (Hunter *et al.*, 1982), and cerebral infarction distal to a carotid dissection has been reported (Pope *et al.*, 1988).

Carotid dissection and rupture within the cavernous sinus leads to a carotid-cavernous fistula in some patients. One of Graf's (1965) patients had a very tortuous, dilated, internal carotid artery ipsilateral to the carotid-cavernous fistula. Several years later, at autopsy, she had multiple arterial aneurysms but no evidence of an intracavernous carotid aneurysm (Imahori *et al.*, 1969). Another patient with a carotid-cavernous fistula died from a dissection of the abdominal aorta; an autopsy revealed multiple smaller dissections in the abdomen, but the carotid-cavernous fistula was clearly caused by a true aneurysm with an interruption of the internal elastic lamina (Lach *et al.*, 1987). Dissection of intra-abdominal, pelvic, intrathoracic, cervical, and intracranial carotid arteries often follows diagnostic or therapeutic angiography and is a major cause of morbidity and mortality with these procedures.

Segmental narrowing of the lumen is the classic angiographic sign of arterial dissection (Schievink *et al.*, 1990), but subtle narrowing may be difficult to demonstrate in patients with tortuous vessels (Graf, 1965). Distinguishing an arterial dissection from a true aneurysm can be difficult (Edwards and Taylor, 1969). Because of the risk of angiography in EDS patients, the need for an arteriogram must be weighed carefully. Magnetic resonance angiography may be less accurate but is undoubtedly safer.

Despite justifiable concern about the risk of arterial manipulation and angiography in these patients, balloon occlusion has been successful in some patients (Fox *et al.*, 1988; Kashiwagi *et al.*, 1993). Surgery is also difficult because the arteries are friable and difficult to suture (Edwards and Taylor, 1969; Krog *et al.*, 1983).

Summary

Patients with EDS type IV have abnormal production of type III collagen, the major collagen type found in blood vessels. The cerebrovascular complications include intracranial aneurysms, arterial rupture, carotid-cavernous fistulae, and arterial dissections. The intracranial internal carotid artery is the most common site for an aneurysm, and rupture of the internal carotid artery within the cavernous sinus can create a direct carotid-cavernous fistula. The fragile arteries make angiography and surgery difficult, but some patients have had successful surgery or endovascular treatment.

REFERENCES

Beighton, P. 1993. *The Ehlers-Danlos syndromes. Heritable Disorders of Connective Tissue*, ed. P. Beighton. St. Louis, MO: Mosby-Year Book, Inc., pp. 189–251.

Beighton, P., and Thomas, M. L. 1969. The radiology of the Ehlers-Danlos syndrome. *Clin Radiol*, **20**, 354–61.

Bergqvist, D. 1996. Ehlers-Danlos type IV syndrome. A review from a vascular surgical point of view. *Eur J Surg*, **162**, 163–70.

Byers, P. H. 1994. Ehlers-Danlos syndrome: recent advances and current understanding of the clinical and genetic heterogeneity. *J Invest Dermatol*, **103S**, 47–52.

Byers, P. H. 1995. Ehlers-Danlos syndrome type IV: a genetic disorder in many guises. *J Invest Dermatol*, **105**, 311–3.

Byers, P. H., Holbrook, K. A., McGillivray, B., MacLeod, P. M., and Lowry, R. B. 1979. Clinical and ultrastructural heterogeneity of Type IV Ehlers-Danlos syndrome. *Hum Genet*, **47**, 141–50.

Chuman, H., Trobe, J. D., Petty, E. M., *et al.* 2002. Spontaneous direct carotid-cavernous fistula in Ehlers-Danlos syndrome type IV: two case reports and a review of the literature. *J Neuroophthalmol*, **22**, 75–81.

Cikrit, D. F., Glover, J. R., Dalsing, M. C., and Silver, D. 2002. The Ehlers-Danlos specter revisited. *Vasc Endovasc Surg*, **36**, 213–7.

Cikrit, D. F., Miles, J. H., and Silver, D. 1987. Spontaneous arterial perforation: the Ehlers-Danlos specter. *J Vasc Surg*, 5, 248–55.

Debrun, G. M., Aletich, V. A., Miller, N. R., and DeKeiser, R. J. W. 1996. Three cases of spontaneous direct carotid cavernous fistulas associated with Ehlers-Danlos syndrome type IV. *Surg Neurol*, **46**, 247–52.

Desal, H. A., Toulgoat, F., Raoul, S., *et al.* 2005. Ehlers-Danlos syndrome type IV and recurrent carotid-cavernous fistula: review of the literature, endovascular approach, technique and difficulties. *Neuroradiology*, **47**, 300–4.

Driscoll, S. H. M., Gomes, A. S., and Machleder, H. I. 1984. Perforation of the superior vena cava: a complication of digital angiography in Ehlers-Danlos syndrome. *Am J Radiol*, **142**, 1021–2.

Edwards, A., and Taylor, G. W. 1969. Ehlers-Danlos syndrome with vertebral artery aneurysm. *Proc Roy Soc Med*, **62**, 734–5.

Finney, L. H., Roberts, T. S., and Anderson, R. E. 1976. Giant intracranial aneurysm associated with Marfan's syndrome. Case report. *J Neurosurg*, **45**, 342–7.

Forlodou, P., de Kersaint-Gilly, A., Pizzanelli, J., Viarouge, M. P., and Auffray-Calvier, E. 1996. Ehlers-Danlos syndrome with a spontaneous caroticocavernous fistula occluded by detachable balloon: case report and review of literature. *Neuroradiology*, **38**, 595–7.

Fox, R., Pope, F. M., Narcisi, P., et al. 1988. Spontaneous carotid cavernous fistula in Ehlers-Danlos syndrome. *J Neurol Neurosurg Psychiatr*, **51**, 984–6.

Freeman, R. K., Swegle, J., and Sise, M. J. 1996. The surgical complications of Ehlers-Danlos syndrome. *Am Surg*, **62**, 869–73.

Germain, D. P., and Herrera-Guzman, Y. 2004. Vascular Ehlers-Danlos syndrome. *Ann Genet*, **47**, 1–9.

Gilchrist, D., Schwarze, U., Shields, K., MacLaren, L., Bridge, P. J., and Byers, P. H. 1999. Large kindred with Ehlers-Danlos syndrome type IV due to a point mutation (G571S) in the COLA1 gene of type III procollagen: low risk of pregnancy complications and unexpected longevity in some affected relatives. *Am J Med Genet*, **82**, 305–11.

Graf, C. J. 1965. Spontaneous carotid-cavernous fistula. *Arch Neurol*, **13**, 662–72.

Grond-Ginsbach, C., Schnippering, H., Hausser, I., *et al.* 2002. Ultrastructural connective tissue aberrations in patients with intracranial aneurysms. *Stroke*, **33**, 2192–6.

Hainsworth, P. J., and Mendelow, A. D. 1991. Giant intracranial aneurysm associated with Marfan's syndrome: a case report. *J Neurol Neurosurg Psychiatr*, **54**, 471–2.

Halbach, V. V., Higashida, R. T., Dowd, C. F., Barnwell, S. L., and Hieshima, G. B. 1990. Treatment of carotid-cavernous fistulas associated with Ehlers-Danlos syndrome. *Neurosurgery*, **26**, 1021–7.

Hamano, K., Kuga, T., Takahashi, M., *et al.* 1998. The lack of type III collagen in a patient with aneurysms and an aortic dissection. *J Vasc Surg*, **28**, 1104–6.

Horowitz, M. B., Purdy, P., Valentine, R. J., and Morrill, K. 2000. Remote vascular catastrophes after neurovascular interventional therapy for type 4 Ehlers-Danlos syndrome. *AJNR Am J Neuroradiol*, **21**, 974–6.

Hunter, G. C., Malone, J. M., Moore, W. S., Misiorowski, D. L., and Chvapil, M. 1982. Vascular manifestations in patients with Ehlers-Danlos syndrome. *Arch Surg*, **117**, 495–8.

Imahori, S., Bannerman, R. M., Graf, C. J., and Brennan, J. C. 1969. Ehlers-Danlos syndrome with multiple arterial lesions. *Am J Med*, **47**, 967–77.

Kanner, A. A., Maimin, S., and Rappaport, Z. H. 2000 Treatment of spontaneous carotid-cavernous fistula in Ehlers-Danlos syndrome by transvenous occlusion with Guglielmi detachable coils. Case report and review of the literature. *J Neurosurg*, **93**, 689–92.

Kashiwagi, S., Tsuchida, E., Goto, K., et al. 1993. Balloon occlusion of a spontaneous carotid-cavernous fistula in Ehlers-Danlos syndrome type IV. *Surg Neurol*, **39**, 187–90.

Krog, M., Almgren, B., Eriksson, I., and Nordstrom, S. 1983. Vascular complications in the Ehlers-Danlos syndrome. *Acta Chir Scand*, **149**, 279–82.

Kuivaniemi, H., Prokop, D. J., Wu, Y., et al. 1993. Exclusion of mutations in the gene for type III collagen (COL3A1) as a common cause of intracranial aneurysms or cervical artery dissections: results from sequence analysis of the coding sequences of type III collagen from 55 unrelated patients. *Neurology*, **43**, 2652–8.

Lach, B., Nair, S. G., Russell, N. A., and Benoit, B. G. 1987. Spontaneous carotid-cavernous fistula and multiple arterial dissections in type IV Ehlers-Danlos syndrome. *J Neurosurg*, **66**, 462–7.

Matsuda, M., Matsuda, I., Handa, H., and Okamoto, K. 1979. Intracavernous giant aneurysm associated with Marfan's syndrome. *Surg Neurol*, **12**, 119–21.

McKusick, V. A. 1972. *Heritable Disorders of Connective Tissue*. St. Louis, MO: C. V. Mosby Company.

Mirza, F. H., Smith, P. L., and Lim, W. N. 1979. Multiple aneurysms in a patient with Ehlers-Danlos syndrome: angiography without sequelae. *Am J Radiol*, **132**, 993–5.

North, K. N., Whiteman, D. A. H., Pepin, M. G., and Byers, P. H. 1995. Cerebrovascular complications in Ehlers-Danlos syndrome type IV. *Ann Neurol*, **38**, 960–4.

Oderich, G. S., Panneton, J. M., Bower, T. C., et al. 2005. The spectrum of management and clinical outcome of Ehlers-Danlos syndrome type IV: a 30-year experience. *J Vasc Surg*, **42**, 98–106.

Peaceman, A. M., and Cruikshank, D. P. 1987. Ehlers-Danlos syndrome and pregnancy: association of type IV disease with maternal death. *Obstet Gynecol*, **69**, 428–31.

Pepin, M., Schwartze, U., Superti-Furga, A., and Byers, P. H. 2000. Clinical and genetic features of Ehlers-Danlos syndrome type IV, the vascular type. *N Engl J Med*, **342**, 673–80.

Pollock, J. S., Custer, P. L., Hart, W. M., Smith, M. E., and Fitzpatrick, M. M. 1997. Ocular complications in Ehlers-Danlos syndrome type IV. *Arch Ophthalmol*, **115**, 416–9.

Pope, F. M., Narcisi, P., Nicholls, A. C., Liberman, M., and Oorthuys, J. W. 1988. Clinical presentations of Ehlers-Danlos syndrome type IV. *Arch Dis Child*, **63**, 1016–25.

Roach, E. S. 1989. Congenital cutaneovascular syndromes. In *Handbook of Clinical Neurology: Vascular Diseases Volume 11*, ed. P. J. Vinken, G. W. Bruyn, H. L. Klawans, and J. F. Toole. Amsterdam: Elsevier, pp. 443–62.

Rubinstein, M. K., and Cohen, N. H. 1964. Ehlers-Danlos syndrome associated with multiple intracranial aneurysms. *Neurology*, **14**, 125–32.

Schievink, W. I. 1997. Genetics of intracranial aneurysms. *Neurosurgery*, **40**, 651–63.

Schievink, W. I., Limburg, M., Oorthuys, J. W., Fleury, P., and Pope, F. M. 1990. Cerebrovascular disease in Ehlers-Danlos syndrome type IV. *Stroke*, **21**, 626–32.

Schievink, W. I., Piepgras, D. G., Earnest F. IV, and Gordon, H. 1991. Spontaneous carotid-cavernous fistulae in Ehlers-Danlos syndrome type IV. *J Neurosurg*, **74**, 991–8.

Schoolman, A., and Kepes, J. J. 1967. Bilateral spontaneous carotid-cavernous fistulae in Ehlers- Danlos syndrome. *J Neurosurg*, **26**, 82–6.

Sheiner, N. M., Miller, N., and Lachance, C. 1985. Arterial complications of Ehlers-Danlos syndrome. *J Cardiovasc Surg*, **26**, 291–6.

Stehbens, W. E., Delahunt, B., and Hilless, A. D. 1989. Early berry aneurysm formation in Marfan's syndrome. *Surg Neurol*, **31**, 200–2.

Zimmerman, C. F., Batjer, H. H., Purdy, P., Samson, D., Kopitnik, T., and Carstens, G. J. 1994. Ehlers-Danlos syndrome type IV: neuro-ophthalmic manifestations and management. *Ophthalmology*, **101S**, 133.

23 PROGERIA

E. Steve Roach, Irena Anselm, N. Paul Rosman, and Louis R. Caplan

Introduction

Progeria is a rare condition characterized by premature aging beginning in very early life and invariably ending in premature death. The term *progeria* is derived from *pro* meaning before and *geras* meaning old age. The original report of this condition was by Jonathan Hutchinson (1886). Hastings Gilford (1904) later restudied Hutchinson's two patients and dubbed the disorder progeria. Thus, progeria is often been called the Hutchinson–Gilford progeria syndrome (HGPS) after these early observers. Clinical manifestations involve the skin and appendages, the joints, and blood vessels causing coronary and cerebrovascular disease during youth (DeBusk, 1972).

Based on clinical descriptions and, more recently, genetic analyses, several *progeroid syndromes* have been defined in addition to progeria itself (Hofer *et al.*, 2005). The manifestations of these conditions vary, but each has some clinical features that resemble physiologic aging (Navarro *et al.*, 2006) and a variable risk of stroke. Progeroid disorders fall into two main categories: (1) disorders resulting from mutations of the LMNA gene coding for the nuclear membrane protein lamin A (e.g. progeria and mandibuloacral dysplasia [MAD]), and (2) disorders resulting from abnormal DNA repair (e.g. Werner syndrome).

Genetics of progeroid syndromes

Progeria is caused by a mutation of the LMNA gene on chromosome 1q (Delgado *et al.*, 2002; Eriksson *et al.*, 2003). The LMNA gene encodes lamin A and C, filamentous structural proteins found in the nuclear lamina (Caoska *et al.*, 2004; Fong, *et al.*, 2006; Huang, *et al.*, 2005). A mutation within exon 11 of LMNA accounts for about 80% of the individuals with progeria (McClintock *et al.*, 2006). In progeria, the LMNA mutation results in the accumulation of a lipid-modified (farnesylated) prelamin A (*progerin*), impairing the nuclear membrane function (Fong, *et al.*, 2006). The LMNA mutation often arises from the paternally derived allele (D'Apice *et al.*, 2004), although this is not always the case (Wuyts *et al.*, 2005).

Occasional siblings who are homozygous for an LMNA mutation confirm the existence of an autosomal recessive form of progeria (Plasilova *et al.*, 2004), and other affected siblings result from germline mosaicism (Rosman *et al.*, 2001; Wyuts *et al.*, 2005). Milder phenotypes could result from somatic mosaicism.

MAD, like progeria, results from a mutation of the lamin A/C gene (Novelli *et al.*, 2002). However, the Wiedemann-Rautenstrauch syndrome does not result from an LMNA mutation (Cao and Hegele, 2003).

The Werner syndrome gene (WRN) on the short arm of chromosome 8 encodes a 1432-amino-acid DNA helicase (Goddard *et al.*, 1996; Gray *et al.*, 1997; Ichikawa *et al.*, 1997). The DNA helicase family unwinds double-stranded DNA and thus plays a role in DNA replication and repair, recombination, and transcription (Gray *et al.*, 1997; Huang *et al.*, 1998). Dysfunction of the Werner syndrome gene leads to genomic instability, accounting for the frequency of neoplasia in this condition. The Werner syndrome protein is expressed in all areas of the brain and is present in both glia and neurons (Gee *et al.*, 2002).

A few patients with atypical Werner syndrome do not have a WRN mutation and instead have an LMNA mutation (Chen *et al.*, 2003; Csoka *et al.*, 2004). This confirms the genetic heterogeneity of Werner syndrome and illustrates why clinical diagnosis is sometimes difficult.

Clinical findings of progeria

The estimated incidence of progeria is about 1 in 4 million births (Hennekam, 2006). The signs of progeria are often first noted during the first year or two of life (Sarkar and Shinton, 2001). At birth, some babies show scleroderma-like skin, especially over the abdomen. Poor weight gain and retarded growth become evident early (Hennekam, 2006). The head and facial appearance is characteristic – the head looks relatively large for the face. The scalp veins are often prominent. The head is usually bald or has scant hair (Figure 23.1). Alopecia is always present by adolescence, and eyebrows and eyelashes often become sparse. The nose is narrow and beaked. The ears and mandible are small, and the teeth are crowded together. The ears often protrude laterally. The voice is typically high-pitched (DeBusk, 1972; Feingold, 1980).

Children with progeria have severe growth retardation, and sexual maturation does not usually occur. Subcutaneous fat is scanty, and the skin is lax. Superficial veins are prominent. The nails are small and dystrophic. Bone and joint abnormalities are usually present. The bones are thinner than normal, and fractures are common. The distal clavicles show thinning and resorption of bone. The ribs are thin. There is progressive loss of bone from the distal phalanges. The joints are enlarged and have limited mobility. Coxa valga is common. The bow-legged appearance gives the patients a characteristic "horse riding stance."

Uncommon Causes of Stroke, 2nd edition, ed. Louis R. Caplan. Published by Cambridge University Press. © Cambridge University Press 2008.

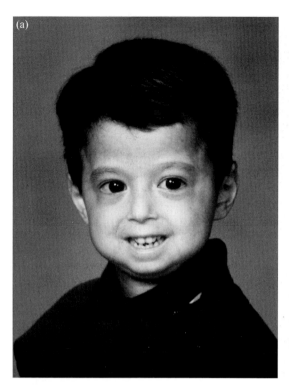 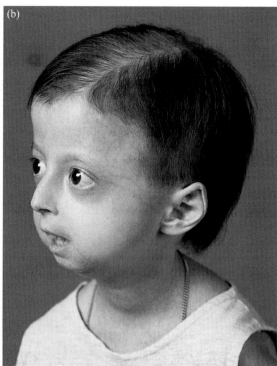

Figure 23.1 A boy with premature aging and multiple brain infarctions. A. Portrait at age 3, before his first stroke, shows slightly dysmorphic facial features but normal subcutaneous tissue and scalp hair. B. By age 8, his hair loss, stooped posture, and loss of subcutaneous fat make him appear prematurely aged. (Reproduced with permission from Miller and Roach, 1999.)

Most children with progeria develop premature severe vascular disease. Coronary artery disease and myocardial infarction are common, and heart disease is the leading cause of death (DeBusk, 1972; Dyck *et al.*, 1987). The median age at death is 13.4 years (McKusick, 1988). Although most patients with progeria die during the second decade, some less severely affected individuals survive until middle age (Ogihara *et al.*, 1986).

Cerebrovascular disease plays an important role in the morbidity of progeria (Figure 23.2). Dyck and colleagues (1987) reported a girl with progeria who had episodes of right hemiplegia at ages 7 and 9 years. She also had recurrent vertigo. Angiography showed occlusion of the left internal carotid artery and severe vertebrobasilar arterial disease. She developed angina pectoris at age 9 and had a myocardial infarct at age 11. Coronary angiography showed severe premature coronary artery occlusive disease (Dyck *et al.*, 1987).

Green (1981) reported a patient with progeria who had cerebral aneurysms. Progeria was diagnosed at age 6 years because of the characteristic features. At age 22, she developed pain in the right eye, headache, and right ophthalmoplegia. Angiography showed a very large aneurysm of the right internal carotid artery within the cavernous sinus. She also had a left internal carotid artery aneurysm on the extracranial portion of the artery just before penetration into the skull base.

Naganuma *et al.* (1990) described a boy who, at age 7 years, had transient ischemic attacks and developed a right hemiplegia. Cranial CT showed multiple cerebral infarcts. Angiography showed occlusion of the left internal carotid artery and occlusive vertebral

artery disease. Wagle and colleagues (1992) reported an 8-year-old girl who had a stroke with left hemiplegia. She had been diagnosed as having progeria at age 14 months because of her characteristic body habitus and clinical features. Brain MRI showed an infarct in the distribution of the superior division of the right middle cerebral artery. Echocardiography, magnetic resonance angiography (MRA), and extracranial Duplex ultrasonography did not reveal a cardiac or cervicocranial vascular cause of the embolic stroke.

A 4-year-old boy developed headaches, drooling, and right arm weakness, then a month later had a right-sided seizure and right hemiparesis (Smith *et al.*, 1993). His cranial MRI showed an acute left posterior parietal infarct, bilateral subdural fluid collections, and diffuse abnormalities involving the white matter and basal ganglia. The cervical, internal carotid arteries and the origins of the vertebral arteries were occluded, and there was extensive collateral circulation. He later had transient left limb weakness and biparietal and right frontal lobe infarcts (Smith *et al.*, 1993). Matsuo *et al.* (1994) reported a 7-year-old boy who had a right putaminal infarct shown on brain MRI. He later developed coronary artery disease, but no vascular studies were reported.

One 5-year-old boy with progeria developed left-sided seizures followed by left hemiparesis (Rosman *et al.*, 2001). His cranial MRI confirmed bilateral parietal infarcts, and his MRA showed severe stenosis of the left internal carotid artery and stenosis of the cavernous portion of the right internal carotid artery. An echocardiogram showed a possible aortic valve vegetation or thrombus and a small patent foramen ovale. He was anticoagulated with heparin then warfarin. Three months later he had multiple focal seizures

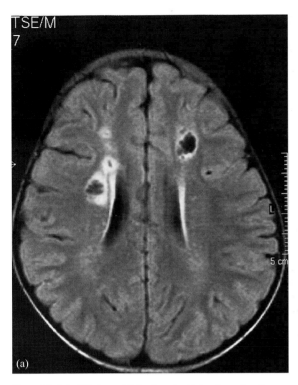 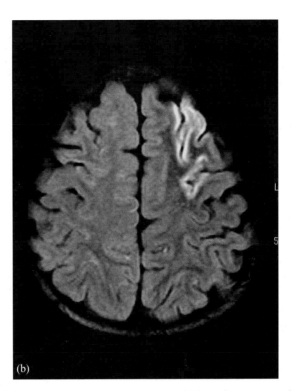

Figure 23.2 A. MRI shows bilateral cerebral infarctions of various ages. B. Later MRI after an episode of hemiplegia and aphasia depicts a new infarction of the frontal lobe. (Reproduced with permission from Miller and Roach, 1999.)

of the right arm followed by temporary right hemiparesis. Two months later right-sided seizures recurred, and an MRA showed occlusion of the right internal carotid artery within the siphon.

The occlusive vascular disease in progeria probably most often affects the cervical carotid and vertebral arteries, but the intracranial large arteries may also be involved. The chronic basal ganglia and white matter changes found on brain imaging raise the possibility of concurrent penetrating artery disease. There is little information about the pathological nature of the occlusive vascular lesions.

Clinical features of Werner syndrome

Werner syndrome is an autosomal recessive disorder characterized by cataract formation, scleroderma, and subcutaneous calcifications, a beak-like nose, and the features of premature aging such as graying of hair, senile macular degeneration, osteoporosis, and atherosclerosis (Epstein *et al.*, 1966). In 1904, Otto Werner in his doctoral thesis described the findings in four siblings who had premature aging (Herrero, 1980; Werner, 1904). Werner's patients were short and had a senile appearance. Cataracts and hair graying appeared during their third decade of life. They developed atrophic hyperkeratotic ulcerated skin, mostly over the hands and feet, and their skeletal limb muscles showed marked atrophy. We now recognize that diabetes, hypogonadism, and retinitis pigmentosa are also usually present. Cataracts are posterior cortical, subcapsular, and bilateral (Herrero, 1980). Liver dysfunction, hyperuricemia, and hyperlipidemia are often present.

Individuals with Werner syndrome appear 20–30 years older than their actual age. The face is thin, and the sharp angle of the

bridge of the nose gives it a beaked appearance. Most patients have a high-pitched voice due to a variety of vocal cord abnormalities. The muscles of the extremities are usually severely atrophied. Patients with Werner syndrome have a striking predilection for developing noncarcinomatous tumors. Meningiomas and neural sheath sarcomas are found within the central nervous system. The age at death averages about 48 years (range 30–63) (Herrero, 1980). Patients with Werner syndrome develop accelerated atherosclerosis, and the aorta and great vessels are often calcified. Often there is heavy calcification of the mitral and/or the aortic valves (Tokunaga *et al.*, 1976). Death is often from malignancies, diabetic coma, myocardial infarction, or liver failure.

Although Werner syndrome has been called adult progeria, the age of onset, clinical features, and length of survival are quite different from those of progeria (Perloff and Phelps, 1958). As with progeria, death from cardiac disease is more common than stroke-related death. Individuals with Werner syndrome have a higher frequency of malignancies than do patients with progeria.

Other progeroid syndromes

MAD is another autosomal recessive disorder that features alopecia and short stature, along with clavicular and mandibular hypoplasia, stiff joints, and persistently open cranial sutures (Palotta and Morgese, 1984; Zina *et al.*, 1981). MAD is also due to a mutation of the LMNA gene (Novelli *et al.*, 2002) that results in the accumulation of lamin A precursor protein, alteration of the nuclear architecture, and chromatin disorganization (Filesi *et al.*, 2005).

The Wiedemann-Rautenstrauch syndrome, sometimes called neonatal progeria, typically manifests from birth and features delayed development, poor growth, alopecia, and lipoatrophy. It is not caused by a mutation of LMNA (Cao and Hegele, 2003).

Treatment

Given the severity of large artery pathology in patients with progeroid syndromes, it is probably reasonable to use antiplatelet agents. Additionally, several reported patients, including two of the authors' patients, seem to have fared well for a time on anticoagulation with warfarin. However, there are too few patients with progeroid disorders to allow strong recommendations about stroke therapy in these individuals.

Although there is currently no means to effectively halt the progression of progeria, preliminary studies in mice suggest a possible benefit from the use of a farnesyltransferase inhibitor (Fong *et al.*, 2006; Yang *et al.*, 2006).

REFERENCES

Cao, H., and Hegele, R. A. 2003. LMNA is mutated in Hutchinson-Gilford progeria (MIM 176670) but not in Wiedemann-Rautenstrauch progeroid syndrome (MIM 264090). *J Hum Genet*, **48**, 271–4.

Chen, L., Lee, L., Kudlow, B. A., *et al.* 2003. LMNA mutations in atypical Werner's syndrome. *Lancet*, **362**, 440–5.

Csoka, A. B., Cao, H., Sammak, P. J., *et al.* 2004. Novel lamin A/C gene (LMNA) mutations in atypical progeroid syndromes. *J Med Genet*, **41**, 304–8.

D'Apice, M. R., Tenconi, R., Mammi, I., and Novelli, G. 2004. Paternal origin of LMNA mutations in Hutchinson-Gilford progeria. *Clin Genet*, **65**, 52–4.

DeBusk, F. L. 1972. The Hutchinson–Gilford progeria syndrome. *J Pediatr*, **80**, 697–724.

Delgado Luengo, W., Rojas Martinez, A., Ortiz Lopez, R., *et al.* 2002. Del(1)(q23) in a patient with Hutchinson-Gilford progeria. *Am J Med Genet*, **113**, 298–301.

Dyck, J. D., David, T. E., Burke, B., Webb, G. D., Henderson, M. A., and Fowler, R. S. 1987. Management of coronary artery disease in Hutchinson–Gilford syndrome. *J Pediatr*, **111**, 407–10.

Epstein, C. J., Martin, G. M., Schultz, A. L., and Motulsky, A. G. 1966. Werner syndrome. A review of its symptomatology, pathologic features, genetics and relationship to the natural aging process. *Medicine*, **45**, 177–221.

Eriksson, M., Brown, W. T., Gordon, L. B., *et al.* 2003. Recurrent de novo point mutations in human lamin A cause Hutchinson-Gilford progeria syndrome. *Nature*, **423**, 293–8.

Feingold, M. 1980. Progeria (Hutchinson–Gilford syndrome). In *Neurogenetic Directory Part ll. Handbook of Clinical Neurology*, **vol. 43**, ed. P. J. Vinken, G. W. Bruyn, and H. Klawans. Amsterdam: North Holland Publishing Company, pp. 465–6.

Filesi, I., Gullotta, F., Lattanzi, G., *et al.* 2005. Alterations of nuclear envelope and chromatin organization in mandibuloacral dysplasia, a rare form of laminopathy. *Physiol Genom*, **23**, 150–8.

Fong, L. G., Frost, D., Meta, M., *et al.* 2006. A protein farnesyltransferase inhibitor ameliorates disease in a mouse model of progeria. *Science*, **311**, 1621–3.

Gee, J., Ding, Q., and Keller, J. N. 2002. Analysis of Werner's expression within the brain and primary neuronal culture. *Brain Res*, **940**, 44–48.

Gilford, H. 1904. Progeria: a form of senilism. *Practitioner*, **73**, 188–217.

Goddard, K. A. B., Yu, C. E., Oshima, J., *et al.* 1996. Toward localization of the Werner syndrome gene by linkage dysequilibrium and ancestral haplotyping: lessons learned from analysis of 35 chromosome 8p11.1–21.1 markers. *Am J Hum Genet*, **58**, 1286–302.

Gray, M. D., Shen, J. C., Kamath-Loeb, A. S., *et al.* 1997. The Werner syndrome protein is a DNA helicase. *Nat Genet*, **17**, 100–3.

Green, L. N. 1981. Progeria with carotid artery aneurysms. Report of a case. *Arch Neurol*, **38**, 659–61.

Hennekam, R. C. 2006. Hutchinson-Gilford progeria syndrome: review of the phenotype. *Am J Med Genet A*, **140**, 2603–24.

Herrero, F. A. 1980. Neurological manifestations of hereditable connective tissue disorders. In *Neurological Manifestations of Systemic Diseases Part II.*

Handbook of Clinical Neurology, **vol. 39**, ed. P. J. Vinken, G. W. Bruyn, and H. L. Klawans. Amsterdam: North Holland Publishing Company, pp. 379–418.

Hofer, A. C., Tran, R. T., Aziz, O. Z., *et al.* 2005. Shared phenotypes among segmental progeroid syndromes suggest underlying pathways of aging. *J Gerontol A Biol Sci Med Sci*, **60**, 10–20.

Huang, S., Baomin, L., Gray, M. D., Oshima, J., Saira, M., and Campisi, J. 1998. The premature ageing syndrome protein WRN, is a 3'–>5' exonuclease. *Nat Genet*, **20**, 114–6.

Huang, S., Chen, L., Libina, N., *et al.* 2005. Correction of cellular phenotypes of Hutchinson-Gilford progeria cells by RNA interference. *Hum Genet*, **118**, 444–50.

Hutchinson, J. 1886. Congenital absence of hair and mammary glands with an atrophic condition of the skin and its appendages in a boy whose mother had been almost wholly bald from alopecia areata from the age of 6. *Trans Med Chir Soc Edinburgh*, **69**, 473–7.

Ichikawa, K., Yamabe, Y., Imamura, O., *et al.* 1997. Cloning and characterization of a novel gene, WS-3, in human chromosome 8p11-p12. *Gene*, **189**, 277–87.

Matsuo, S., Takeuchi, Y., Hayashi, S., Kinugasa, A., and Sawada, T. 1994. Patient with unusual Hutchinson-Gilford syndrome (progeria). *Pediatr Neurol*, **10**, 237–40.

McClintock, D., Gordon, L. B., and Djabali, K. 2006. Hutchinson-Gilford progeria mutant lamin A primarily targets human vascular cells as detected by an anti-Lamin A G608G antibody. *Proc Natl Acad Sci U S A*, **103**, 2154–9.

McKusick, V. 1988. *Mendelian Inheritance in Man*, 8th edn. Baltimore: Johns Hopkins University Press. p. 630.

Miller, V. S., and Roach, E. S. 1999. Neurocutaneous syndromes. In *Neurology in Clinical Practice*, 3rd edn, ed. W. G. Bradley, *et al.* Boston: Butterworth-Heinemann.

Naganuma, Y., Konishi, T., and Hongou, K. 1990. A case of progeria syndrome with cerebral infarction. *No To Hattatsu*, **22**, 71–6.

Navarro, C. L., Cau, P., and Levy, N. 2006. Molecular bases of progeroid syndromes. *Hum Mol Genet*, **15 Spec No 2**, R151–61.

Novelli, G., Muchir, A., Sangiuolo, F., *et al.* 2002. Mandibuloacral dysplasia is caused by a mutation in LMNA-encoding lamin A/C. *Am J Hum Genet*, **71**, 426–31.

Ogihara, T., Hata, T., Tanaka, K., Fukuchi, K., Tabuchi, Y., and Kamahara, Y. 1986. Hutchinson–Gilford progeria syndrome in a 45-year-old man. *Am J Med*, **81**, 135–8.

Palotta, R., and Morgese, G. 1984. Mandibular dysplasia: a rare progeroid syndrome. Two brothers confirm autosomal recessive inheritance. *Clin Genet*, **26**, 133–8.

Perloff, J. K., and Phelps, E. T. 1958. A review of Werner's syndrome with a report of the second autopsied case. *Ann Intern Med*, **48**, 1205–20.

Plasilova, M., Chattopadhyay, C., Pal, P., *et al.* 2004. Homozygous missense mutation in the lamin A/C gene causes autosomal recessive Hutchinson-Gilford progeria syndrome. *J Med Genet*, **41**, 609–14.

Rosman, N. P., Anselm, I., and Bhadelia, R. A. 2001. Progressive intracranial vascular disease with strokes and seizures in a boy with progeria. *J Child Neurol*, **16**, 212–5.

Sarkar, P. K., and Shinton, R. A. 2001. Hutchinson-Gilford progeria syndrome. *Postgrad Med J*, **77**, 312–17.

Smith, A. S., Wiznitzer, M., and Karaman, B. A. 1993. MRA detection of vascular occlusion in a child with progeria. *Am J Neuroradiol*, **14**, 441–3.

Tokunaga, M., Mori, S., Sato, K., Nakamura, K., and Wakamatsu, E. 1976. Postmortem study of a case of Werner's syndrome. *J Am Geriatr Soc*, **24**, 407–11.

Wagle, W. A., Haller, J. S., and Cousins, J. P. 1992. Cerebral infarction in progeria. *Pediatr Neurol*, **8**, 476–7.

Werner, O. 1904. *Uber Katarakt in Verbindung mit Sklerodermis*. Thesis. Kiel, Germany, Kiel, Schmidt und Klaunig.

Wuyts, W., Biervliet, M., Reyniers, E., D'Apice, M. R., Novelli, G., and Storm, K. 2005. Somatic and gonadal mosaicism in Hutchinson-Gilford progeria. *Am J Med Genet A*, **135**, 66–8.

Yang, S. H., Meta, M., Qiao, X., *et al.* 2006. A farnesyltransferase inhibitor improves disease phenotypes in mice with a Hutchinson-Gilford progeria syndrome mutation. *J Clin Invest*, **116**, 2115–21.

Zina, A. M., Cravaior, A., and Bundino, S. 1981. Familial mandibulocranial dysplasia. *Br J Dermatol*, **105**, 719–23.

24 MELAS AND OTHER MITOCHONDRIAL DISORDERS

Lorenz Hirt

Introduction

Mitochondria are the site of oxidative phosphorylation, the major source of the energy substrate adenosine 5'-triphosphate (ATP) in eukaryotic cells. Mitochondrial dysfunction resulting from mutations of mitochondrial DNA (mtDNA) or of nuclear genes coding for proteins involved in the respiratory chain may affect multiple systems and typically organs with high energy requirements such as the brain and skeletal muscles. One of the clinical presentations of mitochondrial dysfunction in the brain is acute focal deficits closely resembling strokes. Stroke-like episodes have most frequently been reported in MELAS (mitochondrial encephalomyopathy, lactic acidosis, and stroke-like episodes), a multisystemic syndrome associated with mutations of mtDNA.

The mitochondrial genome consists of a 16.5-kilobase circular DNA molecule located within the mitochondrion, present in a large, tissue-dependent copy number. MtDNA is maternally transmitted and encodes mitochondrial transfer RNAs (tRNAs), ribosomal RNAs (rRNAs), and 13 proteins of the approximately 80 proteins involved in the respiratory chain (Anderson *et al.*, 1981; Brandon *et al.*, 2004; DiMauro, 1999; DiMauro and Moraes, 1993). The remaining respiratory chain proteins are encoded by nuclear DNA, synthesized in the cytoplasm, and transported to the mitochondria, as are all other proteins found in the mitochondria (e.g. mtDNA polymerase, mitochondrial superoxide dismutase). MtDNA is exposed to free radicals generated by the respiratory chain, and DNA repair mechanisms are less efficient in the mitochondrion than in the nucleus. MtDNA is therefore more prone to mutations than is nuclear DNA. MtDNA mutations may therefore cause respiratory chain dysfunction and ATP depletion, and tissues with high energy expenditure (e.g. brain and muscle) are more at risk of not being able to meet their energy demands. Numerous mtDNA mutations have been identified since 1988 in association with human diseases. Mutations have been found in tRNA, rRNA, and protein-encoding genes. Several mutations in nuclear genes encoding proteins involved in the respiratory chain have also been identified in patients with mitochondrial dysfunction (Bourgeron *et al.*, 1995; Triepels *et al.*, 1999), but not so far in MELAS syndrome.

An interesting feature of mtDNA mutations is heteroplasmy. MtDNA is present in a large copy number within the mitochondrion, and wild-type and mutated mtDNA molecules commonly coexist within one cell. The proportions of mutated and wild-type mtDNA vary between cells and between tissues. If the proportion of mutated mtDNA exceeds a certain threshold, the normal functioning of the cell is disturbed. The threshold above which a functional impairment becomes apparent depends on the tissue. For instance, in a symptomatic mitochondrial myopathy, the ratio typically exceeds 50% of total mtDNA in affected muscle. The degree of heteroplasmy varies from one tissue to another within one individual, and the distribution of the mutation throughout the organism plays a part in determining the phenotype. There is poor correlation between abundance of mutant mtDNA in blood or other peripheral tissues and neurological phenotype (Hirt *et al.*, 1996). The distribution of the mutation in tissues varies between individuals and participates in the wide phenotypic variability encountered in mtDNA mutation-associated diseases, but other unknown factors, for example genetic and environmental, are likely to affect the phenotypic expression of a mutation. With time, the degree of heteroplasmy may vary, due to a better survival of cells with a low degree of heteroplasmy, or to an altered replication speed of the mutated mtDNA molecules.

During the normal aging process, spontaneous mtDNA mutations accumulate and slowly impair mitochondrial function. This age-related phenomenon may favor the appearance of a phenotype. Following early reports of the association of stroke with mitochondrial myopathy (Bogousslavsky *et al.*, 1982; Kuriyama *et al.*, 1984; Skoglund, 1979), the acronym MELAS was introduced in 1984 (Pavlakis *et al.*, 1984), defining a multisystemic syndrome most often associated with a maternally inherited mtDNA point mutation (A to G transition) at position 3243 within the tRNALeu(UUR) encoding gene (Goto *et al.*, 1990). The second most common mutation associated with MELAS lies in the same gene (Goto *et al.*, 1991). Table 24.1 lists the mtDNA mutations associated with the MELAS syndrome.

Clinical presentation

MELAS syndrome affects young patients, and its most striking clinical finding is stroke-like episodes, occurring as early as the teenage years, with transient or permanent hemianopia, cortical blindness, aphasia, or hemiparesis. Fever and infections have been reported as possible triggering factors for stroke-like episodes (Sue *et al.*, 1998). Episodic vomiting, sudden episodes of headache, and seizures are frequent in MELAS patients. Blood lactate levels are increased because of a dysfunction in the respiratory chain, with resulting inhibition of the citric acid cycle and accumulation of pyruvate and lactate. Most commonly, MELAS is associated with an mtDNA point mutation at position 3243 within the

Uncommon Causes of Stroke, 2nd edition, ed. Louis R. Caplan. Published by Cambridge University Press. © Cambridge University Press 2008.

Table 24.1 Mutations associated with stroke in mitochondrial encephalomyopathy

Mutation	Affected gene	Phenotype	References
mtDNA A3243G	tRNALeu(UUR)	MELAS	(Goto et al., 1990)
mtDNA T3271C	tRNALeu(UUR)	MELAS	(Goto et al., 1991)
mtDNA 3260	tRNALeu(UUR)	MELAS	(Nishino et al., 1996)
mtDNA deletion		MELAS	(Zupanc et al., 1991)
mtDNA A11084G	ND4	MELAS	(Lertrit et al., 1992)
mtDNA T9957C	COX III	MELAS	(Manfredi et al., 1995)
mtDNA G13513A	ND5	MELAS	(Santorelli et al., 1997)
mtDNA A8356C	tRNALys	MERRFMELAS overlap	(Zeviani et al., 1993)
mtDNA T7512	tRNASer(UCN)	MERRFMELAS overlap	(Nakamura et al., 1995)
mtDNA T3308C	ND1	MELAS and bilateral striatal necrosis	(Campos et al., 1997)
mtDNA T8993G	ATPase 6	NARP, Leigh syndrome	(Uziel et al., 1997)

Table 24.2 Clinical features associated with the mtDNA A3243G mutation

Clinical features	References
MELAS syndrome	(Goto et al., 1990)
Diabetes mellitus	(Gerbitz et al., 1995; Reardon et al., 1992)
Hearing impairment	(Majamaa et al., 1998; Morgan-Hughes et al., 1995)
Epilepsy	(Majamaa et al., 1998)
Short stature	(Majamaa et al., 1998)
Progressive external ophthalmoplegia	(Majamaa et al., 1998)
Pigmentary retinopathy	(Sue et al., 1997)
Ataxia	(Damian et al., 1995; Majamaa et al., 1998)
Basal ganglia calcification	(Majamaa et al., 1998; Morgan-Hughes et al., 1995)
Hypertrophic cardiomyopathy	(Majamaa et al., 1998; Morgan-Hughes et al., 1995)
Cognitive decline	(Majamaa et al., 1998)
Myoclonus Epilepsy Associated with Ragged-Red Fibers (MERRF)	(Folgero et al., 1995)
Ischemic colitis	(Hess et al., 1995)
Nephropathy	(Damian et al., 1995)
Leigh syndrome	(Sue et al., 1999)

tRNALeu(UUR) encoding gene. This mutation is transmitted in a maternal mode of inheritance. It is always heteroplasmic, suggesting that the presence of wild-type DNA is required for survival. Other mutations reported in association with the MELAS syndrome are listed in Table 24.1 and discussed below. Because mitochondrial diseases have considerable phenotypic and genotypic heterogeneity, siblings of MELAS patients carrying the 3243 mutation may present a different phenotype of the mutation, such as mitochondrial myopathy or diabetes and deafness (Hirt et al., 2001). Many different phenotypes, alone or in various combinations, have been reported with this mutation (Table 24.2). A population survey in a Finnish province with 245 201 inhabitants has, for the first time, established the prevalence of the mitochondrial 3243 A to G mutation in an adult population to 16/100 000 (Majamaa et al., 1998). This mutation therefore is classified as a frequent genetic anomaly. The most frequent phenotype in this survey is not the MELAS syndrome, but short stature, hearing impairment, and cognitive decline.

A list of other clinical features and syndromes reported with the mtDNA 3243 A to G transition is provided in Table 24.2 and includes muscle involvement with ophthalmoparesis and palpebral ptosis due to myopathy of the extrinsic eye muscles. Muscle biopsy shows a mitochondrial myopathy with ragged-red fibers (Gomori's trichrome staining), cytochrome c oxidase-negative fibers, and a reduced respiratory chain activity (complexes I, III, and/or IV). Overlaps between different mitochondrial syndromes are common.

Brain imaging

Neuroradiological features of six kindreds carrying the MELAS tRNALeu(UUR) 3243 A to G mutation have been reported (Sue et al., 1998). The most common feature visible on CT and by MRI was symmetrical calcifications of the basal ganglia (in 14 of 22 patients) (Figure 24.1). These calcifications always involved the globus pallidus, and were also seen in the caudate, putamen, and thalamus. None of the patients with those calcifications had clinical features suggesting basal ganglia dysfunction. Other findings included focal lesions and cerebellar and cerebral atrophy. Focal hypodensities by CT were seen in nine patients, mainly in the occipital and parietal lobes, and in both cerebellar hemispheres in one patient. In four patients, lesions were not confined to the vascular territory of one large artery. This observation strongly suggests that stroke-like episodes in MELAS do not result

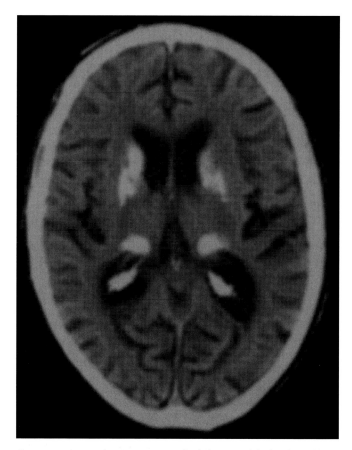

Figure 24.1 CT scan showing symmetrical calcifications of the basal ganglia in a patient bearing the mtDNA A3243G mutation. The patient was suffering from diabetes and deafness and from a late-onset myopathy. (Courtesy of Professor Philippe Maeder.)

from an arterial occlusion, but from a different mechanism, probably metabolic failure. Vascular imaging, when performed, does not show arterial or venous occlusions or stenosis in the great majority of patients. By CT, lesions involved gray and white matter. In the acute stage, there was enhancement with intravenous contrast, and mass effect was also seen. By MRI, there was an increase in the T2 signal, mainly within the cortex. All patients with focal hypodensities had a history of stroke-like episodes.

Brain imaging in mitochondrial disorders was also reviewed by Haas and Dietrich (2004). Cortical hypodensities seen in MELAS syndrome by CT do not correspond to vascular territories. There are reports both of hyper- and hypoperfusion within these cerebral lesions. Blood vessels are patent. There is an increased signal intensity in the acute phase by T2-weighted imaging and fluid-attenuated inversion recovery (FLAIR) that declines with time leading to an area of atrophy or of altered signal intensity. Lesions may migrate. The diffusion-weighted imaging (DWI) signal is increased, and there are reports both of increased and decreased apparent diffusion coefficient (ADC). Nuclear magnetic resonance (NMR) spectroscopy reveals increased lactate levels within the lesions. Leukoencephalopathy has been reported in rare cases (Haas and Dietrich, 2004). In summary, CT scanning

reveals basal ganglial calcifications and cortical hypodensities. MRI shows increased T2 and FLAIR signals in the cortical lesions that decline with time. Both increased and reduced ADC signals have been reported, and there is an increased lactate signal by NMR spectroscopy.

Stroke in other mitochondrial syndromes

Stroke-like episodes have been reported to be associated with other mtDNA mutations (Table 24.1). These mutations are point mutations lying within tRNA-encoding genes or within protein-encoding genes, or are deletions encompassing several genes, showing that all these different genetic anomalies can cause a similar dysfunction of the mitochondrion resulting in stroke. In many instances, a patient's clinical presentation is a combination of features of two or more syndromes. A MELAS-MERRF (myoclonic epilepsy with ragged-red fibers) has been reported with point mutations at positions 8356 and 7512 (Nakamura *et al.*, 1995; Zeviani *et al.*, 1993). Stroke has been reported in association with an mtDNA deletion in two siblings in an overlap between the MELAS and Kearns-Sayre syndromes (Zupanc *et al.*, 1991). Both showed a pigmentary retinopathy, progressive external ophthalmoplegia, neurosensorial hearing loss, and lactic acidosis with diabetes in one individual and hypoparathyroidism in the other.

Diagnostic evaluation

The clinical evaluation includes a careful family history, searching for other phenotypes of the mitochondrial 3243 A to G mutation (e.g. diabetes and deafness). Brain imaging can show calcifications of the basal ganglia and focal lesions in the occipital and parietal lobes that are not usually restricted to a vascular territory. NMR spectroscopy may be useful to detect increased lactate levels. Blood lactate measurement (resting or after exercise) is useful, as is a muscle biopsy (modified Gomori's trichrome staining, cytochrome *c* oxidase and succinate, NADH-reductase histochemistry) with measurement of the respiratory chain activity. The diagnosis can be confirmed by mtDNA analysis (muscle biopsy, blood, or buccal epithelial cell sample).

Treatment

Various approaches have been tried including dietary measures, administration of redox compounds, and vitamins and coenzymes, but because of the rarity of the MELAS syndrome, reports of treatment are anecdotal and sometimes controversial. Published therapies include coenzyme Q10 (Abe *et al.*, 1999), sodium dichloroacetate (Pavlakis *et al.*, 1998; Saitoh *et al.*, 1998), nicotinamide (Majamaa *et al.*, 1997), and coadministration of cytochrome *c*, vitamin B1, and B2 (Tanaka *et al.*, 1997).

Discussion

The function of the mtDNA is to encode proteins participating in the respiratory chain, and many mtDNA mutations affect respiratory chain activity. The most likely origin of stroke-like episodes is a sudden metabolic failure in neuronal tissue with a high proportion of mutant mtDNA, with loss of function and transient or permanent cellular damage, perhaps triggered by fever or infection. This would be consistent with the observation that lesions in some cases are not confined to a single vascular territory, implying that the lesion does not result from the occlusion of blood vessels (Sue *et al.*, 1998).

Alternatively, there are reports of involvement of smooth muscle cells within the arterial wall, with a high rate of mutated DNA in a case of ischemic colitis associated with the 3243 mutation (Hess *et al.*, 1995). Lesions of the arterial wall cause narrowing or occlusion of the arterial lumen with resulting mesenteric ischemia, but this has never been observed in the brain. Anomalies of blood clotting have not been reported in MELAS patients.

Experimental evidence links mitochondria to neuronal death: mitochondria participate in intracellular calcium buffering, and in calcium signaling processes, early steps of apoptosis involve the mitochondria (Green and Reed, 1998). An mtDNA mutation affecting the respiratory chain may affect calcium signaling, free radical production, or apoptosis regulation in the mitochondrion and thereby promote cell death. Cytochrome *c*, for instance, signals apoptosis when released from the mitochondria, and many pro- or antiapoptotic members of the Bcl2 family of proteins are located in the mitochondria. Knowledge of mitochondrial biology is evolving rapidly. Mitochondria are dynamic; they change very rapidly, and within seconds they can fuse (mitochondrial fusion) or divide (mitochondrial fission). Fusion and fission are important during development, during apoptosis, and probably also in disease (Chan, 2006). MtDNA mutations are frequently heteroplasmic. It is likely that mitochondrial fusion induces a mixing of mutant and wild-type DNA molecules, and of mutant and wild-type gene products within mitochondria, allowing maintenance of mitochondrial function (Chan, 2006). A deeper knowledge of mitochondrial biology will hopefully lead to a more complete understanding of the pathogenesis of mitochondrial diseases such as MELAS.

Acknowledgments

I am grateful to Melanie Price for helpful comments.

REFERENCES

Abe, K., Matsuo, Y., Kadekawa, J., Inoue, S., and Yanagihara, T. 1999. Effect of coenzyme Q10 in patients with mitochondrial myopathy, encephalopathy, lactic acidosis, and stroke-like episodes (MELAS): evaluation by noninvasive tissue oximetry. *J Neurol Sci*, **162**(1), 65–8.

Anderson, S., Bankier, A. T., Barrell, B. G., *et al.* 1981. Sequence and organization of the human mitochondrial genome *Nature*, **290**, 457–65.

Bogousslavsky, J., Perentes, E., Deruaz, J. P., and Regli, F., 1982. Mitochondrial myopathy and cardiomyopathy with neurodegenerative features and multiple brain infarcts. *J Neurol Sci*, **55**, 351–7.

Bourgeron, T., Rustin, P., Chretien, D., *et al.* 1995. Mutation of a nuclear succinate dehydrogenase gene results in mitochondrial respiratory chain deficiency. *Nat Genet*, **11**, 144–9.

Brandon, M. C., Lott, M. T., Nguyen, K. C., *et al.* 2004. MITOMAP: a human mitochondrial genome database–2004 update. *Nucleic Acids Res*, **33**, D611–3.

Campos, Y., Martin, M. A., Rubio, J. C., Gutierrez del Olmo, M. C., Cabello, A., and Arenas, J., 1997. Bilateral striatal necrosis and MELAS associated with a new T3308C mutation in the mitochondrial ND1gene. *Biochem Biophys Res Commun*, **238**, 323–5.

Chan, D. C. 2006. Mitochondria: dynamic organelles in disease, aging, and development. *Cell*, **125**, 1241–52.

Damian, M. S., Seibel, P., Reichmann, H., *et al.* 1995. Clinical spectrum of the MELAS mutation in a large pedigree. *Acta Neurol Scand*, **92**, 409–15.

DiMauro, S., 1999. Mitochondrial encephalomyopathies: back to Mendelian genetics. *Ann Neurol*, **45**, 693–4.

DiMauro, S., and Moraes, C. T. 1993. Mitochondrial encephalomyopathies. *Arch Neurol*, **50**, 1197–208.

Folgero, T., Torbergsen, T., and Oian, P., 1995. The 3243 MELAS mutation in a pedigree with MERRF. *Eur Neurol*, **35**, 168–71.

Gerbitz, K. D., van den Ouweland, J. M., Maassen, J. A., and Jaksch, M., 1995. Mitochondrial diabetes mellitus: a review. *Biochim Biophys Acta*, **1271**, 253–60.

Goto, Y., Nonaka, I., and Horai, S., 1991. A new mtDNA mutation associated with mitochondrial myopathy, encephalopathy, lactic acidosis and stroke-like episodes (MELAS). *Biochim Biophys Acta*, **1097**, 238–40.

Goto, Y., Nonaka, I., and Horai, S., 1990. A mutation in the tRNA(Leu)(UUR) gene associated with the MELAS subgroup of mitochondrial encephalomyopathies. *Nature*, **348**, 651–3.

Green, D. R., and Reed, J. C., 1998. Mitochondria and apoptosis. *Science*, **281**, 1309–12.

Haas, R., and Dietrich, R., 2004. Neuroimaging of mitochondrial disorders. *Mitochondrion*, **4**, 471–90.

Hess, J., Burkhard, P., Morris, M., Lalioti, M., Myers, P., and Hadengue, A., 1995. Ischaemic colitis due to mitochondrial cytopathy. *Lancet*, **346**, 189–90.

Hirt, L., Magistretti, P. J., Bogousslavsky, J., Boulat, O., and Borruat, F. X., 1996. Large deletion (7.2 kb) of mitochondrial DNA with novel boundaries in a case of progressive external ophthalmoplegia. *J Neurol Neurosurg Psychiatry*, **61**, 422–3.

Hirt, L., Marechal, C., Ghika, J. A., Magistretti, P. J., and Bogousslavsky, J., 2001. Ocular mitochondrial myopathy evolving late in life into a disabling proximal myopathy associated with the mitochondrial DNA 3243A to G mutation. *J Neurol*, **248**, 332–3.

Kuriyama, M., Umezaki, H., Fukuda, Y., *et al.* 1984. Mitochondrial encephalomyopathy with lactate-pyruvate elevation and brain infarctions. *Neurology*, **34**, 72–7.

Lertrit, P., Noer, A. S., Jean-Francois, M. J., *et al.* 1992. A new disease-related mutation for mitochondrial encephalopathy lactic acidosis and strokelike episodes (MELAS) syndrome affects the ND4 subunit of the respiratory complex I. *Am J Hum Genet*, **51**, 457–68.

Majamaa, K., Moilanen, J. S., Uimonen, S., *et al.* 1998. Epidemiology of A3243G, the mutation for mitochondrial encephalomyopathy, lactic acidosis, and strokelike episodes: prevalence of the mutation in an adult population. *Am J Hum Genet*, **63**, 447–54.

Majamaa, K., Rusanen, H., Remes, A., and Hassinen, I. E., 1997. Metabolic interventions against complex I deficiency in MELAS syndrome. *Mol Cell Biochem*, **174**, 291–6.

Manfredi, G., Schon, E. A., Moraes, C. T., *et al.* 1995. A new mutation associated with MELAS is located in a mitochondrial DNA polypeptide-coding gene. *Neuromuscul Disord*, **5**, 391–8.

Morgan-Hughes, J. A., Sweeney, M. G., Cooper, J. M., *et al.* 1995. Mitochondrial DNA (mtDNA) diseases: correlation of genotype to phenotype. *Biochim Biophys Acta*, **1271**, 135–40.

Nakamura, M., Nakano, S., Goto, Y., *et al.* 1995. A novel point mutation in the mitochondrial tRNA(Ser(UCN)) gene detected in a family with MERRF/MELAS overlap syndrome. *Biochem Biophys Res Commun*, **214**, 86–93.

Nishino, I., Komatsu, M., Kodama, S., Horai, S., Nonaka, I., and Goto, Y., 1996. The 3260 mutation in mitochondrial DNA can cause mitochondrial myopathy, encephalopathy, lactic acidosis, and strokelike episodes (MELAS). *Muscle Nerve*, **19**, 1603–4.

Pavlakis, S. G., Kingsley, P. B., Kaplan, G. P., Stacpoole, P. W., O'Shea, M., and Lustbader, D., 1998. Magnetic resonance spectroscopy: use in monitoring MELAS treatment. *Arch Neurol*, **55**, 849–52.

Pavlakis, S. G., Phillips, P. C., DiMauro, S., De Vivo, D. C., and Rowland, L. P., 1984. Mitochondrial myopathy, encephalopathy, lactic acidosis, and strokelike episodes: a distinctive clinical syndrome. *Ann Neurol*, **16**, 481–8.

Reardon, W., Ross, R. J., Sweeney, M. G., *et al*. 1992. Diabetes mellitus associated with a pathogenic point mutation in mitochondrial DNA. *Lancet*, **340**, 1376–9.

Saitoh, S., Momoi, M. Y., Yamagata, T., Mori, Y., and Imai, M., 1998. Effects of dichloroacetate in three patients with MELAS. *Neurology*, **50**, 531–4.

Santorelli, F. M., Tanji, K., Kulikova, R., *et al*. 1997. Identification of a novel mutation in the mtDNA ND5 gene associated with MELAS. *Biochem Biophys Res Commun*, **238**, 326–8.

Skoglund, R. R., 1979. Reversible alexia, mitochondrial myopathy, and lactic acidemia. *Neurology*, **29**, 717–20.

Sue, C. M., Bruno, C., Andreu, A. L., et al. 1999. Infantile encephalopathy associated with the MELAS A3243G mutation. *J Pediatr*, **134**, 696–700.

Sue, C. M., Crimmins, D. S., Soo, Y. S., *et al*. 1998. Neuroradiological features of six kindreds with MELAS tRNA(Leu) A2343G point mutation: implications for pathogenesis. *J Neurol Neurosurg Psychiatry*, **65**, 233–40.

Sue, C. M., Mitchell, P., Crimmins, D. S., Moshegov, C., Byrne, E., and Morris, J. G., 1997. Pigmentary retinopathy associated with the mitochondrial DNA 3243 point mutation. *Neurology*, **49**, 1013–7.

Tanaka, J., Nagai, T., Arai, H., *et al*. 1997. Treatment of mitochondrial encephalomyopathy with a combination of cytochrome C and vitamins B1 and B2. *Brain Dev*, **19**, 262–7.

Triepels, R. H., van den Heuvel, L. P., Loeffen, J. L., *et al*. 1999. Leigh syndrome associated with a mutation in the NDUFS7 (PSST) nuclear encoded subunit of complex I. *Ann Neurol*, **45**, 787–90.

Uziel, G., Moroni, I., Lamantea, E., *et al*. 1997. Mitochondrial disease associated with the T8993G mutation of the mitochondrial ATPase 6 gene: a clinical, biochemical, and molecular study in six families. *J Neurol Neurosurg Psychiatry*, **63**, 16–22.

Zeviani, M., Muntoni, F., Savarese, N., *et al*. 1993. A MERRF/MELAS overlap syndrome associated with a new point mutation in the mitochondrial DNA tRNA(Lys) gene. *Eur J Hum Genet*, **1**, 80–7.

Zupanc, M. L., Moraes, C. T., Shanske, S., Langman, C. B., Ciafaloni, E., and DiMauro, S., 1991. Deletion of mitochondrial DNA in patients with combined features of Kearns-Sayre and MELAS syndromes. *Ann Neurol*, **29**, 680–3.

25 STURGE-WEBER SYNDROME

E. Steve Roach, Jorge Vidaurre, and Khaled Zamel

Introduction

Sturge-Weber syndrome is characterized by a facial cutaneous nevus (port-wine stain) and a leptomeningeal angioma, often found ipsilateral to the facial lesion. Frequent additional findings include mental retardation, epileptic seizures, contralateral hemiparesis and hemiatrophy, homonymous hemianopia, and glaucoma. However, the clinical features and their severity are quite variable, and patients with the cutaneous nevus and seizures but with normal intelligence and no focal neurologic deficit are common (Uram and Zubillaga, 1982).

The syndrome occurs sporadically, but there is some evidence that somatic mosaicism may play a role in its pathogenesis (Huq *et al.*, 2002). It occurs in all races and has no predilection for either sex. Sturge-Weber syndrome (encephalofacial angiomatosis) remains an enigmatic disorder that is rarely difficult to diagnose, but frequently hard to predict or treat effectively because of the highly variable nature of the clinical manifestations and the lack of effective treatment for some of its more devastating features.

Cutaneous manifestations

The nevus characteristically involves the forehead and upper eyelid, but it commonly affects both sides of the face and may extend onto the trunk and extremities (Figure 25.1). Patients whose nevus involves only the trunk or the maxillary or mandibular area (but not the upper face) have little risk of an intracranial angioma (Enjolras *et al.*, 1985; Tallman *et al.*, 1991; Uram and Zubillaga, 1982). Although the facial angioma is obvious in most children from birth, occasional patients have the characteristic neurologic and radiographic features of Sturge-Weber syndrome without the skin lesion (Crosley and Binet, 1978; Sen *et al.*, 2002). More often, the typical cutaneous angioma is present without any evidence of an intracranial lesion (Morelli, 1999). Even the children with classic Sturge-Weber syndrome usually have normal neurologic function at first, and it is not always easy to identify which neonates have an intracranial angioma.

The leptomeningeal angioma is typically ipsilateral to a unilateral facial nevus, but bilateral brain lesions occur in at least 15% of patients, including some with a unilateral cutaneous nevus (Boltshauser *et al.*, 1976). The extent of the cutaneous lesion correlates poorly with the severity of neurologic impairment (Uram and Zubillaga, 1982), although children with an extensive cutaneous lesion are more likely to have bilateral brain angiomas. Children with bilateral brain lesions have a greater risk of neurologic

impairment and tend to have an earlier onset of seizures (Bebin and Gomez, 1988).

The location of the port-wine nevus of Sturge-Weber syndrome has traditionally been linked to the distribution of the trigeminal nerve branches, but the occurrence of facial and leptomeningeal angiomas can be better explained by the common embryological derivation of these two regions.

Occasionally the port-wine nevus is extensive, involving parts of the trunk and extremities in addition to the face. Patients with extensive cutaneous lesions and limb hypertrophy have been separately classified as displaying Klippel-Trenaunay-Weber syndrome (Meyer, 1979), but if their cutaneous lesion involves the upper face, their neurological picture may be identical to that of Sturge-Weber syndrome.

Ophthalmologic findings

Glaucoma is a common problem in patients with a port-wine nevus near the eye, whether or not they manifest the intracranial disease characteristic of Sturge-Weber syndrome (Chen and Young, 2005; Stevenson *et al.*, 1974). Sullivan *et al.* (1992) found glaucoma in 36 of 51 patients (71%); 26 of these patients developed glaucoma by age 2 years. Buphthalmos and amblyopia are present in some newborns, evidently due to an anomalous anterior chamber angle (Cibis *et al.*, 1984). In other patients, the glaucoma becomes symptomatic later, and untreated leads to progressive blindness (Sujansky and Conradi, 1995a). Therefore, periodic measurement of intraocular pressure is mandatory regardless of the patient's age, particularly when the nevus is near the eye. The intracranial angioma is frequently in the occipital region and, not surprisingly, visual field defects are common.

Neurologic manifestations

Epileptic seizures, mental retardation, and focal neurological deficits are the primary neurologic abnormalities of Sturge-Weber syndrome (Roach and Bodensteiner, 1999). Headache seems to be common as well (Kossoff *et al.*, 2005). Transient neurological deficits in patients with Sturge-Weber syndrome could be related either to seizure activity or to vascular dysfunction. Differentiating postictal changes from vascular deficits can be challenging, and it is likely that the two mechanisms co-exist in many individuals with Sturge-Weber syndrome. Ictal electroencephalography

Uncommon Causes of Stroke, 2nd edition, ed. Louis R. Caplan. Published by Cambridge University Press. © Cambridge University Press 2008.

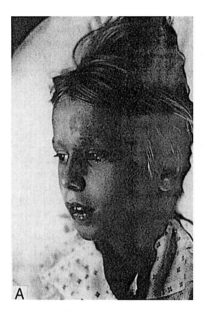 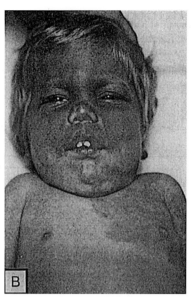

Figure 25.1 A. Classic distribution of the port-wine nevus of Sturge-Weber syndrome on the upper face and eyelid. **B**. Another patient's nevus involved both sides of his face and extends onto the trunk and arm. (From Roach and Riela, 1995, with permission.)

may be helpful in determining the etiology of the episodes (Jansen *et al.*, 2004).

Maria et al. (1998a) describe 119 stroke-like episodes (with either transient or permanent symptoms) in 14 of 20 Sturge-Weber patients. Seizures and hemiparesis typically develop acutely during the first or second year of life, often during a febrile illness. The age when symptoms begin and the overall clinical severity are highly variable, but onset of seizures prior to age 2 tends to increase the likelihood of future mental retardation and refractory epilepsy (Sujansky and Conradi, 1995a). Patients with refractory seizures are much more likely to be mentally retarded, whereas patients who have never had seizures are typically normal (Roach and Bodensteiner, 1999). The age of seizure onset may also correlate with motor function. In one report, children whose epilepsy developed before 1 year of age were more likely to have hemiparesis (Bourgeois *et al.*, 2007). In a series of 52 adults with Sturge-Weber syndrome, 65% had "neurologic deficits" including stroke, hemiparesis, spasticity, and/or weakness (Sujansky and Conradi, 1995b). In another report, 81% of children with Sturge-Weber about to undergo hemispherectomy for intractable epilepsy had hemiparesis contralateral to the planned surgery site (Kossoff *et al.*, 2002), no doubt reflecting an increased willingness to do surgery on children who already have hemiparesis, but perhaps also an indication that frequent seizures could contribute to the weakness.

Intracranial hemorrhage rarely occurs in Sturge-Weber patients. Cushing in 1906 described three patients that he assumed had spontaneous hemorrhage, but all three had acutely developed seizures and weakness, fairly typical of the pattern seen during the initial neurologic deterioration in children without hemorrhage. Even with operative or postmortem examination of the brain in two of these patients, no direct evidence of hemorrhage was found (Cushing, 1906). Anderson and Duncan (1974) presented one adult with subarachnoid hemorrhage attributed to Sturge-Weber syndrome. Microscopic hemorrhages are mentioned in autopsy series but probably have limited clinical significance.

Seizures occur in 72–80% of Sturge-Weber patients with unilateral lesions and in 93% of patients with bihemispheric involvement (Bebin and Gomez, 1988; Oakes, 1992). Focal motor seizures or generalized tonic-clonic seizures are most typical of Sturge-Weber syndrome initially, but infantile spasms, myoclonic seizures, and atonic seizures occur (Chevrie *et al.*, 1988; Miyama and Goto, 2004). The first few seizures are often focal, even in patients who later develop generalized tonic-clonic seizures or infantile spasms. Older children and adults are more likely to have complex partial seizures or focal motor seizures. Some patients continue to have daily seizures after the initial deterioration despite various daily anticonvulsant medications, whereas others have long seizure-free intervals, sometimes even without medication, punctuated by clusters of seizures (Chevrie *et al.*, 1988; Roach and Bodensteiner, 1999).

Hemiparesis often develops acutely in conjunction with the initial flurry of seizure activity. Although often attributed to postictal weakness, hemiparesis may be permanent or persist much longer than the few hours typical of a postictal deficit. Other patients suddenly develop weakness without seizures, either as repeated episodes of weakness similar to transient ischemic attacks or as a single stroke-like episode with persistent deficit (Garcia *et al.*, 1981). Children who develop hemiparesis early in life often have arrested growth in the weak extremities. Other focal neurologic deficits depend on the anatomic site and the extent of the intracranial vascular lesion.

Because the occipital region is frequently involved, visual field deficits are common (Aicardi and Arzimanoglou, 1991). Patients with glaucoma are doubly at risk because they may become amblyopic in one or both eyes from the glaucoma plus they have a superimposed visual field loss from the cortical lesion (Cheng, 1999).

Early development is usually normal, but mental deficiency eventually develops in about half of Sturge-Weber patients (Aicardi and Arzimanoglou, 1991; Uram and Zubillaga, 1982). Only 8% of the patients with bilateral brain involvement are intellectually normal (Bebin and Gomez, 1988). The degree of intellectual impairment ranges from mild to profound. Behavioral abnormalities are often a problem, even in patients who are not mentally retarded.

Mechanisms of neurological deterioration

Neurologic function at birth is typically normal, but most children with Sturge-Weber syndrome eventually develop seizures that are often difficult to control, especially during an acute illness (Roach and Bodensteiner, 1999). Some children undergo saltatory deterioration via a series of discrete episodes of neurologic dysfunction (Garcia et al., 1981), and episodic neurologic deficits can occur even without overt seizure activity (Alexander and Norman, 1960). Although the mechanism of neurologic deterioration in Sturge-Weber patients is debated, several different factors probably contribute. Frequent epileptic seizures surely cause additional impairment in some children, because children with refractory seizures from a variety of other causes also deteriorate. Also important are the extent and location of the vascular lesion in the brain: children with an extensive lesion often have more difficulty controlling seizures and have more intellectual impairment.

Although hemiparesis is often attributed to postictal weakness, in some patients the hemiparesis clearly begins before the onset of seizures. In patients with both hemiparesis and seizures, it is often difficult to be certain which came first. Some patients undergo saltatory deterioration of neurologic function, and others display episodic neurologic dysfunction without obvious seizures. It has been suggested that both of these phenomena result from repeated venous thromboses (Garcia et al., 1981). Perfusion imaging following onset of symptoms demonstrates venous phase impairment in the region of the angioma (Lin et al., 2006), and actual thrombosis of the deep veins can be demonstrated in a few patients (Slasky et al., 2006). Venous thrombosis could also explain the typical first episode of neurologic dysfunction: the clinical picture at the time of the initial deterioration resembles the pattern seen with venous thromboses from other causes. However, a similar pattern of episodic dysfunction without seizures could result from elevated venous pressure without actual thrombosis of the veins.

Abnormal cerebral blood flow in children with Sturge-Weber syndrome was described many years ago, although the exact nature of these vascular abnormalities is still debated (Riela et al., 1985). Chronic hypoxia of the cerebral cortex adjacent to the angioma resulting from reduced blood flow has been postulated, and increased metabolic requirements during seizures could potentiate the oxygen deficit (Aicardi and Arzimanoglou, 1991). A vascular steal phenomenon in the affected areas during seizures, leading to critical ischemia in adjacent areas, was suggested in a recent report using subtraction ictal single photon emission computed tomography (SPECT) coregistered to MRI (Namer et al., 2005). Decreased glucose utilization in the affected cerebral hemisphere was also shown in positron emission tomography (PET) studies. These and similar studies suggest that chronically reduced perfusion could contribute to cerebral hemiatrophy in patients with Sturge-Weber syndrome (Duncan et al., 1995).

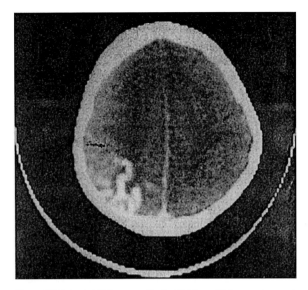

Figure 25.2 Cranial CT from a patient with Sturge-Weber syndrome shows a gyriform pattern of calcification in the parieto-occipital region. (From Garcia et al., 1981, with permission.)

Diagnostic evaluation

Most of the children with facial port-wine nevi do not have an intracranial angioma (Enjolras et al., 1985), and neuroimaging studies and other tests help to distinguish the children with Sturge-Weber syndrome from those with an isolated cutaneous lesion. Neuroimaging, electroencephalography, and functional testing with PET and SPECT may also help to define the extent of the intracranial lesion for possible epilepsy surgery (Chiron et al., 1989; Chugani et al., 1989).

Although gyral calcification is a classic feature of Sturge-Weber syndrome, this "tram track" appearance is not always present (Akpinar, 2004). Bilateral calcification is common (Boltshauser et al., 1976). Calcification often becomes more apparent as the patient becomes older but is sometimes already present at birth (McCaughan et al., 1975; Yeakley et al., 1992). Intracranial calcification can be demonstrated much earlier with computed cranial tomography (Figure 25.2) than with standard skull films.

Cerebral atrophy is more apparent with MRI than with CT (Chamberlain et al., 1989). In addition to cortical atrophy, MRI sometimes demonstrates accelerated myelination in very young Sturge-Weber patients (Jacoby et al., 1987; Maria et al., 1999). MRI with gadolinium (Figure 25.3) effectively demonstrates the abnormal intracranial vessels in Sturge-Weber patients (Benedikt et al., 1993); currently this is the best test to determine intracranial involvement. In children with suspected Sturge-Weber syndrome but no MRI evidence of abnormal vascular contrast enhancement, three-dimensional time-of-flight magnetic resonance venography may increase the chances of detecting the leptomeningeal angioma (Juhasz and Chugani, 2007). Dynamic magnetic resonance perfusion studies in individuals with Sturge-Weber syndrome suggest that hypoperfusion is predominantly from impaired venous drainage but that the most severely affected regions sometimes also show arterial perfusion deficiency (Lin et al., 2006).

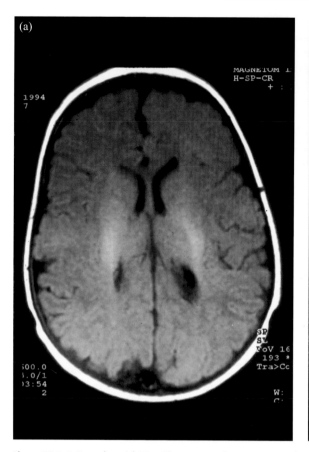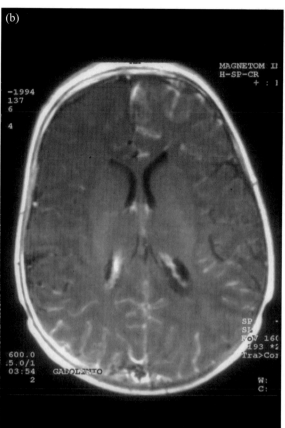

Figure 25.3 **A**. Normal cranial MRI without contrast from a patient with Sturge-Weber syndrome. **B**. After the addition of gadolinium contrast, abnormal veins in the left frontal and bilateral posterior areas become apparent along with a right leptomeningeal lesion.

Functional imaging with PET indicates reduced brain glucose utilization adjacent to the leptomeningeal lesion but often extending beyond the area of abnormality depicted by CT or MRI (Chugani *et al.*, 1989; Maria *et al.*, 1999). Glucose utilization tends to be reduced after the first year of life (Chugani *et al.*, 1989), although PET activation studies suggest that these abnormal areas retain some functional responsiveness (Muller *et al.*, 1997). SPECT typically shows reduced cerebral perfusion even in regions of the brain with normal glucose uptake (Chiron *et al.*, 1989; Maria *et al.*, 1998b). As with PET, the area with abnormal perfusion shown with SPECT is often more extensive than the abnormality seen with CT or MRI (Chiron *et al.*, 1989; Griffiths *et al.*, 1997; Maria *et al.*, 1998b).

Cerebral arteriography is no longer routinely required for the evaluation of Sturge-Weber syndrome, but it may be helpful in atypical patients or prior to surgery for epilepsy. The veins are typically more abnormal than the arteries (Probst, 1980). Occasional patients have evidence of arterial occlusion, and the homogeneous blush of the intracranial angioma is sometimes present (Poser and Taveras, 1957). The superficial cortical veins are reduced in number (Figure 25.4), and the deep draining veins are dilated and tortuous (Farrell *et al.*, 1992).

Failure of the sagittal sinus to opacify after ipsilateral carotid injection may be secondary to thrombosis of the superficial cortical veins (Bentson *et al.*, 1971), and the abnormal deep venous

channels probably have a similar origin as they form collateral conduits for nonfunctioning cortical veins (Probst, 1980).

Pathology

The parietal and occipital lobes are affected more often than the frontal lobes. The leptomeninges are thickened and discolored by increased vascularity. Angiomatous vessels may obliterate the subarachnoid space, and the tortuous deep-draining veins that are seen radiographically can also be seen in pathologic specimens (Wohlwill and Yakovlev, 1957). Microscopically these vessels are primarily thin-walled veins of variable size (Di Trapani *et al.*, 1982; Wohlwill and Yakovlev. 1957). Angiomatous vessels sometimes extend into the superficial brain parenchyma, and the ipsilateral choroid plexus is often involved. Microscopic abnormalities are frequently found in normal looking areas adjacent to the visible malformation, and some vessels are narrowed or occluded by progressive hyalinization and subendothelial proliferation (Norman and Schoene, 1977; Wohlwill and Yakovlev, 1957).

Cerebral atrophy adjacent to the angioma is typical. In some patients, the atrophy becomes progressively more severe in early childhood before eventually stabilizing. Other children, particularly those with mild clinical features, may not develop visible

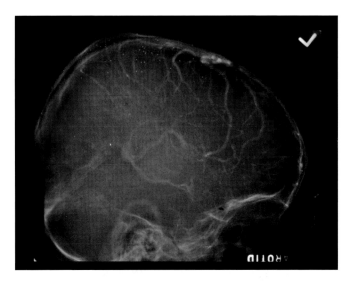

Figure 25.4 Venous phase of the left internal carotid angiogram of a patient with Sturge-Weber syndrome. Note the paucity of superficial cortical veins posteriorly and the prominent deep venous system. (From Garcia et al., 1981, with permission.)

atrophy at all. Microscopic features include neuronal loss and gliosis, which, like angioma itself, usually extends beyond the area of obvious abnormality.

The typical gyriform calcification results from deposition of calcium within the outer cortical layers (Di Trapani et al., 1982; Wohlwill and Yakovlev, 1957). Norman and Schoene (1977) found that the foci of calcium typically lie adjacent to a blood vessel, and Di Trapani et al. (1982) believe that the calcium is deposited in an intravascular mucopolysaccharide substance before shifting into the brain parenchyma adjacent to the vessel. Chronic venous stasis with anoxic damage of the nearby cortex has been postulated as the mechanism for inducing cortical calcifications.

It has been suggested that vascular lesions found in Sturge-Weber are not static lesions, but constitute dynamic structures. Immunohistochemical analyses have demonstrated elevated nuclear hypoxia-inducible factor (HIF) protein level in the abnormal vessels. HIF is known to induce vascular endothelial growth factor (VEGF) (Comati et al., 2007).

Treatment

Treatment of Sturge-Weber syndrome is problematic. The syndrome is rare and its manifestations so variable that controlled trials to evaluate therapy are difficult. The majority of patients with Sturge-Weber syndrome at some point develop seizures, and seizure control can markedly improve their quality of life. Careful attention to dosing schedules and periodic monitoring of serum anticonvulsant levels help to ensure the best possible control of seizures. Complete seizure control with medication is possible in some patients. Ville et al. (2002) advocate starting antiepileptic medications even before the onset of seizures, an intriguing approach that requires further study.

Hemispherectomy sometimes improves seizure control and may promote more normal intellectual development

(Ogunmekan et al., 1989). There is still debate about the role of epilepsy surgery for Sturge-Weber syndrome. Some physicians recommend limiting resective surgery to patients whose seizures fail to respond to an adequate trial of anticonvulsants, much the same approach that is applied to other children with epilepsy (Roach et al., 1994). Others suggest a more aggressive approach based on the premise that early resection of the vascular lesion allows better development (Lee et al., 2001). Nevertheless, most physicians are uncomfortable recommending surgery for a patient who has not yet developed seizures or for one whose seizures are fully controlled with medication, and there is also understandable reluctance to resect a still functional portion of the brain and cause a deficit (Arzimanoglou and Aicardi, 1992; Bruce, 1999). Thus surgery is often reserved for individuals with severe refractory seizures who already have clinical dysfunction of the area to be removed (e.g. hemiparesis or hemianopia). Although bilateral brain involvement may make it difficult to identify a single epileptic focus, successful surgery still can be done in some individuals with bilateral disease (Tuxhorn et al., 2002).

Patients with less extensive lesions should have a limited resection (rather than a complete hemispherectomy) that preserves as much normal brain as possible (Aicardi and Arzimanoglou, 1991; Bye et al., 1989), and corpus callosum section may be a useful alternative for some patients (Rappaport, 1988).

Daily aspirin has been tried in an effort to prevent recurrent vascular thrombosis that may cause neurologic deterioration (Garcia et al., 1981; McCaughan et al., 1975). One more recent study suggested that low-dose aspirin (2 mg/kg/day) may reduce the frequency of stroke-like episodes with Sturge-Weber syndrome (Maria et al., 1998a). Controlled studies with aspirin present the same difficulties as with hemispherectomy, and until more information is available, routine use of aspirin can not be enthusiastically endorsed. It is reasonable to use aspirin in individuals with repeated clinical episodes suggesting transient ischemic attacks (Cambon et al., 1987; Garcia et al., 1981) or for patients with bihemispheric disease for whom surgery is not a reasonable option. Low-dose daily aspirin seems to be well tolerated in children, although the optimum dose has not been established.

Periodic monitoring of intraocular pressure is an important aspect of management that is easily overlooked in patients who have no initial ocular findings. Glaucoma may be present at birth, or symptoms may arise later. Occasionally patients develop glaucoma only after several years, so yearly ophthalmologic examination with intraocular pressure measurement is recommended. Patients who develop ocular pain or visual symptoms should be promptly re-evaluated.

The patient's appearance can be dramatically improved by pulsed-dye laser treatment, although it is not often possible to completely obliterate the lesion (Nguyen et al., 1998). Early treatment is preferable because the skin lesions tend to hypertrophy with time and thereafter require more extensive treatment (Morelli, 1999). Pulsed-dye laser treatment of port-wine lesions has been reviewed in detail (Morelli, 1999). Some physicians reserve cosmetic procedures for those patients with reasonably good neurological function.

REFERENCES

Aicardi, J., and Arzimanoglou, A. 1991. Sturge-Weber syndrome. *Int Pediatr*, **6**, 129–34.

Akpinar, E. 2004. The tram-track sign: cortical calcifications. *Radiology*, **231**, 515–6.

Alexander, G. L., and Norman, R. M. 1960. *Sturge-Weber Syndrome*. Bristol: John Wright and Sons Ltd.

Anderson, F. H., and Duncan, G. W. 1974. Sturge-Weber disease with subarachnoid hemorrhage. *Stroke*, **5**, 509–11.

Arzimanoglou, A., and Aicardi, J. 1992. The epilepsy of Sturge-Weber syndrome: clinical features and treatment in 23 patients. *Acta Neurol Scand (Suppl)*, **140**, 18–22.

Bebin, E. M., and Gomez, M. R. 1988. Prognosis in Sturge-Weber disease: comparison of unihemispheric and bihemispheric involvement. *J Child Neurol*, **3**, 181–4.

Benedikt, R. A., Brown, D. C., Walker, R., Ghaed, V. N., Mitchell, M., and Geyer, C. A. 1993. Sturge-Weber syndrome: cranial MR imaging with Gd-DTPA. *AJNR Am J Neuroradiol*, **14**, 409–15.

Bentson, J. R., Wilson, G. H., and Newton, T. H. 1971. Cerebral venous drainage pattern of the Sturge-Weber syndrome. *Radiology*, **101**, 111–8.

Boltshauser, E., Wilson, J., and Hoare, R. D. 1976. Sturge-Weber syndrome with bilateral intracranial calcification. *J Neurol Neurosurg Psychiatr*, **39**, 429–35.

Bourgeois, M., Crimmins, D. W., De Oliveira, R. S., *et al.* 2007. Surgical treatment of epilepsy in Sturge-Weber syndrome in children. *J Neurosurg*, **106**, 20–8.

Bruce, D. A. 1999. Neurosurgical aspects of Sturge-Weber syndrome. In *Sturge-Weber Syndrome*. eds. J. B. Bodensteiner, and E. S. Roach. Mt. Freedom, NJ: Sturge-Weber Foundation, pp. 39–42.

Bye, A. M., Matheson, J. M., and Mackenzie, R. A. 1989. Epilepsy surgery in Sturge-Weber syndrome. *Aust N Z J Ophthalmol*, **25**, 103–5.

Cambon, H., Truelle, J. L., Baron, J. C., Chiras, J., Tran Dinh, S., and Chatel, M. 1987. Focal chronic ischemia and concomitant migraine: an atypical form of Sturge-Weber angiomatosis? *Rev Neurol*, **143**, 588–94.

Chamberlain, M. C., Press, G. A., and Hesselink, J. R. 1989. MR imaging and CT in three cases of Sturge-Weber syndrome: prospective comparison. *Am J Neuroradiol*, **10**, 491–6.

Chen, T. C., and Young, L. H. 2005. Sturge-Weber syndrome (choroidal hemangioma and glaucoma). *J Pediatr Ophthalmol Strabismus*, **42**, 320.

Cheng, K. P. 1999. Ophthalmologic manifestations of Sturge-Weber syndrome. In *Sturge-Weber Syndrome*. eds. J. B. Bodensteiner, and E. S. Roach. Mt. Freedom, NJ: Sturge-Weber Foundation, pp. 17–26.

Chevrie, J. J., Specola, N., and Aicardi, J. 1988. Secondary bilateral synchrony in unilateral pial angiomatosis: successful surgical management. *J Neurol Neurosurg Psychiatr*, **15**, 95–8.

Chiron, C., Raynaud, C., Tzourio, N., *et al.* 1989. Regional cerebral blood flow by SPECT imaging in Sturge-Weber disease: an aid for diagnosis. *J Neurol Neurosurg Psychiatr*, **52**, 1402–9.

Chugani, H. T., Mazziotta, J. C., and Phelps, M. E. 1989. Sturge-Weber syndrome: a study of cerebral glucose utilization with positron emission tomography. *J Pediatr*, **114**, 244–53.

Cibis, G. W., Tripathi, R. C., and Tripathi, B. J. 1984. Glaucoma in Sturge-Weber syndrome. *Ophthalmology*, **91**, 1061–71.

Comati, A., Beck, H., Halliday, W., Snipes, G. J, Plate, K. H., and Acker, T. 2007. Upregulation of hypoxia- inducible factor (HIF)-1 alpha and HIF-2 alpha in leptomeningeal vascular malformations of Sturge-Weber syndrome. *J Neuropathol Exp Neurol*, **66**, 86–97.

Crosley, C. J., and Binet, E. F. 1978. Sturge-Weber Syndrome–presentation as a focal seizure disorder without nevus flammeus. *Clin Pediatr*, **17**, 606–9.

Cushing, H. 1906. Cases of spontaneous intracranial hemorrhage associated with trigeminal nevi. *JAMA*, **47**, 178–83.

Di Trapani, G., Di Rocco, C., Abbamondi, A. L., Caldarelli, M., and Pocchiari, M. 1982. Light microscopy and ultrastructural studies of Sturge-Weber disease. *Brain*, **9**, 23–36.

Duncan, D. B., Herholz, K., Pietrzk, U., and Heiss, W. D. 1995. Regional cerebral blood flow and metabolism in Sturge-Weber disease. *Clin Nucl Med*, **20**, 522–3.

Enjolras, O., Riche, M. C., and Merland, J. J. 1985. Facial port-wine stains and Sturge-Weber syndrome. *Pediatrics*, **76**, 48–51.

Farrell, M. A., Derosa, M. J., Curran, J. G., *et al.* 1992. Neuropathologic findings in cortical resections (including hemispherectomies) performed for the treatment of intractable childhood epilepsy. *Acta Neuropathol*, **83**, 246–59.

Garcia, J. C., Roach, E. S., and Mclean, W. T. 1981. Recurrent thrombotic deterioration in the Sturge-Weber syndrome. *Child's Brain*, **8**, 427–33.

Griffiths, P. D., Boodram, M. B., Blaser, S., Armstrong, D., Gilday, D. L., and Harwood-Nash, D. 1997. 99mTechnetium HMPAO imaging in children with the Sturge-Weber syndrome: a study of nine cases with CT and MRI correlation. *Neuroradiology*, **39**, 219–24.

Huq, A. H., Chugani, D. C., Hukku B., and Serajee, F. J. 2002 Evidence of somatic mosaicism in Sturge-Weber syndrome. *Neurology*, **59**, 780–2.

Jacoby, C. G., Yuh, W. T., Afifi, A. K., Bell, W. E., Schelper, R. L., and Sato, Y. 1987. Accelerated myelination in early Sturge-Weber syndrome demonstrated by MR imaging. *J Comput Assist Tomogr*, **11**, 226–31.

Jansen, F. E., Van Der Worp, H. B., and Van Huffelen, A. 2004. Sturge-Weber syndrome and paroxysmal hemiparesis: epilepsy or ischaemia? *Dev Med Child Neurol*, **46**, 783–6.

Juhasz, C., and Chugani, H. T. 2007. An almost missed leptomeningeal angioma in Sturge-Weber syndrome. *Neurology*, **68**, 243.

Kossoff, E., Buck, C., and Freeman, J. 2002. Outcomes of 32 hemispherectomies for Sturge-Weber syndrome worldwide. *Neurology*, **59**, 1735–8.

Kossoff, E. H., Hatfield, L. A., Ball, K. L., and Comi, A. M. 2005. Comorbidity of epilepsy and headache in patients with Sturge-Weber syndrome. *J Child Neurol*, **20**, 678–82.

Lee, J. S., Asano, E., Muzik, O., *et al.* 2001. Sturge-Weber syndrome: correlation between clinical course and FDG PET findings. *Neurology*, **57**, 189–95.

Lin, D. D., Barker, P. B., Hatfield, L. A., and Comi, A. M. 2006. Dynamic MR perfusion and proton MR spectroscopic imaging in Sturge-Weber syndrome: correlation with neurological symptoms. *J Magn Reson Imaging*, **24**, 274–81.

Maria, B. L., Neufeld, J. A., Rosainz, L. C., *et al.* 1998a. Central nervous system structure and function in Sturge-Weber syndrome: evidence of neurologic and radiologic progression. *J Child Neurol*, **13**, 606–18.

Maria, B. L., Hoang, K. N., Robertson, R. L., Barnes, P. D., Drane, W. E., and Chugani, H. T. 1999. Imaging brain structure and function in Sturge-Weber syndrome. In *Sturge-Weber Syndrome*. eds. J. B. Bodensteiner, and E. S. Roach. Mt. Freedom, NJ: Sturge-Weber Foundation, pp. 43–69.

Maria, B. L., Neufeld, J. A., Rosainz, L. C., *et al.* 1998b. High prevalence of bihemispheric structural and functional defects in Sturge-Weber syndrome. *J Child Neurol*, **13**, 595–605.

McCaughan, R. A., Ouvrier, R. A., De Silva, K., and McLaughlin, A. 1975. The value of the brain scan and cerebral arteriogram in the Sturge-Weber syndrome. *Proc Aust Assoc Neurol*, **12**, 185–90.

Meyer, E. 1979. Neurocutaneous syndrome with excessive macrohydrocephalus (Sturge-Weber/Klippel-Trenaunay syndrome). *Neuropadiatrie*, **10**, 67–75.

Miyama, S., and Goto, T. 2004. Leptomeningeal angiomatosis with infantile spasms. *Pediatr Neurol*, **31**, 353–6.

Morelli, J. G. 1999. Port-wine stains and the Sturge-Weber syndrome. In *Sturge-Weber Syndrome*. eds. J. B. Bodensteiner, and E. S. Roach. Mt. Freedom, NJ: Sturge-Weber Foundation, pp. 11–6.

Muller, R. A., Chugani, H. T., Muzik, O., Rothermel, R. D., and Chakraborty, P. K. 1997. Language and motor functions activate calcified hemisphere in patients with Sturge-Weber syndrome: a positron emission tomography study. *J Child Neurol*, **12**, 431–7.

Namer, I. J., Battaglia, F., Hirsch, E., Constantinesco, A., and Marescaux, C. 2005. Subtraction ictal SPECT co-registered to MRI (SISCOM) in Sturge-Weber syndrome. *Clin Nucl Med*, **30**, 39–40.

Nguyen, C. M., Yohn, J. J., Huff, C., Weston, W. L., and Morelli, J. G. 1998. Facial port wine stains in childhood: prediction of the rate of improvement as a function of the age of the patient, size and location of the port wine stain and the number of treatments with the pulsed dye (585 nm) laser. *Br J Dermatol*, **138**, 821–5.

Norman, M. G., and Schoene, W. C. 1977. The ultrastructure of Sturge-Weber disease. *Acta Neuropathol*, **37**, 199–205.

Oakes, W. J. 1992. The natural history of patients with the Sturge-Weber syndrome. *Pediatr Neurosurg*, **18**, 287–90.

Ogunmekan, A. O., Hwang, P. A., and Hoffman, H. J. 1989. Sturge-Weber-Dimitri disease: role of hemispherectomy in prognosis. *Can J Neurol Sci*, **16**, 78–80.

Poser, C. M., and Taveras, J. M. 1957. Cerebral angiography in encephalo-trigeminal angiomatosis. *Radiology*, **68**, 327–36.

Probst, F. P. 1980. Vascular morphology and angiographic flow patterns in Sturge-Weber angiomatosis. *Neuroradiology*, **20**, 73–8.

Rappaport, Z. H. 1988. Corpus callosum section in the treatment of intractable seizures in the Sturge-Weber syndrome. *Child's Nerv Syst*, **4**, 231–2.

Riela, A. R., Stump, D. A., Roach, E. S., McLean, W. T., and Garcia, J. C. 1985. Regional cerebral blood flow characteristics of the Sturge-Weber syndrome. *Pediatr Neurol*, **1**, 85–90.

Roach, E. S., and Bodensteiner, J. B. 1999. Neurologic manifestations of Sturge-Weber syndrome. In *Sturge-Weber Syndrome*. eds. J. B. Bodensteiner, and E. S. Roach. Mt. Freedom, NJ: Sturge-Weber Foundation, pp. 27–38.

Roach, E. S., and Riela, A. R. 1995. *Pediatric Cerebrovascular Disorders*. New York: Futura.

Roach, E. S., Riela, A. R., Chugani, H. T., Shinnar, S., Bodensteiner, J. B., and Freeman, J. 1994. Sturge-Weber syndrome: recommendations for surgery. *J Child Neurol*, **9**, 190–3.

Sen, Y., Dilber, E., Odemis, E., Ahmetogly, A., and Aynaci, F. M. 2002. Sturge-Weber syndrome in a 14-year-old girl without facial naevus. *Eur J Pediatr*, **161**, 505–6.

Slasky, S. E., Shinnar, S., and Bello, J. A. 2006 Sturge-Weber syndrome: deep venous occlusion and the radiologic spectrum. *Pediatr Neurol*, **35**, 343–7.

Stevenson, R. F. 1974. Unrecognized ocular problems associated with port-wine stain of the face in children. *Can Med Assoc J*, **111**, 953–4.

Sujansky, E., and Conradi, S. 1995a. Sturge-Weber syndrome: age of onset of seizures and glaucoma in the prognosis for affected children. *J Child Neurol*, **10**, 49–58.

Sujansky, E., and Conradi, S. 1995b. Outcome of Sturge-Weber syndrome in 52 adults. *Am J Med Genet*, **57**, 35–45.

Sullivan, J., Clarke, M. P., and Morin, J. D. 1992. The ocular manifestations of the Sturge-Weber syndrome. *J Pediatr Ophthalmol Strabismus*, **29**, 349–56.

Tallman, B., Tan, O. T., Morelli, J. G., *et al.* 1991. Location of port-wine stains and the likelihood of ophthalmic and/or central nervous system complications. *Pediatrics*, **87**, 323–7.

Tuxhorn, I. E., and Pannek, H. W. 2002. Epilepsy surgery in bilateral Sturge-Weber syndrome. *Pediatr Neurol*, **26**, 394–7.

Uram, M., and Zubillaga, C. 1982. The cutaneous manifestations of Sturge-Weber syndrome. *J Clin Neuroophthalmol*, **2**, 245–8.

Ville, D., Enjolras, O., Chiron, C., and Dulac, O. 2002. Prophylactic antiepileptic treatment in Sturge-Weber disease. *Seizure*, **11**, 145–50.

Wohlwill, F. J., and Yakovlev, P. I. 1957. Histopathology of meningo-facial angiomatosis (Sturge-Weber's disease). *J Neuropathol Exp Neurol*, **16**, 341–64.

Yeakley, J. W., Woodside, M., and Fenstermacher, M. J. 1992. Bilateral neonatal Sturge-Weber-Dimitri disease: CT and MR findings. *Am J Neuroradiol*, **13**, 1179–82.

Introduction

Von Hippel-Lindau (VHL) disease is an autosomal dominant disorder with a 95% penetrance at age 60 years and incomplete expression (Latif *et al.*, 1993) that is characterized by the development of various benign and malignant tumors and cysts. The major tumors and cysts are hemangioblastoma (HB) in the central nervous system (CNS), retinal hemangioblastoma (RA), pheochromocytoma (Pheo), renal cell carcinoma (RCC), renal cyst, pancreatic cystadenoma, and pancreatic neuroendocrine tumors.

HB, the most characteristic CNS lesions, are highly vascular tumors comprising approximately 3% of all tumors of the CNS (Neumann *et al.*, 1989). The familial forms comprise anywhere from 5.3% to 11.8% of cases according to the literature (Couch *et al.*, 2000; Huson *et al.*, 1986; Resche *et al.*, 1993). They occur predominantly in the cerebellum and spinal cord, but they have been found throughout the CNS. The tumors also occur as a sporadic entity (Richard *et al.*, 1994). Because of their vascular nature, these tumors harbor a risk of hemorrhage that can occur spontaneously, intraoperatively, or postoperatively. Although intracranial hemorrhage is confined to small series and case reports, it forms an important part of the subject matter of this chapter. To our knowledge, there are no reported cases or series of acute brain ischemia as a direct complication of VHL.

Historically, the first case of HB was described at autopsy in 1872 by Hughlings Jackson. Von Hippel first described an RA in 1904; subsequently, the association of visceral and cerebral lesions with RAs was observed in 1926 by Lindau (Rengachary, 1985). The term "hemangioblastoma" was coined by Bailey and Cushing in 1928 to delineate all vascular tumors of the CNS and to differentiate from primary vascular malformations. Contentious issues regarding HBs include uncertain histogenesis, factors predictive of tumor recurrence, factors predictive of multifocal disease, and cumulative morbidity of central and retinal lesions are under investigation.

Genetics

The VHL tumor suppressor gene, which is located on chromosome 3p25–26, is responsible for this disease (Humphrey *et al.*, 1996; Kaelin *et al.*, 1998). The VHL gene was identified by Zbar *et al.* (1996) by positional cloning, and the authors then identified the germline mutations in the VHL. Following identification of the VHL gene, there was remarkable progress in molecular genetics and molecular diagnosis of VHL disease and also in the understanding of the molecular basis of the pathogenesis of VHL-associated disorders. The major cause underlying the development of the disease is inactivation of the VHL tumor suppressor protein and subsequent loss of the function of the VHL protein, and Elongin B, C (VBC) complex (Kaelin, 2002; Stolle *et al.*, 1998). This results in dysfunction of the ubiquitination of hypoxia-inducible factors (HIF) and other proteins for the VBC complex. The failure in the degradation of HIFs is an important step in the development of highly vascular tumors. The highly vascular nature of tumors may be explained by the fact that, under normal conditions, the VHL gene product (pVHL) negatively regulates the hypoxia-inducible messenger RNA (mRNA) encoding vascular endothelial growth factor (VEGF) (Wizigmann-Voos *et al.*, 1995). Loss of pVHL leads to an inappropriate accumulation of this mRNA and results in dramatic upregulation of VEGF in stromal cells and its corresponding receptors VEGFR-1 and VEGFR-2 in tumor endothelial cells (Wizigmann-Voos *et al.*, 1995). It is thought that this signaling pathway plays a crucial role in the angiogenesis and cyst formation of these tumors (Figure 26.1). In addition, the pVHL is a protein that plays a role in regulating extracellular matrix formation and regulating the ability of cells to exit the cell cycle.

Clinical classification of VHL disease

VHL was clinically classified into two types of diseases – with or without Pheo – in the initial classification of this disease. Those without Pheo are categorized as VHL type 1 disease. Those with Pheo are categorized as VHL type 2 disease. VHL type 2 disease is further classified into three categories: type 2A, type 2B, and type 2C (Couch *et al.*, 2000; Shuin *et al.*, 2006). Type 2A VHL has Pheo with other HBs in the CNS, but not with RCC. Type 2B has Pheo, RCCs, and other CNS tumors. A recent notion is that type 2C disease has only Pheo, with no other disease. Only a few mutations for VHL type 2C have been identified. A low risk of RCC and neuroendocrine pancreatic tumor is associated with type 2A and a high risk with type 2B (Linehan *et al.*, 1995). In addition, some individuals who have the same type present with a life-threatening disease with multiple tumors and considerable reduction of life span, whereas other patients have only a few manifestations of

VHL Mutation → Altered VHL protein and Elongin B,C complex → Altered degradation of HIF→ ↑VEGF,↑ VEGFR1,↑VEGFR2 → Development of highly vascular tumor

Figure 26.1 Schematic illustration of the pathogenesis of VHL disease.

Uncommon Causes of Stroke, 2nd edition, ed. Louis R. Caplan. Published by Cambridge University Press. © Cambridge University Press 2008.

the disease with no impairment of quality of life. Chuvash poly-cythemia is a rare type of the disease that is caused by VHL gene inactivation at a specific point of the VHL protein, and does not result in a tumor, but rather in polycythemia (Ang *et al.*, 2002).

Clinical criteria for the diagnosis of VHL disease

The following criteria are used for the diagnosis of VHL disease (Richard *et al.*, 2000; Shuin *et al.*, 2006):

1. Patients with a positive family history of VHL disease who develop HBs in the CNS or RAs, RCC, Pheo, pancreatic tumors or cysts, or epididymal cystadenoma. However, epididymal cystadenomas alone are not considered a diagnostic criterion because of their high incidence in the general population

2. Patients without a family history of VHL disease, but who develop HBs or RAs in combination with other tumors, such as RCC, Pheo, pancreatic tumors or cysts, or epididymal cystadenoma

In the majority of VHL disease-affected patients (80%), there is a demonstrative multigenerational family history, and only one of the manifestations of the disease is necessary for the clinical diag-nosis (Horton *et al.*, 1976; Zbar *et al.*, 1996). There is, however, a considerable intrafamilial and interfamilial phenotypic variability in disease presentation (Green, 1986; Lamiell *et al.*, 1989; Maddock *et al.*, 1996; Maher *et al.*, 1990; Richard *et al.*, 1998). In isolated "cryptic" cases (20% of cases), possibly indicating a de novo muta-tion, two manifestations, including one CNS or RA, are required for diagnosis (Hes *et al.*, 2000).

Genetic testing for VHL disease

Once diagnosed, an investigation to identify the mutation in the VHL gene can benefit family members. If the proband's mutation can be identified, its presence or absence in family members at risk can then define his or her status. Genetic testing for muta-tions in the VHL gene requires complete sequencing of the coding regions, Southern blot analysis, and fluorescence *in situ* hybridiza-tion (FISH), which has proved 70% sensitivity in the laboratory (Shuin *et al.*, 2006).

Clinical presentation

Isolated HBs in the CNS develop from childhood at an age <10 years or early in the teens until the age of 30 years In VHL dis-ease, HB presents in early adulthood (ages 20–40 years). It devel-ops as type 1 or type 2A VHL disease in 70% of VHL patients. According to a Japanese series, the mean age of patients with germline mutations suggestive of VHL disease did not differ from that of the general group (Shuin *et al.*, 2006). Overall, men are more commonly affected with HB, with a male-to-female ratio of 1.5:1.

The most common sites for HB development are the cerebellum (83%–95%), spinal cord (3.2–13%), and medulla oblongata (2.1%). Multiple spinal HBs in VHL disease have also been described (Boker *et al.*, 1984). The symptoms of this disease are largely explained by the expansion of the tumor in the cranial space or

the spinal cord. With posterior fossa HB, headache is the most common presenting symptom. Associated vomiting when present suggests raised intracranial pressure. Other symptoms are ataxia and gait disturbance (Round Table: Infratentorial Hemangioblas-tomas, 1985; Constans *et al.*, 1986). Rare symptoms include abnor-mal head attitudes and the so called cerebellar "fits" characterized by drop attacks with or without deterioration of consciousness, opisthotonic posturing, and varying degrees of respiratory com-promise. In one series, an abnormal neurological examination was found in 87.7% of cases (Huson *et al.*, 1986). Polycythemia with overproduction of erythropoietin is associated with a high level of HIFs in tumors.

In general, HBs accompanying VHL disease account for 5%–30% of cerebellar HBs and 80% of spinal HBs, indicating that HBs in VHL disease tend to originate in more unusual regions of the CNS (Sora *et al.*, 2001). In contrast, some data showed that patients in whom a germline mutation was evidenced may harbor a solitary cerebellar lesion (Shuin *et al.*, 2006). Totally asymptomatic VHL gene carriers are estimated at approximately 4% (Neumann *et al.*, 1989).

The proportion of primary symptomatic HBs associated with VHL disease is estimated at 10%–40%, and in approximately 40% of patients with VHL, HB is the first manifestation of the disease (Sora *et al.*, 2001). The true proportion of HB associated with VHL dis-ease, in any case, seems to be underestimated, given the fact that molecular genetic analysis was not performed in all patients with CNS HB without evidence of family history or other VHL disease-related lesions.

Diagnostic investigations

Detailed investigation starts with a thorough physical examina-tion bearing in mind all potential manifestations of VHL disease. In addition to neurological examination including fundoscopy, abdominal and genital examination are most pertinent. Labo-ratory investigation should include red cell count, hemoglobin, hematocrit, serum epinephrine and norepinephrine, and a 24-hour urinary analysis for vanillylmandelic acid and catecholamine levels.

HBs are diagnosed by MRI of the brain and the spinal cord (Figure 26.2). The MRI is the examination of choice for diagno-sis. MRI of the entire neuraxis should be performed for all patients with the diagnosis of an HB to rule out multiple hemangiomas. MRI is recommended at least once a year for patients older than 10 years with VHL. HBs have a typical appearance of an extraor-dinarily bright-enhancing, well-circumscribed mass often associ-ated with a cyst. Cystic lesions appear hypointense on T1-weighted and hyperintense in T2-weighted images with minimal edema and a mural nodule that enhances intensely with intravenous gadolin-ium. Solid HBs typically enhance homogenously with gadolinium. Vascular flow voids of prominent vessels may also be seen. Dif-ferential diagnoses of a typical single lesion on MRI are pilocytic astrocytoma (children), pleomorphic astrocytoma (uncommon in post fossa), or metastasis (rarely with cyst). Cerebral CT typi-cally shows a hypodense cyst with an isodense, noncalcified mural nodule on the part of the cyst closest to a pial surface and has a

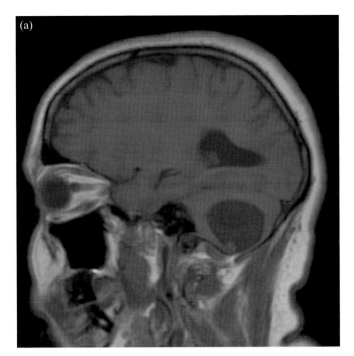
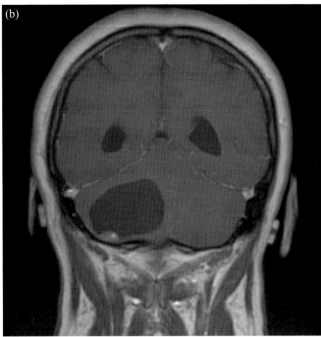

Figure 26.2 a. Non-enhanced sagittal MRI shows a cystic lesion in the posterior fossa compatible with HB. **b**. Coronal MRI with gadolinium depicts the bright nodular enhancement associated with the large cystic component, as a typical feature of posterior fossa HB. (Courtesy of Professor P. Maeder, Department of Radiology, Centre Hospitalier Universitaire Vaudois, Lausanne.)

complementary nature in the diagnosis of posterior fossa HBs, especially in cases with hemorrhage (Cornell *et al.*, 1979; Zimmerman *et al.*, 1980).

Before the introduction of MRI, angiography was essential to establish the diagnosis of HB (Di Chiro *et al.*, 1982; Kitaoka *et al.*, 1981). With increasing MRI experience, the indication for angiography has become increasingly debatable; angiography is an invasive investigation, can result in some complications, and its clinical utility is ambiguous (Heiserman *et al.*, 1994; Willinsky *et al.*, 2003). Conventional digital subtraction angiography should be used very selectively (not for diagnostic but for preoperative management of cases with very large and solid HB). Figure 26.3 shows in detail the large vascular pedicle that may be of mixed pial dural origin and often an early draining vein indicating AV shunting. Large solid HBs with high flow may mimic arteriovenous malformations. Note that the radiological absence of a typical cystic component raises the real possibility of a metastatic RCC in view of the known association of these lesions; however, the two can be readily differentiated histologically. The radiological work-up for extra CNS lesions are discussed elsewhere (Levine *et al.*, 1982).

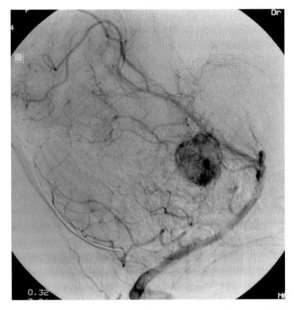

Figure 26.3 Selective lateral vertebral angiography showing a highly vascular mass typical of HB. (Courtesy of Professor P. Maeder, Department of Radiology, Centre Hospitalier Universitaire Vaudois, Lausanne.)

Proposal for apparently sporadic CNS HB

Patients in whom a sporadic CNS HB is detected should undergo a screening protocol: ophthalmological examination, blood work and urinary catecholamine evaluation, whole neuraxis MRI, abdominal ultrasound or CT, and an interview with a geneticist. If there is a negative pedigree analysis and absence of clinical and radiological evidence of VHL disease, they might undergo a DNA analysis if they give informed consent. If the DNA analysis is not affected, there is no need for periodic monitoring. If affected, the patient should have periodic monitoring (neuraxis MRI, abdominal ultrasound, and ophthalmic examination every year), and family members should have a DNA analysis. If their DNA is also affected, they should be screened for VHL and monitored periodically.

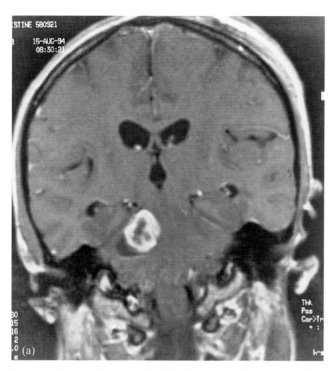 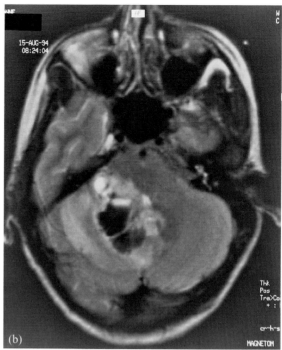

Figure 26.4 T1-weighted coronal MRI (**a**) showing a markedly enhancing lesion in the right superior cerebellar peduncle that presented with vermian and subarachnoid hemorrhage. Note also the associated cyst suggestive of HB. T2-weighted axial MRI (**b**) showing the typical finding of an acute hemorrhage. (Courtesy of Professor P. Maeder, Department of Radiology, Centre Hospitalier Universitaire Vaudois, Lausanne.)

Stroke and VHL

Presentation of HBs with a stroke syndrome is rare despite their highly vascular nature (Figure 26.4), and the risk of hemorrhage associated with them is not yet known.

The risk of clinically apparent intracranial or intramedullary subarachnoid or parenchymal hemorrhage is decidedly uncommon and accounted for only 2% in one series (Resche *et al.*, 1993). Twelve studies report spontaneous hemorrhage (intraparenchymal or subarachnoid) in patients with HBs. The tumor size was not stated in all studies and ranged from 1.5 to 5 cm (mean 2.3 cm) (Cervoni *et al.*, 1995; Glasker and Van Velthoven, 2005; Minami *et al.*, 1998; Wakai *et al.*, 1984; Yu *et al.*, 1994). A 0.0024 risk of spontaneous hemorrhage per person per year was calculated according to a recent German study (Glasker and Van Velthoven, 2005). The most important point of interest is the size of the lesions that bled. The average diameter was 2.7 cm in the literature review. Most HBs are much smaller than this. Wanebo *et al.* (2003) recently published size measures of a large series of 279 cerebellar and 385 spinal HBs. The mean diameter was calculated retrospectively from the published data: an average of 1.1 cm for cerebellar HBs and 0.85 cm for spinal HBs (Wanebo *et al.*, 2003). The lesion size associated with spontaneous hemorrhage appears to be larger. The same observation was made for patients with severe postoperative hemorrhage, in which the tumors were even larger.

Depending on the localization and the extent of the spontaneous hemorrhage, the patients' symptoms are different. Decreased level of consciousness, nausea, vomiting, generalized seizures, and focal neurological deficits are stated as possible symptoms. Case fatalities following acute hemorrhage have also been described (Adegbite *et al.*, 1983; Kikuchi *et al.*, 1994).

It seems that the risk of hemorrhage, whether spontaneous or postoperative, might be determined by the size of the tumors. This could be explained by the high blood flow through these lesions. Similar pathophysiological mechanisms as in arteriovenous malformations take place, and the partial transmission of the arterial pressure to the venous side, together with the high flow, eventually causes structural changes that lead to vascular vulnerability.

The high percentage of subarachnoid hemorrhage (68% in one of series) described can be explained by the superficial location of medullary HBs in cases of spinal cord HB (Berlis *et al.*, 2003; Cerejo *et al.*, 1990; Dijindjian *et al.*, 1978; Irie *et al.*, 1998; Kormos *et al.*, 1980), whereas cerebellar HBs tend to bleed intraparenchymally.

Recently, an association of VHL disease affecting the CNS with a ruptured intracranial aneurysm as the initial presentation was described in a young patient (Sharma and Jha, 2006). A possible causal relationship between a mutation in the VHL tumor suppressor gene and the aneurysm formation was suggested.

Hemorrhage and management

A patient presenting with a hemorrhage in the posterior fossa warrants an emergency neurosurgical admission. Urgent surgical evacuation of the hematoma and the underlying HB may be life saving and is particularly indicated in these rare instances of acute hemorrhage. These patients with VHL tend to present at a younger age than most with spontaneous intracerebral hemorrhage, and most have a good overall prognosis in the absence of RCC. With regard to the lesion itself, surgical resection is the treatment of choice for symptomatic HBs (with or without hemorrhage) as a complete resection is possible in almost all cases. At surgery, the lesions usually appear as highly vascular nodules and usually abut the leptomeninges. Surgical attack of cystic lesions should be targeted only at the enhancing mural nodule, and the cystic wall should be resected only in those rare purely cystic lesions without evidence of a mural nodule at the time of surgery. Further details of surgical technique are beyond the scope of this chapter and are found elsewhere (Vernet and de Tribolet, 1999).

Postoperative mortality of cerebellar HB has been reported as high as 16% (higher for solid tumors). This percentage may be explained in part by the multisystem nature of the disease and the multitude of potential complications. Of particular surgical relevance is difficulty with control of systemic blood pressure as a previously unsuspected Pheo is unmasked under general anesthesia. It is also known that resection of one lesion may lead to the development of other previously quiescent tumors (Miyagami and Katayama, 2004). This lends credence to a policy of observing and not operating on asymptomatic lesions. These patients should be subjected to a full evaluation. A very recent study by the National Institutes of Health (NIH) suggests that even unqualified radiographic progression should not be used as an indication for treatment because HBs exhibit a stuttering growth pattern and do not require treatment for long intervals. Some threshold values were presented for tumor size and/or tumor and cyst growth rates to be used to predict symptom formation and future need for treatment (Ammerman et al., 2006).

In early postoperative hemorrhage, a mechanism known from arteriovenous malformation surgery may be applicable. A process known as normal perfusion pressure breakthrough means that the vascular bed in brain adjacent to an arteriovenous malformation is chronically exposed to decreased pressure and, as a result of chronic hypoxia, loses its normal autoregulatory response and becomes maximally vasodilated. Swelling from edema and hemorrhage can occur after removal of the shunt if this dysautoregulated vascular bed is exposed to normal perfusion pressure.

Considerable intraoperative blood loss generally can be avoided, even in large tumors, by respecting the tumor surface and circumscribing coagulation of all feeding vessels. However, when an HB is not primarily suspected from the MRI scan, the surgeon might enter the tumor and significant blood loss might follow. Usually the imaging and intraoperative features of HBs are unambiguous; however, HBs in unusual locations could present some diagnostic difficulty.

Because large solid HBs of the CNS harbor a significant risk of perioperative and postoperative hemorrhage, angiography and eventual preoperative embolization might be considered in large tumors and we suggest in very specific cases with large and solid tumors. Several authors have performed embolization of HBs with ambiguous results and, in some cases, posterior fossa swelling requiring emergency craniotomy (Eskridge et al., 1996; Tampieri et al., 1993; Vazquez-Anon et al., 1997). Therefore, whether to perform angiography and eventually embolization in these vascular tumors remains a matter of debate.

In general, large solid HBs can cause fatal spontaneous or postoperative hemorrhage and should be managed with this complication in mind. Conversely, HBs with a diameter smaller than 1.5 cm are associated with virtually no risk of hemorrhage. Thus, angiography is not indicated in patients with small HBs.

The role of radiotherapy or radiosurgery is limited and has been recommended for nonresectable or recurrent tumors of the high cervical cords and medulla (Smalley et al., 1990). In a recent series of 14 patients with VHL disease, 50% of patients developed further disease by 5 years (Rajaraman et al., 2004). Although radiosurgery is a useful palliative measure, its efficacy is limited by the tendency of further disease to develop or progress intracranially. Management of extra-CNS lesions is beyond the scope of this chapter; however, it plays a crucial role in the treatment and prognosis of this disease.

Prognosis

Survival depends largely on the presence of visceral lesions and especially RCC (25%–40% of VHL cases). Multiple CNS HBs, the association of retinal and CNS lesions, and onset of the disease before the age of 30 years are predictors of poor prognosis. The development of an adjacent primary lesion must be considered in cases of recurrence after total resection.

Conclusion

In younger patients who present with spontaneous intracerebral hemorrhage, particularly in the posterior fossa, one may add HB as part of the differential diagnosis. The possibility of VHL syndrome should be kept in mind in the context of (1) multiple cerebral lesions, (2) progressive visual loss with retinal lesions, or (3) suggestive family history.

Screening for VHL disease following the diagnosis of a cerebral HB is indispensable given the high risk of associated lesions with hereditary forms. The most commonly associated lesions are cerebellar HBs and RAs, so the diagnosis of VHL disease can occasionally be made on fundoscopy following the discovery of a typical posterior fossa HB. If the tumors are small and asymptomatic, the patient's clinical condition should be carefully watched until the appearance of any symptoms. The best treatment for this tumor is surgical resection. If the tumor is difficult to remove from its primary site, it can sometimes be treated with radiosurgery. The long-term outcome with radiosurgery treatment is still uncertain, however.

Direct genetic testing is available for patients affected with VHL disease in whom the majority of germline mutations can be detected. This mutational analysis has proved to be of important prognostic significance, and gene testing has become an important tool in the management of VHL disease. Novel treatment strategies at a molecular level will be developed according to a better understanding of the VHL gene product. Recent clinical advances have improved outcomes for patients with CNS HBs and emphasized the importance of early detection of VHL disease for more precocious and effective treatment of the several associated conditions. Similarly, it is important to recognize affected asymptomatic family members who could benefit by early detection of associated VHL lesions. Conversely, the exclusion of family members who are not gene carriers as at-risk subjects reduces the economic and psychological burden of tiring clinical and instrumental screening and monitoring protocols.

Thus the importance of early diagnosis and long-term follow-up cannot be overemphasized to recognize affected individuals and high-risk groups. In this way, one can avoid complications and treat lesions at an earlier presymptomatic stage, leading to a better quality of life and improved long-term prognosis.

REFERENCES

Adegbite, A. B., Rozdilsky, B., and Varughese, G. 1983. Supratentorial capillary hemangioblastoma presenting with fatal spontaneous intracerebral hemorrhage. *Neurosurgery*, **12**, 327–30.

Ammerman, J. A., Lonser, L. L., Dambrosia, J., Butman, J. A., and Oldfield, E. H. 2006. Long-term natural history of hemangioblastomas in patients with von Hippel-Lindau disease: implications for treatment. *J Neurosurg*, **105**, 248–55.

Ang, S. O., Chen, H., Hirota, K., *et al.* 2002. Disruption of oxygen homeostasis underlies congenital Chuvash polycythemia. *Nat Genet*, **32**, 614–21.

Berlis, A., Schumacher, M., Spreer, J., Neumann, H. P., and van Velthoven, V. 2003. Subarachnoid haemorrhage due to cervical spinal cord haemangioblastomas in a patient with von Hippel-Lindau disease. *Acta Neurochir (Wien)*, **145**, 1009–13; discussion 1013.

Boker, D. K., Wassmann, H., and Solymosi, L. 1984. Multiple spinal hemangioblastomas in a case of Lindau's disease. *Surg Neurol*, **22**, 439–43.

Cerejo, A., Vaz, R., Feyo, P. B., and Cruz, C. 1990. Spinal cord hemangioblastoma with subarachnoid hemorrhage. *Neurosurgery*, **27**, 991–3.

Cervoni, L., Franco, C., Celli, P., and Fortuna, A. 1995. Spinal tumors and subarachnoid hemorrhage: pathogenetic and diagnostic aspects in 5 cases. *Neurosurg Rev*, **18**, 159–62.

Constans, J. P., Meder, F., Maiuri, F., Donzelli, R., Spaziante, R., and de Divitiis, E. 1986. Posterior fossa hemangioblastomas. *Surg Neurol*, **25**, 269–75.

Cornell, S. H., Hibri, N. S., Menezes, A. H., and Graf, C. J. 1979. The complementary nature of computed tomography and angiography in the diagnosis of cerebellar hemangioblastoma. *Neuroradiology*, **17**, 201–5.

Couch, V., Lindor, N. M., Karnes, P. S., Michels, V. V. 2000. von Hippel-Lindau disease. *Mayo Clin Proc*, **75**, 265–72.

Di Chiro, G., Rieth, K. G., Oldfield, E. H., Tievsky, A. L., Doppman, J. L., and Davis, D. O. 1982. Digital subtraction angiography and dynamic computed tomography in the evaluation of arteriovenous malformations and hemangioblastomas of the spinal cord. *J Comput Assist Tomogr*, **6**, 655–70.

Dijindjian, M., Djindjian, R., Houdart, R., and Hurth, M. 1978. Subarachnoid hemorrhage due to intraspinal tumors. *Surg Neurol*, **9**, 223–9.

Eskridge, J. M., McAuliffe, W., Harris, B., Kim, D. K., Scott, J., and Winn, H. R. 1996. Preoperative endovascular embolization of craniospinal hemangioblastomas. *AJNR Am J Neuroradiol*, **17**, 525–31.

Glasker, S., and van Velthoven, V. 2005. Risk of hemorrhage in hemangioblastomas of the central nervous system. *Neurosurgery*, **57**, 71–6; discussion 71–6.

Green, J. R. 1986. VHL disease in a Newfoundland kindred. *Can Med Assoc J*, **134**, 133–46.

Heiserman, J. E., Dean, B. L., Hodak, J. A., *et al.* 1994. Neurologic complications of cerebral angiography. *AJNR Am J Neuroradiol*, **15**, 1401–7; discussion 1408–11.

Hes, F. J., McKee, S., Taphoorn, M. J., *et al.* 2000. Cryptic von Hippel-Lindau disease: germline mutations in patients with haemangioblastoma only. *J Med Genet*, **37**, 939–43.

Horton, W. A., Wong, V., and Eldridge, R. 1976. Von Hippel-Lindau disease: clinical and pathological manifestations in nine families with 50 affected members. *Arch Intern Med*, **136**, 769–77.

Humphrey, J. S., Klausner, R. D., and Linehan, W. M. 1996. von Hippel-Lindau syndrome: hereditary cancer arising from inherited mutations of the VHL tumor suppressor gene. *Cancer Treat Res*, **88**, 13–39.

Huson, S. M., Harper, P. S., Hourihan, M. D., Cole, G., Weeks, R. D., and Compston, D. A. 1986. Cerebellar haemangioblastoma and von Hippel-Lindau disease. *Brain*, **109**, 1297–310.

Irie, K., Kuyama, H., and Nagao, S. 1998. Spinal cord hemangioblastoma presenting with subarachnoid hemorrhage. *Neurol Med Chir (Tokyo)*, **38**, 355–8.

Kaelin, W. G., Iliopoulos, O., Lonergan, K. M., and Ohh, M. 1998. Functions of the von Hippel-Lindau tumour suppressor protein. *J Intern Med*, **243**, 535–9.

Kaelin, W. G. Jr. 2002. Molecular basis of the VHL hereditary cancer syndrome. *Nat Rev Cancer*, **2**, 673–82.

Kikuchi, K., Kowada, M., Sasaki, J., and Yanagida, N. 1994. [Cerebellar hemangioblastoma associated with fatal intratumoral hemorrhage: report of an autopsied case]. *No Shinkei Geka*, **22**, 593–7.

Kitaoka, K., Ito, T., Tashiro, K., Abe, H., Tsuru, M., and Miyasaka, K. 1981. [Vertebral angiography of cerebellar hemangioblatoma -tumor stain, tumor circulation, CT and angiography in diagnosis (author's transl)]. *No Shinkei Geka*, **9**, 37–49.

Kormos, R. L., Tucker, W. S., Bilbao, J. M., Gladstone, R. M., Bass, A. G. 1980. Subarachnoid hemorrhage due to a spinal cord hemangioblastoma: case report. *Neurosurgery*, **6**, 657–60.

Lamiell, J. M., Salazar, F. G., and Hsia, Y. E. 1989. von Hippel-Lindau disease affecting 43 members of a single kindred. *Medicine (Baltimore)*, **68**, 1–29.

Latif, F., Tory, K., Gnarra, J., *et al.* 1993. Identification of the von Hippel-Lindau disease tumor suppressor gene. *Science*, **260**, 1317–20.

Levine, E., Collins, D. L., and Horton, W. A. 1982. CT scanning of the abdomen in von-Hippel Lindau disease. *Am J Radiol*, **139**, 505–10.

Linehan, W. M., Lerman, M. I., and Zbar, B. 1995. Identification of the von Hippel-Lindau (VHL) gene. Its role in renal cancer. *JAMA*, **273**, 564–70.

Maddock, I. R., Moran, A., Maher, E. R., *et al.* 1996. A genetic register for von Hippel-Lindau disease. *J Med Genet*, **33**, 120–7.

Maher, E. R., Yates, J. R., Harries, R., *et al.* 1990. Clinical features and natural history of von Hippel-Lindau disease. *Q J Med*, **77**, 1151–63.

Minami, M., Hanakita, J., Suwa, H., Suzui, H., Fujita, K., and Nakamura, T. 1998. Cervical hemangioblastoma with a past history of subarachnoid hemorrhage. *Surg Neurol*, **49**, 278–81.

Miyagami, M., and Katayama, Y. 2004. Long term prognosis of hemangioblastoma of the central nervous system: clinical and immunohistochemical study in relation to recurrence. *Brain Tumor Pathol*, **21**, 75–82.

Neumann, H. P., Eggert, H. R., Weigel, K., Friedburg, H., Wiestler, O. D., and Schollmeyer, P. 1989. Hemangioblastomas of the central nervous system. A 10-year study with special reference to von Hippel-Lindau syndrome. *J Neurosurg*, **70**, 24–30.

Rajaraman, C., Rowe, J. G., Walton, L., Malik, I., Radatz, M., and Kemeny, A. A. 2004. Treatment options for von Hippel-Lindau's haemangioblastomatosis: the role of gamma knife stereotactic radiosurgery. *Br J Neurosurg*, **18**, 338–42.

Rengachary, S. S. 1985. Hemangioblastoma. In *Neurosurgery*, eds. R. H. Wilkins and S. S Rangachary. New York: McGraw-Hill.

Resche, F., Moisan, J. P., Mantoura, J., *et al.* 1993. Haemangioblastoma, haemangioblastomatosis, and von Hippel-Lindau disease. *Adv Tech Stand Neurosurg*, **20**, 197–304.

Richard, S., Beigelman, C., Gerber, S., *et al.* 1994. [Does hemangioblastoma exist outside von Hippel-Lindau disease?] *Neurochirurgie*, **40**, 145–54.

Richard, S., Campello, C., Taillandier, L., Parker, F., and Resche, F. 1998. Haemangioblastoma of the central nervous system in von Hippel-Lindau disease. French VHL Study Group. *J Intern Med*, **243**, 547–53.

Richard, S., David, P., Marsot-Dupuch, K., Giraud, S., Beroud, C., and Resche, F. 2000. Central nervous system hemangioblastomas, endolymphatic sac tumors, and von Hippel-Lindau disease. *Neurosurg Rev*, **23**, 1–22; discussion 23–4.

Round Table: Infratentorial Hemangioblastomas. 1985. *Neurochirurgie*, **31**, 91–149.

Sharma, M. S., and Jha, A. N. 2006. Ruptured intracranial aneurysm associated with von Hippel Lindau syndrome: a molecular link? *J Neurosurg (2 Suppl Pediatrics)*, **104**, 90–3.

Shuin, T., Yamasaki, I., Tamura, K., Okuda, H., Furihata, M., and Ashida, S. 2006. von Hippel-Lindau disease: molecular pathological basis, clinical criteria, genetic testing, clinical features of tumors and treatment. *Jpn J Clin Oncol*, **36**, 337–43.

Smalley, S. R., Schomberg, P. J., Earle, J. D., Laws, E. R. Jr., Scheithauer, B. W., and O'Fallon, J. R. 1990. Radiotherapeutic considerations in the treatment of hemangioblastomas of the central nervous system. *Int J Radiat Oncol Biol Phys*, **18**, 1165–71.

Sora, S., Ueki, K., Saito, N., Kawahara, N., Shitara, N., and Kirino, T. 2001. Incidence of von Hippel-Lindau disease in hemangioblastoma patients: the University of Tokyo Hospital experience from 1954–1998. *Acta Neurochir (Wien)*, **143**, 893–6.

Stolle, C., Glenn, G., Zbar, B., *et al.* 1998. Improved detection of germline mutations in the von Hippel-Lindau disease tumor suppressor gene. *Hum Mutat*, **12**, 417–23.

Tampieri, D., Leblanc, R., and TerBrugge, K. 1993. Preoperative embolization of brain and spinal hemangioblastomas. *Neurosurgery*, **33**, 502–5; discussion 505.

Vazquez-Anon, V., Botella, C., Beltran, A., Solera, M., and Piquer, J. 1997. Preoperative embolization of solid cervicomedullary junction hemangioblastomas: report of two cases. *Neuroradiology*, **39**, 86–9.

Vernet, O., and de Tribolet, N. 1999. Posterior fossa hemangioblastoma. In *Operative Neurosurgery, 1ˢᵗ edn*, eds. A. Kaye and P. M. Black. Oxford, UK: WB Saunders, pp. 635–40.

Wakai, S., Inoh, S., Ueda, Y., and Nagai, M. 1984. Hemangioblastoma presenting with intraparenchymatous hemorrhage. *J Neurosurg*, **61**, 956–60.

Wanebo, J. E., Lonser, R. R., Glenn, G. M., and Oldfield, E. H. 2003. The natural history of hemangioblastomas of the CNS in patients with VHL disease. *J Neurosurg*, **98**, 82–94.

Willinsky, R. A., Taylor, S. M., TerBrugge, K., Farb, R. I., Tomlinson, G., and Montanera, W. 2003. Neurologic complications of cerebral angiography: prospective analysis of 2899 procedures and review of the literature. *Radiology*, **227**, 522–8.

Wizigmann-Voos, S., Breier, G., Risau, W., and Plate, K. H. 1995. Up-regulation of vascular endothelial growth factor and its receptors in von Hippel-Lindau disease-associated and sporadic hemangioblastomas. *Cancer Res*, **55**, 1358–64.

Yu, J. S., Short, M. P., Schumacher, J., Chapman, P. H., and Harsh, G. R. 1994. Intramedullary hemorrhage in spinal cord hemangioblastoma. Report of two cases. *J Neurosurg*, **81**, 937–40.

Zbar, B., Kishida, T., Chen, F., *et al.* 1996. Germline mutations in the von Hippel-Lindau disease (VHL) gene in families from North America, Europe, and Japan. *Hum Mutat*, **8**, 348–57.

Zimmerman, R. A., Bilaniuk, L. T. 1980. Computed tomography of acute intratumoral hemorrhage. *Radiology*, **135**, 355–9.

ANEURYSMS

Taro Kaibara and Roberto C. Heros

Overview

The rupture of a cerebral arterial aneurysm, often with devastating clinical results, is a well-documented cause of hemorrhagic stroke. These aneurysms are dilatations of the walls of major cerebral arteries, typically located at branch points, and are categorized by their shape or etiology. Rupture of these aneurysms classically results in bleeding into the basal subarachnoid cisterns (subarachnoid hemorrhage [SAH]), often with extension into the ventricular cavities. Clinical manifestations are related to the initial hemorrhage and its subsequent complications such as vasospasm and hydrocephalus. In unruptured aneurysms, symptoms related to aneurysmal mass effect and thromboembolism and resultant ischemia can occur.

Saccular aneurysms

Prevalence and incidence

Although the exact figure is somewhat controversial, the prevalence of intracranial aneurysms in the general population is relatively high. Review of autopsy and radiographic studies suggest that between 2% and 4% of people harbor intracranial aneurysms (Rinkel et al., 1998). In contrast, the incidence of SAH from ruptured saccular aneurysms is relatively low, estimated at between 6 and 11 per 100 000 persons per year, or approximately 1 per 10 000, (Mayberg et al., 1994; Weir, 1987). Given the low rupture-to-prevalence rate, demonstrating that most aneurysms do not rupture, much effort has been spent on attempting to determine what aneurysms are at the greatest risk of bleeding.

Gender and age at rupture

It is clear that the risk of having an aneurysm rupture increases with age (Pakarinen, 1967; Phillips et al., 1980; Weir, 1987; Wiebers et al., 1987). Combined data of several studies indicate that ruptures peak in the fifth and sixth decade of life, with approximately 50% of all ruptures occurring during these two decades. In one review, the incidence in the first decade was <1%, 2% in the second, 6% in the third, 15% in the fourth, 26% in the fifth, 28% in the sixth, 16% in the seventh, and 6% in the eighth (Pakarinen, 1967). There is also a slight overall female predilection (56%) for aneurysmal rupture. However, this is borne out only after the fifth decade, prior to which men have a slight preponderance. Interestingly, men appear to be more prone to aneurysms of the anterior communicating artery whereas the converse is true for carotid artery aneurysms (Weir, 1987).

Familial aneurysms

The clustering of intracranial aneurysms in families is well reported in the literature and is likely more common than has been appreciated (Ronkainen et al., 1993; Sakai et al., 1974; Schievink et al., 1994). Approximately 7%–20% of patients with a ruptured aneurysm have a first- or second-degree relative with an intracranial aneurysm (ISUIA, 1998; Norrgard et al., 1987; Ronkainen et al., 1993; Schievink et al., 1994), and among first-degree relatives of a patient with a ruptured aneurysm, the risk of having a ruptured intracranial aneurysm is approximately four times higher than in the general population (Schievink, 1997). The role of screening for aneurysms in family members is not determined. It is recommended by some (Leblanc et al., 1994; Obuchowski et al., 1995), whereas others feel the yield will be too low (MRA Study Group, 1999; Raaymakers, 1999). A reasonable recommendation is to screen with non-invasive methodology (magnetic resonance angiography [MRA] or three-dimensional CT angiography) late teenage and adult first-degree relatives in families where two or more first-degree relatives have been proven to have a cerebral aneurysm (Heros, 2006). Genetic linkage studies are underway to attempt to identify genes that may underlie the development and rupture of intracranial aneurysms (Broderick et al., 2005; Ruigrok et al., 2004, 2005).

Multiplicity

More common in women, multiple aneurysms are present in approximately 14%–24% of patients with aneurysms based on large series (ISUIA, 1998; Sahs et al., 1969; Suzuki, 1979). In patients with multiple aneurysms, two are present in 77%, three in 15%, and four or more in 8% (Suzuki, 1979). In patients with two aneurysms, 47% had them on opposite sides, 21% had them on the same side, 29% had one in the midline and one on the side, and 3% had both midline (Sahs et al., 1969).

Determination of which aneurysm ruptured may occasionally be challenging, and the localization of blood on CT imaging is often helpful. Aneurysm characteristics such as irregularity of shape (Nehls et al., 1985), size (Wood, 1964), local vasospasm, intra-aneurysmal thrombus, or focal neurological findings may be of further assistance.

Uncommon Causes of Stroke, 2nd edition, ed. Louis R. Caplan. Published by Cambridge University Press. © Cambridge University Press 2008.

Natural history

Ruptured

The ruptured intracranial aneurysm with SAH has been well investigated in the neurological literature (Haley *et al.*, 1992; Kassell and Drake, 1982; Pakarinen, 1967; Sahs *et al.*, 1969). Rupture of an aneurysm is associated with a very high degree of morbidity and mortality. It is estimated that approximately one-third of patients die or are severely disabled by the initial hemorrhage. Of the survivors, 50% will die or be severely disabled due to rebleed, vasospasm, or complications of treatment, and only 50% will make a good functional survival (Kassell and Drake, 1982). The last cooperative study reported that the risk of rerupture was greatest in the first 24 hours, at 4.1%, and was 1.5% per day for the next few days with an approximate risk of 20% at 2 weeks (Kassell and Torner, 1983). The poor prognosis for patients with a ruptured aneurysm provides the impetus for aggressive therapeutic management.

Unruptured

Asymptomatic unruptured aneurysms are found as incidental lesions on CT, MR, or conventional contrast cerebral angiography performed for rupture of a different aneurysm, for unrelated symptoms, or for routine screening. Unruptured aneurysms have been the subject of intense scrutiny and discussion by several authors (ISUIA, 1998, 2003; Juvela *et al.*, 1993, 2000; Wiebers *et al.*, 1981, 1987; Yasui *et al.*, 1997), and our understanding of their behavior continues to evolve. The recent international study of unruptured intracranial aneurysms included retrospective (ISUIA, 1998) and prospective (ISUIA, 2003) components and enrolled more than 6600 patients. This controversial study suggests that the risk of rupture is lower than previously believed and that an unruptured aneurysm in a patient with no prior history of SAH (group 1) behaves differently than one in a patient with prior hemorrhage from a different aneurysm (group 2). In group 1 patients the risk of rupture was 0.05% per year for aneurysms smaller than 10 mm, 1% per year for those larger than 10 mm, and 6% per year in those larger than 25 mm. Higher risk was also predicted for posterior communicating, basilar apex, posterior cerebral, and vertebrobasilar aneurysms. In group 2 patients the risk of rupture in <10-mm aneurysms was 10 times higher at 0.5% per year; however, basilar apex was the only location associated with increased risk (ISUIA, 1998). The prospective arm of this multicenter trial enrolled 4060 patients from 61 centers, with a mean follow-up of 3.9 years. This study suggests an overall incidence of 0.8% per year risk of rupture, which was more in keeping with, although still lower than, other published data (Jane *et al.*, 1985, Juvela *et al.*, 2000; Tsutsumi *et al.*, 2000). Given the high prevalence of intracranial aneurysms in the general population and the high risk of poor outcome following rupture, the management of the unruptured, asymptomatic aneurysm is a current topic of debate (Dumont *et al.*, 2002; Riina and Spetzler, 2002; Tummala *et al.*, 2005; Wiebers *et al.*, 2003).

Clinical syndromes

SAH

While most intracranial aneurysms remain silent until rupture, the clinical syndrome of aneurysmal SAH is distinct and characteristic. Despite the classic history of the sudden onset of an explosive headache, often recalled as the worst headache of the patient's life, misdiagnoses such as migraine, flu, sinusitis, hypertension, etc., are common (Ostergaard, 1991; Schievink *et al.*, 1988). Furthermore, as many as half of patients describe an acute but slight headache in the weeks preceding rupture, suggestive of a warning, or sentinel, hemorrhage (Leblanc, 1987; Ostergaard, 1991; Sahs *et al.*, 1969; Waga *et al.*, 1975). Depending upon the severity of the hemorrhage, menigismus, loss of consciousness, lethargy, nausea, vomiting, sixth nerve palsies, papilledema, and subhyaloid retinal hemorrhages may be found. A generalized seizure, although dramatic and occurring in up to 25% of patients, does not appear to be a predictor of outcome or of late epilepsy (Hart *et al.*, 1981). Major focal deficits at onset are rare except when there is associated intracerebral hemorrhage.

Intracerebral hemorrhage

Significant parenchymal hemorrhage occurs in approximately 40% of patients with a ruptured aneurysm (Hauerberg *et al.*, 1994). Most frequently it is accompanied by some degree of SAH, which suggests that the origin of the intracerebral hemorrhage was a ruptured aneurysm. Occasionally, the intracerebral hemorrhage occurs without associated SAH, but even in these cases a ruptured aneurysm may frequently be suspected by the location of the hemorrhage. For example, temporal lobe or frontal lobe hemorrhages that appear to originate from the sylvian fissure are very suggestive of a ruptured middle cerebral aneurysm, deep frontal hemorrhages that appear to arise from the general area of the top of the carotid bifurcation suggest a ruptured carotid bifurcation aneurysm, basal frontal hemorrhages reaching the anterior communicating region are very suggestive of an anterior communicating aneurysm, and "butterfly" hemorrhages into both medial frontal lobes are virtually pathognemonic of a ruptured pericallosal aneurysm.

Stroke-like apoplectic clinical syndromes occur with aneurysmal intracerebral hemorrhage and correspond to the affected area. Lateralized focal neurologic deficits are most common with intraparenchymal hemorrhages due to middle cerebral aneurysms. When the hemorrhage involves the temporal lobe, it can lead rapidly to herniation, and it is important to recognize an aneurysm as the possible source of the hemorrhage because, in these cases, emergency surgical evacuation can be life-saving, but it should be accompanied by treatment of the aneurysm to avoid the very high risk of a rehemorrhage, which is very common if the hematoma is evacuated and the aneurysm is left unsecured. Remarkable clinical recoveries can occur from prompt evacuation of an intratemporal hemorrhage even in patients in deep coma with unilateral pupillary dilatation.

Intraventricular hemorrhage

Intraventricular hemorrhage from rupture of an aneurysm is observed in approximately 13%–28% of patients, with the responsible aneurysm being located at the anterior cerebral (40%), internal carotid (25%), middle cerebral (21%), and vertebrobasilar (14%) arteries (Mohr et al., 1983). This study also showed that the degree of ventricular dilatation correlated with the outcome. Certain aneurysms are associated with specific patterns of intraventricular blood. Anterior communicating artery or upper basilar artery aneurysms may rupture into the third ventricle whereas distal posterior inferior cerebellar artery aneurysms often rupture into the fourth ventricle (Yeh et al., 1985). In contrast, acute subdural hematoma occurred in only 2% of patients with SAH and, as expected, was associated with a high degree of mortality (50%) (Weir et al., 1984).

Brain ischemia

Brain ischemia manifested as transient ischemic attack or cerebral infarction is a rare but well-documented presentation of a previously undetected intracranial aneurysm. This is the presentation in 3–11% of patients with intracranial aneurysms (ISUIA, 1998; Nagashima et al., 1993; Qureshi et al., 2000; Weibers et al., 1987) and is diagnosed when ischemic symptoms are attributable to the vascular territory distal to the location of the aneurysm and when other more common causes of cerebral ischemia are excluded. In a review of 41 reported cases, the typical ischemic symptoms included motor deficit (47%), dysphasia (23%), sensory loss (11%), and visual field abnormality (9%). Responsible aneurysms were most commonly located on the internal carotid artery (40%) and middle cerebral artery (37%) (Qureshi et al., 2000). Although thromboembolism from large or giant aneurysms appears to be more common (Antunes and Correll, 1976; Brownlee et al., 1995; Sakaki et al., 1980; see Figure 27.1), this phenomenon can certainly occur with any size aneurysm, with the average being 12.5 mm (Kato et al., 2005; Qureshi et al., 2000). Experimental work utilizing radiolabeled platelets has confirmed that thrombus may form within aneurysmal sacs and may subsequently embolize (Sutherland et al., 1982). Another study showed that a higher aneurysm sac-to-orifice ratio results in intra-aneurysmal hemodynamics favoring thrombus formation (Black and German, 1960). Although the clinical course of an aneurysm causing ischemic symptoms appears to be more benign than previously believed (Qureshi et al., 2000), it is likely poorer than that of an asymptomatic unruptured aneurysm and should therefore be appropriately treated (Kato et al., 2005; Nanda and Vannemreddy, 2006).

Mass effect

The most familiar clinical presentation attributable to aneurysmal mass effect is that of third nerve palsy. Classically this manifests with pain, oculomotor palsy, mydriasis, and/or ptosis (Feely and Kapoor, 1987; Raja, 1972; Soni, 1974). However, the full spectrum of third nerve function has been implicated including painless, complete, or incomplete oculomotor paresis with or without pupil sparing, ptosis, etc. (Tummala et al., 2001). Thus an aneurysm should be suspected and ruled out in any patient with new-onset third nerve dysfunction.

Mass effect related to giant (>25 mm) aneurysms present very similarly to neoplastic mass lesions; giant vertebrobasilar aneurysms may present with brainstem compression, cerebellar signs, or lower cranial nerve palsies; giant ophthalmic and anterior communicating aneurysms may cause a variable degree of visual loss; giant middle cerebral artery aneurysms may cause seizures or hemiparesis; and cavernous sinus aneurysms may present with retro-orbital pain and a cavernous sinus syndrome. Despite their significant size and often surrounding edema, most giant aneurysms still present with hemorrhage (Pia and Zierski, 1982). Unruptured aneurysms presenting with mass effect may have a rupture risk as high as 6% per year (Wiebers et al., 1987), commanding their prompt treatment.

Although focal clinical syndromes from aneurysmal mass effect usually develop gradually in a fashion more suggestive of a tumor, they can be sudden and stroke-like, presumably from acute expansion related perhaps to intramural hemorrhage or acute partial intra-aneurysmal thrombosis.

Vasospasm

Vasospasm is an important and still incompletely understood consequence of SAH from a ruptured aneurysm. Currently vasospasm has surpassed rebleeding as the most important complication after rupture of an aneurysm. Because general consensus nowadays is to secure the aneurysm early after rupture with either open microsurgery or endovascular occlusion, rebleeding, although still observed in the early hours after SAH, has acquired secondary importance in terms of responsibility for morbidity and mortality. The most important cause of morbidity and mortality after SAH is the initial hemorrhage itself; however, after the initial hemorrhage is survived, vasospasm is now the most dangerous consequence of SAH. We still have only incomplete understanding of the cellular and molecular mechanisms responsible for vasospasm; however, it has become very clear that the amount of blood (the thickness of the clot) within the basal subarachnoid space is the most important determinant of vasospasm (Fisher et al., 1980; Mizukami et al., 1982). This has great clinical importance because a simple early CT scan can be used as a very accurate predictor of vasospasm; with very few exceptions, it is only patients who have thick clots in the subarachnoid basal cisterns that develop significant clinical vasospasm. Furthermore, vasospasm is usually maximal in those areas where the basal clot is the thickest. The importance of this is that prophylactic treatments such as intravascular volume expansion and perhaps some hemodilution and hypertension can be used prophylactically in anticipation of vasospasm in those patients at high risk.

Although angiographic vasospasm is detectable in perhaps as many as 60%–70% of patients after SAH, only about 20% of these patients become clinically symptomatic. The clinical syndrome of vasospasm is delayed, usually becoming manifest sometime between the 4th day and 12th day after SAH. Usually the syndrome

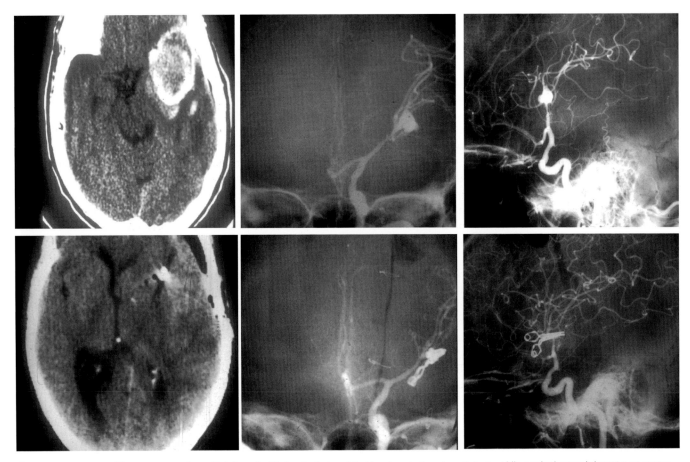

Figure 27.1 A 45-year-old woman presenting with left cerebral ischemic stroke related to a largely thrombosed giant middle cerebral artery bifurcation aneurysm. **Top row, left to right**: preoperative CT scan, anteroposterior and lateral carotid arteriograms showing mass effect and thrombosis of the aneurysm. **Bottom row, left to right**: similar postoperative CT scan, anteroposterior and lateral carotid arteriograms showing clipping of the aneurysm and resection of the aneurysmal mass.

develops slowly over a period of several hours to 1 or 2 days; however, clinical evolution can be rather rapid and simulate a stroke. It is common to see a slight increase in temperature and in the white blood count 1 or 2 days before the onset of clinical vasospasm. Hyponatremia, another common complication of SAH, is also frequently detected in these patients before the clinical onset of symptoms. It is important to recognize that this hyponatremia is due to excessive renal loss of sodium and consequent intravascular volume depletion as a result of excessive secretion of natriuretic factors secondary to hypothalamic derangement. Therefore, these patients need to be treated with volume repletion rather than with water restriction, which can exacerbate the ischemic consequences of vasospasm. The clinical syndrome of vasospasm is often heralded by an increase in the severity of headache and confusion and a gradually decreasing level of consciousness. Focal deficits can develop rapidly or in a more delayed fashion, but usually the full syndrome is apparent in a day or two if not treated clinically. Focal deficits usually correspond to arterial territories where maximal angiographic vasospasm is evident. Consequent decrease in cerebral perfusion pressure can lead to cerebral infarction if the patient is left untreated and in the worst cases despite maximal treatment.

For years now, the most effective and established treatment for clinical vasospasm has been the rapid and vigorous institution of what has become colloquially known as "triple-H-therapy" consisting of hypervolemia, hypertension (which frequently is artificially induced with vasopressors), and hemodilution (which often occurs naturally as a result of volume expansion with colloids or crystalloids without concomitant blood transfusions). When this therapy fails to reverse the clinical syndrome, endovascular angioplasty (mechanical dilatation of the arteries in spasm by balloons) and/or intra-arterial infusions of vasodilators such as calcium channel blockers or papaverine has now been established as a very effective treatment.

One of the complexities of vasospasm from the clinical point of view is that frequently we have a mixture of marginally perfused areas in the brain, which are not yet fully infarcted and which respond to volume expansion and increased perfusion pressure, and frankly infarcted areas where such therapy can be expected not to be effective and to be possibly detrimental. The balance between areas already infarcted and marginally perfused areas at risk determines whether hypervolemic hypertensive therapy is continued or not; this of course is an area that requires exquisite clinical judgment aided by imaging studies and, if available, other physiologic forms of monitoring such as blood flow determinations by a variety of methods, microdialysis, etc.

Other aneurysms

Infectious

Aneurysms related to infections are uncommon but well recognized. Well over 200 cases of infectious brain aneurysms have been reported (Baldwin *et al.*, 1994), with those due to bacteria far outnumbering those due to fungal infections. Classically, these aneurysms are a result of emboli from vegetative bacterial endocarditis. They generally are peripheral in location, where infective emboli are likely to occur, and frequently are multiple. The reported incidence is as high as 10% in patients with endocarditis (Bohmfalk *et al.*, 1978; Weir, 1987). The most common organisms isolated are *Streptococcus*, *Staphylococcus*, and *Enterococcus*, followed by *Neisseria*, *Pseudomonas*, and *Corynebacterium*. The resolution of infectious aneurysms is well documented; however, their formation and rupture during and/or following antibiotic therapy is also reported (Barrow and Prats, 1990; Bohmfalk *et al.*, 1978; Cantu *et al.*, 1966; Frazee *et al.*, 1980). As aneurysm size and number may fluctuate over time, close monitoring with serial angiography is warranted regardless of treatment. Factors to consider in deciding to surgically treat an infectious aneurysm include the neurological/medical condition of the patient, treatment of endocarditis, progression/development of aneurysms on antibiotics, accessibility of the aneurysm, and the presence of multiple aneurysms. The onset of a stroke-like syndrome in a patient with known or suspected infective endocarditis calls for investigation to rule out a mycotic aneurysm. Most often these strokes will be found to be due to embolic arterial occlusion, but the finding of an aneurysm (which in this setting can be presumed to be mycotic) may call for urgent surgical therapy.

In contrast, fungal infectious aneurysms have a uniformly poor outcome with a >90% mortality rate. In their review of the literature, Baldwin *et al.* (1994) noted that only two patients with fungal infectious aneurysms have survived, both having been operated on. No patient treated conservatively survived. These aneurysms are commonly related to extension of localized infection from the skull and air sinuses, with *Aspergillus* being the most common pathogen followed by *Candida albicans*. Others include mucormycosis, phycomycetosis, cryptococcosis, and coccidiomycosis. Given the 100% mortality with conservative treatment, aggressive surgical treatment is warranted in medically stable patients.

Fusiform

Fusiform dolichoectatic aneurysms are elongated dilatations of arteries, often growing to large proportions, commanding descriptions such as "megadolichoectatic." These aneurysms are generally believed to be due to atherosclerosis with disruption of the internal elastic membrane (Goldstein and Tibbs, 1981); however,

some hypothesize that arterial dissection may be the initial insult leading to formation (Anson *et al.*, 1996; Day *et al.*, 2003). Fusiform aneurysms are common in both the anterior circulation, specifically, the internal carotid and middle cerebral arteries as well as the vertebrobasilar circulation. A broad spectrum of clinical presentation exists (Anson *et al.*, 1996). Mass effect and compression can result in almost any cranial neuropathy, including diplopia, trigeminal neuralgia, oculomotor paresis, facial numbness and/or weakness, and glossopharyngeal neuralgia. Large aneurysms can cause brainstem dysfunction and even obstructive hydrocephalus (Nishizaki *et al.*, 1985; Rozario *et al.*, 1978).

Thrombosis in the aneurysm can result in ischemia related to main vessel occlusion (Little *et al.*, 1981), distal emboli (Maruyama *et al.*, 1989; Steel *et al.*, 1982), or perforator occlusion or distortion (Hirsh and Gonzalez, 1979; Nishizaki *et al.*, 1985). Rupture of these aneurysms occurs in 20%–40% (Anson *et al.*, 1996; Little *et al.*, 1981) and with less frequency than with similar size saccular aneurysms (Drake, 1975). Treatment of these lesions is a formidable challenge to even the most accomplished of surgeons and must be tailored to each patient with careful consideration of several key factors. These include location, anatomical features such as length and size of ectasia, involvement of perforating vessels, presence of collateral vessels, symptomatology (i.e. mass effect vs. ischemia vs. rupture). Surgical strategies include direct treatment (i.e. direct clipping, clip reconstruction, and aneurysm resection; see Figure 27.2) or indirect treatment (i.e. proximal vessel occlusion with or without revascularization, aneurysm trapping with or without revascularization, and wrapping). Endovascular techniques are gradually gaining popularity in the treatment of these aneurysms. In a recent series of 40 patients, those with anterior circulation aneurysms fared better than those with posterior circulation aneurysms. Ninety percent of patients with anterior circulation aneurysms had a good outcome, whereas this number was 65% in patients with posterior circulation aneurysms (Anson *et al.*, 1996).

Although strokes secondary to extracranial arterial dissections are a separate topic, we would like to point out here that intracranial dissections, which are frequently called "dissecting aneurysms," are a frequent cause of both hemorrhagic and ischemic stroke (Caplan *et al.*, 1988; Hart and Easton, 1983; Mokri *et al.*, 1988). Curiously, most patients present with either ischemic syndromes, which are usually of abrupt stroke-like onset, or hemorrhage. Rarely these two clinical presentations can co-exist or follow each other by a short period of time. Hemorrhage is particularly common with vertebral dissecting aneurysms but can occur with any intracranial dissecting aneurysm. Hemorrhage is common in intracranial dissections because the dissection plane is usually through the media or subadventitial layers as opposed to extracranial dissections, which usually occur at a subintimal plane and rarely if ever lead to hemorrhage.

Vertebral dissections can simulate a number of vertebro-basilar stroke syndromes including the lateral medullary infarct from occlusion of the posterior inferior cerebellar artery. Occasionally the dissection may involve or extend into the basilar artery

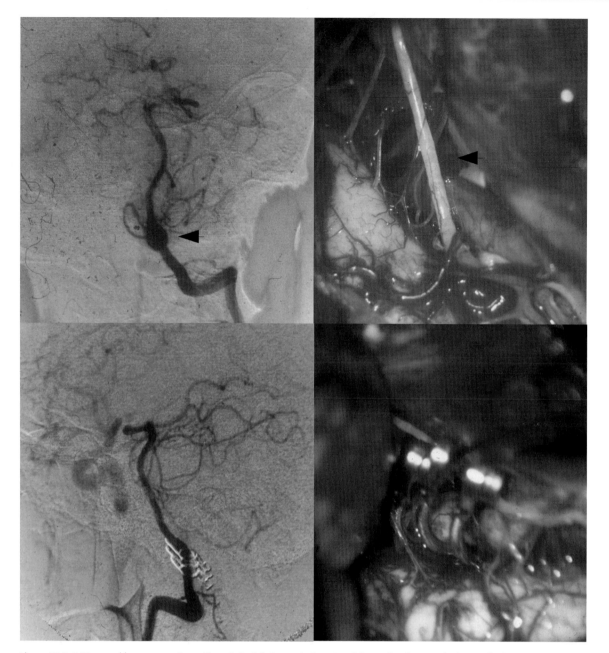

Figure 27.2 A 53-year-old man presenting with posterior inferior cerebellar artery infarct related to vertebral artery fusiform aneurysm. **Top row**: vertebral arteriogram and intraoperative photograph showing aneurysmal dilatation of the vertebral artery (*arrowhead*). **Bottom row**: vertebral arteriogram and intraoperative photograph demonstrating obliteration of aneurysm and preservation of vertebral artery lumen with three fenestrated clips placed in a "picket-fence" fashion. See color plate.

causing a variety of pontine and posterior circulation ischemic syndromes (Caplan *et al.*, 1995; Hart and Easton, 1983; Mokri *et al.*, 1988). Carotid artery dissections extending into, as well as those originating within, the middle cerebral artery lead to typical ischemic stroke syndromes of the middle cerebral territory. When patients present with purely ischemic symptoms without evidence of hemorrhage, the treatment of choice is anti-coagulation which, although recommended, is always administered with some hesitation given the fact that these dissecting aneurysms can bleed; however, hemorrhage after ischemic presentation, as indicated above, is unusual.

Associated diseases

Polycystic kidney disease

Autosomal dominant polycystic kidney disease (PKD) has long been known to be associated with intracranial aneurysms (Brown, 1951). PKD is prevalent, affecting between 1 in 400 to 1 in 1000 persons (Fick and Gabow, 1994). In these patients, intracranial aneurysm are 4–5 times more common than in the general population, and are found in approximately 8% of these patients (Pirson *et al.*, 2002). The incidence of rupture is roughly five times greater than in the general population, and is estimated at 1 per 2000

(Schievink *et al.*, 1992). Screening with CT angiography or MRA is recommended for patients with PKD (Chapman *et al.*, 1992; Pirson *et al.*, 2002). Two genes have been implicated. PKD1 (85%, chromosome 16) and PKD2 (15%, chromosome 4) produce Polycystin1 and Polycystin2, respectively. These are expressed in vascular smooth muscle cells, adjacent endothelial cells, and elastic tissue of normal adult elastic arteries and are implicated in the structural integrity of vessels (Pirson *et al.*, 2002).

Connective tissue disorders

Marfan's syndrome affects 1 in 10 000 to 20 000 people. It is recognized by tall stature, arachnodactyly, and anterior chest deformity. Aortic and mitral valve insufficiency and aortic dissection and rupture can cause sudden death. The arterial defect is characterized by cystic medial necrosis and disruption of elastic fibers (Stehbens *et al.*, 1989), and aneurysms of both saccular and fusiform nature have been described (Finney *et al.*, 1976; Schievink *et al.*, 1994). The implicated gene FBN-1 encodes for a glycoprotein, Fibrillin-1, a component of microfibrils (Ramirez *et al.*, 1999; Sakai *et al.*, 1986). Microfibrils are an important constituent of the extracellular matrix and are found in elastic and non-elastic tissues throughout the body. In elastic arteries, it is expressed in all three layers. Although large series do not exist, the incidence of intracranial aneurysms in Marfan's patients is approximately 6.5% (Schievink, 1999).

Ehlers-Danlos syndrome type IV is rare, affecting 1 in 50 000 to 1 in 500 000 (Byers, 1995). It is characterized by hypermobility of the joints and easy bruising, with life-threatening problems arising from aneurysmal dilation, dissection, or spontaneous rupture of medium and large sized vessels of the body because of a deficiency of type III collagen, encoded by the *COL3A1* gene on chromosome 2 (Byers, 1995; Pope *et al.*, 1975), and an important component of distensible organs of the body, such as blood vessels and viscera. Intracranial aneurysms, carotid cavernous fistulae, and undetermined spontaneous intracranial hemorrhage have all been described in patients with Ehlers-Danlos (Graf, 1965; North *et al.*, 1995; Rubenstein and Cohen, 1964; Schoolman and Kepes, 1967). All invasive procedures, treatment or diagnostic, are associated with high complication rates, greatly limiting treatment options.

Conclusions

Intracranial aneurysms are not a rare cause of both hemorrhagic and ischemic stroke. Although the initial and most serious manifestation of an intracranial aneurysm, SAH, does not typically result in focal neurologic deficits, several complications of ruptured or unruptured aneurysms can lead to focal neurologic deficits, which may develop suddenly in a stroke-like fashion. This is most often seen as a result of intracerebral hemorrhage from the initial rupture of the aneurysm. Cerebral vasospasm after SAH is another common cause of stroke-like, focal deficits. Thromboembolism from the dislodgement of an intra-aneurysmal clot is a less frequent cause of ischemic stroke. Although focal neurologic syndromes from mass effect from unruptured aneurysms usually develop gradually, they can occur abruptly in a stroke-like fashion,

probably from acute intra-aneurysmal thrombosis and/or intramural hemorrhage within the aneurysm leading to acute aneurysmal expansion. Intracranial dissecting aneurysms and fusiform dolichoectatic aneurysms can produce stroke-like ischemic syndromes from occlusion of large branches such as the posterior inferior cerebellar artery in cases of vertebral dissection or from occlusion of the origin of perforating arteries such as occurs frequently when these aneurysms involve the basilar artery or the middle cerebral artery. Finally, a mycotic aneurysm should always be suspected in patients with proven or presumed bacterial endocarditis who develop a stroke. Although most frequently this stroke would be due to occlusive thromboembolism, the frequency of mycotic aneurysms in this setting is high enough to justify aggressive diagnostic and therapeutic interventions.

REFERENCES

Anson, J. A., Lawton, M. T., and Spetzler, R. F. 1996. Characteristics and surgical treatment of dolichoectatic and fusiform aneurysms. *J Neurosurg*, **84**, 185–93.

Antunes, J. L., and Correll, J. W. 1976. Cerebral emboli from intracranial aneurysms. *Surg Neurol*, **6**, 7–10.

Baldwin, H. Z., Zabramski, J. M., and Spetzler, R. F. 1994. Infectious intracranial aneurysms. In *Neurovascular Surgery*, eds. L. P. Carter, and R. F. Spetzler. New York: McGraw-Hill.

Barrow, D. L., and Prats, A. R. 1990. Infectious intracranial aneurysms: comparison of groups with and without endocarditis. *Neurosurgery*, **27**, 562–72.

Black, S. P. W., and German, W. J. 1960. Observations on the relationship between the volume and the size of the orifice of experimental aneurysms. *J Neurosurg*, **17**, 984.

Bohmfalk, G. L., Story, J. L., Wissinger, J. P., and Brown, W. E. Jr. 1978. Bacterial intracranial aneurysm. *J Neurosurg*, **48**, 369–82.

Broderick, J. P., Sauerbeck, L. R., Foroud, T., *et al.* 2005. The Familial Intracranial Aneurysm (FIA) study protocol. *BMC Med Genet*, **6**, 17.

Brown, R. A. 1951. Polycystic disease of the kidneys and intracranial aneurysms. The etiology and interrelationship of these conditions: review of recent literature and report of seven cases in which both conditions coexisted. *Glasgow Med J*, **32**, 333–48.

Brownlee, R. D., Tranmer, B. I., Sevick, R. J., Karmy, G., and Curry, B. J. 1995. Spontaneous thrombosis of an unruptured anterior communicating artery aneurysm. An unusual cause of ischemic stroke. *Stroke*, **26**, 1945–9.

Byers, P. H. 1995. Ehlers-Danlos syndrome type IV: a genetic disorder in many guises. *J Invest Dermatol*, **105**, 311–3.

Cantu, R. C., LeMay, M., and Wilkinson, H. A. 1966. The importance of repeated angiography in the treatment of mycotic-embolic intracranial aneurysms. *J Neurosurg*, **25**, 189–93.

Caplan, L. R., Baquis, G. D., Pessin, M. S., *et al.* 1988. Dissection of the intracranial vertebral artery. *Neurology*, **38**, 868–77.

Chapman, A. B., Rubinstein, D., Hughes, R., *et al.* 1992. Intracranial aneurysms in autosomal dominant polycystic kidney disease. *N Engl J Med*, **327**, 916–20.

Day, A. L., Gaposchkin, C. G., Yu, C. J., Rivet, D. J., and Dacey, R. G. Jr. 2003. Spontaneous fusiform middle cerebral artery aneurysms: characteristics and a proposed mechanism of formation. *J Neurosurg*, **99**, 228–40.

Drake, C. G. 1975. Ligation of the vertebral (unilateral or bilateral) or basilar artery in the treatment of large intracranial aneurysms. *J Neurosurg*, **43**, 255–74.

Dumont, A. S., Lanzino, G., and Kassell, N. F. 2002. Unruptured aneurysms. *J Neurosurg*, **96**, 52–6.

Feely, M., and Kapoor, S. 1987. Third nerve palsy due to posterior communicating artery aneurysm: the importance of early surgery. *J Neurol Neurosurg Psychiatr*, **50**, 1051–2.

Fick, G. M., Gabow, P. A. 1994. Natural history of autosomal dominant polycystic kidney disease. *Annu Rev Med*, **45**, 23–9.

Finney, L. H., Roberts, T. S., and Anderson, R. E. 1976. Giant intracranial aneurysm associated with Marfan's syndrome. Case report. *J Neurosurg*, **45**, 342–7.

Fisher, C. M., Kistler, J. P., and Davis, J. M. 1980. Relation of cerebral vasospasm to subarachnoid hemorrhage visualized by computerized tomographic scanning. *Neurosurgery*, **6**, 1–9.

Frazee, J. G., Cahan, L. D., and Winter, J. 1980. Bacterial intracranial aneurysms. *J Neurosurg*, **53**, 633–41.

Goldstein, S. J., Tibbs, P. A. 1981. Recurrent subarachnoid hemorrhage complicating cerebral arterial ectasia. Case report. *J Neurosurg*, **55**, 139–42.

Graf, C. J. 1965. Spontaneous carotid-cavernous fistula. Ehlers-Danlos syndrome and related conditions. *Arch Neurol*, **13**, 662–72.

Haley, E. C. Jr., Kassell, N. F., and Torner, J. C. 1992. The International Cooperative Study on the Timing of Aneurysm Surgery. The North American experience. *Stroke*, **23**, 205–14.

Hart, R. G., Byer, J. A., Slaughter, J. R., Hewett, J. E., and Easton, J. D. 1981. Occurrence and implications of seizures in subarachnoid hemorrhage due to ruptured intracranial aneurysms. *Neurosurgery*, **8**, 417–21.

Hart, R. G., and Easton, J. D. 1983. Dissections of cervical and cerebral arteries. *Neurol Clin*, **1**, 155–82.

Hauerberg, J., Eskesen, V., and Rosenorn, J. 1994. The prognostic significance of intracerebral haematoma as shown on CT scanning after aneurysmal subarachnoid haemorrhage. *Br J Neurosurg*, **8**, 333–9.

Heros, R. C. 2006. *Clin Neurosurg*, In press.

Hirsh, L. F., and Gonzalez, C. F. 1979, Fusiform basilar aneurysm simulating carotid transient ischemic attacks. *Stroke*, **10**, 598–601.

International Study of Unruptured Intracranial Aneurysms Investigators (ISUIA). 1998. Unruptured intracranial aneurysms–risk of rupture and risks of surgical intervention. *N Engl J Med*, **339**, 1725–33.

Jane, J. A., Kassell, N. F., Torner, J. C., and Winn, H. R. 1985. The natural history of aneurysms and arteriovenous malformations. *J Neurosurg*, **62**, 321–3.

Juvela, S. 2002. Natural history of unruptured intracranial aneurysms: risks for aneurysm formation, growth, and rupture. *Acta Neurochir Suppl*, **82**, 27–30.

Kassell, N. F., and Drake, C. G. 1982. Timing of aneurysm surgery. *Neurosurgery*, **10**, 514–9.

Kassell, N. F., and Torner, J. C. 1983. Aneurysmal rebleeding: a preliminary report from the Cooperative Aneurysm Study. *Neurosurgery*, **13**, 479–81.

Kato, M., Kaku, Y., Okumura, A., Iwama, T., and Sakai, N. 2005. Thrombosed unruptured cerebral aneurysm causing brain infarction followed by subarachnoid hemorrhage–case report. *Neurol Med Chir (Tokyo)*, **45**, 472–5.

Leblanc, R. 1987. The minor leak preceding subarachnoid hemorrhage. *J Neurosurg*, **66**, 35–9.

Leblanc, R., Worsley, K. J., Melanson, D., and Tampieri, D. 1994. Angiographic screening and elective surgery of familial cerebral aneurysms: a decision analysis. *Neurosurgery*, **35**, 9–18.

Little, J. R., St. Louis, P., Weinstein, M., and Dohn, D. F. 1981. Giant fusiform aneurysm of the cerebral arteries. *Stroke*, **12**, 183–8.

The Magnetic Resonance Angiography in Relatives of Patients with Subarachnoid Hemorrhage Study Group. (MRA Study Group) 1999. Risks and benefits of screening for intracranial aneurysms in first-degree relatives of patients with sporadic subarachnoid hemorrhage. *N Engl J Med*, **341**, 1344–50.

Maruyama, M., Asai, T., Kuriyama, Y., *et al.* 1989. Positive platelet scintigram of a vertebral aneurysm presenting thromboembolic transient ischemic attacks. *Stroke*, **20**, 687–90.

Mayberg, M. R., Batjer, H. H., Dacey, R., *et al.* 1994. Guidelines for the management of aneurysmal subarachnoid hemorrhage. A statement for healthcare professionals from a special writing group of the Stroke Council, American Heart Association. *Stroke*, **25**, 2315–28.

Mizukami, M., Kawase, T., Usami, T., and Tazawa, T. 1982. Prevention of vasospasm by early operation with removal of subarachnoid blood. *Neurosurgery*, **10**, 301–7.

Mohr, G., Ferguson, G., Khan, M., *et al.* 1983. Intraventricular hemorrhage from ruptured aneurysm. Retrospective analysis of 91 cases. *J Neurosurg*, **58**, 482–7.

Mokri, B., Houser, O. W., Sandok, B. A., and Piepgras, D. G. 1988. Spontaneous dissections of the vertebral arteries. *Neurology*, **38**, 880–5.

Nagashima, M., Nemoto, M., Hadeishi, H., Suzuki, A., and Yasui, N. 1993. Unruptured aneurysms associated with ischaemic cerebrovascular diseases. Surgical indication. *Acta Neurochir (Wien)*, **124**, 71–8.

Nanda, A., and Vannemreddy, PS. 2006. Cerebral ischemia as a presenting feature of intracranial aneurysms: a negative prognostic indicator in the management of aneurysms. *Neurosurgery*, **58**, 831–7.

Nehls, D., G., Flom, R. A., Carter, L. P., and Spetzler, R. F. 1985. Multiple intracranial aneurysms: determining the site of rupture. *J Neurosurg*, **63**, 342–8.

Nishizaki, T., Tamaki, N., Matsumoto, S., and Fujita, S. 1985. Multiple giant fusiform aneurysms with hydrocephalus. *Surg Neurol*, **24**, 101–4.

Norrgard, O., Angquist, K. A., Fodstad, H., Forsell, A., and Lindberg, M. 1987. Intracranial aneurysms and heredity. *Neurosurgery*, **20**, 236–9.

North, K. N., Whiteman, D. A., Pepin, M. G., and Byers, P. H. 1995. Cerebrovascular complications in Ehlers-Danlos syndrome type IV. *Ann Neurol*, **38**, 960–4.

Obuchowski, N. A., Modic, M. T., and Magdinec, M. 1995. Current implications for the efficacy of noninvasive screening for occult intracranial aneurysms in patients with a family history of aneurysms. *J Neurosurg*, **83**, 42–9.

Ostergaard, J. R. 1991. Headache as a warning symptom of impending aneurysmal subarachnoid haemorrhage. *Cephalalgia*, **11**, 53–5.

Pakarinen, S. 1967. Incidence, aetiology, and prognosis of primary subarachnoid haemorrhage. A study based on 589 cases diagnosed in a defined urban population during a defined period. *Acta Neurol Scand*, **43**(**Suppl 29**), 1–28.

Phillips, L. H. 2nd, Whisnant, J. P., O'Fallon, W. M., and Sundt, T. M. Jr. 1980. The unchanging pattern of subarachnoid hemorrhage in a community. *Neurology*, **30**, 1034–40.

Pia, H. W., and Zierski, J. 1982. Giant cerebral aneurysms. *Neurosurg Rev*, **5**, 117–48.

Pirson, Y., Chauveau, D., and Torres, V. 2002. Management of cerebral aneurysms in autosomal dominant polycystic kidney disease. *J Am Soc Nephrol*, **13**, 269–76.

Pope, F. M., Martin, G. R., Lichtenstein, J. R., *et al.* 1975. Patients with Ehlers-Danlos syndrome type IV lack type III collagen. *Proc Natl Acad Sci U S A*, **72**, 1314–6.

Qureshi, A. I., Mohammad, Y., Yahia, A. M., *et al.* 2000. Ischemic events associated with unruptured intracranial aneurysms: multicenter clinical study and review of the literature. *Neurosurgery*, **46**, 282–9; discussion 289–90.

Raaymakers, T. W. 1999. Aneurysms in relatives of patients with subarachnoid hemorrhage: frequency and risk factors. MARS Study Group. Magnetic resonance angiography in relatives of patients with subarachnoid hemorrhage. *Neurology*, **53**, 982–8.

Raja, I. A. 1972. Aneurysm-induced third nerve palsy. *J Neurosurg*, **36**, 548–51.

Ramirez, F., Gayraud, B., and Pereira, L. 1999. Marfan syndrome: new clues to genotype-phenotype correlations. *Ann Med*, **31**, 202–7.

Riina, H. A., and Spetzler, R. F. 2002. Unruptured aneurysms. *J Neurosurg*, **96**, 61–2.

Rinkel, G. J., Djibuti, M., Algra, A., and van Gijn, J. 1998. Prevalence and risk of rupture of intracranial aneurysms: a systematic review. *Stroke*, **29**, 251–6.

Ronkainen, A., Hernesniemi, J., and Ryynanen, M. 1993. Familial subarachnoid hemorrhage in east Finland, 1977–1990. *Neurosurgery*, **33**, 787–96.

Rozario, R. A., Levine, H. L., and Scott, R. M. 1978. Obstructive hydrocephalus secondary to an ectatic basilar artery. *Surg Neurol*, **9**, 31–4.

Rubinstein, M. K., and Cohen, N. H. 1964. Ehlers-Danlos syndrome associated with multiple intracranial aneurysms. *Neurology*, **14**, 125–32.

Ruigrok, Y. M., Rinkel, G. J., and Wijmenga, C. 2005. Genetics of intracranial aneurysms. *Lancet Neurol*, **4**, 179–89.

Ruigrok, Y. M., Seitz, U., Wolterink, S., *et al.* 2004. Association of polymorphisms and pairwise haplotypes in the elstin gene in Dutch patients with subarachnoid hemorrhage from non-familial aneurysms. *Stroke*, **35**, 2064–8.

Sahs, A. L., Perret, G. E., Locksley, H. B., and Nishioka, H., eds. *Intracranial Aneurysms and Subarachnoid Hemorrhage: A Cooperative Study*. Philadelphia: JB Lippincot, 1969.

Sakai, L. Y., Keene, D. R., and Engvall, E. 1986. Fibrillin, a new 350-kd glycoprotein, is a component of extracellular microfibrils. *J Cell Biol*, **103**(**6 Pt 1**), 2499–509.

Sakai, N., Sakata, K., Yamada, H., *et al.* 1974. Familial occurrence of intracranial aneurysms. *Surg Neurol*, **2**, 25–9.

Sakaki, T., Kinugawa, K., Tanigake, T., *et al.* 1980. Embolism from intracranial aneurysms. *J Neurosurg*, **53**, 300–4.

Schievink, W. I. 1997. Intracranial aneurysms. *N Engl J Med*, **336**, 28–40.

Schievink, W. I. 1999. Marfan syndrome and intracranial aneurysms. *Stroke*, **30**, 2767–8.

Schievink, W. I., Bjornsson, J., and Piepgras, D. G. 1994. Coexistence of fibromuscular dysplasia and cystic medial necrosis in a patient with Marfan's syndrome and bilateral carotid artery dissections. *Stroke*, **25**, 2492–6.

Schievink, W. I., Mokri, B., Piepgras, D. G., and Gittenberger-de Groot, A. C. 1996. Intracranial aneurysms and cervicocephalic arterial dissections associated with congenital heart disease. *Neurosurgery*, **39**, 685–9.

Schievink, W. I., Schaid, D. J., Rogers, H. M., Piepgras, D. G., and Michels, V. V.1994. On the inheritance of intracranial aneurysms. *Stroke*, **25**, 2028–37.

Schievink, W. I., Torres, V. E., Piepgras, D. G., and Wiebers, D. O. 1992. Saccular intracranial aneurysms in autosomal dominant polycystic kidney disease. *J Am Soc Nephrol*, **3**, 88–95.

Schievink, W. I., van der Werf, D. J., Hageman, L. M., and Dreissen, J. J. 1988. Referral pattern of patients with aneurysmal subarachnoid hemorrhage. *Surg Neurol*, **29**, 367–71.

Schoolman, A., Kepes, J. J. 1967. Bilateral spontaneous carotid-cavernous fistulae in Ehlers-Danlos syndrome. Case report. *J Neurosurg*, **26**, 82–6.

Soni, S. R. 1974. Aneurysms of the posterior communicating artery and oculomotor paresis. *J Neurol Neurosurg Psychiatr*, **37**, 475–84.

Steel, J. G., Thomas, H. A., and Strollo, P. J. 1982. Fusiform basilar aneurysm as a cause of embolic stroke. *Stroke*, **13**, 712–6.

Stehbens, W. E., Delahunt, B., and Hilless, A. D. 1989. Early berry aneurysm formation in Marfan's syndrome. *Surg Neurol*, **31**, 200–2.

Sutherland, G. R., King, M. E., Peerless, S. J., *et al.* 1982. Platelet interaction within giant intracranial aneurysms. *J Neurosurg*, **56**, 53–61.

Suzuki, J. 1979. Multiple aneurysms: treatment. In *Cerebral Aneurysms: Advances in Diagnosis and Therapy*, eds. H. W. Pia, C. Langmaid, and J. Zierski. Berlin: Springer-Verlag, pp. 352–63.

Torner, J., Adams, H. P. Jr., Feinberg, W., *et al.* 1994. Guidelines for the management of aneurysmal subarachnoid hemorrhage. A statement for healthcare professionals from a special writing group of the Stroke Council, American Heart Association. *Circulation*, **90**, 2592–605.

Tsutsumi, K., Ueki, K., Morita, A., and Kirino, T. 2000. Risk of rupture from incidental cerebral aneurysms. *J Neurosurg*, **93**, 550–3.

Tummala, R. P., Baskaya, M. K., and Heros, R. C. 2005. Contemporary management of incidental intracranial aneurysms. *Neurosurg Focus*, **18**, e9.

Tummala, R. P., Harrison, A., Madison, M. T., and Nussbaum, E. S. 2001. Pseudomyasthenia resulting from a posterior carotid artery wall aneurysm: a novel presentation: case report. *Neurosurgery*, **49**, 1466–8.

Waga, S., Otsubo, K., and Handa, H. 1975. Warning signs in intracranial aneurysms. *Surg Neurol*, **3**, 15–20.

Weir, B. 1987. *Aneurysms Affecting the Central Nervous System*. Baltimore: Williams & Wilkins.

Weir, B., Myles, T., Kahn, M., *et al.* 1984. Management of acute subdural hematomas from aneurysmal rupture. *Can J Neurol Sci*, **11**, 371–6.

Wiebers, D. O., Whisnant, J. P., Huston, J. 3rd, *et al.*; 2003. International Study of Unruptured Intracranial Aneurysms Investigators. 2003. Unruptured intracranial aneurysms: natural history, clinical outcome, and risks of surgical and endovascular treatment. *Lancet*, **362**, 103–10.

Wiebers, D. O., Whisnant, J. P., and O'Fallon, W. M. 1981. The natural history of unruptured intracranial aneurysms. *N Engl J Med*, **304**, 696–8.

Wiebers, D. O., Whisnant, J. P., Sundt, T. M. Jr., and O'Fallon, W. M. 1987. The significance of unruptured intracranial saccular aneurysms. *J Neurosurg*, **66**, 23–9.

Wood, E. H. 1964. Angiographic identification of the ruptured lesion in patients with multiple cerebral aneurysms. *J Neurosurg*, **21**, 182–98.

Yasui, T., Kishi, H., Sakamoto, H., *et al.* 1997. Vertebral artery occlusion after subarachnoid hemorrhage from a dissecting aneurysm of the vertebral artery: case report. *Surg Neurol*, **47**, 149–52.

Yeh, H. S., Tomsick, T. A., and Tew, J. M. Jr. 1985. Intraventricular hemorrhage due to aneurysms of the distal posterior inferior cerebellar artery. Report of three cases. *J Neurosurg*, **62**, 772–5.

Taro Kaibara and Roberto C. Heros

Introduction

The dramatic descriptions by Harvey Cushing regarding his experiences operating on "angiomas" of the brain reflected the initial sense of futility in the treatment of arteriovenous malformations (AVMs). Although Cushing and Bailey (1928) and Dandy (1928) published personal case series, it was the development of cerebral angiography in 1927 (Moniz, 1927) that initiated our modern understanding and treatment of AVMs.

AVMs are complex vascular lesions that typically present with hemorrhage or seizures. Classically there is no normal intervening brain within an AVM, and the lack of a capillary bed results in fistulous, rapid shunting of blood from the arterial to the venous system. This creates a sump-like effect that may result in relative ischemia of the surrounding brain, or may cause venous congestion and ischemia through arterialization of the normal venous drainage of the brain. These flow-related effects may be responsible for the focal neurological deficits occasionally observed in patients with an AVM. These congenital lesions occur throughout the brain; however, they most often are located supratentorially (90%), and often project in a funnel-like fashion to a ventricular surface deep within the cerebrum.

The earliest successful operations of AVMs were reported by Olivecrona and Riives (1948), who successfully removed 81 AVMs with "only" a 9% mortality, and Yasargil (1987), who identified and reviewed 500 surgically treated patients with AVMs between 1932 and 1957. Even in these early cases, the importance of AVM size upon outcome was recognized, noting a 5% mortality in small AVMs compared to a 10% mortality for moderate-sized lesions. With the gradual development and advancement of microsurgical techniques and technology, including the surgical microscope and bipolar cautery, AVMs can now be treated with low morbidity and practically no mortality (Drake, 1979; Heros *et al.*, 1990, 1993; Malis, 1979; Parkinson and Bachers, 1980; Penfield and Erickson, 1941; Spetzler and Martin, 1986; Tamaki *et al.*, 1991; Yasargil, 1969, 1988).

Natural history

A clear understanding of the natural history of the disease is critical in the management of AVMs. AVMs are approximately one-tenth as common as aneurysms. The prevalence of AVM from autopsy studies is estimated at 0.5–0.8% (Martin and Vinters, 1995), whereas the incidence of hemorrhage from AVM is estimated at approximately

1 per 100 000 population (Perret and Nishioka, 1966; Schoenberg *et al.*, 1988).

Several studies have evaluated in detail the risk of hemorrhage in patients harboring AVMs. An important population study from Finland reported by Ondra *et al.* (1990) followed 163 AVM patients for a mean period of 23.7 years (77% greater than 20 years), with a male-to-female ratio of 3:2. The mean age at presentation was 33 years; 71% presented with hemorrhage, and 24% with seizures. Interestingly, the results showed a 4% per year risk of hemorrhage, regardless of presentation, i.e. hemorrhage or not. The average time to rehemorrhage was 7.7 years, and the annual morbidity rate was 2.7%, with a mortality rate of 1%. Approximately 23% of the patients died during the follow-up as a result of the AVM. The average age at death from AVM was 44 years compared to the country's average of 73 years. Other large series also report similar hemorrhage rates. Brown *et al.* (1996) reported a series of 168 patients without a history of previous hemorrhage. A yearly bleeding rate of 2.2% was observed over a mean follow-up of 8.2 years. A retrospective review by Crawford *et al.* (1986) including 217 AVM patients with an average follow-up of 10.4 years reported a yearly bleeding rate of 3.4%. There was a slight increase in hemorrhage risk for the first 6 months after a hemorrhage, following which it returned to the baseline risk. The significant cumulative hemorrhage rate was well demonstrated by Graf *et al.* (1983) who found that the risk of bleeding was 2% at 1 year, 14% at 5 years, and 31% at 10 years. The risk of rebleeding is 6%–7% during the 6 months subsequent to the initial hemorrhage, after which the risk falls to the same level of 3%–4% per year found in patients with unruptured AVMs (Crawford *et al.*, 1986; Ondra *et al.*, 1990).

At times AVMs are recognized before hemorrhage, usually during evaluation of patients with headaches or seizures. Most older series did not separate the frequency of hemorrhage according to whether the patients had already had a hemorrhage or not. A new study ARUBA is now underway to determine the risk of a first hemorrhage in patients with AVMs who have had no prior evidence of bleeding.

Clinical syndromes

Intracerebral hemorrhage

The single most common mode of presentation of an AVM is hemorrhage, usually intraparenchymal. On CT scans, the hemorrhage may not always be diagnostic of AVM; however, a cone-shaped lesion based at the periphery, intralesional calcifications, or unusual patterns of lobar and/or intraventricular hemorrhage may be clues to an underlying AVM. With intravenous contrast, the nidus with associated feeding arteries or dilated veins may be visible; with high-flow lesions, there are frequently venous varices that show as hyperdense, enhancing lesions. AVMs present with hemorrhage in approximately 71%–77% of patients (Ondra et al., 1990; Yasargil, 1988).

The stroke-like clinical syndrome of intracerebral hemorrhage from AVM is indistinguishable from that of hemorrhagic stroke from any other cause. Patients with supratentorial AVMs typically present with hemiplegia/paresis with or without speech deficits and/or visual field deficits depending on the location of the AVM. Patients with deep AVMs can present with striking focal deficits without major impairment of consciousness when the hemorrhage is small and can also present with acute hydrocephalus when the hemorrhage ruptures into the ventricle. Patients with cerebellar AVMs can present with a rapidly evolving clinical syndrome typical of cerebellar hemorrhage from other causes. If the hemorrhage remains small and is confined to the cerebellum, they can be minimally symptomatic or present only focal cerebellar findings; however, with larger hemorrhages, brainstem compression manifesting initially by the typical findings of ipsilateral peripheral facial palsy and gaze paralysis can develop rapidly.

A peculiar difficulty with intraparenchymal hemorrhages related to AVMs is that, if they require emergency surgical evacuation, as frequently happens with cerebellar and temporal lobe hemorrhages, exquisite judgment must be exercised as to what to do with the AVM. In general, we prefer to gently and carefully evacuate as much of the hemorrhage as is necessary to relieve intracranial hypertension without being aggressive and without making any attempt to remove the AVM except in those patients that bleed from a very small superficial AVM that can easily be removed at the time of removal of the hemorrhage. With more complex AVMs, the excision of the AVM itself should be performed on an elective basis, usually delaying the surgery for 2–4 weeks to allow the brain to relax, the reactive hyperemia that accompanies the hemorrhage to subside, and further careful angiographic definition of the AVM to take place.

Subarachnoid hemorrhage

Although it is not unusual for AVMs to result in some degree of subarachnoid hemorrhage usually accompanying a more significant intracerebral hemorrhage, it is rare, in the senior author's opinion, to have an AVM present mostly with basal subarachnoid hemorrhage, as aneurysms do. Of course, AVMs are frequently (10%–20% incidence) accompanied by intracranial aneurysms in feeding arteries, and these aneurysms can be quite proximal and result in typical basal subarachnoid hemorrhage like any other ruptured aneurysm. In these cases, it is relatively easy to recognize that the hemorrhage was from the aneurysm and not from the AVM; therefore, the aneurysm should be treated urgently in the same manner as any other ruptured saccular aneurysm. Not infrequently, the hemorrhage occurs in the general area of the AVM where there can also be either prenidal or intranidal aneurysms, and in these cases,

it is frequently very difficult or impossible to determine whether the AVM or the aneurysm bled. Careful clinical judgment must be exercised in the design of treatment strategies in these patients.

Except in those cases of rupture of an aneurysm associated with an AVM, the senior author has rarely observed the typical syndrome of clinical vasospasm developed in relation to a hemorrhage from an AVM. We have no doubt that this can occur, but it certainly must be very rare, and vasospasm is not generally one of the important clinical considerations after hemorrhage from an AVM.

Seizures

Seizures are the second most common presentation of AVMs. They are reported fairly consistently, accounting for 18%–33% of AVM presentations (Drake, 1979; Heros et al., 1990; Ondra et al., 1990; Yasargil, 1988). Crawford et al. (1986) found significantly larger (6 cm) AVMs in those patients presenting with seizures. They also observed that younger age was a risk for developing seizures, the incidence of which decreased with age. Waltimo (1973) also suggested that larger AVMs are more likely to cause seizures. There is nothing distinct about seizures caused by AVMs, and the clinical manifestations of theses seizures correspond to the location of the AVM; for example, typical complex partial seizures occur commonly with AVMs that involve the temporal lobe (see Figure 28.1).

Ischemia

In the absence of significant hemorrhage, explanations for the progression of neurologic deficit or dysfunction related to an AVM has been attributed to mass effect, recurrent microhemorrhages, ischemia, and steal (see Figure 28.2). The concept of steal-related symptoms from an AVM was first raised by Norlen (1949), who noted that the perilesional brain demonstrated increased filling on angiography following resection of the AVM. These findings provide support for the theory of normal perfusion breakthrough, which attempts to explain the phenomenon of postoperative edema and/or hemorrhage after the excision of high-flow AVMs (Spetzler et al., 1978). The incidence of patients presenting with vascular steal is unclear. In Drake's series, 3% (5 of 166 patients) presented with symptoms attributed to steal. Yasargil (1988) reported that 11% of patients without hemorrhage presented with neurological deficits, and Brown et al. (1996) observed that 8% of 146 patients presented with ischemic symptoms. Several studies have attempted to show the steal phenomenon. Intraoperative angiogram and cerebral blood flow (CBF) measurements have shown high flows in malformations that decrease with increasing distance from the AVM (Feindel et al., 1971). Transcranial Doppler (TCD) studies show abnormally high velocities (increased blood flow) and low pulsatility index (decreased vascular resistance) in the major arteries supplying an AVM (Diehl et al., 1994; Lindegaard et al., 1986; Manchola et al., 1993; Mast, Mohr, Thompson, et al., 1995; Schwartz and Hennerici, 1986). This was exemplified in a patient with a left frontal AVM fed mainly by the left anterior cerebral artery. TCD showed a two-times

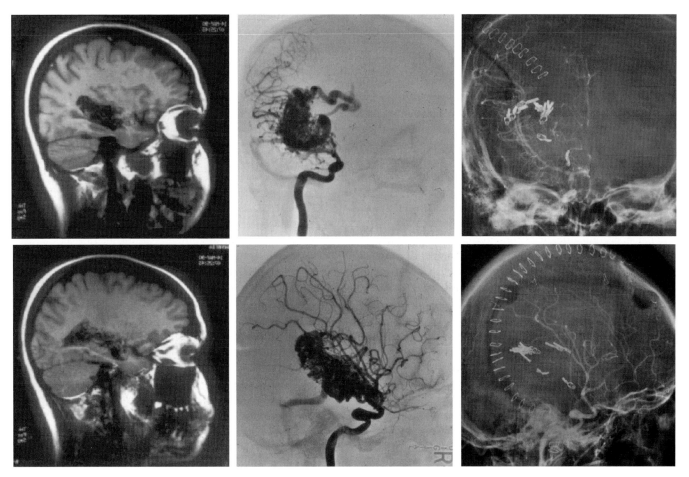

Figure 28.1 A 26-year-old man presenting with seizures. Sagittal MRI (*left column*) and anteropostero (*middle column top*) and lateral (*middle column bottom*) showing high-grade AVM of the right insula/temporal lobe. Postoperative arteriograms (*right column*) show complete resection of the AVM.

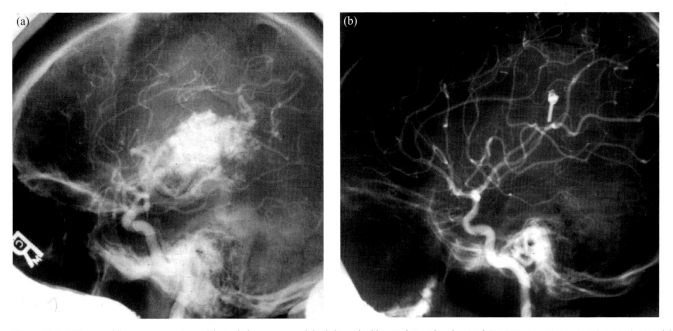

Figure 28.2 A 30-year-old woman presenting with steal phenomenon of the left cerebral hemisphere related to a sylvian AVM seen on preoperative arteriogram (**a**). Postoperative arteriogram (**b**) shows complete resection of AVM with resolution of ischemic symptoms.

normal velocity in the anterior cerebral arteries whereas in the contralateral and ipsilateral middle cerebral arteries (MCAs; i.e. unrelated vessels), velocities were two-thirds and one-half normal, respectively (Schwartz and Hennerici, 1986). In contrast, Mast, Mohr, Osipov, *et al.* (1995) found no significant difference in the velocities or pulsatility index in the feeding arteries of AVM patients with steal symptoms compared to AVM patients without steal; however, they did not measure flows in other, non-AVM-related vessels. Xenon-CT provides some supportive data for AVM-related changes in regional blood flow. AVM patients can have a significant decrease in blood flow to gray and white matter adjacent to an AVM (Okabe *et al.*, 1983). Interestingly the contralateral gray matter contains decreased flow and in the contralateral white matter flow usually remains unchanged. There was significant increase in blood flow in the ipsilateral hemisphere and the contralateral gray matter following resection of the AVM. Using single photon emission computed tomography (SPECT), Batjer *et al.* (1988) quantified "steal" by calculating a steal "index," which they defined as the ratio of the blood flow in the ipsilateral area of hypoperfusion to the total brain flow. An increasing steal index in AVM patients was correlated with progressive neurologic deficit.

Although acute stroke-like ischemic events do occur in patients with AVMs, they are distinctly unusual. Generally these ischemic syndromes develop in a slow, progressive manner. More acute syndromes can occur as a result of spontaneous thrombosis of feeding arteries, which can occur rarely in isolation or occasionally in relation to thrombosis of the entire AVM, which has been documented to occur spontaneously in rare cases. In some patients with stroke-like acute deterioration, venous thrombosis, usually occurring in the previously arterialized venous outflow system after resection of an AVM, has been implicated (Heros *et al.*, 1993).

Migraine

The co-existence of typical "classical" migrainous syndromes and AVMs is more than coincidental. Although the frequency with which this occurs is not well known, it has become clear that when patients with classical migraine are found to have an AVM, that AVM usually involves the occipital lobe. Interestingly, as has been pointed out by Troost and Newton (1975), when patients with AVMs have symptoms of classical migraine, these symptoms are almost always unilateral, corresponding to the visual field contralateral to the AVM, and the headache is ipsilateral to the AVM. In fact, it is recommended that in patients in whom the migraine is always on the same side with visual symptoms consistently in the contralateral field, an AVM should be suspected and appropriate imaging should be obtained to exclude such a lesion (Troost and Newton, 1975).

Headaches

Headaches are common in patients with AVMs. Frequently they are nonspecific and well tolerated. However, occasionally they are severe and progressive both in frequency and severity. The latter are usually related to large AVMs that cause increased intracranial pressure, venous hypertension, or both. Severe focal headaches can also occur as a result of dilatation of meningeal feeding arteries in those AVMs that have significant meningeal supply. The importance of recognizing these focal headaches is that even when the AVM cannot be "cured" by surgical excision or complete obliteration with radiosurgery or embolization, the patient can be palliated and the headaches frequently improve markedly with embolization of the meningeal feeders.

Increased intracranial pressure/venous hypertension

We cover these under the same heading because frequently the clinical syndrome manifested by these patients is identical and it is difficult for the clinician to define the cause as either increased intracranial pressure or venous hypertension because frequently both co-exist. This problem is seen mostly with large, high-flow AVMs that produce widespread retrograde arterialization of the normal venous drainage system of the brain. These patients present frequently with headaches that can be progressive in frequency and severity, as indicated above. They can also present with generalized "cerebral dysfunction" with impairment of cognitive function, memory, intellectual output, general stamina, etc. Treatment considerations in these patients are difficult because the AVMs are usually large and complex and may not be amenable to surgical excision. Palliative embolization is frequently helpful in these patients.

Hydrocephalus

Hydrocephalus can occur in patients with AVMs for several reasons. In some patients, multiple small hemorrhages that reach the ventricles or the subarachnoid space are the cause. Of course, a large hemorrhage can result in acute hydrocephalus as mentioned earlier, and this must be treated by emergency ventriculostomy until such time as a permanent shunt is possible, depending on the gradual clearing of blood from the cerebrospinal fluid (CSF). Hydrocephalus can also occur from obstruction of normal CSF pathways by dilated venous varices. This usually occurs with deep, high-flow AVMs and again, treatment in these patients is difficult but usually entails symptomatic treatment of the hydrocephalus with a standard ventricular peritoneal shunt. In patients with posterior fossa AVMs that become symptomatic and have hydrocephalus, it is sometimes difficult to know whether the symptoms, such as progressive gait difficulty and ataxia, are due to the effects of the lesion on the cerebellum itself or from hydrocephalus. When in doubt, the hydrocephalus should be treated because its treatment is relatively straightforward, usually with ventricular peritoneal shunting, although in those cases caused by obstruction of the aqueduct of Sylvius by a venous varix, an endoscopic third ventriculostomy can be considered.

Treatment considerations

The management of AVMs of the brain is a complicated process that requires a neurologist and/or neurosurgeon to understand clearly a large number of issues related to the AVM, the patient, and the available treatment modalities. Treatment options include observation, stereotactic radiation (radiosurgery), embolization, surgery, or a combination of these modalities. Most importantly, experienced cerebrovascular neurosurgeons should be able to appropriately consider the various factors applicable to each of the treatment options, and recommend a "best" available treatment plan for a given patient. Clearly, every AVM, patient, and surgeon's experience is unique, and thus it is impossible to generate a treatment protocol or formula, and each patient must be considered individually.

Several grading systems have been proposed in assessing AVMs (Luessenhop and Gennarelli, 1977; Pellettieri *et al.*, 1979; Shi and Chen, 1986; Spetzler and Martin, 1986). The most widely utilized system is that of Spetzler and Martin (1986). Points are assigned for certain characteristics (location, deep venous drainage, and size) with the sum being the grade of the AVM. Lesions in eloquent brain are assigned a value of 1 and non-eloquent: zero; presence of deep venous drainage: 1 and no deep venous drainage: zero; size <3 cm: 1, 3–6 cm: 2, and > 6 cm: 3. The utility of this system has been shown by the consistency in predicting the morbidity and mortality associated with surgical treatment of AVMs across independent investigators (Heros *et al.*, 1990; Martin and Vinters, 1995; Spetzler and Martin, 1986).

Imaging characteristics

CT scan, MRI, and conventional contrast cerebral angiography are the standard essential diagnostic tools utilized in planning the treatment of an AVM. A CT scan is generally the screening tool used to investigate patients with neurologic symptoms. In patients harboring an AVM, CT may show hemorrhage, calcifications, hyperdensity, mass effect, hydrocephalus, location of the AVM, and presence of sequelae related to unruptured or ruptured AVMs. The addition of intravenous contrast may show feeding arteries, veins, and nidus. MRI provides further information regarding anatomic localization and topographic relationships between AVM vessels, nidus, and nervous structures as well as evidence of previous hemorrhage (Leblanc *et al.*, 1987; Smith *et al.*, 1988). MR angiography presently remains inferior to conventional contrast cerebral angiography. Angiography provides information crucial to treatment such as identification in various planes and projections of the feeding arteries, nidus, venous drainage patterns, and any associated lesions such as large varices or aneurysms. The recruitment of perforating arteries such as deep thalamoperforators may be identified by an angiogram; this is a characteristic often associated with too great a risk to consider surgical treatment. Flow velocity through an AVM, with implications for postoperative brain swelling or hemorrhage, can also be estimated by angiography. Furthermore, functional studies such as functional MRI, positron emission tomography, and magnetoencephalography are occasionally used to provide further information regarding the eloquence of brain directly adjacent to an AVM; this is occasionally useful in determining the risk of surgical resection and may dictate treatment modality (Bambakidis *et al.*, 2001).

Patient-related factors

The age, general medical health, neurological health, and occupation of the patient with an AVM are all key factors to consider in the decision process (Heros *et al.*, 1993; Heros and Tu, 1987). Any management decision must weigh the risks of treatment against the risks of hemorrhage over the patient's lifetime. The cumulative lifetime hemorrhage risk, assuming a life expectancy of 70 years and an annual hemorrhage risk of 2%–4%, can be predicted by the formula: lifetime risk = 105 – present age (Brown, 2000; Kondziolka *et al.*, 1995). Thus more aggressive management is recommended in younger patients with a very high cumulative risk. Fortunately, these patients also have a higher tolerance of surgical morbidity. Risks of surgery must also be considered in the context of a patient's occupation or lifestyle; for example, a significant risk of hemianopia may be unacceptable to a pilot or a surveyor but tolerated in others.

AVM-related factors

Cerebellar, brainstem, and supratentorial deep nuclear (i.e. basal ganglia and thalamic) AVMs appear to have a higher propensity for bleeding than do hemispheric AVMs (Drake, 1979; Fleetwood *et al.*, 2003; Yasargil, 1988). It is estimated that basal ganglia/thalamic AVMs hemorrhage at a rate 9.8% per year (Fleetwood *et al.*, 2003), with a very high morbidity; 86% develop hemiparesis or hemiplegia. As might be expected, the surgical treatment of AVMs in these locations is also associated with high risks, requiring careful consideration of all treatment options.

Although controversial, smaller sized AVMs may have a higher rate of bleeding (Waltimo, 1973), attributed to higher measured intra-arterial pressures in small AVMs (Spetzler *et al.*, 1992). Han *et al.* (2003) estimated that large AVMs (grade IV and V) bleed at a rate of only 1.5% per year; however, other series fail to correlate AVM size to hemorrhage risk (Brown *et al.*, 1988; Marks *et al.*, 1990). Generally, larger AVMs are associated with a higher degree of surgical morbidity.

Venous drainage patterns are important in planning AVM treatment. AVMs with a single draining vessel (Albert *et al.*, 1990) or the presence of deep venous drainage are associated with increased frequency of bleeding (Nataf *et al.*, 1997). Deep venous drainage, however, may be useful at surgery, as these vessels are protected in the depths of the cavity until the final stages of resection. Stenosis of a draining vein likely increases the risk of AVM bleeding (Miyasaka *et al.*, 1992) and represents a relatively strong indication for surgical treatment.

As discussed above, aneurysms can occur separate from, proximally on a feeding vessel (prenidal), or within the nidus (intranidal) in up to 20% of patients with AVMs. Although their significance is uncertain, prenidal aneurysms may increase the risk for intracerebral hemorrhage (Brown *et al.*, 1990). The impact of an AVM-associated aneurysm on the treatment decision process remains unclear.

Surgeon-related factors

Surgeon experience is crucial in the technical aspects of surgical resection of an AVM and, possibly most importantly, in the decision process in the management of an AVM. Comprehensive management requires an experienced surgeon, endovascular therapist, radiologist, operating room team, and intensive care staff. All but the simplest grade I and II AVMs should be treated by an experienced cerebrovascular surgeon and team in a center treating AVMs on a regular basis.

Treatment options

Embolization

Endovascular occlusion of vessels supplying an AVM may be helpful in making surgical resection less difficult. This is achieved by occluding deep arterial pedicles or perforating arteries that are inaccessible during early stages of resection and are often fragile and difficult to coagulate. Staged occlusion of deep or large feeding pedicles in a high-flow AVM may decrease the risk of postoperative brain swelling or hemorrhage (Martin et al., 2000). Overall, however, embolization is associated with a relatively high risk of morbidity and mortality (Deruty et al., 1996; Frizzel and Fisher, 1995; Nozaki et al., 2000; Wickholm et al., 1996). This can be due to infarct from occlusion of non-AVM or en passage vessels, occlusion of draining veins, or guidewire perforations and hemorrhages (Martin et al., 2000; Taylor et al., 2004). The frequency of serious complications appears to be, in part, related to aggressive attempts at complete endovascular obliteration. In general it is our recommendation that embolization be used judiciously to eliminate difficult-to-access feeding vessels to aid surgical resection or decrease flow through a very high-flow AVM prior to treatment or for palliation of intractable symptoms such as headache, bruit, or progressive neurologic deficit in "unresectable" AVMs. Partial embolization of a large or "unresectable" AVM does not decrease the future risk of hemorrhage (Han et al., 2003).

Surgery

Surgery for an AVM results in immediate elimination of risk of AVM hemorrhage and is generally recommended in a young or healthy patient with a low-grade AVM (i.e. grade I, II, and most grade III), particularly in the presence of venous outflow stenosis, cerebellar location, intractable seizures, or intractable headaches. Occasionally symptomatic grade IV and rarely grade V AVMs are excised, although surgical morbidity is expected to be higher. Surgery for AVM is elective. Even in a patient presenting with hemorrhage and mass effect requiring evacuation, a controlled craniotomy with passive evacuation of the clot is performed, and resection of the AVM is performed later electively as discussed above. The surgical resection of grade I–III AVMs carries a low risk of morbidity and mortality (<10%), consistent across many surgeons (Hamilton and Spetzler, 1994; Heros et al., 1990; Morgan et al., 2003; Pik and Morgan, 2000; Sisti et al., 1993).

Radiosurgery

Obliteration rates of AVMs treated with stereotactic radiation treatment are clearly higher in smaller AVMs (Friedman et al., 1995). Although reporting is inconsistent, the obliteration rate is roughly 80% for lesions less than approximately 3 cm (Friedman, 1997; Pollock et al., 1998, 2003; Steinberg et al., 1991). However, this typically does not occur for up to 2 years after radiation, during which time the patient has the same hemorrhage risk as an untreated AVM. Thus radiosurgery is generally recommended in a patient with a small (3 cm) AVM located in eloquent brain, such as speech or motor cortex, basal ganglia, thalamus, etc., when surgical risk is deemed unacceptable (Heros, 2002; Heros and Korosue, 1990; Sasaki et al., 1998).

Observation

The natural history of AVMs is relatively well-defined except for those malformations that are discovered before bleeding. We are able to recommend, with some confidence, observation for certain AVMs. These include deep brainstem, basal ganglial, or thalamic AVMs too large for radiosurgery, and most grade IV and almost all grade V AVMs.

Conclusions

Brain AVMs are complex cerebrovascular lesions capable of protean symptomatology. They are an infrequent, but serious cause of stroke that often occurs in young people. Most commonly, they result in hemorrhagic stroke by bleeding into the parenchyma of the brain. Much less commonly, they result in subarachnoid hemorrhage. Ischemic stroke is distinctly uncommon with cerebral AVMs but occurs occasionally due to retrograde thrombosis of feeding arteries frequently associated with complete or partial thrombosis of the AVM. Even less commonly, retrograde venous occlusion can result in a stroke-like syndrome, but this usually occurs only after excision or embolization of the high-flow AVM with antegrade thrombosis of the previously arterialized, high-flow venous drainage of the AVM. Of course, seizures can also sometimes mimic ischemic symptoms, and they are the second most common clinical manifestation of cerebral AVMs. AVMs, particularly when they are located in the occipital lobe, can result in classical migranous syndromes, which can at times also be confused with ischemic symptoms.

The natural history of cerebral AVMs is well known because of long follow-up data on large numbers of patients who were untreated. In general, the risk of future hemorrhage is about 2%–4% per year and, of these hemorrhages, about one-third result in significant morbidity, and 1 in 10 are fatal. This risk of future hemorrhage appears to be the same for an AVM that has never bled as for an AVM that bled for more than 6 months previously. Therefore, treatment should be considered in all patients with cerebral AVMs, particularly if they are young, even if the AVM is asymptomatic. The three treatment modalities available to patients with cerebral AVMs – embolization, radiosurgery, and surgical excision – should be carefully considered in each patient and should not be thought of as being interchangeable. The clinician has an obligation to determine the "best" form of treatment for each patient depending on the characteristics of the AVM, factors related to the patient, and of course, the experience of the treating team. Frequently, these treatment alternatives can be used in combination to reduce the overall morbidity of the treatment plan in any one patient. Small and medium-sized AVMs in non-eloquent brain should be surgically excised with or without embolization with the expectation that morbidity in experienced hands should be very low. Small AVMs (<3 cm) in eloquent brain or in deep structures of the brain that would require approach through eloquent brain, should generally be treated with radiosurgery. Observation should be considered for larger lesions that are not amenable to radiosurgery and are located in eloquent areas of the brain. Embolization is rarely curative but can be used to advantage to reduce the risk of subsequent surgery. Partial embolization does not reduce the future risk of hemorrhage; therefore, we do not recommend it as a palliative procedure or as a preradiosurgical procedure.

REFERENCES

Albert, P., Saldago, H., Polaoina, M., *et al.* 1990. A study on the venous drainage of 150 cerebral arteriovenous malformations as related to haemorrhagic risks and size of the lesion. *Acta Neurochir*, **103**, 30–4.

Bambakidis, N. C., Sunshine, J. L., Faulhaber, P. F., *et al.* 2001. Functional evaluation of arteriovenous malformations. *Neurosurg Focus*, **11**, e2.

Batjer, H. H., Devous, M. D. Sr., Seibert, G. B., *et al.* 1988. Intracranial arteriovenous malformation: relationships between clinical and radiographic factors and ipsilateral steal severity. *Neurosurgery*, **23**, 322–8.

Brown, R. D. 2000. Simple risk predictions for arteriovenous malformation hemorrhage. *Neurosurgery*, **46**, 1024.

Brown, R. D., Weibers, D. O., Forbes, G., *et al.* 1988. The natural history of unruptured intracranial arteriovenous malformations. *J Neurosurg*, **68**, 352–7.

Brown, R. D., Weibers, D. O., and Forbes, G. S. 1990. Unruptured intracranial aneurysms and arteriovenous malformations: frequency of intracranial hemorrhage and relationship of lesions. *J Neurosurg*, **73**, 859–63.

Brown, R. D., Weibers, D. O., Torner, J. C., and O'Fallon, W. M. 1996. Incidence and prevalence or intracranial vascular malformations in Olmsted County, Minnesota, 1965 to 1992. *Neurology*, **46**, 949–52.

Crawford, P. M., West, C. R., Chadwick, D. W., and Shaw, M. D. M. 1986. Arteriovenous malformations of the brain: the natural history in unoperated patients. *J Neurol Neurosurg Psychiatr*, **49**, 1–10.

Cushing, H., and Bailey, P. 1928. Tumors arising from the blood vessels of the brain. Angiomatous malformations and hemangioblastomas, vol III. Springfield, IL: Thomas.

Dandy, W. 1928. Arteriovenous aneurysms of the brain. *Arch Surg*, **17**, 715–93.

Deruty, R., Pelissou-Guyotat, I., Amat, D., *et al.* 1996. Complications after multidisciplinary treatment of cerebral arteriovenous malformations. *Acta Neurochir*, **138**, 119–31.

Diehl, R. R., Henkes, H., Nahser, H. C., Kuhne, D., and Berlit, P. 1994. Blood flow velocity and vasomotor reactivity in patients with arteriovenous malformations. A transcranial Doppler study. *Stroke*, **25**, 1574–80.

Drake, C. G. 1979. Cerebral arteriovenous malformations: considerations for and experience with surgical treatment in 166 cases. *Clin Neurosurg*, **26**, 145–208.

Feindel, W., Yamamoto, Y. L., Hodge, C. P. 1971. The cerebral microcirculation in man: analysis by radioisotopic microregional flow measurement and fluorescein angiography. *Clin Neurosurg*, **18**, 225–46.

Fleetwood, I. G., Marcellus, M. L., Levy, R. P., Marks, M. P., and Steinberg, G. K. 2003. Deep arteriovenous malformations of the basal ganglia and thalamus: natural history. *J Neurosurg*, **98**, 747–50.

Friedman, W. A. 1997. Radiosurgery versus surgery for arteriovenous malformations: the case for radiosurgery. *Clin Neurosurg*, **45**, 18–20.

Friedman, W. A., Bova, F. J., and Mendenhall, W. M. 1995. Linear accelerator radiosurgery for arteriovenous malformations: the relationship of size to outcome. *J Neurosurg*, **82**, 180–9.

Frizzel, R. T., and Fisher, W. S. 1995. Cure, morbidity, and mortality associated with embolization of brain arteriovenous malformations: a review of 1246 patients in 32 series of a 35-year period. *Neurosurgery*, **37**, 1031–40.

Graf, C. J., Perret, G. E., and Torner, J. C. 1983. Bleeding from cerebral arteriovenous malformations as part of their natural history. *J Neurosurg*, **58**, 331–7.

Hamilton, M. G., and Spetzler, R. F. 1994. The prospective application of a grading system for arteriovenous malformations. *Neurosurgery*, **34**, 2–7.

Han, P. P., Ponce, F. A., and Spetzler, R. F. 2003. Intention-to-treat analysis of Spetzler-Martin grades IV and V arteriovenous malformations: natural history and treatment paradigm. *J Neurosurg*, **98**, 3–7.

Heros, R. C. 2002. Treatment of arteriovenous malformations: gamma knife surgery. *J Neurosurg*, **97**, 753–4.

Heros, R. C., and Korosue, K. 1990. Radiation treatment of cerebral arteriovenous malformations. *N Engl J Med*, **323**, 127–9.

Heros, R. C., Korosue, K., and Diebold, P. M. 1990. Surgical excision of cerebral arteriovenous malformations: late results. *Neurosurgery*, **26**, 570–7.

Heros, R. C., Morcos, J., and Korosue, K. 1993. Arteriovenous malformations of the brain. Surgical management. *Clin Neurosurg*, **40**, 139–73.

Heros, R. C., and Tu, Y. K. 1987. Is surgical therapy needed for unruptured arteriovenous malformations? *Neurology*, **37**, 279–86.

Kondziolka, D., McLaughlin, M. R., and Kestle, J. R. 1995. Simple risk predictions for arteriovenous malformation hemorrhage. *Neurosurgery*, **37**, 851–5.

Leblanc, R., Levesque, M., Comair, Y., and Ethier, R. 1987. Magnetic resonance imaging of cerebral arteriovenous malformations. *Neurosurgery*, **21**, 15–20.

Lindegaard, K. F., Grolimund, P., Aaslid, R., and Nornes, H. 1986. Evaluation of cerebral AVM's using transcranial Doppler ultrasound. *J Neurosurg*, **65**, 335–44.

Luessenhop, A. J., and Gennarelli, T. A. 1977. Anatomical grading of supratentorial arteriovenous malformations for determining operability. *Neurosurgery*, **1**, 30–5.

Malis, L. I. 1979. Microsurgery for spinal cord arteriovenous malformations. *Clin Neurosurg*, **26**, 543–69.

Manchola, I. F., De Salles, A. A., Foo, T. K., *et al.* 1993. Arteriovenous malformation hemodynamics: a transcranial Doppler study. *Neurosurgery*, **33**, 556–62.

Marks, M. P., Lane, B., Steinberg, G. K., and Chang, P. J. 1990. Hemorrhage in intracerebral arteriovenous malformations: angiographic determinants. *Radiology*, **176**, 807–13.

Martin, N. A., Khanna, R., Doberstein, C., and Bentson, J. 2000. Therapeutic embolization of arteriovenous malformations: the case for and against. *Clin Neurosurg*, **46**, 295–318.

Martin, N. A., Vinters, H. V. 1995. Arteriovenous malformations. In *Neurovascular Surgery*, eds. L. P. Carter, and R. F. Spetzler. New York: McGraw-Hill.

Mast, H., Mohr, J. P., Osipov, A., *et al.* 1995. 'Steal' is an unestablished mechanism for the clinical presentation of cerebral arteriovenous malformations. *Stroke*, **26**, 1215–20.

Mast, H., Mohr, J. P., Thompson, J. L., *et al.* 1995. Transcranial Doppler ultrasonography in cerebral arteriovenous malformations. Diagnostic sensitivity and association of flow velocity with spontaneous hemorrhage and focal neurological deficit. *Stroke*, **26**, 1024–7.

Miyasaka, Y., Yada, K., Ohwada, T., *et al.* 1992. An analysis of the venous drainage system as a factor in hemorrhage from arteriovenous malformations. *J Neurosurg*, **76**, 239–43.

Moniz, E. 1927. L'encephalographie arterielle: son importance dans la localisation des tumeurs cerebrales. *Rev Neurol (Paris)*, **2**, 72–90.

Morgan, M. K., Winder, M., Little, N. S., Finfer, S., and Ritson, E. 2003. Delayed hemorrhage following resection of an arteriovenous malformation in the brain. *J Neurosurg*, **99**, 967–71.

Nataf, F., Meder, J. F., and Roux, F. X. 1997. Angioarchitecture associated with haemorrhage in cerebral arteriovenous malformations: a prognostic statistical model. *Neuroradiology*, **39**, 52–8.

Norlen, G. 1949. Arteriovenous aneurysms of the brain; report of ten cases of total removal of the lesion. *J Neurosurg*, **6**, 475–94.

Nozaki, K., Hashimoto, N., Miyamoto, S., and Kikuchi, H. 2000. Resectability of Spetzler-Martin grade IV and V cerebral arteriovenous malformations. *J Clin Neurosci*, **7**(**Suppl 1**), 78–81.

Okabe, T., Meyer, J. S., Okayasu, H., *et al.* 1983. Xenon-enhanced CT CBF measurements in cerebral AVM's before and after excision. Contribution to pathogenesis and treatment. *J Neurosurg*, **59**, 21–31.

Olivecrona, H., and Riives, J. 1948. Arteriovenous aneurysms of the brain: their diagnosis and treatment. *Arch Neurol Psychiatry*, **59**, 567–603.

Ondra, S. L., Troupp, H., George, E. D., and Schwab, K. 1990. The natural history of symptomatic arteriovenous malformations of the brain: a 24 year follow-up assessment. *J Neurosurg*, **73**, 387–91.

Parkinson, D., and Bachers, G. 1980. Arteriovenous malformations. Summary of 100 consecutive supratentorial cases. *J Neurosurg*, **53**, 285–99.

Pellettieri, L., Carlsson, C. A., Grevsten, S., Norlen, G., and Uhlemann, C. 1979. Surgical versus conservative treatment of intracranial arteriovenous malformations. A study in surgical decision-making. *Acta Neurochir*, (**Suppl**) **29**, 1–86.

Penfield, W., and Erickson, T. 1941. *Epilepsy and Cerebral Llocalization*. Springfield, IL: Charles C. Thomas, 1941.

Perret, G., and Nishioka, H. 1966. Report on the cooperative study of intracranial aneurysms and subarachnoid hemorrhage. Section IV. Arteriovenous malformations. An analysis of 545 cases of cranio-cerebral arteriovenous malformations and fistulae reported to the cooperative study. *J Neurosurg*, **25**, 467–90.

Pik, J. H., and Morgan, M. K. 2000. Microsurgery for small arteriovenous malformations of the brain: results in 110 consecutive patients. *Neurosurgery*, **47**, 571–5.

Pollock, B. E., Flickinger, J. C., Lundsford, L. D., Maitz, A., and Kondziolka, D. 1998. Factors associated with successful arteriovenous malformation radiosurgery. *Neurosurgery*, **42**, 1239–47.

Pollock, B. E., Gorman, D. A., and Coffey, R. J. 2003. Patient outcome after arteriovenous malformation radiosurgical management: results based on a 5- to 14- year follow-up study. *Neurosurgery*, **52**, 1291–7.

Sasaki, T., Kurita, H., Saito, I., *et al.* 1998. Arteriovenous malformations in the basal ganglia and thalamus: management and results in 101 cases. *J Neurosurg*, **88**, 285–92.

Schwartz, A., and Hennerici, M. 1986. Noninvasive transcranial Doppler ultrasound in intracranial angiomas. *Neurology*, **36**, 626–35.

Shi, Y. Q., and Chen, X. C. 1986. A proposed scheme for grading intracranial arteriovenous malformations. *J Neurosurg*, **65**, 484–9.

Sisti, M. B., Koder, A., and Stein, B. M. 1993. Microsurgery for 67 intracranial arteriovenous malformations less than 3 cm in diameter. *J Neurosurg*, **79**, 653–60.

Smith, H. J., Strother, C. M., Kikuchi, Y., *et al.* 1988. MR imaging in the management of supratentorial intracranial AVMs. *AJR Am J Roentgenol*, **150**, 1143–53.

Spetzler, R. F., Hargraves, R. W., McCormick, P. W., *et al.* 1992. Relationship of perfusion pressure and size to risk of hemorrhage from arteriovenous malformations. *J Neurosurg*, **76**, 918–23.

Spetzler, R. F., and Martin, N. A. 1986. A proposed grading system for arteriovenous malformations. *J Neurosurg*, **65**, 476–83.

Spetzler, R. F., Wilson, C. B., Weinstein, P., *et al.* 1978. Normal perfusion pressure breakthrough theory. *Clin Neurosurg*, **25**, 651–72.

Steinberg, G. K., Fabricant, J. I., Marks, M. P., *et al.* 1991. Stereotactic helium ion Bragg peak radiosurgery for intracranial arteriovenous malformations. Detailed clinical and neurologic outcome. *Stereotact Funct Neurosurg*, **57**, 36–49.

Tamaki, N., Ehara, K., Lin, T. K., *et al.* 1991. Cerebral arteriovenous malformations: factors influencing the surgical difficulty and outcome. *Neurosurgery*, **29**, 856–61.

Taylor, C. L., Dutton, K., Rappard, G., *et al.* 2004. Complications of preoperative embolization of cerebral arteriovenous malformations. *J Neurosurg*, **100**, 810–2.

Troost, B. T., and Newton, T. H. 1975. Occipital lobe arteriovenous malformations. Clinical and radiologic features in 26 cases with comments on differentiation from migraine. *Arch Ophthalmol*, **93**, 250–6.

Waltimo, O. 1973. The relationship of size, density and localization of intracranial arteriovenous malformations to the type of initial symptom. *J Neurol Sci*, **19**, 13–9.

Wickholm, G., Lundqvist, C., and Svendsen, P. 1996. Embolization of cerebral arteriovenous malformations: part I – technique, morphology, and complications. *Neurosurgery*, **39**, 448–57.

Yasargil, M. G. 1969. *Microsurgery Applied to Neurosurgery*. Stuttgart, West Germany: George Thieme Verlag.

Yasargil, M. G. 1987. *Microneurosurgery*, volume IIIA: AVM of the brain, history, embryology, pathological considerations, hemodynamics, diagnostic studies, microsurgical anatomy. Stuttgart, West Germany: George Thieme Verlag.

Yasargil, M. G. 1988. *Microneurosurgery*, volume IIIB: AVM of the brain, clinical considerations, general and special operative techniques, surgical results, non-operated cases, cavernous and venous angiomas, neuroanesthesia. Stuttgart, West Germany: George Thieme Verlag.

Philippe Metellus, Siddharth Kharkar, Doris Lin, Sumit Kapoor, and Daniele Rigamonti

Introduction

Cavernous malformations (CMs) are angiographically occult vascular malformation considered as congenital anomalies of the brain. The first comprehensive review by Voigt and Yasargil (1976) provided a good overview of the knowledge of CMs in the 1970s with special references to epidemiology, diagnosis, and clinical findings. Over the past two decades numerous articles on CMs have been published, and our knowledge of this pathology has considerably evolved (Awad and Robinson, 1993; Moriarity, Clatterbuck, and Rigamonti, 1999; Simard et al., 1986). There is now general agreement on the diagnosis and pathology of CMs, but controversies still persist in the recent literature concerning their natural history and dynamic nature. Recent literature concerning the genetics of CMs and their biology with special reference to angiogenesis and cellular proliferation has provided new clues to the pathogenesis and pathophysiology of these malformations.

The therapeutic management of CMs, particularly in those located within highly functional areas of the brain, remains a source of debate, and the place of conservative management, surgical removal, and radiosurgery has still to be defined.

We address in this chapter a review of the pertinent literature on CMs regarding epidemiology, genetics, pathology, clinical findings, and therapeutic management with special emphasis placed upon the natural bleeding risk of these malformations.

Terminology and pathologic classification

In 1846 the term "cavernous" as applied to a vascular lesion of the brain was used for the first time by Rokitansky. In 1853, Luschka et al. reported a case of so-called cavernous vascular brain tumor with a detailed macroscopic description, but histopathology of CM was first described in 1863 by Virchow (Luschka, 1854; Rokitansky, 1846; Virchow, 1864–1865). Crawford and Russel (1956) first coined the term "cryptic" vascular malformation in reference to small, clinically "latent" vascular lesions, some of which were angiographically occult, that resulted in either apoplectic cerebral hemorrhage or signs of a growing mass lesion. Later, the term "angiographically occult vascular malformations" was introduced by many investigators (Dillon, 1997; McCormick et al., 1968; Ogilvy and Heros, 1988; Roberson et al., 1974). The terms "occult" and "cryptic" are now more or less synonymous, and refer to vascular malformations that have in common angiographic invisibility and a distinct appearance on MRI (Dillon, 1997). There is not wide agreement on terminology, as there is no consensus on the precise pathology or pathophysiology of these lesions.

The most widely accepted classification of cerebral vascular malformation was published by McCormick and colleagues (McCormick et al., 1968; McCormick and Nofzinger, 1966). They described four types of cerebral vascular malformations: arteriovenous malformations (AVMs), CMs, capillary telangiectasies, and venous malformations. Venous malformations have also been referred to as venous angiomas, but they are now properly called developmental venous anomalies (DVAs). McCormick's system divided central nervous system (CNS) vascular malformations based on both gross and microscopic pathological features, including the architecture of involved vessels and their relationship with the surrounding parenchyma (McCormick et al., 1968; McCormick and Nofzinger, 1966). The coexistence of two or more of these types in the same patient or even in the same lesion has been well documented (Awad et al., 1993; Chang et al., 1997; Rigamonti et al., 1988, 1991; Roberson et al., 1974; Robinson et al., 1991). Transitional forms between CM and capillary telangiectasia have been identified (Rigamonti et al., 1991). The existence of these transitional lesions raises the possibility that CM and capillary telangectasia represent a spectrum within a single pathological entity (Rigamonti et al., 1991).

CMs of the brain are now defined as hamartomatous vascular lesions with specific characteristics. Macroscopically they appear as well-circumscribed lesions with a reddish purple, multilobulated appearance resembling a mulberry. Microscopically they can be clearly distinguished from other vascular malformations due to specific features that will be described in more detail below. Current nomenclature includes terms such as cavernoma, cavernous angioma, cavernous hemangioma, and CM, which are used synonymously (Zabramski et al., 1999).

Epidemiology

Incidence and prevalence

No reliable study reflects the true incidence and prevalence of CMs in the population. From large series based on necropsy and/or MRI, the overall incidence reported in the general population varies from 0.1% to 0.9% (Del Curling et al., 1991; McCormick, 1966; Rigamonti et al., 1996; Robinson et al., 1991; Zabramski et al., 1999). Clinically, symptomatic lesions seem to be less common (Cantu et al., 2005; Del Curling et al., 1991; McLaughlin et al.,

Uncommon Causes of Stroke, 2nd edition, ed. Louis R. Caplan. Published by Cambridge University Press. © Cambridge University Press 2008.

1998; Moriarity, Clatterbuck, and Rigamonti, 1999; Robinson *et al.*, 1991). They constitute 8%–15% of all vascular malformations (Del Curling *et al.*, 1991; Kim *et al.*, 1997; Labauge *et al.*, 2000; Moriarity, Clatterbuck, and Rigamonti, 1999; Porter *et al.*, 1999; Robinson *et al.*, 1991). The incidence of CMs found before death is clearly linked to the development of imaging modalities. In the angiography era, only a few CMs were diagnosed clinically, and the relation of incidence between CMs and AVMs was estimated as 1:20 (Johnson *et al.*, 1993). Although Vaquero, Cabezudo, and Leunda, (1983) noted that only 44% of CMs were detected preoperatively by CT scan, this imaging modality has been responsible for a significant increase in their diagnosis. The advent and the widespread use of MRI represented considerable progress in CM imaging diagnosis. According to large MRI-based retrospective studies, there is an incidence rate of 0.47% (Del Curling *et al.*, 1991) or 0.39% (Robinson *et al.*, 1991), whereas an Australian study reported a 0.9% prevalence (Sage *et al.*, 1993).

Age

The range of age varies between neonates and the ninth decade, with a median of 34 years (Robinson and Awad, 1993). The highest incidence seems to occur between the third and fifth decades (Hsu *et al.*, 1993). The mean age of large series varies between 32.2 and 37.6 (Abdulrauf, Kaynar, and Awad, 1999; Amin-Hanjani and Ogilvy, 1999; Bertalanffy *et al.*, 1992, 2002; Del Curling *et al.*, 1991; Kim *et al.*, 1997; Kondziolka, Lunsford, and Kestle, 1995; Moriarity, Wetzel, Clatterbuck, *et al.*, 1999; Porter *et al.*, 1999; Robinson *et al.*, 1991, 1993). Maraire and Awad (1995) found that one-fourth of the patients in the various series were children, which is consistent with the findings of Mottolese *et al.*, 2001. Among 172 pediatric patients, Cavalheiro and Braga (1999) noted two age peaks: one during the first year of life and the other between the ages of 12 and 16 years.

Sex distribution

An equal distribution is observed in both sexes even if some authors report a female predominance in patients between 30 and 60 years (Giombini and Morello, 1978; Hsu *et al.*, 1993; Otten *et al.*, 1989; Simard *et al.*, 1986; Wakai *et al.*, 1985; Yamasaki *et al.*, 1986). Among 1240 cases collected by Hahn (1999) in which the sex distribution was mentioned, 644 (52%) were female and 596 (48%) were male.

Location

Supratentorial lesions account for 63%–81% of the total (Abdulrauf, Kaynar, and Awad, 1999; Aiba *et al.*, 1995; Amin-Hanjani and Ogilvy, 1999; Bertalanffy *et al.*, 1992, 2002; Del Curling *et al.*, 1991; Kim *et al.*, 1997; Moriarity, Wetzel, Clatterbuck, *et al.*, 1999; Otten *et al.*, 1989; Porter *et al.*, 1999; Robinson *et al.*, 1991, 1993). Most commonly frontal and temporal, they tend to be located cortically or subcortically in more than 50% of cases and less frequently paraventricular, in the basal ganglia, the lateral ventricle, and the thalamus (Chadduck *et al.*, 1985; Coin *et al.*, 1977; Namba,

1983; Numaguchi *et al.*, 1977; Pau and Orunesu, 1979; Reyns *et al.*, 1999; Simard *et al.*, 1986; Tatagiba *et al.*, 1991; Yamasaki *et al.*, 1986). Posterior fossa CMs constitute 7.8%–35.8% of all cases, and the brainstem is the most common site of involvement in this compartment representing 9%–35% of all CNS cases (de Oliveira *et al.*, 2006; Fritschi *et al.*, 1994; Kondziolka, Lunsford, and Kestle, 1995; Porter *et al.*, 1999; Simard *et al.*, 1986). Fritschi *et al.* (1994) described the location of the pontine lesions as being close to the surface of the fourth ventricle in 50%, extending into one of the cerebellar peduncles in 30%, and localized deeply in the pons in 20%. Of the mesencephalic lesions, more than 60% were located in the tectum. Among 1311 cases, Hahn (1999) found that 899 lesions (68.6%) were located supratentorially, 339 (25.8%) infratentorially, and 73 lesions (5.5%) were in the spinal cord. The lesion side was documented in 902 cases, revealing no evident side predilection (Hahn, 1999).

CMs are also found in less frequent locations such as the third ventricle (Harbaugh *et al.*, 1984; Lavyne and Patterson, 1983; Ogawa *et al.*, 1990; Pozzati *et al.*, 1981), the pineal region (Fukui *et al.*, 1983; Lombardi *et al.*, 1996; Occhiogrosso *et al.*, 1983; Vaquero *et al.*, 1980), or extra-axially. Extra-axial CMs are relatively rare. (Biondi *et al.*, 2002; Goel *et al.*, 2003; Lewis *et al.*, 1994; Lombardi *et al.*, 1994; Okada *et al.*, 1977; Vogler and Castillo, 1995). Their most common location is in the middle cranial fossa near the cavernous sinus (Biondi *et al.*, 2002). Other localizations such as tentorium cerebelli, dura mater of the vertex, cerebellopontine angle, Meckel's cave, or anterior cranial fossa have been described (Bordi *et al.*, 1991; Fehlings and Tucker, 1988; Hyodo *et al.*, 2000; Isla *et al.*, 1989; Lewis *et al.*, 1994; Moritake *et al.*, 1985). These lesions have also been reported in the sella turcica and the optic chiasm. The involvement of some cranial nerves has also been described (Cobbs and Wilson, 2001; Lombardi *et al.*, 1994; Sundaresan *et al.*, 1976; Yamada *et al.*, 1986). Extension in the skull has been reported, and intraosseous CMs of the skull are well known (Heckl *et al.*, 2002a, 2002b; Voelker *et al.*, 1998).

Familiality (hereditary) and multiplicity

CMs occur in two forms: a sporadic or nonhereditary form, in which patients tend to have a single isolated lesion; and a familial form characterized by the presence of multiple lesions, the number of which is strongly correlated to patients' age (Denier, Goutagny, LaBauge, *et al.*, 2004; Denier *et al.*, 2006; Labauge *et al.*, 1998; Rigamonti *et al.*, 1988; Zabramski *et al.*, 1994). Although a familial form of CMs has been suspected since the 1930s, it was believed to account for only a small fraction of all cases of CMs before the introduction of MRI (Clark, 1970; Kufs, 1928; Michael and Levin, 1936). In a review of 24 patients with histologically verified CMs, Rigamonti *et al.* (1988) found that 54% of patients with CMs have a strong family history consistent with a hereditary pattern of development.

The familial form appears to be more frequent in Hispanics. (Denier, Goutagny, LaBauge, *et al.*, 2004; Denier *et al.*, 2006; Gunel *et al.*, 1995, 1996a, 1996b; Hayman *et al.*, 1982; Rigamonti *et al.*, 1988; Zabramski *et al.*, 1994). The proportion of the familial form is less frequent in Caucasians who represent approximately 20% of cases (Denier, Goutagny, LaBauge, *et al.*, 2004; Denier *et al.*, 2006; Gunel *et al.*, 1996b; Labauge *et al.*, 1998). Clinical and neuroradiological studies conducted before the identification of the cerebral CMs genes helped to delineate some of the main features of this condition, namely its autosomal dominant pattern of inheritance and its incomplete clinical penetrance. These studies also showed the intrafamilial and interfamilial variability of familial CMs (Couteulx *et al.*, 2002; Denier, Goutagny, LaBauge, *et al.*, 2004; Denier *et al.*, 2006; Eerola *et al.*, 2000; Labauge *et al.*, 1998, 1999; Rigamonti *et al.*, 1988).

In their clinical analysis of all previously documented cases, Voigt and Yasargil (1976) reported a multiple lesion incidence in 13.4%. An incidence of 9.9% was found in a large autopsy study (Otten *et al.*, 1989), and it was between 10% and 21% in large MRI studies (Del Curling *et al.*, 1991; Kim *et al.*, 1997; Kondziolka, Lunsford, and Kestle, 1995; Porter *et al.*, 1999; Robinson *et al.*, 1991). The frequency of cases with multiple lesions varies widely between sporadic (nonfamilial) and hereditary (familial) forms (Hsu *et al.*, 1993; Rigamonti *et al.*, 1988). In the latter, 50%–93% of patients harbor multiple lesions (Labauge *et al.*, 2000), whereas in sporadic forms 10%–33% of multiples lesions have been reported (Clatterbuck *et al.*, 2000; Gunel et al., 1995, 1996a, 1996b). In a study that analyzed the MRI features of 68 patients, Clatterbuck *et al.* (2000) found more than 228 CMs in their population of 24 men and 44 women. In this series, multiple lesions were present in 11 of 13 familial cases (84.6%) and in 14 of the 55 sporadic cases (25.4%) (Clatterbuck *et al.*, 2000).

Radiation-induced lesions

The use of radiation therapy as a primary treatment modality or as an adjuvant therapy is increasing in patients harboring CNS lesions. Although radiation therapy is an effective therapeutic option in many situations, it is now becoming clear that there are some long-term sequelae associated with this treatment. De novo formation of CMs after brain irradiation, most of which occur in the pediatric population, is observed with an increasing frequency (Nimjee *et al.*, 2006). There is a propensity for these lesions to occur in males, and they are most frequently encountered in patients who have undergone irradiation for medulloblastomas, gliomas, and acute lymphoblastic leukemia (Nimjee *et al.*, 2006). Nimjee *et al.* (2006) compiled data from all 76 reported patients in whom de novo CMs formed after brain irradiation. They found that the mean age of patients at the time of irradiation was 11.7 years and that the mean latency period before detection of the CMs was 8.9 years. These patients received a mean radiation dose of 60.5 Gy. Most of these patients were asymptomatic at the time of diagnosis, and the most common presenting symptom in symptomatic patients was a seizure. During follow-up, 37 (48.7%) of 76 patients had a hemorrhagic event and 54% had surgical intervention (Nimjee *et al.*, 2006). Because there is a propensity for radiation-induced CMs to hemorrhage, a close monitoring of these lesions is warranted. More exceptional cases of de novo CMs forming in the spinal cord after irradiation have been reported. Although they appear with equal frequency at the cervical and thoracic levels,

they are rare in the lumbar region (Jabbour *et al.*, 2004; Maraire *et al.*, 1999; Yoshino *et al.*, 2005).

Although there are several hypotheses (vascular and connective tissue changes in stroma, cell swelling, vessel lumen dilatation, and exaggerated fibrosis, hyalization, and mineralization) to explain why these lesions occur, to date the pathophysiological mechanisms underlying radiation-induced CM formation are not clearly understood.

Genetics

Familial (hereditary) condition

Kufs (1928) first suggested that the transmission and development of CMs might be genetically influenced. These early suspicions were supported by a limited number of subsequent reports (Bicknell *et al.*, 1978; Clark, 1970; Combelles *et al.*, 1983; Hayman *et al.*, 1982; Kidd and Cummings, 1947; Michael and Levin, 1936) until the pioneering work of Rigamonti *et al.* (1988) was published. They found in 13 patients (54% of their population) of six unrelated families of Mexican-Americans a positive family history with a high incidence of multiple lesions on T2-weighted (T2WI) MRI constituting the hallmarks of the familial form of CMs that seems to be transmitted in an autosomal dominant fashion (Rigamonti *et al.*, 1988). Since then, an increasing number of reports have confirmed the more frequent incidence than previously reported of the familial form of CMs, especially among Hispanics, and genetic predisposition has been recognized to be important in their pathophysiology (Gangemi *et al.*, 1990; Gunel *et al.*, 1996a; Labauge *et al.*, 1998; Mason *et al.*, 1988; Steichen-Gersdorf *et al.*, 1992; Zabramski *et al.*, 1994). Analysis of linkage in Hispanic American kindreds has revealed genetic homogeneity, with linkage to CCM1 locus at 7q21–22 (Dubovsky *et al.*, 1995; Gunel *et al.*, 1995; Marchuk *et al.*, 1995). In this population, there is strong evidence of a founder mutation that accounts for virtually all inherited and many apparently sporadic cases (Gunel *et al.*, 1996a). Studies in this population have demonstrated a delayed and incomplete penetrance of the disease among known gene carriers (Gunel *et al.*, 1996a). In 1998, Craig *et al.* (1998) found two additional cerebral CM loci (CCM 2 at 7p15–13 and CCM3 at 3p25.2–27) in 20 non-Hispanic Caucasian kindreds. Linkage to the three loci (CCM1, CCM2, and CCM3) could account for inheritance of cerebral CMs in all of the kindreds studied (Craig *et al.*, 1998). They also showed a genetic heterogeneity of inherited non-Hispanic Caucasian patients harboring cerebral CMs with the following distribution: 40% CCM1, 20% CCM2, and 40% CCM3 (Craig *et al.*, 1998).

Clinical penetrance in familial cerebral CM is reported to be incomplete (Craig *et al.*, 1998; Denier, Goutagny, LaBauge, *et al.*, 2004; Denier *et al.*, 2006). In a French survey of 163 consecutively recruited cerebral CM families, 333 CCM1/CCM2/CCM3 mutation carriers were analyzed, and clinical penetrance was found to be 62% (Denier *et al.*, 2006). In another North American survey of non-Hispanic kindred, Craig *et al.* (1998) found a symptomatic disease penetrance in CCM1, CCM2, and CCM3 mutation carriers of 88%, 100%, and 63%, respectively. Neuroimaging penetrance of cerebral CMs was considered much higher and complete or almost complete. However, an increasing number of normal MRIs in mutation carriers is reported. Recently, Denier, Labauge, Brunereau, *et al.* (2004) found up to 13% of T2WI MRIs to be normal in 76 asymptomatic CCM1 mutation carriers and five (6.6%) normal gradient-echo MRI. These findings, combined with the incomplete clinical penetrance, strongly suggest that the familial nature of cerebral CM may be overlooked in some patients.

CCM1 has been identified as the Krev Interaction Trapped 1 (KRIT-1) gene (Laberge-le Couteulx *et al.*, 1999; Sahoo *et al.*, 1999). KRIT-1, a protein of unknown function so far, was previously identified through a yeast two-hybrid screen designed to identify proteins interacting with Rap1 A, a small Ras-like GTPase protein (Serebriiskii *et al.*, 1997). KRIT-1 encodes a 736 amino-acid protein containing four ankyrin domains, a FERM domain, and a C-terminal portion interacting with Rap1 A, a small ras-like GTP-ase and ICAP1α, a modulator of β1 integrin signal transduction pathway, as well as with CCM2 protein (Frischmeyer and Dietz, 1999; Serebriiskii *et al.*, 1997; Zawistowski *et al.*, 2002, 2005; Zhang *et al.*, 2001). The KRIT-1 protein, the product of the KRIT-1 gene, has been found in vascular endothelium, astrocytes, and pyramidal cells of the adult brain (Guzeloglu-Kayisli *et al.*, 2004). The essential function of this protein is shown in KRIT-1 knockout mice, which die at mid-gestation of vascular pathology suggesting an essential role in arterial morphogenesis (Whitehead *et al.*, 2004). Recently, eight additional exons have been described among which are four coding exons. This novel N-terminal region of KRIT-1 has been shown to contain an NPXY motif required for interaction of KRIT-1 with the integrin-binding protein ICAP1α (Zawistowski *et al.*, 2002). Integrin molecules are transmembrane receptor proteins that play a critical role in endothelial cell-cell and cell-extracellular matrix (ECM) interactions as well as in endothelial cell migration and lumen formation during angiogenesis (Bloch *et al.*, 1997; Brooks, 1996a, 1996b; Gamble *et al.*, 1999). The ICAP1α has been identified to bind avidly to the β1 integrin cytoplasmic domain (Zhang *et al.*, 2001).

In a mutational analysis of 206 families with cerebral CMs, Laurans *et al.* (2003) showed that all mutations were nonsense mutations, frame-shift mutations predicting premature termination, or splice-site mutations located throughout the KRIT-1 gene, suggesting that these are genetic-loss-function mutations. These genetic findings in conjunction with the clinical phenotype are consistent with a two-hit model for the occurrence of cerebral CMs. Mutations of the KRIT-1 gene result in complete loss of KRIT-1/ICAP1α interaction (Zawistowski *et al.*, 2002). Most mutations in the KRIT-1 gene responsible for familial CM result in early stop codons and truncated protein synthesis, suggesting a defect in ICAP1α-mediated ECM interaction as a possible contributor to cerebral CM pathogenesis (Dashti *et al.*, 2006).

Gunel *et al.* (2002) showed that KRIT-1 encodes a microtubule-associated protein, possibly responsible for microtubule targeting. Furthermore, interaction of KRIT-1 with Rap1a and ICAPP1α-integrin suggests that KRIT-1 may help modulate the cytoskeleton, and thus shape endothelial cell morphology and function in response to cell-matrix and cell-cell interactions. Gunel *et al.*

(2002), propose that the loss of this targeting mechanism would lead to abnormal endothelial tube development and the subsequent appearance of cerebral CMs.

The CCM2 locus has been identified as the MGC4607 gene located on 7p15–13 and encoding the phosphotyrosine binding (PTB) domain protein malcavernin (Liquori *et al.*, 2003; Zawistowski *et al.*, 2005), the murine ortholog of which was characterized as a mitogen-activated protein kinase (MAPK) scaffold named osmosensing scaffold for MEKK3 (OSM). The OSM is involved in the cellular response to osmotic insults, and is required for MEKK3-mediated activation of p38 in response to cellular stress (Uhlik *et al.*, 2003). It is known that p38 is one of several intracellular kinases that transduce signals essential for vascular remodeling and maturation (Issbrucker *et al.*, 2003; Jackson *et al.*, 1998; Tanaka *et al.*, 1999). The p38 kinase negatively regulates endothelial cell survival, proliferation, and differentiation in fibroblast growth factor 2-stimulated angiogenesis (Matsumoto *et al.*, 2002). McMullen *et al.* (2005) showed cell cycle arrest in endothelial cells transfected with an upstream activator of p38 MAPK. The same cells have increased migration, with alterations in the actin ultrastructure and enhanced lamellipodia. Further evidence for a regulatory capacity for p38 in angiogenesis is provided by its critical role in mural cell recruitment during neovascularization in the rat aorta model of angiogenesis (Zhu *et al.*, 2003).

Using in situ hybridization, Seker *et al.* (2006) found significant colocalization of CCM2 with CCM1 messenger RNA in embryonal and postnatal mice. This was confirmed at the protein expression level, with both proteins present in arterial endothelium as well as in pyramidal neurons and the foot processes of astrocytes. Co-immunoprecipitation and fluorescence resonance energy transfer studies showed that the CCM1 and CCM2 gene products interact with each other (Zawistowski *et al.*, 2005). In much the same way that CCM1 and β1 integrin interact with ICAP1α, this interaction is dependent on the PTB domain of CCM2 and is inhibited by a familial CCM2 missense mutation, suggesting that loss of this interaction may be another step in the pathogenesis of familial CMs (Zawistowski *et al.*, 2005). In the same way, Zhang *et al.* (2007) reported recently that KRIT-1 interacts with malcavernin through its NPXY motifs and may shuttle it through the nucleus via its nuclear localization signal and nuclear export signals, thereby regulating its cellular function. The parallel expression and mutual binding of CCM1 and CCM2 suggest that they may function through the same regulatory pathways in CM formation. Moreover, CCM1, CCM2, and MEKK3 bind in a ternary complex, suggesting that the pathways are not simply parallel but probably converge.

Approximately 40% of kindred with familial CMs show linkage to the CCM3 locus (Craig *et al.*, 1998). The CCM3 locus has been identified as the programmed cell death 10 (PDCD10) gene located on 3q25.2–27 (Bergametti *et al.*, 2005). The PDCD10 gene codes for a 212 amino acid protein lacking any known domains. PDCD10 gene, also called "TFAR15," was initially identified by screening for genes differentially expressed during the induction of apoptosis, which is an essential process in arterial morphogenesis, in the TF-1 premyeloid cell line (Busch *et al.*, 2004; Wang *et al.*, 1999). Interestingly, apoptosis in smooth-muscle cells has been shown to be mediated by a β1 integrin signaling cascade, providing a possible link with CCM1 and CCM2 in the formation of cerebral CMs (Wernig *et al.*, 2003). The PDCD10 gene is highly conserved in both vertebrates and invertebrates. Its implication in cerebral CMs strongly suggests that it is a new player in vascular morphogenesis and/or remodeling.

Taken together, these data clearly show that cerebral CMs constitute a formidable Mendelian model of stroke characterized by focal abnormalities in small intracranial blood vessels leading to hemorrhage and strokes and/or seizures. The exact mechanism of familial CM pathogenesis is still unknown. Mutation at three distinct loci (CCM1, CCM2, and CCM3) has been shown in cases of familial cerebral CM, and interaction between CCM1 and CCM2 in cell signaling has been reported (Zawistowski *et al.*, 2005). Whether CCM3 is also implicated in this pathway remains to be determined. The roles of these three CCM proteins in the formation and maintenance of cerebral vessels, the genetics mechanisms that lead to cerebral CMs, and the factors that influence their number and growth are still quite obscure. Analysis of animal models (Plummer *et al.*, 2004, 2006; Whitehead *et al.*, 2004) involving one or more of these CCM proteins will be of great help in understanding the initial steps involved in the appearance of cerebral CMs as well as to identify modifying genetic or environmental factors that are important for clinical care.

Genotype-phenotype correlations in familial cerebral CMs patients

There are genotype-phenotype correlations among the different familial forms of cerebral CMs. Craig *et al.* (1998) found that the penetrance of symptomatic disease among patients harboring CCM1, CCM2, and CCM3 was 88%, 100%, and 63%, respectively (Craig *et al.*, 1998). These differences were not explained by differences in age or gender in the families of gene carriers, and none of the asymptomatic gene carriers in this analysis was younger than 20 years. Denier, Labauge, Brunereau, *et al.* (2004) analyzed clinical features of 202 KRIT-1 mutation carriers in 64 cerebral CM families and found that clinical penetrance was 62%.

Denier *et al.* (2006) conducted a detailed clinical, neuroradiological, and molecular analysis of 163 consecutively recruited cerebral CM families. A deleterious mutation was found in 128 probands, and 333 mutation carriers were identified. They found that, in the CCM3 group, the proportion of patients with onset of symptoms before the age of 15 years was significantly higher and that in this group the most common initial presentation was hemorrhage. They also found that the number of lesions on gradient-echo sequence was significantly lower in the CCM2 group and that the number of these lesions increased, significantly, more rapidly with age in CCM1 than in CCM2 patients (Denier *et al.*, 2006).

Sporadic (nonhereditary) condition

The sporadic form of cerebral CMs cannot be distinguished by phenotype from the familial form. Some authors investigated the role that mutations at the CCM1 locus play in sporadic cerebral CMs and the prevalence of occult familial forms among symptomatic CM patients (Reich *et al.*, 2003; Verlaan *et al.*, 2002; Verlaan,

Laurent, Rouleau, *et al.*, 2004; Verlaan, Laurent, Sure, *et al.*, 2004). Reich *et al.* (2003) screened the DNA of 72 consecutive patients with CMs and found that none of the patients showed a mutation at the CCM1 site. They concluded that mutations in KRIT-1 are seldom a cause of sporadic cerebral CMs. Verlaan, Laurent, Sure, *et al.*. (2004) analyzed 35 patients with sporadic cerebral CMs, 14 with multiple lesions and 21 with a single lesion. They found no CCM1 mutation in the single lesion group but 29% of CCM1 mutations in the multiple lesion group, suggesting that sporadic cases with multiple lesions seem to harbor CCM1 mutations in approximately the same proportion as do familial cases (Verlaan, Laurent, Sure, *et al.*, 2004). These findings are consistent with those of others who found that sporadic cases harboring multiple lesions are affected by a hereditary form of the disease because 75% of them have an asymptomatic parent with cerebral CMs lesion on MRI, due to the incomplete clinical penetrance of this condition (Labauge *et al.*, 1998; Rigamonti *et al.*, 1988).

Pathobiology

Histology

CMs are well-circumscribed lesions that consist of closely packed, enlarged, capillary-like vessels, without intervening parenchyma. On gross examination, CMs are dark red to purple, multilobulated masses, often described has having a "mulberry-like" appearance (Kondziolka, Lunsford, and Kestle, 1995; Rigamonti *et al.*, 1996; Zabramski *et al.*, 1994). Lesions may range in size from a few millimeters to several centimeters in diameter. Microscopically, CMs are characterized by a complex of markedly dilated vascular channels (caverns) arranged in a back-to-back pattern with little or no intervening parenchyma (Davis and Robertson, 1997; Hsu *et al.*, 1993; Maraire and Awad, 1995; Rigamonti *et al.*, 1988, 1996; Robinson *et al.*, 1991; Tomlinson *et al.*, 1994; Zabramski *et al.*, 1994). Histologically, the vascular channels closely resemble dilated capillaries, but the walls of the vessels are distinguished from classical telangiectasies that display enormous variations in size. These walls are composed wholly of collagen and are lined with a single layer of endothelial cells. Any cells within the lesion are macrophages, usually laden with iron pigment.

Thrombosis and organization may lead to a considerable production of reticulin fibrils, and cholesterin crystals are frequently a sequel to thrombosis (Russel and Rubinstein, 1989). The main pathological features of CMs (Maraire and Awad, 1995) are sinusoidal spaces lined by a single layer of endothelium, separated by a collagenous stroma devoid of elastin and smooth muscle, lack of intervening brain parenchyma, possible inclusion of satellite-like projections into the adjacent brain and evidence of prior microhemorrhage, hemosiderin discoloration, and hemosiderin-filled macrophages in the surrounding parenchyma. They may appear thickened and hyalinized in some areas but do not contain elastin or smooth muscle.

Examination often indicates past thrombosis with varying degrees of organization, calcification, cysts, and cholesterol crystals. A gliomatous reaction may be present in the surrounding parenchyma, and sometimes they are associated with capillary telangiectasias (Hsu *et al.*, 1993; Zabramski *et al.*, 1994, 1999). Rigamonti *et al.* (1991) found a 35% incidence of brain parenchyma between the abnormally dilated vascular channels in the centers of the cavernous lesions they studied and concluded that capillary telangiectasia and CMs may represent two pathological extremes within the same vascular malformation category. CMs are sometimes associated with DVAs but this issue will be detailed later.

Ultrastructural characteristics

The ultrastructural appearance of CMs is that of endothelial cell-lined cavern walls composed of an amorphous material lacking organized collagen. In 2001, Clatterbuck, Eberhart, Crain, *et al.* (2001) suggested that ultrastructural and immunocytochemical evidence of an incompetent blood–brain barrier was related to the pathophysiology of CMs. Examination of the ultrastructure of their specimens showed endothelium lined vascular sinusoids embedded in a dense collagenous matrix and a paucity of any other cell type. They reported that CMs vascular sinusoids differed from normal cerebral microvessels in important ways. The basal lamina underlying the endothelial cells was often multilaminar and bordered the dense collagenous matrix directly. There were no ensheathing pericytes, smooth muscle cells, or astrocytic processes bordering the microvascular units. Immunocytochemistry for glial fibrillary acidic protein (GFAP) confirmed that astrocytic processes reached the border of these CMs but did not extend beyond the brain–CM interface. They also noted gaps between endothelial cells lining the channels of the CMs (Clatterbuck, Eberhart, Crain, *et al.* 2001).

Wong et al. (2000) described poorly formed tight junctions with gaps between endothelial cells and vascular channels embedded in an amorphous matrix lacking organized collagen. They concluded that the gaps between endothelial cells and the poorly organized "cavern" walls contribute to microhemorrhages. These findings support the observations of Clatterbuck, Eberhart, Crain, *et al.* (2001) and provide clues in the understanding of the pathophysiology of CMs. More recently, Tu *et al.* (2005) reported ultrastructural analysis of 13 CMs specimens and showed, besides the typical previously reported findings of poorly formed endothelial junction and subendothelial support in the vessel walls, that deficiencies occurred in the nonhemorrhagic lesions, including the frequent presence of fenestrae and the absence of basal lamina. In particular, they found that nonhemorrhagic lesions were different from the hemorrhagic ones, in which commonly noted large vesicles are bordered on their lumen by thin plasma membranes. They also found that primary CMs differ from recurrent ones, in which endothelial cells are immature and active in differentiation (Tu *et al.*, 2005).

Biology of growth and angiogenesis

The potential of CMs to grow was mentioned in 1928 by Cushing and Bailey, who observed an increase in size of vascular tumors without clearly differentiating between CMs and hemangioblastoma. Voigt and Yasargil (1976) and others confirmed this characteristic of CMs in up to 38% of patients with intracranial lesions

(Bertalanffy *et al.*, 1991; Clatterbuck *et al.*, 2000; Fritschi *et al.*, 1994; Gangemi *et al.*, 1993; Maraire and Awad, 1995; Pozzati, Acciarri, Tognetti, *et al.*, 1996; Pozzati *et al.*, 1989; Simard *et al.*, 1986; Yamasaki *et al.*, 1986; Zimmerman *et al.*, 1991). Although the biological progression of cavernous angiomas is well recognized, the mechanisms of enlargement and growth are still debated and include: 1) gross hemorrhage with acute expansion and acute mass effect or repeated intralesional hemorrhage and thrombosis, with expansion of a hemorrhagic cyst cavity (Pozzati, Acciarri, Tognetti, *et al.*, 1996); 2) chronic hemorrhage with repeated re-endothelialization of hemorrhagic cavities, growth of new blood vessels as part of the organization of the hematoma, and the laying down of additional fibrous scar tissue (Maraire and Awad, 1995; Pozzati, Acciarri, Tognetti, *et al.*, 1996; Schefer *et al.*, 1991); 3) intraluminal thrombosis with organization and recanalization (Tomlinson *et al.*, 1994); 4) budding of new capillaries as reactive angiogenesis with new vessel formation and coalescence, so-called hemorrhagic angiogenic proliferation (Maraire and Awad, 1995; Notelet *et al.*, 1997; Pozzati, Acciarri, Tognetti, *et al.*, 1996; Sure, Butz, Schlegel, *et al.*, 2001); and 5) formation of an enhancing membrane similar to the membrane of a chronic subdural hematoma as a result of recurrent hemorrhages from sinusoids of the malformation and from the neocapillary network of the cyst membrane with osmotic effects (Steiger *et al.*, 1987).

Recent publications on the biology of CMs led to the hypothesis that these lesions should be classified as slowly growing vascular neoplasms rather than true developmental vascular malformations (Hashimoto *et al.*, 2000; Kilic *et al.*, 2000; Notelet *et al.*, 1997; Sonstein *et al.*, 1996). Clinical reports on the de novo formation of CMs with radiotherapy (Detwiler *et al.*, 1998; Gaensler *et al.*, 1994; Larson *et al.*, 1998; Maraire *et al.*, 1999; Pozzati, Giangaspero, Marliani, *et al.*, 1996) and without radiotherapeutic induction (Ciricillo *et al.*, 1994) for both familial and sporadic CMs prompted discussion on whether CMs are developmental or acquired and whether these lesions bear a proliferating and/or neoplastic capacity (Brunereau *et al.*, 2000; Detwiler *et al.*, 1997, 1998; Larson *et al.*, 1998; Massa-Micon *et al.*, 2000; Pozzati, Acciarri, Tognetti, *et al.*, 1996; Pozzati, Giangaspero, Marliani, *et al.*, 1996; Rosahl *et al.*, 1998).

Recent immunohistochemical studies have investigated the expression of angiogenic and proliferative markers in cerebral vascular malformations (Abdulrauf, Malik, and Awad, 1999; Hashimoto *et al.*, 2000; Kilic *et al.*, 2000; Sure *et al.*, 2004, 2005; Sure, Butz, Schlegel, *et al.*, 2001; Sure, Butz, Siegel, *et al.*, 2001). Such investigations contribute to the understanding of the proliferative and angioneogenetic mechanisms that are operative during the development of CMs.

The processes of new vessel genesis during embryonic development (vasculogenesis) and the sprouting of vessels from pre-existing vascular beds during organogenesis and in pathological processes, such as inflammation, wound healing, and tumor growth (angiogenesis), have been studied extensively (Bobik and Campbell, 1993; Clauss *et al.*, 1990; Folkman and Klagsbrun, 1987; Keep and Jones, 1990; Krum *et al.*, 1991; Risau, 1990). Several factors have been identified that mediate endothelial cell and other vascular wall element proliferation, migration, adhesion, and permeability. Vascular endothelial growth factor (VEGF), a glycoprotein initially identified as vascular permeability factor, promotes angiogenesis and possesses unique features of endothelial cell target specificity. It also promotes the permeability of vascular beds through leakage at intercellular junctions, possesses unique features of endothelial cell target specificity, and is associated with a number of pathological processes (Berkman *et al.*, 1993; Clauss *et al.*, 1990; de Vries *et al.*, 1992; Ferrara *et al.*, 1991, 1992; Gospodarowicz *et al.*, 1989; Jakeman *et al.*, 1992; Keck *et al.*, 1989; Leung *et al.*, 1989; Senger *et al.*, 1993, 1997). Another factor, bFGF has been shown to be a powerful mediator of endothelial and fibroblast proliferation (Gospodarowicz *et al.*, 1987, 1988; Paulus *et al.*, 1990; Rifkin and Moscatelli, 1989; Schweigerer *et al.*, 1987; Tsuboi *et al.*, 1990; Vlodavsky *et al.*, 1991).

In an immunohistochemical study, Rothbart *et al.* (1996) found immunostaining of VEGF and bFGF in four of five cases of CMs. They also found no expression of laminin in any CMs, whereas laminin was expressed in AVMs. By contrast, fibronectin expression was more prominent in CMs.

The basement membrane of vascular beds contains varying amounts of fibronectin and laminin (matrix proteins) (Garbisa and Negro, 1984; Kittelberger *et al.*, 1990; Krum *et al.*, 1991; Risau and Lemmon, 1988). These proteins are thought to contribute to the structural integrity of the vessel wall, anchoring endothelial cells to the underlying internal elastic and smooth muscle layers (Dejana *et al.*, 1987; Krum *et al.*, 1991; Risau and Lemmon, 1988). During vasculogenesis and angiogenesis, immature vessels are associated with nonadherent proliferating endothelium in a fibronectin-rich matrix deficient in laminin expression, whereas more mature vessels with adherent nonproliferating endothelium express laminin more consistently and contain scant fibronectin in their matrix. This suggests that CMs have more immature proliferating vessels than AVMs. There is weaker expression of structural protein (collagen IV and alpha smooth muscle actin) in CMs than in AVMs. These findings are consistent with the poorly formed subendothelial support reported in ultrastructural analysis (Clatterbuck, Eberhart, Crain, *et al.*, 2001). New angiogenesis in CMs has now been often noted, confirming the expression of angiogenic factors in most cases and the poor expression of structural protein. VEGF has been reported to be expressed in 40%–97% of CMs. The expression of VEGF receptors (FLT-1 and FLK-1) has also been reported in several studies (Jung *et al.*, 2003; Kilic *et al.*, 2000; Sure *et al.*, 2004, 2005; Sure, Butz, Schlegel, *et al.*, 2001; Zhao *et al.*, 2003).

Maiuri *et al.* (2006) reported the analysis of angiogenic and growth factors in 43 cases of CMs. They found expression of VEGF in 83% of cases and of transforming growth factor alpha (TGF-α), a dimeric protein that regulates angiogenesis by stimulating the formation of blood vessels in 54% of cases. Two other studies reported the expression of the α-isomer of TGF in 97% and 100% of specimens, but no study assessed the difference between isomers of TGF (Kilic *et al.*, 2000; Zhao *et al.*, 2003). Maiuri *et al.* (2006) also found expression of tenascin in 84% of cases. Tenascin, a glycoprotein of ECM, is expressed during embryonic life and is absent in the normal brain. Evidence of this growth factor has been found in the vessels of anaplastic gliomas, and is considered a marker of vascular proliferation for intracerebral growing lesions (Zagzag and

Capo, 2002). Viale *et al.* (2002) also found expression of tenascin-c in 100% of cases in their series. These findings support the growth potential of CMs.

A protein isolated from human platelets, platelet-derived growth factor (PDGF), stimulates the proliferation of connective and neuroglial cells and may play an important role in angiogenesis (Lamszus *et al.*, 2004). The expression of PDGF has been described in some brain tumors. Maiuri *et al.* (2006) reported its expression in 95% of cases in their series. The fact that CMs strongly express growth factors involved in angiogenesis and ECM formation might indicate a growth potential of these vascular malformations. Table 29.1 summarizes the expression of different proliferative and angiogenic factors as well as some structural proteins CMs among larger series.

The proliferative indices PCNA and Ki-67 have also been assessed in several studies (Kilic *et al.*, 2000; Maiuri *et al.*, 2006; Notelet *et al.*, 1997; Sure *et al.*, 2004, 2005; Sure, Butz, Schelegel, *et al.*, 2001; Tirakotai *et al.*, 2006; Zhao *et al.*, 2003). PCNA positivity has been reported in 85% (Notelet *et al.*, 1997) and 86% (Sure *et al.*, 2005) of cases in two series and Ki-67 positivity in 19% (Maiuri *et al.*, 2006) and 38% (Sure *et al.*, 2005) of cases in two adult series and significantly more often in a pediatric series (Tirakotai *et al.*, 2006). The different expression of PCNA and Ki-67 may be explained by the difference of their half-lives (Sure *et al.*, 2005).

Local hypoxia contributes to neoangiogenesis (Sure *et al.*, 2004; Zagzag *et al.*, 2000). Recently, Sure *et al.* (2004) first investigated the expression of HIF-1α in cerebral CMs. They identified HIF-1α as a protein involved in the biological process of angiogenesis in almost half of their cerebral CMs (48.1%) (Sure *et al.*, 2004).

Apoptosis is known to be involved in the development and malignant progression of brain gliomas. It is regulated by the balance between antiapoptotic proteins (bcl-2 and bcl-XL) and proapoptotic proteins, which may activate the caspases (Maiuri *et al.*, 2006). Three reports detailed the role of apoptosis in CMs (Cheng *et al.*, 1999; Maiuri *et al.*, 2006; Takagi *et al.*, 2000). Takagi *et al.* (2000) found caspase-3 immunoreactivity in all five CMs in their series. Cheng *et al.*, (1999) found increased expression of the antiapoptotic protein bcl-2 in 10 CMs, and Maiuri *et al.* (2006) found bcl-2 positivity in 10 (23.3%) of 43 specimens, all of them displaying an aggressive clinical course. These findings are consistent with the recent identification of the CCM3 gene (PDCD10), which encodes a protein that has been related to apoptosis (Bergametti *et al.*, 2005).

Maiuri *et al.* (2006) analyzed the reactive normal brain tissue adjacent to CMs and found expression of tenascin, TGF-α, and PDGF, although at a rate significantly lower (20%–27.5%) than that found in the CM tissue. The expression of these growth factors may reflect the gliotic reaction of the adjacent brain to repeated hemorrhages. Nevertheless, VEGF was not expressed in the reactive brain tissue, as was reported by Kilic *et al.*, 2000.

Researchers have also investigated the natural history of cerebral CMs, both the sporadic and familial forms (Aiba *et al.*, 1995; Clatterbuck *et al.*, 2000; Del Curling *et al.*, 1991; Houtteville, 1997; Kim *et al.*, 1997; Kondziolka, Lunsford, and Kestle, 1995; Labauge *et al.*, 2000, 2001; Porter *et al.*, 1997). Some factors associated with clinical and radiological progression have been identified such as

Table 29.1 Proliferative and angiogenic factors and structural proteins expression in CMs literature Review

Authors	Nb CMs	PCNA % of cases	MIB-1 % of cases	VEGF % of cases	VEGF receptors % of cases	bFGF % of cases	PDGF % of cases	TGF % of cases	HIF-1α % of cases	Tenascin % of cases	Apoptotic protein % of cases	Matrix proteins (staining)	Structural proteins
Rothbart et al., 1996	5	–	–	80%	–	80%	–	–	–	–	–	Laminin +/− Fibronectin +++	Weak expression of collagen IV and SMA in the medium compared to AVM
Notelet et al., 1997	42	85%	–	–	–	–	–	–	–	–	–	–	–
Cheng et al., 1999	10	–	–	–	–	–	–	–	–	–	100% (bcl-2)	–	–
Kilic et al., 2000	10	–	0%	90%	–	100%	–	100% (α)	–	–	–	Laminin +/− Fibronectin +++	Weak expression of collagen IV and SMA in the medium compared to AVM
Viale et al., 2002	16	–	–	–	–	–	–	–	–	100%	–	–	–
Zhao et al., 2003	70	0%	–	97%	63% (Flt-1)	–	–	97% (α)	–	–	–	–	–
Sure et al., 2005	56	86%	38%	41%	71% (Flk-1)	–	–	–	48%	–	–	–	–
Maiuri et al., 2006	43	–	18.6%	83.7%	–	–	95.4%	97% (β)	–	83.7%	23.3% (bcl-2)	–	–

α = isomer α of TGF; β = isomer β of TGF

age, large size with mass effect, familial occurrence, documented change in size, de novo appearance, and hemorrhagic episode. They confirm that some cases show a more aggressive course. However, even if familial forms seem to have a more aggressive behavior, factors associated with this more aggressive course have yet to be determined.

Whether the familial occurrence and the more aggressive clinical course of some brain CMs can be correlated with differences in the expression of growth factors and proliferative indices has been poorly investigated (Maiuri *et al.*, 2006; Sure *et al.*, 2005). Sure *et al.* (2005) found no correlation between clinical factors and biological markers but did not correlate these markers specifically to CMs with an aggressive course. Jung *et al.* (2003) found that VEGF serum levels increased during the dynamic period and became normal during the steady and resolved stages of a CM that had a progressive course. These authors speculated that the endothelial proliferation induced by VEGF was an important element in the development of brain CMs.

Maiuri *et al.* (2006), among 43 patients harboring cerebral CMs, 32 with a stable and sporadic form and 11 with more aggressive behavior, found a higher rate of positive TGF-α expression in the aggressive group, whereas the expression of VEGF, PDGF, and tenascin showed no differences between the two groups. In contrast, they found that more aggressive CMs had a significantly higher expression of TGF-α, PDGF, and tenascin in the perilesional reactive brain parenchyma, whereas VEGF expression was found in all but two cases in both stable and aggressive lesions. They also found both the Ki-67 labeling index and bcl-2 to be absent in the group of stable lesions, whereas it was positive in 8 (72.7%) of the 11 more aggressive CMs. Tirakotai *et al.* (2006) found the immunoreactivity of MIB-1 to occur significantly more often in children than in adults. Given that pediatric CMs seem to have more aggressive behavior than do adult CMs, this might indicate an actual prognostic value of Ki-67 expression. However, these findings have yet to be confirmed because Sure *et al.* did not find any difference between clinical features in patients with positive or negative Ki-67 and because Cheng *et al.* (1999) found bcl-2 positivity in all of their patients.

The strong expression of some biological markers involved in angiogenesis, proliferation, ECM formation, and apoptosis in brain CMs shows that they are dynamic lesions with growth potential, even when they are observed as stable lesions with an indolent course. VEGF is an important growth factor involved in the progression of brain gliomas, where it is correlated with tumor aggressiveness and neovascularization. Nevertheless, its role in the progression of cavernous angiomas remains controversial, and whether it reflects a nonspecific pathological reaction to intracranial hemorrhage rather than a true endothelial proliferation remains unclear. Moreover, whether more evolutive CMs are associated with a significantly higher expression of Ki-67 and bcl-2 has to be analyzed further. Finally, the possibility that the perilesional brain parenchyma surrounding aggressive CMs expresses some growth factors such as TGF-α, PDGF, and tenascin at a significantly higher rate than is found in stable and more indolent lesions should be investigated in larger series. This would per-

haps indicate that the perilesional tissue may be predisposed and recruited for further growth and progression of the CM.

Natural history and risk of hemorrhage

Dynamic mature

There is growing evidence that, in both sporadic and familial forms, CMs are lesions of dynamic nature. Studies have been conducted to assess the actual dynamic mature of CMs (Bertalanffy *et al.*, 2002; Fritschi *et al.*, 1994; Maraire *et al.*, 1999; Moriarity, Clatterbuck, and Rigamonti, 1999; Nimjee *et al.*, 2006; Pozzati, Acciarri, Tognetti, *et al.*, 1996) but few were especially dedicated to radiological assessement (Clatterbuck *et al.*, 2000; Kim *et al.*, 1997; Labauge *et al.*, 2000, 2001) (Table 29.2). Kim *et al.* (1997) first reported the MRI changes of CMs in a retrospective study of 62 patients harboring 108 lesions. They noted modification of these lesions both in size and signal intensity. To understand imaging-documented changes in CMs over time, Clatterbuck *et al.* (2000) analyzed the MRI signal characteristics of 114 CMs found in 68 patients who were followed prospectively. They showed that, during a follow-up interval of 18 months, 22% of lesions were stable in volume, 43% increased, and 35% decreased in size. Over a longer interval of serial imaging (mean 26 months), only 10% of lesions were stable in volume, 35% increased, and 55% decreased in volume. The overall trend was for CMs slowly to decrease in size (Clatterbuck *et al.*, 2000). Interestingly, the clinically relevant hemorrhage rate reported over the same time period in these patients was much less: 3.1% per patient per year (Moriarity, Wetzel, Clatterbuck, *et al.*, 1999). Even though the decrease in volume can be explained by resorption and organization of an intralesional or extralesional hematoma, the increase in volume, however, is probably due not only to hemorrhage but also to another process, namely cell growth disorder. Clatterbuck *et al.* (2000) also showed that the observed changes in MRI characteristics were common; they proposed an ordered scheme in which lesions generally progress from type I to type II and then to the type III MRI characteristics described by Zabramski *et al.* (1994) with the age of blood products they contain. In 2000, Labauge *et al.* (2000) reported a retrospective MRI study of 40 patients with cerebral CMs over a mean follow-up period of 3.2 years. They showed that CMs changed in both size and signal during the follow-up period and that the changes in signal intensity suggested a continuum between the different types of CMs (Clatterbuck *et al.*, 2000; Labauge *et al.*, 2000).

De novo lesions

De novo genesis of CMs has recently been established as a part of their natural history. New lesions have been described after both whole brain radiation and stereotactic irradiation as well as along a needle biopsy tact (Detwiler *et al.*, 1998; Gaensler *et al.*, 1994; Larson *et al.*, 1998; Maraire *et al.*, 1999; Ogilvy *et al.*, 1993; Pozzati, Giangaspero, Marliani *et al.*, 1996). De novo formation of CMs without radiotherapeutic induction for both familial and sporadic cases is a well-known phenomenon

Table 29.2 Patient characteristics literature review

Authors	No. of pts	No. of CMs	Mean Age	Male / Female (%)	Location				Fam. form	Multiple CMs (% cases)	Init. sympt. Hem.	Seizure	HA	Focal deficit	Incid.
					Hemisph.	Deep seated	Brain stem	Cerebellum							
Del Curling et al., 1991	32	76	37.6	53/47	86%		14%		Nc	18.7%	Nc	50%	34%	22%	19%
Robinson et al., 1991	66	76	34.6	54/46	72.3%	5.3%	10.5%	11.9%	Nc	9.1%	18.7%	51.5%	30.3%	45.5%	13.6%
Zabramski et al., 1994	31	128*	25	58/42	83%	9%	4%	4%	100%	84%	Nc	38.7%	51.6%	9.7	38.7%
Aiba et al., 1995	110	Nc	36	24/76	60%$	12%$	10%$	18%$	Nc	Nc	56.4%	22.7%$	Nc	Nc	20.9%
Kondziolka et al., 1995	122	Nc	37.3	49/51	48%**	17%	35%	–	Nc	20%	Nc	23%	15%	Nc	Nc
Kim et al., 1997	62	108	32.2	61/39	63%	10%	21%	6%	Nc	21%	Nc	40.8%	6%	40.2%	13%
Porter et al., 1997	173	Nc	37.5	51/49	56.7%	7.5%	30%	5.8%	Nc	17.9%	25.4%	35.8%	6.4%	20.2%	12.1%
Moriarty et al., 1999	68	>228	34.6	35/65	70%	11%	14%	5%	19%	37	13%	49%	65%	46%	1.5%
Labauge et al., 2000	40	232	Nc	52/48	75.8%		24.2%		100%	93%	45%	30%	Nc	Nc	12.5%
Labauge et al., 2001	33	234	40.8	42/58	86%		14%		100%	85%	–	–	–	–	100%
Brainstem CMs series					Mes.	Pons	Med.	>1 level							
Fritschi et al., 1994	139	Nc	31.8	49/51	14%	62%	5%	24%	Nc	Nc	88%	0%	14%	100%	0%
Porter et al., 1999	100	103	37	38/62	16%	39%	16%	29%	14%	24%	97%	3%	36%	97%	3%
Kupersmith et al., 2001	37	Nc	37.5	41/59	32%	35%	11%	22%	0%	8.1%	73%	0%	43%	95%	5%
Wang et al., 2003	137	141	33.5	58/42	15%	61%	13%	11%	Nc	9.5%	Nc	Nc	Nc	Nc	Nc
Ferroli et al., 2005	52	Nc	38.5	50/50	11%%	60%	13%	16%	Nc	13%	96.2%	Nc	Nc	96.2%	3.8%
Bruneau et al., 2006	22	22	39.8	68/32	14%	50%	9%	27%	Nc	0%	100%	0%	Nc	100%	0%

Notes: HA, Headaches; Nc, not communicated/indicated/provided.

* Only in 21 patients with complete follow-up data.

$ % in a subset of the population (50 patients) who have presented hemorrhage at presentation or during follow-up.

$ This percentage concerns only patients with seizure but without symptomatic hemorrhage at diagnosis.

** Including cerebellum cases.

(Bertalanffy *et al.*, 2002; Brunereau *et al.*, 2000; Ciricillo *et al.*, 1994; Detwiler *et al.*, 1997; Fender *et al.*, 2000; Massa-Micon *et al.*, 2000; Pozzati, Acciarri, Tognetti, *et al.*, 1996; Rosahl *et al.*, 1998). Such new lesions were first reported in patients with the familial form (Zabramski *et al.*, 1994). Detwiler *et al.* (1997) later described a patient with no family history of this disease or a history of treatment with cranial radiation, which invalidates the assumption that CMs are always congenital lesions. Zabramski *et al.* (1994) in a prospective study of 21 patients with the familial form of CMs found de novo lesions in 29% of patients at a rate of 0.4 lesions per patient per year. These results are consistent with those of Labauge *et al.* (2000), who found in a retrospective study of 40 familial Cavernous malformations affected patients during a follow-up period of 38.4 months, 11 patients with de novo lesions (27.5%). In a study of 33 familial cases prospectively followed over a period of 25.2 months, Labauge *et al.* (2001) found new lesions in 30% of cases at the same incidence rate reported by Zabramski *et al.* (1994), 0.4% per patient per year. An important feature of this study was the systematic use of gradient-echo MR sequences for all patients, thus decreasing the possibility of false-positive cases. Kim *et al.* (1997), in a retrospective study of 68 patients, reported 4% of new lesions during a follow-up period of 22.4 months. They did not report the proportion of familial cases, but the frequency of multiple lesions (21%) was consistent with a rather sporadic series. Clatterbuck *et al.* (2000) reported in 68 patients comprising 13 familial forms 4.4% of de novo lesions over a follow-up period of 62.4 months. However, since the time of their analysis, a new case of de novo lesion has been reported in one patient leading the frequency of de novo lesions to 15% in their familial forms. These findings clearly demonstrate a trend toward a greater incidence of de novo lesions in familial forms but confirm the actual occurrence of de novo lesions in sporadic cases.

The origin and the cause of new lesion formation are obscure. A common finding in three previous studies of familial forms is the MR appearance of de novo lesions (Labauge *et al.*, 2000, 2001; Zabramski *et al.*, 1994). These lesions are seen mainly as hypointense signals on T2WI images or hypointense signals on gradient-echo sequences corresponding to type III and IV in the classification described by Zabramski *et al.* (1994). In the study of Labauge *et al.* (2001), 86% of the 30 new lesions detected during the follow-up period were of type IV appearance. The nature of these lesions seen as hypointense signals remains poorly understood. They may be true new lesions or small malformations, initially undetectable on MRI. Appearance of these lesions on serial MRI with gradient-echo sequences suggests that they are true new lesions. The histological correlation of these hypointense signals is not established. They may be telangiectasias or small CMs (Rigamonti *et al.*, 1991). The natural history and the ultimate behavior of hypointense lesions are not well known. Of the 154 type IV CMs reported in the study of Labauge *et al.* 2001, none presented as a hemorrhage and only one turned to type II. Similarly, in the study of Zabramski *et al.* (1994), these lesions remained uniformly silent. These features suggest that, in familial CMs, two different types of lesion are observed: true CMs, seen as types I and II on MRI, and related vascular malformations, seen as types III and

IV, which may represent the precursor state of the familial form of CMs.

The possibility that de novo lesions, represent pre-existing radiologically undetectable lesions, cannot be excluded. However, the sensitivity of gradient-echo MRI sequences and the growing number of reports on the proliferating and/or neoplastic capacity of CMs (Kilic *et al.*, 2000; Maiuri *et al.*, 2006; Notelet *et al.*, 1997; Rothbart *et al.*, 1996; Zabramski *et al.*, 1994) favors the hypothesis of development of de novo lesions in the natural history of CMs both in their familial and sporadic form. This is an important issue given that some authors calculate a "retrospective" hemorrhagic rate assuming that the lesions are present at birth (Del Curling *et al.*, 1991; Fritschi *et al.*, 1994; Kim *et al.*, 1997; Kupersmith *et al.*, 2001; Porter *et al.*, 1999; Wang *et al.*, 2003). Indeed, the acknowledgment of de novo appearance of CM invalidates this approach, which may underestimate by an unknown factor the true incidence of bleeding.

Risk of hemorrhage

Bleeding rate

Knowledge of the natural history of CMs is important in clinical practice, because decisions on further treatment recommendations are based to a great extent on the estimated risk of further morbidity in each patient. Reports have appeared during the past 10 years dealing with retrospective and prospective analysis of the natural history of CMs (Del Curling *et al.*, 1991; Fritschi *et al.*, 1994; Kondziolka, Lunsford, and Kestle, 1995; Kupersmith *et al.*, 2001; Labauge *et al.*, 2000, 2001; Maraire and Awad, 1995; Moriarity, Clatterbuck, and Rigamonti, 1999; Moriarity, Wetzel, Clatterbuck, *et al.*, 1999; Porter *et al.*, 1997, 1999; Pozzati, Acciarri, Tognetti, *et al.*, 1996; Robinson *et al.*, 1991; Zabramski *et al.*, 1994). The risk of hemorrhage for CMs is lower than that of AVMs. But definition of the hemorrhagic rate is complicated by the considerable heterogeneity regarding the terminology and definition of hemorrhage and the methods of calculating bleeding rates across series. The variability of hemorrhage patterns from a CM is reflected by the great variety of terms used in the literature to describe the bleeding event from the CM. Some commonly used terms are "overt hemorrhage," "symptomatic hemorrhage," "microhemorrhage," "intralesional or perilesional ooze or diapedesis," "extralesional hemorrhage," or "subclinical hemorrhage" (Aiba *et al.*, 1995; Fritschi *et al.*, 1994; Kondziolka, Lunsford, and Kestle, 1995; Labauge *et al.*, 2000; Moriarity, Clatterbuck, and Rigamonti, 1999; Pozzati, Acciarri, Tognetti, *et al.*, 1996; Robinson and Awad, 1993; Robinson *et al.*, 1991; Zabramski *et al.*, 1994).

Because of uncertainty regarding the definition of hemorrhage and to assess what is of greatest import to the patient, Porter *et al.* (1997) reported "event rates" (neurological deterioration regardless of neuroradiological findings) rather than hemorrhagic rates in their series of 173 patients. The clinical significance of hemorrhage depends not only on the severity of the bleeding but also on the location of the lesion. Even large hematomas occurring in noneloquent areas of the brain may cause little or no neurological symptoms, and conversely, even small intralesional or extralesional hematomas within the brainstem or other functional areas

Retrospective rates:	Prospective rates:
1) Retrospective patient-year bleeding rate:	**1) Prospective patient-year bleeding rate:**
Number of bleeding episodes since birth	*Number of bleeding episodes after detection of CM*
Mean age of patients X Number of patients	*Mean duration of Follow-up after detection X Number of patients*
2) Retrospective lesion-year bleeding rate:	**2) Prospective lesion-year bleeding rate:**
Number of bleeding episodes since birth	*Number of bleeding episodes after detection of CM*
Mean age of patients X Number of lesions	*Mean duration of Follow-up after detection X Number of lesions*

Figure 29.1 Calculation modalities of CMs bleeding rate.

may cause severe neurological deficits. Therefore, it seems reasonable to combine the clinical signs and symptoms with objective radiographic evidence of extralesional hemorrhage for the calculation of a clinically meaningful hemorrhage rate (Moriarity, Clatterbuck, and Rigamonti, 1999; Moriarity, Wetzel, Clatterbuck, et al., 1999).

There are mainly two ways that calculated bleeding rates in a population have been reported – the annual per-patient rate and the annual per-lesion rate. The data quantified in terms of "patient-year" are determined by the sum of follow-up duration in years for each patient in a prospective way and by the sum of each patient's age in years in a retrospective way, assuming that the lesion is present at birth. Similarly, data quantified in terms of "lesion-year" are determined by the sum of the lesions multiplied by the follow-up period for each patient in a prospective way and by the sum of each patient's age in years in a retrospective way (see Figure 29.1). However, another confusion has been created by using either the total number of hemorrhage events, observed in the population of a study, or the number of patients who have presented with a hemorrhagic event to calculate the annual bleeding rate per patient. Among 40 patients with familial form, Labauge et al. (2000) reported a prospective annual bleeding rate of 16.5% per patient per year (21 hemorrhages in 14 patients over a 127 patient-year period = $21/127 = 0.165$). The same authors later cited this study as showing an annual bleeding rate of 11% per patient per year ($14/127 = 0.11$) (Labauge et al., 2001). Kondziolka, Lunsford, and Kestle, (1995), calculating the prospective risk of hemorrhage among 122 patients with a mean follow-up period of 2.8 years (a 341.6 patient-year interval), found 9 hemorrhagic events in 7 patients and reported an annual bleeding rate of 2.63% ($9 / 341.6$) per patient per year. Similarily, Moriarty, Wetzel, Clatterbuck, et al. (1999) in a prospective study of 68 patients over a mean follow-up period of 62 months ($62 \times 68 \sim 352.9$ patient-year follow-up period) found 11 hemorrhagic events in 7 patients leading to a prospective hemorrhage rate of 3.1% ($11 / 352.9 = 0.031$) per patient-year. The data shown in Table 29.3 and quantified in "patient-year" for all the series are calculated by dividing the number of hemorrhagic events (not the number of patients with hemorrhagic events) by the prospective or retrospective patient-years of observation.

Retrospective annual hemorrhage rates, assuming that the lesion is present since birth, have been reported in a range of 0.25%–2.3% per patient-year in sporadic and mixed series (Aiba et al., 1995; Del Curling et al., 1991; Kim et al., 1997; Kondziolka, Lunsford, and Kestle, 1995). Prospective annual hemorrhage rates have been reported in a range of 0.8%–3.1% per patient-year in sporadic and mixed series (Aiba et al., 1995; Kondziolka, Lunsford, and Kestle, 1995; Moriarity, Wetzel, Clatterbuck, et al., 1999; Porter et al., 1997; Robinson et al., 1991) and in a range of 4.3%–16.5% per patient-year in familial series (Labauge et al., 2000, 2001; Zabramski et al., 1999).

Annual hemorrhage rates in term of lesion-year whether prospectively or retrospectively assessed have been reported in a range of 0.1%–1.4% in sporadic and mixed series and in a range of 0.7%–2.5% per lesion-year in familial CMs series. Thus when calculated in a "lesion-year" way, the observed rate of hemorrhage in familial CMs do not differ from those reported in sporadic cases. These data suggest that each CM in a familial form has the same hemorrhage rate as single (and therefore sporadic) CMs. As most patients with familial CMs have multiple lesions (84%–93%), the reported hemorrhage rate per patient is higher (Clatterbuck et al., 2000; Labauge et al., 2000, 2001; Zabramski et al., 1994).

Rebleeding rates have been poorly reported. Given that the mean follow-up period, in studies where the bleeding rates are assessed prospectively, is quite short (ranging from 25 to 62 months), the rebleeding rate when calculated was 0% (Labauge et al., 2001; Moriarity, Wetzel, Clatterbuck, et al., 1999; Robinson et al., 1991; Zabramski et al., 1994). Kim et al. (1997) in a retrospective series found a rebleeding rate of 3.8% per patient-year for patients treated medically and a rate of 7.8% for patients treated by gamma knife radiosurgery.

Brainstem CMs

Hemorrhage is the most common clinical presentation in brainstem CMs, accounting for 73%–97% of cases (Fritschi et al., 1994; Kupersmith et al., 2001; Porter et al., 1999; Wang et al., 2003). The reported bleeding rates in brainstem CMs series (mostly sporadic forms), range from 3.3%–6.3% patient-year and are higher than the rates found in supratentorial series supporting that location constitutes a predictive factor for hemorrhage (Aiba et al., 1995; Labauge, 2000; Porter et al., 1997; Robinson et al., 1991). All the reported bleeding rates were calculated retrospectively and so were probably underestimated. Fritschi et al. (1994) reported a rate of bleeding of 4.3% patient-year. Wang et al. (2003) reported the highest estimated bleeding rate of 6.3% per patient-year in a series of 137 patients harboring 141 brainstem CMs (Table 29.3). Unlike CMs in other locations, the rebleeding rate of brainstem lesions is significantly higher than in their supratentorial counterparts. Most series found previous hemorrhage to be associated with a higher risk of rebleeding. Fritschi et al. (1994), Porter et al.

Table 29.3 Natural history of CMs literature review

Authors	No. of pts	No. of CMs	Assessment of bleeding rate	Bleeding rate / patient / year	Bleeding rate / lesion / year	De novo lesion (% / patients)	Rebleeding rate / patient / year	Changes in size (% / patients)	Changes in signal (% / patients)	Mean FU (months)
Del Curling et al., 1991	32	76	Retrospective	0.25%	0.1%	Nc	0%	Nc	Nc	8.5
Robinson et al., 1991	66	76	Prospective	0.8%	0.7%	Nc	0%	8.6%§	88.6%§	26
Zabramski et al., 1994	31	128	Prospective	13% 6.5%**	2% 1.1%**	29%	0%	19%	38%	26.4
Aiba et al., 1995	110	Nc	Prospective	0.39%† Nc$	Nc† 22.9$%	Nc	11.1%£	Nc	Nc	56.4
Kondziolka et al., 1995	122	Nc	Prospective	2.63% / 0.6%† 4.5%$	Nc	Nc	Nc	Nc	Nc	34
Kim et al., 1997	62	108	Retrospective	2.3%	1.4%	4%	3.8%§§ 7.8%$$	4%	28%	22.4
Porter PJ, et al., 1997	173	Nc	Prospective	1.6% 4.2%#	Nc	Nc	Nc	Nc	Nc	46
Moriarity et al., 1999	68	>228	Prospective	3.1%	Nc	4.4%	0%	90%##	Nc	62.4
Labauge et al., 2000	40	232	Prospective	16.5%	2.5%	27.5%	Nc	22.5%	27.5%	38.4
Labauge et al., 2001	33	234	Prospective	4.3%	0.7%	30%	0%	9.1%	3%	25.2
Brainstem CMs series										
Fritschi et al., 1994	139	Nc	Retrospective	4.3%	Nc	Nc	21%	21%	Nc	30
Porter et al., 1999	100	103	Retrospective	5%	Nc	Nc	30%	Nc	Nc	35
Kupersmith et al., 2001	37	Nc	Retrospective	2.8% 0.44%††	Nc	Nc	5.1% 14.2% ††	33%	Nc	59
Wang et al., 2003	137	141	Retrospective	6.3%	Nc	Nc	60%	Nc	Nc	52
Ferroli et al., 2005	52	52	Retrospective	3.8%	3.8%	Nc	34.7%	Nc	Nc	51
Bruneau et al., 2006	22	22	Retrospective	2.68%	2.68%	Nc	17.7%	Nc	Nc	45

Notes: Nc, not communicated/indicated/provided; FU, follow-up.

§ Results from a subgroup of 35 patients with serial MRI review.

* Only in 21 patients with complete follow-up data.

† Patient group with prior hemorrhage.

$ Patient group with no prior hemorrhage.

** Symptomatic bleeding rate.

§§ Annual rebleeding rate per person for patients treated medically.

$$ Annual rebleeding rate per person for patients treated by radiosurgery.

"Event rate" definition of Porter, PJ, et al. 1997.

Data from the article of Clatterbuck et al. on the same series of patients.

£ Only for brainstem lesions.

†† Extralesional bleeding and rebleeding rates.

(1997) and Wang *et al.* (2003) reported rebleeding rates of 21%, 30%, and 60% per patient-year, respectively.

Predictors of hemorrhage

Predictive factors for intracranial hemorrhage in patients harboring CMs is a critical issue because the optimal therapeutic management of such lesions is tailored according to the bleeding risk. Data regarding predictors of hemorrhage in patients affected by CMs varies considerably (Aiba *et al.*, 1995; Clatterbuck *et al.*, 2000; Del Curling *et al.*, 1991; Fritschi *et al.*, 1994; Kondziolka, Lunsford, and Kestle, 1995; Kupersmith *et al.*, 2001; Labauge *et al.*, 2000, 2001; Maiuri *et al.*, 2006; Maraire and Awad, 1995; Moriarity, Clatterbuck, and Rigamonti, 1999; Porter *et al.*, 1997; Pozzati, Acciarri, Tognetti, *et al.*, 1996; Zabramski *et al.*, 1994) (Table 29.4). Several authors calculated annualized bleeding rate as related to the patient age and sex, size, location, and multiplicity of the lesion, and previous hemorrhage events, although not all factors were analyzed by each author. Table 29.4 summarizes the published results.

Robinson *et al.* (1991) commented that the bleeding may be higher in women and in brainstem lesions. Others also found a female preponderance of bleeding risk (Aiba *et al.*, 1995; Moriarity, Wetzel, Clatterbuck, *et al.*, 1999; Pozzati, Acciarri, Tognetti, *et al.*, 1996), suggesting that endocrine factors may influence hemorrhage tendencies, because some bleeding episodes in women occurred during pregnancy (Aiba *et al.*, 1995; Robinson *et al.*, 1991). These observations are supported by investigations that detected estrogen receptors in a few women who had CMs (Porter *et al.*, 1999). Another study found no impact of gender on bleeding occurrence (Del Curling *et al.*, 1991; Kondziolka, Lunsford, and Kestle, 1995).

The location of the CMs may also play an important role, although some studies found no differences. Porter *et al.* (1997) found infratentorial and deep-seated lesions to be significantly correlated to a higher bleeding rate. Their results concur with those of Aiba *et al.* (1995), Labauge *et al.* (2000), and Robinson *et al.* (1991) but contrast with those of other series (Del Curling *et al.*, 1991; Kondziolka, Lunsford, and Kestle, 1995; Zabramski *et al.*, 1994). Location is clearly a significant predictive factor of hemorrhage (Fritschi *et al.*, 1994; Kupersmith *et al.*, 2001; Porter *et al.*, 1999; Wang *et al.*, 2003).

Zabramski *et al.* (1994) and Aiba *et al.* (1995) reported a considerably higher bleeding incidence in patients who had previous hemorrhages. The high frequency, rapidity, and gravity of hemorrhagic recurrences after a first intracranial hemorrhage from a cerebral CM have also been stressed by Duffau *et al.* (1997). This factor failed to show any influence in other series (Moriarity, Wetzel, Clatterbuck, *et al.*, 1999; Porter *et al.*, 1997).

Association with DVAs

Mixed or transitional vascular malformations were described in the early 1990s raising the possibility that these lesions might represent a wide continuum of progression of a single pathological entity. Several authors reported the coexistence of these different vascular malformations (Ciricillo *et al.*, 1994; Clatterbuck, Elmaci, and Rigamonti, 2001; Hirsh, 1981; Maeder *et al.*, 1998; Ogilvy and Heros, 1988; Porter *et al.*, 1999; Rigamonti *et al.*, 1990, 1991; Rigamonti and Spetzler, 1988; Sheehan *et al.*, 2002). The most common mixed vascular malformations reported are CMs associated with DVAs (Topper *et al.*, 1999). The natural history, the biological behavior, as well as the management of such mixed lesions remain unclear. Most authors agree that microsurgical resection of CMs protects efficiently against future bleeding and that resection of the associated DVA may result in a clinically significant venous infarction, and controversies exist about whether DVAs are involved in the induction of CMs (Awad *et al.*, 1993; Ciricillo *et al.*, 1994; Wilson, 1992; Wurm *et al.*, 2005).

DVAs are congenital anomalies of normal venous drainage consisting in a number of dilated, radially arranged medullary veins resembling a "caput medusae" surrounded by normal parenchyma converging into a single large draining vein (Abe *et al.*, 1998, 2003; Perrini and Lanzino, 2006; Topper *et al.*, 1999; Wurm *et al.*, 2005). DVAs represent the most frequent intracranial vascular malformation, accounting for more than 60% of them (Martin *et al.*, 1984). Autopsy- and MRI-based studies have shown DVAs occurring in the population with a prevalence of 3% (McLaughlin *et al.*, 1998). An association between CMs and DVA was first reported by Roberson *et al.* (1974). Since then, an increasing number of cases have been reported. However there is an important discrepancy in the reported frequency of this association, because it ranges from 2.1% to 100% across series (Wurm *et al.*, 2005). Based on MRI findings, Abdulrauf, Kaynar, and Awad (1999) identified 24% of DVA-CM associations in 55 patients with CMs. Similarly, Wurm *et al.* (2005) found that 25.8% of CMs were associated with DVA in 58 patients. Porter *et al.* (1999), among 86 surgically treated lesions, reported an incidence of associated DVA of 100%, whereas their preoperative MRI showed DVAs only in 32% of 73 explored cases. These findings suggest that MRI-based detection of DVAs may underestimate their true incidence (see Figure 29.2). However, in series by Wurm *et al.* (2005) only one case of surgically found DVA was missed by the preoperative MRI assessment leading the sensitivity of this technique to 93.3%.

Venous angiomas are angiographically demonstrated venous anomalies with a caput medusae-like appearance; however, angiographically occult venous angiomas have been described by Abe *et al.* (2003), who have suggested a distinction between these two types of angiomas. They found angiographically occult venous angiomas to contain compactly arranged venous channels with no smooth muscle layer and angiographically detectable DVAs to be composed of dilated thin-walled vessels diffusely distributed in the normal white matter. They also reported that, when associated with CMs, surgical resection of the latter form, namely DVAs, was associated with venous infarction, whereas the former one could be resected safely (Abe *et al.*, 2003).

Isolated DVAs are usually benign, and most remain clinically silent. Recent clinical studies on the natural history of cerebral venous malformations support the indolent course of these lesions with an estimated annual symptomatic bleeding risk of 0.22% (Garner *et al.*, 1991) and 0.34% (McLaughlin *et al.*, 1998). Rigamonti *et al.* (1990) reported two hemorrhage episodes among 30 patients harboring DVAs, but the coexistence of a CM was pathologically

Table 29.4 Bleeding risk in CM patients

Authors	No. of pts	No. of CMs	Age	Sex	Clinical presentation	Size of lesion	Type of lesion	No. of lesions	Location	Previous vs. nonprevious hemorrhage (annual bleeding rates)
Del Curling et al., 1991	32	76	Nc	Ns	Nc	Nc	Nc	Nc	Ns	Nc
Robinson et al., 1991	66	76	Ns	Females	Nc	Ns	Nc	Nc	Ns	Nc
Zabramski et al., 1994	31	128*	Younger pts	Nc	Nc	Nc	Nc	Nc	Nc	Nc
Aiba et al., 1995	110	Nc	Younger pts	Females	Nc	Nc	Nc	Ns	Ns	22.9% lesion / yr vs. 0.39% pt / yr
Kondziolka et al., 1995	122	Nc	Ns	Ns	Nc	Nc	Nc	Nc	Ns	4.5% vs. 0.6% pt / yr
Kim et al., 1997	62	108	Nc	Nc	Nc	Nc	IIIB*	Nc	Nc	Nc
Porter et al., 1997	173	Nc	Nc	Ns	Focal deficit + hemorrhage	Nc	Nc	Ns	Deep lesions (10.6% vs. 0% pt / yr)	Ns
Moriarity et al., 1999	68	>228	Nc	Females	Nc	Nc	Nc	Ns	Nc	Ns
Labauge et al., 2000	40	232	Nc	Ns	Nc	Ns	I	Ns	Infratentorial (5.1% vs. 1.9% lesion / yr)	Nc
Labauge et al., 2001	33	234	Nc	Ns	Nc	Nc	II	Ns	Nc	Na
Brainstem CMs series										
Fritschi et al., 1994	139	Nc	Ns	Ns	Nc	Nc	Nc	Nc	Nc	Yes
Porter et al., 1999	100	103	Nc	Ns	Nc	Nc	Nc	Nc	Nc	Yes
Kupersmith et al., 2001	37	37	Younger pts	Ns	Ns	Nc	Nc	Na	Ns	Ns**
Wang et al., 2003	137	141	Nc	Females	Nc	Nc	Nc	Nc	Na	Yes

Notes: ns, not significant; na, not applicable; nc, not communicated/indicated/provided.

* Type IIIB in the modified classification of Kim *et al.* (1997) in fact corresponds to type IV of the well-accepted classification of Zabramski *et al.* (1994).

** Kupersmith *et al.* (2001) found no significant difference in the previous hemorrhage group but extralesional bleeding and rebleeding rates were significantly different (0.44% vs. 14.2% / les / yr).

confirmed in two cases, suggesting that aggressive courses of DVAs are more likely to be related to an underlying associated occult vascular malformation.

Several authors suggested that patients with CM-associated DVA have a more aggressive course (Abdulrauf, Kaynar, and Awad, 1999; Awad *et al.*, 1993; Ciricillo *et al.*, 1994; Kamezawa *et al.*, 2005; Wurm *et al.*, 2005). Abdulrauf, Kaynar, and Awad (1999), in a retrospective series of 55 patients with CMs, found that 38% of those with an isolated CM presented with hemorrhage, whereas 62% of those with an associated DVA bled. Because of the small number of cases, the difference between these two groups did not reach signifi-

cance. Wurm *et al.* (2005) reported a bleeding rate of 93.3% among 15 patients (mean age 38.7 years) who had CMs associated with a DVA. This rate is far higher than that reported in the natural history of CMs. These findings strongly support the theory that patients with coexistent DVA are more likely to bleed than are those with CMs alone.

Several studies suggest that CMs are active lesions with endothelial proliferation and neoangiogenesis responsible for their dynamic behavior characterized by growth, regression, and de novo formation (Abdulrauf, Kaynar, and Awad, 1999; Hashimoto *et al.*, 2000; Kilic *et al.*, 2000; Maiuri *et al.*, 2006; Notelet

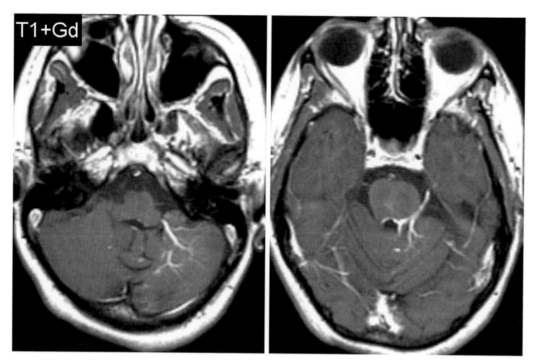

Figure 29.2 T1 post-contrast MRI appearance of a DVA in the posterior fossa.

et al., 1997; Sure et al., 2004, 2005; Sure, Butz, Shlegel, et al., 2001; Sure, Butz, Siegel, et al., 2001). The association of different intracranial vascular malformations and the pathological heterogeneity within lesions also support the assumption of a common origin of distinct vascular malformations (Awad et al., 1993; Naff et al., 1998; Rigamonti et al., 1990; Wilson, 1992; Wurm et al., 2005). Although a DVA is a congenital lesion, any associated malformation might be a dynamically acquired anomaly. The alteration in blood flow of venous malformations with hemodynamic turbulence, progressive obstruction, venous hypertension, and diapedesis of blood cells through leaky capillaries could stimulate angiogenetic factors and so promote the development of associated malformations (Bertalanffy et al., 2002; Ciricillo et al., 1994; Clatterbuck, Elmaci, and Rigamonti, 2001; Little et al., 1990; Wilson, 1992; Wurm et al., 2005), with some forms constituting transitional forms or precursors of other lesions (Mullan et al., 1996; Rigamonti et al., 1990). These hypotheses are supported by Wurm et al. (2005), who found in 15 patients operated on for CMs associated with DVA and in whom the large draining vein was left untouched, three recurrent lesions of different histological type – three AVMs in two patient and a capillary telangectasia in one. Altogether, these findings support the concept that DVAs are congenital lesions leading to mixed and then different intracranial vascular malformations, which can be considered as a wide continuum of progression of a single pathological process.

The prevailing opinion is that DVAs constitute anomalous venous drainage of normal brain tissue. The usual recommendation is to spare DVAs during surgery to avoid venous infarction (Abdulrauf, Kaynar, and Awad, 1999; Amin-Hanjani and Ogilvy, 1999; Awad et al., 1993; Perrini and Lanzino, 2006; Porter et al.,

1999). Postoperative brain swelling and infarction are reported after partial or total coagulation of a DVA with a subsequent occasional fatal outcome (Porter et al., 1999; Rigamonti and Spetzler, 1988). Spontaneous thrombosis of a DVA has been found to be associated with a nonhemorrhagic infarction in one report (Konan et al., 1999), but sparing of a large draining vein of a DVA during surgery can lead to an incomplete resection of the CMs. Porter et al. (1999) reported that almost all recurrences in their series were due to a voluntarily incomplete resection to preserve the DVA. In contrast to Abe et al. (2003), Wurm et al. (2005) proposed the coagulation and division of the transcerebral vein of the DVA to prevent the recurrence or the de novo appearance of vascular malformations and claimed that this method does not necessarily result in brain swelling and hemorrhagic infarction. They do not recommend this approach for infratentorial DVAs in which disruption of the draining vein has been more often reported to be catastrophic (Porter et al., 1999). They also note that there may be patients in whom the DVA is the sole drainage for the surrounding brain, but they did not suggest imaging techniques to identify them preoperatively. To date, there are no reliable diagnostic criteria that could predict whether the resection of DVAs associated with CMs will cause postoperative morbidity, and most authors still recommend a conservative surgery regarding the large draining vein.

Clinical presentation

Symptoms related to cerebrovascular malformations can present acutely or may have an insidious onset. Presentation is related to intrinsic growth, bleeding, thrombosis, or perilesional iron depositions and perilesional atrophy. Owing to heterogeneity in size, location, and propensity of bleeding, CMs may cause a wide spectrum of clinical symptoms, with frequent changes over time such as repeated exacerbation of symptoms and alternating periods of remission. CMs occasionally simulate multiple sclerosis due to fluctuating progressive neurological deficits (Vrethem et al., 1997) and sometimes also trigeminal neuralgia (Shimpo, 2000). The clinical syndromes have been divided into the broad categories of seizures, focal neurological deficits, and hemorrhage. The latter will be discussed in more detail in the section on natural history.

Epileptic seizures constitute the most frequent clinical presenting symptom of patients with CMs and occur in 40%–50% of patients (Del Curling et al., 1991; Kim et al., 1997; Moriarity, Wetzel, Clatterbuck, et al., 1999; Porter et al., 1997; Robinson et al., 1991; Zabramski et al., 1994). The estimated risk of a patient developing seizures is reported to range from 1.5% to 4.8% patient-years in different series (Kondziolka, Lunsford, and Kestle, 1995; Moriarity, Wetzel, Clatterbuck, et al., 1999; Robinson et al., 1991). The overall incidence of epilepsy in patients with cerebral CMs varies between 35% and 70% of symptomatic lesions and is associated with recurrent seizures that are drug-resistant in 40% of patients (Ryvlin et al., 1995). According to Cohen et al. (1995), 41%–59% of symptomatic CMs will eventually present with seizures. About 4% of refractory partial epilepsies are thought to be symptomatic of a CM.

Awad and Robinson (1993) found seizure frequencies of 50%–70% in CMs, 20%–40% in AVMs, and 10%–30% in gliomas. The mechanism of epilepsy generation by CMs has not been elucidated. The deposition of hemoglobin breakdown products may result in abnormal presence of intracellular iron salts that are proven potent epileptogenic agents when applied on a rat cortex (Ryvlin et al., 1995; Steiger et al., 1987; Willmore et al., 1978). Other theories including glutamate uptake by astrocytes in the perilesional parenchyma (Wagner et al., 1998) and elevated serine and glycine levels in the peripheral zones of CMs (von Essen et al., 1996).

Excision of the lesions improves seizure control in most patients (Awad and Robinson, 1993). Moran et al. (1999) concluded from a systematic review of the literature that outcome was poorer in cases with longer duration of seizures at the time of surgery. In supratentorial lesions, not only the malformation itself but also the surrounding hemosiderin-loaded gliotic rim should be removed to avoid the recurrence of seizures, but some authors performing only mesionectomy have reported good results (Casazza et al., 1996). Awad and Robinson (1993) noted that the visualized lesion may not necessarily be responsible for the seizure disorder, and therefore sufficient preoperative electroencephalographic evaluation should be performed in order to confirm the responsible region.

While most reports claim good outcomes with surgery (Amin-Hanjani and Ogilvy, 1999; Bertalanffy et al., 1992, 2002; Moran et al., 1999; Zevgaridis et al., 1996), very few recommend radiosurgery for treatment of epilepsy associated with cavernous angiomas (Regis et al., 2000; Zhang et al., 2000). Régis et al. (2000), in a retrospective study that included 49 patients with CM-related epilepsy, reported good seizure control when good electroclinical correlation existed between CM location and epileptogenic zone. Others doubt that

radiosurgery is a valuable therapeutic tool in a large number of patients (Goodman, 2000).

Focal neurological deficits are less frequent and are present in 10%–40% of cases in global series, but are more frequent in brainstem lesions. They may be transient, progressive, recurrent, or fixed (Maraire and Awad, 1995). Headache presentation occurs in a range of 6%–52% (Del Curling et al., 1991; Kim et al., 1997; Kondziolka, Lunsford, and Kestle, 1995; Porter et al., 1997; Robinson et al., 1991; Zabramski et al., 1999) but was described in up to 65% of patients in a recent series (Moriarity, Wetzel, Clatterbuck, et al., 1999). Much of the variability relates to the multifactorial and subjective nature of headache as well as to differences between studies soliciting complaints.

Thirteen to 56% of CMs present with a clinically symptomatic hemorrhage. Incidental detection of CMs represents about 20% of the diagnosis pattern ranging from 1.5% to 40% of cases (Aiba et al., 1995; Del Curling et al., 1991; Kim et al., 1997; Labauge et al., 2000; Moriarity, Wetzel, Clatterbuck, et al., 1999; Porter et al., 1997; Robinson et al., 1991; Zabramski et al., 1994). CMs are now being detected frequently by chance in individuals who undergo MRI studies for unrelated problems (Requena et al., 1991; Robinson et al., 1991; Sage et al., 1993).

Brainstem CMs should be considered separately from supratentorial lesions. Brainstem CMs account for about 20% of brain CMs. Age at clinical presentation and sex distribution do not differ from CMs at other locations. Brainstem CMs often present with a sudden onset of symptoms and a high neurological deficit rate. In the series reported by Fritschi et al. (1994), all 139 patients were symptomatic at diagnosis, 88% presented with an initial symptomatic hemorrhage, and 14 patients who presented in a comatose state died from their hemorrhage. Porter et al. (1999 and Kupersmith et al. (2001) have reported two other studies of brainstem CMs, including 100 and 37 cases, respectively. The patients were symptomatic at diagnosis in 97% (Porter et al., 1999) and 95% (Kupersmith et al., 2001), and presented an initial symptomatic hemorrhage in 97% (Porter et al., 1999) and 73% (Kupersmith et al., 2001), respectively.

Radiology of cavernous angiomas

Angiography was the first imaging study used to detect cerebrovascular malformations. Several studies showed that CMs produce no or little pathological changes on angiography (Lobato et al., 1988; Rigamonti et al., 1987). In the review of Simard et al. (1986), it was noted that angiography was performed in 83% of patients, and a negative angiogram was found in 27%. Among pathologic angiograms, 77% showed only an avascular area, whereas venous pooling, capillary blush, or neovascularization was present in 20% (Simard et al., 1986). Today, digital subtraction angiography is considered an unnecessary diagnostic tool in diagnosing CMs. To exclude a mixed lesion with arteriovenous shunts or for designing the surgical approach, angiography may be quite helpful because it shows exactly the venous drainage pattern at the surface of the brain.

CT may be the first diagnostic imaging performed in a patient with acute clinical symptoms, and it does show the bony structure

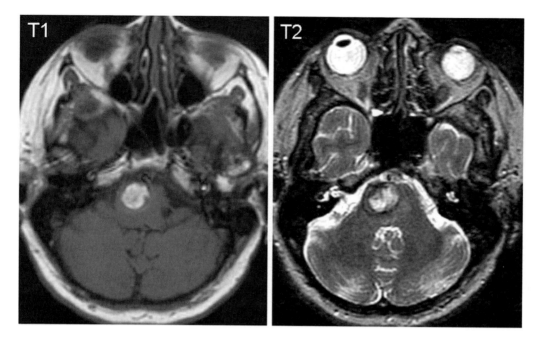

Figure 29.3.a. 58-year-old women presenting with two recent syncopal episodes due to a right pontine CM that has recently bled (type I lesion). T1- and T2-weighted MRIs show a hemorrhagic lesion in the right pons with central hyperintensity indicating extracellular methemoglobin. A darker rim is evident on T2-weighted image reflecting older blood products (hemosiderin). There is very minimal surrounding edema and mass effect.

of the skull base for posterior fossa and especially brainstem CMs. The most sensitive and therefore most important imaging study is MRI, with particularly high sensitivity of gradient-echo sequences (Labauge *et al.*, 1998, 2001) and high-resolution blood oxygenation level–dependent venography (Lee *et al.*, 1999). Rigamonti *et al.* (1987) were among the first to describe in detail the MRI features of CMs. They compared the angiographic, CT, and MRI appearances of CMs and showed clearly superior accuracy of MRI. Whereas CT showed only 14 lesions in 10 patients, T2WI MRIs showed 27 distinct lesions (Rigamonti *et al.*, 1987). Others reviewed the MRI appearances of CMs (Rapacki *et al.*, 1990; Rigamonti *et al.*, 1991; Schefer *et al.*, 1991).

Zabramski *et al.* (1994) first divided CMs into four types based on pathological correlation and MRI signal characteristics (see Figure 29.3a). Type I lesions had a hyperintense core on T1WI due to the presence of methemoglobin, and so are visualized on CT scans. On T2WI, they display a hyper- (methemoglobin) or hypointense (as the hematoma ages methemoglobin is rapidly broken down and converted to hemosiderin and ferritin) core with a surrounding hypointense rim. This type corresponds pathologically with a sub-acute hemorrhage surrounded by a rim of hemosiderin-stained macrophages and gliotic brain tissue. CMs are considered type I until the T1WI core sigsnal becomes iso- or hypointense (see Figure 29.3a).

Type II lesions have a reticulated mixed signal intensity core on T1WI and a reticulated mixed signal intensity core with a surrounding hypointense rim on T2WI. Pathologically these lesions correspond to loculated areas of hemorrhage and thrombosis of varying age, surrounding by gliotic and hemosiderin-stained brain tissue. In large lesions, calcification may be seen (see Figure 29.3b).

Type III lesions have an iso- or hyopintense signal on T1WI and a hypointense signal with a hypointense rim that magnifies the size of the lesion on T2WI. With gradient-echo sequences that are more sensitive than T2 sequences, the lesions have a hypointense signal with greater magnification than T2WI. They correspond to chronic resolved hemorrhage, with hemosiderin staining within and around the lesion (see Figure 29.3c). Type IV lesions are poorly seen or not visualized at all on T1WI and T2WI, and have a punctate hypointense signal on gradient-echo sequences. Two types of lesions have been pathologically shown in this type IV group of lesions – CMs and telangectasies (Rigamonti *et al.*, 1991; Zabramski *et al.*, 1994) (see Figure 29.3d).

Zabramski *et al.* (1994) reported that signs and symptoms were seen almost exclusively in patients with type I and II lesions ("active lesions"). In 15 of their patients with type I and II lesions, 93% were symptomatic. Zabramski *et al.* (1994) reported as did Labauge *et al.* (2001) that de novo lesions considered as clinically silent lesions most often had type III or type IV features.

Owing to the morphologic variability of CMs, a number of other lesions have a similar appearance on MRI and they may also have similar clinical patterns that mimick CMs. These include hemor-rhagic neoplasms such as brain metastases, meningiomas, low-grade or even high-grade gliomas, inflammatory lesions such as cysticercosis and other chronic granulomas, and rare intracranial lesions such as lipomas and hamartomas (Steinberg and Marks, 1993).

Treatment

With evolving knowledge of the natural history of CMs, the risks of operative intervention should be balanced against the risks

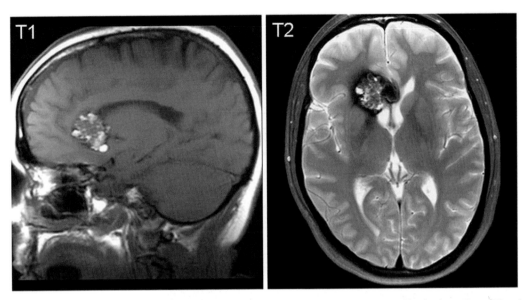

Figure 29.3. b. An incidental type II cavernoma diagnosed in a 41-year-old women presenting with migraine. . T1- and T2-weighted MRIs show a reticulated (mulberry-like) appearance with mixed signal intensity within the core of a CM in the right frontal lobe (type II lesion). There is prominent T2 dark hemosiderin rim. There is no associated edema or mass effect.

of expectant management. Although microsurgical resection of symptomatic CMs is well established (Maraire and Awad, 1995; Mathiesen *et al.*, 2003; Porter *et al.*, 1999; Tung *et al.*, 1990) controversy remains regarding surgical treatment of CMs in eloquent locations. Stereotactic radiosurgery has been shown to obliterate cerebral AVMs with a high success rate and a low morbidity rate (Lunsford *et al.*, 1991; Steiner *et al.*, 1992). Following this experience with AVMs, radiosurgery has also been used to treat CMs, but its efficacy remains in doubt (Amin-Hanjani *et al.*, 1998; Chang *et al.*, 1998; Karlsson *et al.*, 1998; Kondziolka, Lunsford, Flickinger, *et al.* 1995; Regis *et al.*, 2000).

Conservative management

Patients with an established diagnosis of cerebral CM who present without gross hemorrhage, seizures, or other specific symptoms are candidates for clinical observation and repeated imaging. Non-operative management should be considered in patients with multiple asymptomatic lesions, purely incidental lesions, or solitary type III lesion located deeply (basal ganglia, thalamus, insula, and brainstem) or within high-function areas (central sulcus) (Maraire and Awad, 1995). Medical treatment is indicated in patients with only epileptic seizures (Bertalanffy *et al.*, 1992; Casazza *et al.*, 1996; Maraire and Awad, 1995; Robinson *et al.*, 1991). The patients managed conservatively should be monitored clinically and radiologically with sequential MRI studies. In case of gross hemorrhage, neurological deterioration, or change in size, surgery should be reconsidered.

Surgery for supratentorial CMs

Several surgical series and numerous case series report the outcomes of surgical treatment for CMs with varying but generally good results (Acciarri *et al.*, 1993; Giombini and Morello, 1978; Scott *et al.*, 1992; Tagle *et al.*, 1986; Vaquero, Leunda, Martinez, *et al.*, 1983)., Estimates of surgical risk are often derived from small series and case reports, the latter of which are especially subject to bias selection. Such estimates may not reflect the risk associated with the full range of operable lesions and may lack the conformity of data gathered from a single institution.

Indications and patient selection for surgery

Because the indication for surgery depends to a great extent upon the surgical accessibility and resectability of the lesion, preoperative diagnostic imaging plays a major role in decision-making. Patient selection and indications for surgery have gradually changed over time. During the 1980s, there was consensus among authors that the majority of readily accessible supratentorial CMs that caused medically intractable epilepsy, recurrent overt hemorrhage, and severe focal or progressive neurological deficit should be resected (Bertalanffy *et al.*, 1992; Giombini and Morello, 1978; Pozzati *et al.*, 1981; Simard *et al.*, 1986). Now, considering the high cumulative risk of bleeding, there is a tendency to extend the indication for surgery to young patients with mild or nondisabling symptoms harboring solitary type I or II CM and particularly in childbearing-age women before pregnancy (Amin-Hanjani *et al.*, 1998; Chaskis and Brotchi, 1998; Maraire and Awad, 1995).

In patients who have multiple lesions, there is a consensus that only symptomatic lesions are considered for surgery (Amin-Hanjani *et al.*, 1998; Chaskis and Brotchi, 1998; Maraire and Awad, 1995). More problematic are lesions located either within cortical or subcortical eloquent areas and within other functionally important regions such as the basal ganglia and thalamus (Amin-Hanjani *et al.*, 1998; Duffau *et al.*, 1997; Mehdorn *et al.*, 1998; Steinberg *et al.*, 2000) or those located within the third ventricle, the

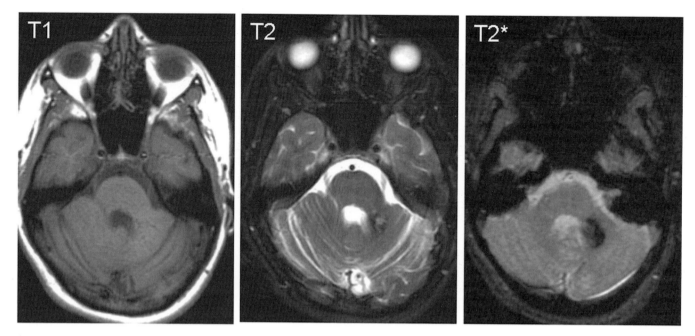

Figure 29.3. c. A 24-year-old woman who had one episode of headache, difficulty walking, nausea, and vomiting due to cerebellar hemorrhage 2 months ago. Follow-up MRI shows a CM in the left middle cerebellar peduncle that is inconspicuous on T1WI image (isointense to adjacent parenchyma) with mild T2 hyperintense core and T2 dark rim (pattern of type III lesion). This lesion is exaggerated on the T2WI (susceptibility-weighted) gradient echo image with a "blooming" artifact.

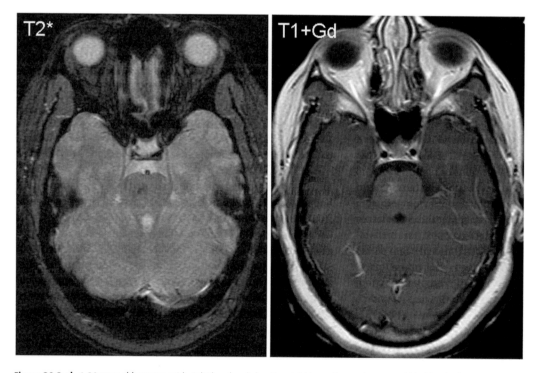

Figure 29.3. d. A 30-year-old woman with right hand and shooting right leg pain, weakness, and bladder dysfunction. T2WI gradient echo image shows an ill-defined hypointense lesion in the right pons, and this lesion demonstrates faint, brush-like enhancement, without associated mass effect or edema. It is not visualized in any other sequences. This is a characteristic pattern of a capillary telangiectasia or a type IV lesion.

corpus callosum, the cingulate gyrus, the paraventricular and paratrigonal regions, or the deep temporal area (Shah and Heros, 1993). However, these reports showed that lesions within all such locations can be removed safely and with acceptable morbidity.

Surgical management

The following factors play an important role in the timing of surgery: the presence or absence of hemorrhage, the presence or absence of intractable seizures, the acuteness and the mass effect of hemorrhage, the patient's clinical condition, and the referral pattern. Owing to considerable variability in these factors, no unanimous recommendations exist, and each clinical scenario requires a distinct management approach (Maraire and Awad, 1995).

The surgical technique includes precise preoperative planning especially for CMs located in critical areas, based on neuroimaging and technical adjuncts such as frameless stereotactic guidance, intraoperative ultrasonography, integrated neuronavigation with functional MRI, and/or electrophysiological monitoring (Duffau et al., 1997). Shah and Heros (1993) described the various surgical approaches used for exposing superficial or deep-seated supratentorial cavernomas. Criteria for assessing surgical outcome are the completeness of lesion removal, the presence of transient or permanent neurological morbidity, and control of seizures. Treatment results must also be judged against the known or assumed natural history of the disease (Maraire and Awad, 1995). Excellent surgical results have been achieved in superficial lesions of both eloquent and non-eloquent areas and in many patients with lesions in critical locations such as the basal ganglia and thalamus. Surgery improves the control of seizure with 50%–90% postoperative seizure-free patients without anticonvulsivant therapy (Awad and Jabbour, 2006; Del Curling et al., 1991; Giombini and Morello, 1978; Robinson et al., 1991). Well-recognized predictive factors of postoperative poor outcome in patients with associated epilepsy are the duration of symptoms, particularly when seizures have been present for more than 12 months (Yeh et al., 1993), the number of seizures particularly if more than five, the age at onset of epilepsy, the lower the age the higher the risk, and the sex – women have more risk of postoperative seizures. In those patients, additional excision of the epileptogenic surrounding brain should be considered in order to control intractable epilepsy.

Surgery for brainstem CMs

The surgery of brainstem CMs remains debatable. Brainstem CMs represent a formidable surgical treatment challenge because of their location within parenchyma responsible for critical neurological function, rendering them much more difficult to remove without significant morbidity than in other locations. Advances in microsurgical techniques, preoperative neuroimaging planning, and the use of technical adjuncts have enabled the successful extirpation of deep-seated and brainstem lesions (Fritschi et al., 1994; Ojemann et al., 1993; Ojemann and Ogilvy, 1999; Sakai et al., 1991; Symon et al., 1991; Zimmerman et al., 1991). In experienced hands, the surgical resection of brainstem CMs is feasible with a low morbidity. Some authors advocate conservative expectation, according to the natural history of the malformation (Esposito et al., 2003; Kupersmith et al., 2001). However, there is evidence that the hemorrhage rate of brainstem cavernomas is up to 30 times greater than at other brain locations (Boecher-Schwarz et al., 1996; Del Curling et al., 1991; Fritschi et al., 1994; Kondziolka, Lunsford, Flickinger, et al., 1995; Porter et al., 1997; Robinson et al., 1991; Zabramski et al., 1994). Owing to anatomical reasons, hemorrhage within the brainstem is more likely to produce severe neurological deficits than cavernomas in other locations (Fritschi et al., 1994; Kondziolka, Lunsford, and Kestle, 1995). Finally, patients who have a brainstem CM that has already bled are more likely to have repeated hemorrhages than are patients with malformations in other locations (Aiba et al., 1995; Fritschi et al., 1994; Kondziolka, Lunsford, and Kestle, 1995; Mizoi et al., 1992; Porter et al., 1997). For these reasons, surgical resection remains an important therapeutic option in the management of brainstem CMs.

Patient selection and indications for surgery

Surgical indications must be guided by the natural history of the pathology and results of treatment applied. Considering the high incidence of permanent morbidity associated with resection of brainstem cavernomas and the lack of large-scale data concerning the natural history of this subgroup of lesions, it remains problematic to define generally accepted and established criteria for patient selection and surgery in patients harboring brainstem CMs.

Surgical exposure of intrinsic brainstem lesions that do not reach the ventricular or pial surface of the brainstem may result in unacceptable neurological consequences and is therefore not recommended (Steinberg et al., 2000). For lesions in the floor of the fourth ventricle, surgical indications are usually limited to exophytic lesions. Porter et al. (1999) recommended that surgery of intrinsic pontine lesions located in the paramedian floor of the fourth ventricle should be only undertaken for actively deteriorating patients. Only patients who had clinically symptomatic hemorrhaging with neurological symptoms are considered good candidates for surgical therapy. Surgery is generally not recommended if the patient comes for consultation several months after normalization of the neurological examination, even after multiple episodes of bleeding, because the risk of postoperative worsening equals the risk of neurological impairment if the CMs rebleed (Bruneau et al., 2006). The incidental finding of a brainstem CM is not an indication for surgery. Some authors state that they would operate only on patients who have had at least two bleeding episodes (Batjer, 1998; Solomon, 2000). Bricolo (2000) mentioned operating also on asymptomatic patients with brainstem cavernomas. The outcome of surgery depends not only on clinical and morphological features in a specific patient harboring a brainstem CM, but also on the operative judgement of the neurosurgeon, who basically relies on his experience and surgical skill. Because the latter criterion cannot be quantified, the debate about the threshold for surgical intervention will continue in the future.

Surgical management

Together with establishing the indication for surgery, the goals of the surgical procedure must be clearly defined as well. The main goals of surgery are clearly summarized by Porter *et al.* (1999): 1) To prevent rebleeding, which implies total removal of the lesion; 2) to minimize damage to the surrounding normal brainstem parenchyma, which implies designing a special and individually tailored approach in each patient; and 3) to preserve an associated venous anomaly.

The appropriate timing for surgery is also debated. Fahlbusch and colleagues (Fahlbusch and Strauss, 1991; Fahlbusch *et al.*, 1990, 1991) suggested waiting 4–6 weeks after the hemorrhagic event; during this time period the patient's condition usually stabilizes, the hematoma becomes organized, and there is less reactive gliosis. Others wait more than 7 weeks (Sindou *et al.*, 2000). However most authors advocate early surgery in brainstem CMs within 1 month after bleeding (Bruneau *et al.*, 2006). They claim that the hematoma creates the surgical approach and that removal of the fresh clot after extralesional hemorrhage or removal of a larger cavernoma after intralesional hemorrhage releases the mass effect on brainstem nuclei and tracts and thus improves the neurological condition. They also note that when hematoma organizes over time, fibroses, and is surrounded by glial scarring and calcifications, the well-demarcated dissection plane may be compromised and surgical resection becomes more difficult (Fahlbusch *et al.*, 1990; Ferroli *et al.*, 2005, 2006; Mathiesen *et al.*, 2003; Steinberg *et al.*, 2000; Wang *et al.*, 2003).

In the largest study, Wang *et al.* (2003) advocated early surgery and operated after 1 or 2 weeks of corticosteroid administration with good results. Mathiesen *et al.* (2003) favor early surgery based on a study of cavernomas located within the thalamus, basal ganglia, and brainstem. When comparing patients operated on within 1 month after the last ictus with those operated on later, they observed a statistically significant risk of transient neurological deterioration when operated on later, an immediate improvement only after early surgery, and permanent deficits only after late surgery. Samii *et al.* (2001) found no differences in the final outcome when patients had surgery within 3 months posthemorrhage or later, even though they observed fewer motor deficits in patients operated on earlier.

Until the end of the 1980s, very few neurosurgeons dared to operate within the brainstem. With the increasing number of published reports describing surgical removal of intrinsic brainstem lesions, the necessity of defining "safe entry zones" to the brainstem became obvious. Kyoshima and coworkers first addressed this issue systematically describing two "safe entry zones" into the brainstem through a suboccipital approach via the floor of the fourth ventricle, namely the "suprafacial and infrafacial triangles" (Kyoshima *et al.*, 1993). However, Strauss *et al.* (1997) noted one shortcoming of the Kyoshima *et al.* (1993) work: that they strictly relied upon external landmarks. Considering the anatomical variability of these landmarks, Strauss *et al.* (1997) performed a morphometric investigation of the rhomboid fossa. They also emphasized the importance of identifying distorted or displaced superficial anatomical structures by direct electrical stimulation and thus described what they consider "safe surgical corridors" (Strauss *et al.*, 1997).

Many authors suggest a paramedian (supracollicular or infracollicular) incision of the rhomboid fossa in order to avoid damage to the longitudinal fascicle (Boecher-Schwarz *et al.*, 1996; Cantore *et al.*, 1999; Fahlbusch *et al.*, 1990; Kyoshima *et al.*, 1993; Steinberg *et al.*, 2000); others advocate a midline incision to spare the dorsal or dorsolateral vascular supply of the pontomedullary region (Bouillot *et al.*, 1996; Konovalov *et al.*, 2000; Symon *et al.*, 1991). Some less frequent reports discuss incision of the brainstem at other locations (Bouillot *et al.*, 1996; Konovalov *et al.*, 2000; Porter *et al.*, 1999; Symon *et al.*, 1991; Zimmerman *et al.*, 1991).

Definition of safe entry zones to the brainstem is important only in those few cases in which the brainstem surface is apparently healthy with no bulging and no discoloration, so that the lesion cannot be seen directly (Lewis and Tew, 1994). When there is an evident dark blue area corresponding to the bulging hematoma, the entry zone depends on this exact site because no or little parenchyma covers the lesion (Cantore *et al.*, 1999; Sindou *et al.*, 2000).

Results of surgery in brainstem CMs in terms of clinical outcome are usually good when operated on by experienced teams (Fritschi *et al.*, 1994; Porter *et al.*, 1999; Wang *et al.*, 2003) (Table 29.5). Fritschi *et al.* (1994) reviewed prior reports and noted that 84% of patients recovered completely with no or minimal disability after surgery. In the largest series published to date, Wang *et al.* (2003) observed that 89.2% of patients returned to work, and Porter *et al.* (1999) reported that 87% of the patients were the same or better at the last follow-up review. The results achieved in brainstem CM surgery improve with increasing experience and with increasing neuroimaging and dissection techniques (Bertalanffy *et al.*, 2002).

The morbidity observed in a significant number of patients postoperatively is caused by manipulation or edema of critical brainstem parenchyma, and this includes various degrees of internuclear ophthalmoplegia, worsening of hemiparesis, facial or abducens paresis, gaze palsy, facial, truncal, and/or extremity numbness, dysphagia, dysarthria, gait ataxia, etc. A high mortality rate was reported in the largest series comprising 86 surgically treated patients (Porter *et al.*, 1999), but others have also reported fatal outcome after surgery for brainstem cavernomas (Bouillot *et al.*, 1996; Cantore *et al.*, 1999; Pechstein *et al.*, 1997; Zimmerman *et al.*, 1991).

Radiosurgery of CMs

Radiosurgical treatment of CMs remains controversial. Considering the high surgical risk in patients with deep-seated cavernomas, radiosurgery was introduced as a reasonable alternative in analogy to the successful radiosurgical treatment of AVMs. However, controversial results have been obtained in reported series. A latency interval of a minimum 2 or 3 years is commonly accepted to appreciate the results of radiosurgery in AVMs (Amin-Hanjani *et al.*, 1998; Kondziolka, Lunsford, Flickinger, *et al.*, 1995). The main goal of radiosurgical treatment should be a significant reduction in bleeding risk, especially after a latency period of 2 years. Whether the same effect obtained in AVM can be achieved also in low-flow

Table 29.5 Brainstem CMs treated surgically literature review

Authors	No. of pts	Preoperative bleeding rate	Gross total removal	Clinical outcome	Transient neurological impairment	Permanent neurological impairment	Recurrence	Recurrent bleeding	Mortality	Mean FU (months)
Fritschi et al., 1994	93	4.3%	82.5%	Total recovery 40% Min. disabled 44% Mod. disabled 15% Sev. disabled 1%	–	–	2%	2%	0%	30.3
Porter et al., 1999	86	5%	99%	Improved or unchanged 88% Worsened 12%	35%	10%	2.4%	0%	3.5%	35
Samii et al., 2001	36	4.7%	100%	No to min. disabled 65% Mod. disabled 21% Sev. disabled 14%	New CN 47% New SM deficit 42%	–	0%	0%	0%	21.5
Wang et al., 2003	137	6.3%	96%	Improved or unchanged 72% Worsened 28%	27.7%	–	–	2.3%	0%	52
Mathiesen et al., 2003	29	–	86%	Improved 80% Unchanged or worsened 20%	69%	20%	–	14%	0%	54
Ferroli et al., 2005	52	3.8%	100%	Improved or unchanged 81% Worsened 19%	56%	19%	–	0%	1.9%	51
Bruneau et al., 2006	22	2.68%	86.4%	Improved 90.8% Worsened 4.6% Lost of follow-up 4.6%	39%	8.6%	–	4.5%	4.5%	50

Notes: FU, follow-up; CN, cranial nerve; SM, sensorimotor.

malformations, such as CMs, has still to be proven. In contrast to AVMs, no imaging test exists to confirm obliteration of the lesion, and an obvious end point in evaluating the treatment results does not exist (Karlsson et al., 1998). The only way of assessing the efficacy of the treatment is clinical observation of hemorrhage rates before and after treatment (Mitchell et al., 2000). Close clinical follow-up and absence of new episodes of bleeding is an indication but not a confirmation of the absence of residual hemorrhagic risk (Chaskis and Brotchi, 1998). Among the most important issues related to the radiosurgical treatment of CMs is the question of whether radiosurgery has any important effect on these lesions compared with their natural history and provides sufficient protection from recurrent and clinically significant hemorrhage.

Gamma-knife treatment may have a greater risk of morbidity compared with AVM radiosurgery even when correcting for lesion size and location (Amin-Hanjani et al., 1998; Karlsson et al., 1998; Pollock et al., 2000) (Table 29.6). A high incidence of neurological sequelae caused either by radiation necrosis or by post-treatment hemorrhage and fatalities have been reported (Amin-Hanjani

et al., 1998; Chang et al., 1998). Unlike for patients with deep AVMs, microsurgical resection can be performed safely for some patients with deep CMs (Porter et al., 1999; Steinberg et al., 2000). Surgical excision with modern neurosurgical techniques not only prevents future bleeding but also has acceptable morbidity. Only patients with repeated bleeding episodes due to a CM in a location that precludes surgery without prohibitive risk and patients with poor clinical condition that contraindicates surgery should be considered for radiosurgery.

Conclusions

CMs are more common than previously appreciated and are found without symptoms in a significant number of patients. Familial cases have been recognized to constitute 30%–50% of cases (Moriarity, Clatterbuck, and Rigamonti, 1999). Familial CMs are transmitted as an autosomal dominant trait with incomplete clinical and radiological penetrance and have intrafamilial and interfamilial variability. By genetic linkage analyses, three cerebral CM loci

Table 29.6 Radiosurgery and CMs literature review

Authors	No. of pts	Mean age (yr)	Location	Bleeding rate		Mean max. dose	Rad.-Relat. compl.	Decrease in size (%)	Perm. Neurol. Seq.	Type of radio-surgery	Mortality	Mean FU (years)
				Before RS	After RS							
Kondziolka et al. 1995	47	39	83% deep 17% hemis.	32%	8.8% (years 1–2); 1.1% (after 2 yrs)	32 Gy	26%	21%	4%	GK	0%	3.6
Amin-Hanjani et al., 1998	73			17.4%	22.5% (years 1–2); 4.5% (after 2 yrs)		16%		16%	Proton beam	3%	5.4
Chang et al., 1998	57		Nc	Nc	9.4% (years 1–3); 1.6% (after 3 yrs)	33 Gy	10.5%	13.6%	1.7%	Helium ion beam LINAC	3.5%	7.5
Karlsson et al., 1998	22		59% deep 41% hemis.	Nc	10–12% (years 1–4); 5% (after 4 years)	32 Gy	27%		22.7%	GK	0%	6.9
Pollock et al., 2000	17	45	100% deep	13%	3.7%	34 Gy	16.6%		5.5%	GK	0%	4.5
Mitchell et al., 2000	18	31.6	83% deep 17% hemis.	24.8%	8.8% (years 1–2); 2.9% (after 2 yrs)	31 Gy	59%	42.7%	41%	GK	0%	4.2
Hasegawa et al., 2002	82	37.7	84% deep 16% hemis.	34%	12.3% (years 1–2); 0.76% (after 2 years)	30 Gy	13.4%	45%	Nc	GK	0%	4.3
Liscak et al., 2005	112	42	45% deep 55% hemis.	2%	1.6%		20.5%		4.5%	GK	0%	4
Liu et al., 2005	125	Nc	71% deep 29% hemis.	Nc	10.3% (years 1–2); 3.3% (after 2 years)	Nc	13.1%		2.5%	GK	0%	5.4
Kim et al., 1997	65	37.6	62% deep 38% hemis.	Nc	Nc	Nc	26%	27 Gy	Nc	GK	0%	3.5

have been assigned to chromosome 7p, 7q, and 3q. They account for all familial forms of CM, thus constituting a formidable mendelian model of stroke (Craig *et al.*, 1998). The three genes corresponding to each loci have been identified (Bergametti *et al.*, 2005). There is growing evidence that these lesions (sporadic or familial) are dynamic and change with time. This is supported by recognition of de novo lesions and by many biological studies on the proliferative and angiogenic potential of CMs (Denier *et al.*, 2006; Maiuri *et al.*, 2006).

The bleeding rates of CMs are lower than previously reported and likely lie between the lowest retrospective rates (0.25%–2.3%) (Del Curling *et al.*, 1991; Kim *et al.*, 1997) and the highest prospective rates (0.8%–16.5%) (Aiba *et al.*, 1995; Kondziolka, Lunsford, and Kestle, 1995; Labauge et al., 2000, 2001; Moriarity, Wetzel, Clatterbuck, *et al.*, 1999; Robinson *et al.*, 1991; Zabramski *et al.*, 1994). Although histologically identical, CMs located in different parts of the CNS have different natural histories. The outcome of these patients depends on the location of the lesion and the history of prior hemorrhage. These facts make an understanding of the regional behavior of CMs essential in making wise management decisions.

REFERENCES

Abdulrauf, S. I., Kaynar, M. Y., and Awad, I. A. 1999. A comparison of the clinical profile of cavernous malformations with and without associated venous malformations. *Neurosurgery*, **44**, 41–6; discussion 46–7.

Abdulrauf, S. I., Malik, G. M., and Awad, I. A. 1999. Spontaneous angiographic obliteration of cerebral arteriovenous malformations. *Neurosurgery*, **44**, 280–7; discussion 287–8.

Abe, M., Hagihara, N., Tabuchi, K., Uchino, A., and Miyasaka, Y. 2003. Histologically classified venous angiomas of the brain: a controversy. *Neurol Med Chir (Tokyo)*, **43**, 1–10; discussion 11.

Abe, T., Singer, R. J., Marks, M. P., *et al.* 1998. Coexistence of occult vascular malformations and developmental venous anomalies in the central nervous system: MR evaluation. *AJNR Am J Neuroradiol*, **19**, 51–7.

Acciarri, N., Padovani, R., Giulioni, M., Gaist, G., and Acciarri, R. 1993. Intracranial and orbital cavernous angiomas: a review of 74 surgical cases. *Br J Neurosurg*, **7**, 529–39.

Aiba, T., Tanaka, R., Koike, T., *et al.* 1995. Natural history of intracranial cavernous malformations. *J Neurosurg*, **83**, 56–9.

Amin-Hanjani, S., and Ogilvy, C. S. 1999. Overall surgical results of occult vascular malformations. *Neurosurg Clin N Am*, **10**, 475–83.

Amin-Hanjani, S., Ogilvy, C. S., Candia, G. J., Lyons, S., and Chapman, P. H. 1998. Stereotactic radiosurgery for cavernous malformations: Kjellberg's experience with proton beam therapy in 98 cases at the Harvard Cyclotron. *Neurosurgery*, **42**, 1229–36; discussion 1236–8.

Awad, I., and Jabbour, P. 2006. Cerebral cavernous malformations and epilepsy. *Neurosurg Focus*, **21**, e7.

Awad, I. A., Robinson, J. R. 1993. In *Cavernous Malformations*, eds. I. A. Awad, and D. L. Barrow. Park Ridge, IL: American Association of Neurological Surgeons, pp. 49–63.

Awad, I. A., Robinson, J. R., Jr., Mohanty, S., and Estes, M. L. 1993. Mixed vascular malformations of the brain: clinical and pathogenetic considerations. *Neurosurgery*, **33**, 179–88; discussion 188.

Batjer, H. H. 1998. Comment: Risks of surgical management for cavernous malformations of the nervous system. *Neurosurgery*, **42**, 1227.

Bergametti, F., Denier, C., Labauge, P., *et al.* 2005. Mutations within the programmed cell death 10 gene cause cerebral cavernous malformations. *Am J Hum Genet*, **76**, 42–51.

Berkman, R. A., Merrill, M. J., Reinhold, W. C., *et al.* 1993. Expression of the vascular permeability factor/vascular endothelial growth factor gene in central nervous system neoplasms. *J Clin Invest*, **91**, 153–9.

Bertalanffy, H., Benes, L., Miyazawa, T., *et al.* 2002. Cerebral cavernomas in the adult. Review of the literature and analysis of 72 surgically treated patients. *Neurosurg Rev*, **25**, 1–53; discussion 54–5.

Bertalanffy, H., Gilsbach, J. M., Eggert, H. R., and Seeger, W. 1991. Microsurgery of deep-seated cavernous angiomas: report of 26 cases. *Acta Neurochir (Wien)*, **108**, 91–9.

Bertalanffy, H., Kuhn, G., Scheremet, R., and Seeger, W. 1992. Indications for surgery and prognosis in patients with cerebral cavernous angiomas. *Neurol Med Chir (Tokyo)*, **32**, 659–66.

Bicknell, J. M., Carlow, T. J., Kornfeld, M., Stovring, J., and Turner, P. 1978. Familial cavernous angiomas. *Arch Neurol*, **35**, 746–9.

Biondi, A., Clemenceau, S., Dormont, D., *et al.* 2002. Intracranial extra-axial cavernous (HEM) angiomas: tumors or vascular malformations? *J Neuroradiol*, **29**, 91–104.

Bloch, W., Forsberg, E., Lentini, S., et al. 1997. Beta 1 integrin is essential for teratoma growth and angiogenesis. *J Cell Biol*, **139**, 265–78.

Bobik, A., and Campbell, J. H. 1993. Vascular derived growth factors: cell biology, pathophysiology, and pharmacology. *Pharmacol Rev*, **45**, 1–42.

Boecher-Schwarz, H. G., Grunert, P., Guenthner, M., Kessel, G., and Mueller-Forell, W. 1996. Stereotactically guided cavernous malformation surgery. *Minim Invasive Neurosurg*, **39**, 50–5.

Bordi, L., Pires, M., Symon, L., and Cheesman, A. D. 1991. Cavernous angioma of the cerebello-pontine angle: a case report. *Br J Neurosurg*, **5**, 83–6.

Bouillot, P., Dufour, H., Roche, P. H., et al. 1996. [Angiographically occult vascular malformations of the brain stem. Apropos of 25 cases]. *Neurochirurgie*, **42**, 189–200; discussion 200–1.

Bricolo, A. 2000. Comment on: Functional results after microsurgical resection of brainstem cavernous malformations: retrospective study of a 12 patient series and review of the recent literature. *Acta Neurochir (Wien)*, **137**, 34–7.

Brooks, P. C. 1996a. Cell adhesion molecules in angiogenesis. *Cancer Metastasis Rev*, **15**, 187–94.

Brooks, P. C. 1996b. Role of integrins in angiogenesis. *Eur J Cancer*, **32A**, 2423–9.

Bruneau, M., Bijlenga, P., Reverdin, A., *et al.* 2006. Early surgery for brainstem cavernomas. *Acta Neurochir (Wien)*, **148**, 405–14.

Brunereau, L., Levy, C., Laberge, S., Houtteville, J., and Labauge, P. 2000. De novo lesions in familial form of cerebral cavernous malformations: clinical and MR features in 29 non-Hispanic families. *Surg Neurol*, **53**, 475–82; discussion 482–3.

Busch, C. R., Heath, D. D., and Hubberstey, A. 2004. Sensitive genetic biomarkers for determining apoptosis in the brown bullhead (Ameiurus nebulosus). *Gene*, **329**, 1–10.

Cantore, G., Missori, P., and Santoro, A. 1999. Cavernous angiomas of the brain stem. Intra-axial anatomical pitfalls and surgical strategies. *Surg Neurol*, **52**, 84–93; discussion 93–4.

Cantu, C., Murillo-Bonilla, L., Arauz, A., *et al.* 2005. Predictive factors for intracerebral hemorrhage in patients with cavernous angiomas. *Neurol Res*, **27**, 314–8.

Casazza, M., Broggi, G., Franzini, A., *et al.* 1996. Supratentorial cavernous angiomas and epileptic seizures: preoperative course and postoperative outcome. *Neurosurgery*, **39**, 26–32; discussion 32–4.

Cavalheiro, S., and Braga, F. M. 1999. Cavernous hemangiomas. In *Pediatric Neurosurgery*, eds. M. Choux, C. Di Rocco, A. D. Hockley, and M. L. Walker. London: Churchill Livingstone, pp. 691–701.

Chadduck, W. M., Binet, E. F., Farrell, F. W. Jr., Araoz, C. A., and Reding, D. L. 1985. Intraventricular cavernous hemangioma: report of three cases and review of the literature. *Neurosurgery*, **16**, 189–97.

Chang, S. D., Levy, R. P., Adler, J. R. Jr., *et al.* 1998. Stereotactic radiosurgery of angiographically occult vascular malformations: 14-year experience. *Neurosurgery*, **43**, 213–20; discussion 220–1.

Chang, S. D., Steinberg, G. K., Rosario, M., Crowley, R. S., and Hevner, R. F. 1997. Mixed arteriovenous malformation and capillary telangiectasia: a rare subset of mixed vascular malformations. Case report. *J Neurosurg*, **86**, 699–703.

Chaskis, C., and Brotchi, J. 1998. The surgical management of cerebral cavernous angiomas. *Neurol Res*, **20**, 597–606.

Cheng, L., Liang, J., and Tang, S. 1999. [The study on the role of apoptosis suppressive gene bcl-2 in the pathogenesis of hemangioma]. *Zhonghua Zheng Xing Shao Shang Wai Ke Za Zhi*, **15**, 35–6.

Ciricillo, S. F., Dillon, W. P., Fink, M. E., and Edwards, M. S. 1994. Progression of multiple cryptic vascular malformations associated with anomalous venous drainage. Case report. *J Neurosurg*, **81**, 477–81.

Clark, J. V. 1970. Familial occurrence of cavernous angiomata of the brain. *J Neurol Neurosurg Psychiatr*, **33**, 871–6.

Clatterbuck, R. E., Eberhart, C. G., Crain, B. J., and Rigamonti, D. 2001. Ultrastructural and immunocytochemical evidence that an incompetent blood-brain barrier is related to the pathophysiology of cavernous malformations. *J Neurol Neurosurg Psychiatr*, **71**, 188–92.

Clatterbuck, R. E., Elmaci, I., and Rigamonti, D. 2001. The juxtaposition of a capillary telangiectasia, cavernous malformation, and developmental venous anomaly in the brainstem of a single patient: case report. *Neurosurgery*, **49**, 1246–50.

Clatterbuck, R. E., Moriarity, J. L., Elmaci, I., *et al.* 2000. Dynamic nature of cavernous malformations: a prospective magnetic resonance imaging study with volumetric analysis. *J Neurosurg*, **93**, 981–6.

Clauss, M., Gerlach, M., Gerlach, H., *et al.* 1990. Vascular permeability factor: a tumor-derived polypeptide that induces endothelial cell and monocyte procoagulant activity, and promotes monocyte migration. *J Exp Med*, **172**, 1535–45.

Cobbs, C. S., and Wilson, C. B. 2001. Intrasellar cavernous hemangioma. Case report. *J Neurosurg*, **94**, 520–2.

Cohen, D. S., Zubay, G. P., and Goodman, R. R. 1995. Seizure outcome after lesionectomy for cavernous malformations. *J Neurosurg*, **83**, 237–42.

Coin, C. G., Coin, J. W., and Glover, M. B. 1977. Vascular tumors of the choroid plexus: diagnosis by computed tomography. *J Comput Assist Tomogr*, **1**, 146–8.

Combelles, G., Blond, S., Biondi, A., *et al.* 1983. [Familial forms of intracranial cavernous hemangioma. Apropos of 5 cases in 2 families]. *Neurochirurgie*, **29**, 263–9.

Couteulx, S. L., Brezin, A. P., Fontaine, B., Tournier-Lasserve, E., and Labauge, P. 2002. A novel KRIT-1/CCM1 truncating mutation in a patient with cerebral and retinal cavernous angiomas. *Arch Ophthalmol*, **120**, 217–8.

Craig, H. D., Gunel, M., Cepeda, O., *et al.* 1998. Multilocus linkage identifies two new loci for a mendelian form of stroke, cerebral cavernous malformation, at 7p15–13 and 3q25.2–27. *Hum Mol Genet*, **7**, 1851–8.

Crawford, J. V., and Russel, D. S. 1956. Cryptic arteriovenous and venous hamartomas of the brain. *J Neurol Neurosurg Psychiatr*, **19**, 1–11.

Cushing, H., and Bailey, P. 1928. *Tumours arising from the blood vessels of the brain. Angiomatous malformations and hemangioblastomas.* Springfield: Thomas.

Dashti, S. R., Hoffer, A., Hu, Y. C., and Selman, W. R. 2006. Molecular genetics of familial cerebral cavernous malformations. *Neurosurg Focus*, **21**, e2.

Davis, R. L., and Robertson, D. M. 1997. *Textbook of Neuropathology.* Baltimore: Williams & Wilkins, pp. 785–822.

de Oliveira, J. G., Rassi-Neto, A., Ferraz, F. A., and Braga, F. M. 2006. Neurosurgical management of cerebellar cavernous malformations. *Neurosurg Focus*, **21**, e11.

de Vries, C., Escobedo, J. A., Ueno, H., et al. 1992. The fms-like tyrosine kinase, a receptor for vascular endothelial growth factor. *Science*, **255**, 989–91.

Dejana, E., Colella, S., Languino, L. R., *et al.* 1987. Fibrinogen induces adhesion, spreading, and microfilament organization of human endothelial cells in vitro. *J Cell Biol*, **104**, 1403–11.

Del Curling, O. Jr., Kelly, D. L. Jr., Elster, A. D., and Craven, T. E. 1991. An analysis of the natural history of cavernous angiomas. *J Neurosurg*, **75**, 702–8.

Denier, C., Goutagny, S., Labauge, P., *et al.* 2004. Mutations within the MGC4607 gene cause cerebral cavernous malformations. *Am J Hum Genet*, **74**, 326–37.

Denier, C., Labauge, P., Bergametti, F., *et al.* 2006. Genotype-phenotype correlations in cerebral cavernous malformations patients. *Ann Neurol*, **60**, 550–6.

Denier, C., Labauge, P., Brunereau, L., *et al.* 2004. Clinical features of cerebral cavernous malformations patients with KRIT-1 mutations. *Ann Neurol*, **55**, 213–20.

Detwiler, P. W., Porter, R. W., Zabramski, J. M., and Spetzler, R. F. 1997. De novo formation of a central nervous system cavernous malformation: implications for predicting risk of hemorrhage. Case report and review of the literature. *J Neurosurg*, **87**, 629–32.

Detwiler, P. W., Porter, R. W., Zabramski, J. M., and Spetzler, R. F. 1998. Radiation-induced cavernous malformation. *J Neurosurg*, **89**, 167–9.

Dillon, W. P. 1997. Cryptic vascular malformations: controversies in terminology, diagnosis, pathophysiology, and treatment. *AJNR Am J Neuroradiol*, **18**, 1839–46.

Dubovsky, J., Zabramski, J. M., Kurth, J., *et al.* 1995. A gene responsible for cavernous malformations of the brain maps to chromosome 7q. *Hum Mol Genet*, **4**, 453–8.

Duffau, H., Capelle, L., Sichez, J. P., *et al.* 1997. Early radiologically proven rebleeding from intracranial cavernous angiomas: report of 6 cases and review of the literature. *Acta Neurochir (Wien)*, **139**, 914–22.

Eerola, I., Plate, K. H., Spiegel, R., *et al.* 2000. KRIT-1 is mutated in hyperkeratotic cutaneous capillary-venous malformation associated with cerebral capillary malformation. *Hum Mol Genet*, **9**, 1351–5.

Esposito, P., Coulbois, S., Kehrli, P., *et al.* 2003. [Place of the surgery in the management of brainstem cavernomas. Results of a multicentric study]. *Neurochirurgie*, **49**, 5–12.

Fahlbusch, R., and Strauss, C. 1991. [Surgical significance of cavernous hemangioma of the brain stem]. *Zentralbl Neurochir*, **52**, 25–32.

Fahlbusch, R., Strauss, C., and Huk, W. 1991. Pontine-mesencephalic cavernomas: indications for surgery and operative results. *Acta Neurochir Suppl (Wien)*, **53**, 37–41.

Fahlbusch, R., Strauss, C., Huk, W., *et al.* 1990. Surgical removal of pontomesencephalic cavernous hemangiomas. *Neurosurgery*, **26**, 449–56; discussion 456–7.

Fehlings, M. G., and Tucker, W. S. 1988. Cavernous hemangioma of Meckel's cave. Case report. *J Neurosurg*, **68**, 645–7.

Fender, L. J., Lenthall, R. K., and Jaspan, T. 2000. De novo development of presumed cavernomas following resolution of E. coli subdural empyemas. *Neuroradiology*, **42**, 778–80.

Ferrara, N., Houck, K. A., Jakeman, L. B., Winer, J., and Leung, D. W. 1991. The vascular endothelial growth factor family of polypeptides. *J Cell Biochem*, **47**, 211–8.

Ferrara, N., Winer, J., and Henzel, W. J. 1992. Pituitary follicular cells secrete an inhibitor of aortic endothelial cell growth: identification as leukemia inhibitory factor. *Proc Natl Acad Sci U S A*. **89**, 698–702.

Ferroli, P., Casazza, M., Marras, C., *et al.* 2006. Cerebral cavernomas and seizures: a retrospective study on 163 patients who underwent pure lesionectomy. *Neurol Sci*, **26**, 390–4.

Ferroli, P., Sinisi, M., Franzini, A., *et al.* 2005. Brainstem cavernomas: long-term results of microsurgical resection in 52 patients. *Neurosurgery*, **56**, 1203–12; discussion 1212–4.

Folkman, J., and Klagsbrun, M. 1987. Angiogenic factors. *Science*, **235**, 442–7.

Frischmeyer, P. A., and Dietz, H. C. 1999. Nonsense-mediated mRNA decay in health and disease. *Hum Mol Genet*, **8**, 1893–900.

Fritschi, J. A., Reulen, H. J., Spetzler, R. F., and Zabramski, J. M. 1994. Cavernous malformations of the brain stem. A review of 139 cases. *Acta Neurochir (Wien)*, **130**, 35–46.

Fukui, M., Matsuoka, S., Hasuo, K., Numaguchi, Y., and Kitamura, K. 1983. Cavernous hemangioma in the pineal region. *Surg Neurol*, **20**, 209–15.

Gaensler, E. H., Dillon, W. P., Edwards, M. S., *et al.* 1994. Radiation-induced telangiectasia in the brain simulates cryptic vascular malformations at MR imaging. *Radiology*, **193**, 629–36.

Gamble, J., Meyer, G., Noack, L., *et al.* 1999. B1 integrin activation inhibits in vitro tube formation: effects on cell migration, vacuole coalescence and lumen formation. *Endothelium*, **7**, 23–34.

Gangemi, M., Maiuri, F., Donati, P., *et al.* 1990. Familial cerebral cavernous angiomas. *Neurol Res*, **12**, 131–6.

Gangemi, M., Maiuri, F., Donati, P. A., and Sigona, L. 1993. Rapid growth of a brain-stem cavernous angioma. *Acta Neurol (Napoli)*, **15**, 132–7.

Garbisa, S., and Negro, A. 1984. Macromolecular organization and functional architecture of basement membranes. *Appl Pathol*, **2**, 217–22.

Garner, T. B., Del Curling, O. Jr., Kelly, D. L. Jr., and Laster, D. W. 1991. The natural history of intracranial venous angiomas. *J Neurosurg*, **75**, 715–22.

Giombini, S., and Morello, G. 1978. Cavernous angiomas of the brain. Account of fourteen personal cases and review of the literature. *Acta Neurochir (Wien)*, **40**, 61–82.

Goel, A., Muzumdar, D., and Sharma, P. 2003. Extradural approach for cavernous hemangioma of the cavernous sinus: experience with 13 cases. *Neurol Med Chir (Tokyo)*, **43**, 112–8; discussion 119.

Goodman, R. R. 2000. Comment on: Radiosurgery for epilepsy associated with cavernous malformation: retrospective study in 49 patients. *Neurosurgery*, **47**, 1097.

Gospodarowicz, D., Abraham, J. A., and Schilling, J. 1989. Isolation and characterization of a vascular endothelial cell mitogen produced by pituitary-derived folliculo stellate cells. *Proc Natl Acad Sci U S A*, **86**, 7311–5.

Gospodarowicz, D., Ferrara, N., Haaparanta, T., and Neufeld, G. 1988. Basic fibroblast growth factor: expression in cultured bovine vascular smooth muscle cells. *Eur J Cell Biol*, **46**, 144–51.

Gospodarowicz, D., Ferrara, N., Schweigerer, L., and Neufeld, G. 1987. Structural characterization and biological functions of fibroblast growth factor. *Endocr Rev*, **8**, 95–114.

Gunel, M., Awad, I. A., Anson, J., and Lifton, R. P. 1995. Mapping a gene causing cerebral cavernous malformation to 7q11.2-q21. *Proc Natl Acad Sci U S A*, **92**, 6620–4.

Gunel, M., Awad, I. A., Finberg, K., et al. 1996a. A founder mutation as a cause of cerebral cavernous malformation in Hispanic Americans. *N Engl J Med*, **334**, 946–51.

Gunel, M., Awad, I. A., Finberg, K., et al. 1996b. Genetic heterogeneity of inherited cerebral cavernous malformation. *Neurosurgery*, **38**, 1265–71.

Gunel, M., Laurans, M. S., Shin, D., et al. 2002. KRIT-1, a gene mutated in cerebral cavernous malformation, encodes a microtubule-associated protein. *Proc Natl Acad Sci U S A*, **99**, 10677–82.

Guzeloglu-Kayisli, O., Amankulor, N. M., Voorhees, J., et al. 2004. KRIT-1/cerebral cavernous malformation 1 protein localizes to vascular endothelium, astrocytes, and pyramidal cells of the adult human cerebral cortex. *Neurosurgery*, **54**, 943–9; discussion 949.

Hahn, M. 1999. Kavernome des zentralen Nervensystems.111 eigene Fälle und Metaanalyse von 1361 Literaturfällen. Medical thesis. Germany: University of Heidelberg.

Harbaugh, R. E., Roberts, D. W., and Fratkin, J. D. 1984. Hemangioma calcificans. Case report. *J Neurosurg*, **60**, 417–9.

Hasegawa, T., McInerney, J., Kondziolka, D., et al. 2002. Long-term results after stereotactic radiosurgery for patients with cavernous malformations. *Neurosurgery*, **50**, 1190–7.

Hashimoto, T., Emala, C. W., Joshi, S., et al. 2000. Abnormal pattern of Tie-2 and vascular endothelial growth factor receptor expression in human cerebral arteriovenous malformations. *Neurosurgery*, **47**, 910–8; discussion 918–9.

Hayman, L. A., Evans, R. A., Ferrell, R. E., et al. 1982. Familial cavernous angiomas: natural history and genetic study over a 5-year period. *Am J Med Genet*, **11**, 147–60.

Heckl, S., Aschoff, A., and Kunze, S. 2002a. Cavernomas of the skull: review of the literature 1975–2000. *Neurosurg Rev*, **25**, 56–62; discussion 66–7.

Heckl, S., Aschoff, A., and Kunze, S. 2002b. Cavernous hemangioma of the temporal muscle. *Neurosurg Rev*, **25**, 63–65; discussion 66–7.

Hirsh, L. F. 1981. Combined cavernous-arteriovenous malformation. *Surg Neurol*, **16**, 135–9.

Houtteville, J. P. 1997. Brain cavernoma: a dynamic lesion. *Surg Neurol*, **48**, 610–4.

Hsu, F. P. K., Rigamonti, D., and Huhn, S. L. 1993. Epidemiology of cavernous malformations. In *Cavernous Malformations*, eds. I. A. Awad, and D. L. Barrow. Park Ridge, IL: American Association of Neurological Surgeons, pp. 13–23.

Hyodo, A., Yanaka, K., Higuchi, O., Tomono, Y., and Nose, T. 2000. Giant interdural cavernous hemangioma at the convexity. Case illustration. *J Neurosurg*, **92**, 503.

Isla, A., Roda, J. M., Alvarez, F., et al. 1989. Intracranial cavernous angioma in the dura. *Neurosurgery*, **25**, 657–9.

Issbrucker, K., Marti, H. H., Hippenstiel, S., et al. 2003. p38 MAP kinase–a molecular switch between VEGF-induced angiogenesis and vascular hyperpermeability. *FASEB J*, **17**, 262–4.

Jabbour, P., Gault, J., Murk, S. E., and Awad, I. A. 2004. Multiple spinal cavernous malformations with atypical phenotype after prior irradiation: case report. *Neurosurgery*, **55**, 1431.

Jackson, J. R., Bolognese, B., Hillegass, L., et al. 1998. Pharmacological effects of SB 220025, a selective inhibitor of P38 mitogen-activated protein kinase, in angiogenesis and chronic inflammatory disease models. *J Pharmacol Exp Ther*, **284**, 687–92.

Jakeman, L. B., Winer, J., Bennett, G. L., Altar, C. A., and Ferrara, N. 1992. Binding sites for vascular endothelial growth factor are localized on endothelial cells in adult rat tissues. *J Clin Invest*, **89**, 244–53.

Johnson, P. C., Wascher, T. M., Golfinos, J., and Spetzler, R. F. 1993. Definition and pathological features. In *Cavernous Malformations*, eds. I. A. Awad, and D. L. Barrow. Park Ridge,: AANS, pp. 1–11.

Jung, K. H., Chu, K., Jeong, S. W., et al. 2003. Cerebral cavernous malformations with dynamic and progressive course: correlation study with vascular endothelial growth factor. *Arch Neurol*, **60**, 1613–8.

Kamezawa, T., Hamada, J., Niiro, M., et al. 2005. Clinical implications of associated venous drainage in patients with cavernous malformation. *J Neurosurg*, **102**, 24–8.

Karlsson, B., Kihlstrom, L., Lindquist, C., Ericson, K., and Steiner, L. 1998. Radiosurgery for cavernous malformations. *J Neurosurg*, **88**, 293–7.

Keck, P. J., Hauser, S. D., Krivi, G., et al. 1989. Vascular permeability factor, an endothelial cell mitogen related to PDGF. *Science*, **246**, 1309–12.

Keep, R. F., and Jones, H. C. 1990. Cortical microvessels during brain development: a morphometric study in the rat. *Microvasc Res*, **40**, 412–26.

Kidd, H. A., and Cummings, J. M. 1947. Cerebral angiomata in an Icelandic family. *Lancet*, **1**, 747–8.

Kilic, T., Pamir, M. N., Kullu, S., et al. 2000. Expression of structural proteins and angiogenic factors in cerebrovascular anomalies. *Neurosurgery*, **46**, 1179–91; discussion 1191–2.

Kim, D. S., Park, Y. G., Choi, J. U., Chung, S. S., and Lee, K. C. 1997. An analysis of the natural history of cavernous malformations. *Surg Neurol*, **48**, 9–17; discussion 17–8.

Kittelberger, R., Davis, P. F., and Stehbens, W. E. 1990. Distribution of type IV collagen, laminin, nidogen and fibronectin in the haemodynamically stressed vascular wall. *Histol Histopathol*, **5**, 161–7.

Konan, A. V., Raymond, J., Bourgouin, P., et al. 1999. Cerebellar infarct caused by spontaneous thrombosis of a developmental venous anomaly of the posterior fossa. *AJNR Am J Neuroradiol*, **20**, 256–8.

Kondziolka, D., Lunsford, L. D., Flickinger, J. C., and Kestle, J. R. 1995. Reduction of hemorrhage risk after stereotactic radiosurgery for cavernous malformations. *J Neurosurg*, **83**, 825–31.

Kondziolka, D., Lunsford, L. D., and Kestle, J. R. 1995. The natural history of cerebral cavernous malformations. *J Neurosurg*, **83**, 820–4.

Konovalov, A., Samii, M., Porter, R. W., et al. 2000. Brainstem cavernoma. *Surg Neurol*, **54**, 418–21.

Krum, J. M., More, N. S., and Rosenstein, J. M. 1991. Brain angiogenesis: variations in vascular basement membrane glycoprotein immunoreactivity. *Exp Neurol*, **111**, 152–65.

Kufs, H. 1928. Über die heredofamiliäre Angiomatose des Gehirns und der Retina, ihre Beziehungen zueinander und zur Angiomatose der Haut. *Z Neurol Psychiatrie*, **113**, 651–86.

Kupersmith, M. J., Kalish, H., Epstein, F., et al. 2001. Natural history of brainstem cavernous malformations. *Neurosurgery*, **48**, 47–53; discussion 53–4.

Kyoshima, K., Kobayashi, S., Gibo, H., and Kuroyanagi, T. 1993. A study of safe entry zones via the floor of the fourth ventricle for brain-stem lesions. Report of three cases. *J Neurosurg*, **78**, 987–93.

Labauge, P., Brunereau, L., Laberge, S., and Houtteville, J. P. 2001. Prospective follow-up of 33 asymptomatic patients with familial cerebral cavernous malformations. *Neurology*, **57**, 1825–8.

Labauge, P., Brunereau, L., Levy, C., Laberge, S., and Houtteville, J. P. 2000. The natural history of familial cerebral cavernomas: a retrospective MRI study of 40 patients. *Neuroradiology*, **42**, 327–32.

Labauge, P., Enjolras, O., Bonerandi, J. J., et al. 1999. An association between autosomal dominant cerebral cavernomas and a distinctive hyperkeratotic cutaneous vascular malformation in 4 families. *Ann Neurol*, **45**, 250–4.

Labauge, P., Laberge, S., Brunereau, L., et al. 1998. Hereditary cerebral cavernous angiomas: clinical and genetic features in 57 French families. Societe Francaise de Neurochirurgie. *Lancet*, **352**, 1892–7.

Laberge-le Couteulx, S., Jung, H. H., Labauge, P., *et al.* 1999. Truncating mutations in CCM1, encoding KRIT-1, cause hereditary cavernous angiomas. *Nat Genet*, **23**, 189–93.

Lamszus, K., Heese, O., and Westphal, M. 2004. Angiogenesis-related growth factors in brain tumors. *Cancer Treat Res*, **117**, 169–90.

Larson, J. J., Ball, W. S., Bove, K. E., Crone, K. R., and Tew, J. M. Jr. 1998. Formation of intracerebral cavernous malformations after radiation treatment for central nervous system neoplasia in children. *J Neurosurg*, **88**, 51–6.

Laurans, M. S., DiLuna, M. L., Shin, D., *et al.* 2003. Mutational analysis of 206 families with cavernous malformations. *J Neurosurg*, **99**, 38–43.

Lavyne, M. H., and Patterson, R. H. Jr. 1983. Subchoroidal trans-velum interpositum approach to mid-third ventricular tumors. *Neurosurgery*, **12**, 86–94.

Lee, B. C., Vo, K. D., Kido, D. K., *et al.* 1999. MR high-resolution blood oxygenation level-dependent venography of occult (low-flow) vascular lesions. *AJNR Am J Neuroradiol*, **20**, 1239–42.

Leung, D. W., Cachianes, G., Kuang, W. J., Goeddel, D. V., and Ferrara, N. 1989. Vascular endothelial growth factor is a secreted angiogenic mitogen. *Science*, **246**, 1306–9.

Lewis, A. I., and Tew, J. M. Jr. 1994. Management of thalamic-basal ganglia and brain-stem vascular malformations. *Clin Neurosurg*, **41**, 83–111.

Lewis, A. I., Tew, J. M. Jr., Payner, T. D., and Yeh, H. S. 1994. Dural cavernous angiomas outside the middle cranial fossa: a report of two cases. *Neurosurgery*, **35**, 498–504; discussion 504.

Liquori, C. L., Berg, M. J., Siegel, A. M., *et al.* 2003. Mutations in a gene encoding a novel protein containing a phosphotyrosine-binding domain cause type 2 cerebral cavernous malformations. *Am J Hum Genet*, **73**, 1459–64.

Liscak, R., Vladyka, V., Simonova, G., Vymazal, J., and Novotny, J. Jr. 2005. Gamma knife surgery of brain cavernous hemangiomas. *J Neurosurg*, **102(Suppl)**, 207–13.

Little, J. R., Awad, I. A., Jones, S. C., and Ebrahim, Z. Y. 1990. Vascular pressures and cortical blood flow in cavernous angioma of the brain. *J Neurosurg*, **73**, 555–9.

Liu, K. D., Chung, W. Y., Wu, H. M., *et al.* 2005. Gamma knife surgery for cavernous hemangiomas: an analysis of 125 patients. *J Neurosurg*, **102(Suppl)**, 81–6.

Lobato, R. D., Perez, C., Rivas, J. J., and Cordobes, F. 1988. Clinical, radiological, and pathological spectrum of angiographically occult intracranial vascular malformations. Analysis of 21 cases and review of the literature. *J Neurosurg*, **68**, 518–31.

Lombardi, D., Giovanelli, M., and de Tribolet, N. 1994. Sellar and parasellar extra-axial cavernous hemangiomas. *Acta Neurochir (Wien)*, **130**, 47–54.

Lombardi, D., Scheithauer, B. W., Villani, R. M., Giovanelli, M., and de Tribolet, N. 1996. Cavernous haemangioma of the pineal region. *Acta Neurochir (Wien)*, **138**, 678–83.

Lunsford, L. D., Kondziolka, D., Flickinger, J. C., *et al.* 1991. Stereotactic radiosurgery for arteriovenous malformations of the brain. *J Neurosurg*, **75**, 512–24.

Luschka, H. 1854. Cavernöse Blutgeschwulst des Gehirnes. *Virchows Archiv*, **6**, 458–70.

Maeder, P., Gudinchet, F., Meuli, R., and de Tribolet, N. 1998. Development of a cavernous malformation of the brain. *AJNR Am J Neuroradiol*, **19**, 1141–3.

Maiuri, F., Cappabianca, P., Gangemi, M., *et al.* 2006. Clinical progression and familial occurrence of cerebral cavernous angiomas: the role of angiogenic and growth factors. *Neurosurg Focus*, **21**, e3.

Maraire, J. N., Abdulrauf, S. I., Berger, S., Knisely, J., and Awad, I. A. 1999. De novo development of a cavernous malformation of the spinal cord following spinal axis radiation. Case report. *J Neurosurg*, **90**, 234–8.

Maraire, J. N., and Awad, I. A. 1995. Intracranial cavernous malformations: lesion behavior and management strategies. *Neurosurgery*, **37**, 591–605.

Marchuk, D. A., Gallione, C. J., Morrison, L. A., *et al.* 1995. A locus for cerebral cavernous malformations maps to chromosome 7q in two families. *Genomics*, **28**, 311–4.

Martin, N. A., Wilson, C. B., and Stein, B. M. 1984. Venous and cavernous malformations. In *Intracranial Arteriovenous Malformations*, eds. C. B. Wilson, and B. M. Stein. Baltimore: Williams & Wilkins, pp. 234–245.

Mason, I., Aase, J. M., Orrison, W. W., *et al.* 1988. Familial cavernous angiomas of the brain in an Hispanic family. *Neurology*, **38**, 324–6.

Massa-Micon, B., Luparello, V., Bergui, M., and Pagni, CA. 2000. De novo cavernoma case report and review of literature. *Surg Neurol*, **53**, 484–7.

Mathiesen, T., Edner, G., and Kihlstrom, L. 2003. Deep and brainstem cavernomas: a consecutive 8-year series. *J Neurosurg*, **99**, 31–7.

Matsumoto, T., Turesson, I., Book, M., *et al.* 2002. p38 MAP kinase negatively regulates endothelial cell survival, proliferation, and differentiation in FGF-2-stimulated angiogenesis. *J Cell Biol*, **156**, 149–60.

McCormick, W. F. 1966. The pathology of vascular ("arteriovenous") malformations. *J Neurosurg*, **24**, 807–16.

McCormick, W. F., Hardman, J. M., and Boulter, T. R. 1968. Vascular malformations ("angiomas") of the brain, with special reference to those occurring in the posterior fossa. *J Neurosurg*, **28**, 241–51.

McCormick, W. F., Nofzinger, J. D. 1966. "Cryptic" vascular malformations of the central nervous system. *J Neurosurg*, **24**, 865–75.

McLaughlin, M. R., Kondziolka, D., Flickinger, J. C., Lunsford, S., and Lunsford, L. D. 1998. The prospective natural history of cerebral venous malformations. *Neurosurgery*, **43**, 195–200; discussion 200–1.

McMullen, M. E., Bryant, P. W., Glembotski, C. C., Vincent, P. A., and Pumiglia, K. M. 2005. Activation of p38 has opposing effects on the proliferation and migration of endothelial cells. *J Biol Chem*, **280**, 20995–1003.

Mehdorn, H. M., Barth, H., Buhl, R., Nabavi, A., and Weinert, D. 1998. Intracranial cavernomas: indications for and results of surgery. *Neurol Med Chir (Tokyo)*, **38** Suppl, 245–9.

Michael, J. C., and Levin, P. M. 1936. Multiple telangiectases of the brain: a discussion of hereditary factors in their development. *Arch Neurol Psychiatr*, **36**, 514.

Mitchell, P., Hodgson, T. J., Seaman, S., Kemeny, A. A., and Forster, D. M. 2000. Stereotactic radiosurgery and the risk of haemorrhage from cavernous malformations. *Br J Neurosurg*, **14**, 96–100.

Mizoi, K., Yoshimoto, T., and Suzuki, J. 1992. Clinical analysis of ten cases with surgically treated brain stem cavernous angiomas. *Tohoku J Exp Med*, **166**, 259–67.

Moran, N. F., Fish, D. R., Kitchen, N., *et al.* 1999. Supratentorial cavernous haemangiomas and epilepsy: a review of the literature and case series. *J Neurol Neurosurg Psychiatr*, **66**, 561–8.

Moriarity, J. L., Clatterbuck, R. E., and Rigamonti, D. 1999. The natural history of cavernous malformations. *Neurosurg Clin N Am*, **10**, 411–7.

Moriarity, J. L., Wetzel, M., Clatterbuck, R. E., *et al.* 1999. The natural history of cavernous malformations: a prospective study of 68 patients. *Neurosurgery*, **44**, 1166–71; discussion 1172–3.

Moritake, K., Handa, H., Nozaki, K., and Tomiwa, K. 1985. Tentorial cavernous angioma with calcification in a neonate. *Neurosurgery*, **16**, 207–11.

Mottolese, C., Hermier, M., Stan, H., *et al.* 2001. Central nervous system cavernomas in the pediatric age group. *Neurosurg Rev*, **24**, 55–71; discussion 72–3.

Mullan, S., Mojtahedi, S., Johnson, D. L., and Macdonald, R. L. 1996. Cerebral venous malformation-arteriovenous malformation transition forms. *J Neurosurg*, **85**, 9–13.

Naff, N. J., Wemmer, J., Hoenig-Rigamonti, K., and Rigamonti, D. R. 1998. A longitudinal study of patients with venous malformations: documentation of a negligible hemorrhage risk and benign natural history. *Neurology*, **50**, 1709–14.

Namba, S. 1983. Extracerebral cavernous hemangioma of the middle cranial fossa. *Surg Neurol*, **19**, 379–88.

Nimjee, S. M., Powers, C. J., and Bulsara, K. R. 2006. Review of the literature on de novo formation of cavernous malformations of the central nervous system after radiation therapy. *Neurosurg Focus*, **21**, e4.

Notelet, L., Houtteville, J. P., Khoury, S., Lechevalier, B., and Chapon, F. 1997. Proliferating cell nuclear antigen (PCNA) in cerebral cavernomas: an immunocytochemical study of 42 cases. *Surg Neurol*, **47**, 364–70.

Numaguchi, Y., Fukui, M., Miyake, E., *et al.* 1977. Angiographic manifestations of intracerebral cavernous hemangioma. *Neuroradiology*, **14**, 113–6.

Occhiogrosso, M., Carella, A., D'Aprile, P., and Vailati, G. 1983. Brain-stem hemangioma calcificans. Case report. *J Neurosurg*, **59**, 150–2.

Ogawa, A., Katakura, R., and Yoshimoto, T. 1990. Third ventricle cavernous angioma: report of two cases. *Surg Neurol*, **34**, 414–20.

Ogilvy, C. S., and Heros, R. C. 1988. Angiographically occult intracranial vascular malformations. *J Neurosurg*, **69**, 960–2.

Ogilvy, C. S., Moayeri, N., and Golden, J. A. 1993. Appearance of a cavernous hemangioma in the cerebral cortex after a biopsy of a deeper lesion. *Neurosurgery*, **33**, 307–9; discussion 309.

Ojemann, R. G., Crowell, R. M., and Ogilvy, C. S. 1993. Management of cranial and spinal cavernous angiomas (honored guest lecture). *Clin Neurosurg*, **40**, 98–123.

Ojemann, R. G., and Ogilvy, C. S. 1999. Microsurgical treatment of supratentorial cavernous malformations. *Neurosurg Clin N Am*, **10**, 433–40.

Okada, J., Hara, M., and Takeuchi, K. 1977. Dural haemangioma with extracranial component. *Acta Neurochir (Wien)*, **36**, 111–5.

Otten, P., Pizzolato, G. P., Rilliet, B., and Berney, J. 1989. [131 cases of cavernous angioma (cavernomas) of the CNS, discovered by retrospective analysis of 24535 autopsies]. *Neurochirurgie*, **35**, 82–3, 128–31.

Pau, A., and Orunesu, G. 1979. Vascular malformations of the brain in achondroplasia. Case report. *Acta Neurochir (Wien)*, **50**, 289–92.

Paulus, W., Grothe, C., Sensenbrenner, M., *et al.* 1990. Localization of basic fibroblast growth factor, a mitogen and angiogenic factor, in human brain tumors. *Acta Neuropathol (Berl)*, **79**, 418–23.

Pechstein, U., Zentner, J., Van Roost, D., and Schramm, J. 1997. Surgical management of brain-stem cavernomas. *Neurosurg Rev*, **20**, 87–93.

Perrini, P., and Lanzino, G. 2006. The association of venous developmental anomalies and cavernous malformations: pathophysiological, diagnostic, and surgical considerations. *Neurosurg Focus*, **21**, e5.

Plummer, N. W., Gallione, C. J., Srinivasan, S., *et al.* 2004. Loss of p53 sensitizes mice with a mutation in Ccm1 (KRIT-1) to development of cerebral vascular malformations. *Am J Pathol*, **165**, 1509–18.

Plummer, N. W., Squire, T. L., Srinivasan, S., *et al.* 2006. Neuronal expression of the Ccm2 gene in a new mouse model of cerebral cavernous malformations. *Mamm Genome*, **17**, 119–28.

Pollock, B. E., Garces, Y. I., Stafford, S. L., *et al.* 2000. Stereotactic radiosurgery for cavernous malformations. *J Neurosurg*, **93**, 987–91.

Porter, P. J., Willinsky, R. A., Harper, W., and Wallace, M. C. 1997. Cerebral cavernous malformations: natural history and prognosis after clinical deterioration with or without hemorrhage. *J Neurosurg*, **87**, 190–7.

Porter, R. W., Detwiler, P. W., Spetzler, R. F., *et al.* 1999. Cavernous malformations of the brainstem: experience with 100 patients. *J Neurosurg*, **90**, 50–8.

Pozzati, E., Acciarri, N., Tognetti, F., Marliani, F., and Giangaspero, F. 1996. Growth, subsequent bleeding, and de novo appearance of cerebral cavernous angiomas. *Neurosurgery*, **38**, 662–9; discussion 669–70.

Pozzati, E., Gaist, G., Poppi, M., Morrone, B., and Padovani, R. 1981. Microsurgical removal of paraventricular cavernous angiomas. Report of two cases. *J Neurosurg*, **55**, 308–11.

Pozzati, E., Giangaspero, F., Marliani, F., and Acciarri, N. 1996. Occult cerebrovascular malformations after irradiation. *Neurosurgery*, **39**, 677–82; discussion 682–4.

Pozzati, E., Giuliani, G., Nuzzo, G., and Poppi, M. 1989. The growth of cerebral cavernous angiomas. *Neurosurgery*, **25**, 92–7.

Rapacki, T. F., Brantley, M. J., Furlow, T. W. Jr., *et al.* 1990. Heterogeneity of cerebral cavernous hemangiomas diagnosed by MR imaging. *J Comput Assist Tomogr*, **14**, 18–25.

Regis, J., Bartolomei, F., Kida, Y., *et al.* 2000. Radiosurgery for epilepsy associated with cavernous malformation: retrospective study in 49 patients. *Neurosurgery*, **47**, 1091–7.

Reich, P., Winkler, J., Straube, A., Steiger, H. J., and Peraud, A. 2003. Molecular genetic investigations in the CCM1 gene in sporadic cerebral cavernomas. *Neurology*, **60**, 1135–8.

Requena, I., Arias, M., Lopez-Ibor, L., *et al.* 1991. Cavernomas of the central nervous system: clinical and neuroimaging manifestations in 47 patients. *J Neurol Neurosurg Psychiatr*, **54**, 590–4.

Reyns, N., Assaker, R., Louis, E., and Lejeune, J. P. 1999. Intraventricular cavernomas: three cases and review of the literature. *Neurosurgery*, **44**, 648–54; discussion 654–5.

Rifkin, D. B., and Moscatelli, D. 1989. Recent developments in the cell biology of basic fibroblast growth factor. *J Cell Biol*, **109**, 1–6.

Rigamonti, D., Drayer, B. P., Johnson, P. C., *et al.* 1987. The MRI appearance of cavernous malformations (angiomas). *J Neurosurg*, **67**, 518–24.

Rigamonti, D., Hadley, M. N., Drayer, B. P., *et al.* 1988. Cerebral cavernous malformations. Incidence and familial occurrence. *N Engl J Med*, **319**, 343–7.

Rigamonti, D., Hsu, F. P. K., and Monsein, L. H. 1996. Cavernous malformations and related lesions. In *Neurosurgery*, eds. R. H. Wilkins, and S. S. Rengachary. New York: McGraw-Hill, pp. 2503–8.

Rigamonti, D., Johnson, P. C., Spetzler, R. F., Hadley, M. N., and Drayer, B. P. 1991. Cavernous malformations and capillary telangiectasia: a spectrum within a single pathological entity. *Neurosurgery*, **28**, 60–4.

Rigamonti, D., and Spetzler, R. F. 1988. The association of venous and cavernous malformations. Report of four cases and discussion of the pathophysiological, diagnostic, and therapeutic implications. *Acta Neurochir (Wien)*, **92**, 100–5.

Rigamonti, D., Spetzler, R. F., Medina, M., *et al.* 1990. Cerebral venous malformations. *J Neurosurg*, **73**, 560–4.

Risau, W. 1990. Angiogenic growth factors. *Prog Growth Factor Res*, **2**, 71–9.

Risau, W., and Lemmon, V. 1988. Changes in the vascular extracellular matrix during embryonic vasculogenesis and angiogenesis. *Dev Biol*, **125**, 441–50.

Roberson, G. H., Kase, C. S., and Wolpow, E. R. 1974. Telangiectases and cavernous angiomas of the brainstem: "cryptic" vascular malformations. Report of a case. *Neuroradiology*, **8**, 83–9.

Robinson, J. R., and Awad, I. A. 1993. Clinical spectrum and natural course. In *Cavernous Malformations*, eds. I. A. Awad, and D. L. Barrow. Park Ridge, IL: American Association of Neurological Surgeons, pp. 25–36.

Robinson, J. R., Awad, I. A., and Little, J. R. 1991. Natural history of the cavernous angioma. *J Neurosurg*, **75**, 709–14.

Robinson, J. R. Jr., Awad, I. A., Masaryk, T. J., and Estes, M. L. 1993. Pathological heterogeneity of angiographically occult vascular malformations of the brain. *Neurosurgery*, **33**, 547–54; discussion 554–5.

Rokitansky, C. F. 1846. *Handbuch der allgemeinen pathologischen anatomie*. ed. B. I., Braunmüller. Vienna: Seidel.

Rosahl, S. K., Vorkapic, P., Eghbal, R., Ostertag, H., and Samii, M. 1998. Ossified and de novo cavernous malformations in the same patient. *Clin Neurol Neurosurg*, **100**, 138–43.

Rothbart, D., Awad, I. A., Lee, J., *et al.* 1996. Expression of angiogenic factors and structural proteins in central nervous system vascular malformations. *Neurosurgery*, **38**, 915–24; discussion 924–5.

Russel, D. S., and Rubinstein, L. J. 1989. *Pathology of Tumours of the Nervous System*. Baltimore: Williams & Wilkins, pp. 727–65.

Ryvlin, P., Mauguiere, F., Sindou, M., Froment, J. C., and Cinotti, L. 1995. Interictal cerebral metabolism and epilepsy in cavernous angiomas. *Brain*, **118** (Pt 3), 677–87.

Sage, M. R., Brophy, B. P., Sweeney, C., *et al.* 1993. Cavernous haemangiomas (angiomas) of the brain: clinically significant lesions. *Australas Radiol*, **37**, 147–55.

Sahoo, T., Johnson, E. W., Thomas, J. W., *et al.* 1999. Mutations in the gene encoding KRIT-1, a Krev-1/rap1a binding protein, cause cerebral cavernous malformations (CCM1). *Hum Mol Genet*, **8**, 2325–33.

Sakai, N., Yamada, H., Tanigawara, T., *et al.* 1991. Surgical treatment of cavernous angioma involving the brainstem and review of the literature. *Acta Neurochir (Wien)*, **113**, 138–43.

Samii, M., Eghbal, R., Carvalho, G. A., and Matthies, C. 2001. Surgical management of brainstem cavernomas. *J Neurosurg*, **95**, 825–32.

Schefer, S., Valavanis, A., and Wichmann, W. 1991. [MRT morphology and classification of cerebral cavernomas]. *Radiologe*, **31**, 283–8.

Schweigerer, L., Neufeld, G., Friedman, J., *et al.* 1987. Capillary endothelial cells express basic fibroblast growth factor, a mitogen that promotes their own growth. *Nature*, **325**, 257–9.

Scott, R. M., Barnes, P., Kupsky, W., and Adelman, L. S. 1992. Cavernous angiomas of the central nervous system in children. *J Neurosurg*, **76**, 38–46.

Seker, A., Pricola, K. L., Guclu, B., *et al.* 2006. CCM2 expression parallels that of CCM1. *Stroke*, **37**, 518–23.

Senger, D. R., Claffey, K. P., Benes, J. E., *et al.* 1997. Angiogenesis promoted by vascular endothelial growth factor: regulation through alpha1beta1 and alpha2beta1 integrins. *Proc Natl Acad Sci U S A*, **94**, 13612–7.

Senger, D. R., Van de Water, L., Brown, L. F., *et al.* 1993. Vascular permeability factor (VPF, VEGF) in tumor biology. *Cancer Metastasis Rev*, **12**, 303–24.

Serebriiskii, I., Estojak, J., Sonoda, G., Testa, J. R., and Golemis, E. A. 1997. Association of Krev-1/rap1a with KRIT-1, a novel ankyrin repeat-containing protein encoded by a gene mapping to 7q21–22. *Oncogene*, **15**, 1043–9.

Shah, M. V., and Heros, R. C. 1993. Microsurgical treatment of supratentorial lesions. In *Cavernous Malformations*, eds. I. A. Awad, and D. L. Barrow. Park Ridge, IL: American Association of Neurological Surgeons, pp. 101–16.

Sheehan, J., Lunsford, L. D., Kondziolka, D., and Flickinger, J. 2002. Development of a posterior fossa cavernous malformation associated with bilateral venous anomalies: case report. *J Neuroimaging*, **12**, 371–3.

Shimpo, T. 2000. Trigeminal neuralgia in pontine cavernous angioma. *J Neurol*, **247**, 139.

Simard, J. M., Garcia-Bengochea, F., Ballinger, W. E. Jr., Mickle, J. P., and Quisling, R. G. 1986. Cavernous angioma: a review of 126 collected and 12 new clinical cases. *Neurosurgery*, **18**, 162–72.

Sindou, M., Yada, J., and Salord, F. 2000. Functional results after microsurgical resection of brain stem cavernous malformations (retrospective study of a 12 patient series and review of the recent literature). *Acta Neurochir (Wien)*, **142**, 843–52; discussion 852–3.

Solomon, R. A. 2000. Comment on: Microsurgical resection of brainstem, thalamic, and basal ganglia angiographically occult vascular malformation. *Neurosurgery*, **46**, 270.

Sonstein, W. J., Kader, A., Michelsen, W. J., *et al.* 1996. Expression of vascular endothelial growth factor in pediatric and adult cerebral arteriovenous malformations: an immunocytochemical study. *J Neurosurg*, **85**, 838–45.

Steichen-Gersdorf, E., Felber, S., Fuchs, W., Russeger, L., and Twerdy, K. 1992. Familial cavernous angiomas of the brain: observations in a four generation family. *Eur J Pediatr*, **151**, 861–3.

Steiger, H. J., Markwalder, T. M., and Reulen, H. J. 1987. Clinicopathological relations of cerebral cavernous angiomas: observations in eleven cases. *Neurosurgery*, **21**, 879–84.

Steinberg, G. K., Chang, S. D., Gewirtz, R. J., and Lopez, J. R. 2000. Microsurgical resection of brainstem, thalamic, and basal ganglia angiographically occult vascular malformations. *Neurosurgery*, **46**, 260–70; discussion 270–1.

Steinberg, G. K., and Marks, M. P. 1993. Lesions mimicking cavernous malformations. In *Cavernous Malformations*, eds. I. A. Awad, and D. L. Barrow. Park Ridge, IL: American Association of Neurological Surgeons, pp. 151–62.

Steiner, L., Lindquist, C., Adler, J. R., *et al.* 1992. Outcome of radiosurgery for cerebral AVM. *J Neurosurg*, **77**, 823.

Strauss, C., Lutjen-Drecoll, E., and Fahlbusch, R. 1997. Pericollicular surgical approaches to the rhomboid fossa. Part I. Anatomical basis. *J Neurosurg*, **87**, 893–9.

Sundaresan, N., Eller, T., and Ciric, I. 1976. Hemangiomas of the internal auditory canal. *Surg Neurol*, **6**, 119–21.

Sure, U., Battenberg, E., Dempfle, A., *et al.* 2004. Hypoxia-inducible factor and vascular endothelial growth factor are expressed more frequently in embolized than in nonembolized cerebral arteriovenous malformations. *Neurosurgery*, **55**, 663–9; discussion 669–70.

Sure, U., Butz, N., Schlegel, J., *et al.* 2001. Endothelial proliferation, neoangiogenesis, and potential de novo generation of cerebrovascular malformations. *J Neurosurg*, **94**, 972–7.

Sure, U., Butz, N., Siegel, A. M., *et al.* 2001. Treatment-induced neoangiogenesis in cerebral arteriovenous malformations. *Clin Neurol Neurosurg*, **103**, 29–32.

Sure, U., Freman, S., Bozinov, O., *et al.* 2005. Biological activity of adult cavernous malformations: a study of 56 patients. *J Neurosurg*, **102**, 342–7.

Symon, L., Jackowski, A., and Bills, D. 1991. Surgical treatment of pontomedullary cavernomas. *Br J Neurosurg*, **5**, 339–47.

Tagle, P., Huete, I., Mendez, J., and del Villar, S. 1986. Intracranial cavernous angioma: presentation and management. *J Neurosurg*, **64**, 720–3.

Takagi, Y., Hattori, I., Nozaki, K., Ishikawa, M., and Hashimoto, N. 2000. DNA fragmentation in central nervous system vascular malformations. *Acta Neurochir (Wien)*, **142**, 987–94.

Tanaka, K., Abe, M., and Sato, Y. 1999. Roles of extracellular signal-regulated kinase 1/2 and p38 mitogen-activated protein kinase in the signal transduction of basic fibroblast growth factor in endothelial cells during angiogenesis. *Jpn J Cancer Res*, **90**, 647–54.

Tatagiba, M., Schonmayr, R., and Samii, M. 1991. Intraventricular cavernous angioma. A survey. *Acta Neurochir (Wien)*, **110**, 140–5.

Tirakotai, W., Fremann, S., Soerensen, N., *et al.* 2006. Biological activity of paediatric cerebral cavernomas: an immunohistochemical study of 28 patients. *Childs Nerv Syst*, **22**, 685–91.

Tomlinson, F. H., Houser, O. W., Scheithauer, B. W., *et al.* 1994. Angiographically occult vascular malformations: a correlative study of features on magnetic resonance imaging and histological examination. *Neurosurgery*, **34**, 792–9; discussion 799–800.

Topper, R., Jurgens, E., Reul, J., and Thron, A. 1999. Clinical significance of intracranial developmental venous anomalies. *J Neurol Neurosurg Psychiatr*, 67, 234–8.

Tsuboi, R., Sato, Y., and Rifkin, D. B. 1990. Correlation of cell migration, cell invasion, receptor number, proteinase production, and basic fibroblast growth factor levels in endothelial cells. *J Cell Biol*, **110**, 511–7.

Tu, J., Stoodley, M. A., Morgan, M. K., and Storer, K. P. 2005. Ultrastructural characteristics of hemorrhagic, nonhemorrhagic, and recurrent cavernous malformations. *J Neurosurg*, **103**, 903–9.

Tung, H., Giannotta, S. L., Chandrasoma, P. T., and Zee, C. S. 1990. Recurrent intraparenchymal hemorrhages from angiographically occult vascular malformations. *J Neurosurg*, **73**, 174–80.

Uhlik, M. T., Abell, A. N., Johnson, N. L., *et al.* 2003. Rac-MEKK3-MKK3 scaffolding for p38 MAPK activation during hyperosmotic shock. *Nat Cell Biol*, **5**, 1104–10.

Vaquero, J., Cabezudo, J. M., and Leunda, G. 1983. Cystic cavernous haemangiomas of the brain. *Acta Neurochir (Wien)*, **67**, 135–8.

Vaquero, J., Carrillo, R., Cabezudo, J., *et al.* 1980. Cavernous angiomas of the pineal region. Report of two cases. *J Neurosurg*, **53**, 833–5.

Vaquero, J., Leunda, G., Martinez, R., and Bravo, G. 1983. Cavernomas of the brain. *Neurosurgery*, **12**, 208–10.

Verlaan, D. J., Davenport, W. J., Stefan, H., *et al.* 2002. Cerebral cavernous malformations: mutations in KRIT-1. *Neurology*, **58**, 853–7.

Verlaan, D. J., Laurent, S. B., Rouleau, G. A., and Siegel, A. M. 2004. No CCM2 mutations in a cohort of 31 sporadic cases. *Neurology*, **63**, 1979.

Verlaan, D. J., Laurent, S. B., Sure, U., *et al.* 2004. CCM1 mutation screen of sporadic cases with cerebral cavernous malformations. *Neurology*, **62**, 1213–5.

Viale, G. L., Castellani, P., Dorcaratto, A., *et al.* 2002. Occurrence of a glioblastoma-associated tenascin-C isoform in cerebral cavernomas and neighboring vessels. *Neurosurgery*, **50**, 838–42; discussion 842.

Virchow, R. L. 1864–1865. Angiome. In: *Die krankhaften Geschwülste, Band 3*, ed. R. L. Virchow. Berlin: Hirschwald.

Vlodavsky, I., Fuks, Z., Ishai-Michaeli, R., *et al.* 1991. Extracellular matrix-resident basic fibroblast growth factor: implication for the control of angiogenesis. *J Cell Biochem*, **45**, 167–76.

Voelker, J. L., Stewart, D. H., and Schochet, S. S. Jr. 1998. Giant intracranial and extracranial cavernous malformation. Case report. *J Neurosurg*, **89**, 465–9.

Vogler, R., and Castillo, M. 1995. Dural cavernous angioma: MR features. *AJNR Am J Neuroradiol*, **16**, 773–5.

Voigt, K., and Yasargil, M. G. 1976. Cerebral cavernous haemangiomas or cavernomas. Incidence, pathology, localization, diagnosis, clinical features and treatment. Review of the literature and report of an unusual case. *Neurochirurgia (Stuttg)*, **19**, 59–68.

von Essen, C., Rydenhag, B., Nystrom, B., *et al.* 1996. High levels of glycine and serine as a cause of the seizure symptoms of cavernous angiomas? *J Neurochem*, **67**, 260–4.

Vrethem, M., Thuomas, K. A., and Hillman, J. 1997. Cavernous angioma of the brain stem mimicking multiple sclerosis. *N Engl J Med*, **336**, 875–6.

Wagner, K. R., Xi, G., Hua, Y., *et al.* 1998. Early metabolic alterations in edematous perihematomal brain regions following experimental intracerebral hemorrhage. *J Neurosurg*, **88**, 1058–65.

Wakai, S., Ueda, Y., Inoh, S., and Nagai, M. 1985. Angiographically occult angiomas: a report of thirteen cases with analysis of the cases documented in the literature. *Neurosurgery*, **17**, 549–56.

Wang, C. C., Liu, A., Zhang, J. T., Sun, B., and Zhao, Y. L. 2003. Surgical management of brain-stem cavernous malformations: report of 137 cases. *Surg Neurol*, **59**, 444–54; discussion 454.

Wang, Y. G., Liu, H. T., Zhang, Y. M., and Ma, D. L. 1999. cDNA cloning and expression of an apoptosis-related gene, human TFAR-15 gene. *Sci China C Life Sci*, **42**, 323–329.

Wernig, F., Mayr, M., and Xu, Q. 2003. Mechanical stretch-induced apoptosis in smooth muscle cells is mediated by beta1-integrin signaling pathways. *Hypertension*, **41**, 903–11.

Whitehead, K. J., Plummer, N. W., Adams, J. A., Marchuk, D. A., and Li, D. Y. 2004. Ccm1 is required for arterial morphogenesis: implications for the etiology of human cavernous malformations. *Development*, **131**, 1437–48.

Willmore, L. J., Sypert, G. W., Munson, J. V., and Hurd, R. W. 1978. Chronic focal epileptiform discharges induced by injection of iron into rat and cat cortex. *Science*, **200**, 1501–3.

Wilson, C. B. 1992. Cryptic vascular malformations. *Clin Neurosurg*, **38**, 49–84.

Wong, J. H., Awad, I. A., and Kim, J. H. 2000. Ultrastructural pathological features of cerebrovascular malformations: a preliminary report. *Neurosurgery*, **46**, 1454–9.

Wurm, G., Schnizer, M., and Fellner, F. A. 2005. Cerebral cavernous malformations associated with venous anomalies: surgical considerations. *Neurosurgery*, **57**, 42–58; discussion 42–58.

Yamada, T., Nishio, S., Matsunaga, M., Fukui, M., and Takeshita, I. 1986. Cavernous haemangioma in the oculomotor nerve. A case report. *J Neurol*, **233**, 63–4.

Yamasaki, T., Handa, H., Yamashita, J., *et al.* 1986. Intracranial and orbital cavernous angiomas. A review of 30 cases. *J Neurosurg*, **64**, 197–208.

Yeh, H. S., Tew, J. M. Jr., and Gartner, M. 1993. Seizure control after surgery on cerebral arteriovenous malformations. *J Neurosurg*, **78**, 12–8.

Yoshino, M., Morita, A., Shibahara, J., and Kirino, T. 2005. Radiation-induced spinal cord cavernous malformation. Case report. *J Neurosurg*, **102**, 101–4.

Zabramski, J. M., Henn, J. S., and Coons, S. 1999. Pathology of cerebral vascular malformations. *Neurosurg Clin N Am*, **10**, 395–410.

Zabramski, J. M., Wascher, T. M., Spetzler, R. F., *et al.* 1994. The natural history of familial cavernous malformations: results of an ongoing study. *J Neurosurg*, **80**, 422–32.

Zagzag, D., and Capo, V. 2002. Angiogenesis in the central nervous system: a role for vascular endothelial growth factor/vascular permeability factor and tenascin-C. Common molecular effectors in cerebral neoplastic and non-neoplastic "angiogenic diseases". *Histol Histopathol*, **17**, 301–21.

Zagzag, D., Zhong, H., Scalzitti, J. M., *et al.* 2000. Expression of hypoxia-inducible factor 1alpha in brain tumors: association with angiogenesis, invasion, and progression. *Cancer*, **88**, 2606–18.

Zawistowski, J. S., Serebriiskii, I. G., Lee, M. F., Golemis, E. A., and Marchuk, D. A. 2002. KRIT-1 association with the integrin-binding protein ICAP-1: a new direction in the elucidation of cerebral cavernous malformations (CCM1) pathogenesis. *Hum Mol Genet*, **11**, 389–96.

Zawistowski, J. S., Stalheim, L., Uhlik, M. T., *et al.* 2005. CCM1 and CCM2 protein interactions in cell signaling: implications for cerebral cavernous malformations pathogenesis. *Hum Mol Genet*, **14**, 2521–31.

Zevgaridis, D., van Velthoven, V., Ebeling, U., and Reulen, H. J. 1996. Seizure control following surgery in supratentorial cavernous malformations: a retrospective study in 77 patients. *Acta Neurochir (Wien)*, **138**, 672–7.

Zhang, J., Clatterbuck, R. E., Rigamonti, D., Chang, D. D., and Dietz, H. C. 2001. Interaction between KRIT-1 and icap1alpha infers perturbation of integrin beta1-mediated angiogenesis in the pathogenesis of cerebral cavernous malformation. *Hum Mol Genet*, **10**, 2953–60.

Zhang, J., Rigamonti, D., Dietz, H. C., and Clatterbuck, R. E. 2007. Interaction between KRIT-1 and malcavernin: implications for the pathogenesis of cerebral cavernous malformations. *Neurosurgery*, **60**, 353–9; discussion 359.

Zhang, N., Pan, L., Wang, B. J., *et al.* 2000. Gamma knife radiosurgery for cavernous hemangiomas. *J Neurosurg*, **93 Suppl 3**, 74–7.

Zhao, Y., Mao, Y., Zhou, L. F., and Zhang, Y. L. 2003. [Immunohistochemical study on central nervous system cavernous hemangiomas]. *Zhonghua Yi Xue Za Zhi*, **83**, 544–7.

Zhu, W. H., Han, J., and Nicosia, R. F. 2003. Requisite role of p38 MAPK in mural cell recruitment during angiogenesis in the rat aorta model. *J Vasc Res*, **40**, 140–8.

Zimmerman, R. S., Spetzler, R. F., Lee, K. S., Zabramski, J. M., and Hargraves, R. W. 1991. Cavernous malformations of the brain stem. *J Neurosurg*, **75**, 32–9.

30 CEREBROVASCULAR MANIFESTATIONS OF NEUROFIBROMATOSIS

Krassen Nedeltchev and Heinrich P. Mattle

General considerations

Neurofibromatosis (NF) is an autosomal dominant disorder encompassing a broad spectrum of distinct genetic defects with overlapping clinical features. *Neurofibromatosis type 1* (NF1, formerly known as von Recklinghausen's disease or peripheral NF) and *neurofibromatosis type 2* (NF2, also known as bilateral acoustic or central NF) are best distinguished because each has distinctive clinical features and genetic origins on different chromosomes.

NF1 is caused by a mutation on chromosome 17q11.2, the gene product being *neurofibromin* (a guanosine triphosphatase [GTPase]-activating enzyme). Café-au-lait spots, peripheral neurofibromas, and Lisch nodules are the clinical manifestations of NF1 that most consistently occur in the majority of affected patients. NF2 is caused by a mutation on chromosome 22q12.2. The gene product called *merlin* is a cytoskeletal protein. NF2 is characterized by multiple intracranial tumors, especially vestibular schwannomas and meningiomas. Recently, a third form called *schwannomatosis* has been recognized. Multiple schwannomas (rather than neurofibromas) occur, and the vestibular nerve is spared. Six other, extremely rare, forms are also recognized (Allanson *et al.*, 1985; Ars *et al.*, 1998; Griffiths *et al.*, 1983; Hashemian, 1952; Rodriguez and Berthrong, 1966).

Occlusive and aneurysmal lesions in thymic and renal arteries of a patient with NF1 were first described in an autopsy study by Reubi (1944). Cerebrovascular manifestations are not rare in NF1. Recently, there have been two case reports on vascular pathologies in NF2 (Lesley *et al.*, 2004; Ryan *et al.*, 2005). To date, vascular manifestations of other types of NF have not been reported. Therefore, the following synopsis focuses on the main genetic, clinical, pathological, and radiological features of NF1.

Epidemiology

NF1 constitutes 90% of all types of neurofibromatoses with an incidence of 1 in 3000–4000 live births (Huson *et al.*, 1989). This makes it the most common phakomatosis (i.e. neurocutaneous syndrome). Population prevalence has predominantly been determined in Caucasian populations, but patients from all ethnic and racial groups have been reported in the literature.

Hereditability and genetics

All major surveys confirm an autosomal dominant mode of inheritance, which means that only one copy of the mutated gene needs to be inherited to pass NF1 to the next generation. Approximately half of the patients are the first affected persons in their families. In these cases, somatic mutations occur due to miscopying events during cell division with clonal expansion of the mutated viable cells. Mutations occuring very early in the embryogenesis (i.e. before tissue differentiation) are more generalized than are those taking place at a later stage (Hall, 2000).

The NF1 gene has one of the highest new mutation rates in humans (Viskochil, 1998). Accordingly, it was speculated that a significant proportion of patients with NF1 who have that somatic mutation in which the gonad is spared are rare (Littler and Morton, 1990). Nevertheless, localized or segmental NF1 is not uncommon, suggesting that somatic mutations can occur at all stages of embryogenesis. The diagnosis of a somatic mosaicism has implications for genetic counseling, as the risk to offspring may be lower than 50%.

The gene locus for NF1 is on chromosome 17 and codes for *neurofibromin*, a polypeptide of 2818 amino acids. Neurofibromin is expressed in neurons, oligodendrocytes, Schwann cells, the adrenal medulla, and white blood cells (Daston *et al.*, 1992). The NF1 gene is considered to be a tumor suppressor gene, because loss-of-function mutations have been associated with the occurrence of benign and malignant tumors in neural crest–derived tissues in patients with NF1 (Coleman *et al.*, 1995). Sequence analysis of the full-length NF1 gene revealed a portion that codes for a 360-amino-acid peptide with structural and functional similarities to some GTPase-activating proteins (Xu *et al.*, 1990). These proteins have the ability to stimulate cell proliferation or differentiation. The large size of the entire gene product in relation to the small portion conferring GTPase-activating activity suggests that other domains may have entirely different and, as yet, unknown functions (Marchuk and Collins, 1994). Recent studies have shown neurofibromin to positively regulate intracellular cyclic adenosine monophosphate (cAMP) in mammalian neurons (Tong *et al.*, 2002). Mutations in different regions of the NF1 gene and environmental factors could further contribute to the variability of disease expression.

Pathological findings

Reubi (1944) originally described two main types of vascular lesions in the thymic and renal arteries of a patient with NF1: an occlusive intimal form affecting small arteries and an aneurysmal form with replacement of the muscular wall with fibrohyaline thickening in arterioles of 0.1–1 mm. Salyer and Salyer (1974)

Uncommon Causes of Stroke, 2nd edition, ed. Louis R. Caplan. Published by Cambridge University Press. © Cambridge University Press 2008.

found peculiar arterial lesions in 7 of 18 autopsy cases of NF at the Johns Hopkins Hospital. They proposed that the pathogenesis of the arterial lesions was proliferation of Schwann cells within arteries with secondary degenerative changes, e.g. fibrosis, resulting in lesions with various appearances. Further cases of "vascular neurofibromatosis" affected the abdominal aorta (Stanley and Fry, 1981), the mesenteric arteries (Zochodne, 1984), or visceral and muscle arteries, or presented with multiple arterial aneurysms and venous thrombosis (Lehrnbecher *et al.*, 1994). Tomsick *et al.* (1976) described two patients with intracranial occlusive arterial disorder. Overall, there is a great variation of number, type, and severity of the vascular disorders in NF1. Vascular anomalies may involve extra- or intracranial arteries (Hoffmann *et al.*, 1998; Sasaki *et al.*, 1995). Occlusive arterial disorders or aneurysms may be present in the carotid or vertebral arteries, quite often combined with arteriovenous fistulae (Schievink and Piepgras, 1991).

The pathogenesis of the vascular lesions is controversial. In the patient reported by Lehrnbecher *et al.* (1994) the proliferating cells seemed to have originated from myoblasts or myofibroblasts and not, as has been speculated, from Schwann cells. Hamilton and Friedman (2000) suggested that NF1 might result from an alteration of neurofibromin function in blood vessel endothelial and smooth muscle cells. Riccardi (2000) supported the view that endothelial injury and its repair may also play a role in NF1 vasculopathy.

Clinical vascular manifestations

The cerebrovascular manifestations of NF1 include cerebral ischemia, intracranial hematoma, and subarachnoidal hemorrhage. Stroke can occur at any age, but more than half of the reported cases were children or young adults. Familial occurrence of arterial occlusive disease is uncommon (Erickson *et al.*, 1980). Both first-ever and recurrent strokes have been reported. Recurrent strokes can occur in the same or in different territories. Every large or medium-sized artery can be affected, and some patients have multiple stenoses of intracranial vessels combined with stenoses or occlusion of extracranial vessels (Gebarski *et al.*, 1983; Pellock *et al.*, 1980). Hemispheric territorial infarction is the most common stroke manifestation (de Kersaint-Gilly *et al.*, 1980; Gilly *et al.*, 1982; Levisohn *et al.*, 1978; Pellock *et al.*, 1980). Lacunar strokes are less frequent (Creange *et al.*, 1999). Ocular involvement may present with retinal ischemia (Tholen *et al.*, 1998) or global ocular ischemia (Barral and Summers, 1996).

A classical manifestation is laterocervical hematoma as a result of an aneurysm of the vertebral artery or another neck artery. A large vertebral aneurysm may present with a brachial plexus lesion or even medullary compression with para- or tetraparesis. Intracranial aneurysms may be saccular or fusiform. The circle of Willis is the most common location, but also more distal vessels such as the posterior choroid artery may be affected (Leone *et al.*, 1982). Intracranial aneurysms commonly present as subarachnoid hemorrhage (Bergouignan and Arne, 1951). Fusiform aneurysm of the intrapetrosal part of the carotid artery may be associated with sphenoid wing dysplasia or cause abducens nerve palsy (Steel *et al.*, 1994). It is unclear how much the risk of

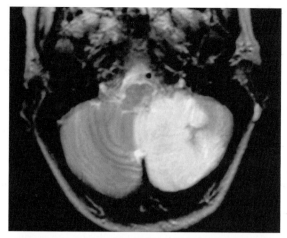

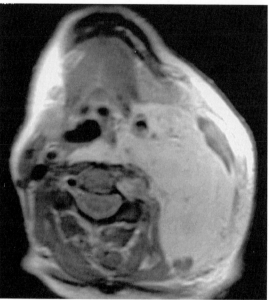

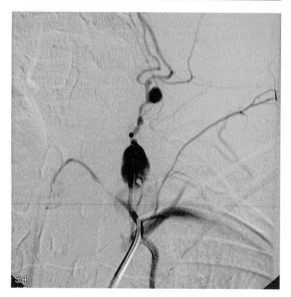

Figure 30.1 Angiogram showing an aneurysmal dilatation and irregular narrowing over a long distance of the left vertebral artery in a patient with a posterior inferior cerebellar artery (PICA) infarction in the absence of other cerebrovascular risk factors. (Courtesy of A. Carruzzo and J. Bogousslavsky.)

developing an aneurysm in NF1 is increased and whether screening of asymptomatic patients is useful.

Diagnosis

The radiological findings of NF1 are nonspecific, although in the appropriate clinical setting when the index of clinical suspicion is high, a fairly confident diagnosis can be made. Angiography remains the golden standard for providing information on vascular aneurysms, occlusions, and arteriovenous fistulae (Figure 30.1). Vascular abnormalities of the intra- and extracranial vasculature are depicted well with time-of-flight magnetic resonance angiography (TOF-MRA) and contrast-enhanced MRA. Color duplex and spectral Doppler ultrasonography are also useful diagnostic modalities for revealing the vascular complications of NF1.

Typical findings of occlusive arterial disorder include focal concentric stenosis, irregular narrowing over a long distance (resembling fibromuscular dysplasia), and hypoplasia without luminal narrowing over a long distance (Leone *et al.*, 1982). In contrast to atherosclerotic stenoses, occlusive arterial disease in NF1 does not occur at sites of maximal flow turbulence, like the origin of vertebral artery or the carotid bifurcation. Vertebral arteries are particularly prone to develop arteriovenous fistulae. In this case, the fistula can be combined with stenoses and pseudoaneurysmal dilatation of the feeding arterial vessel.

Probably because occlusive disorders progress slowly, extensive collateral pathways may develop. In case of bilateral carotid stenoses and/or occlusions, moyamoya-like changes are almost invariably found at angiography. In many cases of proximal stenoses of intracranial arteries, collateralization from the external carotid artery through leptomeningeal anastomoses to the circle of Willis can be observed.

Treatment

Medical stroke treatment and prevention studies in NF are missing. Therefore, we would manage stroke in NF similar to stroke of atheromatous origin.

Neurosurgical revascularization in patients with moyamoya syndrome has been shown to reduce the risk of first-ever and recurrent stroke and transient ischemic attack (TIA) (Scott *et al.*, 2004).

Surgery or angioplasty can be performed to minimize the natural risk of hemorrhage in patients with aneurysms or arteriovenous fistulae, especially in those originating from the vertebral artery (Negoro *et al.*, 1990; Siddhartha *et al.*, 2003). In many patients who have arteriovenous fistula, endovascular treatment is technically demanding because of multiple and tortuous feeding arteries allowing only partial embolization. In such instances, surgery is still necessary after endovascular treatment (Latchaw *et al.*, 1980). Because affected vessels are prone to rupture, massive hemorrhage is a feared complication of both surgical and endovascular treatment.

REFERENCES

Allanson, J. E., Hall, J. G., and Van Allen, M. I. 1985. Noonan phenotype associated with neurofibromatosis. *Am J Med Genet*, **21**, 457–62.

Ars, E., Kruyer, H., Gaona, A., *et al.* 1998. A clinical variant of neurofibromatosis type 1: familial spinal neurofibromatosis with a frameshift mutation in the NF1 gene. *Am J Hum Genet*, **62**, 834–41.

Barral, J. L., and Summers, C. G. 1996. Ocular ischemic syndrome in a child with moyamoya disease and neurofibromatosis. *Surv Ophthalmol*, **40**, 500–4.

Bergouignan, M., and Arne, L. 1951. A propos des anévrysmes des artères cérébrales associés à d'autres malformations. *Acta Neurol et Psychiat Belgica*, **51**, 529–35.

Coleman, S. D., Williams, C. A., and Wallace, M. R. 1995. Benign neurofibromas in type 1 neurofibromatosis (NF1) show somatic deletions on NF1 gene. *Nat Genet*, **11**, 90–2.

Creange, A., Zeller, J., Rostaing-Rigattieri, S., *et al.* 1999. Neurological complications of neurofibromatosis type 1 in adulthood. *Brain*, **122**, 473–81.

Daston, M. M., Scrable, H., Nordlund, M., *et al.* 1992. Protein product of the neurofibromatosis type 1 gene is expressed at highest abundance in neurons, Schwann cells and oligodendrocytes. *Neuron*, **8**, 415–28.

de Kersaint-Gilly, A., Zenthe, L., Dabouis, G., *et al.* 1980. Abnormalities of the intracerebral vasculature in a case of neurofibromatosis. *J Neuroradiol*, **7**, 193–8.

Erickson, R. P., Woolliscroft, J., and Allen, R. J. 1980. Familial occurrence of intracranial arterial occlusive disease (Moyamoya) in neurofibromatosis. *Clin Genet*, **18**, 191–6.

Gebarski, S. S., Gabrielsern, T. O., Knake, J. E., and Latack, J. T. 1983. Posterior circulation intracranial arterial occlusive disease in neurofibromatosis. *Am J Neuroradiol*, **4**, 1245–6.

Gilly, R., Elbaz, N., Langue, J., and Raveau, J. 1982. Sténoses artérielles cérébrales multiples et progressives, sténose d l'artère rénale et maladie de Recklinghausen. *Pédiatrie*, **38**, 523–30.

Griffiths, D. F. R., Williams, G. T., and Williams, E. D. 1983. Multiple endocrine neoplasia associated with von Recklinghausen's disease. *Brit Med J*, **287**, 1341–3.

Hall, J. G. 2000. Review and hypotheses: somatic mosaicism: observations related to clinical genetics. *Am J Hum Genet*, **43**, 355–63.

Hamilton, S. J., and Friedman, J. M. 2000. Insights into the pathogenesis of neurofibromatosis 1 vasculopathy. *Clin Genet*, **58**, 341–4.

Hashemian, H. 1952. Familial fibromatosis of small intestine. *Brit J Surg*, **40**, 346–50.

Hoffmann, K. T., Hosten, N., Liebig, T., Schwarz, K., and Felix, R. 1998. Giant aneurysm of the vertebral artery in neurofibromatosis type 1: report of a case and review of the literature. *Neuroradiology*, **40**, 245–8.

Huson, S. M., Compston, D. A., Clark, P., and Harper, P. S. 1989. A genetic study of von Recklinghausen neurofibromatosis in south east Wales. I. Prevalence, fitness, mutation rate, and effect of parental transmission on severity. *J Med Genet*, **26**, 704–11.

Latchaw, R. E., Harris, R. D., Chou, S. N., and Gold, L. H. A. 1980. Combined embolization and operation in the treatment of cervical arteriovenous malformations. *Neurosurgery*, **6**, 131–7.

Lehrnbecher, T., Gassel, A. M., Rauh, V., Kirchner, T., and Huppertz, H. I. 1994. Neurofibromatosis presenting as a severe systemic vasculopathy. *Eur J Pediatr*, **153**, 107–9.

Leone, R. G., Schatzki, S. C., and Wolpow, E. R. 1982. Neurofibromatosis with extensive intracranial arterial occlusive disease. *Am J Neuroradiol*, **3**, 572–6.

Lesley, W. S., Thomas, M. R., and Abdulrauf, S. I. 2004. N-butylcyanoacrylate embolization of a middle meningeal artery aneurysm in a patient with neurofibromatosis type 2. *Am J Neuroradiol*, **25**, 1414–6.

Levisohn, P. M., Mikhael, M. A., and Rothman, S. M. 1978. Cerebrovascular changes in neurofibromatosis. *Dev Med Child Neurol*, **20**, 789–93.

Littler, M., and Morton, N. E. 1990. Segregation analysis of peripheral neurofibromatosis. *J Med Genet*, **27**, 307–10.

Marchuk, D. A., and Collins, F. S. 1994. Molecular genetics of neurofibromatosis 1. In *The Neurofibromatoses. A Pathogenetic and Clinical Overview*, eds, S. M. Huson, and R. A. C. Hughes. London: Chapman and Hall, pp. 23–49.

Negoro, M., Nakaya, T., Terashima, K., and Sugita, K. 1990. Extracranial vertebral artery aneurysm with neurofibromatosis. Endovascular treatment by detachable balloon. *Neuroradiology*, **31**, 533–6.

Pellock, J. M., Kleinman, P. K., McDonald, B. M., and Wixson, D. 1980. Hypertensive stroke with neurofibromatosis. *Neurology*, **30**, 656–9.

Reubi, F. 1944. Les vaisseaux et les glandes endocrines dans la neurofibromatose. *Z Path u Bakt*, **7**, 168.

Riccardi, V. M. 2000. The vasculopathy of NF1 and histogenesis control genes. *Clin Genet*, **58**, 345–7.

Rodriguez, H. A., and Berthrong, M. 1966. Multiple primary intracranial tumors in von Recklinghausen's neurofibromatosis. *Arch Neurol*, **14**, 467–75.

Ryan, A. M., Hurley, M., Brennan, P., and Moroney, J. T. 2005. Vascular dysplasia in neurofibromatosis type 2. *Neurology*, **65**, 163–4.

Salyer, W. R., and Salyer, D. C. 1974. The vascular lesions of neurofibromatosis. *Angiology*, **25**, 510–9.

Sasaki, J., Miura, S., Ohishi, H., and Kikuchi, K. 1995. Neurofibromatosis associated with multiple intracranial vascular lesions: stenosis of the internal carotid artery and peripheral aneurysm of the Heubner's artery; report of a case. *No Shinkei Geka*, **23**, 813–7.

Schievink, W. I., and Piepgras, D. G. 1991. Cervical vertebral artery aneurysms and arteriovenous fistulae in neurofibromatosis type 1: case reports. *Neurosurgery*, **29**, 760–5.

Scott, R. M., Smith, J. L., Robertson, R. L., *et al.* 2004. Long-term outcome in children with moyamoya syndrome after cranial revascularization by pial synangiosis. *J Neurosurg*, **100(2 Suppl Pediatrics)**, 142–9.

Siddhartha, W., Chavhan, G. B., Shrivastava, M., and Limaye, U. S. 2003. Endovascular treatment for bilateral vertebral arteriovenous fistulas in neurofibromatosis 1. *Australas Radiol*, **47**, 457–61.

Stanley, J. C., and Fry, W. J. 1981. Pediatric renal artery occlusive disease and renovascular hypertension: etiology, diagnosis, and operative treatment. *Arch Surg*, **116**, 669–76.

Steel, T. R., Bentivoglio, P. B., and Garrick, R. 1994. Vascular neurofibromatosis affecting the internal carotid artery: a case report. *Brit J Neurosurg*, **8**, 233–7.

Tholen, A., Messmer, A. P., and Landau, K. 1998. Peripheral retinal vascular occlusive disorder in a young patient with neurofibromatosis 1. *Retina*, **18**, 184–6.

Tomsick, T. A., Lukin, R. R., Chambers, A. A., and Benton, C. 1976. Neurofibromatosis and intracranial arterial occlusive disease. *Neuroradiology*, **11**, 229–34.

Tong, J., Hannan, F., Zhu, Y., Bernards, A., and Zhong, Y. 2002. Neurofibromin regulates G protein-stimulated adenylyl cyclase activity. *Nat Neurosci*, **5**, 95–6.

Viskochil, D. H. 1998. Gene structure and expression. In Neurofibromatosis Type 1 from Genotype to Phenotype, eds. M. Upadhyaya, and D. N. Cooper. Oxford: Bios Scientific Publishers, pp. 39–53.

Xu, G., O'Connell, P., Viskochil, D. H., *et al.* 1990. The neurofibromatosis type 1 gene encodes a protein related to GAP. *Cell*, **62**, 599–608.

Zochodne, D. 1984. Von Recklinghausen's vasculopathy. *Am J Med Sci*, **287**, 64–5.

31 MENKES DISEASE (KINKY HAIR DISEASE)

John H. Menkes

This X-linked disorder of copper metabolism was first described in 1962 by Menkes and associates (1962).

Molecular genetics and bochemical pathology

The characteristic feature of Menkes disease (MD), as expressed in the human infant, is a maldistribution of body copper, so that it accumulates to abnormal levels in a form or location that renders it inaccessible for the synthesis of various copper enzymes (Cox, 1999; Danks *et al.*, 1972). The basic gene defect is a mutation in *ATP7A*, a gene mapped to the long arm of the X-chromosome (Xq12-q13) and encoding a highly evolutionarily conserved P-type ATP protein (ATP7A) essential for the translocation of metal cations across cellular membranes (Moller *et al.*, 1996). At basal copper levels ATP7A is localized to the trans-Golgi network, the sorting station for proteins exiting from the Golgi apparatus (Andrews, 2001). ATP7A contains six copper-binding sites, and receives copper ions with assistance of the cytosolic copper chaperone Atox1 (Paulsen *et al.*, 2006). ATP7A is involved in the transport of copper to copper-requiring enzymes synthesized within the secretory compartments. At increased intra- and extracellular copper concentrations, ATP7A shifts to the cytosolic vesicular compartments and to the plasma membrane, where it mediates copper efflux (Cobbold *et al.*, 2003; Goodyer *et al.*, 1999; Paulsen *et al.*, 2006).

ATP7A has considerable structural homology with *ATP7B*, the gene whose defect is responsible for Wilson disease, in the 3′ two-thirds of the gene, but there is much divergence between them in the 5′ one-third (Harrison and Dameron, 1999). *ATP7A* is expressed in most tissues, including brain, but not in liver. Numerous mutations have been recognized. These include point mutations and deletions, and it appears as if almost every family has its own private mutation (Moller *et al.*, 2000). As yet there is no good correlation between the type of mutation and the severity of the clinical course.

As a consequence of the defect in ATP7A, copper becomes inaccessible for the synthesis of ceruloplasmin, superoxide dismutase, and a variety of other copper-containing enzymes, notably ascorbic acid oxidase, peptidylglycine alpha-amidating monooxygenase (PAM), cytochrome oxidase, dopamine ß-hydroxylase (DBH), and lysyl hydroxylase. Most of the clinical manifestations can be explained by the low activities of these copper-containing enzymes. Patients absorb little or no orally administered copper.

When the metal is given intravenously, patients develop a prompt increase in serum copper and ceruloplasmin (Bucknall *et al.*, 1973). Copper levels are low in liver and brain, but are elevated in several other tissues, notably intestinal mucosa, muscle, spleen, and kidney. The copper content of cultured fibroblasts, myotubes, or lymphocytes derived from patients with MD is several times greater than control cells; however, the kinetics of copper uptake in these cells are normal (van den Berg *et al.*, 1990).

Pathology

Because of the defective activity of the various copper-containing enzymes, a variety of pathologic changes are set into motion. Arteries are tortuous, with irregular lumens and a frayed and split intimal lining. In the aorta, the elastin fibers are disrupted, fragmented, and are wider than normal (Figure 31.1). Unsulfated and sulfated chondroitins are deposited within elastin fibers, whereas heparin sulfate, a constituent of normal elastin fibers, is significantly reduced (Pasquali-Ronchetti *et al.*, 1994). These abnormalities reflect a failure in elastin formation and collagen cross-linking caused by dysfunction of the key enzyme for this process, copper-dependent lysyl hydroxylase.

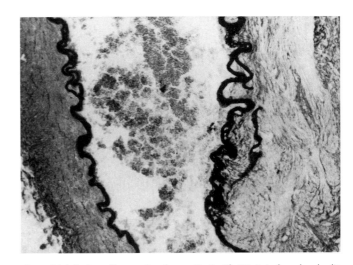

Figure 31.1 Section of large artery from patient with MD. Note frayed and split internal elastic lamina.

Uncommon Causes of Stroke, 2nd edition, ed. Louis R. Caplan. Published by Cambridge University Press. © Cambridge University Press 2008.

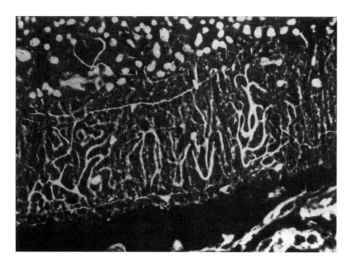

Figure 31.2 Cerebellum in MD. Note "weeping willow" formation of cerebellar molecular layer (Bodian 500×). (Reproduced with permission of Dr. D. Troost, Department of Neuropathology, University of Amsterdam, Amsterdam.)

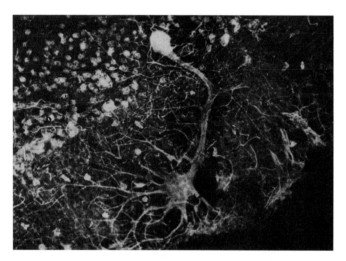

Figure 31.3 Cerebellum in MD. Purkinje cell with "Medusa Head" formation (Bodian 500×). (Reproduced with permission of Dr. D. Troost, Department of Neuropathology, University of Amsterdam, Amsterdam.)

Changes within the brain result from vascular lesions, copper deficiency, or a combination of the two. El Meskini *et al.* (2007) proposed that the inability of mutant ATP7A to support axon outgrowth contributes to neurodegeneration, and that some of the abnormalities seen in MD are the result of age-dependent developmental defects. Extensive focal degeneration of gray matter occurs, with neuronal loss, gliosis, and an associated axonal degeneration in white matter. Cellular loss is prominent in the cerebellum. Here, Purkinje cells are hard hit; many are lost, and others show abnormal dendritic arborization (weeping willow) (Figure 31.2) and perisomatic processes. Focal axonal swellings are observed also (Figure 31.3) (Danks *et al.*, 1972; Menkes *et al.*, 1962). Electron microscopy often shows a marked increase in the number of mitochondria in the perikaryon of Purkinje cells, and to a lesser degree in the neurons of the cerebral cortex and basal ganglia (Menkes *et al.*, 1962). Mitochondria are enlarged, and intramito-chondrial electron-dense bodies are present. The pathogenesis of these changes is controversial.

Clinical manifestations

MD is a rare disorder; its frequency has been estimated at 1 in 114 000 to 1 in 250 000 live births (Tønnesen *et al.*, 1991).

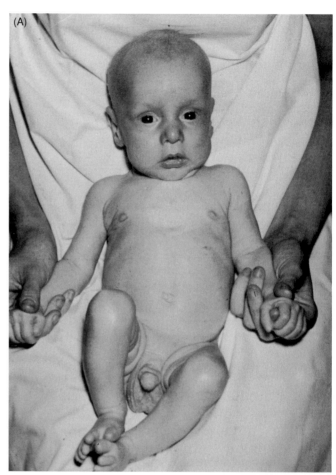

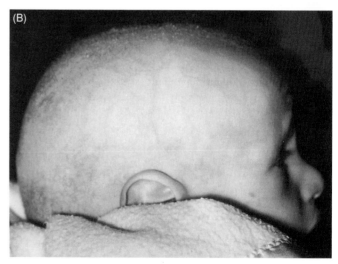

Figure 31.4 A. Typical facies of one of the original infants with MD (kinky hair disease). **B**. Sparse and poorly pigmented hair in a patient with MD.

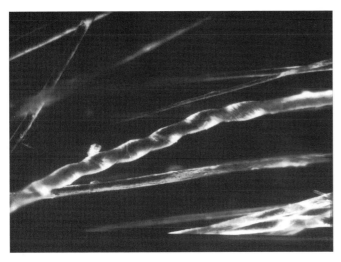

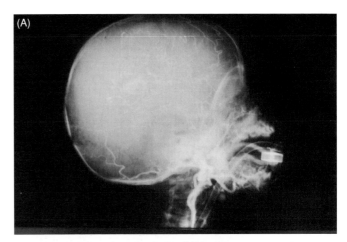

Figure 31.5 Microscopic images of scalp hair in MD. Note the characteristic "corkscrew" twisting of pili torti.

Baerlocher and Nadal (1988) provided a comprehensive review of the clinical features. In the classic form of the illness, symptoms appear during the neonatal period. Babies show hypothermia, poor feeding, and impaired weight gain. Seizures soon become apparent. Marked hypotonia, poor head control, and progressive deterioration of all neurologic functions are seen. The face has a cherubic appearance with a depressed nasal bridge and reduced facial movements (Figure 31.4, A and B) (Grover *et al.*, 1979). There also is gingival enlargement and delayed eruption of primary teeth. The optic discs are pale, and microcysts of the pigment epithelium are seen (Seelenfreund *et al.*, 1968). The most striking finding is the appearance of the scalp hair; it is colorless and friable. Examination under the microscope reveals a variety of abnormalities, most often pili torti (twisted hair) (Figure 31.5), monilethrix (varying diameter of hair shafts), and trichorrhexis nodosa (fractures of the hair shaft at regular intervals) (Menkes *et al.*, 1962).

On angiography or magnetic resonance (MR) angiography, a striking and progressive intracranial and extracranial vascular tortuosity is apparent (Figure 31.6, A and B) (Kim and Suh, 1997). Similar changes are seen in the systemic vasculature. Aneurysms are not unusual. They can involve the internal jugular vein (Grange *et al.*, 2005) and the brachial (Godwin *et al.*, 2006), lumbar, and iliac arteries (Adaletli *et al.*, 2005).

PAM, another copper-dependent enzyme, is required for removal of the carboxy-terminal glycine residue characteristic of numerous neuroendocrine peptide precursors (e.g. gastrin, cholecystokinin, vasoactive intestinal peptide, corticotropin-releasing hormone, thyrotropin-releasing hormone, calcitonin, vasopressin). Failure to amidate these precursors can result in marked reduction of their bioactivity (Steveson *et al.*, 2003).

Radiography of long bones reveals metaphyseal spurring and a diaphyseal periosteal reaction, reminiscent of scurvy (Wesenberg *et al.*, 1968). The urinary tract is not spared. Hydronephrosis, hydroureter, and bladder diverticula are common (Wheeler and Roberts, 1976). As a consequence of the defective activity of DBH, plasma and cerebrospinal fluid (CSF) catecholamine levels are abnormal in MD patients at all stage of life, including the pre-

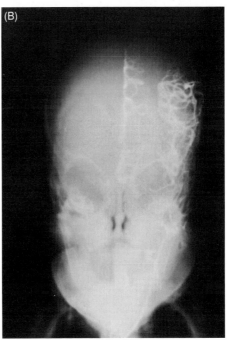

Figure 31.6 Right carotid angiogram of a 5-month-old infant with MD. The films show tortuous and anomalous middle cerebral artery vessels. In addition, there was marked tortuosity of the superior aspect of the cervical portion of the internal carotid artery in the early arterial phase. **A**. Lateral view. **B**. Anterior-posterior view. (Reproduced with permission of Dr. John Gwinn, Department of Radiology, Children's Hospital, Los Angeles.)

natal period. DOPA (dihydroxyphenylacetic acid) and dopamine are elevated, and dihydroxyphenyl glycol, the deamination product of norepinephrine, is reduced (Kaler *et al.*, 1993). Assay of these compounds can be used for neonatal diagnosis (Kaler *et al.*, 2008).

Neuroimaging discloses cerebral atrophy and bilateral ischemic lesions in deep gray matter, or in the cortical areas, the consequence of brain infarcts (Hsich *et al.*, 2000). Asymptomatic subdural hematomas are almost invariable, and when these occur in conjunction with a skull fracture, the diagnosis of nonaccidental trauma is frequently considered (Menkes, 2001; Ubhi *et al.*, 2000). Electroencephalograms (EEGs) show multifocal paroxysmal discharges or hypsarrhythmia. Visually evoked potentials are of low amplitude or completely absent (Ferreira *et al.*, 1998).

The course is usually inexorably downhill, but the rate of neurologic deterioration varies considerably. There are recurrent infections of the respiratory and urinary tracts, and sepsis and meningitis are fairly common. I have seen a patient in his 20s, and numerous patients have been reported whose clinical manifestations are less severe than those seen in the classic form of MD, and it appears likely that a continuum in disease severity exists. The correlation between the severity of phenotype and the type of mutation is not good, and variable clinical expressions for identical mutations have been observed (Borm *et al.*, 2004; Tümer *et al.*, 2003).

Diagnosis

The clinical history and the appearance of the infant should suggest the diagnosis. Serum ceruloplasmin and copper levels are normally low in the neonatal period and do not reach adult levels until 1 month of age. Therefore, measurements of plasma dopamine and other neurochemicals are required for an early diagnosis (Kaler *et al.*, 2008). The diagnosis can best be confirmed by demonstrating the intracellular accumulation of copper and decreased efflux of Cu^{64} from cultured fibroblasts (Tümer and Horn, 1997). The increased copper content of chorionic villi has been used for first-trimester diagnosis of the disease (Tümer and Horn, 1997). These analyses require considerable expertise, and only few centers can perform them reliably.

In heterozygotes, areas of pili torti constitute between 30% and 50% of the hair. Less commonly, skin depigmentation is present. Carrier detection by measuring the accumulation of radioactive copper in fibroblasts is possible, but is not very reliable (Tümer and Horn, 1997). The full neurodegenerative disease, accompanied by chromosome X/2 translocation, has been encountered in girls (Kapur *et al.*, 1987).

Treatment

Copper supplementation, using daily injections of copper-histidine, appears to be the most promising treatment. Parenterally administered copper corrects the hepatic copper deficiency and restores serum copper and ceruloplasmin levels to normal. The effectiveness of treatment in arresting or reversing neurologic symptoms probably depends on whether some activity of the copper-transporting enzyme ATP7A has been preserved, and whether copper supplementation has been initiated promptly (Christodoulou *et al.*, 1998; Tümer and Horn, 1997). Therefore, it is advisable to begin copper therapy as soon as the diagnosis is established if the child has good neurologic function, and to continue therapy until it becomes evident that cerebral degeneration cannot be arrested. The use of intracerebroventricular copper-histidine is being explored (Lem *et al.*, 2007).

REFERENCES

Adaletli, I., Omeroglu, A., Kurugoglu, S., *et al.* 2005. Lumbar and iliac artery aneurysms in Menkes' disease: endovascular cover stent treatment of the lumbar artery aneurysm. *Pediatr Radiol*, **35**, 1006–9.

Andrews, N. C. 2001. Mining copper transport genes. *Proc Nat Acad Sci USA*, **98**, 6543–5.

Baerlocher, K., and Nadal, D. 1988. Das Menkes-Syndrom. *Ergeb Inn Mediz*, **57**, 79–144.

Borm, B., Moller, L. B., Hausser, I., *et al.* 2004. Variable clinical expression of an identical mutation in the ATP7 A gene for Menkes disease/occipital horn syndrome in three affected males in a single family. *J Pediatr*, **145**, 119–21.

Bucknall, W. E., Haslam, R. H., and Holtzman, N. A. 1973. Kinky hair syndrome: response to copper therapy. *Pediatrics*, **52**, 653–7.

Christodoulou, J., Danks, D. M., Sarkar, B., *et al.* 1998. Early treatment of Menkes disease with parenteral copper-histidine: long-term follow-up of four treated patients. *Am J Med Genet*, **76**, 154–64.

Cobbold, C., Coventry, J., Ponnambalam, S., and Monaco, A. P. 2003. The Menkes disease ATPase (ATP7A) is internalized via a Rac-1 regulated, clathrin and caveolae-independent pathway. *Hum Mol Genet*, **12**, 1523–33.

Cox, D. W. 1999. Disorders of copper transport. *Br Med Bull*, **55**, 544–55.

Danks, D. M., Campbell, P. E., Stevens, B. J., *et al.* 1972. Menkes' kinky hair syndrome: an inherited defect in copper absorption with widespread effects. *Pediatrics*, **50**, 188–201.

El Meskini, R., Crabtree, K. L., Cline, L. B., *et al.* 2007. ATP7A (Menkes protein) functions in axonal targeting and synaptogenesis. *Mol Cell Neurosci*, **34**, 409–21.

Ferreira, R. C., Heckenlively, J. R., Menkes, J. H., and Bateman, J. B. 1998. Menkes disease. New ocular and electroretinographic findings. *Ophthalmology*, **105**, 1076–8.

Godwin, S. C., Shawker, T., Chang, B., and Kaler, S. G. 2006. Brachial artery aneurysms in Menkes disease. *J Pediatr*, **149**, 412–5.

Goodyer, I. D., Jones, E. E., Monaco, A. P., and Francis, M. J. 1999. Characterization of the Menkes protein copper-binding domains and their role in copper-induced protein relocalization. *Hum Mol Genet*, **8**, 1473–8.

Grange, D. K., Kaler, S. G., Albers, G. M., *et al.* 2005. Severe bilateral panlobular emphysema and pulmonary arterial hypoplasia: unusual manifestations of Menkes disease. *Am J Med Genet A*, **139**, 151–5.

Grover, W. D., Johnson, W. C., and Henkin, R. I. 1979. Clinical and biochemical aspects of trichopoliodystrophy. *Ann Neurol*, **5**, 65–71.

Harrison, M. D., and Dameron, C. T. 1999. Molecular mechanisms of copper metabolism and the role of the Menkes disease protein. *J Biochem Mol Toxicol*, **13**, 93–106.

Hsich, G. E., Robertson, R. L., Irons, M., *et al.* 2000. Cerebral infarction in Menkes' disease. *Pediatr Neurol*, **23**, 425–8.

Kaler, S. G., Goldstein, D. S., Holmes, C., *et al.* 1993. Plasma and cerebrospinal fluid neurochemical pattern in Menkes disease. *Ann Neurol*, **33**, 171–5.

Kaler, S. G., Holmes, C. S., Goldstein, D. S., *et al.* 2008. Neonatal diagnosis and treatment of Menkes disease. *NEJM*, **358**, 605–14.

Kapur, S., Higgins, J. V., Delp, K., and Rogers, B. 1987. Menkes' syndrome in a girl with X-autosome translocation. *Am J Hum Genet*, **26**, 503–10.

Kim, O. H., and Suh, J. H. 1997. Intracranial and extracranial MR angiography in Menkes disease. *Pediatr Radiol*, **27**, 782–4.

Lem, K. E., Brinster, L. R., Tjurmina, O., *et al.* 2007. Safety of intracerebroventricular copper histidine in adult rats. *Mol Genet Metab*, (In Press).

Menkes, J. H. 2001. Subdural haematoma, non-accidental head injury or . . .? *Eur J Paediatr Neurol*, **5**, 175–6.

Menkes, J. H., Alter, M., Weakley, D., *et al.* 1962. A sex-linked recessive disorder with growth retardation, peculiar hair, and focal cerebral and cerebellar degeneration *Pediatrics*, **29**, 764–79.

Moller, J. V., Juul, B., and Le Maire, M. 1996. Structural organization, ion transport, and energy transduction of P-type ATP-ases. *Biochem Biophys Acta*, **1286**, 1–51.

Moller, L. B., Tumer, Z., Lund, C., *et al.* 2000. Similar splice-site mutations of the ATP7 A gene lead to different phenotypes: classical Menkes disease or occipital horn syndrome. *Am J Hum Genet*, **66**, 1211–20.

Pasquali-Ronchetti, I., Baccarani-Contri, M., Young, R. D., *et al.* 1994. Ultrastructural analysis of skin and aorta from a patient with Menkes disease. *Exp Mol Pathol*, **61**, 36–57.

Paulsen, M., Lund, C., Akram, Z., *et al.* 2006. Evidence that translation reinitiation leads to a partially function Menkes protein containing two copper-binding sites. *Am J Hum Genet*, **79**, 214–29.

Seelenfreund, M. H., Gartner, S., Vinger, P. E. 1968. The ocular pathology of Menkes' disease. *Arch Ophthalmol*, **80**, 718–20.

Steveson, T. C., Ciccotosto, G. D., Ma, X. M., *et al.* 2003. Menkes protein contributes to the function of peptidylglycine alpha-amidating monooxygenase. *Endocrinology*, **144**, 188–200.

Tønnesen, T., Kleijer, W. J., and Horn, N. 1991. Incidence of Menkes disease. *Hum Genet*, **86**, 408–10.

Tümer, Z., Bir Moller, L., and Horn, N. 2003. Screening of 383 unrelated patients affected with Menkes disease and finding of 57 gross deletions in ATP7A. *Hum Mutat*, **22**, 457–64.

Tümer, Z., and Horn, N. 1997. Menkes disease: recent advance and new aspects. *J Med Genet*, **34**, 265–74.

Ubhi, T., Reece, A., and Craig, A. 2000. Congenital skull fracture as a presentation of Menkes disease. *Dev Med Child Neurol*, **42**, 347–8.

van den Berg, G. J., Kroon, J. J., Wijburg, F. A., *et al.* 1990. Muscle cell cultures in Menkes' disease: copper accumulation in myotubes. *J Inherit Metab Dis*, **13**, 207–11.

Wesenberg, R. L., Gwinn, J. L., and Barnes, G. R. 1968. Radiologic findings in the kinky hair syndrome. *Radiology*, **92**, 500–6.

Wheeler, E. M., and Roberts, P. F. 1976. Menke's steely hair syndrome. *Arch Dis Child*, **51**, 269–74.

WYBURN-MASON SYNDROME

Stephen D. Reck and Jonathan D. Trobe

Wyburn-Mason syndrome (WMS), also known as the Bonnet-Dechaume-Blanc syndrome, is a rare nonhereditary phakomatosis characterized by congenital retinal, orbital, and brainstem (usually midbrain) arteriovenous malformations (AVMs), and, less frequently, facial AVMs (Bonnet *et al.*, 1937; Théron *et al.*, 1974; Wyburn-Mason, 1943). The combination of a retinal and intracranial AVM has traditionally been required to make the diagnosis of WMS, but there are patients with multiple orbital, facial, and brainstem AVMs without retinal AVMs that probably represent the same disorder (Danis and Appen, 1984; Kim *et al.*, 1998; Ponce *et al.*, 2001).

Historical features

Bonnet *et al.* (1937) first noted the combination of retinal and intracranial AVMs in 1937, but the eponym derives from the more comprehensive 1943 report of Wyburn-Mason of 27 patients with retinal AVMs, 22 of whom also had intracranial AVMs (Wyburn-Mason, 1943). The retinal lesion consists of a markedly dilated and tortuous arteriole contiguous to a similar vein involving the optic disc and retina (Brown, 1999; Selhorst, 1998) (Figures 32.1–32.3). The intracranial lesion consists of dilated vascular channels, often with arteriovenous shunts. The AVMs are usually unilateral and deeply located, and often involve the optic chiasm, hypothalamus, basal ganglia, and mudbrain (Théron *et al.*, 1974) (Figure 32.1).

The syndrome is often first identified by finding the retinal abnormality on a routine ophthalmologic examination. Before the development of noninvasive brain imaging, intracranial AVMs were typically discovered after they had bled and become symptomatic. With the increased availability of noninvasive brain imaging, intracranial AVMs are now often detected even if they do not produce any symptoms and signs.

Recognition of the association between the retinal and intracranial lesions is important because it may allow early identification of the associated intracranial and facial AVMs (Selhorst, 1998). Notably, however, the prevalence of intracranial AVMs in cases with retinal AVMs is not well defined (Beck and Jenesen, 1958; Brown, 1999; 1961; Font and Ferry, 1972; Wyburn-Mason, 1943). Théron *et al.* (1974) observed that of the 80 cases reported to have retinal AVMs before 1974, 25 (31%) also had intracranial AVMs, and 10 (12%) had facial AVMs.

Pathophysiology

WMS is believed to result from a disturbance occurring before the seventh gestational week in the vascular mesoderm shared by the optic cup and the anterior neural tube. In this early period, this vascular plexus differentiates into the hyaloid vascular system and the vascular supply of the midbrain (Selhorst, 1998).

Clinical manifestations

Retinal AVMs

Retinal AVMs usually do not grow or bleed, and are usually not responsible for significant visual loss (Brown, 1999; Lee, 1998) (Figure 32.1, A and B). In three cases reported with a follow-up of 2–15 years (de Keizer and van Dalen, 1981; Gulick and Taylor, 1978; Muthukumar and Sundaralingam, 1998), the ocular findings remained stable without treatment. However, Effron *et al.* (1985) reported a case of neovascular glaucoma resulting from retinal ischemia from retinal arteriovenous shunting. There are several reports of patients presenting with decreased visual acuity and progressive optic neuropathy from accompanying orbitocranial AVMs (Ausburger *et al.*, 1980; Brown *et al.*, 1973; Danis and Appen, 1984; Effron *et al.*, 1985; Kim *et al.*, 1998; Muthukumar and Sundaralingam, 1998).

Intracranial AVMs

The morbidity in this syndrome usually comes from the associated intracranial AVMs (Figure 32.1, A–D). Reports of 25 Wyburn-Mason patients contained diagnostic imaging or autopsy information sufficient to confirm the diagnosis (Ausburger *et al.*, 1980; Brodsky and Hoyt, 2002; Brodsky *et al.*, 1987; Brown *et al.*, 1973; Chakravarty and Chatterjee, 1990; Chan *et al.*, 2004; Danis and Appen, 1984; de Keizer and van Dalen, 1981; Effron *et al.*, 1985; Gibo *et al.*, 1989; Gulick and Taylor, 1978; Kim *et al.*, 1998; Lalonde *et al.*, 1979; Morgan *et al.*, 1985; Muthukumar and Sundaralingam, 1998; Ponce *et al.*, 2001; Reck *et al.*, 2005; Théron *et al.*, 1974; Wyburn-Mason, 1943). These cases presented with vision loss in 18 (72%), headache in 6 (24%), spontaneous nose or jaw bleeding in 6 (24%), hemiparesis in 4 (16%), and seizure, proptosis, unconsciousness, and routine ophthalmoscopic detection of a retinal AVM in 1 case each.

Among the 10 of these 25 reported patients whose intracranial AVMs were adequately followed (range, 1–17 years; average, 6 years), 5 were not treated. One patient presented with a retinal

Uncommon Causes of Stroke, 2nd edition, ed. Louis R. Caplan. Published by Cambridge University Press. © Cambridge University Press 2008.

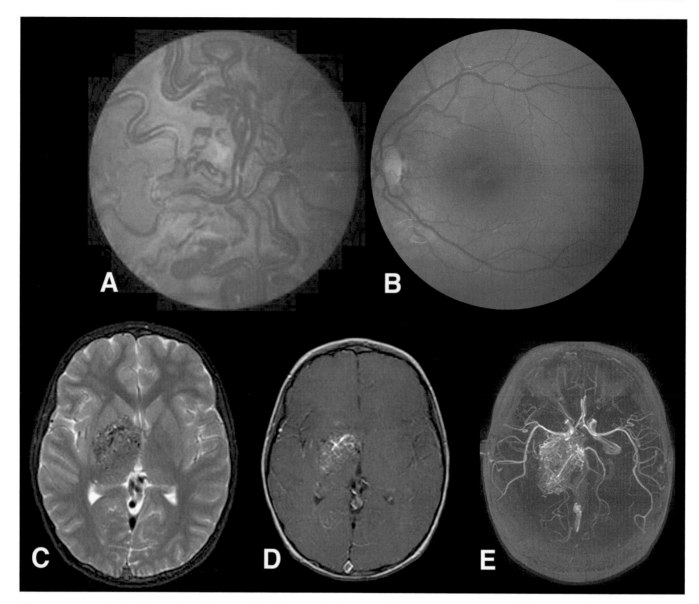

Figure 32.1 WMS. **A**. Fundus photograph of the right eye shows tortuous arteriovenous anastomoses centered over the optic disc and extending to the equator of the eye. **B**. Fundus photograph of the left eye is normal. **C**. T2-weighted axial MRI with fat suppression shows flow voids in the right basal ganglia and thalamus, consistent with a large AVM. **D**. Enhanced T1-weighted axial MRI shows high signal in areas of anomalous vessels. **E**. Three-dimensional reformatted magnetic resonance angiogram, viewed from above, shows an AVM. See color plate. (Reprinted with permission from Reck, S. D., Zacks, D. N., and Eibschitz-Tsimhoni, M. 2005. Retinal and intracranial arteriovenous malformations: Wyburn-Mason syndrome. *J Neuro-Ophthalmol*, **25**, 205–8.)

AVM and died 1 year later of intracranial hemorrhage at the age of 9 years (Chan *et al.*, 2004); one patient had increased hemiparesis after 15 years; one patient had increased hemianopia 12 years after recovering from a coma induced by spontaneous subarachnoid hemorrhage; and two patients were unchanged after 1 and 2 years.

Review of the reported cases of WMS does not permit firm conclusions regarding the natural history of the asymptomatic intracranial AVMs. There is no evidence that they have a natural history different from intracranial AVMs unassociated with retinal AVMs, but they tend to be more extensive and deeper than the average isolated intracranial AVM.

Treatment

Of the 25 reported patients with imaging or autopsy information sufficient to confirm the diagnosis of WMS, five received treatment and were followed. One patient presented with decreased vision (20/15 right eye, and 20/100 left eye) and headache and underwent excision of an orbital and parachiasmal AVM. After 4 years, this patient was blind in the left eye and developed a small nasal visual field defect in the right eye (Danis and Appen, 1984). One patient underwent excision of a suprasellar AVM after several spontaneous subarachnoid hemorrhages and had slight visual field loss after 1 year (Gibo *et al.*, 1989). One patient presented with

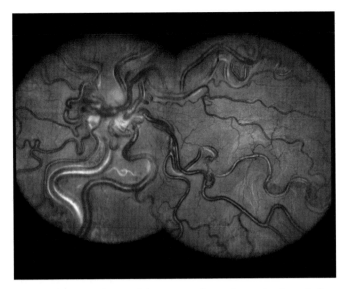

Figure 32.2 Fundus photograph from a second case of WMS showing retinal AVM. (Kellogg Eye Center, Department of Ophthalmology and Visual Sciences, University of Michigan.)

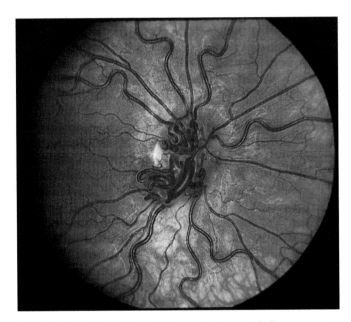

Figure 32.3 Fundus photograph from a third case of WMS. (Kellogg Eye Center, Department of Ophthalmology and Visual Sciences, University of Michigan.)

decreased vision (20/400 right eye, 20/20 left eye) and underwent radiation therapy for a suprasellar AVM. Vision had improved at 2-year follow-up (20/200 right eye and 20/20 left eye) (Brown *et al.*, 1973). One patient underwent pan-retinal laser photocoagulation for neovascular glaucoma and was blind in that eye at 20-month follow-up (Effron *et al.*, 1985). One patient underwent external carotid artery ligation followed by subtotal maxillary resection for a facial AVM that was complicated by severe hemorrhage requiring ligation of the ipsilateral internal carotid artery, resulting in incomplete hemiplegia at a 17-year follow-up (Ausburger *et al.*, 1980).

Because of their size and location, WMS AVMs are usually not amenable to surgical removal or radiosurgery. Embolization carries an increased risk because these lesions share a blood supply with vital brainstem structures. Therefore, patients are usually left untreated until the AVMs bleed, at which time heroic measures may be necessary (Brown *et al.*, 1988).

REFERENCES

Ausburger, J. T., Goldberg, R. E., Shields, J. A., *et al.* 1980. Changing appearance of retinal arteriovenous malformation. *Albrecht Von Graefes Arch Klin Exp Ophthalmol*, **215**, 65–70.

Beck, K., and Jenesen, O. A. 1958. Racemose haemangioma of the retina; two additional cases, including one with defects of the visual fields as a complication of arteriography. *Acta Ophthalmol*, **36**, 769–81.

Beck, K., and Jenesen, O. A. 1961. On the frequency of co-existing racemose haemangiomata of the retina and brain. *Acta Psychiatr Scand*, **36**, 47–56.

Bonnet, P., Dechaume, J., and Blanc, E. 1937. L'anévrysme cirsoïde de la rétine (anévrysme recémeux): ses relations avec l'anéurysme cirsoïde de la face et avec l'anévrysme cirsoïde du cerveau. *J Med Lyon*, **18**, 165–78.

Brodsky, M. C., and Hoyt, W. F. 2002. Spontaneous involution of retinal and intracranial arteriovenous malformation in Bonnet-Dechaume-Blanc syndrome. *Br J Ophthalmol*, **86**, 360–1.

Brodsky, M. C., Hoyt, W. F., Higashida, R. T., *et al.* 1987. Bonnet-Dechaume-Blanc syndrome with large facial angioma. *Arch Ophthalmol*, **105**, 854–5.

Brown, D. G., Hilal, S. K., and Tenner, M. S. 1973. Wyburn-Mason syndrome. Report of two cases without retinal involvement. *Arch Neurol*, **28**, 67–9.

Brown, G. C. 1999. Congenital retinal arteriovenous communications (racemose hemangiomas). In *Retina-Vitreous-Macula*, eds. D. R. Guyer, L. A. Yannuzzi, S. Chang, *et al.* Philadelphia: WB Saunders Co., pp. 1172–4.

Brown, R. D. Jr., Wiebers, D. O., Forbes, G., *et al.* 1988. The natural history of unruptured intracranial arteriovenous malformations. *J Neurosurg*, **68**, 352–7.

Chakravarty A, Chatterjee S. Retino-cephalic vascular malformation. *J Assoc Physicians India* 1990; 38: 941–3.

Chan, W. M., Yip, N. K., and Lam, D. S. 2004. Wyburn-Mason syndrome. *Neurology*, **62**, 99.

Danis, R., and Appen, R. E. 1984. Optic atrophy and the Wyburn-Mason syndrome. *J Clin Neuroophthalmol*, **4**, 91–5.

de Keizer, R. J., and van Dalen, J. T. 1981. Wyburn-Mason syndrome subcutaneous angioma extirpation after preliminary embolisation. *Doc Ophthalmol*, **50**, 263–73.

Effron, L., Zakov, Z. N., and Tomsak, R. L. 1985. Neovascular glaucoma as a complication of the Wyburn-Mason syndrome. *J Clin Neuroophthalmol*, **5**, 95–8.

Font, R. I., and Ferry, A. P. 1972. The phakomatoses. *Int Ophthalmol Clin*, **12**, 1–50.

Gibo, H., Watanabe, N., Kobayashi, S., *et al.* 1989. Removal of an arteriovenous malformation in the optic chiasm. A case of Bonnet-Dechaume-Blanc syndrome without retinal involvement. *Surg Neurol*, **31**, 142–8.

Gulick, A. W., and Taylor, W. B. 1978. A case of basal-cell carcinoma in a patient with the Wyburn-Mason syndrome. *J Dermatol Surg Oncol*, **4**, 85–6.

Kim, J., Kim, O. H., Suh, J. H., *et al.* 1998. Wyburn-Mason syndrome: an unusual presentation of bilateral orbital and unilateral brain arteriovenous malformation. *Pediatr Radiol*, **28**, 161.

Lalonde, G., Duquette, P., Laflamme, P., *et al.* 1979. Bonnet-Dechaume-Blanc syndrome. *Can J Ophthalmol*, **14**, 47–50.

Lee, A. G. 1998. Tumors and hamartomas of blood vessels. In *Walsh and Hoyt Clinical Neuro-Ophthalmology*, 5th edn, eds. N. R. Miller, and N. J. Newman. Baltimore: Williams & Wilkins, pp. 2266–8.

Morgan, M. K., Johnston, I. H., and de Silva, M. 1985. Treatment of ophthalmofacial-hypothalamic arteriovenous malformation (Bonnet-Dechaume-Blanc syndrome). Case report. *J Neurosurg*, **63**, 794–6.

Muthukumar, N., and Sundaralingam, M. 1998. Retinocephalic vascular malformation: Case report. *Br J Neurosurg*, **12**, 458–60.

Ponce, F. A., Han, P. P., Spetzler, R. F., *et al.* 2001. Associated arteriovenous malformation of the orbit and brain: a case of Wyburn-Mason syndrome without retinal involvement. Case report. *J Neurosurg*, **95**, 346–9.

Reck, S. D., Zacks, D. N., and Eibschitz-Tsimhoni, M. 2005. Retinal and intracranial arteriovenous malformations: Wyburn-Mason syndrome. *J Neuro-Ophthalmol*, **25**, 205–8.

Selhorst, J. B. 1998. Phacomatoses. In *Walsh and Hoyt Clinical Neuro-Ophthalmology*, 5th edn., eds. N. R. Miller, and N. J. Newman. Baltimore: Williams and Wilkins, pp. 2725–9.

Théron, J., Newton, T. H., and Hoyt, W. F. 1974. Unilateral retinocephalic vascular malformations. *Neuroradiology*, **7**, 185–96.

Wyburn-Mason, R. 1943. Arteriovenous aneurysm of mid-brain and retina, facial naevi, and mental changes. *Brain*, **66**, 163–203.

PART III: VASCULAR CONDITIONS OF THE EYES, EARS, AND BRAIN

33 EALES RETINOPATHY

Valérie Biousse

Introduction

Henry Eales, in 1880, described a syndrome of recurrent vitreous hemorrhages associated with abnormal retinal veins and peripheral retinal capillary dropout in young men (Biswas *et al.*, 2002). There is now good evidence that the condition described by Eales as a specific disease entity is rather a retinopathy that can be found in a variety of vascular retinal conditions (Biswas *et al.*, 2002; Duker *et al.*, 1998; Goldberg, 1971; Karam *et al.*, 1999; Mizener *et al.*, 1997). This is why the terms "Eales retinopathy" or "Eales disease" are only rarely used. Most authors prefer "retinal neovascularization," which is usually classified as "idiopathic" or "secondary."

Clinical manifestations of "Eales retinopathy"

So-called "Eales retinopathy" associates peripheral retinal changes often described as "vasculitis," peripheral capillary non-perfusion (retinal ischemia), and retinal or optic nerve neovascularization (secondary to chronic retinal ischemia) resulting in vitreous hemorrhage and retinal detachment (Figure 33.1). This variety of retinal findings explains why visual symptoms are non-specific. Patients may be asymptomatic and the retinal vascular changes found only during a routine funduscopic examination, or they may have devastating visual loss from vitreous hemorrhage and retinal detachment secondary to neovascularization (Biswas *et al.*, 2002; Dastur and Singhal, 1976).

So-called "Eales disease" affects most often young adults, is usually bilateral, and is more common in the Middle East and in India where it has been associated with tuberculosis (Biswas *et al.*, 2002).

The list of disorders associated with such retinopathy is extensive. During the past 20 years, numerous syndromes have been reported with the ophthalmic features of so-called "Eales retinopathy." Some of these syndromes are associated with lesions of the central nervous system, explaining why Eales retinopathy is considered an "uncommon cause of stroke" by some authors (Dastur and Singhal, 1976). However, this should be interpreted with caution because other, perhaps better known, entities may be the cause of the retinopathy and the central nervous system lesions. For example, systemic inflammatory disorders such as systemic lupus erythematosus, sarcoidosis, and ulcerative colitis can present with similar findings (Biswas *et al.*, 2002; Duker *et al.*, 1998; Karam *et al.*, 1999; Mizener *et al.*, 1997). Peripheral

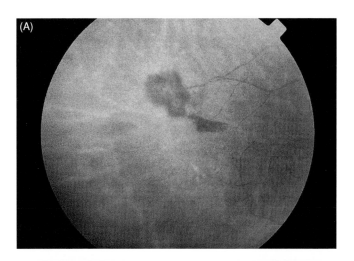

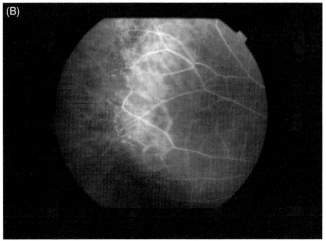

Figure 33.1 A. Peripheral retinal neovascularization shown on fundus photo. **B**. Retinal fluorescein angiogram.

retinal neovascularization without inflammation is seen in sickle cell disease, diabetic retinopathy, retinopathy of prematurity, familial exudative vitreoretinopathy, hyperviscosity syndromes, and other hypercoagulable states (Biswas *et al.*, 2002; Goldberg, 1971). In addition, pars planitis (often associated with multiple sclerosis or other inflammatory or infectious disorders) and rare vascular retinal syndromes such as idiopathic retinal vasculitis, aneurysms, and neuroretinitis (IRVAN syndrome) (Chang *et al.*, 1995; Hammond *et al.*, 2004) or Susac syndrome (O'Halloran *et al.*, 1998) have been included in previous reports of Eales disease.

Neurologic findings

Many of the disorders responsible for peripheral retinal neovascularization also involve the central nervous system. Therefore, various neurologic findings have been reported in so-called Eales disease, including meningitis, encephalitis, cerebral vasculitis, brain infarctions and hemorrhages, cerebral venous thrombosis, and white matter diseases. These manifestations are nonspecific and are related to the underlying neurologic disorder.

Treatment

There is no specific treatment except for that of the underlying disorder. The treatment of the retinopathy is limited to stimulating regression of neovascularization by applying laser photocoagulation to the nonperfused retina. Vitrectomy is indicated for nonclearing vitreous hemorrhage, extensive retinal neovascularization, epiretinal membrane, and traction retinal detachment (Biswas *et al.*, 2002; Dehghan *et al.*, 2005).

REFERENCES

Biswas, J., Sharma, T., Gopal, L., *et al.* 2002. Eales disease–an update. *Surv Ophthalmol*, **47**, 197–214.

Chang, T. S., Aylward, G. W., Davis, J. L., *et al.* 1995. The retinal vasculitis study group. Idiopathic retinal vasculitis, aneurysms, and neuro-retinitis. *Ophthalmology*, **102**, 1089–97.

Dastur, D. K., and Singhal, B. 1976. Eales' disease with neurological involvement. Part 2. Pathology and pathogenesis. *J Neurol Sci*, **27**, 323–45.

Dehghan, M. H., Ahmadieh, H., Soheilian, M., *et al.* 2005. Therapeutic effects of laser photocoagulation and/or vitrectomy in Eales' disease. *Eur J Ophthalmol*, **15**, 379–83.

Duker, J. S., Brown, G. C., and McNamara, J. A. 1998. Proliferative sarcoid retinopathy. *Ophthalmology*, **95**, 1680–6.

Goldberg, M. F. 1971. Natural history of untreated proliferative sickle retinopathy. *Arch Opthalmol*, **85**, 428–33.

Hammond, M. D., Ward, T. P., Katz, B., *et al.* 2004. Elevated intracranial pressure associated with idiopathic retinal vasculitis, aneurysms, and neuroretinitis syndrome. *J Neuro-Ophthalmol*, **24**, 221–4.

Karam, E. Z., Muci-Mendoza, R., and Hedges, T. R. III. 1999. Retinal findings in Takayasu's arteritis. *Acta Ophthalmol Scand*, **77**, 209–13.

Mizener, J. B., Podhajsky, P., and Hayreh, S. S. 1997. Ocular ischemic syndrome. *Ophthalmology*, **104**, 859–64.

O'Halloran, H. S., Pearson, P. A., Lee, W. B., Susac, J. O., and Berger, J. R. 1998. Microangiopathy of the brain, retina and cochlea (Susac Syndrome). *Ophthalmology*, **105**, 1038–44.

34 ACUTE POSTERIOR MULTIFOCAL PLACOID PIGMENT EPITHELIOPATHY

Marc D. Reichhart

General considerations and pathophysiology

Acute posterior multifocal placoid pigment epitheliopathy (APMPPE), first recognized by J. Donald Gass 40 years ago (Gass, 1968, 2003a), is an ophthalmologic syndrome rather than a specific entity, characterized by "multiple cream-colored placoid lesions" located in the posterior pole "lying at the level of the pigment epithelium and choroids" (see Figure 34.1). Gass reported on three young women presenting painless acute visual loss, with persistent lesions of the retinal pigment epithelium despite visual acuity remission, and hence proposed the term of acute posterior multifocal placoid pigment epitheliopathy, believing that it represented a primary disease of the retinal pigment epithelium. He highlighted an association with tuberculosis (positive tuberculin test, two cases; familial history, one case), which was confirmed later (Anderson *et al.*, 1996). The pathognomic signs of APMPPE are typically seen on fluorescein angiography, and its hallmarks are particularly evident using indocyanine green angiography (Dhaliwal *et al.*, 1993; Howe *et al.*, 1995; Park *et al.*, 1995b; Stanga *et al.*, 2003).

Questions have been raised whether APMPPE was a primary disorder of the retinal pigment epithelium (Gass, 1968, 2003a), a vasculitis of the choriocapillaries (Deutman *et al.*, 1972; Hedges *et al.*, 1979), a choroidal vasculitis (Spaide *et al.*, 1991), or a partial choroidal occlusive vasculitis (Park *et al.*, 1995a) with secondary lesions of the retinal pigment epithelium (Jones, 1995). Fluorescein angiography in APMPPE shows early hypofluorescence of the placoid lesion with gradual accumulation of fluorescein within the retinal pigment epithelium; this hypofluorescence failed to discriminate whether the choroid or the retinal pigment epithelium was primarily involved (Stanga *et al.*, 2003). Angiography with indocyanine green confirmed choroidal hypofluorescence secondary to choroidal vascular occlusion, related to occlusive vasculitis (Howe *et al.*, 1995; Stanga *et al.*, 2003; Uyama *et al.*, 1999). Later hyperfluorescence is seen because of the secondary retinal pigment epithelium damage, whereas with resolution of the placoid lesion, there are persistent areas of choroidal hypoperfusion (Howe *et al.*, 1995; Stanga *et al.*, 2003; Uyama *et al.*, 1999).

By comparing fundoscopic signs (multifocal posterior pole lesions vs. diffuse changes) and clinical courses (spontaneous remission vs. recurrent disease), a continuum probably exists between APMPPE and Harada disease (Jones, 1995; Wright *et al.*, 1978). A patient with recurrent APMPPE with late-onset central nervous system (CNS) involvement and aseptic meningitis (see Patient 4, Table 34.1) has been reported (Kersten *et al.*,

1987). Furthermore, a patient with Harada diseases and recurrent APMPPE was published (Furusho *et al.*, 2001). Even in APMPPE patients without CNS involvement, cerebrospinal fluid (CSF) analysis may show increased white blood cell (WBC) content, comprising mainly lymphocytes (Bullock and Fletcher, 1977). For these reasons, APMPPE has been classified by some authorities as an inflammatory or an autoimmune cause of the true uveomeningeal syndrome (Table 34.2), together with Vogt-Koyanagi syndrome and Harada disease (VKH syndrome), Behçet syndrome, sarcoidosis, and Wegener granulomatosis (Brazis *et al.*, 2004). Regarding its cerebrovascular complications, APMPPE may be considered a vasculitis with posterior chorioretinitis and rarely CNS involvement, such as stroke and cerebral vasculitis (Ferro, 1998). Even if APMPPE presents most often as an isolated ocular choroidal vasculitis, a growing body of evidences suggests that it can be associated with a systemic vasculitic process, including the CNS. Like other vasculitis, it can be secondary to or associated with the following disorders, which are summarized in Table 34.2.

Infectious/post-infectious – i.e. streptococcus (Deutman *et al.*, 1972) of group A (Lowder *et al.*, 1996), tuberculosis (Anderson *et al.*, 1996; Deutman *et al.*, 1972), and positive tuberculin skin tests (Brown *et al.*, 1973; Gass, 1968, 1983, 2003a; Schubert *et al.*, 1988), syphilis (Gass *et al.*, 1990), Lyme disease (Bodine *et al.*, 1992; Toenjes *et al.*, 1989), *Schistosoma mansoni* (Dickinson *et al.*, 1990), toxoplasmosis (Annesley *et al.*, 1973; Kirkham *et al.*, 1972),

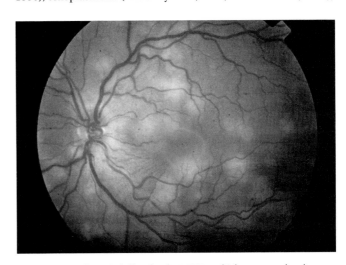

Figure 34.1 Fundoscopic hallmarks of APMPPE: multiple creamy colored (white), flat, and discrete placoid, without clear-cut margins, lesions at the level of the retinal pigment epithelium. (Courtesy of F.-X Borruat, MD, Hôpital Jules Gonin, Lausanne, Switzerland.)

Table 34.1 Patient number, source (first author, year), and case or patient number for series, demographic data, headache and meningeal signs, clinical pattern of CNS insult, radiological and CSF features, latencies between diagnosis of APMPPE and CNS insult, outcome and therapy of 23 patients with PACNS and/or cerebrovascular diseases (CVDs)

Pt No.1st author, Year (Pt/case n°)	Age Sex Race	Headache Meningeal signs	Clinical pattern of CNS insult	CT, MRI, Angiography Muscle biopsy (MB) Other findings (necropsy)	CSF WBC/mL	CSF protein mg/L	APMPPE-to-CNS insult Latency	Outcome, therapy
1) Holt et al., 1976 Case 1	22 M w	Headache Photophobia Nausea Vomiting	Bilateral MCA TIAs	Normal Tc-99 CT-scan; Signs of vasculitis of B M3-MCA branches (angiogram) PACNS	177	1810	Inaugural	Good CS
2) Sigelman et al., 1979	18 M w	Headache Vomiting "Migraine"	L homonymous hemianopia	R occipital stroke (CT + Tc-99 CT-scan); Signs of vasculitis on angiogram PACNS	5	520 (330 IgG)	Inaugural	Good No CS
3) Smith et al., 1983	25 M w	Headache Photophobia Stiff neck	L homonymous hemianopia And hemihypesthesia	R occipital stroke (CT-scan) Signs of vasculitis (MCA, ACA), R PCA occlusion on angiogram PACNS	100	3000	7 weeks	Good CS
4) Kersten et al., 1987	30 M w	Headache Stiff neck	Vertigo, downbeat nystagmus/ ocular flutter ataxia, tremor	Normal CT (2) and angiogram (on CS); symptomatology recurrence after 5 years suspected PACNS	151	1440 OP 20 cm H$_2$0	5 years	Good CS
5) Wilson et al., 1988	24 M w	Headache nausea	Coma, corticospinal tract sign, tonic seizure, brain death	Gray matter ischemia + edema, B parietal > frontal + occipital (tonsillar herniation); GANS (Langhans'cells at necropsy)	0 (120 RBC)	660 OP 15 cm H$_2$0	6 weeks	Died despite CS
6) Weinstein et al., 1988	23 M w	Headache	R hand clumsiness, leg dysesthesia, dysarthria; L homonymous hemianopia	L subacute striatocapsular and R acute occipital strokes (CT); R occipital hemorrhage (MRI); Vasculitis signs on angiogram PACNS	19 8 RBC	330	4 weeks 12 weeks	Persistent hemianopia, Memory impairment CS
7) Smith in: Weinstein 1988	32 M w	No	R homonymous hemianopia	L occipital stroke (CT) Signs of vasculitis on angiogram PACNS	ND	ND	4 weeks	Partial resolution despite CS
8) Hammer et al., 1989	25 F w	Headache	Coma, hemiplegia	B ischemic strokes of ACA + MCA (CT); angiogram ND; suspected PACNS (necropsy refused)	ND	ND	5 weeks	Died despite CS
9) Stoll et al., 1991	54 M w	Headache Flu-like symptoms	Dysarthria, L hemiparesis, ataxia, B pyramidal signs	Multiple deep WM + pontine and L thalamus hyperintensities (MRI); Vasculitis of basal arteries (angiogram); subcortical PACNS	18	670	14 weeks	Good CS + AZA

Table 34.1 *(cont.)*

Pt No.1st author, Year (Pt/case n°)	Age Sex Race	Headache Meningeal signs	Clinical pattern of CNS insult	CT, MRI, Angiography Muscle biopsy (MB) Other findings (necropsy)	CSF WBC/mL	CSF protein mg/L	APMPPE-to-CNS insult Latency	Outcome, therapy
10) Bodiguel 1992	35 M w	Headache Flu-like symptoms	Dysarthria, R hemiparesis	L posterior limb of internal capsule + corpus callosum strokes, subcortical frontal + parietal lesions (MRI);N angiogram; sarcoidosis	75 66 RBC	650 +IgG Intrathecal production	5 weeks	Good CS
11) Bewermeyer *et al.*, 1993 Althaus, *et al.*, pt. 2 1993	27 M w	Flu-like Symptoms Photophobia	Horizontal nystagmus, dysarthria, stupor L spastic hemiparesis	R pontine infarct (MRI); N angiogram; Brain stem hypoperfusion (PET); Systemic vasculitis on MB (T-cells around small vessels)	55	360	24 weeks	Good CS + AZA
12) Althaus, *et al.*, 1993 1993 Case 1	54 M w	Flu-like symptoms	Dysarthria, L hemiparesis, B pyramidal signs	B WM, thalamus, pons lesions-MRI. Vasculitis of basal arteries (angiogram); Subcortical PACNS	ND	ND	12 weeks	Good CS + AZA
13) Comu *et al.*, 1996 Case 1	23 F h	Headache	Stupor, R hemiplegia, aphasia; L hemidysesthesia Seizures, L hemiparesis	B parietal, occipital (2nd hemorrhagic) + L putaminal ischemic strokes (MRI); N angiogram (suspected PACNS); R parietal acute stroke (MRI)	60	450	3 weeks 8 weeks 12 weeks	R hemianopia CS + CYC
14) Engelinus 1999	21 M w	Headache	Headache, R inferior homonymous quadrantanopsia	Normal CT-scan (suspected L parieto-occipital stroke and PACNS)	8	ND	Inaugural	Not known (3 months) CS
15) Reinthal 2001	29 M w	Headache Flu-like symptoms	Tetraparesis, four-limbs dysesthesia, B Corticospinal tract signs (Babinski)	Demyelinating lesions of L medulla oblongata, R paraventricular and nucleus caudatus (MRI);	40	1630 Without Intrathecal production	12 weeks	Good CS
16) O'Halloran *et al.*, 2001 Pt. 1	16 M w	Headache "migraine"	Seizure, L hemi-hypesthesia, confusion	R fronto-parietal hypodensities B parietal hemorrhages (MRI) Superior sagittal sinus thrombosis (angiogram); N brain biopsy	28	850 OP 39 cm H$_2$0	48 weeks	Good, CS, Craniotomia AC
17) O'Halloran *et al.*, 2001 Pt. 2	25 M w	Headache Viral meningitis	R hemiparesis Sphincter dysfunction	Normal MRI, CNS arteritis on angiogram PACNS	ND	ND	20 weeks	Good (5 years) CS CYC
18) O'Halloran *et al.*, 2001 Pt. 3	36 M w	Flu-like symptoms	Transient and chronic L hemidysesthesia	Thalamic and WM T2-WI signal abnormalities (MRI)	NK	880	4 weeks	Good, CS
19) O'Halloran, *et al.*, 2001 Pt 8	51 M w	NK	L superior homonymous quadrantanopia	Multiple R temporal strokes (MRI) PACNS	NK	NK	Inaugural	Good, CS
20) O'Halloran *et al.*, 2001 Pt. 9	49 M w	Headache Flu-like symptoms	Aphasia, confusion	N CT et MRI Suspected PACNS	NK	NK	Inaugural	Good, CS

(cont.)

Table 34.1 (*cont.*)

Pt No.1st author, Year (Pt/case n°)	Age Sex Race	Headache Meningeal signs	Clinical pattern of CNS insult	CT, MRI, Angiography Muscle biopsy (MB) Other findings (necropsy)	CSF WBC/mL	CSF protein mg/L	APMPPE-to-CNS insult Latency	Outcome, therapy
21) Al Kawi, *et al.*, 2004	33 M a	No	Conduction aphasia, R homonymous hemi-tanopia	L temporo-parietal (MCA) + occipital (PCA) ischemic strokes (MRI);signs of vasculitis (L MCA) on angiogram; PACNS	ND	ND	8 weeks	Good CS AC
22) Bugnone *et al.*, 2006	20 F w	Headache Photophobia phonophobia	dysphasia, R sensori-motor hemisyndrome headache	Increased signal intensity in the deep WM; acute R caudate nucleus head, old post. corpus callosum strokes (MRI); suspected subcortical PACNS	ND	ND	6 weeks 12 weeks (acute stroke)	Good, Inaugural CS (short Course)
23) De Vries 2006	23 M w	Headache	L sensori-motor hemisyndrome Tonic-clonic status epilepticus	L MCA and R PCA infarcts, L MCA occlusion, R PCA stenosis; GANS (Langhans cells) Multisystemic granuloma (necropsy)	ND	ND	0.5 week	Death

CS = corticosteroids; AZA = azathioprine; CYC = cyclophosphamide; B = bilateral; R = right; L =left; MB = muscle biopsy; ND = not done; NK= not known; Pt = Patient; w = white; b = black; h = half-cast (native American); a = Asian; CAT = computed axial tomography; Tc-99 CT-scan = dynamic Technecium CT-scan; GANS = granulomatous angiitis of the CNS; PACNS= primary angiitis of the CNS; OP = opening pressure on spinal tap; ACA = anterior cerebral artery; AC = anticoagulation therapy; WM = white-matter.

Epstein-Barr virus (Ryan and Maumenee, 1972), adenovirus (Azar *et al.*, 1975; Thomson and Roxburgh, 2003), mumps (Borruat *et al.*, 1998), and VZV (post-infectious) (Holt *et al.*, 1976).

Vaccination – i.e. complicating swine flu (Hector, 1978), hepatitis B (Brézin *et al.*, 1995), and meningococcal (Yang *et al.*, 2005) vaccines.

Inflammatory – i.e. lymphadenopathy found in 14%–22% of cases in series (Holt *et al.*, 1976; Lyness and Bird, 1984; Ryan and Maumenee, 1972) and isolated (Caccavale and Mignemi, 2001; Dick *et al.*, 1988; Laatikainen and Immonen, 1988; Uthman *et al.*, 2003), nephritis (Laatikainen and Immonen, 1988), Wegener's (Chiquet *et al.*, 1999), systemic granulomatosis (de Vries *et al.*, 2006), sarcoidosis (Bodiguel *et al.*, 1992; Dick *et al.*, 1988; Foulds and Damato, 1986; see Chapter 52), Crohn's disease (Gass, 1983), ulcerative colitis (Di Crecchio *et al.*, 2001), and thyroiditis (Jacklin, 1977).

Autoimmune diseases – i.e. poststreptococcal syndrome with erythema nodosum (Caccavale and Mignemi, 2001), systemic lupus erythematosus (Kawaguchi *et al.*, 1990; Matsuo *et al.*, 1987; see Chapter 45), anticardiolipin antibodies (Uthman *et al.*, 2003), juvenile-onset rheumatoid arthritis (Bridges *et al.*, 1995), and Graves-Basedow's disease (Ruiz Vinals *et al.*, 2002).

Paraneoplastic syndrome – i.e. renal cell carcinoma (Parmeggiani *et al.*, 2004).

Other rare conditions – i.e. lead intoxication (Schubert *et al.*, 1988), antimicrobial agents hypersensitivity reaction (Lyness and Bird, 1984), which is debatable (infectious vs. drug reaction), and hemophagocytic syndrome (Suzuki *et al.*, 2002).

The fact that it has been reported in the following vasculitic entities strongly support the hypothesis that APMPPE is caused by a choroidal occlusive vasculitis: necrotizing systemic arteritis including polyarteritis nodosa (PAN) (Hsu *et al.*, 2003) and small vessel vasculitis ("micro-PAN") with positive pANCA antibody (Matsuo *et al.*, 2002; see Chapter 43), and erythema nodosum (Caccavale and Mignemi, 2001; Deutman *et al.*, 1972; Uthman *et al.*, 2003; Van Buskirk *et al.*, 1971). In one series, urinary casts were found in patients with APMPPE, raising the hypothesis of a concomitant renal and choroidal microangiopathic vasculitis (Priluck *et al.*, 1981). Proven histopathological signs of vasculitis on muscle biopsy have been reported in one patient with APMPPE and pontine infarct (Table 34.1): Patient 11 (Bewermeyer *et al.*, 1993), also published as Case 2 in Althaus *et al.* (1993). Two additional APMPPE patients showed typical signs of granulomatous angiitis of the CNS with giant cells (Langerhans) on necropsy (Table 34.1, Patient 5) (Wilson *et al.*, 1988), and Patient 23 (de Vries *et al.*, 2006), who had evidences of multisystemic granulomatous arteritic injuries. Finally, human leukocyte antigen (HLA) mapping of families with APMPPE emphasized HLA DR2 (and B7) to be associated with an

Table 34.2 Conditions or diseases associated with APMPPE (see text for references)

Infectious/postinfectious
Streptococcus, including A type
Tuberculosis
Positive tuberculin skin test
Syphilis
Lyme disease
Schistosomiasis (mansoni)
Toxoplasmosis
Epstein-Barr virus (infectious mononucleosis)
Adenovirus
Mumps
Varicella zoster virus (VZV): postinfectious

Vaccinations
Swine flu
Hepatitis B
Meningococcus

Inflammations
Lymphadenopathy
Subacute thyroiditis (De Quervain's)
Nephritis
Wegener's and systemic granulomatosis
Sarcoidosis
Crohn's disease and ulcerative colitis

Autoimmune diseases
Poststreptococcal syndrome
Systemic lupus erythematosus
Anticardiolipin antibodies
Juvenile onset rheumatoid arthritis
Graves-Basedow's disease (hyperthyroidism)

Vasculitis
Polyarteritis nodosa
Small vessel vasculitis
Erythema nodosum
Pontine stroke with vasculitis signs on muscle biopsy
Granulomatous angiitis of the CNS (GANS) with systemic involvement (Langerhans cells)
GANS (Langerhans cells)
Primary angiitis of the CNS (PACNS) with and without stroke

Paraneoplastic syndrome
Clear renal cell carcinoma

Other conditions
Hemophagocytic syndrome
Lead intoxication
Antimicrobial drugs: sulfamethoxazole + trimethoprim, tetracycline, not specified

increased risk of recurrent diseases (Kim *et al.*, 1995; Wolf *et al.*, 1990b) and also reinforce the hypothesis of an immunologically mediated choroidal vasculitis process causing APMPPE.

According to Park *et al.* (1995a), partial choroidal occlusive vasculitis causing APMPPE and its associated vasculitic processes secondary to some aforementioned previously reported disorders –

i.e. granulomatous angiitis of the CNS (Wilson *et al.*, 1988), sarcoidosis (Dick *et al.*, 1988), schistosomiasis (Dickinson *et al.*, 1990), positive tuberculin tests suggestive of tuberculosis (Brown *et al.*, 1973; Gass, 1968, 2003a), and systemic vasculitis documented on muscle biopsy in one stroke-patient (Althaus *et al.*, 1993; Bewermeyer *et al.*, 1993) – might be all explained by delayed type hypersensitivity (type IV) reactions.

The neuro-ophthalmological manifestations of APMPPE include papillitis and optic neuritis with Marcus Gunn pupil (Frohman *et al.*, 1987; Jacklin, 1977; Jenkins *et al.*, 1973; Kirkham *et al.*, 1972; O'Halloran *et al.*, 2001; Savino *et al.*, 1974; Schubert *et al.*, 1988; Wolf *et al.*, 1990a), whereas its neuro-otological features encompass tinnitus, hearing loss, and vertigo (Clearkin and Hung, 1983; Holt *et al.*, 1976). The following neurological complications in patients with APMPPE have been reported: headache without meningitis (16%–50%) (Foulds and Damato, 1986; Holt *et al.*, 1976; Ryan and Maumenee, 1972) or associated with aseptic meningitis (Bullock and Fletcher, 1977; Comu *et al.*, 1996; Fishman *et al.*, 1977) confirmed on CSF analysis showing lymphocytic pleiocytosis (range, 56–70 WBC/mL), elevated protein level (>800 mg/L) (Bullock and Fletcher, 1977), and elevated mononuclear WBC (range 61–89 per mL) with hyperproteinorachia (range 460–540 mg/L) (Patients 2 and 3) (Comu *et al.*, 1996) (but conversely CSF analysis may give normal results) (Holt *et al.*, 1976); multiple sclerosis (MS)-like diseases (Patients 5–7) (O'Halloran *et al.*, 2001), pseudotumor cerebri (Patient 4) (O'Halloran *et al.*, 2001); "meningoencephalitis" (Hammer *et al.*, 1989; Holt *et al.*, 1976; Jones, 1995; Kersten *et al.*, 1987; Ryan and Maumenee, 1972; Sigelman *et al.*, 1979; Smith *et al.*, 1983; Weinstein *et al.*, 1988; Wilson *et al.*, 1988); and vasculitis of the CNS with or without stroke (Brazis *et al.*, 2004; Comu *et al.*, 1996; Ferro, 1998; Jones, 1995).

Most published so-called meningoencephalitis case-reports (Hammer *et al.*, 1989; Holt *et al.*, 1976; Jones, 1995; Kersten *et al.*, 1987; Sigelman *et al.*, 1979; Smith *et al.*, 1983; Weinstein *et al.*, 1988; Wilson *et al.*, 1988) represent cases of APMPPE associated with vasculitis of the CNS. Conversely, only one previously published case (Case 5) of true (meningo-)encephalitis has been reported (Ryan and Maumenee, 1972). Indeed, APMPPE, together with Buergers disease (thromboangiitis obliterans; see Chapter 5) and Susac's syndrome (retino-cochlear encephalopathy; see Chapter 35), are reputed exceptional forms of apparently primary angiitis of the CNS (PACNS) (Zuber *et al.*, 1999; see Cshapter 35), which is the most appropriate term (Lie, 1997).

Although CNS complications of APMPPE are extremely rare, 23 patients with APMPPE and associated CNS vasculitis and/or cerebrovascular disorders, including ischemic and secondary hemorrhagic strokes and lobar hemorrhages related to cerebral venous thrombosis (CVT), have been published to date (Al Kawi *et al.*, 2004; Althaus *et al.*, 1993; Bewermeyer *et al.*, 1993; Bodiguel *et al.*, 1992; Bugnone *et al.*, 2006; Comu *et al.*, 1996; de Vries *et al.*, 2006; Engelinus *et al.*, 1999; Hammer *et al.*, 1989; Holt *et al.*, 1976; Kersten *et al.*, 1987; O'Halloran *et al.*, 2001; Reinthal *et al.*, 2001; Sigelman *et al.*, 1979; Smith *et al.*, 1983; Stoll *et al.*, 1991; Weinstein *et al.*, 1988; Wilson *et al.*, 1988). These 23 cases will be analyzed in the following section.

Nosology, clinical and paraclinical features of APMPPE

From a nosologic ophthalmological point of view, APMPPE is now classified as one of the multifocal choroidopathy syndromes (Jampol and Becker, 2003), together with the acute zonal occult outer retinopathy complex also described by Gass (1993, 2000), which comprises other specific but sometimes overlapping entities (for details, see Gass, 1993, 2000, 2003b; Jampol and Becker, 2003). APMPPE affects young white adults (mean age, 26.5 years; range 11–66 years) without gender predilection (Jones, 1995). As compared with the two other "uveo-cerebral vasculitic syndromes," the major differences are the following: Eales disease (see Chapter 33), an angiitis also confined to retinal arteries (neovascular proliferation, vitreous hemorrhage) and less often affecting cerebral arteries with stroke, affects young men (range 20–40 years) from India and the Middle East (Biswas et al., 2001; Gordon et al., 1988; Jimenez et al., 2003; Katz et al., 1991; Kumaravelu et al., 2002; Misra et al., 1996), whereas Susac's syndrome (see Chapter 35), a microangiopathy of the retina, cochlea, and brain, which involves the corpus callosum, affects predominantly young women (mean 30 years) (O'Halloran et al., 1998; Susac, 2004; Susac et al., 1979, 2003). APMPPE presents with rapid decreased central vision, while the yellow-white multiple placoid lesions affect the macula (Foulds and Damato, 1986; Holt et al., 1976; Williams and Mieler, 1989), and is characterized by acute and/or subacute visual blurring, scotomas, or metamorphopsia (Jones, 1995).

The ophthalmoscopic hallmarks of APMPPE consist of cream-colored, flat, and discrete placoid, without clear-cut marginal lesions at the level of the retinal pigment epithelium, masking the fundus view of the underlying choroids, which typically involve the macula but are never seen anterior to the equator (Jones, 1995) (see Figure 34.1). Both eyes are involved, either simultaneously or sequentially within a few days (Foulds and Damato, 1986; Holt et al., 1976; Jones, 1995; Williams and Mieler, 1989), and recurrence, possibly related to the presence of HLA antigen DR2, is rare (Kim et al., 1995; Lyness and Bird, 1984; Wolf et al., 1990b). Although the retinal pigment epithelium changes are definitive, the visual prognosis is usually good (Williams and Mieler, 1989), although some other long-term studies (6–8 years) showed that two-thirds of patients had paracentral scotomas and persistent blurred vision with metamorphopsia (Wolf et al., 1991) and that 57% of them showed full recovery of visual acuity (Roberts and Mitchell, 1997).

Fluorescein or indocyanine green (Dhaliwal et al., 1993; Howe et al., 1995; Park et al., 1995b; Stanga et al., 2003; Uyama et al., 1999;) angiographic studies show typical choroidal hypofluorescence underneath the active lesions (early stage) and further bright staining (late stage) (Jones, 1995). Associated ocular findings include anterior and/or posterior uveitis, retinal vasculitis, papillitis, Marcus-Gunn pupil (see above), retinal serous detachment, edema, hemorrhages, episcleritis, central retinal vein occlusion, and subretinal neovascularization (Jones, 1995; Williams and Mieler, 1989). More than one-third of patients have prodromic flu-like symptoms (fever, malaise, headache, dizziness, myalgia, arthralgia, upper respiratory tract infection, chills, sore throat) before APMPPE onset (mean, 41%) (Comu et al., 1996; Dick et al., 1988; Foulds and Damato, 1986; Holt et al., 1976; Howe et al., 1995; Laatikainen and Immonen, 1988; Lyness and Bird, 1984; O'Halloran et al., 2001; Priluck et al., 1981; Roberts and Mitchell, 1997; Ryan and Maumenee, 1972; Savino et al., 1974; Uthman et al., 2003; Williams and Mieler, 1989).

Analysis of 23 patients with APMPPE and PACNS and/or CVDs

The fact that CVDs occur in patients with APMPPE strongly supports the thesis that it represents a particular "uveo-cerebral vasculitic syndrome," like Eales disease and the syndrome of Susac. APMPPE shares some common features other than CVDs (i.e. small infarcts for Susac's syndrome), with Eales disease (retinal capillary nonperfusion, multiple sclerosis-like disease, cerebral white matter involvement) (Biswas et al., 2001; see Chapter 33), and with the syndrome of Susac (hearing loss, corpus callosum involvement, multiple sclerosis-like disorder, deep white matter lesions; see Chapter 35) (O'Halloran et al., 1998; Susac et al., 2003). Susac himself believed that his syndrome was a form of primary angiitis of the CNS, and emphasizes that there are microinfarctions of the cortex, white matter, and leptomeninges on brain biopsies (Susac, 2004). The first published stroke patient (Patient 1; see Table 34.1 for the analysis of the 23 cases following) with APMPPE (Holt et al., 1976) was a 22-year-old man who, 3 weeks after a flu-like episode, developed bilateral middle cerebral artery (MCA) transient ischemic attacks (TIAs) (aphasia, right-side paresis; numbness and/or weakness of left arm). Tc-99 brain scan was normal (1973), but carotid angiograms showed "attenuation, lumen irregularity, and abrupt termination of various small opercular branches and distal cortical vessels of the bilateral MCAs," and CSF analysis showed a pleiocytosis (Table 34.2). The neurological symptoms improved before the initiation of corticosteroids (3 weeks later). Another Tc-99 and rudimentary computed axial tomography-proven (1979) occipital infarct (contralateral hemianopia) in an 18-year-old (migrainous) man with APMPPE was published (Sigelman et al., 1979); again, carotid angiography showed multiple focal narrowing of MCA branches, whereas hyperproteinorachia with mild pleiocytosis were found on CSF. The first CT proven (occipital) stroke was further reported by Smith et al. (1983). All three cases fulfilled the criteria for the diagnosis of primary angiitis of the CNS (Lie, 1997). The fourth case (Patient 4) has been mistaken in the literature for recurrent APMPPE-associated meningoencephalitis with an exceptional long time interval of 5 years (Kersten et al., 1987). However, the CSF analysis gave negative results for bacterial, fungal, and viral cultures, although it showed 151 WBCs with a predominance of lymphocytes. CT scan and electroencephalogram (EEG) were normal, and corticosteroids (oral prednisone 100 mg/day) were initiated for a "presumed CNS vasculitis," which produced a "dramatic improvement" of the patient's symptoms. As soon as prednisone was tapered, her symptoms recurred, corticosteroids were re-initiated (prednisone 30 mg/day), and the patient experienced abnormal movements (chorea). The second EEG showed bursts of diffuse slowing, and repeated spinal taps gave normal findings (4 WBC/mL), including cytology, and extensive repeated infection research (extended to Cryptococcus and tuberculosis), tuberculin skin test, and Lyme serologies were negative, as were antinuclear antibodies. The patient could not be weaned from corticosteroid treatment for 10 months, and a conventional four-vessel angiogram performed on steroid treatment was normal.

To date, 20 additional cases with APMPPE and primary angiitis of the CNS (or CNS vasculitis in the setting of systemic vasculitis or sarcoidosis) and/or CVDs have been published (Al Kawi et al., 2004; Althaus et al., 1993; Bewermeyer et al., 1993; Bodiguel et al., 1992; Bugnone et al., 2006; Comu et al., 1996; de Vries et al., 2006; Engelinus et al., 1999; Hammer et al., 1989; O'Halloran et al., 2001; Reinthal et al., 2001; Stoll et al., 1991; Weinstein et al., 1988; Wilson et al., 1988), including one patient (Patient 7, Table 34.1) reported by personal communication from C. H. Smith to J. M. Weinstein (Weinstein et al., 1988). Their demographic data (age, gender, ethnical APMPPE origin), headache and/or meningeal signs, clinical pattern of CNS insult, radiological and MB or necropsy findings, CSF analysis results (WBC/mL, protein content), latencies between diagnosis of APMPPE and CNS insult, outcome, and therapy are summarized in Table 34.1. Compared with patients with isolated APMPPE (Jones, 1995), APMPPE patients with CNS complications are slightly older (mean 30 ± 11 vs. 26.5 years), are usually men (20 cases, 87%) contrary to the aforementioned near equal male-to-female ratio for patients with APMPPE without CNS involvement, and are usually white (21/23, 91%); noteworthy, the two remaining cases were half-cast native American and Asian, respectively.

Overall, patients showed the following classical prodromic symptoms at the time of APMPPE diagnosis: headache in nearly three-quarters (17, 74%) and flu-like symptoms in near one-third (7, 30%). However, concomitant signs of meningeal irritation (nausea, vomiting, photophobia, stiff neck) were also present in nearly one-third (7, 30%), whereas signs of aseptic meningitis with elevated WBC (mean, 61 WBC/mL; range 5–177) were confirmed in 86% of patients who underwent spinal tap (12/14), except patients 5 and 18. Only one patient showed elevated red blood cells (RBC) (Patient 5) (Wilson et al., 1988). Furthermore, all but one (Patient 14) (Engelinus et al., 1999) (93%, 13/14) showed signs of blood-brain barrier disruption with elevated protein content (mean, 1019 mg/L; range 330–3000 mg/L). Overall, these findings are consistent with the diagnosis of PACNS. The CNS insult was inaugural in five cases (22%, 5/23), whereas the mean latency from diagnosis of APMPPE to CNS involvement was 11 weeks (range 0.5–48 weeks) in 17 cases (74%), with three of them recurrent CNS lesions: one recurrence within 12 weeks in Patient 6 (Weinstein et al., 1988) and 22 (Bugnone et al., 2006), and two recurrences at 8 and 12 weeks, respectively, in Patient 13 (Case 1) (Comu et al., 1996). The remaining patient (Patient 4) (Kersten et al., 1987) had an exceptionaly long latency of 5 years.

The APMPPE-associated CVDs consisted in CVT with bilateral parietal hemorrhagic strokes with increased intracranial pressure

(ICP) in one case (4%) (Patient 16, Case 1) (O'Halloran et al., 2001), with favorable outcome following craniotomy and anticoagulation therapy, whereas brain biopsy gave normal results. Two other patients developed bilateral diffuse hemispheric ischemic infarctions with elevated ICP leading to death despite corticosteroid therapy, related to confirmed granulomatous angiitis of the CNS (Patient 5) (Wilson et al., 1988), and suspected primary angiitis of the CNS (Patient 8) (Hammer et al., 1989). Another patient with bilateral hemispheric ischemic infarcts correlating with confirmed granulomatous angiitis of the CNS died in the setting of multisystemic granulomatous involvement (de Vries et al., 2006). Overall, the mortality of the present series was 13% (3/23).

Overall, cortical territorial strokes occurred in nearly two-thirds of patients (70%, 16/23). The most frequent cortical arterial territory involved in this series was the posterior cerebral artery (PCA), with occipital ischemic strokes (homonymous hemianopia) found in more than one-third of patients (39%, 9/23), and which occurred as isolated infarcts in one-third of them: Patient 2 (Sigelman et al., 1979), Patient 3 (Smith et al., 1983), and Patient 7 reported by Smith in Weinstein et al. (1988). Two cases developed secondary hemorrhagic occipital strokes: Patient 6 (Weinstein et al., 1988) and Patient 13 (Case 1) (Comu et al., 1996). The remaining six patients had associated MCA territory (Patients 5, 13, 14, 21, and 23) or deep infarcts (Patients 6 and 13).

Territorial MCA ischemic infarcts, found in 30% of cases (7/23), occurred isolated (temporal) in only one patient (Patient 19) (O'Halloran et al., 2001), and were multiple (Patients 14, 21, and 23), or multiple and bilateral (Patients 5, 8, and 13); were associated with PCA (Patients 5, 13, 14, 21, and 23) or anterior cerebral artery (ACA) (Patient 8); and were deep (Patient 13) ischemic strokes in the remaining cases. Bilateral MCA TIAs occurred in only one case (Patient 1) (Holt et al., 1976). The pattern of deep infarcts occurred in 39% of cases (9/23), involving the deep white matter in three-quarters (77%, 7/9) (Patients 6, 9, 10, 12, 15, 18, and 22), and comprising striatocapsular infarction in four (Patients 6, 13, 15, and 22), pontine (Patients 9, 11, and 12) or thalamic (Patients 9, 12, and 18) ischemic stroke in three cases each, and bulbar (Patient 15) or corpus callosum (Patient 22) infarct in one case each. Two of them had associated PCA (Patient 6) and both MCA and PCA (Patient 13) territorial strokes.

Regarding the etiology of CVD complications in the present series, the diagnosis of primary angiitis of the CNS (Patients 4, 8, 13, 14, and 20) and the subcortical type of primary angiitis of the CNS (Patients 15, 18, and 22) could only be suspected in one-third of cases (8/23), because MRI, angiography, histology, and CSF were not available. In 57% of cases (13/23), the diagnosis of vasculitis of the CNS was confirmed by abnormal conventional angiogram in 77% (10/13), by brain biopsy in two (Patients 5 and 23), and by muscle biopsy in the remaining case (Patient 11). The vasculitis of the CNS subtype were the following: primary angiitis of the CNS (Patients 1, 2, 3, 6, 7, 17, and 21) in near half (54%, 7/13), subcortical PACNS (Patients 9 and 12), and true granulomatous angiitis of the CNS with Langerhans cells on brain histology (Patients 5 and 23) in two cases each, and aspecific vasculitis (Patient 11) in the remaining patient. Two of them showed signs of a more multisystemic vasculitic process: Patient 11 showed signs of vasculitis

(T cell-mediated) on muscle biopsy (Althaus *et al.*, 1993; Bewermeyer *et al.*, 1993), whereas Patient 23 had a multisystemic granulomatous angiitis with Langhans cells on autopsy (de Vries *et al.*, 2006). One patient (Patient 10) had probable sarcoidosis (Bodiguel *et al.*, 1992) (see Chapter 13), whereas no specific cause for the CVT could be found in Patient 16 with APMPPE (O'Halloran *et al.*, 2001).

All but two patients (Patients 2 and 23) received corticosteroid therapy, including the latter patient with CVT, with additional azathioprine in three (Patients 9, 11, and 12), cyclophosphamide (Patients 13 and 17) or anticoagulation therapy (Patients 16 and 21) in two cases each. Among the 20 survivors (80%), 80% of them (16/20; total, 70%, 16/23) showed a favorable outcome without neurological deficits, whereas three had partial resolution of symptoms (Patients 6, 7, and 13), including two cases with persistent hemianopia (Patients 6 and 13). The remaining patient (Patient 14) had an unknown outcome.

Conclusion

APMPPE, a rare multifocal choroidopathy syndrome characterized by choroidal occlusive vasculitis, affects young white adults (mean, 27 years old) and presents with blurring of vision after a flu-like episode. Various etiologies have been found (infectious/postinfectious; vaccinations; inflammations; autoimmune diseases; vasculitis; paraneoplastic syndrome). The main differences with the two other "uveo-cerebral vasculitic syndrome" are the following: Eales diseases, an angiitis confined to retinal arteries involves rarely cerebral arteries, affects young men (range 20–40 years) from India and the Middle East, whereas Susac's syndrome, a microangiopathy of the retina, cochlea, and brain with frequent corpus callosum small infarctions, affects young women (mean 30 years). The neurological complications of APMPPE are headache, aseptic meningitis, encephalitis, multiple sclerosis-like disease, and pseudotumor cerebri. CVDs associated with APMPPE consist of ischemic cortical strokes (70%) involving the PCA (39%) and the MCA (30%), and deep infarcts (39%) with striatocapsular infarctions in nearly half of them. CVTs with lobar hemorrhages are rare (4%). Vasculitis of the CNS, found in more then half of cases (57%), confirmed by abnormal angiogram in three-quarters of them, comprises primary angiitis of the CNS (half of cases), subcortical primary angiitis of the CNS, and granulomatous angiitis of the CNS with Langerhans cells in 15% each. Elevated WBC (mean, 61 WBC/mL) and increased protein content (mean, 1 g/L) were found in 86% and 93% of patients who underwent spinal tap, respectively. These CVDs and vasculitis of the CNS were the initial findings in 22% of cases, and appeared at a mean of 3 months after the diagnosis of APMPPE in 74% of patients. Classical prodromic symptoms such as headache and flu-like symptoms occurred in 74% and 30% of cases, respectively. Noteworthy, and contrary to patients with isolated APMPPE, these patients with vascular complications of the CNS were predominantly men (87%). On corticosteroids in 91% of patients and additional immunosuppressive therapy (azathioprine, cyclophosphamide) in a minority of them, the outcome was favorable in 70% of patients, whereas persistent neurological deficits (hemi-anopia) and mortality were found in 13% of patients each, respectively.

REFERENCES

Al Kawi, A., Wang, D. Z., Kishore, K., and Kattah, J. C. 2004. A case of ischemic cerebral infarction associated with acute posterior multifocal placoid pigment epitheliopathy, CNS vasculitis, vitamin B(12) deficiency and homocysteinemia. *Cerebrovasc Dis*, **18**, 338–9.

Althaus, C., Unsold, R., Figge, C., and Sundmacher, R. 1993. Cerebral complications in acute posterior multifocal placoid pigment epitheliopathy. *Ger J Ophthalmol*, **2**, 150–4.

Anderson, K., Patel, K. R., Webb, L., and Dutton, G. N. 1996. Acute posterior multifocal placoid pigment epitheliopathy associated with pulmonary tuberculosis (letter). *Br J Ophthalmol*, **80**, 186.

Annesley, W. H., Tomer, T. L., and Shields, J. A. 1973. Multifocal placoid pigment epitheliopathy. *Am J Ophthalmol*, **76**, 511–8.

Azar, P., Gohd, R. S., Waltman, D., and Gitter, K. A. 1975. Acute posterior multifocal placoid pigment epitheliopathy associated with adenovirus type 5 infection. *Am J Ophthalmol*, **80**, 1003–5.

Bewermeyer, H., Nelles, G., Huber, M., *et al.* 1993. Pontine infarction in acute posterior multifocal placoid pigment epitheliopathy. *J Neurol*, **241**, 22–6.

Biswas, J., Raghavendran, R., Pinakin, G., and Arjundas, D. 2001. Presumed Eales' disease with neurologic involvement: report of three cases. *Retina*, **21**, 141–5.

Bodiguel, E., Benhamou, A., Le Hoang, P., and Gautier, J. C. 1992. Infarctus cérébral, épithéliopathie en plaques et sarcoïdose. *Rev Neurol (Paris)*, **148**, 746–51.

Bodine, S. R., Marino, J., Camisa, T. J., and Salvate, A. J. 1992. Multifocal choroiditis with evidence of Lyme disease. *Ann Ophthalmol*, **24**, 169–73.

Borruat, F. X., Piguet, B., and Herbort, C. P. 1998. Acute posterior multifocal placoid pigment epitheliopathy following mumps. *Ocul Immunol Inflamm*, **6**, 189–93.

Brazis, P. W., Stewart, M., and Lee, A. G. 2004. The uveo-meningeal syndromes. *Neurologist*, **10**, 171–84.

Brézin, A. P., Massin-Korobelnik, P., Boudin, M., Gaudric, A., and LeHoang, P. 1995. Acute posterior multifocal placoid pigment epitheliopathy after hepatitis B vaccine. *Arch Ophthalmol*, **113**, 297–300.

Bridges, W. J., Saadeh, C., and Gerald, R. 1995. Acute posterior multifocal placoid pigment epitheliopathy in a patient with systemic-onset juvenile rheumatoid arthritis: treatment with cyclosporin A and prednisone. *Arthritis Rheum*, **38**, 446–7.

Brown, M., Eberdt, A., and Ladas, G. 1973. Pigment epitheliopathy in a patient with mycobacterium infection. *J Ped Ophthalmol*, **10**, 278–81.

Bugnone, A. N., Hartker, F., Shapiro, M., Pineless, H. S., and Velez, G. 2006. Acute and chronic brain infarcts on MR imaging in a 20-year-old woman with acute posterior multifocal placoid pigment epitheliopathy. *AJNR Am J Neuroradiol*, **27**, 67–9.

Bullock, J. D., and Fletcher, R. L. 1977. Cerebrospinal fluid abnormalities in acute posterior multifocal placoid pigment epitheliopathy. *Am J Ophthalmol*, **84**, 45–9.

Caccavale, A., and Mignemi, L. 2001. Fluorescein and indocyanine green angiography findings in a case of poststreptococcal syndrome with erythema nodosum and posterior uveitis. *Retina*, **21**, 669–72.

Chiquet, C., Lumbroso, L., Denis, P., *et al.* 1999. Acute posterior multifocal placoid pigment epitheliopathy associated with Wegener's granulomatosis. *Retina*, **19**, 309–13.

Clearkin, L. G., and Hung, S. O. 1983. Acute posterior multifocal placoid pigment epitheliopathy associated with transient hearing loss. *Trans Ophthalmol Soc UK*, **103**, 562–4.

Comu, S., Verstraeten, T., Rinkoff, J. S., and Busis, N. A. 1996. Neurological manifestations of acute posterior multifocal placoid pigment epitheliopathy. *Stroke*, **27**, 996–1001.

de Vries, J. J., den Dunnen, W. F., Timmerman, E. A., Kruithof, I. G., and De Keyser, J. 2006. Acute posterior multifocal placoid pigment epitheliopathy with cerebral vasculitis: a multisystem granulomatous disease. *Arch Ophthalmol*, **124**, 910–3.

Deutman, A. F., Oosterhuis, J. A., Boen-Tan, T. N., and Aan De Kerk, A. L. 1972. Acute posterior multifocal placoid pigment epitheliopathy. Pigment epitheliopathy or choriocapillaritis. *Br J Ophthalmol*, **56**, 863–74.

Dhaliwal, R. S., Maguire, A. M., Flower, R. W., and Arribas, N. P. 1993. Acute posterior multifocal placoid pigment epitheliopathy. An indocyanine green angiographic study. *Retina*, **13**, 317–25.

Di Crecchio, L., Parodi, M. B., Saviano, S., and Ravalico, G. 2001. Acute posterior multifocal placoid pigment epitheliopathy and ulcerative colitis: a possible association. *Acta Ophthalmol Scand*, **79**, 319–21.

Dick, D. J., Newman, P. K., Richardson, J., Wilkinson, R., and Morley, A. R. 1988. Acute posterior multifocal placoid pigment epitheliopathy and sarcoidosis. *Br J Ophthalmol*, **72**, 74–7.

Dickinson, A. J., Rosenthal, A. R., and Nicholson, K. G. 1990. Inflammation of the retinal pigment epithelium: a unique presentation of ocular schistosomiasis. *Br J Ophthalmol*, **74**, 440–2.

Engelinus, F., Rasquin, F., Blecic, S., and Zanen, A. 1999. [Placoid pigment epitheliopathy and cerebral vasculitis: a clinical case]. *Bull Soc Belge Ophthalmol*, **274**, 41–6.

Ferro, J. M. 1998. Vasculitis of the central nervous system. *J Neurol*, **245**, 766–76.

Fishman, G. A., Baskin, M., and Jednock, N. 1977. Spinal fluid pleocytosis in acute posterior multifocal placoid pigment epitheliopathy. *Ann Ophthalmol*, **9**, 36.

Foulds, W. S., and Damato, B. E. 1986. Investigations and prognosis in the retinal pigment epitheliopathies. *Aust N Z J Ophthalmol*, **14**, 301–11.

Frohman, L. P., Klug, R., Bielory, L., Patti, J. C., and Noble, K. G. 1987. Acute posterior multifocal placoid pigment epitheliopathy with unilateral retinal lesions and bilateral disk edema. *Am J Ophthalmol*, **104**, 548–50.

Furusho, F., Imaizumi, H., and Takeda, M. 2001. One case of Harada disease complicated by acute posterior multifocal placoid pigment epitheliopathy-like recurrence in both eyes. *Jpn J Ophthalmol*, **45**, 117–8.

Gass, J. D. 1993. Acute zonal occult outer retinopathy. Donders Lecture: The Netherlands Ophthalmological Society, Maastricht, Holland, June 19, 1992. *J Clin Neuroophthalmol*, **13**, 79–97.

Gass, J. D. 2000. The acute zonal outer retinopathies. *Am J Ophthalmol*, **130**, 655–7.

Gass, J. D. 2003a. Acute posterior multifocal placoid pigment epitheliopathy. 1968. *Retina*, **23**, 177–85.

Gass, J. D. 2003b. Are acute zonal occult outer retinopathy and the white spot syndromes (AZOOR complex) specific autoimmune diseases? *Am J Ophthalmol*, **135**, 380–1.

Gass, J. D., Braunstein, R. A., and Chenoweth, R. G. 1990. Acute syphilitic posterior placoid chorioretinitis. *Ophthalmology*, **97**, 1288–97.

Gass, J. D. M. 1968. Acute posterior multifocal placoid pigment epitheliopathy. *Arch Ophthalmol*, **80**, 177–85.

Gass, J. D. M. 1983. Acute posterior multifocal placoid pigment epitheliopathy: a long-term follow up. In *Management of Retinal Vascular and Macular Disorder*, eds. S. L. Fine, and L. Owens. Baltimore, MD: Williams and Wilkins Co., pp. 176–81.

Gordon, M. F., Coyle, P. K. and Golub, B. 1988. Eales' disease presenting as stroke in the young adult. *Ann Neurol*, **24**, 264–6.

Hammer, M. E., Grizzard, W. S., and Travies, D. 1989. Death associated with acute multifocal placoid pigment epitheliopathy. *Arch Ophthalmol*, **107**, 170–1.

Hector, R. E. 1978. Acute posterior multifocal posterior pigment epitheliopathy. *Am J Ophthalmol*, **86**, 424–5.

Hedges, T. R. III, Sinclair, S. H., and Gragoudas, E. S. 1979. Evidence for vasculitis in acute posterior multifocal placoid pigment epitheliopathy. *Ann Ophthalmol*, **11**, 539–42.

Holt, W. S., Regan, C. D. J., and Trempe, C. 1976. Acute posterior multifocal placoid pigment epitheliopathy. *Am J Ophthalmol*, **81**, 403–12.

Howe, L. J., Woon, H., Graham, E. M., et al. 1995. Choroidal hypoperfusion in acute posterior multifocal placoid pigment epitheliopathy. *Ophthalmology*, **102**, 790–8.

Hsu, C. T., Harlan, J. B., Goldberg, M. F., and Dunn, J. P. 2003. Acute posterior multifocal placoid pigment epitheliopathy associated with a systemic necrotizing vasculitis. *Retina*, **23**, 64–8.

Jacklin, H. N. 1977. Acute posterior multifocal placoid pigment epitheliopathy and thyroiditis. *Arch Ophthalmol*, **95**, 995–7.

Jampol, L. M., and Becker, K. G. 2003. White spot syndromes of the retina: a hypothesis based on the common genetic hypothesis of autoimmune/inflammatory disease. *Am J Ophthalmol*, **135**, 376–9.

Jenkins, R. B., Savino, P. J., Pilkerton, A. R. 1973. Placoid pigment epitheliopathy with swelling of the optic disks. *Arch Neurol*, **29**, 204–5.

Jimenez, P. E., Marsal, C., Velazquez, J. M., and Alvarez, A. 2003. [Eales' disease with bilateral brain strokes and jaw-closing dystonia]. *Neurologia*, **18**, 750–3.

Jones, N. P. 1995. Acute posterior multifocal placoid pigment epitheliopathy. *Br J Ophthalmol*, **79**, 384–9.

Katz, B., Wheeler, D., Weinreb, R. N., and Swenson, M. R. 1991. Eales' disease with central nervous system infarction. *Ann Ophthalmol*, **23**, 460–3.

Kawaguchi, Y., Hara, M., Hirose, T., et al. 1990. A case of SLE complicated with multifocal posterior pigment epitheliopathy. *Ryumachi*, **30**, 396–402.

Kersten, D. H., Lessell, S., and Carlow, T. J. 1987. Acute posterior multifocal placoid pigment epitheliopathy and late-onset meningo-encephalitis. *Ophthalmology*, **94**, 393–6.

Kim, R. Y., Holz, F. G., Gregor, Z., and Bird, A. C. 1995. Recurrent acute multifocal placoid pigment epitheliopathy in two cousins. *Am J Ophthalmol*, **119**, 660–2.

Kirkham, T. H., Ffytche, T. J., and Sanders, M. D. 1972. Placoid pigment epitheliopathy with retinal vasculitis and papillitis. *Br J Ophthalmol*, **56**, 875–80.

Kumaravelu, S., Johri, S., Mukherji, J. D., Poduval, R. G., and Bhandari, N. K. 2002. Eales' disease with neurological manifestations. *J Assoc Physicians India*, **50**, 596–8.

Laatikainen, L. T., and Immonen, I. J. 1988. Acute posterior multifocal placoid pigment epitheliopathy in connection with acute nephritis. *Retina*, **8**, 122–4.

Lie, J. T. 1997. Classification and histopathologic spectrum of central nervous system vasculitis. *Neurol Clin*, **15**, 805–19.

Lowder, C. Y., Foster, R. E., Gordon, S. M., and Gutman, F. A. 1996. Acute posterior multifocal placoid pigment epitheliopathy after acute group A streptococcal infection. *Am J Ophthalmol*, **122**, 115–7.

Lyness, A. L., and Bird, A. C. 1984. Recurrences of acute posterior multifocal placoid pigment epitheliopathy. *Am J Ophthalmol*, **98**, 203–7.

Matsuo, T., Horikoshi, T., and Nagai, C. 2002. Acute posterior multifocal placoid pigment epitheliopathy and scleritis in a patient with pANCA-positive systemic vasculitis. *Am J Ophthalmol*, **133**, 566–8.

Matsuo, T., Nakayama, T., Koyama, T., and Matsuo, N. 1987. Multifocal pigment epithelial damages with serous retinal detachment in systemic lupus erythematosus. *Ophthalmologica*, **195**, 97–102.

Misra, U. K., Jha, S., Kalita, J., and Sharma, K. 1996. Stroke – a rare presentation of Eales' disease. A case report. *Angiology*, **47**, 73–6.

O'Halloran, H. S., Berger, J. R., Lee, W. B., et al. 2001. Acute multifocal placoid pigment epitheliopathy and central nervous system involvement: nine new cases and a review of the literature. *Ophthalmology*, **108**, 861–8.

O'Halloran, H. S., Pearson, P. A., Lee, W. B., Susac, J. O., and Berger, J. R. 1998. Microangiopathy of the brain, retina, and cochlea (Susac syndrome). A report of five cases and a review of the literature. *Ophthalmology*, **105**, 1038–44.

Park, D., Schatz, H., McDonald, H. R., and Johnson, R. N. 1995a. Acute multifocal posterior placoid pigment epitheliopathy: a theory of pathogenesis. *Retina*, **15**, 351–2.

Park, D., Schatz, H., McDonald, H. R., and Johnson, R. N. 1995b. Indocyanine green angiography of acute multifocal posterior placoid pigment epitheliopathy. *Ophthalmology*, **102**, 1877–83.

Parmeggiani, F., Costagliola, C., D'Angelo, S., et al. 2004. Clear cell renal cell carcinoma associated with bilateral atypical acute posterior multifocal placoid pigment epitheliopathy. *Oncology*, **66**, 502–9.

Priluck, I. A., Robertson, D. M., and Buettner, H. 1981. Acute posterior multifocal placoid pigment epitheliopathy. Urinary findings. *Arch Ophthalmol*, **99**, 1560–2.

Reinthal, E. K., Schlote, T., and Zierhut, M. 2001. [Neurological complications in acute posterior multifocal placoid pigment epitheliopathy (APMPPE)–a review with case report]. *Klin Monatsbl Augenheilkd*, **218**, 756–62.

Roberts, T. V., and Mitchell, P. 1997. Acute posterior multifocal placoid pigment epitheliopathy: a long-term study. *Aust N Z J Ophthalmol*, **25**, 277–81.

Ruiz Vinals, A. T., Buil Calvo, J. A., Martinez, G. O., and Castilla, C. M. 2002. [Acute posterior multifocal placoid pigment epitheliopathy associated with Graves-Basedow's disease]. *Arch Soc Esp Oftalmol*, **77**, 381–4.

Ryan, S. J., and Maumenee, A. E. 1972. Acute posterior multifocal placoid pigment epitheliopathy. *Am J Ophthalmol*, **74**, 1066–74.

Savino, P. J., Weinberg, R. J., Yassin, J. G., and Pilkerton, A. R. 1974. Diverse manifestations of acute posterior multifocal placoid pigment epitheliopathy. *Am J Ophthalmol*, **77**, 659–62.

Schubert, H. D., Lucier, A. C., and Bosley, T. M. 1988. Pigmentary epitheliopathy, disc edema, and lead intoxication. *Retina*, **8**, 154–7.

Sigelman, J., Behrens, M., and Hilal, S. 1979. Acute posterior multifocal placoid pigment epitheliopathy associated with cerebral vasculitis and homonymous hemianopia. *Am J Ophthalmol*, **88**, 919–24.

Smith, C. H., Savino, P. J., Beck, R. W., Schatz, N. J., and Sergott, R. C. 1983. Acute posterior multifocal placoid pigment epitheliopathy and cerebral vasculitis. *Arch Neurol*, **40**, 48–50.

Spaide, R. F., Yanuzzi, L. A., and Slakter, J. 1991. Choroidal vasculitis in acute posterior multifocal placoid pigment epitheliopathy. *Br J Ophthalmol*, **75**, 685–7.

Stanga, P. E., Lim, J. I., and Hamilton, P. 2003. Indocyanine green angiography in chorioretinal diseases: indications and interpretation: an evidence-based update. *Ophthalmology*, **110**, 15–21.

Stoll, G., Reiners, K., Schwartz, A., *et al.* 1991. Acute posterior multifocal placoid pigment epitheliopathy with cerebral involvement. *J Neurol Neurosurg Psychiatr*, **54**, 77–9.

Susac, J. O. 2004. Susac's syndrome. *AJNR Am J Neuroradiol*, **25**, 351–2.

Susac, J. O., Hardman, J. M., and Selhorst, J. B. 1979. Microangiopathy of the brain and retina. *Neurology*, **29**, 313–6.

Susac, J. O., Murtagh, F. R., Egan, R. A., *et al.* 2003. MRI findings in Susac's syndrome. *Neurology*, **61**, 1783–7.

Suzuki, S., Mizota, A., and chi-Usami, E. 2002. A case of hemophagocytic syndrome with retinal changes resembling acute posterior multifocal placoid pigment epitheliopathy. *Retina*, **22**, 219–22.

Thomson, S. P., and Roxburgh, S. T. 2003. Acute posterior multifocal placoid pigment epitheliopathy associated with adenovirus infection (letter). *Eye*, **17**, 542–4.

Toenjes, W., Mielke, U., Schmidt, H. J., Haas, A., and Holzer, G. 1989. Akute multifokale plakoide Pigmentepitheliopathie mit entzuendlichem Liquorbefund. Sonderform einer Borreliose? *Dtsch med Wschr*, **114**, 793–5.

Uthman, I., Najjar, D. M., Kanj, S. S., and Bashshur, Z. 2003. Anticardiolipin antibodies in acute multifocal posterior placoid pigment epitheliopathy. *Ann Rheum Dis*, **62**, 687–8.

Uyama, M., Matsunaga, H., Matsubara, T., *et al.* 1999. Indocyanine green angiography and pathophysiology of multifocal posterior pigment epitheliopathy. *Retina*, **19**, 12–21.

Van Buskirk, E. M., Lessell, S., and Friedman, E. 1971. Pigmentary epitheliopathy and erythema nodosum. *Arch Ophthalmol*, **85**, 369–72.

Weinstein, J. M., Bresnik, G. H., Bell, C. L., *et al.* 1988. Acute posterior multifocal placoid pigment epitheliopathy associated with cerebral vasculitis. *J Clin Neuroophthalmol*, **8**, 195–201.

Williams, D. F., and Mieler, W. F. 1989. Long-term follow-up of acute multifocal posterior placoid pigment epitheliopathy. *Br J Ophthalmol*, **73**, 985–90.

Wilson, C. A., Choromokos, E. A., and Sheppard, R. 1988. Acute posterior multifocal placoid pigment epitheliopathy and cerebral vasculitis. *Arch Ophthalmol*, **106**, 796–800.

Wolf, M. D., Alward, W. L., and Folk, J. C. 1991. Long-term visual function in acute posterior multifocal placoid pigment epitheliopathy. *Arch Ophthalmol*, **109**, 800–3.

Wolf, M. D., Folk, J. C., and Goeken, N. E. 1990a. Acute posterior multifocal pigment epitheliopathy and optic neuritis in a family. *Am J Ophthalmol*, **110**, 89–90.

Wolf, M. D., Folk, J. C., Panknen, C. A., and Goeken, N. E. 1990b. HLA-B7 and HLA-DR2 antigens and acute posterior multifocal placoid pigment epitheliopathy. *Arch Ophthalmol*, **108**, 698–700.

Wright, B. E., Bird, A. C., and Hamilton, A. M. 1978. Placoid pigment epitheliopathy and Harada's disease. *Br J Ophthalmol*, **62**, 609–21.

Yang, D. S., Hilford, D. J., and Conrad, D. 2005. Acute posterior multifocal placoid pigment epitheliopathy after meningococcal C conjugate vaccine. *Clin Experiment Ophthalmol*, **33**, 219–21.

Zuber, M., Blustajn, J., Arquizan, C., *et al.* 1999. Angiitis of the central nervous system. *J Neuroradiol*, **26**, 101–17.

35 MICROANGIOPATHY OF THE RETINA, INNER EAR, AND BRAIN: SUSAC'S SYNDROME

Isabel Lestro Henriques, Julien Bogousslavsky, and Louis R. Caplan

First reports and eponyms

Two young women with a multifocal nonembolic occlusion of the retinal arteries, with brain involvement classified as probable disseminated lupus erythematosus were described in 1973 by Pfaffenbach and Hollenhorst. Other partial forms of what is nowadays considered Susac's syndrome were described in patients with retinal vascular occlusions and bilateral sensorineural hearing loss, but with no brain involvement (Delaney and Torrisi, 1976). The complete clinical triad of encephalopathy, deafness, and retinal artery branch occlusions was first reported in 1979 by Susac, including one patient observed in 1975 by Susac and another submitted by Selhorst. With the contribution of the neuropathologist Hardiman, they reported these patients as having a microangiopathy of the brain and retina (Susac et al., 1979).

During the 1980s, a total of 13 new patients were reported with similar descriptions (Bogousslavsky et al., 1989; Coppeto et al., 1984; Heiskala et al., 1988; MacFadyen et al., 1987; Mass et al., 1988; Monteiro et al., 1985). Until then, all patients were women of childbearing age. The first description of a male patient appeared in 1996 referring to a 29-year-old man who presented with a triad and a comparable outcome concerning clinical and laboratory evaluation (Ballard et al., 1996). Early reports of similar syndromes, confined only to two systems (inner ear and retina or retina and brain), were published, but it is not certain if they represent the same entity with atypical (incomplete) presentation or a different disease (Delaney and Torrisi, 1976; McCabe, 1979; Pfaffenbach and Hollenhorst, 1973; Susac et al., 1979).

Different designations of what is supposed to be the same clinical entity have been used. After it was designated as microangiopathy of the brain and retina, Coppeto et al. (1984) referred to it as an arterial occlusive retinopathy and encephalopathy. Mass et al. (1988) designated it as RED-M (Retinopathy, Encephalopathy, Deafness-associated Microangiopathy) syndrome, and Bogousslavsky et al. (1989) as retinocochleocerebral arteriolopathy. Schwitter et al. (1992) referred to it as SICRET (Small Infarction of Cochlear, Retinal, and Encephalic Tissue) syndrome. Since 1994, after the review of the syndrome by Susac in Neurology (Susac, 1994), the eponym Susac's syndrome is generally used in publications.

Clinical features

Prototypic case

A Caucasian woman of childbearing age with no significant previous history develops a subacute neurological syndrome with a triad of diffuse encephalopathy, neurosensory auditory dysfunction, and retinal involvement, without evidence of systemic illness. The course of the disease is self-limited, with three clinical bursts of disease activity, and achieves a "steady state" after 2 years with minimal neurological deficit including neurosensorial hearing deficit. No more bursts are observed, and deficits are stable in the long-term follow-up. Repeated laboratory data are negative for systemic diseases including connective tissue disease, procoagulant states, infection, demyelinating disease, neoplasia, and current mechanisms of cerebral and retinal ischemia.

Clinical presentation

The triad of encephalopathy, hearing loss, and retinal artery branch occlusions usually develops in patients without any remarkable previous medical history. However, previous behavioral disturbances and personality changes a few weeks or months before the onset of other symptoms can be found, as well as headache that can be the presenting symptom. Diffuse encephalopathy with difficulties in auditory and visual perception are common (Bogousslavsky et al., 1989), and a smoother onset is also observed with the involvement of the brain, inner ear, and retina not always simultaneous. Psychiatric and cognitive disturbances, multifocal neurological symptoms, memory loss, and confusion can rapidly progress to dementia.

Most published patients (more than 80) are Caucasian women, although Asian, South American, and Australian patients are also described (Murata et al., 2000; Saw et al., 2000; Skacel et al., 2000). Age of patients varies between 8 and 58 years, but most of the patients are 20–40 years old when diagnosis is made (Delaney and Torrisi, 1976; Susac et al., 2007). Table 35.1 summarizes the main clinical features.

Encephalopathy

In one-quarter of patients, the first attack is preceded by slowly progressive personality and mental changes (Susac, 1994).

Uncommon Causes of Stroke, 2nd edition, ed. Louis R. Caplan. Published by Cambridge University Press. © Cambridge University Press 2008.

Table 35.1 Common clinical signs in Susac's syndrome
Eye; Branch retinal arteriolar occlusions
Hearing loss: Neurosensory, bilateral
Encephalopathy: Personality / behavioral changes / headache
Long tract signs

Table 35.2 Diagnostic criteria in Susac's syndrome
Neurosensory hearing loss*
Retinal branch arteriolar occlusion**
Encephalopathy
Central callosal MRI lesions***

* Bilateral neurosensory hearing loss, in low and medium frequencies.

** Bilateral distal retinal branch arteriolar occlusions with arterial narrowing, and microvascular lesions showing increased vascular permeability.

*** Supports the diagnosis when only two of the triad features are present.

Cognitive dysfunction is characterized by short-term memory loss and periods of apathy or disorientation. Prodromal symptoms of encephalopathy include headache and psychiatric features such as slowly progressive personality changes, with indifference, mood changes, eating disorders, bizarre behavior, or hallucinations (MacFadyen *et al.*, 1987). Neuropsychological testing in one man suggested diffuse cerebral dysfunction, with presumed prominent involvement of reciprocal diencephalic-cortical projections (Ballard *et al.*, 1996). Primitive reflexes may also be present as well as long tract signs. Ataxic gait, pseudobulbar speech, dysmetria, hyperactive tendon reflexes, Babinski's sign, and nystagmus of vestibular or nonvestibular origin are the most commonly referred motor signs. Cranial nerve palsies (III, VI, VII), hemidysesthesia, urinary incontinence, and hemiparesis are less frequent. Generalized tonic-clonic seizures and myoclonus may also occur.

Retinopathy and hearing loss

In Susac's syndrome, diagnostic signs involve the retina. In most patients, the abnormalities are readily seen through an ordinary ophthalmoscope. Some retinal arteries are amputated whereas others are severely narrowed. The thickened arterial walls produce a "light-streaking" effect. Multiple bilateral retinal branch occlusions can coexist. Fundoscopic examination shows arteriolar occlusions with narrowing of arterioles, as well as signs of other ischemic changes in the affected vascular area, such as edema and increased vascular permeability (Figures 35.1 and 35.2). The macula may show a cherry-red appearance (Coppeto *et al.*, 1984). Fluorescein angiography is often helpful in showing the vascular

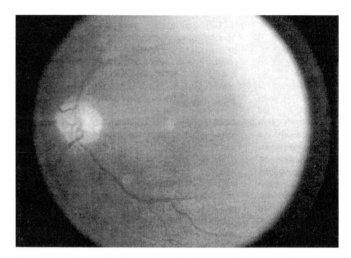

Figure 35.2 Left optic fundus: perimacular edema and arteriolar occlusion.

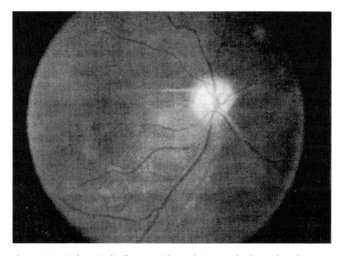

Figure 35.1 Right optic fundus: arteriolar occlusions and submacular edema.

occlusions and leaking into the retina. When the occlusions are limited to the peripheral branches of the retinal artery, there may be no visual loss and fundoscopy may be normal.

Auditory and visual involvement may not occur at the same time in the course of the disease, and may be delayed in relation to motor dysfunction. Auditory dysfunction consists of a progressive difficulty in perceiving low- to medium-frequency sounds, with uni- or bilateral involvement, or it might be asymptomatic and only found in the audiogram. Vertigo, nausea, and tinnitus may also occur; vertigo is most likely from microinfarction in the vestibular labyrinth (Ballard *et al.*, 1996). The loss of low- and moderate-frequency tones is thought to result from microinfarction of the apical portions of the cochlea, which are supplied by end arterioles of the inner ear (Monteiro *et al.*, 1985). Suggested diagnostic criteria are given in Table 35.2.

Bursts and "steady state"

The initial symptoms generally improve with or without treatment. Weeks or months later, a second "burst" (subacute worsening of symptoms) may occur, leading to further deterioration. After each burst, there is a tendency towards remission, but the degree of recovery is variable. On fundoscopy, it is occasionally possible to observe a partial reopening of previously occluded artery branches

(Wildemann *et al.*, 1996); on MRI, at least one patient showed disappearance of hypersignal images on T2, 2 years after onset (Mala *et al.*, 1998). The reported number of symptomatic worsenings was between 1 and 8 times, appearing with an interval of 1–34 months between attacks.

A "final stage" is often achieved at after a period varying from 1 to 8 years, although one reported patient had a recurrence after 18 years (Petty *et al.*, 2001). Most patients spontaneously improve, but it is common that they remain with some degree of handicap (commonly gait difficulties and auditory and visual deficits) that stays stable for the rest of their lives. These deficits vary from slight pyramidal signs to complete dependency upon others. Although the natural history of the condition is unknown, the disease seems to have a self-limited multiphasic course, in most instances.

Pathology and pathogenesis

Pathology

Pathological specimens were obtained from frontal cortical white matter biopsies and from autopsies (Petty *et al.*, 2001). Pathological material showed the presence of microinfarcts in the territories of the end arterioles of the brain (both in white and gray matter), the retina, and the inner ear (Bogousslavsky *et al.*, 1989; Gordon *et al.*, 1991; Heiskala *et al.*, 1988; Monteiro *et al.*, 1985). The most significant findings include multiple foci of necrosis in the cerebral cortex and white matter, with loss of neurons, axons, and myelin, as well as diffuse proliferation of hypertrophied astrocytes in the white matter, especially around the small vessels. The walls of small arterioles were thickened and surrounded by an abnormal reticulin network. The normal capillary network was destroyed and replaced by fragmented material, with thickened arteriolar segments staining intensely for laminin and fibronectin. These findings suggested the concept of a new type of brain, inner ear, and retinal microangiopathy (Heiskala *et al.*, 1988). Minimal nonspecific periarteriolar chronic inflammatory cell infiltration with or without microinfarcts (Petty *et al.*, 2001). Electronic microscopy showed very thick basal lamina in the capillary walls. There was no evidence of amyloid angiopathy. Some of these biopsies were performed after different treatments were prescribed, including steroids, so the interpretation of the minimal perivascular inflammation changes may have been influenced by prior treatment.

Pathology of other organs showed no associated disease except for microangiopathy in muscle biopsy specimens (Ballard *et al.*, 1996; Petty *et al.*, 2001); in all other patients, the arteriopathy was circumscribed to a cephalic localization. Cerebral biopsies are described in Table 35.3.

Mechanism of arteriolar occlusion

Small-vessel diseases are responsible for a large amount of ischemic and hemorrhagic strokes as well as encephalopathies including Susac's syndrome. However, in Susac's syndrome, all pathological evidence converges to the presence of a typical lesion, the arteriolar occlusion, but the exact mechanism of occlusion

Table 35.3 Brain biopsies in Susac's syndrome
Case 1: Sclerosis of the media and adventitial and cortical vessels, consistent with a "healed" angiitis.
Case 2: Numerous microinfarcts (500-μm maximum diameter) in the gray matter. No evidence for inflammation. Small vessels with muscular walls present within most of the infarcts, possibly precapillary arterioles. Reactive astrocytic gliosis associated with the infarcts. No infarct in white matter. Leptomeninges without abnormality.
Case 3: Microinfarcts in the white and gray matter (500-μm maximum diameter) with loss of neurons, axons, and myelin and proliferation of hypertrophic astrocytes. Walls of several small arterioles were thick and surrounded by an abnormal reticulin network and occasional lymphocytes. Normal capillary network was destroyed and replaced by fragmented material reactive to antibodies for laminin and fibronectin. Electronic microscopy showed a thick basal lamina.
Case 4: Moderate gliosis with neuronal loss, suggesting chronic hypoxic changes. Slightly thickened blood vessels, possibly only cortical tissue involved. No amyloid deposits, fibrosis, or hyalinosis was present.
Case 5: Foci of necrosis and minimal perivascular infiltration of small blood vessels by mononuclear cells.
Case 6: Mild arteriolar wall sclerosis without vasculitis in leptomeningeal and small cortical arterioles.
Case 7: Chronic organizing multifocal microinfarcts in the white matter, in association with focal acute ischemic neuronal necrosis in the gray matter.*
Case 8: Microinfarcts of different ages with tiny foci of eosinophilic ischemic neurons in the cerebral cortex and perivascular rarefaction, breakdown of axons and accumulation of foamy macrophages in the white matter.

* Muscle biopsy showed inflammatory and occlusive microangiopathy.

is unknown. There is no evidence supporting a true vasculitis, although the clinical evolution with fluctuations could suggest it. There has been no evidence for a coagulopathy except in one female heterozygote for the factor V Leyden mutation and another one with a protein S deficiency (Cafferty *et al.*, 1994). The Leyden mutation occurs in about 5% of the population and, although associated with thrombosis, is not associated with microangiopathy.

The localization of the infarcts, limited to the brain, eye, and ear, may be related to the common embryologic origin of these tissues (Monteiro *et al.*, 1985), with a common endothelium and similar barriers like the blood-brain barrier, where antigens might act and cause delayed arteriolar occlusion. Most arguments favor a disease of the vascular wall as an etiology for this syndrome (Mala *et al.*, 1998).

Pathological findings suggest a specific vascular disease of small arterial vessels. Retinal fluorescence angiography is also consistent with the hypothesis of microvascular lesions that cause increased vascular permeability, and the mechanism of arterial occlusion is more consistent with thrombosis rather than embolism. Recent pathological studies have shown endothelial changes that are typical of an antiendothelial cell injury syndrome. Elevated levels of Factor VIII and von Willebrand factor antigen may reflect the endothelial perturbation.

Pathogenesis

Although the etiopathogenesis of this entity remains unknown, several hypotheses have been considered. The first reports showed clinical similarities with central nervous system vasculitis, and a diagnosis of cerebral systemic lupus erythematosus (SLE) was proposed (MacFadyen et al., 1987; Pfaffenbach and Hollenhorst, 1973), but no reported case fulfilled the criteria for SLE.

Another hypothesis was that of an immune-mediated process. Increase in cerebrospinal fluid (CSF) protein content, erythrocyte sediment rate, and in the Leu 3a/Leu 2a ratio (with a decrease in Leu 7) in the first patient of Bogousslavsky et al. (1989), suggested an immunological dysfunction, despite the negativity of all other immunological markers. Intra-arterial thrombosis and occlusion could be induced by circulating immune complexes. A process directed primarily against the small vessels through antibodies against the endothelial antigens is plausible, but antibodies directed against endothelial antigens were not observed in human models of vasculitic syndromes (Coppeto et al., 1984; Moore and Cupps, 1983).

The hypothesis of an atypical viral infection, triggering subsequent pathological or immunological changes, has also been proposed. This theory was supported by the case of an anencephalic fetus from a mother who became pregnant 2 months after the first burst of the disease. She had a sore throat and skin rash with fever before the development of the first signs (Coppeto et al., 1984).

An iatrogenic origin linked to fenfluramine has also been suggested. Fenfluramine is an anorectic drug that can injure serotoninergic neurons and cause a transient decrease in dopamine turnover in the rat brain (Zaczek et al., 1990). This drug was taken by both patients of Schwitter et al. (1992) before the onset of the disease.

Pregnancy in this age group can be just coincidental, but was also thought to be a possible contributing factor. Puerperium is known as a period during which an increased tendency for thrombosis exists (Davidson et al., 1963). No laboratory test supported this theory. In contrast, the reactivation of symptoms in the postpartum period (Patient 2 of Coppeto et al., 1984) is another argument suggesting that an immune-mediated mechanism may be involved.

One patient with Susac's syndrome showed concomitant features of a vasospastic syndrome, including prolonged flow arrest time after cooling shown by microscopic examination of the nail bed, increased resistivity by Doppler in orbital vessels, increased plasma endotelin-1 level, as well as history of cool hands, migraine, and low blood pressure, suggesting that Susac's syndrome might be another manifestation of a widely vasospastic syndrome (Flammer et al., 2001).

The etiology of the disease remains unknown, but the reversibility of some of the lesions is an indirect argument in favor of a nondestructive process (Coppeto et al., 1984). Despite extensive investigation including autopsies, there has never been strong evidence for systemic disease, and the pathogenesis remains unclear.

Diagnosis

Diagnosis is easier when the triad of encephalopathy, hearing loss, and retinal artery occlusion is present. There is mid- to-low-frequency uni- or bilateral sensorineural hearing loss, as well as retinal arterial occlusions without keratoconjunctivitis or uveitis and small increased signal foci in T2-weighted MRI of the brain, in the gray and white matter. The localization of these T2 images in white matter seldom involves the corpus callosum. However, a considerable proportion of patients do not have the clinical triad at the time of onset. Hearing loss can be subclinical and so not recognized. MRI features in the corpus callosum can support the diagnosis in patients with two of the three features of the triad (Susac et al., 2003). Therefore, patients with unexplained encephalopathy should have a careful and thorough fundoscopic examination of the retina, and an audiogram should be performed, in order to exclude this probably underdiagnosed vasculopathy.

Brain imaging

MRI is the neuroimaging study of choice and fluid-attenuated inversion recovery (FLAIR) a sensitive sequence for detecting lesions of Susac's syndrome as well as to show their heterogeneity (Susac et al., 2007; White et al., 2004). Findings include, typically, multiple small hyperintense foci in T2-weighted images and contrast enhancement, in the gray and white matter of supra- and infratentorial structures. Large round lesions (snowballs) and linear ones (spokes) can also dominate MRI findings (Susac et al., 2007).

In a review of the MRI findings in 27 patients, Susac et al. (2003) found multifocal supratentorial white matter lesions that included the corpus callosum in all patients, and there was often involvement of the cerebellum, brachium pontis, and brainstem. The corpus callosal lesions are typically small and involve central fibers with relative sparing of the periphery. Acute callosal lesions that develop during the acute period of symptom worsening are often replaced by a punched out appearance that looks like holes on follow-up MRI scans (Susac et al., 2003; Xu et al., 2004). These central callosal lesions differ from those in demyelinating disease and were considered by some authors to be so specific for Susac's syndrome (Gross amd Eliashar, 2005; Susac et al., 2007) that their existence could support the diagnosis when only two of the triad features are present (Susac et al., 2003, 2007). Leptomeningeal involvement is also present in up to one-third of patients (Gross and Eliashar, 2005).

Serial MRI with diffusion-weighted imaging (DWI) and apparent diffusion coefficients (ADCs) show that size and number of lesions change over time, and that with disease progression ADC in the nonlesional white matter changes from normal to elevated (Susac et al., 2007; White et al., 2004). Cerebral and cerebellar atrophy are also found on later scans.

Fluorescein retinal angiography

Bilateral distal branch retinal occlusions are present in the fluorescein retinal angiography (as well as observed on fundoscopy), which may show the pathognomonic multifocal fluorescence. Gass plaques are frequently present and reflect endothelial damage. Branch occlusions should not be misdiagnosed nor confounded with retinal artery wall plaques. These wall plaques exist together with retinal artery branch occlusions. The plaques locate usually away from retinal bifurcations, at the mid-arteriolar segments (Egan *et al.*, 2003). In some cases, retinal vessel wall hyperfluorescence can be noted days prior to retinal infarction (Notis *et al.*, 1995).

Tonal audiometry

Mid- to low-frequency uni- or bilateral sensorineural hearing loss is the common pattern.

Laboratory data

Although extensively studied, the only common CSF abnormality is an elevated protein content. In some patients the protein content can be quite high. Oligoclonal bands are negative. Immunological laboratory parameters, microbiology, or virology studies are also negative. However, some patients have elevated levels of Factor VIII and von Willebrand factor antigen, probably reflecting the endothelial perturbation (Susac *et al.*, 2007).

Differential diagnosis

Differential diagnosis is extensive. Misdiagnoses include multiple sclerosis, but differential diagnosis must be done with all causes of multifocal neurologic symptoms with hearing and/or visual loss. Because some patients do not have the clinical triad at the time of onset of symptoms, the disease is often underdiagnosed.

Cogan's syndrome

This is a rare clinical syndrome that affects mostly young adults and causes progressive deafness. It is characterized by sudden-onset interstitial keratitis (photophobia, lacrimation, and eye pain) and vestibuloauditory dysfunction, usually bilateral, with tinnitus, acute vertigo episodes, and sensorineural hearing loss. See Chapter 37.

Brown-Vialletto-Van Laere syndrome

Pontobulbar palsy with deafness is a rare disorder with bilateral neurosensorial deafness and cranial disorders including motor components of the lower cranial nerves. Familiar and sporadic cases have been described, and autoimmune mechanisms have also been considered.

Multiple sclerosis

The MRI findings of multiple focal lesions in the corpus callosum and subcortical white matter can be misdiagnosed as multiple sclerosis. Age of onset and sex predominance are similar as well as MRI lesions in the subacute phase, but the CSF does not show typical oligoclonal bands, the number of bursts and the deterioration are usually limited in Susac's syndrome, extending the disease process over a 1- to 3-year period before remission. Chronic lesions on MRI differ from those of multiple sclerosis: lesion size is smaller, number is higher, and location differs. On DWI MRI, new lesions are hyperintense, with reduced ADC. Later, these lesions become hypointense or less prominent on subsequent DWI MRI. Concerning the visual abnormalities, visual fields showed no retrobulbar optic neuropathy or retinal periphlebitis. Hearing loss and arteriolar occlusive retinal disease are rare in multiple sclerosis. Serial DWI and ADC maps may help to differentiate Susac's syndrome from demyelinating disease (Xu *et al.*, 2004).

Acute disseminated encephalomyelitis (ADEM)

When the age of onset is young adulthood, ADEM must be included in the differential diagnosis. ADEM begins abruptly, the lesions are larger, and retinal and auditory findings are rare. The full triad in Susac's syndrome only develops years after the initial clinical presentation (Hahn *et al.*, 2004).

SLE

Seronegative cerebral type SLE was one of the first diagnoses proposed for this syndrome (MacFadyen *et al.*, 1987; Pfaffenbach and Hollenhorst, 1973). There were previous reports of multiple retinal artery occlusions in SLE patients (Bishko, 1972; Coppeto and Lessell, 1977; DuBois, 1974; Estes and Christian, 1971; Gold *et al.*, 1977; Johnson and Richardson, 1968; Kayazawa and Honda, 1981; Wong *et al.*, 1981). Although SLE can cause cerebral and retinal ischemia, retinal involvement is a rare complication of SLE, even more rare when there is CNS involvement. None of the patients had positive anti-nuclear antibody determinations or LE cells.

Polyarteritis nodosa (PAN)

Classic PAN is a multisystem disease involving all the organs except the lung and spleen (Blau *et al.*, 1977; Cupps and Fauci, 1981; Travers *et al.*, 1979). Ocular and auditory deficits may be present (Dick *et al.*, 1972; Moore and Sevel, 1966; Peitersen and Carlson, 1966). CNS abnormalities occur in 20%–40% of patients. Common CNS presentations are diffuse encephalopathy with focal or multifocal brain or spinal cord involvement caused by vasculitis. Symptoms may resolve spontaneously over weeks, and recurrence is unusual. Blurred vision and vision loss are common symptoms of affected choroid or retinal vessels, but more often choroidal. Untreated patients with PAN have only a 13% survival rate at 5 years.

Wegener granulomatosis

Wegener granulomatosis is a systemic necrotizing vasculitis with granulomatous vasculitis of the respiratory tract with or without glomerulonephritis (Fauci and Wolff, 1973; Wolff *et al.*, 1974). Neurologic symptoms occur in 20–50% of untreated patients (Anderson *et al.*, 1975; Drachman, 1963). Involvement of cranial nerves II and VIII is possible by a compressing granuloma or by ischemia. There is no evidence that hearing loss in Susac's syndrome is due to nerve VIII involvement. Slight changes in cognitive function may occur. Seizures, stroke, and encephalopathy are late complications in untreated patients.

Hypersensitivity vasculitis

Hypersensitivity vasculitis, including allergic vasculitis and drug-induced vasculitis, should also be considered. Neurological, as well as inner ear and retinal, involvement is rare. Commonly, skin and small veins are involved. Concerning iatrogenic cases, CNS arteritis has been described in patients with a history of drug abuse; these include anorectic drugs, particularly amphetamines. In angiography, typically beaded arteries appearance is common.

Isolated angiitis of the CNS can have the same early manifestations and CSF changes. Vision loss is possible but related to decompensated papilledema (Susac *et al.*, 1979). Retinal arteriography can be normal. Nevertheless, it is usually a fatal disease, with small artery and vein involvement and a necrotizing vasculitis on brain biopsy. Retinal occlusions are uncommon, and brain biopsy is required for the diagnosis (Cogan, 1969).

CNS infections

Several infections can originate multifocal signs. Posterior fossa meningitis may appear with cranial nerve signs. CSF may help in the diagnosis. Syphilis can occasionally cause retinal periphlebitis and neurological involvement (Delaney and Torrisi, 1976). Labyrinthitis has been reported and is accompanied by hearing loss over months or years.

Cerebral autosomal dominant arteriopathy with subcortical infarcts and leukoencephalopathy (CADASIL)

CADASIL is also a small-vessel disease of the brain that has a hereditary nature, and it is caused by mutations in the *Notch3* gene. Notch genes are now known to be important for endothelial and smooth muscle cells to form arteries and veins (Rigelstein and Nabavi, 2005). CADASIL patients may have retinal changes, but on fundoscopy just foveal telangiectasias do occur. Diagnosis can be made reliably by cerebral MRI, skin biopsy, or genetic testing.

Other

Other differential diagnoses for patients with microangiopathy of the retina, inner ear, and brain, include diseases like Usher's syndrome (retinopathy pigmentosa and labyrinthitis with deafness,

transmitted as a recessive trait), Vogt-Koyanagi-Harada's syndrome (deafness with blindness that results from diffuse exudative choroiditis and retinal detachment), Rocky Mountain spotted fever (that can lead to necrosis of retinal vascular walls), Norrie's disease, or Takayasu's disease (Bruyn and Went, 1964; Delaney and Torrisi, 1976; Haynes *et al.*, 1980; Vernon, 1969; Wilson *et al.*, 1979). Mitochondrial encephalomyopathies with progressive sensorineural hearing loss, like classic or multisystem Kearns-Sayre syndrome, MELAS (mitochondrial myopathy, encephalopathy, lactic acidosis, and stroke-like episodes), or Friedreich ataxia should also be included in the differential diagnosis (Zwirner and Wilichowski, 2001).

Investigations

Patients have been extensively investigated in order to exclude diseases that may mimic some aspects of this syndrome. Apart from routine examinations (biochemistry, hemoleukogram, urinalysis, chest x-ray, echocardiogram), some other investigation is recommended including CSF studies (elevated protein and minimal cell content), cerebral MRI (normal or showing multiple areas of increased signal on T2-weighted images, both in white and gray matter), neuropsychological examination, audiogram (neurosensorial bilateral asymmetrical hearing loss, more intense for low and medium frequencies), brainstem auditory evoked potentials, fundoscopy (peripheral ophthalmoscopy), and retinal angiography (retinal branch arteriolar occlusions frequently bilateral, with artery narrowing and microvascular lesions showing increased vascular permeability).

Laboratory tests, to exclude a vasculitis or infectious disease are also negative. CT scan shows no lesions or discrete to mild generalized atrophy. CT is considered unnecessary when MRI is available.

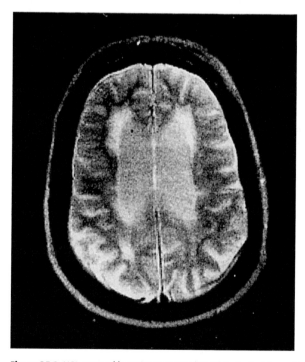

Figure 35.3 MRI: spots of hyperintense signal in subcortical white matter.

Neither CT nor cerebral angiography detect lesions that explain the higher cortical function disorders. The small size of the lesions may be responsible for that (Coppeto *et al.*, 1984) (Figure 35.3). The predominance of microinfarcts in white matter may contribute to the difficulty in the differential diagnosis with multiple sclerosis. On MRI, lesions are enhanced by gadolinium in the subacute phase, and brain atrophy is common in the chronic stadium. Electroencephalogram performed in the encephalopathic phase is diffusely slow (Susac, 1994). Indication for brain biopsy is individual, considering both the lack of knowledge on etiopathogenic mechanisms and on effective treatment. Peripheral ophthalmoscopy is obligatory (Coppeto *et al.*, 1984).

Management

The natural history of the disease is unknown and, because the disease is mainly self-limited, treatment side effects and expected benefit must seriously be taken into account. As it is common in rare diseases, treatment trials are not available, so therapy remains empirical, symptomatic, and based on anecdotal case reports as well as "personal experience." However, corticotherapy and immunosuppressive agents such as cyclophosphamide and azathioprine, plasmapheresis, and intravenous immunoglobulins have been used, based on the presumption that an immune-mediated mechanism may be involved. Calcium channel blockers (nimodipine), anticoagulants, and aspirin may also be useful.

Steroid therapy seems to achieve clinical improvement, at least temporarily, in most patients. Some authors advise corticosteroids as first-line treatment (Petty *et al.*, 2001). Immunosuppressive therapy is used alone or in association with steroids, with some favorable results reported. However, the benefit of prolonged immunosuppressive therapy is not established. The benefit of plasmapheresis, used together with oral cyclophosphamide in patients clinically deteriorating, although not proven can be effective in some cases.

Treatment with anticoagulants is rarely effective. Wildemann *et al.* (1996) reported clinical improvement in a patient with a combined therapy using an antiplatelet drug (ASA) and the calcium antagonist agent nimodipine. A possible mechanism for the effect of nimodipine includes increased cerebral blood flow related to vasodilatation. Improvement with hyperbaric oxygen therapy, together or not with corticoids, was described for visual and hearing symptoms, based on similar results in other sudden-onset vision or hearing losses (Li *et al.*, 1996; Narozny *et al.*, 2004).

Neither the number of patients described nor the severity of individual symptoms permit randomization of therapy. As spontaneous recovery and remission are reported (Susac, 1994), treatment efficacy is even more difficult to evaluate, but might include comparison to placebo. Recent imaging studies emphasize the disruption of white matter connections in the pathogenesis of cognitive impairment in acquired small-vessel diseases, suggesting therapeutic benefits of acetylcholinesterase inhibitors. It is not known if this presumption is applicable for patients with Susac's syndrome.

The main clinical outcome measures for therapeutic interventions should be return of vision, recovery of auditory function, improvement of psychiatric and neurological symptoms, and changes in MRI (O'Halloran *et al.*, 1998).

The only consensus in therapy is rehabilitation, including vestibular rehabilitation and hearing aids, when required. New effective therapeutic approaches are difficult to establish while further knowledge concerning the pathogenesis of the disease is not available.

REFERENCES

Anderson, J. M., Jamieson, D. G., and Jefferson, J. M. 1975. Non-healing granuloma and the nervous system. *Q J Med*, **44**, 309–11.

Ballard, E., Butzer, J. F., and Donders, J. 1996. Susac's syndrome: neuropsychological characteristics in a young man. *Neurology*, **47**, 266–8.

Bishko, F. 1972. Retinopathy in systemic lupus erythematosus. A case report and review of the literature. *Arthritis Rheum*, **15**, 57.

Blau, E. B., Morris, R. F., and Yunis, E. J. 1977. Polyarteritis in older children. *Pediatrics*, **60**, 227–34.

Bogousslavsky, J., Gaio, J. M., Caplan, L. R., *et al.* 1989. Encephalopathy, deafness and blindness in young women: a distinct retinocochleocerebral arteriolopathy? *J Neurol Neurosurg Psychiatry*, **52**, 43.

Bruyn, G. W., and Went, L. N. 1964. A sex-linked heredo-degenerative neurological disorder associated with Leber's optic atrophy: I. Clinical studies. *J Neurol Sci*, **54**, 59–80.

Cafferty, M. S., Notis, C., and Kitei, R. 1994. Retinal artery occlusions, hearing loss and stroke in a 19-year old (abstract). *Neurology*, **44**, A267.

Cogan, D. G. 1969. Retinal and papillary vasculitis. In *The Williem MacKenzie Centenary Symposium on the Ocular Circulation in Health and Disease*, ed. J Cant. St. Louis, MD: CV Mosby, p. 249.

Coppeto, J. R., Currie, J. N., Monteiro, M. L. R., and Lessell, S. 1984. A syndrome of arterial-occlusive retinopathy and encephalopathy. *Am J Ophthalmol*, **98**, 189–202.

Coppeto, J. R., and Lessell, S. 1977. Retinopathy in systemic lupus erythematosus. *Arch Ophthalmol*, **95**, 1580.

Cupps, T. R., and Fauci, A. S. 1981. The vasculitides. In *Major Problems in Internal Medicine*, ed. L. Smith. Philadelphia: WB Saunders, 21:18.

Davidson, E., Tomlin, S., Hoffman, G. S., and Epstein, W. V. 1963. The levels of plasma coagulation factors after trauma and childbirth. *J Clin Pathol*, **16**, 112.

Delaney, W. V., and Torrisi, P. F. 1976. Occlusive retinal vascular disease and deafness. *Am J Ophthalmol*, **82**, 232–6.

Dick, P., Conn, D. L., and Okazaki, H. 1972. Necrotizing angiopathic neuropathy: three dimensional morphology of fiber degeneration related to sites of occluded vessels. *Mayo Clin Proc*, **47**, 461.

Drachman, D. A. 1963. Neurological complications of Wegener's granulomatosis. *Arch Neurol*, **8**, 145.

DuBois, E. L., ed. 1974. *Lupus Erythematosus*, 2nd edn. Los Angeles: University of Southern California Press, p. 323.

Egan, R. A., Ha Nguyen, T., Gass, J. D., *et al.* 2003. Retinal arterial wall plaques in Susac syndrome. *Am J Ophthalmol*, **135**, 483–6.

Estes, D., and Christian, C. L. 1971. The natural history of systemic lupus erythematosus by prospective analysis. *Medicine*, **50**, 85.

Fauci, A. S., and Wolff, S. M. 1973. Wegener's granulomatosis: studies in eighteen patients and a review of the literature. *Medicine*, **52**, 535.

Flammer, J., Kaiser, H., and Haufschild, T. 2001. Susac syndrome: a vasospastic disorder? *Eur J Ophthalmol*, **11**, 175–9.

Gold, D., Feiner, L., and Henkind, P. 1977. Retinal arterial occlusive disease in systemic lupus erythematosus. *Arch Ophthalmol*, **95**, 1580.

Gordon, D. L., Hayreh, S. S., and Adams, H. P. Jr. 1991. Microangiopathy of the brain, retina, and ear: improvement without immunosuppressive therapy. *Stroke*, **22**, 993–7.

Gross, M., and Eliashar, R. 2005. Update on Susac's syndrome. *Curr Opin Neurol*, **18**, 311–4.

Hahn, J. S., Lannin, W. C., and Sarwal, M. M. 2004. Microangiopathy of the brain, retina and inner ear (Susac's syndrome) in an adolescent female presenting as acute disseminated encephalomyelitis. *Pediatrics*, **114**, 276–81.

Haynes, B. F., Kaiser-Kupfer, M. I., Mason, P., and Fauci, A. S. 1980. Cogan syndrome. *Medicine*, **59**, 426–41.

Heiskala, H., Somer, H., Kovanen, J., *et al.* 1988. Microangiopathy with encephalopathy, hearing loss and retinal arteriolar occlusions: two new cases. *J Neurol Sci*, **86**, 239–50.

Johnson, R. T., and Richardson, E. P. 1968. The neurological manifestations of systemic lupus erythematous. *Medicine*, **47**, 337.

Kayazawa, F., and Honda, A. 1981. Severe retinal vascular lesions in systemic lupus erythematous. *Ann Ophthalmol*, **13**, 1291.

Li, H. K., Dejean, B. J., and Tang, R. A. 1996. Reversal of visual loss with hyperbaric oxygen treatment in a patient with Susac syndrome. *Ophthalmology*, **103**, 2091–8.

MacFadyen, D. J., Schneider, R. J., and Chisholm, I. A. 1987. A syndrome of brain, inner ear and retinal microangiopathy. *Can J Neurol Sci*, **14**, 315–8.

Mala, L., Bazard, M. C., Berrod, J. P., Wahl, D., and Raspiller, A. 1998. Petits infarctus rétiniens, cochléaires et cérébraux du sujet jeune, ou "SICRET" syndrome ou syndrome de Susac. *J Fr Ophthalmol*, **21**, 375–80.

Mass, M., Bourdette, D., Bernstein, W., and Hammerstad, J. 1988. Retinopathy, encephalopathy, deafness associated microangiopathy (the RED M syndrome): three new cases. *Neurology*, **38**(**Suppl 1**), 215.

McCabe, B. F. 1979 Autoimmune sensorineural hearing loss. *Ann Otol Rhinol Laryngol*, **88**, 585–9.

Monteiro, M. L. R., Swanson, R. A., Coppeto, J. R., *et al.* 1985. A microangiopathic syndrome of encephalopathy, hearing loss, and retinal arteriolar occlusions. *Neurology*, **35**, 1113–21.

Moore, J., and Sevel, D. 1966. Corneoscleral ulceration in periarteritis nodosa. *Br J Ophthalmol*, **50**, 651.

Moore, P. M., and Cupps, T. R. 1983. Neurological complications of vasculitis. *Ann Neurol*, **14**, 155–67.

Murata, Y., Inada, K., and Negi, A. 2000. Susac syndrome. *Am J Ophthalmol*, **129**, 682–4.

Narozny, W., Sicko, Z., Przewozny, T., *et al.* 2004. Usefulness of high doses of glucocorticoids and hyperbaric oxygen therapy in sudden sensorineural hearing loss treatment. *Otol Neurotol.* **25**, 916–23.

Notis, C. M., Kitei, R. A., Cafferty, M. S., Odel, J. G., and Mitchell, J. P. 1995. Microangiopathy of brain, retina and inner ear. *J Neurophthalmol*, **15**, 1–8.

O'Halloran, H. S., Pearson, P. A., Lee, W. B., Susac, J. O., and Berger, J. R. 1998. Microangiopathy of the brain, retina, and cochlea (Susac syndrome). A report of five cases and a review of the literature. *Ophthalmology*, **105**, 1038–44.

Peitersen, E., and Carlson, B. H. 1966. Hearing impairment as the initial sign of polyarteritis nodosa. *Acta Otolaryngol*, **61**, 189.

Petty, G. W., Matteson, E. L., Younge, B. R., McDonald, T. J., and Wood, C. P. 2001. Recurrence of Susac syndrome (retinocochleocerebral vasculopathy) after remission of 18 years. *Mayo Clin Proc*, **76**, 958–60.

Pfaffenbach, D. D., and Hollenhorst, R. W. 1973. Microangiopathy of the retinal arterioles. *JAMA*, **225**, 480–3.

Rigelstein, E. B., and Nabavi, D. G. 2005. Cerebral small vessels diseases: cerebral microangiopathies. *Curr Opin Neurol*, **18**, 179–88.

Saw, V. P., Canty, P. A., Green, C. M., *et al.* 2000. Susac syndrome: microangiopathy of the retina, cochlea and brain. *Clin Exp Ophthalmol*, **28**, 373–81.

Schwitter, J., Agosti, R., Ott, P., Kalman, A., and Waespe, W. 1992. Small infarctions of cochlear, retinal, and encephalic tissue in young women. *Stroke*, **23**, 903–7.

Skacel, M., Bardy, F. B., Pereira, M. B., and Mendes, M. H. 2000. *Arq Neuropsiquiatr*, **58**, 1128–32.

Susac, J. O. 1994. Susac's syndrome: the triad of microangiopathy of the brain and retina with hearing loss in young women. *Neurology*, **44**, 591–3.

Susac, J. O., Egan, R. A., Rennebohm, R. M., and Lubow, M. 2007. Susac's syndrome: 1975–2005 microangiopathy/autoimmune endotheliopathy. *J Neurol Sci*, 27 [Epub ahead of print].

Susac, J. O., Hardman, J. M., and Selhorst, J. B. 1979. Microangiopathy of the brain and retina. *Neurology*, **29**, 313–6.

Susac, J. O., Murtagh, F. R., Egan, R. A., *et al.* 2003. MRI findings in Susac's syndrome. *Neurology*, **61**, 1783–7.

Travers, R. L., Allison, D. J., Brettle, R. P., and Hughes, G. R. V. 1979. Polyarteritis nodosa: a clinical and angiographic analysis of 17 cases. *Semin Arthritis Rheum*, **8**, 184–9.

Vernon, N. 1969. Usher's syndrome. *J Chronic Dis*, **22**, 133.

White, M. L., Zhang, Y., and Smoker, W. R. 2004. Evolution of lesions in Susac syndrome at serial MR imaging with diffusion-weighted imaging and apparent diffusion coefficient values. *AJNR Am J Neuroradiol*, **25**, 706–13.

Wildemann, B., Schülin, C., Storch-Hagenlocher B, *et al.* 1996. Susac's syndrome: improvement with combined antiplatelet and calcium antagonist therapy. *Stroke*, **1**, 149–50.

Wilson, L. A., Warlow, C. P., and Russell R. W. 1979. Cardiovascular disease in patients with retinal artery occlusion. *Lancet*, **1**, 292–4.

Wolff, S. M., Fauci, A. S., Horn, R. G., and Dale, D. C. 1974. Wegener's granulomatosis. *Ann Intern Med*, **81**, 513–25.

Wong, K., Ai, E., Jones, J. V., and Young, D. 1981. Visual loss as the initial symptom of lupus erythematosus. *Am J Ophthalmol*, **92**, 238.

Xu, M. S., Tan, C. B., Umapathi, T., and Lim, C. C. 2004. Susac syndrome: serial diffusion-weighted MR imaging. *Magn Reson Imaging*, **22**, 1295–8.

Zaczek, R., Battaglia, G., Culp, S., *et al.* 1990. Effects of repeated fenfluramine administration on indices of monoamine function in the rat brain: pharmacokinetic, dose response, regional specificity and time course data. *J Pharmacol Exp Ther*, **253**, 104–12.

Zwirner, P., and Wilichowski, E. 2001. Progressive sensorineural hearing loss in children with mitochondrial encephalomyopathies. *Laryngoscope*, **111**, 515–21.

36 HEREDITARY ENDOTHELIOPATHY WITH RETINOPATHY, NEPHROPATHY, AND STROKE (HERNS)

Joanna C. Jen and Robert W. Baloh

Background

Grand *et al.* (1988) reported an American family with a cerebroretinal vasculopathy (CRV) with recurrent strokes and visual loss due to characteristic retinal capillary abnormalities. Shortly afterward, Gutmann *et al.* (1989) described another American family with a similar syndrome of progressive visual loss and leukoencephalopathy without other organ involvement. In 1997, we reported a large Chinese family that presented with a hereditary vasculopathy similar to CRV with subcortical leukoencephalopathy and retinopathy but that also had renal dysfunction (Jen *et al.*, 1997). Ultrastructural studies identified characteristic alterations of vascular basement membranes not previously described; therefore, the syndrome was named hereditary endotheliopathy with retinopathy, nephropathy, and stroke (HERNS). Finally, Terwindt *et al.* (1998) described a Dutch family with hereditary vascular retinopathy (HVR) with microangiopathy of the retina similar to the above noted families, but without central nervous system involvement. Recently, a genome-wide linkage analysis of the Dutch family with HVR mapped the disease locus to chromosome 3p, which was also consistent with linkage in CRV and HERNS, suggesting that they are allelic syndromes (Ophoff *et al.*, 2001) (Table 36.1). Mutations in TREX1, a gene that codes for a 3′-5′ DNA exonuclease, were found in all of these families (Richards *et al.*, 2007).

Clinical characteristics

HERNS typically begins with progressive visual loss in the third or fourth decade of life followed by focal neurological deficits within 4–10 years. The visual loss begins in the central vision with decreased visual acuity. Blind spots in the visual field are also common. Many affected individuals report long-standing psychiatric symptoms such as depression, anxiety, and paranoia with onset as early as the second decade of life. Stroke-like episodes occur in most, and in some are the presenting symptoms. Often the stroke will progress over several days before reaching its completed stage. Later in the disease, signs of multifocal cortical and subcortical involvement such as dysarthria, hemiparesis, apraxia, ataxia, and dementia are common. More than half of patients report migraine headaches. About half of the patients have evidence of renal dysfunction including azotemia, proteinuria, and hematuria.

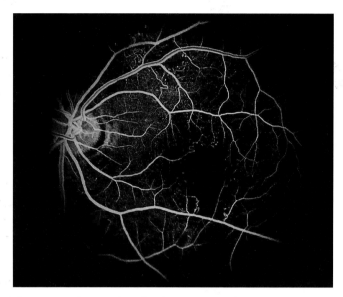

Figure 36.1 Mid-venous phase fluorescein angiogram from Patient 310 in Pedigree 1 demonstrating areas of macular capillary drop-out as well as dilated tortuous telangiectatic vessels and capillary shunts. (Jen *et al.*, 1997, with permission from Lippincott, Williams & Wilkins.)

Diagnosis

Ophthalmologic examination

There is a characteristic retinal vasculopathy that is most prominent in the macular region. Drop-out of macular capillaries may be associated with macular edema. One can typically identify dilated tortuous telangiectatic vessels and capillary shunts. Fluorescein angiograms show juxtafoveolar capillary obliteration with tortuous telangiectatic microaneurysms (Figure 36.1). Peripheral retinopathy including telangiectasia can occur later in the disease process (Cohen *et al.*, 2005).

Neuroimaging

On MRI, multifocal T2 high-signal-intensity lesions in the deep white matter can often be identified at the time of the initial onset of retinal involvement before neurologic symptoms and signs develop (Figure 36.2A). With the onset of focal neurologic deficits, the patient will have contrast-enhancing lesions with surrounding vasogenic edema most commonly in the deep frontoparietal

Table 36.1 Comparison of kindreds with dominantly inherited retinal vasculopathy with cerebral leukodystrophy (RVCL)

Syndrome	Clinical features	Retinal findings	Brain imaging	Vascular pathology
Hereditary endotheliopathy with retinopathy, nephropathy, and stroke (HERNS)	Strokes, retinopathy, nephropathy, migraine, mood disorders, dementia	Telangiectasia, microaneurysms, macular edema, capillary obliteration	Contrast-enhancing white matter lesions with vasogenic edema	Multilaminated basement membranes on electron microscopy
Hereditary cerebroretinal vasculopathy (CRV)	Strokes, visual loss, vasculopathy, dementia	Same	Same	Fibrinoid necrosis without inflammation on light microscopy
Hereditary vascular retinopathy (HVR)	Visual loss, Raynaud's phenomenon, migraine	Same	Same	Not reported

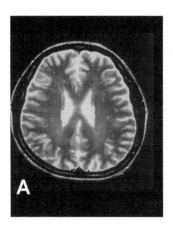 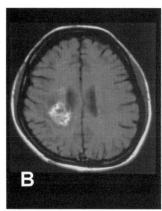 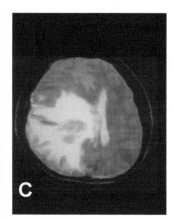 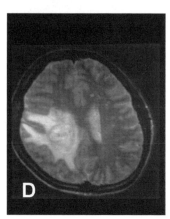

Figure 36.2 Brain MRIs of a patient with HERNS. **A**. Neurologically asymptomatic; multiple small subcortical hyperintense lesions on T2-weighted images. **B**. Slight clumsiness in the left hand and left leg at age 36, contrast-enhancing lesions with surrounding edema in the right frontoparietal subcortical region on T1-weighted images. **C**. Persistent headache with an episode of projectile vomiting but no other neurologic changes; increased size of the lesions with marked edema and mass effect on proton-weighted images. **D**. After 3 days of intravenous dexamethasone (Decadron), decreased edema on proton-weighted images. (Jen *et al.*, 1997, with permission from Lippincott, Williams & Wilkins.)

regions. Larger lesions can act as a space-occupying mass causing herniation of brain structures (Figure 36.2, B and C).

Pathology

On light microscopy, the brain lesions in patients with HERNS appear to be cerebral infarcts with extensive nuclear fragmentation and spongy change, often centered on small blood vessels occluded by fibrin thrombi. Ultrastructural studies show distinctive multilaminated vascular basement membranes in the brain and other tissues including the kidney, stomach, appendix, omentum, and skin (Figure 36.3). Endothelial cell cytoplasm is normal or slightly swollen. There was no evidence of either abnormal mitochondria or accumulation of mitochondria in any tissue examined by electron microscopy.

Pathophysiology

The underlying mechanism of HERNS appears to be a generalized vasculopathy with disruption of the integrity of capillaries

and arterioles. Fluorescein angiograms clearly show retinal vasculopathic changes. That the intracerebral lesions show contrast enhancement on MRI indicates breakdown in the blood-brain barrier. The surrounding edema in a vasogenic pattern also suggests increased capillary permeability. Because the basement membrane is synthesized by endothelial cells, the basement membrane abnormalities seen on electron microscopy probably reflect a primary endothelial injury.

Why should a generalized vasculopathy preferentially affect the brain, the retina, and the kidney? One explanation may be that these organs rely heavily on an intact endothelial barrier to maintain proper function and are particularly "eloquent" when injured. Furthermore, the basis for the regional vulnerability in the brain is intriguing in that the intracranial mass lesions tend to involve the frontoparietal region in both HERNS and CRV.

Treatment

At the present time there is no known treatment that is effective in patients with HERNS. Most patients have been maintained on

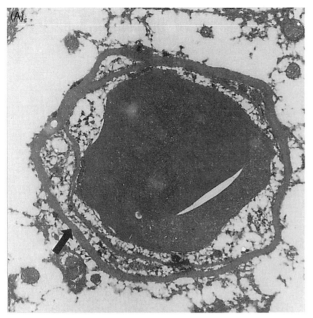

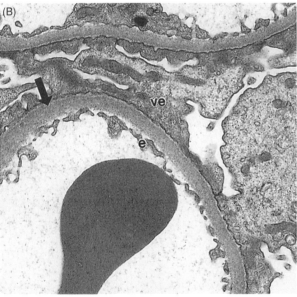

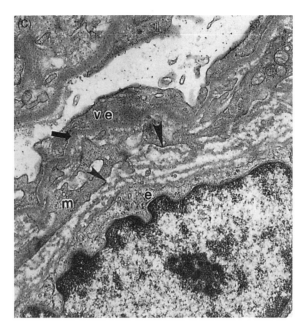

Figure 36.3 Electron microscopic appearance of vascular tissue in HERNS. **A**. Reprocessed specimen from brain from a patient with HERNS with several layers of basement membrane (*arrow*) in cerebral capillary. **B**. Normal glomerular capillary wall. Note uniform appearance and thickness of basement membrane (arrow). e = endothelial cells; ve = visceral epithelial cells. **C**. Glomerular capillary wall from a HERNS patient. The original basement membrane (arrow) beneath visceral epithelial cell (ve), although somewhat wrinkled, approaches a normal appearance. The basement membrane (*arrowheads*) beneath endothelial cell (e) is multilayered. A mesangial cell (m) separates the two basement membranes. (Jen *et al.*, 1997, with permission from Lippincott, Williams & Wilkins.)

aspirin for its antiplatelet action, but there is no indication that this has altered the course of the disease. Resection of a "pseudo-tumor" has not helped in patients who have undergone surgery. Laser treatments have been of little benefit in controlling the retinal vasculopathy. Corticosteroids have been useful to decrease cerebral edema and may even be life-saving in patients with

large edematous lesions (Figure 36.2D). Often patients must be maintained on a maintenance dose of corticosteroids because the edema returns if they are discontinued. Grand *et al.* (1988) and Niedermayer *et al.* (2000) noted the histologic similarities between CRV and delayed radiation-induced cerebral necrosis. Delayed cerebral radiation necrosis appears to result from damage of endothelial cells in small vessels. The observation of similarities between CRV and delayed radiation-induced cerebral necrosis may have important therapeutic implications because anticoagulation may arrest and even reverse endothelial injury due to radiation. However, a trial of anticoagulation in a single patient with HERNS was not beneficial, and bleeding complications developed.

REFERENCES

Cohen, A. C., Kotschet, K., Veitch, A., Delatycki, M. B., and McCombe, M. F. 2005. Novel ophthalmological features in hereditary endotheliopathy with retinopathy, nephropathy and stroke syndrome. *Clin Experiment Ophthalmol*, **33**, 181–3.

Grand, M. G., Kaie, J., Fulling, K., *et al.* 1988. Cerebroretinal vasculopathy, a new hereditary syndrome. *Ophthalmology*, **95**, 649–59.

Gutmann, D. H., Fishbeck, K. H., and Sergott, R. C. 1989 Hereditary retinal vasculopathy with cerebral white matter lesions. *Am J Med Genet*, **34**, 217–20.

Jen, J., Cohen, A. H., Yue, Q., *et al.* 1997. Hereditary endotheliopathy with retinopathy, nephropathy and stroke (HERNS). *Neurology*, **49**, 1322–30.

Niedermayer, I., Graf, N., Schmidbauer, J., Reiche, W., and Feiden, W. 2000. Cerebroretinal vasculopathy mimicking a brain tumor. *Neurology*, **54**, 1878–9.

Ophoff, R. A., DeYoung, J., Service, S. K., *et al.* 2001. Hereditary vascular retinopathy, cerebroretinal vasculopathy, and hereditary endotheliopathy with retinopathy, nephropathy and stroke map to a single locus on chromosome 3p21.1-p21.3. *Am J Hum Genet*, **69**, 447–53.

Richards, A., van den Maagdenberg, A. M., Jen, J. C., *et al.* 2007. C-terminal truncations in human 3′-5′ DNA exonuclease TREX1 cause autosomal dominant retinal vasculopathy with cerebral leukodystrophy. *Nat Genet*, **39**, 1068–70.

Terwindt, G. M., Haan, J., Ophoff, R. A., *et al.* 1998. Clinical and genetic analysis of a large Dutch family with autosomal dominant vascular retinopathy, migraine and Raynaud's phenomenon. *Brain*, **121**, 303–16.

COGAN'S SYNDROME

Olivier Calvetti and Valérie Biousse

Introduction

Cogan's syndrome is a rare multisystem disease first recognized as a separate clinical entity by David Cogan in 1945 (Cogan, 1945). Fewer than 250 cases have been reported in the literature (Grasland *et al.*, 2004). Cogan's syndrome is characterized by nonsyphilitic interstitial keratitis, vestibulo-auditory Menière-like symptoms, and, occasionally, systemic manifestations of vasculitis. In 1980, Haynes *et al.* suggested a diagnosis of "atypical Cogan' syndrome" to account for patients who develop inflammatory ocular disease other than interstitial keratitis (uveitis, scleritis, episcleritis, retinal vasculitis, or optic nerve edema), or if there is more than 2 years between the onset of ophthalmologic symptoms and hearing loss. Although neurologic manifestations are rare, several patients with stroke in the setting of Cogan's syndrome have been reported (Bicknell and Holland, 1978; Gluth *et al.*, 2006; Grasland *et al.*, 2004).

The cause and pathophysiology of Cogan's syndrome remain unknown, although a vasculitic process affecting vessels of all sizes has been described (Vollertsen, 1990). Clinically, vasculitis has been reported to affect the skin, kidneys, distal coronary arteries, central nervous system, and muscles. Autopsies have revealed vasculitis in the dura, brain, gastrointestinal system, kidneys, spleen, aorta, and the coronary arteries (Crawford, 1957; Fisher and Hellstrom, 1961; Vollertsen, 1990). Pathologic examinations of the proximal portion of the aorta in patients with Cogan's syndrome have shown generalized dilatation and narrowing of the coronary arteries in the region of the aortic valve. Microscopic examination of the aorta revealed neutrophils, mononuclear cells, giant cells, destruction of the internal elastic membrane, neovascularization, necrosis, scarring, and fibrotic hypertrophy; similar findings were noted in other vessels as well (Ho *et al.*, 1999; Vollertsen *et al.*, 1986). Autopsy findings reported by H. G. Thomas (1992) included numerous aneurysmal endothelial plaques associated with vasculitis affecting the entire aorta and surrounding ostia, as well as bilateral carotid bifurcation aneurysms.

However, the role of vasculitis in the pathogenesis of the ocular and vestibulo-auditory lesions of Cogan's syndrome remains to be demonstrated. Ishii *et al.* (1995) found no evidence of vasculitis in the blood vessels supplying the inner ear structures in a patient thought to have Cogan's syndrome. The audiovestibular symptoms of autoimmune sensorineural hearing loss are very similar to those of Cogan's syndrome (McCabe, 1979), and it is possible that, in some patients, autoimmune sensorineural hearing loss could be the first symptom of Cogan's syndrome. The presence of autoantibodies against inner ear, endothelial antigens, and cornea found in some patients with Cogan's syndrome adds further evidence for the autoimmune nature of this disease (Harris and Sharp, 1990; Helmchen *et al.*, 1999; Lunardi *et al.*, 2002; Majoor *et al.*, 1992). The presence of antinuclear antibodies (Orsoni *et al.*, 2002), rheumatoid factor (Garcia Callejo *et al.*, 2001), and cytoplasmic autoantibodies against neutrophils (Garcia Callejo *et al.*, 2001; Ikeda *et al.*, 2002) in some patients with Cogan's syndrome lends support to this notion.

The autoimmune hypothesis for sensorineuronal hearing loss and interstitial keratitis in Cogan's syndrome has been further studied (Lunardi *et al.*, 2002). Immunoglobulin G obtained from eight patients with Cogan's syndrome was pooled to screen a random peptide library. Antibodies directed against an immunodominant peptide showing similarity with autoantigens, including SSA/Ro and CD148, which is expressed in the inner ear and on endothelial cells, were identified in all eight patients and none of the controls. After intravenous administration to mice, these autoantibodies were capable of inducing the features of Cogan's syndrome, with tissue damage of the inner ear and endothelial cells, and also corneal involvement.

Clinical manifestations of Cogan's syndrome

The mean age of onset is 25 years, although patients may become symptomatic at any age. Men and women are equally affected. Interstitial keratitis and hearing loss are the most common manifestations. Neurologic manifestations are rare.

Ophthalmologic manifestations

The most common and classic ocular manifestation of Cogan's syndrome is bilateral interstitial keratitis. Interstitial keratitis is a nonsuppurative inflammation characterized by cellular infiltration of the corneal stroma. The inflammation is generally secondary to an immunologic response to a specific antigen. Clinically, interstitial keratitis is characterized by areas of dense, white, stromal necrosis with neovascularization (Figure 37.1). At the time of description of this disorder by Cogan, the most common cause of interstitial keratitis was congenital syphilis, explaining why many authors refer to "non-syphilitic interstitial keratitis." This corneal disorder manifests as insidious visual loss, photophobia, and ocular pain and redness. The diagnosis of interstitial keratitis is easily made on ocular examination with a slit lamp

Uncommon Causes of Stroke, 2nd edition, ed. Louis R. Caplan. Published by Cambridge University Press. © Cambridge University Press 2008.

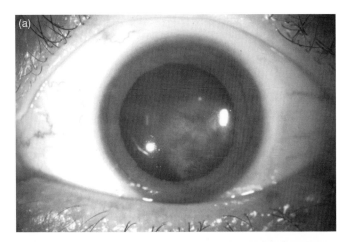

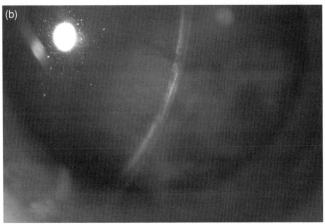

Figure 37.1 a and **b**. Interstitial keratitis in Cogan's syndrome. Slit-lamp examination showing corneal stromal opacities. See color plate.

(Figure 37.1) (Cobo and Haynes, 1984). Initial findings may be subtle, but they worsen over time, with most patients developing deep stromal keratitis with corneal vascularization. Cogan emphasized a characteristic day-to-day fluctuation in the severity of the keratitis, unlike what is seen in patients with congenital syphilis. He also remarked upon the patchy involvement of the cornea, the normal appearance of the posterior cornea, and the absence of striking intraocular inflammation. Some patients do, however, develop uveitis, episcleritis, scleritis, retinal vasculitis, and optic nerve edema; when any of these features are present, the term "atypical Cogan syndrome" is generally used (Haynes *et al.*, 1980). Most patients retain relatively good vision; severe visual loss, usually from complete opacification of the cornea, occurs in only about 5% of patients (Gluth *et al.*, 2006; Grasland *et al.*, 2004; Haynes *et al.*, 1980; Vollertsen *et al.*, 1986).

Vestibulocochlear manifestations

Unlike vision loss that is usually slight, hearing loss in Cogan' syndrome is often severe. Vertigo, tinnitus, and progressive deafness are present in all patients with this disorder. Bilateral asymmetric hearing loss is typically sudden, severe, and often permanent.

It may fluctuate initially with a progressive worsening over time, with more than 50% of patients eventually becoming deaf.

Vestibular manifestations – including vertigo, tinnitus, ataxia, nausea, vomiting, and nystagmus – are present in a large majority of patients with Cogan's syndrome (Bicknell and Holland, 1978; Grasland *et al.*, 2004). About 90% of patients have symptoms of peripheral vestibular dysfunction, 50% have ataxia, and 25% complain of oscillopsia (Bicknell and Holland, 1978; Grasland *et al.*, 2004). Caloric testing usually shows absent or diminished vestibular responses, depending on the time the test is obtained relative to disease onset. The vestibulo-auditory symptoms and signs may occur concomitantly with visual symptoms and signs, or may precede or follow the onset of visual phenomena by as long as 3 months (Bicknell and Holland, 1978; Cobo and Haynes, 1984; Gluth *et al.*, 2006; Grasland *et al.*, 2004; Zeitouni *et al.*, 1993).

Systemic manifestations

More than 50% of patients with Cogan's syndrome have nonspecific systemic manifestations, including headache, fever, weight loss, and fatigue, and about 30% have myalgias and arthralgias (Gluth *et al.*, 2006; Haynes *et al.*, 1980; Vollertsen *et al.*, 1986). About 10% of patients have features of systemic vasculitis, with skin or visceral damage, and about 10% develop aortic insufficiency and associated cardiac disturbances (Vollertsen *et al.*, 1986).

Neurologic manifestations

The frequency of central and peripheral nervous system involvement varies according to the authors from 2% to 5% (Sigal, 1987) to more than 50% of patients with Cogan's syndrome (Bicknell and Holland, 1978), and consists mainly of meningoencephalitis, seizures, and peripheral neuropathy. Patients with encephalopathy, psychosis, cranial neuropathy, myelopathy, and meningitis have been reported (Chynn and Jacobiec, 1996; Majoor *et al.*, 1992; St Clair and McCallum, 1999; Vollertsen *et al.*, 1986). Cerebrovascular involvement is rare (Bicknell and Holland, 1978). Reported cases include cerebral venous sinus thrombosis (Gilbert and Talbot, 1969), posterior inferior cerebellar artery thrombosis (Fair and Levi, 1960; Norton and Cogan, 1959), and multiple cerebellar lesions (Albayram *et al.*, 2001; Calopa *et al.*, 1991; Karni *et al.*, 1991; Manto and Jacguy, 1996). A recent review of 60 patients from the Mayo Clinic (Gluth *et al.*, 2006) described only two patients with a brain infarct (3%). In this series, six patients (10%) had peripheral neuropathy, three patients (5%) had a meningeal process, and three patients (5%) had encephalitis. In 2004, Grasland *et al.* reported 32 personal cases and reviewed 222 previously published cases with a frequency of neurological manifestations of 13% (29 patients). Among their 32 patients, 25 presented with systemic manifestations that occurred within the first 2 months after the onset of the disease and 12 patients presented with neurological manifestations, including headache (six patients), lymphocytic meningitis (seven patients), encephalitis (two patients), and peripheral neuropathy (four patients).

All patients with central nervous system involvement had brain ischemic lesions, often multiple if investigated with an MRI

(Albayram *et al.*, 2001; Calopa *et al.*, 1991; Manto and Jacguy, 1996). A vasculopathy suggesting vasculitis was shown by angiographic findings in one patient (Albayram *et al.*, 2001), and other authors have suggested the presence of circulating immunocomplexes (Manto and Jacquy, 1996) in patients with brain ischemia in the setting of Cogan's syndrome. Rarely, large-artery infarcts from cardiac emboli secondary to valvular disease may also occur in patients with Cogan's syndrome.

Diagnosis of Cogan's syndrome

No laboratory or radiographic test is diagnostic of Cogan's syndrome. The diagnosis is classically suggested by the association of interstitial keratitis with acute-onset sensorineuronal hearing loss in a patient who has a negative laboratory evaluation for syphilis. The most common laboratory abnormality is an elevated erythrocyte sedimentation rate. Other abnormalities include leukocytosis, anemia, and thrombocytosis. Autoantibodies such as rheumatoid factor and nuclear antibodies are usually negative, and are obtained mostly to exclude another autoimmune disease. Lumbar puncture may demonstrate meningitis with elevated protein and pleocytosis, even in the absence of clinical manifestations. Audiography, electronystagmography, and other tests of vestibular function, which are usually abnormal, may be helpful in both diagnosing and following the course of the disease. CT scans may occasionally show intralabyrinthine calcifications, whereas MRIs often show soft tissue obliteration of the membranous labyrinth (Casselman *et al.*, 1994; Helmchen *et al.*, 1998) and may also show multiple lesions of the white matter consistent with cerebral vasculitis (Calopa *et al.*, 1991). Cerebral angiography may demonstrate intracranial vascular abnormalities suggestive of vasculitis (Albayram *et al.*, 2001).

Treatment

The treatment of Cogan's syndrome varies based on the severity of the clinical manifestations. Because of the presumed autoimmune mechanism with vasculitis, most treatments have included steroids and immunosuppressants (Fricker *et al.*, 2006). Because of the rarity of the disease, the treatment is empiric and not based on any formal therapeutic trial (Fricker *et al.*, 2006; Gluth *et al.*, 2006).

Ocular manifestations such as interstitial keratitis are usually controlled by topical corticosteroids (steroid drops) (Haynes *et al.*, 1980; Rabinovitch *et al.*, 1986).

Vestibulocochlear, systemic, and neurologic signs are indications for systemic steroids. An initial dose of 1 mg/kg/d of prednisone is usually recommended, and gradually tapered over 2–6 months. The probability of recovering hearing loss may be higher when corticosteroids are given early in the disease course (Vollertsen *et al.*, 1986). High-dose intravenous steroids are also commonly used in this setting or when neurologic symptoms and signs suggest cerebral vasculitis. When hearing loss is profound and nonresponsive to steroid treatment, cochlear implants may improve hearing (Gluth *et al.*, 2006; Grasland *et al.*, 2004; Orsoni *et al.*, 2002; Pasanisi *et al.*, 2003; Rabinovitch *et al.*, 1986).

Immunosuppressants and intravenous immunoglobulins are occasionally used for patients who have persistent symptoms and signs despite apparently adequate therapy. Patients with severe aortic or cardiac disease may benefit from aortic valve replacement or vascular bypass surgery. The prognosis for vision and for life is generally good, although the prognosis for hearing is guarded because of irreversible changes that occur in the membranous labyrinth over time (Grasland *et al.*, 2004; Zeitouni *et al.*, 1993).

REFERENCES

Albayram, M. S., Wityk, R., Yousem, D. M., and Zinreich, S. J. 2001. The cerebral angiographic findings in Cogan syndrome. *AJNR Am J Neuroradiol*, **22**, 751–4.

Bicknell, J. M., and Holland, J. V. 1978. Neurologic manifestations of Cogan's syndrome. *Neurology*, **28**, 278–81.

Calopa, M., Marti, T., Rubio, F., and Peres, J. 1991. Imagerie par raisonnance magnétique et syndrome de Cogan. *Rev Neurol*, **147**, 161–3.

Casselman, W., Majoor, M. H., and Albers, F. W. 1994. MR of the inner ear in patients with Cogan's syndrome. *AJNR Am J Neuroradiol*, **15**, 131–8.

Chynn, E. W., and Jacobiec, F. A. 1996. Cogan's syndrome: ophthalmic, audiovestibular, and systemic manifestations and therapy. *Int Ophthalmol Clin*, **36**, 61–72.

Cobo, L. M., and Haynes, B. F. 1984. Early corneal findings in Cogan's syndrome. *Ophthalmology*, **1**, 903–7.

Cogan, D. G. 1945. Syndrome of nonsyphilitic interstitial keratitis and vestibuloauditory symptoms. *Arch Ophthalmol*, **33**, 144–9.

Crawford, W. J. 1957. Cogan's syndrome associated with polyarteritis nodosa: a report of three cases. *Pa Med*, **60**, 835–8.

Fair, J. R., and Levi, G.. 1960. Keratitis and deafness. *Am J Ophthalmol*, **49**, 1017–21.

Fisher, E. R., and Hellstrom, H. 1961. Cogan's syndrome and systemic vascular disease. *Arch Pathol*, **72**, 572–92.

Fricker, M., Baumann, A., Wermelinger, F., Villiger, P. M., and Helbling, A. 2007. A novel therapeutic option in Cogan diseases? TNF-alpha blockers. *Rheumatol Int*, **27**, 493–5.

Garcia Callejo, F. J., Costa Alcacer, I., Blay Galaud, L., Sebastian Gil, E., Platero Zamarreno, A. (2001). Inner ear autoimmune disorder: Cogan's syndrome. *An Esp Pediatr*, **55**, 87–91.

Gilbert, W. S., and Talbot, F. J. 1969. Cogan's syndrome: signs of periarteritis nodosa and cerebral venous sinus thrombosis. *Arch Ophthalmol*, **82**, 633–6.

Gluth, M. B., Baratz, K. H., Matteson, E. L., and Driscoll, C. L. W. 2006. Cogan' syndrome: a retrospective review of 60 patients throughout a half century. *Mayo Clin Proc*, **81**, 483–8.

Grasland, A., Pouchot, J., Hachulla, E., *et al.*, for the Study Group for Cogan's syndrome. 2004. Typical and atypical Cogan's syndrome: 32 cases and review of the literature. *Rheumatology*, **43**, 1007–15.

Harris, J. P., and Sharp, P. A. 1990. Inner autoantibodies in patients with rapidly progressive sensorineural hearing loss. *Laryngoscope*, **100**, 516–24.

Haynes, B. F., Kaiser-Kupfer, M. I., Mason, P., *et al.* 1980. Cogan's syndrome: studies in 13 patients, long term follow-up, and a review of the literature. *Medicine*, **59**, 426–41.

Helmchen, C., Arbusow, V., Jager, L., *et al.* 1999. Cogan's syndrome: clinical significance of antibodies against the inner ear and cornea. *Acta Otolaryngol*, **119**, 528–36.

Helmchen, C., Jager, L., Buttner, U., Reiser, M., and Brandt, T. 1998. Cogan's syndrome: high resolution MRI indicator of activity. *J Vestib Res*, **8**, 155–67.

Ho, A. C., Roat, M. I., Venbrux, A., and Hellmann, D. B. 1999. Cogan' syndrome with refractory abdominal aortitis and mesenteric vasculitis. *Rheumatology*, **26**, 1404–7.

Ikeda, I., Okazaki, H., and Minota, S. 2002. Cogan's syndrome with antineutrophil cytoplasmic autoantibody. *Ann Rheum Dis*, **61**, 761–2.

Ishii, T., Watanabe, I., and Suzuki, J. 1995. Temporal bone findings in Cogan's syndrome. *Acta Otolaryngol*, **519**, 118–23.

Karni, A., Sadeh, M., Blatt, I., and Goldhammer, Y. 1991. Cogan's syndrome complicated by lacunar brain infarcts. *J Neurol Neurosurg Psychiatry,* **54**, 169–71.

Lunardi, C., Bason, C., Landry, M., *et al.* 2002. Autoantibodies to inner ear and endothelial antigens in Cogan's syndrome. *Lancet,* **360**, 915–21.

Majoor, M. H., Albers, F. W., van der Gaag, R., Gmelig-Meyling, F., and Huizing, E. H. 1992. Corneal autoimmunity in Cogan's syndrome? Report of two cases. *Ann Otol Rhinol Laryngol,* **101**, 679–84.

Manto, M. U., and Jacquy, J. 1996. Cerebellar ataxia in Cogan syndrome. *J Neurol Sci,* **136**, 189–91.

McCabe, B. F. 1979. Autoimmune sensorineural hearing loss. *Ann Otol,* **88**, 585–9.

Norton, H. W., and Cogan, D. G. 1959. Syndrome of nonsyphilitic interstitial keratitis and vestibuloauditory symptoms: long-term follow-up. *Arch Ophthalmol,* **61**, 695–7.

Orsoni, J. G., Zavota, L., Pellistrini, I., Piazza, F., and Cimino, L. 2002. Cogan syndrome. *Cornea,* **21**, 356–9.

Pasanisi, E., Vincenti, V., Bacciu, A., *et al.* 2003. Cochlear implantation and Cogan syndrome. *Otol Neurotol,* **24**, 601–4.

Rabinovitch, J., Donnenfeld, E. D., and Laibson, P. R. 1986. Management of Cogan's syndrome. *Am J Ophthalmol,* **101**, 494–5.

Sigal, L. H. 1987. The neurologic presentation of vasculitic and rheumatologic syndromes. *Medicine,* **66**, 157–80.

St Clair, E. W., and McCallum, R. M. 1999. Cogan's syndrome. *Curr Opin Rheumatol,* **11**, 47–52.

Thomas, H. G. 1992. Case report: clinical and radiological features of Cogan's syndrome–non syphilitic interstitial keratitis, audiovestibular symptoms, and systemic manifestations. *Clin Radiol,* **45**, 418–21.

Vollertsen, R. S. 1990. Vasculitis and Cogan's syndrome. *Rheum Dis Clin North Am,* **16**, 433–8.

Vollertsen, R. S., McDonald, T. J., Younge, B. R., *et al.* 1986. Cogan's syndrome: 18 cases and a review of the literature. *Mayo Clin Proc,* **61**, 344–61.

Zeitouni, A. G., Tewfik, T. L., and Schloss, M. 1993. Cogan's syndrome: a review of otologic management and 10-year follow-up of a pediatric case. *J Otolaryngology,* **22**, 337–40.

PART IV: DISORDERS INVOLVING ABNORMAL COAGULATION

38 ANTI-PHOSPHOLIPID ANTIBODY SYNDROME

Jose F. Roldan and Robin L. Brey

Introduction

The anti-phospholipid syndrome (APS) was first described in 1983. The major clinical features consist of arterial (Antiphospholipid Antibodies in Stroke Study [APASS] Group, 1990; Cervera et al., 2002; Nojima et al., 1997; Rosove and Brewer, 1992) and venous (Wahl et al., 1998) thrombosis leading to tissue ischemia and placental thrombosis resulting in recurrent fetal loss (Levy et al., 1998; Rand et al., 1997), and thrombocytopenia in the presence of anti-phospholipid antibodies (Hughes, 1983). The research definition for APS has evolved over the years to its current state including moderate to highly positive anti-cardiolipin and anti-beta-2-glycoprotein 1 (anti-b_2GP-I) antibodies present twice at least 12 weeks apart and evidence for a thrombotic event or recurrent fetal loss (Miyakis et al., 2006) (Table 38.1).

Anti-phospholipid antibodies form a heterogeneous family that can be detected using a number of immunoreactivity assays (Table 38.2). As will be discussed in more detail in subsequent sections, some of these appear to lead to a greater risk for clinical manifestations of the APS than can anti-cardiolipin antibodies. Phospholipids are ubiquitous in the plasma membranes of all cells, and can form complexes with phospholipid-binding proteins under certain conditions that may involve cellular activation or injury (Arnout, 1996; Arnout and Vermylen, 1998).

Thrombotic episodes in patients with APS are primarily venous, but if the thrombosis occurs on the arterial side, the brain is affected most often (Hughes, 1983). APS is classified as secondary if it occurs in an individual with systemic lupus erythematosus (SLE) or another collagen disease and primary in the absence of SLE. However, primary and secondary APS are indistinguishable (Cervera et al., 2002; Krnic-Barrie et al., 1997; Shah et al., 1998) with regard to the types of thromboses. There is some evidence that patients with SLE and anti-phospholipid antibodies have a greater recurrent thrombosis risk than do patients with primary APS (Cervera et al., 2002).

The definitive role of anti-phospholipid antibodies in thrombogenesis continues to elude investigators, and not all patients with anti-phospholipid antibodies develop thrombosis. Anti-phospholipid antibodies associated with infection or certain medications are usually transient, contain a more restricted range of phospholipid immunoreactivity, and are not associated with clinical symptoms (Drouvalakis and Buchanan, 1998). Anti-phospholipid antibodies may also be found in otherwise normal people. A prospective blood bank study found that approximately 6.5% of normal subjects had ELISA-detected anti-phospholipid antibody IgG (Vila et al., 1994). Many anti-phospholipid antibody levels normalized with time, though, and no thrombotic events occurred in anti-phospholipid antibody-positive patients during a 12-month period. Krnic-Barrie et al. (1997) described recurrent thromboses after a lengthy quiescent period of many years in some anti-phospholipid antibody-positive patients. A 12-month follow-up period may not be long enough to determine thrombosis risk. Here, we review the history, clinical features, potential pathogenic mechanisms, screening techniques, and treatment of neurological disorders currently associated with APS.

Historical perspectives

Following the description of APS in the early 1980s, the anti-phospholipid antibody screening tests consisted of solid-phase and, later, ELISA techniques that used cardiolipin as the detecting antigen (Loizou et al., 1985). This negatively charged phospholipid, found primarily in the plasma membranes of mitochondria (McNeil et al., 1991), was assumed to be the antigen that anti-phospholipids were directed against. However, it was soon recognized that other anionic phospholipid antigens could better serve in the detection of anti-phospholipid antibodies. Phosphatidylserine, for instance, seemed better at identifying antibodies associated with fetal loss (Levy et al., 1998; Rote et al., 1990) and thrombosis (Inanc et al., 1997; Tuhrim et al., 1999), especially in association with a positive LA (Rote et al., 1990).

Biologically, the concept that these antibodies might target phosphatidylserine in vivo seemed more plausible because it is found in the plasma membrane of all cells and is commonly displayed on the extracellular surface in response to cell injury, activation, and remodeling (McNeil et al., 1991). This was theoretically problematic, though, considering the poor immunogenic properties of lipids (Gharavi and Pierangeli, 1998). Several groups identified the need for a cooperative phospholipid-binding protein in order to detect most, but not all, anti-phospholipid antibodies (Galli et al., 1990; Matsuura et al., 1990; McNeil et al., 1990; Meroni et al., 1998). Considering the substantial immunogenic quality of proteins, the involvement of a phospholipid-binding protein was more biologically sound. Shortly thereafter, coprecipitation and subsequent protein sequencing identified one serological cofactor to be b_2GP-I (Galli et al., 1990; Matsuura et al., 1990). Proteins such as prothrombin, annexin V, protein C, protein S, low-molecular-weight kininogens, and factor XI (Arnout and Vermylen, 1998) have also been shown to bind phospholipids, but b_2GP-I is

Uncommon Causes of Stroke, 2nd edition, ed. Louis R. Caplan. Published by Cambridge University Press. © Cambridge University Press 2008.

Table 38.1 Revised 2006 classification criteria of APS

Clinical criteria

Vascular thrombosis[§, °]

One or more clinical episodes of arterial, venous, or small-vessel thrombosis in any tissue or organ. Thrombosis must be confirmed by objective validated criteria (i.e. unequivocal findings of appropriate imaging studies or histopathology). For histopathologic confirmation, thrombosis should be present without significant evidence of inflammation in the vessel wall.

Pregnancy morbidity

(a) One or more unexplained deaths of a morphologically normal fetus at or beyond the 10th week of gestation with normal fetal morphology documented by ultrasound or by direct examination of the fetus

Or

(b) One or more premature births or a morphologically normal neonate at or before the 34th week of gestation because of: (i) eclampsia or severe pre-eclampsia or (ii) recognized features of placental insufficiency,

Or

(c) Three or more unexplained consecutive spontaneous abortions before the 10th week of gestation with maternal anatomic or hormonal abnormalities and maternal and paternal chromosomal causes excluded.

In studies of populations of patients who have more than one type of pregnancy morbidity, investigators are strongly encouraged to stratify groups of subjects according to a, b, or c above.

Laboratory criteria [*, **]

(a) Lupus anticoagulant (LA) present in plasma on two or more occasions at least 12 weeks apart, detected according to the guidelines of the International Society of Thrombosis and Hemostasis (Scientific Subcommittee on LAs / phospholipid-dependant antibodies)

(b) Anticardiolipin antibody of IgG and/or IgM isotype in serum or plasma, present in medium or high titer (i.e. >40 GPL or MPL, or > the 99th percentile). On two or more occasions at least 12 weeks or more apart, measured by a standardized ELISA.

(c) Anti-b_2GP-I antibody of IgG and/or IgM isotype in serum or plasma (in titer > 99th percentile), present on two or more occasions at least 12 weeks apart, measured by standardized ELISA, according to recommended procedures.

IgG, immunoglobulin G; IgM, immunoglobulin M; ELISA, enzyme-linked immunosorbent assay.

Copied with permission from the authors and publishers (from Miyakis *et al.*, 2006).

[*]Classification of the anti-phospholipid antibody syndrome (AAS) should be avoided if <12 weeks or >5 years separate the positive anti-phospholipid antibody test and the clinical manifestation.

[§]Coexisting inherited or acquired factors for thrombosis are not reasons for excluding patients from AAS trials. However, two subgroups of AAS patients should be recognized, according to: (a) the presence and (b) the absence of additional risk factors for thrombosis. Indicative (but not exhaustive) cases include: age (>55 in men and >65 in women) and the presence of any of the established risk factors for cardiovascular disease (hypertension, diabetes mellitus, elevated low-density lipoprotein or low high-density lipoprotein cholesterol, cigarette smoking, family history of premature cardiovascular disease, body mass index $\geq$30 kg/m^2, microalbuminuria, estimated glomerular filtration rate <60 mL/min, inherited thrombophilias, oral contraceptives, nephrotic syndrome, malignancy, immobilization, and surgery. Thus, patients who fulfill criteria should be stratified according to contributing causes of thrombosis. A thrombotic episode in the past could be considered as a clinical criterion, provided that thrombosis is proved by appropriate diagnostic means and that no alternative diagnosis or cause of thrombosis is found.

[°]Superficial venous thrombosis is not included in the clinical criteria. Generally accepted features of placental insufficiency include: (i) abnormal or nonreassuring fetal surveillance test(s), e.g. a nonreactive nonstress test, suggestive of fetal hypoxemia, (ii) abnormal Doppler flow velocimetry waveform analysis suggestive of fetal hypoxemia, e.g. absent end-diastolic flow in the umbilical artery, (iii) oligohydramnios, e.g. an amniotic fluid index of $\leq$5 cm, or (iv) a postnatal birth weight less than the 10th percentile for the gestational age.

[**]Investigators are strongly advised to classify AAS patients in studies into one of the following categories: I, more than one laboratory criteria present (any combination); IIa, LA present alone; IIb, anticardiolipin antibody present alone; IIc, b_2GP-I antibody present alone.

Table 38.2 Immunoreactivity assays utilized for anti-phospholipid antibody detection

Those whose antigens are
Anionic phospholipids alone
Cardiolipin
Phosphatidylserine
Phosphatidylinositol
b_2GP-I or other protein cofactors alone
Prothrombin
Annexin V
Anionic phospholipids *and* b_2GP-I or other protein cofactors

or phospholipid-dependent coagulation assays
Las

Table 38.3 Factors associated with increased thrombotic risk

Elevated, persistent anti-cardiolipin antibody – IgG titer
Presence of b_2GP-I anti-phospholipid antibodies
Increased LA

Table 38.4 Factors warranting evaluation of anti-phospholipid presence in stroke

Patient <40 years of age
Stroke is recurrent
Thrombocytopenia, fetal loss, or venous thrombosis have been documented
SLE or other connective disease is present

by far the most common and well-characterized protein with this ability (Inanc *et al.*, 1997; McNeil *et al.*, 1991).

Clinical manifestations

Brain ischemia

Brain ischemic events in patients with anti-phospholipid antibodies can occur in any vascular territory. A variety of cardiac valvular lesions have been associated with anti-phospholipid antibodies making cardiac emboli a possible stroke mechanism in some patients. Two-dimensional transthoracic echocardiography is abnormal in one-third of patients, typically demonstrating non-specific left-sided valvular (predominantly mitral) lesions characterized by valve thickening (reviewed in Tenedios *et al.*, 2006). These may represent a potential cardiac source of stroke.

Anti-phospholipid antibodies are well established as risk factors in a first ischemic stroke, but their role in recurrent stroke is less clear (Table 38.3). All (Brey *et al.*, 1990, 2001; Nencini *et al.*, 1992; Singh *et al.*, 2001; Toschi *et al.*, 1998) but one (Blohorn *et al.*, 2002) of the case–controlled and prospective studies that evaluated anti-phospholipid antibodies as a stroke risk factor in young adults (primarily in patients without SLE) showed an increased risk for incident ischemic stroke in young people. The study failed to find an association tested only for anti-cardiolipin antibodies, whereas the other studies evaluated for both anti-cardiolipin antibodies and LA. The presence and magnitude of the ischemic stroke risk associated with anti-phospholipid antibodies in older populations is more evenly split between finding an increased risk and no increased risk; however, of the studies where both anti-cardiolipin antibodies and LA were tested, all but one found an increased risk (reviewed in Brey, 2004). This suggests that anti-phospholipid antibodies may be a more important stroke mechanism in young people whereas, in older populations, other stroke risk factors take on more importance. Alternatively, the presence of LA may be more important in determining stroke risk at any age than are anti-cardiolipin antibodies alone. Most of these studies either excluded cardioembolic disease or did not distinguish between cardioembolic, artery-to-artery embolic, and thrombotic mechanisms. This is an important point, because cardiac valvular

lesions have been reliably associated with anti-phospholipid antibodies (Table 38.4).

Women may be at higher risk for an anti-phospholipid antibody-associated stroke. A recent study of the Framingham cohort and offspring study examined anti-cardiolipin antibodies in both females and males without history of stoke or transient ischemic attack (TIA). They found an increased risk of stroke and TIA for women with high anti-cardiolipin (hazard ratio [HR], 2.6; 95% confidence interval [CI], 1.3–5.4; absolute risk, 3.2%, 95% CI, 2.2–4.3) but not in men (HR, 1.3; 95% CI, 0.7–2.4; absolute risk, 4.5%; 95% CI, 3.0–6.0) (Janardhan *et al.*, 2004).

Two large studies evaluated the risk for recurrent stroke and anti-phospholipid antibodies in young adults (Nencini *et al.*, 1992). One study evaluated both anti-cardiolipin antibodies and LA and found an increase in recurrent stroke risk attributable to anti-phopholipid antibodies. The other, more recent study, which also evaluated for both anti-phospholipid antibodies and LA found no increased recurrent stroke risk (van Goor *et al.*, 2004). Two studies done in pediatric populations, likewise, found no increased stroke risk (Lanthier *et al.*, 2004; Strater *et al.*, 2002).

In the only prospective study of anti-phospholipid antibodies-associated recurrent stroke risk, the APASS group did not find the presences of anti-cardiolipin antibodies or LA to increase the risk of recurrent stroke (Levine *et al.*, 2004). The presence of both anti-cardiolipin antibodies and LA did show a trend towards increased recurrent stroke risk. Neville *et al.* (2003) also found that positivity for both anti-cardiolipin antibodies and LA had a greater odds ratio (OR) for thrombosis than either anti-cardiolipin antibodies or LA alone among 208 patients as compared to matched controls. Another study also found that multiple prothrombotic risk factors in patients with anti-cardiolipin antibodies increased the risk of thrombosis with an OR associated with a previous thrombotic event of 1.46 (95% CI, 1.003–2.134) per each additional prothrombotic risk factor (Hudson *et al.*, 2003). In a small pediatric SLE cohort, positivity for multiple anti-phospholipid antibody subtypes also showed stronger associations with thrombotic events than did single anti-phospholipid antibody tests (Male *et al.*, 2005). This supports the concept that LA and anti-phospholipid antibodies other than cardiolipin may have greater pathophysiologic potential to precipitate thrombosis.

Evidence also suggests that anti-phosphatidyl serine antibodies (aPS) alone may be a strong risk factor for thrombosis, as well. Tuhrim *et al.* (1999) found that aPS were independently associated with first ischemic stroke in the Minorities Risk Factors And Stroke Study (MRFASS). This is the largest ischemic stroke cohort studied to date for anti-phosphatidyl serine antibodies and suggests that anti-phosphatidyl serine antibodies are a potentially important anti-phospholipid antibody marker for ischemic stroke (Tuhrim *et al.*, 1999).

Atsumi *et al.* (2000) studied concordance, sensitivity, and specificity of various anti-phospholipid antibody assays and their isotypes for manifestations of the AAS and presence of the LA. The presence of anti-phosphatidyl serine antibodies had the highest OR (4.39, 95% CI, 2.06–9.38) for the clinical manifestations of AAS, and IgG anti-phosphatidyl serine antibodies correlated strongly with the presence of the LA (OR, 38.2; 95% CI, 13.4–109.1). The presence of anti-phosphatidyl serine antibodies (IgG or IgM) or b_2GP-I (IgG, IgM, or IgA) antibodies improved the specificity for the AAS over anti-cardiolipin antibodies alone. Anti-b_2GP-I antibodies of the IgG class were strongly associated with clinical manifestations of APS (OR, 5.72; 95% CI, 2.31–14.15, $p = .0001$). Furthermore, the relationship of anti-phosphatidyl serine antibodies and b_2GP-I antibodies to the presence of LA was stronger than that for anti-cardiolipin antibodies, including higher sensitivities and specificities. In another study, the positive predictive value (PPV) for anti-phosphatidyl serine antibodies and b_2GP-I was stronger for arterial thrombosis (87%–91%, $p < .001$) than for venous thrombosis (80%–92%, $p = .01$) (Lopez *et al.*, 2004).

The Euro-Phospholipid Project Group began a study of the clinical and immunologic manifestations and patterns of disease expression of AAS among a cohort of 1000 patients in 2002 (Cervera *et al.*, 2002). Primary AAS was present in 53.1% of patients, AAS associated with SLE in 36.2%, AAS associated with "lupus-like" disease in 5.9%, and other diseases in 5.9%. At study entry, deep venous thrombosis was the most common thrombotic manifestation occurring in 317 (31.7%) and stroke was the most common arterial thrombotic manifestation in 135 (13.1%) patients. Cerebrovascular ischemic events were also noted: TIA in 70 (7.0%) and amaurosis fugax in 28 (2.8%) patients. Although some clinical differences existed between primary and secondary AAS patients, none of these included thrombotic manifestations. Although follow-up information is not yet available for this extremely well-characterized cohort, invaluable information about recurrent stroke and other clinical manifestations will be forthcoming, as 10 years of follow-up is planned.

In another European collaborative study (the European Working Party on SLE), the morbidity and mortality in patients with SLE over a 10-year period were studied in a cohort of 1000 patients (Cervera *et al.*, 2003). This is the best study of the risk of thrombotic events and anti-phospholipid antibodies in people with SLE. At the beginning of this study, there were 204 (20.4%) patients with anti-cardiolipin IgG, 108 (10.8%) patients with anti-cardiolipin antibody IgM, and 94 (9.4%) patients with LA. Thromboses were the most common cause of death in the last 5 years of follow-up

and were always associated with AAS (Cervera *et al.*, 2002). The most common thrombotic events in these patients were strokes (11.8%), followed by myocardial infarction (7.4%) and pulmonary embolism (5.9%). This suggests an important role for anti-phospholipid antibodies and recurrent thrombosis in patients with SLE.

When it does occur, recurrent stroke and other thromboembolic events in patients with anti-phospholipid antibodies have been reported both early (within the first year of an index episode of cerebral ischemia) (Levine *et al.*, 1993, 1995) and late (5–10 years) (Krnic-Barrie *et al.*, 1997; Shah *et al.*, 1998). The initial type of thromboembolic event (i.e. arterial, venous, miscarriage) appears to be the most likely type of event to recur in a given patient in some (Rosove and Brewer, 1992) but not all studies (Krnic-Barrie *et al.*, 1997). Shah *et al.* (1998) studied patients with both primary and secondary AAS during a 10-year period and found recurrent thromboembolic events to be common in both groups. In their series of 52 patients with anti-phospholipid antibodies, 9 of 31 (29%) patients with AAS developed recurrent thrombotic episodes and 11 of 21 (52%) patients with anti-phospholipid antibodies but without clinical manifestations developed them during the follow-up period.

Krnic-Barrie *et al.* (1997) retrospectively evaluated 61 patients with primary and secondary AAS for an average of 6.4 years to identify risk factors for the development of recurrent thrombosis. There was no difference between patients with primary and secondary AAS regarding recurrent arterial or venous events (arterial: 55% vs. 38%; venous: 47% vs. 50%). In patients with primary and secondary AAS, recurrent arterial events were associated with Caucasian race and venous events with the puerperium or oral contraceptive use. High titers of anti-cardiolipin antibodies have been associated with recurrent events in patients with primary (Levine *et al.*, 1993, 1995, 1997) and secondary AAS (Alarcon-Segovia *et al.*, 1989; Cervera *et al.*, 2003; Escalante *et al.*, 1995). In a study of 141 patients with secondary AAS related to SLE, the presence of both anti-cardiolipin antibodies and LA were associated with thrombotic events (Nojima *et al.*, 1997). In this study, 84% of patients with an abnormal anti-cardiolipin antibody IgG level and LA had a thrombotic event as compared to 16% with an abnormal anti-cardiolipin antibody IgG only, 9.1% with LA only, and 3.8% with neither. All patients with high levels of anti-cardiolipin antibodies and LA and none of the patients without LA had an arterial thrombosis. The correlation between a high level of anti-cardiolipin antibodies and LA has been previously reported; however, Verro *et al.* (1998) did not find a similar relationship between very high titer and risk for recurrent thrombotic events. Specker *et al.* (1998) have shown that cerebral microemboli detected by transcranial Doppler are found in patients with AAS and that they correlate with a history of brain ischemia. If this technique is validated prospectively, it may provide a powerful approach to assess cerebrovascular thrombosis risk.

There are no data to suggest that the severity of the thromboembolic event, including stroke, influences anti-cardiolipin antibody titer. Anti-cardiolipin antibodies do not appear to be a result of the thrombotic event in the brain (Brey *et al.*, 1990; Levine *et al.*, 1995) or elsewhere (Alarcon-Segovia *et al.*, 1989). In a case-controlled study of patients with giant cell arteritis, the prevalence of abnormal anti-cardiolipin antibody levels was higher in patients with temporal arteritis than in controls (20.7% vs. 2.9%). The prevalence was even higher in patients who also had positive temporal artery biopsies than in temporal arteritis patients with normal biopsies (31.2% vs. 16.7%) (Duhaut et al., 1998). Both anti-cardiolipin antibodies and a positive biopsy were associated with thrombosis in univariate analyses; however, only a positive biopsy remained predictive of thrombosis in multivariate analyses. Furthermore, nearly half of biopsy positive patients with high anti-cardiolipin antibody levels at the time of diagnosis had normal levels when retested after 10 days of corticosteroid treatment. The authors speculate that, in giant cell arteritis, the anti-cardiolipin antibodies produced may be a consequence of severe endothelial damage and have no relationship to thrombosis. No further analyses of anti-cardiolipin antibody subtype or other phospholipid specificities were performed, thus it is possible that nonpathogenic antibodies are formed in this situation, similar to those found in response to drugs or infections (Drouvalakis and Buchanon, 1998).

Stroke mechanisms in patients with anti-phospholipid antibodies

Brain ischemic events can occur in any vascular territory. Cerebral angiography typically demonstrates intracranial branch or trunk occlusion or is normal in about one-third of patients so studied (APASS, 1990). Data from in vitro studies, from experimental animal models, and from clinical studies showing an association of anti-phospholipid antibodies with placental infarction, peripheral, and cerebral venous thrombosis strongly suggest that these antibodies cause stroke through induction of a prothrombotic state. A higher than expected frequency of coronary artery (Klemp et al., 1988) and peripheral arterial (Ciocca et al., 1995) graft occlusion has also been noted in patients with anti-phospholipid antibodies. These clinical observations coupled with recent findings of endothelial cell activation by anti-phospholipid (Del Papa, Guidali, Sala, et al., 1997; Del Papa, Raschi, Catelli, et al., 1997) support the hypothesis that anti-phospholipid antibodies may act in concert with other vascular risk factors that damage endothelial cells.

A variety of cardiac valvular lesions have been associated with anti-phospholipid antibodies making cardiac emboli a potential stroke mechanism in some patients. Echocardiography (primarily two-dimensional, transthoracic) is abnormal in one-third of patients, typically demonstrating nonspecific left-sided valvular (predominantly mitral) lesions, characterized by valve thickening (Ford et al., 1989; Tenedios et al., 2006). These may represent a potential cardiac source of stroke. In a large consecutive autopsy series, a higher incidence of cardiac valvular abnormalities and 'bland' (nonvasculitic) thromboembolic lesions were found in patients with anti-phospholipid antibodies (Ford et al., 1994).

Classic Libman-Sacks verrucous valvular lesions may also be attributable to phenomena associated with AAS. In 1924, Libman and Sacks originally described a "hitherto undescribed form of valvular and mural endocarditis," which would later be attributed to SLE (Gross, 1940; Ziporen et al., 1996). These valvular lesions

are typically clinically silent and are frequently associated with thickened, functionally impaired cardiac valves that are prone to hemodynamic deterioration. The causative mechanisms for this pathology have yet to be defined (for review, see Tenedios et al., 2006). Similar cardiac and endocardial lesions are found in patients with cancer and other debilitating diseases – so-called nonbacterial thrombotic endocarditis. A recent study suggests that there is a significant association between valvular lesions and stroke or TIA in patients with primary AAS but not in patients with both AAS and SLE (Krause et al., 2005).

The origins of atherosclerosis comprise a multifaceted histopathological process. It has been proposed that the oxidative modification of low-density lipoprotein in vivo may be a central contributor to atherogenesis. Therefore, anti-phospholipid antibodies may play a role in atherosclerosis because of a cross-reactivity with oxidized anti-phospholipid antibodies (Matsuura et al., 1998; Vaarala, 1998).

Venous sinus thrombosis

Anti-phospholipid antibodies may be an important factor contributing to cerebral venous sinus thrombosis even in the presence of other potential risk factors for thrombosis (Carhuapoma et al., 1997), including the syndrome of activated protein C resistance due to Factor V Leiden mutation (Deschiens et al., 1996). The onset of cerebral venous sinus thrombosis in patients with anti-phospholipid occurs at a younger age and has more extensive superficial and deep cerebral venous system involvement than does cerebral venous sinus thrombosis without anti-phospholipid antibodies. Headache, papilledema, seizures, focal deficits, coma, and death contribute to the clinical classification of cerebral venous sinus thrombosis, along with pathological identification of hemorrhagic infarction (Ameri and Bousser, 1992). Patients who present with cerebral venous sinus thrombosis typically have headache (85%), long tract signs (35%), cognitive disturbances (25%), and/or visual dysfunction (40%). In addition, a higher rate of postcerebral venous sinus thrombosis headache and more infarctions on brain imaging studies are seen in patients with anti-phospholipid antibodies than in those without them (Carhuapoma et al., 1997).

Sneddon's syndrome and other vascular dementia

Recurrent stroke in patients with livedo reticularis (Sneddon's syndrome) has been associated with anti-phospholipid antibodies (Kalashnikova et al., 1990). The frequency of anti-phospholipid antibodies in patients with Sneddon's syndrome has ranged from 0% to 85% (Kalashnikova et al., 1990; Tourbah et al., 1997; Zelger et al., 1993). This syndrome is also frequently accompanied by dementia, most likely on the basis of multiple infarctions. Sneddon's original patients all had focal neurological deficits that he considered to be "limited and benign," leaving little residual disability (Sneddon, 1965). Subsequent descriptions of the syndrome have revealed a spectrum of clinical neurological manifestations. Zelger et al. (1993) described three stages of neurological involvement: (i) "prodromal" symptoms such as dizziness or headache preceding focal neurological deficits by years;

(ii) recurrent focal neurologic deficits due to recurrent cerebral ischemia, also lasting years; and (iii) progressive cognitive impairment leading to severe dementia. Tourbah *et al.* (1997) retrospectively studied 26 Sneddon's syndrome patients and correlated MRI abnormalities with disability, the presence of cardiovascular risk factors, cardiac valvular abnormalities on echocardiography, and titer of anti-phospholipid antibodies. Disability (defined by memory disturbance or ability to perform activities of daily living) was found in 50% of patients and was severe (consisting of dementia) in more than half of patients with disability. Systemic hypertension was present in 65%, cardiac valvular abnormalities in 61%, and anti-phospholipid antibodies in 42% of patients, with no correlation found between any of these and MRI abnormalities. The presence of disability was correlated with increasing severity of MRI lesions. An anti-phospholipid antibody-associated dementia without the other features of Sneddon's syndrome has also been described. In many patients, this appears to be because of multiple cerebral infarctions. In addition, catastrophic AAS (CAAS) can occasionally be present with an acute organic brain dysfunction characterized by fulminant encephalopathy (Chinnery *et al.*, 1997).

An association between high anti-cardiolipin antibody titers and cognitive dysfunction has been found in patients without SLE or other collagen vascular disease (Cesbron *et al.*, 1997; Chapman *et al.*, 2002; Jacobson *et al.*, 1999; Mosek *et al.*, 2000). For example, Schmidt *et al.* (1995) found subtle neuropsychological dysfunction in otherwise normal elderly people with increased levels of anti-cardiolipin antibody IgG. This correlation with anti-cardiolipin antibody IgG titers was significant despite the lack of evidence of any anatomic abnormalities on MRI or correlation of anti-cardiolipin antibody positivity with MRI. De Moerloose *et al.* (1997) evaluated the prevalence of anti-cardiolipin antibody among 192 elderly patients. The overall prevalence of anti-cardiolipin antibodies was 10.9% and decreased by decade in patients 70–99 years old from 18% to 10% to 7%, whereas the prevalence of antinuclear antibody positivity increased by decade from 22% to 32% to 42%. There was no association between the presence of anti-cardiolipin antibodies and decreased survival. In contrast, and in keeping with previous findings, Cesbron *et al.* (1997) found a trend towards an increased prevalence of anti-cardiolipin antibodies by decade in 1042 elderly subjects between the ages of 60 and 99 years. In addition, high anti-cardiolipin antibody levels were associated with increased physical disability in this population independent of age, gender, visual or hearing abnormalities, Mini-Mental State Examination scores, or history of cerebrovascular or cardiovascular disease. Mosek *et al.* (2000) studied 87 elderly demented and 69 elderly nondemented patients and found that anti-cardiolipin antibody IgG positivity is more frequent in demented patients. In the first study of the relationship between anti-phospholipid and cognitive dysfunction in a non-elderly population, Jacobson *et al.* (1999) found a significant association between anti-cardiolipin antibody IgG levels and cognitive dysfunction.

Anti-phospholipid antibody positivity has been associated with several different patterns of cognitive dysfunction in patients with SLE, depending on the study. Verbal memory deficits, decreased psychomotor speed, and decreased overall productivity have been

significantly correlated to elevated anti-phospholipid antibody levels (Denburg *et al.*, 1997; Hanly *et al.*, 1999; Lerita *et al.*, 2002; McLaurin *et al.*, 2005; Menon *et al.*, 1999). Denburg *et al.* (1997) found LA SLE-positive patients to score significantly lower than LA-negative patients on measures of verbal memory, cognitive flexibility, and psychomotor speed. In addition, cognitive deficits were noted even in patients who had no past or present clinical neuropsychiatric event, suggesting a specific association between antibodies and cognitive functioning.

Menon *et al.* (1999) reported that SLE patients with persistently elevated IgG anti-cardiolipin antibody levels over a period of 2–3 years performed significantly worse than SLE patients with occasionally elevated or never elevated titers on a variety of neuropsychological tests. These results were not observed with anti-DNA antibody titers or C3 levels. Attention and concentration, as well as psychomotor speed, were the domains most affected. Hanly *et al.* (1999) followed 51 female SLE patients over a 5-year period and found that persistent anti-cardiolipin antibody IgG elevations were associated with decreased psychomotor speed, whereas persistent anti-cardiolipin antibody IgA elevations were correlated with problems with executive functioning and reasoning abilities. They also found no association between cognitive deficits and anti-DNA antibodies. McLaurin *et al.* (2005) prospectively studied the relationship between anti-cardiolipin antibodies and anti-b_2GP-I antibodies in 123 SLE patients over 3 years. Factors significantly associated with cognitive decline were persistently positive anti-phospholipid antibody levels, prednisone use, diabetes, higher depression scores, and less education. All of these prospective studies found a relationship between persistently positive anti-cardiolipin antibody IgG levels and cognitive dysfunction, suggesting that sustained exposure to anti-phospholipid antibodies may be required for the development of this manifestation. The underlying pathophysiologic mechanism is not clear, but multiple small ischemic events, vasculopathy leading to diffuse chronic brain ischemia, and direct antibody effects have all been suggested.

Progressive sensorineural hearing loss

Toubi *et al.* (1997) studied the association between anti-cardiolipin antibodies and sudden or progressive sensorineural hearing loss in 30 patients and matched normal controls. None of the control group had anti-cardiolipin antibodies, whereas 27% of the patient group had anti-cardiolipin antibodies in low to moderate titers (Toubi *et al.*, 1997). Of the patients with anti-cardiolipin antibodies, five of eight had sudden deafness. In addition, two of five patients with sudden deafness and anti-cardiolipin antibodies relapsed as compared with none of six patients without them. Naarendorp and Spiera (1998) reported six patients with SLE or a lupus-like syndrome with sudden sensorineural hearing loss, all of whom had anti-cardiolipin antibody or LA. The authors suggest that sudden sensorineural hearing loss may be a previously unrecognized manifestation of AAS and that the mechanism is likely to be vascular, and they speculate that the appropriate treatment for these patients may be anticoagulant therapy. Progressive sensorineural hearing loss has also been described in a patient with CAAS who also met criteria for Susac's syndrome (microangiopathic disorder of unknown pathogenesis presenting with encephalopathy, hearing loss, and branch retinal artery occlusions) (Bucciarelli *et al.*, 2004).

Transient global amnesia

Transient global amnesia, a syndrome of sudden, unexplained memory loss, has been associated with anti-phospholipid antibody immunoreactivity (Montalban *et al.*, 1989; Ortego-Centeno *et al.*, 2006). The etiology of transient global amnesia in patients without anti-phospholipid antibodies is controversial and thought to be related to ischemia or epileptiform activity in bilateral hippocampal areas. As both cerebral ischemia and epilepsy have been associated with anti-phospholipid antibodies, either could play a role in anti-phospholipid antibody-associated transient global amnesia (Ortego-Centeno *et al.*, 2006).

Ocular manifestations

Many reports of stroke and TIA associated with anti-phospholipid antibodies include some patients with ocular ischemia as well (Labutta, 1996; Rafuse and Canny, 1992). The ophthalmologic ischemic manifestations commonly associated with anti-phospholipid antibody include anterior ischemic optic neuropathy, branch and central retinal artery occlusions, cilioretinal artery occlusions, combined artery and vein occlusions, and amaurosis fugax (Labutta, 1996). These manifestations are found in patients with both primary and secondary AAS APS.

Neuroimaging studies

Brain MRI studies in patients with AAS (primary or secondary) have revealed small foci of high signal in subcortical white matter scattered throughout the brain (Molad *et al.*, 1992; Provenzale *et al.*, 1994; Toubi *et al.*, 1995). This type of pattern is seen in many other disease processes and is, as such, nonspecific. The correlation between MRI lesions in patients with antiphospholipid and clinical nervous system symptoms is reported to be high by some investigators (Provenzale *et al.*, 1994; Tietjen *et al.*, 1998; Toubi *et al.*, 1995) and not by others (Sailer *et al.*, 1997; Schmidt *et al.*, 1995). Figure 38.1 illustrates multiple cerebral infarction on brain imaging in a 23-year-old woman with anti-phospholipid antibodies and SLE.

Toubi *et al.* (1995) found anti-phospholipid antibody aPL immunoreactivity in 53/96 (55%) SLE patients with central nervous system (CNS) manifestations as compared to 20/100 (20%) of SLE patients without them. In this study, 53 patients with CNS manifestations underwent MRI and 33 showed high-density lesions that were interpreted as 'suggestive of vasculopathy.' MRI abnormalities were seen more frequently in patients with anti-phospholipid antibody immunoreactivity as compared to those without. Some of these patients with MRI abnormalities had seizures or psychiatric disturbances but not stroke. This suggests that, in some cases, anti-phospholipid antibody-associated neurologic manifestations may be because of an anti-phospholipid

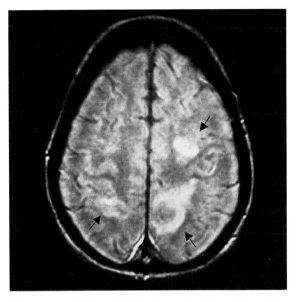

Figure 38.1 Multiple cerebral infarctions on brain imaging in a 23-year-old woman with anti-phospholipid antibodies and SLE.

antibody-brain phospholipid interaction, whereas in others the underlying pathogenic feature may be thrombotic.

Sailer *et al.* (1997) studied 35 SLE patients with inactive SLE using brain MRI and positron emission tomography (PET) imaging, neuropsychological testing, a neurological examination, and serum testing for anti-phospholipid antibodies and anti-neuronal antibodies. Twenty patients had neurological deficits, three had psychiatric symptoms, and 10 had cognitive impairment. No differences in global glucose utilization by PET imaging were seen between SLE patients compared to those without neurological or cognitive abnormalities. On MRI, the number and size of the white matter lesions correlated with the presence of neurological deficit, but were unrelated to the severity of cognitive impairment. Large lesions (≥ 8 mm) were associated with high anti-cardiolipin antibody IgG levels. Tietjen *et al.* (1998) also found an association between MRI lesions and anti-cardiolipin antibody levels in young patients with migraine-associated transient focal neurologic events. In a study evaluating the association between neuropsychological abnormalities and anti-phospholipid antibodies in an elderly population, no association between anti-cardiolipin antibodies and MRI lesions was found, supporting Sailer's findings in the group with cognitive impairment only (Schmidt *et al.*, 1995). Hachulla *et al.* (1998) performed brain MRI in patients with primary and secondary AAS. Both cerebral atrophy and white matter lesions were more common in both groups with respect to control subjects. The number and volume of white matter lesions were increased in patients with primary and secondary AAS who also had neurological symptoms. Only a weak correlation was found between the presence of LA and cerebral atrophy.

In addition to MRI, Specker *et al.* (1998) report the use of the transcranial Doppler technique for the assessment of stroke risk in patients with anti-phospholipid antibodies. Transcranial Doppler has been used to identify microembolic signals, which have been detected in the intracranial circulation of patients with carotid artery disease, artificial heart valves, and coagulopathy, but are infrequently associated with small-vessel disease. They are thought to arise from vascular air bubbles, formed elements, and experimentally induced emboli (Padayachee *et al.*, 1987; Russell *et al.*, 1991; Spencer *et al.*, 1990), and are detected based on the site, degree, extent, and surface of stenosis (Sitzer *et al.*, 1995). The use of transcranial Doppler to detect microembolic signals in AAS is an inexpensive, noninvasive method. It may offer an approach in risk stratification and possibly therapy monitoring in patients with anti-phospholipid antibodies (Brey and Carolin, 1997). Two of the patients with the highest event rates were anti-phospholipid antibody positive, and the rate of microembolic signals correlated with the titer of IgG-anti-cardiolipin antibody, arguing for a pathophysiological association between anti-phospholipid antibodies and microembolic signals.

Potential mechanisms for anti-phospholipid-induced thrombosis

The range of clinical manifestations in AAS might be explained by the breadth of autoantibodies and their characteristics (specificity, affinity/avidity, valency, titer). Consequently, mechanisms may be widely characterized by those involving antibody interference with hemostatic reactions and those involving cell-mediated events (for review, see Roubey, 1998).

A variety of effects on platelets, coagulation proteins, and endothelial cells have been ascribed to anti-phospholipid antibodies, making them not only serological markers for AAS, but direct contributors to the development of thrombosis and other clinical manifestations. b_2GP-I binding to phosphatidyl serine may serve in the identification of apoptotic cells, because cells undergoing apoptosis are known to redistribute phospholipids to expose phosphatidyl serine on the extracellular surface (Casciola-Rosen *et al.*, 1996). In vitro opsonization of apoptotic cells by b_2GP-I antibodies enhances scavenger macrophage binding. With respect to platelet–antibody interactions, Arnout (1996) has drawn attention to the similarities between the pathogenic mechanism for heparin-induced thrombocytopenia and a potential mechanism for anti-phospholipid antibody-induced thrombosis. Heparin-induced thrombocytopenia involves antibody binding of a protein (mainly platelet factor 4) that is bound to heparin, which then interacts with the cellular Fc-gamma receptor to induce activation of a prothrombotic process. There is emerging evidence that anti-phospholipid antibody binding to phospholipid complexes on various cells, including platelets and vascular endothelium, also results in their activation through the Fc-gamma receptor (Meroni *et al.*, 1998). Campbell *et al.* (1995) have demonstrated the induction of a dose-dependent increase in the activation and aggregation of human platelets using antiphospholipid from patients with AAS. This effect appears to be mediated through binding to phosphatidyl serine or b_2GP-I. The feasibility of b_2GP-I binding to endothelial cells is more controversial because they infrequently express large amounts of negatively charged structures at the cell surface. Recent evidence suggests that b_2GP-I may be involved in lipid metabolism and may serve as an endothelial growth factor. Meroni *et al.* (1998) have demonstrated that b_2GP-I

probably binds to endothelial cells through heparin-sulfate proteoglycan, which plays a role in the function of vascular endothelial growth factors.

Both passive and active immunization of normal laboratory mice with either anti-phospholipid antibodies or with b_2GP-I results in the induction of an experimental AAS, including thrombocytopenia, placental infarction and fetal loss, myocardial infarction, and neurological dysfunction (for review, see Ziporen and Shoenfeld, 1998). Some AAS may arise because of infection by common viruses and bacteria (for review, see Gharavi and Pierangeli, 1998). Gharavi *et al.* (1995) showed that pathogenic anti-phospholipid antibodies and anti-b_2GP-I antibody production can be induced following immunization with mutant forms of b_2GP-I containing the anti-phospholipid antibody binding site alone. A subsequent Genebank screen yielded seven proteins with sequence homology to the mutant proteins. Four of the peptides were identified as part of viruses or bacteria to which humans are commonly exposed (human cytomegalovirus and *Bacillus subtilis*). Interestingly, these peptides had a greater ability to bind phospholipids than the mutants they generated. Normal mice immunized with these viral protein fragments developed anti-phospholipid antibodies and developed intrauterine fetal death, spinal cord infarction, and thrombosis (Gharavi *et al.*, 1996), suggesting that infection may well be the trigger for pathogenic anti-phospholipid antibody production (Gharavi and Pierangeli, 1998). A recent report describing APS associated with cytomegalovirus infection illustrates that infection-induced anti-phospholipid antibodies may occasionally be associated with thrombosis (Labarca *et al.*, 1997). In support of this proposal, Vermylen *et al.* (1998) provide corroborative evidence for infective origins of anti-phospholipid antibodies. Varicella-associated neutralizing antibodies against Protein S present clinical resemblance to purpura fulminans, a congenital homozygous protein S deficiency that may exhibit widespread cutaneous thrombosis and necrosis shortly following birth (Marlar and Neumann, 1990). Similar symptoms may arise from IgG and IgM antibodies to protein S in children recovering from varicella infection. Ultimately, common bacterial or viral infection might incite similar mechanisms in humans and yield anti-phospholipid antibody production in AAS.

The possible roll complement activation was demonstrated on mice deficient in C3 and C5. These were resistant to the enhanced thrombosis and endothelial cell activation induced by anti-phospholipid antibodies. Furthermore, the inhibition of C5 activation using anti-C5 monoclonal antibodies prevented thrombosis. (Pierangeli *et al.*, 2005).

Many investigators favor a "two-hit" hypothesis to explain how AAS antiphospholipid might lead to thrombosis; (i) continually circulating AAS antiphospholipid and phospholipid-binding proteins require (ii) a local trigger (i.e. infection, injury, endothelial cell activation) to induce site-specific thrombosis or amplify the thrombotic process (Vaarala, 1998). This hypothesis proposes anti-phospholipid antibody induction of a prothrombotic state in which thrombosis is triggered by an otherwise insufficient local trigger (Roubey, 1998). Thrombosis would require a second triggering factor, so explaining why patients with persistent serum autoantibodies display clotting events only occasionally and in the absence of detectable Ig deposits (Meroni *et al.*, 1998). Although there is some evidence that anti-phospholipid antibodies may actually lead to accelerated atherosclerosis, the majority of evidence favors a prothrombotic mechanism that amplifies thrombosis in certain settings. Pierangeli and Harris (1998) demonstrated larger clot size with a longer time to dissolution in mice administered human anti-phospholipid antibodies compared to control IgG using a pinch-clamp injury model. Taken together, these studies provide important evidence that antibodies to phospholipids and phospholipid-binding proteins like b_2GP-I can cause thrombosis and other antibody-mediated clinical manifestations.

Treatment

Appropriate therapy for cerebrovascular SLE must include the prevention of vasculopathies as well as the minimizing of ischemic damage when it occurs. Unless there is evidence of active inflammation, corticosteroids and immunosuppression are rarely indicated. Acute therapy consists of limiting the extent of damage to the ischemic tissue, rest, antiplatelet agents, and appropriate blood pressure management avoiding tight blood pressure control that may result in hypoperfusion (Navarrete and Brey, 2000).

Treatment of AAS can be directed at thrombo-occlusive events using antithrombotic medications or at modulating the immune response with immunotherapy (Brey, 2004). In the case of thrombotic manifestations, both approaches have been used. There are no data that address the use of any specific treatment strategies for primary prevention of antiphospholipid-associated stroke. The aforementioned Euro-Phospholipid Project Group will also have some information that will shed light on the issue of primary prevention although, in that study, patients are not randomized to a specific treatment (Cervera *et al.*, 2002).

Treatment such as platelet antiaggregant and anticoagulant therapy for secondary stroke prevention have both been used in AAS and in cerebrovascular disease associated with anti-phospholipid antibody immunoreactivity (Crowther *et al.*, 2003; Khamashta *et al.*, 1995; Levine *et al.*, 2004; Rosove and Brewer, 1992). Two groups have retrospective data to suggest that high-intensity warfarin treatment (vs. low- or moderate-intensity warfarin or aspirin treatment) is associated with better outcomes in selected cohorts with various types of thrombotic events (Khamashta *et al.*, 1995; Rosove and Brewer, 1992). Patients reported on in these studies did not have repeat anti-phospholipid antibody testing and would not fulfill current criteria for AAS.

Crowther *et al.* (2003) recently reported the results of the first randomized, double-blind, controlled trial of two different intensities of warfarin treatment on the prevention of recurrent thrombotic events in patients with AAS APS. There were 114 patients enrolled in the study and followed for an average of 2.7 years. The average international normalized ratio (INR) values in the moderate- and high-intensity groups were 2.3 and 3.3, respectively. Recurrent thrombosis occurred in 2/58 (3.4%) patients assigned to moderate-intensity warfarin and in 6/56 (10.7%) patients assigned to receive high-intensity warfarin. There was no difference in recurrent thrombosis or major bleeding rates between the two

groups. These results suggest that high-intensity warfarin treatment is *not* more effective than moderate-intensity treatment in preventing recurrent thrombotic events in patients with AAS. The study did not specifically address the end-point of stroke.

The APASS Group recently completed the first prospective study of the role of antiphospholipid in recurrent ischemic stroke in collaboration with the WARSS group (Levine *et al.*, 2004). This controlled and blinded study was initiated in 1993 and compared the risk of recurrent stroke and other thromboembolic disease over a 2-year follow-up period in patients with ischemic stroke who were randomized to either aspirin therapy (325 mg/day) or warfarin therapy at a dose to maintain the INR between 1.4 and 2.8. The suggested target INR was 2.2. The purpose of the study was to collect information about recurrent stroke rates in antiphospholipid-positive versus antiphospholipid-negative patients controlling for treatment. There were 882 patients randomized to warfarin and 890 patients randomized to aspirin who participated in APASS. No increased risk of thrombotic event was associated with the baseline antiphospholipid in either the warfarin-treated patients (relative risk [RR] 0.97; 95% CI, 0.74–1.27, $p = .82$) or the aspirin-treated patients (RR 0.96; 95% CI, 0.71–1.29, $p = .77$). Patients with baseline positivity for both LA and anti-cardiolipin antibodies tended to have a higher event rate (31.7%) than did patients who were negative on both antibodies (24.0%) – RR 1.36 (95% CI, 0.97–1.92, $p = .07$). There was no difference in major bleeding complications between treatment groups. Thus it appears that, for patients with a positive anti-phospholipid antibody determination at a single time point at the time of ischemic stroke (including low titers of anti-cardiolipin antibodies and/or IgA anti-cardiolipin antibodies), aspirin and warfarin therapy at an INR of approximately 2.0 are equivalent regarding stroke recurrence and major bleeding complications.

CAAS is being recognized as a rare presentation of thrombosis with involvement of the small vasculature and a mortality of about 50%. It resembles a thrombotic thrombocytopenic purpura. Involvement of the CNS is a common feature of CAAS. Its management includes the treatment of the primary cause, which is generally an infectious process and plasma exchange or intravenous IgG for the most severe causes (Vora *et al.*, 2006).

REFERENCES

Alarcon-Segovia, D., Deleze, M., and Oria, C. V. 1989. Antiphospholipid antibodies and the antiphospholipid syndrome in systemic lupus erythematosus: a prospective analysis of 500 consecutive patients. *Medicine*, **68**, 353–65.

Ameri, A., and Bousser, M. G. 1992. Cerebral venous thrombosis. *Neurol Clin*, **10**, 87–111.

Antiphospholipid Antibodies in Stroke Study (APASS) Group. 1990. Clinical and laboratory findings in patients with antiphospholipid antibodies and cerebral ischemia. *Stroke*, **21**, 1268–73.

Arnout, J. 1996. The pathogenesis of antiphospholipid antibody syndrome: hypothesis based on parallelisms with heparin-induced thrombocytopenia. *Thromb Haemost*, **75**, 536–41.

Arnout, J., and Vermylen, J. 1998. Mechanism of action of beta-2-glycoprotein-1-dependent lupus anticoagulants. *Lupus*, **7**, S23–8.

Atsumi, T., Ieko, M., Bertolaccini, M. L., *et al.* 2000. Association of autoantibodies against the phosphatidylserine-prothrombin complex with manifestations of the antiphospholipid syndrome and with the presence of lupus anticoagulant. *Arthritis Rheum*, **43**, 1982–93.

Blohorn, A., Guegan-Massardier, E., Triquenot, A., *et al.* 2002. Antiphospholipid antibodies in the acute phase of cerebral ischaemia in young adults: a descriptive study of 139 patients. *Cerebrovasc Dis*, **13**, 156–62.

Brey, R. L. 2004. Management of the neurological manifestations of APS – what do the trials tell us? *Thromb Res*, **114**, 489–99.

Brey, R. L., Abbott, R. D., Curb, J. D., *et al.* 2001. Beta(2)-glycoprotein 1-dependent anticardiolipin antibodies and risk of ischemic stroke and myocardial infarction: the Honolulu heart program. *Stroke*, **32**, 1701–6.

Brey, R. L., and Carolin, M. K. 1997. Detection of cerebral microembolic signals by transcranial Doppler may be a useful part of the equation in determining stroke risk in patients with antiphospholipid antibody syndrome. *Lupus*, **6**, 621–4.

Brey, R. L., Hart, R. G., Sherman, D. G., and Tegeler, C. T. 1990. Antiphospholipid antibodies and cerebral ischemia in young people. *Neurology*, **40**, 1190–6.

Bucciarelli, S., Cervera, R., Martinez, M., Latorre, X., and Font, J. 2004 Susac's syndrome or catastrophic antiphospholipid syndrome? *Lupus*, **13**, 607–8.

Campbell, A. L., Pierangeli, S. S., Wellhausen, S., and Harris, E. N. 1995. Comparison of the effects of anticardiolipin antibodies from patients with the antiphospholipid antibody syndrome and with syphilis on platelet activation and aggregation. *Thromb Haemost*, **73**, 529–34.

Carhuapoma, J. R., Mitsias, P., and Levine, S. R. 1997. Cerebral venous thrombosis and anticardiolipin antibodies. *Neurology*, **28**, 2363–9.

Casciola-Rosen, L., Rosen, A., Petri, M., and Schlissel, M. 1996. Surface blebs on apoptotic cells are sites of enhanced procoagulant activity implications for coagulation events and antigenic spread in systemic lupus erythematosus. *Proc Natl Acad Sci, USA*, **93**, 1624–9.

Cervera, R., Khamashta, M. A., Font, J., *et al.* 2003. Morbidity and mortality in systemic lupus erythematosus during a 10-year period: a comparison of early and late manifestations in a cohort of 1000 patients. *Medicine*, **82**, 299–308.

Cervera, R., Piette, J. C., Font, J., *et al.* 2002. Antiphospholipid syndrome: clinical and immunologic manifestations and patterns of disease expression in a cohort of 1000 patients. *Arthritis Rheum*, **46**, 1019–27.

Cesbron, J. Y., Amouyel, P., and Masy, E. 1997. Anticardiolipin antibodies and physical disability in the elderly. *Ann Intern Med*, **126**, 1003.

Chapman, J., Abu-Katash, M., Inzelberg, R., *et al.* 2002 Prevalence and clinical features of dementia associated with the antiphospholipid syndrome and circulating anticoagulants. *J Neurol Sci*, **203–204**, 81–4.

Chinnery, P. F., Shaw, P. I., Ince, P. G., Jackson, G. H., and Bishop, R. I. 1997. Fulminant encephalopathy due to the catastrophic primary antiphospholipid syndrome. *J Neurol Neurosurg Psychiatry*, **62**, 300–1.

Ciocca, R. G., Choi, J., and Graham, A. M. 1995. Antiphospholipid antibodies lead to increased risk in cardiovascular surgery. *Am J Surg*, **170**, 198–200.

Crowther, M. A., Ginsberg, J. S., Julian, J., *et al.* 2003. A comparison of two intensities of warfarin for the prevention of recurrent thrombosis in patients with the antiphospholipid antibody syndrome [see comment] [erratum appears in *N Engl J Med*, 2003 Dec 25;349, 2577]. *N Engl J Med*, **349**, 1133–8.

de Moerloose, P., Boehlen, F., and Reber, G. 1997. Prevalence of anticardiolipin and antinuclear antibodies in an elderly hospitalized population and mortality after a 6-year follow-up. *Age Aging*, **27**, 319–21.

Del Papa, N., Guidali, L., Sala, A., *et al.* 1997. Endothelial cells as target for antiphospholipid antibodies. *Arthritis Rheum*, **40**, 551–61.

Del Papa, N., Raschi, E., Catelli, L., *et al.* 1997. Endothelial cells as a target for antiphospholipid antibodies: role of anti-beta-2-glycoprotein 1 antibodies. *Am J Reprod Immunol*, **38**, 212–7.

Denburg, S. D., Carbotte, R. M., Ginsberg, J. S., and Denburg, J. 1997 The relationship of antiphospholipid antibodies to cognitive function in patients with systemic lupus erythematosus. *J Int Neuropsychol Soc*, **3**, 377–86.

Deschiens, M. A., Conard, J., Horellou, M. H., *et al.* 1996. Coagulations studies, factor V Leiden, and anticardiolipin antibodies in 40 cases of cerebral venous sinus thrombosis. *Stroke*, **27**, 1724–30.

Drouvalakis, K. A., and Buchanan, T. T. C. 1998. Phospholipid specificity of autoimmune and drug induced lupus anticoagulants; association of phosphatidylethanolamine reactivity with thrombosis in autoimmune disease. *J Rheumatol*, **25**, 290–5.

Duhaut, P., Berruyer, M., Pinede, L., *et al.* 1998. Anticardiolipin antibodies and giant cell arteritis: a prospective, multicenter case-control study. *Arthritis Rheum*, **41**, 701–9.

Escalante, A., Brey, R. L., Mitchell, B. D., and Dreiner, U. 1995. Accuracy of anticardiolipin antibodies in identifying a history of thrombosis among patients with systemic lupus erythematosus. *Am J Med*, **98**, 559–67.

Ford, S. E., Kennedy, L. A., and Ford, P. M. 1994. Clinico-pathological correlations of antiphospholipid antibodies. *Arch Pathol Lab Med*, **118**, 491–5.

Ford, S. E., Lillicrap, D. M., Brunet, D., and Ford, P. M. 1989. Thrombotic endocarditis and lupus anticoagulant, a pathogenetic possibility for idiopathic rheumatic type valvular heart disease. *Arch Pathol Lab Med*, **113**, 350–3.

Galli, M., Comfurius, P., Maassen, C., *et al.* 1990. Anticardiolipin antibodies (ACA) directed not to cardiolipin but to a plasma protein cofactor. *Lancet*, **335**, 1544–7.

Gharavi, A. E., and Pierangeli, S. S. 1998. Origin of antiphospholipid antibodies: induction of aPL by viral peptides. *Lupus*, **7**, S52–4.

Gharavi, A. E., Tang, H., Gharavi, E. E., Espinoza, L. R., and Wilson, W. A. 1996. Induction of antiphospholipid antibodies by immunization with a viral peptide. *Arthritis Rheum*, **39**, S319.

Gharavi, A. E., Tang, H., Gharavi, E. E., Wilson, W. A., and Espinoza, L. R. 1995. Induction of aPL by immunization with a 15 amino acid peptide. *Arthritis Rheum*, **38**, S296.

Gross, L. 1940. The cardiac lesion in Libman-Sacks disease with a consideration of its relationship to acute diffuse lupus erythematosus. *Am J Pathol*, **16**, 375–408.

Hachulla E., et al. 1998. Cerebral magnetic resonance imaging in patients with or without antiphospholipid antibodies. 1998 *Lupus*, **7**, (2), 124–131.

Hanly, J. G., Hong, C., Smith, S., Fisk, J. D. 1999 A prospective analysis of cognitive function and anticardiolipin antibodies in systemic lupus erythematosus. *Arthritis Rheum*, **42**, 728–34.

Hudson, M., Herr, A. L., Rauch, J., *et al.* 2003. The presence of multiple prothrombotic risk factors is associated with a higher risk of thrombosis in individuals with anticardiolipin antibodies. *J Rheumatol*, **30**, 2385–91.

Hughes, G. R. V. 1983. Thrombosis, abortion, cerebral disease and lupus anticoagulant. *Br Med J*, **187**, 1088–91.

Inanc, M., Radway-Bright, E. L., and Isenberg, D. A. 1997. Beta-2-glycoprotein 1 and anti-beta-2-glycoprotein 1 antibodies: where are we now? *Br J Rheumatol*, **36**, 1247–57.

Jacobson, M. W., Rappaport, L. J., Keenan, P. A., *et al.* 1999. Neuropsychological deficits associated with antiphospholipid antibodies. *J Clin Exp Neuropsychol*, **21**, 251–64.

Janardhan, V., Wolf, P. A., Kase, C. S., *et al.* 2004. Anticardiolipin antibodies and risk of ischemic stroke and transient ischemic attack: the Framingham cohort and offspring study. *Stroke*, **35**, 736–41.

Kalashnikova, L. A., Nasonov, E. L., Kushekbaeva, A. E., and Gracheva, L. A. 1990. Anticardiolipin antibodies in Sneddon's syndrome. *Neurology*, **40**, 464–7.

Khamashta, M. A., Cuadrado, M. J., Mujic, F., *et al.* 1995. The management of thrombosis in the antiphospholipid antibody syndrome. *N Engl J Med*, **332**, 993–7.

Klemp, P., Cooper, R. C., Strauss, F. J., *et al.* 1988. Anticardiolipin antibodies in ischemic heart disease. *Clin Exp Immunol*, **74**, 254–7.

Krause, I., Lev, S., Fraser, A., *et al.* 2005. Close association between valvar heart disease and central nervous system manifestations in the antiphospholipid syndrome. *Ann Rheum Dis*, **64**, 1490–3.

Krnic-Barrie, S., Reister, O., Connor, C., *et al.* 1997. A retrospective review of 61 patients with antiphospholipid syndrome. *Arch Intern Med*, **157**, 2101–8.

Labarca, J. A., Rabagghati, R. M., Radrigan, F. J., *et al.* 1997. Antiphospholipid syndrome associated with cytomegalovirus infection: case report and review. *Clin Infect Dis*, **24**, 197–200.

Labutta, R. J. 1996. Ophthalmic manifestations in the antiphospholipid syndrome. In *The Antiphospholipid Syndrome*, ed. R. A. Asherson, R. Cervera, J. C. Piette, and Y. Shoenfeld. Boca Raton, FL: CRC Press, pp. 213–8.

Lanthier, S., Kirkham, F. J., Mitchell, L. G., *et al.* 2004. Increased anticardiolipin antibody IgG titers do not predict recurrent stroke or TIA in children. *Neurology*, **62**, 194–200.

Lerita, E., Brandt, J., Minor, M., *et al.* 2002 Neuropsychological functioning and its relationship to antiphospholipid antibodies in patients with SLE. *J Clin Exp Neuropsychol*, **24**, 527–33.

Levine, S. R., Brey, R. L., Salowich-Palm, L., Sawaya, K. L., and Havstad, S. 1993. Antiphospholipid antibody associated stroke: prospective assessment of recurrent event risk. *Stroke*, **24**, 188.

Levine, S. R., Brey, R. L., Sawaya, K. L., *et al.* 1995. Recurrent stroke and thrombo-occlusive events in the antiphospholipid syndrome. *Ann Neurol*, **38**, 119–24.

Levine, S. R., Brey, R. L., Tilley, B. C., *et al.* 2004. Antiphospholipid antibodies and subsequent thrombo-occlusive events in patients with ischemic stroke. *JAMA*, **291**, 576–84.

Levine, S. R., Salowich-Palm, L., Sawaya, K. L., *et al.* 1997. IgG anticardiolipin antibody titer > 40 GPL and the risk of subsequent thrombo-occlusive events and death. *Stroke*, **28**, 1660–5.

Levy, R. A., Avvad, E., Olivera, J., and Porto, L. C. 1998. Placental pathology in antiphospholipid syndrome. *Lupus*, **7**, S81–5.

Libman, E., and Sacks, B. 1924. A hitherto undescribed form of valvular and mural endocarditis. *Arch Intern Med*, **33**, 701–37.

Loizou, S., McCrea, J. D., Rudge, A. C., *et al.* 1985. Measurement of anticardiolipin antibodies by an enzyme linked immunosorbent assay (ELISA): standardization and quanitation of results. *Clin Exp Immunol*, **62**, 738–45.

Lopez, L. R., Dier, K. J., Lopez, D., Merrill, J. T., and Fink, C. A. 2004 Anti-β_2-glycoprotein I and antiphosphatidylserine antibodies are predictors of arterial thrombosis in patients with antiphospholipid syndrome. *Am J Clin Pathol*, **121**, 142–9.

Male, C., Foulon, D., Hoogendoorn, H., *et al.* 2005. Predictive value of persistent versus transient antiphospholipid antibody subtypes for the risk of thrombotic events in pediatric patients with systemic lupus erythematosus. *Blood*, **106**, 4152–8.

Marlar, R. A., and Neumann, A. 1990. Neonatal purpura fulminans due to homozygous protein C or protein S deficiencies. *Semin Thromb Hemost*, **16**, 299–309.

Matsuura, E., Igarashi, Y., Fujimoto, M., Ichikawa, K., and Koike, T. 1990. Anticardiolipin cofactors and the differential diagnosis of autoimmune disease. *Lancet*, **336**, 177–8.

Matsuura, E., Kobayashi, K., Yasuda, T., and Koike, T. 1998. Antiphospholipid antibodies and atherosclerosis. *Lupus*, **7(Suppl. 2)**, S135–9.

McLaurin, E. Y., Holliday, S. L., Williams, P., and Brey, R. L. 2005 Predictors of cognitive dysfunction in patients with systemic lupus erythematosus. *Neurology*, **64**, 297–303.

McNeil, H. P., Chesterman, C. N., and Krilis, S. A. 1991. Immunology and clinical importance of antiphospholipid antibodies. *Adv Immunol*, **49**, 193–280.

McNeil, H. P., Simpson, R. J., Chesterman, C. N., and Krilis, S. A. 1990. Antiphospholipid antibodies are directed to a complex antigen that includes a lipid-binding inhibitor of coagulation: b_2-glycoprotein I (apolipoprotein H). *Proc Natl Acad Sci USA*, **87**, 4120–4.

Menon, S., Jameson-Shortall, E., Newman Hall-Craggs, S. P., Chinn, R., and Isenberg, D. A. 1999 A longitudinal study of anticardiolipin antibody levels and cognitive functioning in systemic lupus erythematosus. *Arthritis Rheum*, **42**, 735–41.

Meroni, P. L., Del Papa, N., Raschi, E., *et al.* 1998. b_2 glycoprotein 1 as a co-factor for antiphospholipid reactivity with endothelial cells. *Lupus*, **7(Suppl. 2)**, S44–7.

Miyakis, S., Lockshin, M. D., Atsumi, T., *et al.* 2006. International consensus statement on an update of the classification criteria for definite antiphospholipid syndrome (APS). *J Thromb Haemost*, **4**, 295–306.

Molad, Y., Sidi, Y., Gornish, M., *et al.* 1992. Lupus anticoagulant: correlation with magnetic resonance imaging of brain lesions. *J Rheumatol*, **19**, 556–61.

Montalban, J., Arboix, A., Staub, H., *et al.* 1989. Transient global amnesia and antiphospholipid antibodies. *Clin Exp Rheumatol*, **7**, 85–7.

Mosek, A., Yust, I., Treves, T. A., *et al.* 2000 Dementia and antiphospholipid antibodies. *Dement Geriatr Cogn Disord*, **11**, 36–8.

Naarendorp, M., and Spiera, H. 1998. Sudden sensorineural hearing loss in patients with systemic lupus erythematosus or lupus-like syndromes and antiphospholipid antibodies. *J Rheumatol*, **25**, 589–92.

Navarrete, G., and Brey, R. 2000. Neuropsychiatric systemic lupus erythematosus. *Curr Treat Options Neurol*, **2**, 473–85.

Nencini, P., Baruffi, M. C., Abbate, R., *et al.* 1992. Lupus anticoagulant and anticardiolipin antibodies in young adults with cerebral ischemia. *Stroke*, **23**, 189–93.

Neville, C., Ruach, J., Kassis, J., *et al.* 2003. Thromboembolic risk in patients with high titre anticardiolipin and multiple antiphospholipid antibodies. *Thromb Haemost*, **90**, 108–15.

Nojima, J., Suehisa, E., Akita, N., *et al.* 1997. Risk of arterial thrombosis in patients with anticardiolipin antibodies and lupus anticoagulant. *Br J Haematol*, **96**, 447–50.

Ortego-Centeno, N., Callejas-Rubio, J. L., Fernandez, M. G., and Camello, M. G. 2006. Transient global amnesia in a patient with high and persistent levels of antiphospholipid antibodies. *Clin Rheumatol*, **25**, 407–8.

Padayachee, T. S., Parsons, S., Theobold, R., *et al.* 1987. The detection of microemboli in the middle cerebral artery during cardiopulmonary bypass: a transcranial Doppler ultrasound investigation using membrane and bubble oxygenators. *Ann Thorac Surg*, **44**, 298–302.

Pierangeli, S. S., Girardi, G., Vega-Ostertag, M., *et al.* 2005. Requirement of activation of complement C3 and C5 for antiphospholipid antibody-mediated thrombophilia. *Arthritis Rheum*, **52**, 2120–4.

Pierangeli, S. S., and Harris, E. N. 1998. Antiphospholipid antibodies in an in vivo thrombosis model in mice. *Lupus*, **3**, 247–51.

Provenzale, J. M., Heinz, E. R., Ortel, T. L., *et al.* 1994. Antiphospholipid antibodies in patients without systemic lupus erythematosus: neuroradiologic findings. *Radiology*, **192**, 531–7.

Rafuse, P. E., and Canny, C. L. B. 1992. Initial identification of antinuclear antibody-negative systemic lupus erythematosus on ophthalmic examination: a case report with discussion of the ocular significance of anticardiolipin (antiphospholipid) antibodies. *Can J Ophthalmol*, **27**, 189–93.

Rand, J. H., Wu, X. X., Andree, H. A., *et al.* 1997. Pregnancy loss in the antiphospholipid antibody syndrome – a possible thrombogenic mechanism. *N Engl J Med*, **337**, 154–60.

Rosove, M. H., and Brewer, P. M. C. 1992. Antiphospholipid thrombosis: clinical course after the first thrombotic event in 70 patients. *Ann Intern Med*, **117**, 303–8.

Rote, N. S., Dostal-Johnson, D., and Branch, D. W. 1990. Antiphospholipid antibodies and recurrent pregnancy loss: correlation between the activated partial thromboplastin time and antibodies against phosphatidylserine and cardiolipin. *Am J Obstet Gynecol*, **163**, 575–84.

Roubey, R. A. S. 1998. Mechanisms of autoantibody-mediated thrombosis. *Lupus*, **7(Suppl. 2)**, S114–9.

Russell, D., Madden, K. P., Clark, W. M., Sandset, P. M., and Zivin, J. A. 1991. Detection of arterial emboli using Doppler ultrasound in rabbits. *Stroke*, **22**, 253–8.

Sailer, M., Burchert, W., Ehrenheim, C., *et al.* 1997. Positron emission tomography and magnetic resonance imaging for cerebral involvement in patients with systemic lupus erythematosus. *J Neurol*, **244**, 186–93.

Schmidt, R., Auer-Grumbach, P., Fazekas, F., Offenbacher, H., and Kapeller, P. 1995. Anticardiolipin antibodies in normal subjects. Neuropsychological correlates and MRI findings. *Stroke*, **26**, 749–54.

Shah, N. M., Khamashta, M. A., Atsumi, T., and Hughes, G. R. V. 1998. Outcome of patients with anticardiolipin antibodies: a 10 year follow-up of 52 patients. *Lupus*, **7**, 3–6.

Singh, K., Gaiha, M., Shome, D. K., Gupta, V. K., and Anuradha, S. 2001. The association of antiphospholipid antibodies with ischaemic stroke and myocardial infarction in young and their correlation: a preliminary study. *J Assoc Physicians India*, **49**, 527–9.

Sitzer, M., Muller, W., Siebler, M., *et al.* 1995. Plaque ulceration and lumen thrombus are the main sources of cerebral microemboli in high-grade internal carotid artery stenosis. *Stroke*, **26**, 1231–3.

Sneddon, I. B. 1965. Cerebral vascular lesions in livedo reticularis. *Br J Dermatol*, **77**, 180–5.

Specker, C. H., Perniok, A., Brauckmann, U., Siebler, M., and Schneider, M. 1998. Detection of cerebral microemboli in APS – introducing a novel investigation method and implications of analogies with carotid artery disease. *Lupus*, **7**, S75–80.

Spencer, M. P., Thomas, G. I., Nicholls, S. C., and Sauvage, L. R. 1990. Detection of middle cerebral artery emboli during carotid artery endarterectomy using transcranial Doppler ultrasonography. *Stroke*, **21**, 415–23.

Strater, R., Becker, S., von Eckardstein, A., *et al.* 2002. Prospective assessment of risk factors for recurrent stroke during childhood – a 5-year follow-up study. *Lancet*, **360**, 1540–5.

Tenedios, F., Erkan, D., and Lockshin, M. D. 2006 Cardiac manifestations in the antiphospholipid syndrome. *Rheum Dis Clin North Am*, **32**, 491–507.

Tietjen, G. E., Day, M., Norris, L., *et al.* 1998. Role of anticardiolipin antibodies in young persons with migraine and transient focal neurologic events. *Neurology*, **50**, 1433–40.

Toschi, V., Motta, A., Castelli, C., *et al.* 1998. High prevalence of antiphosphatidylinositol antibodies in young patients with cerebral ischemia of undetermined cause. [see comment]. *Stroke*, **29**, 1759–64.

Toubi, E., Ben-David, J., Kessel, A., Podoshin, L., and Golan, T. D. 1997. Autoimmune aberration in sudden sensorineural hearing loss: association with anticardiolipin antibodies. *Lupus*, **6**, 540–2.

Toubi, E., Khamashta, M. A., Panarra, A., and Hughes, G. R. V. 1995. Association of antiphospholipid antibodies with central nervous system disease in systemic lupus erythematosus. *Am J Med*, **99**, 397–401.

Tourbah, A., Peitte, J. C., Iba-Zizen, M., *et al.* 1997. The natural course of cerebral lesions in Sneddon syndrome. *Arch Neurol*, **54**, 53–60.

Tuhrim, S., Rand, J. H., Wu, X., *et al.* 1999. Antiphosphatidylserine antibodies are independently associated with ischemic stroke. *Neurology*, **53**, 1523–7.

Vaarala, O. 1998. Antiphospholipid antibodies and myocardial infarction. *Lupus*, **7(Suppl. 2)**, S132–4.

van Goor, M. P., Alblas, C. L., Leebeek, F. W., Koudstaal, P. J., and Dippel, D. W. 2004. Do antiphospholipid antibodies increase the long-term risk of thrombotic complications in young patients with a recent TIA or ischemic stroke? *Acta Neurol Scand*, **109**, 410–5.

Vermylen, J., Van Geet, C., and Arnout, J. 1998. Antibody-mediated thrombosis: relation to the antiphospholipid syndrome. *Lupus*, **7**, S63–6.

Verro, P., Levine, S. R., and Tietjen, G. E. 1998. Cerebrovascular ischemic events with high positive anticardiolipin antibodies. *Stroke*, **29**, 2245–53.

Vila, P., Hernandez, M. C., Lopez-Fernandez, M. F., and Batlle, J. 1994. Prevalence, follow-up and clinical significance of the anticardiolipin antibodies in normal subjects. *Thromb Haemost*, **72**, 209–13.

Vora, S. K., Asherson, R. A., and Erkan, D. 2006. Catastrophic antiphospholipid syndrome. *J Intensive Care Med*, **21**, 144–59.

Wahl D. G., *et al.* 1998. Meta-analysis of the risk of venous thrombosis in individuals with antiphospholipid antibodies without underlying autoimmune disease or previous thrombosis. *Lupus*, **7(1)**:15–22.

Zelger, B., Sepp, N., Stockhammer, G., *et al.* 1993. Sneddon's syndrome; a long term follow-up of 21 patients. *Arch Dermatol*, **129**, 437–44.

Ziporen, L., Goldberg, I., Arad, M., *et al.* 1996. Libman-Sacks endocarditis in the antiphospholipid syndrome: immunopathologic findings in deformed heart valves. *Lupus*, **5**, 196–205.

Ziporen, L., and Shoenfeld, Y. 1998. Antiphospholipid syndrome: from patient's bedside to experimental animal models and back to the patient's bedside. *Hematol Cell Ther*, **40**, 175–82.

39 DISSEMINATED INTRAVASCULAR DISEASE

Robert J. Schwartzman and Monisha Kumar

Disseminated intravascular coagulation

Disseminated intravascular coagulation (DIC) is a disorder of clotting caused by a cytokine-induced systemic inflammatory response that results in consumption of platelets, coagulation factors, and tissue factor plasma inhibitors (TFPIs) (Bick, 1992). It culminates in fibrin deposition-mediated thrombosis of vessels in all organ systems (Franchini, 2005; Hanly et al., 2002). It is seen in the setting of:

- sepsis (Gando et al., 1998)
- malignancy (Barbui and Falanga, 2001; Carroll and Binder, 1999; Colman and Rubin, 1990; Donati and Falanga, 2001)
- trauma (Gando, 2001)
- burns (Garcia-Avello et al., 1998)
- obstetric catastrophes (Letsky, 2001; Weiner, 1986)
- hip replacement (Breakwell et al., 1999)
- intravascular hemolysis (Krevans et al., 1957)
- viremia (Persoons et al., 1998)
- prosthetic devices (Bick, 1996)
- Kasabach-Merritt syndrome (Shoji et al., 1998)
- status epilepticus (Felcher et al., 1998)
- catastrophic antiphospholipid syndrome (APS) (Asherson, 1998)
- stroke in the setting of a medical intensive care unit (Wijdicks and Scott, 1998)
- malignant pheochromocytoma (Arai et al., 1998)
- Klippel-Trenaunay-Weber syndrome (Katsaros and Grundfest-Broniatowski, 1998)

Virtually any process that releases tissue factor into the systemic circulation or activates the vascular endothelium to release excitatory cytokines can initiate the process.

General clinical features of DIC

DIC is a syndrome caused by an underlying disease process and is not a disease in and of itself. The extrinsic or tissue factor system is abnormally activated and induces systemic coagulation (Gando et al., 1999). There is usually an early thrombotic phase that causes the deposition of fibrin throughout the small and medium-sized blood vessels of all organ systems. This is followed by consumption of clotting factors and platelets followed by fibrinolysis. Systemic hemorrhage is its most impressive feature. Most patients develop extensive bleeding from previous surgical or venipuncture sites, mucous membranes, or arterial and surgical wounds.

Acrocyanosis of extremities is common, and rarely the nose and genitalia are involved (Baker, 1989; Franchini, 2005). Gram-negative sepsis with hyperhidrosis, hyperventilation, and shock in a hospital setting is the most common presentation (Bick, 1992). Compensated DIC patients often have a solid tumor or connective tissue disease (Bick, 1988; Franchini, 2005). They have $<150\,000$ platelets/mm^3, increased turnover, and decreased survival of clotting factors with increased levels of fibrin degradation products (FDPs) (Bick, 1988). They present with subacute bleeding and thrombosis of small blood vessels rather than hemorrhage (Bick, 1992). They may be asymptomatic (Bick, 1992). The systemic clinical signs and symptoms of DIC are also dependent on the most affected organ system. DIC and sustained systemic inflammatory response syndrome (SIRS) frequently also occur concomitantly after major trauma (Bick, 1988). In this setting, the lung (acute respiratory distress syndrome), heart, and kidney (renal failure) determine the major clinical manifestations.

Pathogenesis of DIC

The four major mechanisms proposed for the initiation and maintenance of DIC are:

- increased generation of thrombin
- activation of inflammatory pathways with release of excitatory cytokines
- depressed fibrinolysis
- altered inhibition of thrombosis (Franchini, 2005)

The overwhelming majority of patients have dramatic and simultaneous activation of the tissue factor/factor VIIa (TF/F VIIa) extrinsic coagulation pathway and the release of inflammatory cytokines (Hanly et al., 2002; Franchini, 2005). Each triggering illness affects one or all of the above noted mechanisms. These mechanisms frequently overlap. Thus activated coagulation enzymes stimulate endothelial cells to produce proinflammatory cytokines, which in turn activate proteases of the extrinsic coagulation cascade.

The result of DIC is widespread coagulation that results in fibrin deposition in medium and small-sized vessels in all organ systems. Occasionally a large vessel is involved. The best studied animal models of DIC use Gram-negative bacterial cell-wall endotoxin that leads to a systemic increase of proinflammatory cytokines (Dempfle, 2004; Franchini, 2005; Wheeler and Bernard, 1999). The most common clinical setting for DIC evokes a systemic inflammatory response that leads to up-regulation and secretion of the

Uncommon Causes of Stroke, 2nd edition, ed. Louis R. Caplan. Published by Cambridge University Press.   © Cambridge University Press 2008.

inflammatory cytokines interleukin (IL)-1, IL-β, and tumor necrosis factor-α (TNF-α) (Conway and Rosenberg, 1988).

The extrinsic clotting cascade is activated during DIC by a complex of TF and F VII. Tissue factor is a tissue membrane glycoprotein that binds its zymogen cofactor to F VII on the cell surface. Activated TF/F VIIa then activates factors X and IX that initiate clotting. Experimental studies have shown that inhibition of the extrinsic pathway blocks endotoxin-induced thrombin generation, which proceeds in the face of intrinsic pathway blockade (Biemond *et al.*, 1995; Pixley *et al.*, 1993). The most likely source of tissue factor in DIC is mononuclear lymphocytes and vascular endothelial cells (Esmon, 2001; Rivers *et al.*, 1975). The expression of tissue factor on these cells is induced by endotoxin and tumor necrosis factor.

The major physiologic anticoagulants antithrombin III, activated protein C, thrombomodulin, and TFPI are down-regulated, reduced in quantity, or dysfunctional during DIC (Hanly *et al.*, 2002). This amplifies thrombin generation and promotes the formation and deposition of fibrin (Esmon, 2001). Decreased antithrombin plasma levels have been demonstrated during sepsis, which is mediated by consumption, enzyme degradation, or impaired synthesis and is the most common cause of DIC (Levi *et al.*, 2004).

Thrombomodulin is an endothelial cell surface receptor that when complexed with thrombin activates the protein anticoagulant protease PC that inhibits factor Va and VIIa. The up-regulated and released IL-1β and TNF-α seen in DIC down-regulate endothelial expression of thrombomodulin and are mechanisms that promotes clotting (Esmon, 2001; Faust *et al.*, 2001). Activated protein C may also inhibit leukocyte activation and inflammatory cytokine secretion (de Jonge *et al.*, 2000). Tissue factor inhibitor dose-dependently blocks coagulation activation independently of effects on cytokine induction or perturbation of the fibrinolytic system in humans (de Jonge E *et al.*, 2000; Maruyama, 1999). It also completely inhibits endotoxin-induced thrombin generation, which supports its involvement in the pathogenesis of DIC (Creasey *et al.*, 1993).

Experimental models of bacteremia and endotoxemia show increased fibrinolytic activity thought to be induced by the release of plasminogen activators from endothelial cells. This early hyperfibrinolytic response is down-regulated by increased levels of plasminogen activator inhibitor type I (PAI-1) (Levi *et al.*, 2003; Suffredini *et al.*, 1989).

Underlying mechanisms that initiate DIC

As noted above, release of IL-1, IL-6, and TNF-α from macrophages, monocytes, and lymphocytes at the site of injury or systemically during sepsis converts the antithrombotic blood vessel endothelium to a prothrombotic surface. Septicemia is the most common clinical condition associated with DIC (Franchini, 2005). There is no difference in its incidence with Gram-negative or Gram-positive organisms. The generalized activation of coagulation is initiated by lipopolysaccharides from the cell membrane and release of endotoxins in the former and bacterial exotoxins (staphylococcal α hemolysin) in the latter, which activate TNF-α

and IL-1 (Dempfle, 2004; Faust *et al.*, 2001; Wheeler and Bernard, 1999). Tissue factor release that occurs with burns and trauma induces systemic activation of inflammatory cytokines that initiates coagulation (Gando, 2001; Levi *et al.*, 2003; Roumen *et al.*, 1993; Sauerwein *et al.*, 1993). The primary mechanisms in these states appear to be the release of constitutively expressed tissue factor from endothelial cells (Gando, 2006). The exact mechanisms of cancer-associated thrombosis have not been elucidated. DIC may be seen in up to 15% of solid and hematologic tumors, particularly acute leukemia (Donati and Falanga, 2001; Furie and Furie, 2006). Possible mechanisms for the high incidence of thrombosis with cancer are:

- release of tissue factor during cancer cell death from chemotherapy
- expression and release of tissue factor by cancer cells
- release of tumor procoagulants and microparticles

Tissue factor microparticles are seen in cancer patients who have thromboembolic complications (Donati and Falanga, 2001). A severe hyperfibrinolytic state occurs with systemic activation of coagulation with promyelocytic leukemia (Barbui and Falanga, 2001). Metastatic malignant cells express both tissue factor and urokinase receptors that are important for neovascularization and clotting (Francis, 1998). Rarely DIC may be the first manifestation of adenocarcinoma of the prostate. Prostate biopsy in this context may exacerbate the coagulation disorder (Navarro *et al.*, 2005). Cancer of the prostate may also present as a consumptive coagulopathy with fibrinolysis (Bern, 2005). DIC occurs in approximately 50% of patients with amniotic fluid embolism, the retained fetus syndrome, and abruptio placentae. Tissue factor release and placental enzymes may activate both the intrinsic and extrinsic systems in this clinical setting (Bick, 1992; Letsky, 2001; Weiner, 1986).

All collagen vascular diseases may present with compensated DIC (Baker, 1989). The common mechanism is postulated to be abnormal physiology of the endothelial cell membrane and its high-affinity thrombin receptor thrombomodulin. Similar mechanisms may apply to some degree in those pathologic processes that affect blood vessels (angiitides, vasculitis sepsis, microangiopathic hemolytic anemia, and viremia) (Boffa and Karmochkine 1998). Activated macrophages and inflammatory cytokines enzymatically cleave thrombomodulin to a soluble fragment that can be followed as a marker of endothelial cell damage.

Vascular malformations such as the Kasabach-Merritt syndrome, Klippel-Trenaunay-Weber syndrome, or aortic aneurysms, may trigger DIC by abnormal platelet activation or direct release of reduced adenosine diphosphate (ADP), membrane phospholipoprotein, or tissue factor into the circulation, which then initiates the clotting cascade (Fernandez-Bustamante and Jimeno, 2005).

Laboratory diagnosis of DIC

The most important component in the diagnosis of DIC is its clinical features and associations with illness that are known to be its cause (Bick, 1992; Hanly *et al.*, 2002). There is a wide differential diagnosis that includes thrombotic thrombocytopenic purpura (TTP), hemolytic uremic syndrome, systemic lupus erythematosus (SLE), catastrophic APS, HELLP, and Evans syndrome. A peripheral blood smear in DIC often shows schistocytes, fragmented red blood cells (RBCs) (50% of patients) that are formed by fibrin RBC adhesion. The platelet count is usually $<80\,000$ mm^3, and large immature platelets and reticulocytosis are seen (Bick, 1992). The same findings may be seen in the other aforementioned components of its differential diagnosis. The classic laboratory features of DIC include prolonged prothrombin time (PT), activated partial thromboplastin time (aPTT), and thrombin time (Franchini, 2005; Schwartzman and Hill, 1982). The prothrombin and aPTT are prolonged in 80% of patients with DIC (Bick, 1992). A caveat is that, in 20% of patients, the PT and PTT may be normal or increased due to circulating activated thrombin and Xa or early degradation products from fibrinolysis (Bick, 1992).

The platelet count is low in the overwhelming majority of DIC patients. It varies from 2000 mm^3 to 100 000 mm^3 in patients with neurologic complications (Schwartzman and Hill, 1982). Platelet function is abnormal due to coating by fibrin fragments and abnormal activation.

DIC serum has increased levels of FDPs and low levels of coagulation inhibitors such as protein C, thrombomodulin, antithrombin III, and TFPI that are either reduced or down-regulated (Yu et al., 2000). Fibrinogen plasma level is not a good index of DIC as it acts as an acute phase reactant and may be normal in all but severe cases (Levi and Ten Cate, 1999). There have been several recently developed scoring systems developed for the diagnosis of DIC. A commonly used system proposed by the subcommittee on DIC of the International Society of Thrombosis and Haemostasis (ISTH) uses an algorithm that consists of:

- platelets
- soluble fibrin monomer/fibrin (FDPs)
- prolonged PT
- fibrinogen level

The sensitivity and specificity of this scoring system are $>90\%$ (Bakhtiari et al., 2004). A new system based on D-dimer, PT, fibrinogen level, and platelet count was found to be effective in predicting mortality (Angstwurm et al., 2006).

A better understanding of the mechanisms underlying DIC has led to an array of specific markers of coagulation that may be more sensitive than those in common laboratory use. A recent study suggests that D-dimer and plasma FDPs offer the most rapid and specific diagnosis of DIC, whereas antithrombin III levels document severity and prognosis (Schwartzman and Hill, 1982). The interest in utilizing physiologic anticoagulants as markers in DIC stems from the observation that all antithrombin III, thrombomodulin, protein C, and TFPIs are decreased during active disease. The fibrinolytic system that converts plasminogen to plasmin by plasminogen activator (t-PA) is impaired in DIC. A postulated mechanism is an increased level of plasma activated inhibitor 1 (PAI-1) during active disease (Roumen et al., 1993). The value of its measurement has not been determined.

The importance of D-dimer is that it is a neoantigen that is formed during thrombin's conversion of fibrinogen to fibrin. The newly generated fibrin is cross-linked by factor XIII. Plasmin cleaves the cross-linked fibrin that generates D-dimer. Monoclonal antibodies against DD-3B6/22 epitope are specific for cross-linked FDPs (Bick, 1992).

Indices of prothrombin conversion to thrombin are the generation of intermediate prothrombin 2 and inactive prothrombin fragments (F1 and 2). Levels of fibrinopeptide A, which are diagnostic of the enzymatic conversion of fibrinogen to fibrin, are not used routinely for diagnosis. New markers such as high-mobility group box (HMGB) protein and others are being evaluated for diagnosis and efficacy in the prognosis of organ failure in DIC patients (Asakura et al., 2006; Hatada et al., 2005). This chromosomal protein is a nuclear DNA-binding protein that is released into the extracellular space from necrotic cells, activated macrophages, and dendritic cells (Hatada et al., 2005). It acts as a proinflammatory cytokine and, when bound to its receptor for advanced glycation end products (RAGE), induces prolonged inflammation, organ failure, septicemia, and death. Another possible prognostic marker in patients with sepsis-induced DIC is deficiency of von Willebrand factor – cleaving protease (ADAMTS13), which is the genetic or autoantibody defect thought to underlie TTP (Ono et al., 2006). The data suggest that deficiency of ADAMTS13 may be associated with sepsis-induced DIC (Ono et al., 2006). Another recently described marker associated with DIC that correlates with the recently described sepsis-related organ failure assessment (SOFA) is granulocyte-derived elastase (GE-XDP) (Matsumoto et al., 2005).

Differential diagnosis of DIC

There are many causes of acute widespread bleeding that affect neurologic patients and must be differentiated from DIC due to therapeutic considerations. These include TTP, SLE with or without the catastrophic APS, primary hyperfibrinolysis, hemolytic uremic syndrome, and obstetrical complications (Rocha et al., 1998).

TTP often presents with neurological signs and symptoms that are seen in more than 90% of patients during the course of the illness (Sadler et al., 2004). The neurological signs derive from infarction of the gray matter. Neurologically, patients have aphasia, hemiparesis, cranial nerve palsies, and headache. Distinguishing neurological features are multifocal deficits that are transient and recurrent. There is associated fever and renal failure in most instances. Most TTP is idiopathic, but in 15% of patients it may be related to bone marrow transplantation, ticlopidine, malignancy, and infection (Sadler et al., 2004). It is one of the few illnesses in medicine characterized by both clotting and bleeding. Almost all patients have a hemolytic anemia of intravascular origin. The peripheral blood smear contains schistocytes with polychromasia and other microangiopathic features. The haptoglobin is low, hemoglobinuria is present, and the direct Coombs test is negative. High levels of low-density lipoprotein are thought to be secondary to mechanical disruption of erythrocytes or body tissue. At diagnosis, platelets are usually 50 000 mm^3. The cause of TTP appears to be a deficiency in a metalloproteinase ADAMTS-13 whose activity is against von Willebrand factor (Sadler et al., 2004).

Hemolytic uremic syndrome is primarily a disease of children but can affect adolescents and young adults. The cause is infection by streptococcus pneumonia and a verotoxin-producing serotype of *Escherichia coli* (usually from poorly cooked meat) or Shigella infection in children (Johnson and Richardson, 1968). In adults, it has been seen during pregnancy and after chemotherapy or mitomycin or cyclosporine administration (George, 2003). It has many overlapping clinical and laboratory features of TTP (George *et al.*, 1998).

The vascular occlusions of active SLE may occur in any organ system and are often multiple and recurrent. Multiple small cortical pial artery infarctions with stroke, seizure, and psychosis as well as transverse myelitis are the most common central nervous system manifestations (Johnson and Richardson, 1968). A compensated form of DIC with diffuse thrombosis and mild bleeding is most often seen with SLE. TTP may be seen in the setting of SLE with thrombosis and microangiopathy (Musio *et al.*, 1998).

APS is often associated with fetal loss, recurrent thrombosis, and morbidity in pregnancy. It is secondary to antiphospholipid antibodies (lupus anticoagulant and anti-cardiolipin) as well as impairment of the fibrinolytic system (Yasuda *et al.*, 2005). In contradistinction to patients with the above-described simple APS that affects large arteries and veins, catastrophic APS causes multiorgan failure. Its mortality is approximately 50%. Thirty percent of these patients develop DIC. The pathologic mechanisms underlying the syndrome are:

- impaired release of t-PA and enhanced release of PAI-1 inhibitor after endothelial activation
- inhibition of fibrinolytic activity from elevated levels of lipoprotein a
- activation of the phospholipid-bound beta (2)-glycoprotein I, which is both a pro- and anticoagulant because of its interaction with phospholipid-binding proteins (coagulants) and protein C (Yasuda *et al.*, 2005). Rarely Evans syndrome (hemolytic anemia and ITP)
- acute fatty liver of pregnancy and multiorgan failure can be confused with DIC (Baron and Baron, 2005; Norton and Roberts, 2006)

Another obstetric complication with widespread bleeding is the HELLP syndrome. This is a severe form of pre-eclampsia that is associated with maternal and perinatal mortality (van Runnard Heimel *et al.*, 2006). It consists of hemolysis, elevated liver enzymes, and a low platelet count, which may mimic DIC.

A fulminant hemorrhagic syndrome that develops during surgery or trauma is often the first sign of a primary fibrinolytic state. Patients bleed from mucous membranes and wounds because of rapid fibrinolysis (Perouansky *et al.*, 1999). The patient's plasma may be clottable by thrombin but redissolves rapidly. Platelet count and function may be normal in the face of a prolonged thrombin, PT, and PTT, depletion of clotting factors, and elevated titers of FDPs with a normal D-dimer. Severe hemorrhagic complications are common as normal fiber monomer polymerization (clot stabilization) is disrupted and fibrin fragments D and E adhere to platelet membranes and disrupt their function (de Haan and van Oeveren, 1998).

Neurological complications of DIC

Most patients with DIC are extremely ill and develop multiorgan system failure from septicemia, cancer, head trauma, hyperpyrexia, and various intoxications. DIC in conjunction with the underlying initiating process often presents with nonfocal coma. The diagnosis should always be suspected if the patient has acrocyanosis; purpura; dusky cyanosis of the nose, ears, and genitalia; and is oozing blood from venipuncture sites and arterial lines. As noted earlier, DIC is not a disease but a consequence of an underlying condition. The neurologic complications that arise in a setting of DIC are hemorrhage in all brain compartments from consumption of coagulation factors and platelets and thrombosis of arteries, arteriole, and venous sinuses of the brain.

The specific neurological complications that occur often during DIC are:

- coma
- depression of mental status and encephalopathy
- subarachnoid hemorrhage
- small and large vessel-related brain infarcts
- embolic infarction from nonbacterial thrombotic heart valve lesions
- anterior and posterior circulation intraparenchymal hemorrhage
- rarely bleeding into nerves, plexi, or the eye (Patchett *et al.*, 1988; Saida *et al.*, 1997)

The cerebrovascular complications in cancer often are due to acute or compensated DIC. Solid tumors are associated with low-grade activation of the clotting cascade, often associated with systemic signs of venous occlusion (Trousseau's sign) (Rogers, 2003). Approximately 15% of an autopsy series evaluating cerebrovascular complications of patients with cancer found a 14% incidence of cerebrovascular disease, 7.4% of which were clinically significant. Nonbacterial thrombotic embolism was found in 18.5% of patients (Graus *et al.*, 1985). Embolic stroke in a setting of adenocarcinoma suggests nonbacterial thrombotic endocarditis (NBTE) (also called marantic endocarditis) that occludes middle cerebral artery distal pial vessels and rarely spinal cord vessels (Kearsley and Tattersall, 1982; Ojeda *et al.*, 1985).

Marantic endocarditis, which may also occur in the setting of any entity associated with DIC, is often verrucous (subleaflet) and is most common on the aortic and mitral valves (Fulham *et al.*, 1994). These platelet fibrin vegetations are often silent as they are subvalvular until they present with a focal neurological deficit.

Recent experimental and clinical experience has demonstrated that intravascular coagulation (microthrombosis) is a major secondary factor in extending the neurologic deficit after traumatic brain injury (Stein and Smith, 2004). The traumatic coagulopathy is not limited to the area of injury, releases tissue thromboplastin that causes intravascular microthrombosis, and is not associated with the apolipoprotein E (ApoE) genotype (Stein *et al.*, 2005).

Amphetamine toxicity (MDMA), methamphetamine 3,4-methylene deoxy-methamphetamine is a serious cause of neurological complications in young patients. Reports describe hyperpyrexia, rhabdomyolysis, neuropsychiatric manifestations, and arteritis in a setting of DIC (White, 2002).

DIC is a major cause of stroke in medical intensive care units and is a frequent complication of a terminally ill patient (Wijdicks and Scott, 1998).

Mechanism-based treatment of DIC

The most important aspect in the treatment of DIC is eliminating the underlying cause (Franchini, 2005; Hanly *et al.*, 2002). Due to a greater understanding both of clotting mechanisms and of the pathophysiology of DIC, the hope is that treatment can be tailored to the specific disordered mechanism of each triggering disease (Levi *et al.*, 2004). Replacement therapy with platelets and coagulation factors is given to those patients with severe bleeding. In general, if the fibrinogen levels are less than 100 mg/dL and platelets are less than 20 000 mm^3 fresh frozen plasma at a dose of 15–20 mg/kg is administered. Platelet transfusion is usually given at 1–2 μ/10 kg of body weight (Franchini, 2005). The danger of increased clotting in the face of active DIC from replacement therapy has not occurred in clinical practice. The use of heparin in active DIC is still controversial (Pernerstorfer *et al.*, 1999; Sakuragawa *et al.*, 1993).

It is now clear that DIC occurs from abnormal activation of the extrinsic clotting system. Inhibition of tissue factor by TFPI seems critical to the process (Bajaj and Bajaj, 1997). Experimental work shows evidence of a benefit in blocking tissue factor in endotoxin-associated thrombin generation, but clear human benefit awaits further trials (Abraham, 2000).

Replenishment of coagulation inhibitors

Antithrombin III is the most important of the thrombin inhibitors. It also inhibits factor Xa and acts as an anti-inflammatory by decreasing interleukin 1 and C-reactive protein (de Jonge *et al.*, 2001; Okajima and Uchiba, 1998). It has a beneficial effect in improving coagulation factors and organ function and decreasing mortality in the majority of DIC clinical trials (Fourrier *et al.*, 2000).

The inflammatory cytokines that are induced in DIC down-regulate endothelial expression of thrombomodulin and impair the thrombomodulin-protein C system. Activated protein C blocks the function of factors Va and VIIIa and thus decreases abnormal clotting during DIC. Consumption of protein C during DIC is a major mechanism in this process (Gluck and Opal, 2004). Studies on the efficacy of activated protein C in severe sepsis and consequent DIC appear promising (Fourrier, 2004; Vincent *et al.*, 2003).

Other agents that are being evaluated for refractory bleeding or specific circumstances that lead to DIC are:

- recombinant factor VII (rF VIIa) for refractory hemorrhagic episodes (Moscardo *et al.*, 2001)
- antifibrinolytic agents for Kasabach-Merritt syndrome and prostate cancer (Avvisati *et al.*, 1989)
- combined blockade of leukocyte/platelet adhesion by anti-selectin antibodies (Norman *et al.*, 2003) to depress tissue inflammations effect on coagulation or administration of IL-10 to decrease activation of inflammatory cytokines (Pajkrt *et al.*, 1997)

- monoclonal antibodies against TNF-α in septic patients (Reinhart and Karzai, 2001)
- inhibition of p38 mitogen-activated protein kinase (MAPK) (a major component of intracellular cascades important in inflammation and coagulation (Branger *et al.*, 2003)
- recombinant chimeric monoclonal antibody (IC14) against human CD 14a receptor for bacterial endotoxins (Verbon *et al.*, 2003)

Great advances have been accomplished in the understanding of the basic mechanisms of DIC. It remains a grave illness, is difficult to treat, and has a high morbidity and mortality, particularly in the presence of neurologic complications (Schwartzman and Hill, 1982).

REFERENCES

Abraham, E. 2000. Tissue factor inhibition and clinical trial results of tissue factor pathway inhibitor in sepsis. *Crit Care Med*, **28(9 Suppl)**, S31–3.

Angstwurm, M. W., Dempfle, C. E., and Spannagl, M. 2006. New disseminated intravascular coagulation score: a useful tool to predict mortality in comparison with Acute Physiology and Chronic Health Evaluation II and Logistic Organ Dysfunction scores. *Crit Care Med*, **34**, 314–20.

Arai, A., Naruse, M., Naruse, K., *et al.* 1998. Cardiac malignant pheochromocytoma with bone metastases. *Intern Med*, **37**, 940–4.

Asakura, H., Wada, H., Okamoto, K., *et al.* 2006. Evaluation of haemostatic molecular markers for diagnosis of disseminated intravascular coagulation in patients with infections. *Thromb Haemost*, **95**, 282–7.

Asherson, R. A. 1998. The catastrophic antiphospholipid syndrome, 1998. A review of the clinical features, possible pathogenesis and treatment. *Lupus*, **7(Suppl 2)**, S55–62.

Avvisati, G., ten Cate, J. W., Buller, H. R., and Mandelli, F. 1989. Tranexamic acid for control of haemorrhage in acute promyelocytic leukaemia. *Lancet*, **2**, 122–4.

Bajaj, M. S., and Bajaj, S. P. 1997. Tissue factor pathway inhibitor: potential therapeutic applications. *Thromb Haemost*, **78**, 471–7.

Baker, W. F. Jr. 1989. Clinical aspects of disseminated intravascular coagulation: a clinician's point of view. *Semin Thromb Hemost*, **15**, 1–57.

Bakhtiari, K., Meijers, J. C., de Jonge, E., and Levi, M. 2004. Prospective validation of the International Society of Thrombosis and Haemostasis scoring system for disseminated intravascular coagulation. *Crit Care Med*, **32**, 2416–21.

Barbui, T., and Falanga, A. 2001. Disseminated intravascular coagulation in acute leukemia. *Semin Thromb Hemost*, **27**, 593–604.

Baron, J. M., Baron, B. W. 2005. Thrombotic thrombocytopenic purpura and its look-alikes. *Clin Adv Hematol Oncol*, **3**, 868–74.

Bern, M. M. 2005. Coagulopathy, following medical therapy, for carcinoma of the prostate. *Hematology*, **10**, 65–8.

Bick, R. L. 1988. Disseminated intravascular coagulation and related syndromes: a clinical review. *Semin Thromb Hemost*, **14**, 299–338.

Bick, R. L. 1992. Disseminated intravascular coagulation. *Hematol Oncol Clin North Am*, **6**, 1259–85.

Bick, R. L. 1996. Alterations of hemostasis associated with surgery, cardiopulmonary bypass surgery and prosthetic devices. In *Disorders of Hemostatsis*, eds. O. D. Ratnoff, and C. Forbes. Philadelphia: WB Saunders, p. 382.

Biemond, B. J., Levi, M., ten Cate, H., *et al.* 1995. Complete inhibition of endotoxin induced coagulation activation in chimpanzees with a monoclonal Fab fragment against factor VII/VIIa. *Thromb Haemost*, **73**, 223–30.

Boffa, M. C., and Karmochkine, M. 1998. Thrombomodulin: an overview and potential implications in vascular disorders. *Lupus*, **7(Suppl 2)**, S120–5.

Branger, J., van den Blink, B., Weijer, S., *et al.* 2003. Inhibition of coagulation, fibrinolysis, and endothelial cell activation by a p38 mitogen-activated protein kinase inhibitor during human endotoxemia. *Blood*, **101**, 4446–8.

Breakwell, L. M., Getty, C. J., and Austin, C. 1999. Disseminated intravascular coagulation in elective primary total hip replacement. *J Arthroplasty*, **14**, 239–42.

Carroll, V. A., and Binder, B. R. 1999. The role of the plasminogen activation system in cancer. *Semin Thromb Hemost,* **25**, 183–97.

Colman, R. W., and Rubin, R. N. 1990. Disseminated intravascular coagulation due to malignancy. *Semin Oncol,* **17**, 172–86.

Conway, E. M., and Rosenberg, R. D. 1988. Tumor necrosis factor suppresses transcription of the thrombomodulin gene in endothelial cells. *Mol Cell Biol,* **8**, 5588–92.

Creasey, A. A., Chang, A. C., Feigen, L., *et al.* 1993. Tissue factor pathway inhibitor reduces mortality from *Escherichia coli* septic shock. *J Clin Invest,* **91**, 2850–60.

de Haan, J., and van Oeveren, W. 1998. Platelets and soluble fibrin promote plasminogen activation causing downregulation of platelet glycoprotein Ib/IX complexes: protection by aprotinin. *Thromb Res,* **92**, 171–9.

de Jonge, E., Dekkers, P. E., Creasey, A. A., *et al.* 2000. Tissue factor pathway inhibitor dose-dependently inhibits coagulation activation without influencing the fibrinolytic and cytokine response during human endotoxemia. *Blood* **95(4)**:1124–9.

de Jonge, E., van der Poll, T., Kesecioglu, J., and Levi, M. 2001. Anticoagulant factor concentrates in disseminated intravascular coagulation: rationale for use and clinical experience. *Semin Thromb Hemost,* **27**, 667–74.

Dempfle, C. E. 2004. Coagulopathy of sepsis. *Thromb Haemost,* **91**, 213–24.

Donati, M. B., and Falanga, A. 2001. Pathogenetic mechanisms of thrombosis in malignancy. *Acta Haematol,* **106**, 18–24.

Esmon, C. T. 2001. Role of coagulation inhibitors in inflammation. *Thromb Haemost,* **86**, 51–6.

Faust, S. N., Levin, M., Harrison, O. B., *et al.* 2001. Dysfunction of endothelial protein C activation in severe meningococcal sepsis. *N Engl J Med,* **345**, 408–16.

Felcher, A., Commichau, C., Cao, Q., *et al.* 1998. Disseminated intravascular coagulation and status epilepticus. *Neurology,* **51**, 629–31.

Fernandez-Bustamante, A., and Jimeno, A. 2005. Disseminated intravascular coagulopathy in aortic aneurysms. *Eur J Intern Med,* **16**, 551–60.

Fourrier, F. 2004. Recombinant human activated protein C in the treatment of severe sepsis: an evidence-based review. *Crit Care Med,* **32(11 Suppl)**, S534.

Fourrier, F., Jourdain, M., and Tournoys, A. 2000. Clinical trial results with antithrombin III in sepsis. *Crit Care Med,* **28(9 Suppl)**, S38–43.

Franchini, M. 2005. Pathophysiology, diagnosis and treatment of disseminated intravascular coagulation: an update. *Clin Lab,* **51**, 633–9.

Francis, J. L. 1998. Laboratory investigation of hypercoagulability. *Semin Thromb Hemost,* **24**, 111–26.

Fulham, M. J., Gatenby, P., and Tuck, R. R. 1994. Focal cerebral ischemia and antiphospholipid antibodies: a case for cardiac embolism. *Acta Neurol Scand,* **90**, 417–23.

Furie, B., and Furie, B. C. 2006. Cancer-associated thrombosis. *Blood Cells Mol Dis,* **36**, 177–81.

Gando, S. 2001. Disseminated intravascular coagulation in trauma patients. *Semin Thromb Hemost,* **27**, 585–92.

Gando, S. 2006. Tissue factor in trauma and organ dysfunction. *Semin Thromb Hemost,* **32**, 48–53.

Gando, S., Nanzaki, S., and Kemmotsu, O. 1999. Disseminated intravascular coagulation and sustained systemic inflammatory response syndrome predict organ dysfunctions after trauma: application of clinical decision analysis. *Ann Surg,* **229**, 121–7.

Gando, S., Nanzaki, S., Sasaki, S., and Kemmotsu, O. 1998. Significant correlations between tissue factor and thrombin markers in trauma and septic patients with disseminated intravascular coagulation. *Thromb Haemost,* **79**, 1111–5.

Garcia-Avello, A., Lorente, J. A., Cesar-Perez, J., *et al.* 1998. Degree of hypercoagulability and hyperfibrinolysis is related to organ failure and prognosis after burn trauma. *Thromb Res,* **89**, 59–64.

George, J. N. 2003. The association of pregnancy with thrombotic thrombocytopenic purpura-hemolytic uremic syndrome. *Curr Opin Hematol,* **10**, 339–44.

George, J. N., Gilcher, R. O., Smith, J. W., *et al.* 1998. Thrombotic thrombocytopenic purpura-hemolytic uremic syndrome: diagnosis and management. *J Clin Apher,* **13**, 120–5.

Gluck, T., and Opal, S. M. 2004. Advances in sepsis therapy. *Drugs,* **64**, 837–59.

Graus, F., Rogers, L. R., and Posner, J. B. 1985. Cerebrovascular complications in patients with cancer. *Medicine (Baltimore),* **64**, 16–35.

Hanly, E. J., Cohn, E. J. Jr., Johnson, J. L., and Peyton, B. D. 2002. DIC: treatment frontiers. *Curr Surg,* **59**, 257–64.

Hatada, T., Wada, H., Nobori, T., *et al.* 2005. Plasma concentrations and importance of High Mobility Group Box protein in the prognosis of organ failure in patients with disseminated intravascular coagulation. *Thromb Haemost,* **94**, 975–9.

Johnson, R. T., and Richardson, E. P. 1968. The neurological manifestations of systemic lupus erythematosus. *Medicine (Baltimore),* **47**, 337–69.

Katsaros, D., and Grundfest-Broniatowski, S. 1998. Successful management of visceral Klippel-Trenaunay-Weber syndrome with the antifibrinolytic agent tranexamic acid (cyclocapron): a case report. *Am Surg,* **64**, 302–4.

Kearsley, J. H., and Tattersall, M. H. 1982. Cerebral embolism in cancer patients. *Q J Med,* **51**, 279–91.

Krevans, J. R., Jackson, D. P., Conley, C. L., and Hartmann, R. C. 1957. The nature of the hemorrhagic disorder accompanying hemolytic transfusion reactions in man. *Blood,* **12**, 834–43.

Letsky, E. A. 2001. Disseminated intravascular coagulation. *Best Pract Res Clin Obstet Gynaecol,* **l15**, 623–44.

Levi, M., de Jonge, E., and van der Poll, T. 2004. New treatment strategies for disseminated intravascular coagulation based on current understanding of the pathophysiology. *Ann Med,* **36**, 41–9.

Levi, M., and Ten Cate, H. 1999. Disseminated intravascular coagulation. *N Engl J Med,* **341**, 586–92.

Levi, M., van der Poll, T., deJonge, E., and ten Cate, H. 2003. Relative insufficiency of fibrinolysis in disseminated intravascular coagulation. *Sepsis,* **3**, 103–9.

Maruyama, I. 1999. Recombinant thrombomodulin and activated protein C in the treatment of disseminated intravascular coagulation. *Thromb Haemost,* **82**, 718–21.

Matsumoto, T., Wada, H., Nobori, T., *et al.* 2005. Elevated plasma levels of fibrin degradation products by granulocyte-derived elastase in patients with disseminated intravascular coagulation. *Clin Appl Thromb Hemost,* **11**, 391–400.

Moscardo, F., Perez, F., de la Rubia, J., *et al.* 2001. Successful treatment of severe intra-abdominal bleeding associated with disseminated intravascular coagulation using recombinant activated factor VII. *Br J Haematol,* **114**, 174–6.

Musio, F., Bohen, E. M., Yuan, C. M., and Welch, P. G. 1998. Review of thrombotic thrombocytopenic purpura in the setting of systemic lupus erythematosus. *Semin Arthritis Rheum,* **28**, 1–19.

Navarro, M., Ruiz, I., Martin, G., Cruz, J. J. 2006. Patient with disseminated intravascular coagulation as the first manifestation of adenocarcinoma of the prostate. Risks of prostatic biopsy. *Prostate Cancer Prostatic Dis,* **9**, 190–1.

Norman, K. E., Cotter, M. J., Stewart, J. B., *et al.* 2003. Combined anticoagulant and antiselectin treatments prevent lethal intravascular coagulation. *Blood,* **101**, 921–8.

Norton, A., and Roberts, I. 2006. Management of Evans syndrome. *Br J Haematol,* **132**, 125–37.

Ojeda, V. J., Frost, F., and Mastaglia, F. L. 1985. Non-bacterial thrombotic endocarditis associated with malignant disease: a clinicopathological study of 16 cases. *Med J Aust,* **142**, 629–31.

Okajima, K., and Uchiba, M. 1998. The anti-inflammatory properties of antithrombin III: new therapeutic implications. *Semin Thromb Hemost,* **24**, 27–32.

Ono, T., Mimuro, J., Madoiwa, S., *et al.* 2006. Severe secondary deficiency of von Willebrand factor cleaving protease (ADAMTS13) in patients with sepsis-induced disseminated intravascular coagulation: its correlation with development of renal failure. *Blood,* **107**, 528–34.

Pajkrt, D., van der Poll, T., Levi, M., *et al.* 1997. Interleukin-10 inhibits activation of coagulation and fibrinolysis during human endotoxemia. *Blood,* **89**, 2701–5.

Patchett, R. B., Wilson, W. B., and Ellis, P. P. 1988. Ophthalmic complications with disseminated intravascular coagulation. *Br J Ophthalmol,* **72**, 377–9.

Pernerstorfer, T., Hollenstein, U., Hansen, J., *et al.* 1999. Heparin blunts endotoxin-induced coagulation activation. *Circulation,* **100**, 2485–90.

Perouansky, M., Oppenheim, A., Sprung, C. L., Eidelman, L. A., and Pizov, R. 1999. Effect of haemofiltration on pathological fibrinolysis due to severe sepsis: a case report. *Resuscitation,* **40**, 53–6.

Persoons, M. C., Stals, F. S., van dam Mieras, M. C., and Bruggeman, C. A. 1998. Multiple organ involvement during experimental cytomegalovirus infection is associated with disseminated vascular pathology. *J Pathol,* **184**, 103–9.

Pixley, R. A., De La Cadena, R., Page, J. D., *et al.* 1993. The contact system contributes to hypotension but not disseminated intravascular coagulation in lethal bacteremia. In vivo use of a monoclonal anti-factor XII antibody to block contact activation in baboons. *J Clin Invest,* **91**, 61–8.

Reinhart, K., and Karzai, W. 2001. Anti-tumor necrosis factor therapy in sepsis: update on clinical trials and lessons learned. *Crit Care Med,* **29(7 Suppl)**, S121–5.

Rivers, R. P., Hathaway, W. E., and Weston, W. L. 1975. The endotoxin-induced coagulant activity of human monocytes. *Br J Haematol,* **30**, 311–6.

Rocha, E., Paramo, J. A., Montes, R., and Panizo, C. 1998. Acute generalized, widespread bleeding. Diagnosis and management. *Haematologica,* **83**, 1024–37.

Rogers, L. R. 2003. Cerebrovascular complications in cancer patients. *Neurol Clin,* **21**, 167–92.

Roumen, R. M., Hendriks, T., van der Ven-Jongekrijg, J., *et al.* 1993. Cytokine patterns in patients after major vascular surgery, hemorrhagic shock, and severe blunt trauma. Relation with subsequent adult respiratory distress syndrome and multiple organ failure. *Ann Surg,* **218**, 769–76.

Sadler, J. E., Moake, J. L., Miyata, T., and George, J. N. 2004. Recent advances in thrombotic thrombocytopenic purpura. *Hematology Am Soc Hematol Educ Program,* 407–23.

Saida, K., Kawakami, H., Ohta, M., and Iwamura, K. 1997. Coagulation and vascular abnormalities in Crow-Fukase syndrome. *Muscle Nerve,* **20**, 486–92.

Sakuragawa, N., Hasegawa, H., Maki, M., Nakagawa, M., and Nakashima, M. 1993. Clinical evaluation of low-molecular-weight heparin (FR-860) on disseminated intravascular coagulation (DIC) – a multicenter co-operative double-blind trial in comparison with heparin. *Thromb Res,* **72**, 475–500.

Sauerwein, R. W., van der Meer, J. W., and Goris, R. J. 1993. Cytokine patterns in patients after major vascular surgery, hemorrhagic shock, and severe blunt trauma. Relation with subsequent adult respiratory distress syndrome and multiple organ failure. *Ann Surg,* **218**, 769–76.

Schwartzman, R. J., and Hill, J. B. 1982. Neurologic complications of disseminated intravascular coagulation. *Neurology,* **32**, 791–7.

Shoji, N., Nakada, T., Sugano, O., Suzuki, H., and Sasagawa, I. 1998. Acute onset of coagulopathy in a patient with Kasabach-Merritt syndrome following transurethral resection of bladder tumor. *Urol Int,* **61**, 115–8.

Stein, S. C., Graham, D. I., Chen, X. H., Dunn, L., and Smith, D. H. 2005. Apo E genotype not associated with intravascular coagulation in traumatic brain injury. *Neurosci Lett,* **387**, 28–31.

Stein, S. C., and Smith, D. H. 2004. Coagulopathy in traumatic brain injury. *Neurocrit Care,* **1**, 479–88.

Suffredini, A. F., Harpel, P. C., and Parrillo, J. E. 1989. Promotion and subsequent inhibition of plasminogen activation after administration of intravenous endotoxin to normal subjects. *N Engl J Med,* **320**, 1165–72.

van Runnard Heimel, P. J., Huisjes, A. J., Franx, A., *et al.* 2006. A randomised placebo-controlled trial of prolonged prednisolone administration to patients with HELLP syndrome remote from term. *Eur J Obstet Gynecol Reprod Biol,* **128**, 187–93.

Verbon, A., Meijers, J. C., Spek, C. A., *et al.* 2003. Effects of IC14, an anti-CD14 antibody, on coagulation and fibrinolysis during low-grade endotoxemia in humans. *J Infect Dis,* **187**, 55–61.

Vincent, J. L., Angus, D. C., Artigas, A., *et al.* 2003. Recombinant Human Activated Protein C Worldwide Evaluation in Severe Sepsis (PROWESS) Study Group. Effects of drotrecogin alfa (activated) on organ dysfunction in the PROWESS trial. *Crit Care Med,* **31**, 834–40.

Weiner, C. P. 1986. The obstetric patient and disseminated intravascular coagulation. *Clin Perinatol,* **l13**, 705–17.

Wheeler, A. P., and Bernard, G. R. 1999. Treating patients with severe sepsis. *N Engl J Med,* **340**, 207–14.

White, S. R. 2002. Amphetamine toxicity. *Semin Respir Crit Care Med,* **23**, 27–36.

Wijdicks, E. F., and Scott, J. P. 1998. Stroke in the medical intensive-care unit. *Mayo Clin Proc,* **73**, 642–6.

Yasuda, S., Bohgaki, M., Atsumi, T., and Koike, T. 2005. Pathogenesis of antiphospholipid antibodies: impairment of fibrinolysis and monocyte activation via the p38 mitogen-activated protein kinase pathway. *Immunobiology,* **210**, 775–80.

Yu, M., Nardella, A., and Pechet, L. 2000. Screening tests of disseminated intravascular coagulation: guidelines for rapid and specific laboratory diagnosis. *Crit Care Med,* **28**, 1777–80.

40

BLEEDING DISORDERS AND THROMBOPHILIA

Dana Védy, Marc Schapira, and Anne Angelillo-Scherrer

Introduction

Cerebral vascular conditions resulting from bleeding, thrombosis, or a combination of both comprise subarachnoid and intracerebral hemorrhage (CH), ischemic stroke (IS), and transient ischemic attack (TIA), as well as cerebral venous and sinus thrombosis (CVST). They are caused by a wide spectrum of blood disorders that include platelet and coagulation defects, thrombophilia, hemoglobin abnormalities, and hematological malignancies. These blood disorders may have an inherited or an acquired origin, or a combination of both.

Because of their various pathological expressions and etiologies, therapeutic and preventive approaches of cerebral disorders resulting from bleeding, thrombosis, or a combination of both need to be specifically adapted to each clinical situation.

After a brief introduction to physiological hemostasis and investigation strategies, this chapter will focus on the various etiologies for CH, IS, TIA, and CVST that are caused by blood disorders. Preventive and therapeutic approaches will be outlined. We have used an evidence-based approach to frame our recommendations when available, based upon guidelines published by medical academic associations and an extensive review of the literature. Based upon the evidence, as well as our own experience, when we concluded that benefits of a particular preventive approach or treatment outweighed risks, we recommended the treatments.

Physiology of hemostasis

Primary hemostasis and blood coagulation lead to clot formation in the case of blood vessel injury. It is a rapid, localized, and well-controlled process. Then, to restore the vessel patency, the clot is removed by fibrinolysis. Primary hemostasis, which is the primary hemostatic response, consists in the formation of a platelet plug that forms in the area of a vessel wall injury and reduces bleeding. After vascular injury, platelets adhere to exposed subendothelial von Willebrand factor (VWF) and collagen through the glycoprotein (GP) Ib/IX/V receptor complex and the GPIa/IIa receptor complex, respectively. Platelet adhesion to the vascular subendothelium induces a series of intracellular signaling events that result in platelet activation. Activated platelets change their shape, secrete their granule contents, produce thromboxane A_2 (TXA$_2$), and aggregate. Recruitment of additional platelets by TXA$_2$, secreted adenosine diphosphate (ADP), and thrombin leads to the formation of a platelet plug that later undergoes further stabilization to prevent its premature disaggregation. Activated platelets also provide cell-surface phospholipid for the assembly of enzyme complexes of the blood coagulation system.

Tissue factor is thought to be the primary initiator of *in vivo* coagulation. Injury to the arterial or venous wall exposes nonvascular tissue factor-expressing cells to blood. Exposed tissue factor initiates the extrinsic pathway of blood coagulation by binding factor VII or activated factor VII (factor VIIa). The tissue factor-factor VIIa complex triggers thrombin generation by activating factor IX and X. Factor IXa binds to factor VIIIa on membrane surfaces to form the tenase (or Xase) complex that activates factor X. Factor Xa propagates coagulation by binding to factor Va on membrane surfaces to form the prothrombinase complex. Factor Xa within this complex activates prothrombin to thrombin. Thrombin converts fibrinogen to fibrin, amplifies its own generation by activating coagulation factors V and VIII, and activates factor XIII, which stabilizes the fibrin clot. In addition, thrombin can activate factor XI, thereby leading to further factor Xa generation. The intrinsic coagulation pathway is important in amplifying the response through "cross-talk" and feedback mechanisms. The blood coagulation cascade is schematically represented in Figure 40.1.

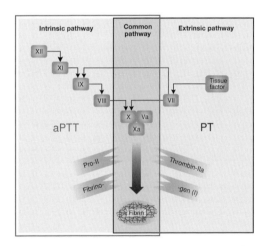

Figure 40.1 Coagulation cascade. Tissue factor initiates the extrinsic pathway of blood coagulation by binding factor VII or activated factor VII. The tissue factor-FVIIa complex triggers thrombin generation by activating factor IX and X. The contact system proteins that include factor XII activate factor XI. Factor IXa forms a complex with its cofactor factor VIIIa and calcium. This complex is the major activator of factor X and is 50 times more active than the tissue factor-FVIIa complex. Once factor Xa is formed by either the extrinsic or the intrinsic pathway, it propagates coagulation by binding to factor Va on membrane surfaces to form the prothrombinase complex. Factor Xa within this complex activates prothrombin to thrombin, and thrombin converts fibrinogen to fibrin. The prothrombin time (PT) assesses the extrinsic and the common coagulation pathways and the activated partial thromboplastin time (aPTT) the intrinsic and the common coagulation pathways.

Uncommon Causes of Stroke, 2nd edition, ed. Louis R. Caplan. Published by Cambridge University Press.   © Cambridge University Press 2008.

Table 40.1 Screening tests of blood coagulation and possible interpretation

PT	aPTT	TT	Fibrinogen	Possible interpretation
↑	Normal	Normal	Normal	Factor VII deficiency (inherited or acquired)
Normal	↑	Normal	Normal	Deficiency of factor VIII, IX, XI, XII[a] or contact factor[a] (prekallikrein, high-molecular-weight kininogen), inherited or acquired; lupus anticoagulant
↑	↑	Normal	Normal	Vitamin K antagonists; vitamin K deficiency; liver disease; inherited or acquired deficiency in factor II, V, X (rare); combined deficiency in factor V and VIII (rare); combined deficiency in vitamin K-dependent factors (II, VII, IX, X), extremely rare
↑	↑	↑	Normal or ↓	Liver disease; DIC; massive transfusion, afibrinogenemia or hypofibrinogenemia (inherited or acquired), dysfibrinogenemia (inherited or acquired)
Normal	Normal	Normal	Normal	Inherited or acquired platelet function disorders, factor XIII deficiency, inherited or acquired disorders of the fibrinolytic system

Notes: PT = prothrombin time, aPTT = activated partial thromboplastin time, TT = thrombin time, ↑ = prolonged, ↓ = decreased. [a] is not responsible for a bleeding phenotype, DIC = disseminated vascular coagulation.

The coagulation cascade transduces a small initiating stimulus into a large fibrin clot. Therefore, action of the coagulation system has to be restrained by the continuous removal of fibrin via the fibrinolytic system and by natural coagulation inhibitors that suppress the generation of thrombin. One of these natural coagulation inhibitors is the tissue factor pathway inhibitor that inhibits the reactions involving tissue factor and factor VIIa. Antithrombin, another natural coagulation inhibitor, inhibits most of the enzymes generated during activation of coagulation. Its physiological role is to limit the coagulation process to sites of vascular injury and to protect the circulation from liberated enzymes. The binding of thrombin to the endothelial cell receptor thrombomodulin induces a change in the enzyme that facilitates conversion by limited proteolysis of circulating protein C to activated protein C (APC). The protein C anticoagulant system provides important control of the coagulation cascade by degrading factors Va and VIIIa, which are required for the production of thrombin. Protein S is a cofactor of protein C in this reaction and acts therefore as a natural coagulation inhibitor. The binding of thrombin to thrombomodulin also inhibits cleavage of fibrinogen and activation of platelets. Thus, the protein C-thrombomodulin pathway acts as a natural anticoagulant mechanism by suppressing excessive action of the coagulation system and also by directly inhibiting thrombin.

Investigation strategies

Bleeding disorders

A history of bleeding is the most reliable predictor of bleeding risk. The personal and family history should be assessed in order to determine whether a bleeding disorder is present, the disorder is inherited or acquired, and whether the bleeding symptoms have been enhanced by an associated medical condition or induced by drugs or dietary supplements. For example, CH may be the result of excessive oral anticoagulation or complicated thrombolysis or antiplatelet drug therapy.

It is important to elicit the type of bleeding and its location, frequency, and precipitating factors. Bleeding can consist of: epistaxis, petechiae, bruises, hematomas, excessive bleeding from minor wounds, oral cavity bleeding, gastrointestinal bleeding, menorrhagia, postpartum hemorrhage, muscle hematomas, hemarthrosis, and/or excessive bleeding after tooth extraction or surgery. The requirement of blood transfusion during a bleeding episode is a criterion of severity. A bleeding score may be used for von Willebrand disease investigation (Tosetto *et al.*, 2006).

Screening laboratory tests include PT, also expressed as the international normalized ratio (INR), aPTT, fibrinogen, the thrombin time (TT), and a platelet count. PT assesses the extrinsic and common coagulation pathways, and the aPTT the intrinsic and common coagulation pathways (Figure 40.1). The INR was developed to follow oral anticoagulation with vitamin K antagonists. TT reflects the action of thrombin on fibrinogen with the formation of fibrin. Logical use of screening tests will suggest possible diagnoses and indicate which specialized tests need to be performed (Table 40.1).

Thrombophilia

A laboratory evaluation for thrombophilia (Table 40.2) is required in the following circumstances: venous thrombosis before 40–50 years of age; unprovoked thrombosis at any age; recurrent thrombosis at any age; unusual sites such as cerebral, mesenteric, portal, or hepatic veins; a positive family history for thrombosis; thrombosis during pregnancy; oral contraceptives; or hormone replacement therapy (HRT). However, when possible, a thrombophilia laboratory profile should be avoided during the acute phase of thrombosis. Investigations for protein C and protein S deficiency are not recommended when the patient is taking a vitamin K antagonist such as warfarin or acenocoumarol or has taken it within the last 4–6 weeks. This is because protein C and S are vitamin K-dependent proteins. Similarly, evaluation for antithrombin deficiency is to be avoided when the patient is being given unfractionated or low-molecular-weight heparin therapy. Interpretation of lupus anticoagulant assays is uncertain when the patient is taking an anticoagulant. Investigation strategies for the antiphospholipid antibodies syndrome are presented in Chapter 12.

Table 40.2 Thrombophilia laboratory tests

Risk factors	First-line tests	Second-line tests	Avoid to perform tests in the following conditions or states
Antithrombin deficiency	Antithrombin activity (heparin cofactor assay)	Antithrombin antigen assay (immunoassay)	Unfractionated heparin or low-molecular-weight heparin administration, liver failure
Protein C deficiency	Protein C activity (clotting assay)	Protein C: amidolytic and immunoassay	Vitamin K antagonists, vitamin K deficiency, liver failure
Protein S deficiency	Free protein S antigen (immunoassay)	Total protein S antigen and APC cofactor activity (clotting assay)	Vitamin K antagonists, vitamin K deficiency, liver failure, pregnancy, oral contraceptives, hormone replacement therapy
Factor V Leiden	APC resistance (APTT-based assay) or factor V Leiden genotyping (PCR)	Factor V Leiden genotyping (PCR)	
G20210 A mutation in the prothrombin gene	Prothrombin genotyping (PCR)		
Lupus anticoagulant	Choose two clot-based assays: i.e., PTT-LA, dRVVT, dPT tests. LA is present when at least one of two tests is positive.		Anticoagulants: heparin affects the PTT-LA, and vitamin K antagonists prolong the dRVVT and the dPT tests; during the 12 weeks following an acute thrombotic event
Anticardiolipin antibodies	Immunoassays for IgM and IgG isotypes		Screen preferably 12 weeks after an acute thrombotic event
Anti-β2-GPI antibodies	Immunoassays for IgM and IgG isotypes		Screen preferably 12 weeks after an acute thrombotic event
Hyperhomocysteinemia	Fasting homocysteinemia		

Notes: aPTT = activated partial thromboplastin time, PCR = polymerase chain reaction, LA = lupus anticoagulant, PTT-LA: a low phospholipid partial thromboplastin time (PTT) designed to detect an LA, dRVVT = dilute Russell viper venom time, dPT = dilute prothrombin time, IgM = immunoglobulin M, IgG = immunoglobulin G.

Antithrombin

Antithrombin is a 58-kd serpin that inhibits procoagulant serine proteases such as thrombin, factor Xa, and factor IXa. Its activity is amplified by heparin and heparin-like molecules that are presented on the surface of endothelial cells (Dahlback, 2000). Antithrombin deficiency may be inherited or acquired, and associated with an increased venous thromboembolism (VTE) risk. Antithrombin activity is measured by a heparin cofactor assay and antithrombin protein concentration by an immunoassay.

Homozygous antithrombin deficiency may cause death *in utero* or in the perinatal period. Two types of inherited antithrombin deficiency exist. Type I (quantitative) is characterized by a reduction in both activity and antigen concentration, whereas type II (qualitative) deficiency is due to a reduction in activity associated with a normal antigen concentration. Patients with antithrombin <60% have a 10-fold increased risk of VTE.

Protein C

Protein C is a serine protease zymogen that belongs to the vitamin K-dependent protein family. It is converted by thrombin in the presence of thrombomodulin to an active serine protease. APC inactivates factors Va and VIIIa, thereby impeding further thrombin generation.

Functional assays measure enzymatic (amidolytic assay) or anticoagulant (clotting assay) activity, and an immunoassay determines protein concentration. Type I (quantitative) deficiency is characterized by a decreased activity in amidolytic and clotting assays and a decreased antigen concentration, whereas type II (qualitative) deficiency is due to a reduction in activity (in amidolytic and clotting assays) associated with a normal antigen concentration. Homozygous protein C deficiency is responsible for a severe phenotype characterized by life-threatening thrombosis at birth and neonatal purpura fulminans comprising necrosis and gangrene. Heterozygous protein C deficiency is suggested by protein C levels <70% and increases the risk of VTE by four- to five-fold.

Protein S

Protein S is vitamin K-dependent and is the cofactor of APC. In plasma, protein S forms inactive complexes with the complement C4b-binding protein, and free protein S constitutes about 40% of the total plasma level. Only free protein S has APC cofactor activity. Immunoassays are used to measure separately free and total protein S. Protein S activity is determined in plasma diluted with protein S-depleted plasma by an aPTT-based assay (clotting assay) in the presence of APC and purified factor Va. Type I deficiency is characterized by low free and total protein S; type II deficiency by normal free protein S and low protein S activity; type III by low free protein S and normal total protein S. Clinical manifestations of protein S deficiency resemble those of protein C deficiency. Protein S deficiency in men and in women >45 years is defined as <65% and <55% in women <45 years. It increases the risk of VTE by four- to five-fold.

APC resistance and factor V Leiden

APC leads to inactivation of factor Va by cleavage. Three APC cleavage sites have been determined on factor V (Arg-306, Arg-506, and Arg-679). The factor V Leiden mutation consists in the replacement at nucleotide 1691 of Arg-506 by glutamine. Because of this mutation, the cleavage of factor Va by APC is impaired and, as factor Va is a cofactor to APC in the inactivation of factor VIIIa, the degradation of factor VIIIa is also reduced (Dahlback and Villoutreix, 2005).

The APC resistance assay is based on an aPTT measurement in the presence or absence of purified APC. Plasma dilution with factor V-deficient plasma augments the specificity for the factor V Leiden mutation and allows testing of patients taking vitamin K antagonists (Tripodi *et al.*, 2003). The results are expressed as APC sensitivity: (aPTT + APC) / (aPTT – APC). A low APC sensitivity ratio defines APC resistance.

Homozygous and heterozygous factor V Leiden mutations are detected by polymerase chain reaction (PCR) amplification of factor V gene. This test is needed to confirm a positive APC resistance test. Heterozygosity for factor V Leiden confers a four- to five-fold increased VTE risk, and homozygosity a 30- to 140-fold risk.

Prothrombin G20210A mutation

Prothrombin is a vitamin K-dependent protein and is activated to thrombin by the prothrombinase complex (Dahlback, 2000). A mutation at nucleotide position 20210 (an adenine instead of a guanine) of the prothrombin gene leads to elevated plasma prothrombin levels, which increase the VTE risk by three- to four-fold (Ventura *et al.*, 2004). The prothrombin mutation is detected by PCR amplification.

Blood disorders causing bleeding in and around the brain

Introduction

Bleeding disorders are rare causes of spontaneous CH in adults. They increase the intracerebral bleeding risk in young and middle-aged individuals (Juvela and Kase, 2006). In the pediatric population with inherited coagulation disorders, CH is an important cause of mortality in the case of head trauma, even minor (Dietrich *et al.*, 1994). In thrombocytopenic children and especially in premature infants, spontaneous and severe hemorrhage may occur at higher platelet counts than in thrombocytopenic adults. The risk of CH and particularly intraventricular hemorrhage is inversely proportional to neonatal gestational age (Manno, 2005).

Bleeding disorders may be inherited or acquired. They include thrombocytopenia and platelet function disorders, coagulation factor deficiencies, excessive anticoagulation, and hemorrhagic complications after thrombolysis. Blood disorders associated with myeloproliferative diseases and disseminated intravascular coagulation (DIC) can cause both bleeding and thrombosis; they are covered in this chapter and in Chapter 39. Heparin-induced thrombocytopenia (HIT), the anti-phospholipid antibody syndrome, and thrombotic thrombocytopenic purpura (TTP), conditions that cause thrombocytopenia but are more frequently responsible for thrombosis than for bleeding, will be discussed in this chapter as well as in Chapters 38 and 41.

Inherited thrombocytopenia

Inherited thrombocytopenia constitutes a small proportion of thrombocytopenias and is suspected after exclusion of the other causes of thrombocytopenia. Several points of triage are identified in order to suspect this disorder: family history of thrombocytopenia, lack of platelet response to autoimmune thrombocytopenia therapies, abnormal size of platelets on blood smear, disproportionate bleeding compared to the number of platelets, onset at birth, associated features like absent radii, and/or persistence of a stable level of thrombocytopenia for years (Cines *et al.*, 2004). CH may be associated. Management depends on the severity of thrombocytopenia and the anticipated natural history of the disorder. It includes platelet transfusion; other hemostatic supports like antifibrinolytic drugs; and allogeneic stem cell transplantation.

Acquired thrombocytopenia in adults

Acquired thrombocytopenia is the most common cause of thrombocytopenia, but a rare cause of CH (Juvela and Kase, 2006). In the absence of a platelet function disorder, spontaneous bleeding may occur when the platelet count is <10–20 G/L. Thrombocytopenia may result from decreased platelet production in cases of bone marrow infiltration by neoplastic cells, acute alcohol toxicity, vitamin B12 and folate deprivation, and infections. It also may be drug-induced.

HIV infection often results in thrombocytopenia (Miguez-Burbano *et al.*, 2005) and idiopathic thrombocytopenic purpura (ITP) occurs in about 40% of HIV-infected patients (Zandman-Goddard and Shoenfeld, 2002). HIV-related thrombocytopenia rarely causes CH, even when platelet counts are low (Shavit and Grenader, 2005). Autoimmune thrombocytopenia also develops in about 2.6% of hepatitis C patients (Giordano *et al.*, 2005). Thrombocytopenia is a common feature of sepsis (Levi, 2005). Its mechanism is probably a combination of impaired platelet production and platelet consumption (Levi, 2005).

ITP is an autoimmune disorder. Thrombocytopenia is caused by autoantibodies directed against platelet antigens that increase the clearance of circulating platelets and decrease platelet production by bone marrow megakaryocytes. Bleeding symptoms including CH are uncommon except in severe ITP (platelets

<30 G/L) (The British Committee for Standards in Haematology, 2003). First-line therapy is usually given when platelet counts are <30 G/L and consists of glucocorticoid therapy 1 mg/kg/day and/or intravenous immunoglobulins (IVG) 2 g/kg for 3–5 days. Splenectomy is considered as second-line therapy and results in durable remission in two-thirds of patients. Recently, rituximab (recombinant anti-CD20 antibody) has been prescribed after failure of glucocorticoids and before splenectomy. However, complete responses appear less frequent and less durable with rituximab than with splenectomy.

Drug-induced thrombocytopenia is common and may be caused by marrow suppression and immune or non-immune thrombocytopenia (Aster, 2005a). In immune-mediated drug-induced thrombocytopenia, platelet counts recover promptly after drug interruption. Glucocorticoid therapy 1 mg/kg/day is administered when platelets are <10 G/L and if bleeding is not severe. In cases of severe bleeding, the treatment combines platelet transfusion with IVG and high-dose glucocorticoids. Severe thrombocytopenia may be associated with quinine, quinidine, and sulfonamide antibiotics. Patients often have petechial hemorrhages and urinary tract or gastrointestinal bleeding. However, CH is rare (Aster, 2005a; Freiman, 1990).

GPIIb/IIIa inhibitors are antiplatelet agents that block the binding of fibrinogen to activated GPIIb/IIIa (Aster, 2005b). Abciximab is sometimes used in the treatment of acute cerebral thromboembolic complications during neuroendovascular procedures (Velat et al., 2006). Acute severe thrombocytopenia may occur within a few hours after the initiation of the drug but may also be delayed 5–8 days after the administration (Aster, 2005b). In most instances, favorable evolution is observed. Bleeding complications are rare, but life-threatening bleeding including CH may occur (The CAPTURE investigators, 1997; Vahdat et al., 2000).

Acquired thrombocytopenia in neonates

The frequency of thrombocytopenia in neonates is estimated to be 1%–4%, and the major risk of severe thrombocytopenia is CH. Fetal thrombocytopenia may also lead to in utero death or porencephaly (Kaplan, 2001).

Neonatal alloimmune thrombocytopenia (NAIT) is the most common cause of severe neonatal thrombocytopenia (Manno, 2005; Williamson et al., 1998). It results from maternal alloimmunization against fetal platelet antigens derived from the father. It may affect the fetus as early as 20 weeks gestational age or the newborn, and the risk of worsening thrombocytopenia increases with each new pregnancy (Kaplan, 2001, 2005; Manno, 2005). In the case of severe thrombocytopenia in a fetus or neonate, CH may occur with subsequent neurological impairment or neonatal and intrauterine death. Neonatal CH occurs in about 10%–30% of patients (Kaplan, 2001; Manno, 2005).

Diagnosis and management
In the first pregnancy, in the case of severe fetal thrombocytopenia, brain hemorrhage or hydrocephalus may be found during a screening prenatal ultrasound, or thrombocytopenia may be diagnosed at birth. In the case of known NAIT, the goal is (for future pregnancies) to anticipate recurrence, and fetal blood is taken at 20 weeks gestation for platelet count and analysis of platelet fetal antigens. If the fetus is affected, IVG (1–2 g/kg) is administered 1–2 times per week to the mother, and a follow-up of fetal blood is performed. If IVG is not effective, glucocorticoids are prescribed to the mother. For delivery, fetal platelet value should be >50 G/L. If the count is lower, platelets should be given in utero before delivery. Newborns with thrombocytopenia <30 G/L should receive IVG or platelet transfusion (platelets from the mother or from a donor whose platelets lack the same antigen as those of the mother), when possible (Manno, 2005).

Immune fetal or neonatal thrombocytopenia due to maternal ITP is severe in 8.9%–14.7%, and intracerebral bleeding occurs in up to 1.5% of infants. Maternal antibodies cross the placenta and induce fetal thrombocytopenia. The infant platelet count is not proportional to the mother's platelet count and is unpredictable. Fetal blood sampling by cordocentesis is not recommended because of a mortality of 1%–2%, at least as high as the risk of intracerebral bleeding (Kaplan, 2001; The British Committee for Standards in Haematology, 2003). IVG is recommended (1 g/kg) in the case of bleeding or platelet count <20 G/L (The British Committee for Standards in Haematology, 2003).

Disorders of platelet function

Disorders of platelet function may be inherited or acquired. Coagulation tests are normal, whereas bleeding time and platelet function assay (PFA)-100 closure time are usually prolonged. Platelet aggregometry may help make a definite diagnosis.

Inherited qualitative platelet disorders are rare diseases that comprise disorders of platelet adhesion, aggregation, and storage pool release. Bleeding symptoms are variable, and the most severe variants of qualitative platelet disorders may cause CH (Brown, 2005). Initial diagnosis of qualitative platelet disorder is based on platelet aggregometry.

Glanzmann's thrombasthenia is a rare autosomal recessive disorder. Whereas platelet count, size, and morphology are normal, there is an absence or a defect in GPIIb/IIIa, and platelets fail to aggregate. Diagnosis is usually made during childhood, especially because of lifelong mucosal bleeding. Intracerebral bleeding may occur, particularly during the neonatal period (Brown, 2005). Bleeding time and PFA-100 closure time are prolonged, and platelet aggregometry shows absent platelet aggregation with all platelet agonists except ristocetin and collagen.

Bernard-Soulier syndrome is characterized by the absence of the GPIb/IX/V complex, which is the principal receptor for the VWF and is characterized by macrothrombocytopenia associated with disproportionate bleeding (Cines et al., 2004).

Whereas inherited platelet disorders are rare, acquired platelet function disorders are common. Platelet function may be affected by drugs such as aspirin, non-aspirin nonsteroidal anti-inflammatory drugs (NSAIDs), and GPIIb/IIIa inhibitors and by systemic disorders like uremia, liver cirrhosis, and myeloproliferative diseases.

Management

In the case of bleeding, platelet transfusion may be required. Desmopressin (DDAVP) is a vasopressin analog that favors release of VWF from tissue stores (mainly endothelial cells) and may be used in acquired platelet disorders such as uremia. Recombinant factor VIIa (rFVIIa) may be used in hemorrhagic complications of inherited or acquired platelet function disorders (Hassan and Kroll, 2005).

Deficiencies of coagulation factors

Inherited deficiencies of coagulation factors

Hemophilia A and B are the most frequent inherited deficiencies of coagulation factors and together with von Willebrand disease (VWD) represent more than 95% of all inherited deficiencies of coagulation factors (Mannucci et al., 2004).

Hemophilia Hemophilia is caused by deficiency of factor VIII (hemophilia A) or factor IX (hemophilia B). The incidence of hemophilia A is 1/10 000 and is five times more frequent than hemophilia B. The transmission is X-linked, and sporadic mutations occur in about 30% of cases without a familial context. The severity of hemophilia depends on factors VIII or IX levels: severe hemophilia, <1%, moderate hemophilia, 1%–5%, and mild hemophilia, 5%–40%. Intracranial bleeding occurs in 2%–14% of hemophiliacs, mainly in severe hemophiliacs. Neonatal hemorrhage may be the first manifestation of hemophilia, and its incidence is about 3% (Brown, 2005). Treatment consists of factor VIII or IX replacement therapy (recombinant products are preferred to plasma concentrates) in case of bleeding or surgery.

Development of an inhibitor, which is an antibody against the coagulant function of the replacement factor, occurs in up to one-third of patients with hemophilia A (Acharya and DiMichele, 2006). It is the most serious therapeutic complication and makes factor VIII or IX replacement therapy ineffective. During an acute bleeding event, based on the inhibitor titer, alternative treatment strategies include high-dose factor VIII or IX for low responders (to saturate existing antibody and provide excessive factor VIII or IX for hemostasis) and bypassing agents like activated prothrombin complex concentrate (FEIBA), rFVIIa, or plasmapheresis/immunoadsorption for high responders. Long-term inhibitor eradication may be achieved with immunotolerance and immunomodulation (Acharya and DiMichele, 2006; Brown, 2005; Gringeri and Mannucci, 2005).

von Willebrand disease VWF is a GP that induces platelet adhesion to the subendothelium and platelet aggregation in the early phases of hemostasis (Sumner and Williams, 2004). VWD is the most common inherited bleeding disorder, and its severity depends on the degree of VWF defect. It is inherited in an autosomal dominant or recessive pattern. Type 1 identifies a partial mild to moderate VWF deficiency. Type 2 is characterized by qualitative defects, and type 3 by an absence of VWF (Federici, 2004; Sumner and Williams, 2004).

The aPTT may be increased because of FVIII deficiency VWF antigen and activity (measured by the ristocetin cofactor assay) may be reduced. The bleeding time and PFA-100 closure time may be prolonged, and ristocetin-induced platelet aggregation may be abnormal. Bleeding is mainly mucocutaneous. Only a few instances of spontaneous intracranial bleeding secondary to VWD are described in the literature (Almaani and Awidi, 1986; Mohri, et al., 1997). Treatment in the case of CH is replacement with VWF-containing factor VIII concentrates (Sumner and Williams, 2004).

Acquired coagulation factor deficiencies

Isolated acquired coagulation factor deficiencies are very uncommon and are often the result of the development of autoantibodies against a coagulation factor, i.e. antibodies directed against factor VIII or IX in acquired hemophilia.

Acquired hemophilia, a rare autoimmune disease caused by antibodies against factor VIII or FIX, often occurs in patients >65 years and is mainly idiopathic, but may also be secondary to neoplasm (lymphoproliferative diseases or solid tumors), autoimmune disease, pregnancy, and intolerance to drug therapy. Severe bleeding episodes occur in 80%–90% of patients with a short-term high mortality rate (10%–25%) (Johansen et al., 2006; Kessler, 2005). CH has been reported (Ries et al., 1995).

The key laboratory findings are a prolonged aPTT associated with a low factor VIII or IX activity and detectable inhibitor by the Bethesda assay. The first target of treatment is to control and prevent acute hemorrhagic complications bypassing agents such as FEIBA or rFVIIa. The second target is to eradicate the autoantibody by immunosuppressive therapy (Johansen et al., 2006; Kessler, 2005).

Acquired multifactorial deficiencies are common and may result from vitamin K deficiency, liver disease, or DIC (discussed in Chapter 39). Vitamin K deprivation impairs post-translation γ-carboxylation of vitamin K-dependent proteins: factor II, VII, IX, and X and protein C and S. It is frequent in neonates to whom vitamin K should be systematically provided to prevent bleeding. In adults, vitamin K deficiency is mainly from malabsorption and vitamin K metabolism impairment by vitamin K antagonists, antibiotics, or rodenticides.

The hepatocyte synthesizes most coagulation factors (except factor VIII and VWF) and coagulation regulation proteins. The γ-carboxylation process of vitamin K-dependent factors is impaired in moderate hepatic failure and particularly in the case of cholestasis (vitamin K malabsorption). In severe hepatic failure, factor V is severely lowered, and hypofibrinogenemia and dysfibrinogenemia occur. Moreover, antithrombin, plasminogen, α-2-antiplasmin, and plasminogen activator inhibitor type I (PAI-1) synthesis is impaired. Hepatic tissue destruction favors fibrin deposition and tissue factor exposition that results in coagulation cascade activation. The impairment of the hepatic clearance of activated factors and t-PA, and reduced hepatic synthesis of PAI-1 and α-2-antiplasmin, results in consumptive coagulopathy and hyperfibrinolysis.

Hemorrhagic complications of oral vitamin K antagonists

The most serious complication associated with oral anticoagulant therapy is life-threatening intracranial bleeding and CH, in particular (about 70% intracerebral and 30% subdural) (Steiner *et al.*, 2006). CH related to vitamin K antagonists accounts for 10%–12% of all intracerebral hemorrhage and is seven- to 10-fold more frequent than in patients who are not receiving vitamin K antagonists (Steiner *et al.*, 2006). The estimated rate of CH related to vitamin K antagonists is about 2–9/100 000 population/year (Steiner *et al.*, 2006) with a mortality of 67% (Rosand *et al.*, 2004). The use of vitamin K antagonists might unmask brain bleeding that would otherwise remain asymptomatic, especially in patients with hypertension and cerebrovascular disease (Hart *et al.*, 2005). Moreover, patients with underlying primary cerebrovascular disease have a higher risk of vitamin K antagonist-related intracranial bleeding (Steiner *et al.*, 2006).

The hemorrhagic risk of vitamin K antagonists is increased by the simultaneous uptake of antiplatelet drugs and drugs that interfere with vitamin K antagonist metabolism like amiodarone, antibiotics, cimetidine, thyroid hormones, miconazole, phenylbutazone, quinidine, and simvastatin (Ansell *et al.*, 2004).

Recommendations for managing elevated INRs or bleeding in patients receiving vitamin K antagonists

1. INR above therapeutic range without bleeding: INR <5: lower dose or omit next dose and then lower doses; INR between 5 and 9: 1–2 mg of vitamin K orally and omit next dose then lower doses; INR >9: 2–5 mg of vitamin K orally, omit next dose and then lower doses (Ansell *et al.*, 2004)
2. Management of vitamin K antagonist-related CH at any INR: rapid reversal of vitamin K antagonists by administration of prothrombin complex concentrates rather than fresh frozen plasma and administration of intravenous rather than oral vitamin K (Ansell *et al.*, 2004; Baglin *et al.*, 2006).

Hemorrhagic complications of thrombolysis

Thrombolysis is performed by intravenous or intra-arterial administration of plasminogen activators like streptokinase, urokinase derivatives, or recombinant tissue plasminogen activator (rt-PA) in order to induce arterial recanalization (Gupta *et al.*, 2006).

CH is the most severe complication of intra-arterial and intravenous thrombolysis for IS. Although less frequent, CH is also an important complication of intravenous thrombolysis in myocardial infarction patients (Trouillas and von Kummer, 2006).

In the report of The National Institute of Neurological Disorders and Stroke (NINDS) controlled study, symptomatic CH is described as "any CT-documented hemorrhage that was temporally related to deterioration in the patient's clinical condition in the judgment of the clinical investigator"; only hemorrhage occurring within 36 hours from treatment onset are considered (The NINDS Study Group, 1995, 1997; Trouillas and von Kummer,

2006). Risk factors for development of symptomatic CH reported in the NINDS rt-PA study are severity at baseline and brain edema or mass effect by CT before treatment. Mortality associated with symptomatic CH is 10-fold higher in the rt-PA group than in the placebo group (17% vs. 21%) (The NINDS Study Group, 1995 and 1997; Trouillas and von Kummer, 2006).

Recommendations for the prevention of thrombolysis complications

Low-molecular-weight heparin should be excluded during the 24 hours after thrombolysis, and unfractionated heparin should be avoided immediately after thrombolysis. Hemostasis analysis should be done before and 2 hours after the start of thrombolysis, with blood count and assay of fibrinogen and fibrinogen/fibrin degradation factors (Trouillas and von Kummer, 2006).

rFVIIa

rFVIIa has been approved for the prevention and treatment of bleeding episodes or in the case of surgery in hemophiliacs with inhibitors and for treatment of bleeding episodes in patients with factor VII deficiency Glanzmann's thrombasthenia. In addition, numerous case reports and studies have described its efficacy in massive bleeding, even in patients without prior coagulopathy. It is thought to enhance hemostasis at the site of injury by activating factor IX and X when complexed to tissue factor and even without the presence of tissue factor (platelet-dependent tissue factor-independent mechanism). Whereas only small amounts of FVII naturally circulate and have very weak enzymatic activity until it binds to tissue factor, administration of a large dose of rFVIIa leads to a huge increase in FVIIa level with faster and higher thrombin generation (Martinowitz and Michaelson, 2005; O'Connell *et al.*, 2006).

Recommendations for the use of rFVIIa in uncontrolled hemorrhage have been proposed by Martinowitz and Michaelson in 2005. The administration of rFVIIa is recommended in any salvageable patient with massive uncontrolled hemorrhage that fails to respond to appropriate surgical measures and blood component therapy. However, before its administration, the following conditions should be fulfilled: fibrinogen level ≥ 0.5 g/L, platelet level ≥ 50 G/L, pH ≥ 7.2 because of a decreased activity of rFVIIa ≤ 7.1, and correction of hypothermia and hypocalcemia. The only absolute contraindication is unsalvageable patients. Relative contraindications include arterial and venous thromboembolic events within the previous 6 months (Martinowitz and Michaelson, 2005).

Mayer and Rincon reported in 2006 on a randomized double-blind, placebo-controlled trial of 399 patients with CH treated with a single dose of rFVIIa or placebo within 4 hours of onset. They found a reduction in hematoma growth and mortality with rFVIIa. However, very recently, Mayer *et al.* (2008) showed that rFVIIa reduces growth of hematoma but does not improve survival and outcome.

The localized activation of coagulation at the site of injury may explain the low rate of thromboembolic events (<0.05% of thromboembolic events in more than 400 000 doses administered to patients with hemophilia) (Martinowitz and Michaelson, 2005).

O'Connell *et al.* (2006) reviewed serious thromboembolic adverse events following rFVIIa administration reported to the U.S. Food and Drug Administration (FDA) adverse event reporting system from 1999 to 2004. Among 99 arterial events (54%), 39 were IS. Among the 42 reports of deep vein thrombosis (23%), cases of retinal vein thrombosis are mentioned, but none of cerebral veins. The median time between the last dose of rFVIIa and the thromboembolic event was about 24 hours. However, in 2004, Aledort studied data from the MedWatch pharmacovigilance program of the FDA that included estimated numbers of infusions available from manufacturers from 1999 to 2002 and reported that CVST is the most common thrombotic event after rFVIIa administration. Recently, Duringer *et al.* (2008) found an increased risk of arterial thromboembolism associated with higher doses of rFVIIa in CH patients.

Blood disorders causing cerebral thrombosis

Introduction

Arterial and venous thrombosis and their complications represent the major cause of morbidity and death in the industrialized countries. The major factors involved in the pathology of thrombosis are injury to the vessel wall, alteration of blood flow, and changes in the composition of the blood. They constitute the triad of Virchow. Arterial thrombosis is mostly associated with atherosclerosis and causes myocardial infarction, IS, and limb gangrene. Thrombi form under conditions of high flow and consist of platelet aggregates held together by small amounts of fibrin. Venous thrombi consist mainly of fibrin and red blood cells and develop under low flow conditions in the deep veins.

The term "thrombophilia" (Egeberg, 1965) was used initially to describe a tendency to venous thrombosis. This term now includes any disorder associated with an increased tendency to thrombosis, either inherited or acquired. Studies on genetic thrombophilia were mainly conducted in patients with venous thrombosis, whereas studies addressing hypercoagulable states and arterial stroke are scarce (Levine, 2005).

Here we will develop the relationship between CVST and IS and inherited and acquired thrombophilia. Preventive approaches and treatment recommendations based upon guidelines and data reported in the literature will also be discussed.

Cerebral venous thrombosis and thrombophilia

Thrombosis of the cerebral veins and sinuses (CVST) most often occurs in young patients; 75% of the adult patients are women (Boncoraglio *et al.*, 2004). The mortality rate ranges between 3% and 10% depending on the series and the period of observation (i.e. perihospitalization vs. follow-up period) (Dentali *et al.*, 2006). An adverse outcome is favored by an age older than 37 years, the presence of focal deficits or altered consciousness at presentation, intracranial hemorrhage, the involvement of cortical veins, and cancer (Dentali *et al.*, 2006). Patients with thrombophilic risk factors also seem to have less favorable outcomes (Appenzeller *et al.*, 2005). A prothrombotic risk factor or another direct cause is identified in about 70–85% of patients. There are various predisposing conditions to CVST: intracranial infections, trauma, hematological

and autoimmune disorders, intracranial neoplasms, vascular malformations, pregnancy, puerperium, and oral contraception (Boncoraglio *et al.*, 2004; Lichy *et al.*, 2006; Ventura *et al.*, 2004). The recurrence rate is similar to lower extremity deep vein thrombosis. Inherited and acquired prothrombotic risk factors will be discussed below.

According to the Canadian Pediatric Ischemic Stroke Registry (CPISR), the incidence of CVST in the pediatric non-neonate population is about 0.25/100 000 children per year, and only 3% of children have idiopathic CVST. Iron-deficiency anemia has been associated with CVST (Belman *et al.*, 1990; Hartfield *et al.*, 1997; Meena *et al.*, 2000; Robetorye and Rodgers, 2001; Sebire *et al.*, 2005), sometimes in association with thrombocytosis. CVST may also occur in the context of β-thalassemia, sickle cell disease, and other chronic anemia. Thrombophilic risk factors were found in 30%–60% of CVST (Belman *et al.*, 1990; Hartfield *et al.*, 1997; Meena *et al.*, 2000; Robetorye and Rodgers, 2001; Sebire *et al.*, 2005). They include antithrombin, protein C, and protein S deficiencies; factor V Leiden; prothrombin gene mutation; and dysfibrinogenemia. Increased factor VIII and thrombomodulin mutation have also been reported. Acquired prothrombotic disorders are more frequent (and sometimes multiple in one child), but their role should still be explored. They include anti-phospholipid antibodies; lupus anticoagulant; APC resistance; acquired deficiencies of antithrombin, protein C, and protein S; and hyperhomocysteinemia (Chan *et al.*, 2003).

Cerebral venous thrombosis and inherited thrombophilia

Deficiency in antithrombin, protein C, and protein S, has been associated with CVST (Dentali *et al.*, 2006). Patients with factor V Leiden mutation have a nine-fold higher risk of CVST (Ventura *et al.*, 2004). Environmental risk factors such as age, oral contraceptive use, pregnancy, postpartum, trauma, and surgery increase the risk of venous thrombosis in patients with factor V Leiden (Robetorye and Rodgers, 2001). Occasionally, APC resistance may occur in the absence of factor V Leiden mutation and may be related to a mutation in the 306 APC cleavage site (factor V Cambridge) (Dahlback, 2005).

Prothrombin G20210A mutation is the most common inherited risk factor associated with CVST (Boncoraglio *et al.*, 2004; Gadelha *et al.*, 2005). The presence of this mutation increases the risk of CVST about 10-fold, particularly in oral contraceptive users (Albers *et al.*, 2004; Ventura *et al.*, 2004).

Cerebral venous thrombosis and acquired thrombophilia

Environmental causes of VTE (Rosendaal, 2005) are often bound to venous stasis, especially in the case of immobilization such as prolonged bed rest, plaster casts, or long-distance travel (>5 hours). Age is one of the most important risk factors for VTE with an incidence 1000-fold higher in the very old than in the very young individual. Multiple trauma is also associated with a high risk of VTE. In the absence of antithrombotic prophylaxis, VTE may occur in more than 50% of patients who undergo surgical interventions. Because of these facts, prophylactic anticoagulation is routinely prescribed. Mechanical causes as head trauma and cranial surgery may also lead to dural sinus damages and thereby to CVST.

Pregnancy is associated with a two- to fourfold higher VTE risk, with an incidence about 0.9 per 1000 deliveries (The British Committee for Standards in Haematology, 2001; Bauer, 2003). During the second and third trimesters of pregnancy, hemodynamic changes leading to progressive venous stasis and increase in APC resistance normally occur and may contribute to an increase in VTE risk (Bauer, 2003; Ginsberg and Bates, 2003). VTE is the major cause of maternal mortality in the developed world (The British Committee for Standards in Haematology, 2001).

VTE risk is higher among pregnant women with inherited thrombophilia. Several studies suggest that antithrombin deficiency is a higher risk-factor for VTE among pregnant women than are the other factors such as protein C and protein S deficiencies (The British Committee for Standards in Haematology, 2001; Rosendaal, 2005). The estimated incidence of VTE among pregnant women with factor V Leiden is about 1/400–500. Moreover, VTE risk is higher in women with a previous VTE event or a family history of VTE (Bauer, 2003). Data reported in the literature from large trials mention a VTE risk three- to fourfold higher in puerperium than in pregnancy, with a higher risk after caesarean section than after vaginal delivery (Bauer, 2003; Ginsberg and Bates, 2003). Other acquired risk factors that are present in two-thirds of pregnant or puerperal patients are age more than 35 years, high parity, intercurrent illness, and immobility (The British Committee for Standards in Haematology, 2001).

Pregnancy and puerperium are associated with an increased risk of CVST. CVST still remains an important cause of maternal mortality and morbidity in developing countries (Masuhr et al., 2004). The U.S. National Hospital Discharge Survey done between 1979 and 1991 has shown that a younger age and cesarean delivery are risk factors that increase the risk of CVST during the peripartum period (Lanska and Kryscio, 2000). There is no additional risk factor in about 25–35% of cases.

The association between malignancy and an increased incidence of VTE is called Trousseau syndrome. The pathogenesis of malignancy-related thrombosis is complex and multifactorial with multiple risk factors leading to a hypercoagulable state.

Cancer patients often show activation of blood coagulation and reduction of fibrinolysis leading to thrombosis. Tumor cells directly increase the risk of thrombosis by the release of humoral factors with procoagulant or fibrinolytic activity. They also interact with host cells including endothelial cells, platelets, and monocytes and thereby promote the activation and release of procoagulant mediators (Lecumberri et al., 2005; Rosendaal, 2005). Large tumors may cause venous obstruction and mechanical thrombosis (Blom et al., 2005; Rosendaal, 2005). The mobility of these patients is decreased, and antineoplastic therapy may have thrombogenic potential. Anticancer agents associated with an increased risk of VTE are L-asparaginase, bevacizumab, bleomycin, carmustine, cisplatin, 5-fluorouracil, mitomycin C, tamoxifen, thalidomide, and derivatives in association with chemotherapy or high-dose dexamethasone (Lee, 2006). Central venous catheters may also promote upper extremity thrombosis (Rosendaal, 2005).

The presence of cancer increases the overall VTE risk about four-fold compared to that in individuals without cancer and the presence of metastasis in solid tumors increases the risk of VTE about 58-fold compared to that in individuals without cancer (Blom et al., 2005; Rosendaal, 2005). Carriers of factor V Leiden or prothrombin G20210A mutation with cancer had a 12- to 17-fold higher risk of developing VTE than did individuals without cancer and without factor V Leiden and prothrombin mutation (Blom et al., 2005).

Acquired deficiencies of natural coagulation inhibitors

Several clinical situations, diseases, and drugs can induce acquired selective or associated deficiency of antithrombin, protein C, and protein S. By accelerated consumption, acute deficiency of antithrombin, protein C, and protein S are found after an ischemic or a thromboembolic event, in the case of DIC or in surgery, shock, and sepsis (Fields and Levine, 2005). Chronic liver disease is associated with insufficient hepatic synthesis of antithrombin, with DIC, antithrombin consumption, and antithrombin loss in ascites. Gastrointestinal loss of antithrombin is favored in inflammatory bowel disease, and antithrombin deficiency may also be observed in renal disease with nephrotic syndrome (Muller, 1992). Free protein S may also be lost in urine, leading to a reduction in circulating levels of free protein S (Siddiqi et al., 1997).

Vitamin K antagonists induce a low level of protein C and protein S, and heparins induce a low level of antithrombin. L-asparaginase, a drug administered in acute lymphoblastic leukemia treatment, inhibits protein synthesis including those involved in coagulation and fibrinolysis. Antithrombin, protein C, and protein S may be lowered favoring the occurrence of VTE (Lee et al., 2000).

Most oral contraceptives consist of a daily dose of a combination of estrogen and progestogen. Estrogens increase the level of procoagulant factors VII, IX, and X and decrease antithrombin and protein S levels, leading to a mild prothrombotic state. Progestogens do not affect the coagulation factor levels, but third-generation progestogens *counteract less* the effects of estrogens than do second-generation progestogens, leading to a prothrombotic state (Rosendaal, 2005).

Data reported in the literature reveal an association between oral contraceptives and CVST, particularly in patients with the prothrombin G20120A mutation (Albers et al., 2004; Gadelha et al., 2005; Ventura et al., 2004). Oral contraceptives are reported to increase the CVST risk by more than 13-fold (Boncoraglio et al., 2004).

Individual risk factors such as age, obesity, and prothrombotic abnormalities increase the risk of VTE when using oral contraceptives (Rosendaal, 2005). Altogether, these data suggest that women with CVST should avoid oral contraceptives and that the use of these agents in women with thrombophilia should be evaluated individually to assess the risk of CVST.

HRT contains either a combination of estrogen and progestin or, in women without a uterus, only estrogen. Although transdermal administration avoids the first-pass effect through the liver, an increased VTE risk has until now not been excluded and is still controversial (Rosendaal, 2005). As for oral contraceptives, individual risk factors such as age, obesity, and factor V Leiden increase the risk of VTE in women who take HRT. Moreover, the risk of recurrence in women with previous VTE is higher in women who use HRT (Rosendaal, 2005).

Tamoxifen and raloxifene are selective estrogen receptor modulators. Tamoxifen is used for the treatment and prevention of breast cancer, and raloxifene is indicated for osteoporosis prevention and treatment. Both are associated with a two- to threefold increased risk of VTE, but the mechanism is not fully understood (Cosman *et al.*, 2005). Most trials have shown that tamoxifen is associated with decreased antithrombin, protein C, and protein S, but increased free protein S, factors VIII and IX, and VWF (Cosman *et al.*, 2005).

Preventive approach and prophylactic/therapeutic anticoagulation recommendations for CVST

CVST

1. Anticoagulation is recommended even in the presence of hemorrhagic infarction. In the acute phase, both unfractionated heparin and low-molecular-weight heparin should be used, and oral vitamin K antagonist anticoagulation is then introduced for 3–6 months (target INR 2–3) (Albers *et al.*, 2004; Sacco *et al.*, 2006).
2. Women with CVST should avoid use of oral contraceptives (Dentali *et al.*, 2006).

CVST and thrombophilia

Patients with a first episode of CVST with antithrombin, protein C, and protein S deficiency; factor V Leiden or prothrombin G20210A gene mutation, or hyperhomocysteinemia (Buller *et al.*, 2004):
• Anticoagulation is recommended for 6–12 months (INR 2–3).
Patients with a first episode of CVST who have antiphospholipid antibodies or who have two or more thrombophilic conditions:
• Anticoagulation is recommended for 12 months (INR 2–3); long-term anticoagulation is suggested (INR 2–3).
Patients with two or more CVST episodes:
• Long-term anticoagulation is suggested (INR 2–3).
Patients with CVST and malignancy:
• Low-molecular-weight heparin for the first 3–6 months of long-term anticoagulation therapy. Long-term anticoagulation is recommended until cancer is resolved.

Pregnancy and postpartum

Single episode of CVST in a patient without long-term anticoagulants (Bates *et al.*, 2004):
• Prophylactic low-molecular-weight heparin/unfractionated heparin and postpartum anticoagulation is recommended.
Single episode of VTE and inherited thrombophilia or strong family history of thrombosis in a patient without long-term anticoagulants:
• Prophylactic dose of low-molecular-weight heparin/unfractionated heparin and postpartum anticoagulation is recommended.

Antithrombin deficiency, compound heterozygotes for prothrombin G20210A and factor V Leiden, and homozygotes for these conditions with a history of CVST:
• Low-molecular-weight heparin intermediate-dose prophylaxis or moderate-dose unfractionated heparin is recommended.
Two or more episodes of CVST and long-term anticoagulation:
• Adjusted-dose of low-molecular-weight heparin/unfractionated heparin and resumption of the long-term anticoagulation postpartum is suggested.
Anti-phospholipid antibody syndrome and VTE with long-term anticoagulation:
• Adjusted-dose low-molecular-weight heparin/unfractionated heparin therapy and resumption of long-term oral anticoagulation therapy postpartum is recommended.

Arterial IS and thrombophilia

Thrombophilia is responsible for about 1%–4% of instances of IS and is more frequent in young adults (Fields and Levine, 2005; Hankey *et al.*, 2001).

Inherited causes of thrombophilia and stroke

Inherited thrombophilia may play a role in childhood IS (Barnes and Deveber, 2005; Kenet *et al.*, 2000; Sacco *et al.*, 2006). Antithrombin, protein C, and protein S deficiencies; APC resistance; plasma homocysteine > 95th percentile; and the mutations factor V Leiden, prothrombin G20210A, and methylene-tetrahydrofolate reductase (MTHFR) C677T are more common in children with a first IS than in healthy children (Haywood *et al.*, 2005). Thrombophilia screening of children with a first arterial IS has been therefore recommended.

Associations between IS and factor V Leiden, MTHFR C677 T, and prothrombin mutation gene have been found in adults (Casas *et al.*, 2004). However, whether factor V Leiden and prothrombin gene mutation are risk factors for IS in adults still remains controversial (Fields and Levine, 2005; Hankey *et al.*, 2001; Lalouschek *et al.*, 2005; Sacco *et al.*, 2006).

The American Heart Association and the American Stroke Association (AHA and ASA) recommend for patients with IS or TIA, with an established inherited thrombophilia (Sacco *et al.*, 2006):

1. evaluation for deep venous thrombosis, which is an indication for short- or long-term therapy
2. full evaluation for alternative mechanisms of stroke
3. in the absence of VTE, long-term anticoagulation or antiplatelet therapy
4. for patients with a history of recurrent thrombotic events, consideration of long-term anticoagulation

Acquired causes of thrombophilia and stroke

Several risk factors increase the risk of IS during the peripartum period: non-white women, cesarean section, and pregnancy-related hypertension. Several other comorbid conditions such as infection, cardiomyopathy, and congestive heart failure also have been associated with IS during pregnancy and puerperium. (Lanska and Kryscio, 2000).

HRT is associated with a higher risk of VTE and is discussed in the acquired causes of thrombophilia and CVST section of this chapter. Data from the Women's Estrogen for Stroke Trial (WEST) fail to show reduction in the risk of ischemic stroke recurrence or death with estradiol and, within the first 6 months of use, the risk of IS was even higher among women randomized to estradiol treatment (Sacco *et al.*, 2006; Viscoli *et al.*, 2001). The Women's Health Initiative (WHI) study, which examined the role of HRT for the primary prevention of cardiovascular disease and IS in post-menopausal women, was stopped because of an increase of vascular events (Rossouw *et al.*, 2002; Sacco *et al.*, 2006). An increased risk of IS also has been shown in women who take HRT and have had a previous hysterectomy (Anderson *et al.*, 2004; Sacco *et al.*, 2006).

According to the AHA and ASA, postmenopausal hormone therapy is not recommended for women with IS or TIA (Sacco *et al.*, 2006).

Patent foramen ovale and thrombophilia

Patent foramen ovale (PFO) is a persistence of an embryonic defect in the interatrial septum and is present in up to 27% of the general population (Sacco *et al.*, 2006). PFO is the most prevalent potential source of cardioembolism in young adults with cryptogenic stroke and is responsible for about 40% of cryptogenic stroke (Hara *et al.*, 2005; Kizer and Devereux, 2005). Although there is only a weak association between thrombophilia and IS in adults, a potential paradoxical VTE in case of PFO should be considered (Sacco *et al.*, 2006).

Pezzini *et al.* (2003) explored the possibility that PFO-related stroke patients may have an underlying hypercoagulable state and found an association between PFO-related stroke patients and the prothrombin G20210A mutation and to a lesser extent with factor V Leiden.

Acquired or inherited thrombophilia associated with CVST and IS

Anti-phospholipid antibody syndrome

Anti-phospholipid antibody syndrome may be associated with both arterial and venous thrombotic events (see Chapter 12).

HIT

There are two types of HIT. HIT type I is a non-immune-mediated thrombocytopenia that occurs in 10–20% of patients with heparin and is associated with slight nonprogressive thrombocytopenia (>100 G/L) without bleeding or thrombosis. The platelet count rises to pretreatment levels within a few days, even if heparin is not discontinued (Kuo and Kovacs, 2005; Menajovsky, 2005).

HIT type II, which is less frequent, consists of an immune-mediated HIT with HIT-associated IgG antibodies that may lead to arterial or venous thrombotic complications. (Menajovsky, 2005). It may be subdivided into three subtypes (Kuo and Kovacs, 2005):

1. latent (HIT-associated IgG-positive but without thrombocytopenia)
2. HIT (with thrombocytopenia)
3. HIT/T (with thrombocytopenia and thrombosis)

Following heparin administration, platelet factor-4 (PF-4) found in the α-granules of the platelets, binds to heparin forming a PF-4-heparin complex leading to platelet activation and to the release of microparticles with procoagulant properties that initiate thrombin generation. HIT occurs in about 3%–5% of patients who are given unfractionated heparin for 5 days or longer and fewer than 1% of patients who are given low-molecular-weight heparin (Davoren and Aster, 2006). HIT diagnosis is first based on clinical presentation; serology and serotonin release assay are useful to corroborate the diagnosis and serology allows to monitor the presence of anti-PF-4 antibodies in patients who may need re-exposure like on-pump open heart surgery (Menajovsky, 2005). The pretest probability can be calculated according to the 4Ts scoring system proposed by Warkentin and Greinacher (2004):

1. thrombocytopenia: usually unexplained fall (>50%) of platelet count
2. timing of onset of platelet fall: usually between 5 and 10 days or in the first day of exposure in the case of recent heparin exposure (past 30 days)
3. thrombosis or other sequelae: proven new thrombosis, skin necrosis, or acute systemic reaction after intravenous unfractionated heparin bolus
4. others causes of platelet fall: none evident

Venous events are four times more common than arterial events. Neurologic complications of HIT are rare and include IS, spinal ischemia, CVST, and transient global amnesia. HIT-related IS may also result from cardiac thrombi. Until now, the incidence of neurologic complications in patients with serologically confirmed diagnosis of HIT has not been studied systematically (Pohl *et al.*, 2000). Pohl *et al.* (2000), reported data from 120 patients with HIT: 11 patients had IS and three had CVST. Hemorrhagic transformation has been found only in patients with CVST and IS (Warkentin and Bernstein, 2003), and primary CH caused by HIT has not been observed. HIT associated with neurologic complications has a poorer prognosis and a higher mortality rate than HIT without central nervous system involvement.

In case of suspected HIT, heparin must be stopped. However, heparin interruption is not sufficient to reverse the process of HIT, and the incidence of HIT-related complications remains high after cessation of heparin. In order to reverse HIT effects and to reduce the risk of thrombotic events, lepirudin or argatroban are prescribed. Danaparoïd may also be used, but in vitro cross-reactivity with HIT antibodies is reported in 10%–20% of patients (Menajovsky, 2005). Coumarin should be avoided during the acute event because of the preferential inhibition of the synthesis of protein C leading to acute skin necrosis and/or progression of VTE or limb gangrene. Vitamin K antagonists should be gradually initiated after the patient has been stabilized and the platelet count has recovered. Anticoagulation should be maintained for 30–60 days after the occurrence of HIT (Davoren and Aster, 2006).

Hyperhomocysteinemia

Homocysteine is formed from methionine after several trans-methylation reactions, and then converted to cysteine in the trans-sulfuration pathway using vitamin B6. When methionine is needed, homocysteine undergoes two remethylations. The remethylation of homocysteine is catalyzed either by betaine-homocysteine methyltransferase in the liver or by methionine synthetase whose cofactor is vitamin B12 and whose substrate is methyltetrahydrofolate in most others tissues. Methylene-tetra-hydrofolate reductase (MTHFR), which is dependent on vitamin B12, catalyzes the formation of methyltetrahydrofolate (Robetorye and Rodgers, 2001). Inhibition of homocysteine metabolism pathways may occur in the case of enzymatic defects or vitamin deficiencies, leading to elevated plasma homocysteine. Accumulation of homocysteine appears to damage the blood vessel wall (Fields and Levine, 2005).

Hyperhomocysteinemia may be acquired in association with smoking, old age, renal failure, vitamin deficiencies (mainly folic acid and vitamin B12), hyperthyroidism, and/or drugs (methotrexate, theophylline, phenytoin). It may also be inherited resulting from genetic disorders affecting the homocysteine metabolism pathway. (Boncoraglio et al., 2004; Fields and Levine, 2005). The most common genetic mutation is a C-to-T substitution at nucleotide 677 (C677T) of the MTHFR gene. Approximately 10%–13% of the Caucasian population are homozygous for this mutation (Cantu et al., 2004), but hyperhomocysteinemia is only rarely observed, indicating that the interaction between genetic and environmental factors is important for the development of hyperhomocysteinemia and that the hereditary metabolic disorder is mainly evident in individuals with poor nutritional status (Cantu et al., 2004). Cystathionine synthase plays a role in the trans-sulfuration pathway of homocysteine, and a genetic mutation of this enzyme may also be a risk factor for IS (Fields and Levine, 2005).

Hyperhomocysteinemia is a known risk factor for idiopathic CVST and IS, especially in young adults and in association with inherited thrombophilia-like procoagulant gene mutations (Boncoraglio et al., 2004). Literature reports show a twofold greater risk of IS associated with hyperhomocysteinemia (Sacco et al., 2006). The Vitamin Intervention from Stroke Prevention Trial randomized in a double-blind controlled trial 3680 patients with noncardioembolic IS and mild-to-moderate hyperhomocysteinemia to receive high-dose or low-dose vitamin therapy (folate, B6, or B12) from September 1996 to December 2003. The risk of IS was related to the level of homocysteine, but there was no reduction in IS rate among patients who took high-dose vitamin (Toole et al., 2004). Although there is no proven clinical benefit of high-dose vitamin therapy for mild to moderate hyperhomocysteinemia, the AHA and ASA encourage patients with IS or TIA, and hyperhomocysteinemia (levels > 10 μmol/L) to take a daily standard multivitamin preparation, given their safety and low cost (Sacco et al., 2006).

Several studies reported in the literature also suggest an increased risk of CVST in patients with hyperhomocysteinemia (Boncoraglio et al., 2004; Cantu et al., 2004; Martinelli et al., 2003). Cantu et al. (2004) suggest that hyperhomocysteinemia and low plasma folate levels are associated with an increased risk of CVST. However, the high incidence of increased risk of CVST in patients with low plasma folate levels may be explained by the low socioeconomic conditions and the deficient nutritional status of the population (Cantu et al., 2004). Martinelli et al. (2003) showed that hyperhomocysteinemia increases the risk of CVST about fourfold. Whether the correction of hyperhomocysteinemia with vitamin therapy will help reduce the risk of recurrent CVST (up to 20% in this study) should be further investigated.

TTP

TTP is characterized by a Coombs-negative hemolytic anemia, thrombocytopenia, petechial hemorrhages, fever, and/or renal and neurological complications. Its underlying pathological mechanism, manifestations, and treatment are discussed in Chapter 41.

Sickle cell anemia

Sickle cell anemia (SCA) is an inherited autosomal disorder resulting from a glutamine-to-valine substitution at codon 6 of the β-globin gene leading to the formation of an abnormal hemoglobin S (HbS) molecule. When HbS is deoxygenated, its interaction with another hemoglobin molecule leads to polymerization of HbS and thereby to a decrease in the red cell deformability ("sickle" shape) favoring vaso-occlusive phenomena (Adams et al., 2003; Bunn, 1997). Moreover, HbS is associated with changes in red cell membrane structure and function, dysregulation of red cell volume, and increased adhesion of red cells to endothelial cells, also leading to vaso-occlusive phenomena (Bunn, 1997). SCA is also associated with chronic hemolysis, resulting in a mild-to-moderate anemia.

SCA and IS in adults

IS is a common complication of sickle cell disease, and its risk is higher with homozygous SS and less pronounced with hemoglobin SC, whereas sickle cell trait hemoglobin AS has little or no elevation of IS rate (Sacco et al., 2006). Although sickle cell disease is considered to be a hypercoagulable state, there is no experience with antiplatelet, anticoagulation, or anti-inflammatory agents for IS prevention. Risk factor identification and reduction can be recommended on the basis of its importance in the general population (Sacco et al., 2006).

The AHA and ASA recommend for adults with SCA, IS, and/or TIA (in addition to general TIA and IS recommendations):

1. regular blood transfusion to reduce HbS to <30%–50% of total hemoglobin
2. hydroxyurea
3. bypass surgery in cases of advanced occlusive disease

SCA and IS in children

Ischemic brain injury (particularly silent brain infarcts) is one of the most common complications of SCA in children, and cognitive disability is a major consequence of microvascular ischemia without clinical IS (Buchanan *et al.*, 2004; Powars, 2000). Twenty-two percent of children with SCA have silent ischemic lesions on brain MRI scans (Buchanan *et al.*, 2004; Golomb, 2005), and repeated clinical ISs occur in two-thirds of untreated children (Powars, 2000). The Cooperative Study of Sickle Cell Disease reported that children with SS SCA who have silent brain infarcts identified at the age of 6 years have a 14-fold increased incidence of subsequent new overt IS (Buchanan *et al.*, 2004; Miller *et al.*, 2001).

Clinical risk factors to predict silent brain infarcts have not yet been established. However, low pain event rate, history of seizures, leukocyte count > 11.8 G/L and the *SEN globin gene haplotype* have been associated with an increased incidence of silent brain infarcts, but their predictive value is unreliable (Buchanan *et al.*, 2004).

Significant risk-factors for overt IS are elevated transcranial Doppler (TCD) measurement and the presence of a silent brain infarct on MRI (Buchanan *et al.*, 2004). The Stroke Prevention Trial in Sickle Cell Anemia (STOP) showed that blood transfusion therapy in patients with increased TCD velocities of the middle cerebral artery or terminal portion of the internal carotid artery could prevent the development of ISs (Adams *et al.*, 1998; Buchanan *et al.*, 2004). The aim of the blood transfusion is to increase total hemoglobin A leading to an improvement of oxygen-carrying capacity and a reduction of cells containing HbS by dilution as well as of the erythropoietic drive in order to maintain an HbS level < 30%. Blood transfusion therapy is recommended as the most important intervention for primary stroke prevention (reducing the onset of stroke in patients with elevated TCD) and secondary stroke prevention in children with sickle cell disease. Until now, there has been no evidence that hydroxyurea is effective for patients with silent brain infarcts (Buchanan *et al.*, 2004).

Aspirin resistance

Antiplatelet therapy (particularly aspirin) reduces by approximately 25% the risk of nonfatal myocardial infarction, nonfatal IS, or vascular death in high-risk patients (Patrono, 2003; Szczeklik *et al.*, 2005). In those patients, European and American guidelines recommend aspirin 75–100 mg/day (Szczeklik *et al.*, 2005). "Aspirin resistance" means the inability of aspirin to protect against thrombotic complications and to reduce platelet function. However, laboratory tests of platelet function are not specific and sensitive enough and are not reproducible enough to quantitatively reflect platelet responsiveness to aspirin. The measurement of whole blood TXA_2 formation and of its metabolite urinary excretion might be the best way to investigate aspirin resistance, because aspirin inhibits more than 95% of the platelet TXA_2 production (Schror *et al.*, 2006; Szczeklik *et al.*, 2005).

The frequency of aspirin resistance is not known, and data from the literature differ substantially in the different groups of patients studied (Szczeklik *et al.*, 2005). Among patients with recurrent IS, 34% were aspirin nonresponders (Grundmann *et al.*, 2003).

A classification of aspirin resistance has been proposed by Weber *et al.* (2002):

1. Type I: failure of aspirin to work *in vivo* but normal inhibition in vitro of platelet aggregation and thromboxane formation: missing compliance. Interference with certain NSAID (ibuprofen, indomethacin) may also be possible.
2. Type II: true resistance due to insufficient platelet response. Inhibition of TXA_2 formation by aspirin might be incomplete at the dose of 100 mg/day in vivo. Therefore, higher doses of aspirin (i.e. 300 mg/day) may be more effective in these patients.
3. Type III: stimulation of platelets by aspirin-insensitive factors or increased platelet sensitivity to platelet agonists like collagen or VWF, or gene polymorphism that may affect platelet function independently from aspirin

Mixed pathologies

In this section, blood disorders associated with both bleeding and thrombosis tendencies are discussed (for DIC, see Chapter 39).

Paroxysmal nocturnal hemoglobinuria

Paroxysmal nocturnal hemoglobinuria is a rare acquired clonal disorder of hematopoiesis resulting from a mutation of the PIG-A gene and leading to red cells, platelets, and neutrophils deficient in all surface proteins (including CD55 and CD59 on the surface of red cells, neutrophils, and CD14, CD16, CD24, CD48, CD52, and CD66 on the surface of neutrophils only) attached to the cell membrane by a glycosylphosphatidylinositol anchor. The absence of these proteins on the red cell membranes leads to an enhanced sensitivity to complement-mediated hemolysis (Audebert *et al.*, 2005; Bagby *et al.*, 2004; Hall *et al.*, 2003; Hillmen *et al.*, 1995). Paroxysmal nocturnal hemoglobinuria is diagnosed by showing by flow cytometry the absence of these proteins on the surface of red cells and neutrophils.

The clinical triad of paroxysmal nocturnal hemoglobinuria is characterized by chronic intravascular hemolysis punctuated by paroxysms with an increase in the intensity of hemolysis and hemoglobinuria, venous thrombosis, and aplastic anemia (Rosse *et al.*, 2004). Myelodysplastic syndrome and acute leukemia may complicate paroxysmal nocturnal hemoglobinuria (Socie *et al.*, 1996).

Venous thrombosis is the most common cause of death in patients with paroxysmal nocturnal hemoglobinuria and especially involves hepatic and cerebral veins (Hall *et al.*, 2003). Large paroxysmal nocturnal hemoglobinuria granulocyte clones (>50%) are predictive of VTE. Indeed, the 10-year risk of VTE was 44% in patients with large paroxysmal nocturnal hemoglobinuria clones and 5.8% in those with small clones (Hall *et al.*, 2003).

Hall *et al.* (2003) showed in patients with large granulocyte clones and platelet count stable or higher than 100 G/L that primary prophylaxis with warfarin (INR 2–3) prevents VTE. Cerebral arterial thrombosis is rare, but isolated life-threatening cases have been reported. (al-Samman *et al.*, 1994; Audebert *et al.*, 2005; von Stuckrad-Barre *et al.*, 2003).

Thrombocytopenia is a common feature of paroxysmal nocturnal hemoglobinuria, and nearly 50% of paroxysmal nocturnal hemoglobinuria patients have platelet counts < 50 G/L. Therefore, serious hemorrhagic events may occur, and paroxysmal nocturnal hemoglobinuria patients with cerebral hemorrhage are reported (Boschetti et al., 2004).

Management

The only way to eradicate paroxysmal nocturnal hemoglobinuria clones is allogeneic stem cell transplantation (Bagby et al., 2004; Boschetti et al., 2004; Socie et al., 1996). Aplastic anemia may respond to immunosuppressive therapy with antilymphocyte globulin and/or cyclosporine. In patients with life-threatening thrombosis, reduced-intensity conditioning allogeneic stem cell transplantation may be considered. Primary antithrombotic prophylaxis should be introduced in selected patients (Rosse et al., 2004).

Chronic myeloproliferative disorders

Myeloproliferative disorders are clonal disorders that include chronic myeloid leukemia, polycythemia vera, essential thrombocytemia, myelofibrosis with myeloid metaplasia, and also, recently, chronic neutrophilic leukemia, chronic eosinophilic leukemia, chronic basophilic leukemia, and systemic mastocytosis (Tefferi, 2006).

Polycythemia vera is characterized by an increased sensitivity of erythroid precursors to erythropoietin and a predominant erythroid hyperplasia. Essential thrombocythemia is associated with an increased sensitivity of megakaryocytes to thrombopoietin and to predominant megakaryocytic hyperplasia (Schafer, 2006).

Polycythemia vera is related in most patients to the recently described JAK2-V617F tyrosine kinase mutations, but only one-half of patients with essential thrombocythemia have these mutations (Campbell and Green, 2005; Campbell et al., 2005). The main cause of morbidity and mortality in polycythemia vera and essential thrombocythemia is thrombosis. Bleeding complications may also occur but are less common (Campbell and Green, 2005; Petrides and Siegel, 2006).

Thrombotic events may occur in 4.1%–9.8% of patients with polycythemia vera with an annual incidence of 2%–9%. There is a lower annual incidence in patients younger than 40 years and a higher frequency in patients older than 70 years. The most important risk factor is the type of therapy, with a higher incidence of thrombosis among patients with phlebotomy than among those treated with hydroxyurea. Moreover, the incidence of thrombosis increases during the 2–3 years before diagnosis of polycythemia vera (Leone et al., 2001).

The prevalence of thrombotic events in patients with essential thrombocythemia is variable in the literature (15%–89%) with an annual incidence of 5%. Thrombosis is more frequent in patients older than 60 years, particularly in those with previous thrombotic events (Campbell and Green, 2005; Harrison, 2005; Leone et al., 2001). Although thrombotic risk is not proportional to platelet count, clinical practice indicates that the incidence of thrombotic events is reduced when platelet counts are lowered (Petrides and Siegel, 2006). An increased risk of thrombosis has been observed with platelet counts >1000 G/L at diagnosis or

above the normal range during treatment. The aim of treatment is to maintain the platelet count <600 G/L (Campbell and Green, 2005; Leone et al., 2001).

Thrombotic events in essential thrombocythemia and polycythemia vera are mainly arterial (50%–70%), and more than 80% of fatal thrombosis in polycythemia vera are arterial (Leone et al., 2001). Arterial thrombotic events in polycythemia vera and essential thrombocythemia occur mainly in large arteries, especially in the cerebrovascular and cardiovascular systems and in the peripheral arterial circulation. Microvascular thrombosis is more common in essential thrombocythemia than in polycythemia vera. Microvascular occlusion may lead to transient neurologic and visual symptoms and signs (Schafer, 2006).

Polycythemia vera is accompanied by a high risk of IS and TIA, with an incidence of about 4–5/year (Koennecke and Bernarding, 2001).

Venous thrombotic events in polycythemia vera and essential thrombocythemia constitute 30%–40% of all thrombotic events associated with these disorders. Cerebral veins are frequently involved (Leone et al., 2001), and cerebral sinus thrombosis has rarely been reported in association with essential thrombocythemia (Arai and Sugiura, 2004). Venous thrombi contain fibrin, erythrocytes, and few platelets (Petrides and Siegel, 2006), and the mechanism of thrombosis includes elevated hematocrit leading to increased whole-blood viscosity and decreased cerebral blood flow.

Treatment

Cytoreduction with hydroxyurea reduces the incidence of thrombosis in essential thrombocythemia, and aspirin reduces the incidence of thrombotic events in polycythemia vera.

Bleeding complications may occur in the case of extreme thrombocytosis (>1500 G/L), and the risk of bleeding is increased by antiplatelet drugs. The mechanism of bleeding is characterized by qualitative platelet abnormalities and especially acquired von Willebrand disease in patients with thrombocytosis (Schafer, 2006). Cerebral bleeding has also been reported in association with polycythemia vera (Friess et al., 2003).

REFERENCES

Acharya, S. S., and DiMichele, D. M. 2006. Management of factor VIII inhibitors. Best Pract Res Clin Haematol, 19, 51–66.

Adams, G. T., Snieder, H., McKie, V. C., et al. 2003. Genetic risk factors for cerebrovascular disease in children with sickle cell disease: design of a case-control association study and genomewide screen. BMC Med Genet, 4, 6.

Adams, R. J., McKie, V. C., Hsu, L., et al. 1998. Prevention of a first stroke by transfusions in children with sickle cell anemia and abnormal results on transcranial Doppler ultrasonography. N Engl J Med, 339, 5–11.

Albers, G. W., Amarenco, P., Easton, J. D., Sacco, R. L., and Teal, P. 2004. Antithrombotic and thrombolytic therapy for ischemic stroke: the Seventh ACCP Conference on Antithrombotic and Thrombolytic Therapy. Chest, 126 (3 Suppl), 483S–512S.

Aledort, L. M. 2004. Comparative thrombotic event incidence after infusion of recombinant factor VIIa versus factor VIII inhibitor bypass activity. J Thromb Haemost, 2, 1700–8.

Almaani, W. S., and Awidi, A. S. 1986. Spontaneous intracranial hemorrhage secondary to von Willebrand's disease. Surg Neurol, 26, 457–60.

al-Samman, M. B., Cuetter, A. C., Guerra, L. G., and Ho, H. 1994. Cerebral arterial thrombosis as a complication of paroxysmal nocturnal hemoglobinuria. *South Med J*, **87**, 765–7.

Anderson, G. L., Limacher, M., Assaf, A. R., *et al.* 2004. Effects of conjugated equine estrogen in postmenopausal women with hysterectomy: the Women's Health Initiative randomized controlled trial. *JAMA*, **291**, 1701–12.

Ansell, J., Hirsh, J., Poller, L., *et al.* 2004. The pharmacology and management of the vitamin K antagonists: the Seventh ACCP Conference on Antithrombotic and Thrombolytic Therapy. *Chest*, **126(3 Suppl)**, 204S–233S.

Appenzeller, S., Zeller, C. B., Annichino-Bizzachi, J. M., *et al.* 2005. Cerebral venous thrombosis: influence of risk factors and imaging findings on prognosis. *Clin Neurol Neurosurg*, **107**, 371–8.

Arai, M., and Sugiura, A. 2004. [Superior sagittal sinus thrombosis as first manifestation of essential thrombocythemia]. *Rinsho Shinkeigaku*, **44**, 34–8.

Aster, R. H. 2005a. Drug-induced immune cytopenias. *Toxicology*, **209**, 149–53.

Aster, R. H. 2005b. Immune thrombocytopenia caused by glycoprotein IIb/IIIa inhibitors. *Chest*, **127(2 Suppl)**, 53S–59S.

Audebert, H. J., Planck, J., Eisenburg, M., Schrezenmeier, H., and Haberl, R. L. 2005. Cerebral ischemic infarction in paroxysmal nocturnal hemoglobinuria report of 2 cases and updated review of 7 previously published patients. *J Neurol*, **252**, 1379–86.

Bagby, G. C., Lipton, J. M., Sloand, E. M., and Schiffer, C. A. 2004. Marrow failure. *Hematology Am Soc Hematol Educ Program*, 318–36.

Baglin, T. P., Keeling, D. M., and Watson, H. G. 2006. Guidelines on oral anticoagulation (warfarin): third edition – 2005 update. *Br J Haematol*, **132**, 277–85.

Barnes, C., and Deveber, G. 2005. Prothrombotic abnormalities in childhood ischaemic stroke. *Thromb Res*, **118**, 67–74.

Bates, S. M., Greer, I. A., Hirsh, J., and Ginsberg, J. S. 2004. Use of antithrombotic agents during pregnancy: the Seventh ACCP Conference on Antithrombotic and Thrombolytic Therapy. *Chest*, **126(3 Suppl)**, 627S–644S.

Bauer, K. A. 2003. Management of thrombophilia. *J Thromb Haemost*, **1**, 1429–34.

Belman, A. L., Roque, C. T., Ancona, R., Anand, A. K., and Davis, R. P. 1990. Cerebral venous thrombosis in a child with iron deficiency anemia and thrombocytosis. *Stroke*, **21**, 488–93.

Blom, J. W., Doggen, C. J., Osanto, S., and Rosendaal, F. R. 2005. Malignancies, prothrombotic mutations, and the risk of venous thrombosis. *JAMA*, **293**, 715–22.

Boncoraglio, G., Carriero, M. R., Chiapparini, L., *et al.* 2004. Hyperhomocysteinemia and other thrombophilic risk factors in 26 patients with cerebral venous thrombosis. *Eur J Neurol*, **11**, 405–9.

Boschetti, C., Fermo, E., Bianchi, P., *et al.* 2004. Clinical and molecular aspects of 23 patients affected by paroxysmal nocturnal hemoglobinuria. *Am J Hematol*, **77**, 36–44.

The British Committee for Standards in Haematology. Investigation and management of heritable thrombophilia. 2001. *Br J Haematol*, **114**, 512–28.

The British Committee for Standards in Haematology. Guidelines for the investigation and management of idiopathic thrombocytopenic purpura in adults, children and in pregnancy. 2003. *Br J Haematol*, **120**, 574–96.

Brown, D. L. 2005. Congenital bleeding disorders. *Curr Probl Pediatr Adolesc Health Care*, **35**, 38–62.

Buchanan, G. R., DeBaun, M. R., Quinn, C. T., and Steinberg, M. H. 2004. Sickle cell disease. *Hematology Am Soc Hematol Educ Program*, 35–47.

Buller, H. R., Agnelli, G., Hull, R. D., *et al.* 2004. Antithrombotic therapy for venous thromboembolic disease: the Seventh ACCP Conference on Antithrombotic and Thrombolytic Therapy. *Chest*, **126(3 Suppl)**, 401S–428S.

Bunn, H. F. 1997. Pathogenesis and treatment of sickle cell disease. *N Engl J Med*, **337**, 762–9.

Campbell, P. J., and Green, A. R. 2005. Management of polycythemia vera and essential thrombocythemia. *Hematology Am Soc Hematol Educ Program*, 201–8.

Campbell, P. J., Scott, L. M., Buck, G., *et al.* 2005. Definition of subtypes of essential thrombocythaemia and relation to polycythaemia vera based on JAK2 V617 F mutation status: a prospective study. *Lancet*, **366**, 1945–53.

Cantu, C., Alonso, E., Jara, A., *et al.* 2004. Hyperhomocysteinemia, low folate and vitamin B12 concentrations, and methylene tetrahydrofolate reductase mutation in cerebral venous thrombosis. *Stroke*, **35**, 1790–4.

The CAPTURE investigators. 1997. Randomised placebo-controlled trial of abciximab before and during coronary intervention in refractory unstable angina: the CAPTURE Study. *Lancet*, **349**, 1429–35.

Casas, J. P., Hingorani, A. D., Bautista, L. E., and Sharma, P. 2004. Meta-analysis of genetic studies in ischemic stroke: thirty-two genes involving approximately 18000 cases and 58000 controls. *Arch Neurol*, **61**, 1652–61.

Chan, A. K., Deveber, G., Monagle, P., Brooker, L. A., and Massicotte, P. M. 2003. Venous thrombosis in children. *J Thromb Haemost*, **1**, 1443–55.

Cines, D. B., Bussel, J. B., McMillan, R. B., and Zehnder, J. L. 2004. Congenital and acquired thrombocytopenia. *Hematology Am Soc Hematol Educ Program*, 390–406.

Cosman, F., Baz-Hecht, M., Cushman, M., *et al.* 2005. Short-term effects of estrogen, tamoxifen and raloxifene on hemostasis: a randomized-controlled study and review of the literature. *Thromb Res*, **116**, 1–13.

Dahlback, B. 2000. Blood coagulation. *Lancet*, **355**, 1627–32.

Dahlback, B. 2005. Blood coagulation and its regulation by anticoagulant pathways: genetic pathogenesis of bleeding and thrombotic diseases. *J Intern Med*, **257**, 209–23.

Dahlback, B., and Villoutreix, B. O. 2005. The anticoagulant protein C pathway. *FEBS Lett*, **579**, 3310–6.

Davoren, A., and Aster, R. H. 2006. Heparin-induced thrombocytopenia and thrombosis. *Am J Hematol*, **81**, 36–44.

Dentali, F., Gianni, M., Crowther, M. A., and Ageno, W. 2006. Natural history of cerebral vein thrombosis: a systematic review. *Blood*, **108**, 1129–34.

Dietrich, A. M., James, C. D., King, D. R., Ginn-Pease, M. E., and Cecalupo, A. J. 1994. Head trauma in children with congenital coagulation disorders. *J Pediatr Surg*, **29**, 28–32.

Diringer, M. N. Skolnick, B. E., Mayer, S. A., *et al.* 2008. Risk of thromboembolic events in controlled trials of rFVIIa in spontaneous intracerebral hemorrhage. *Stroke*, **39**, 850–6.

Egeberg, O. 1965. On the natural blood coagulation inhibitor system. Investigations of inhibitor factors based on antithrombin deficient blood. *Thromb Diath Haemorrh*, **14**, 473–89.

Federici, A. B. 2004. Clinical diagnosis of von Willebrand disease. *Haemophilia*, **10(Suppl 4)**, 169–76.

Fields, M. C., and Levine, S. R. 2005. Thrombophilias and stroke: diagnosis, treatment, and prognosis. *J Thromb Thrombolysis*, **20**, 113–26.

Freiman, J. P. 1990. Fatal quinine-induced thrombocytopenia. *Ann Intern Med*, **112**, 308–9.

Friess, D., Lammle, B., and Alberio, L. 2003. Qualitative platelet defect and thrombohaemorrhagic complications in a patient with polycythaemia vera. Case 10. *Hamostaseologie*, **23**, 138–43.

Gadelha, T., Andre, C., Juca, A. A., and Nucci, M. 2005. Prothrombin 20210 A and oral contraceptive use as risk factors for cerebral venous thrombosis. *Cerebrovasc Dis*, **19**, 49–52.

Ginsberg, J. S., and Bates, S. M. 2003. Management of venous thromboembolism during pregnancy. *J Thromb Haemost*, **1**, 1435–42.

Giordano, N., Amendola, A., Papakostas, P., *et al.* 2005. Immune and autoimmune disorders in HCV chronic liver disease: personal experience and commentary on literature. *New Microbiol*, **28**, 311–7.

Golomb, M. R. 2005. Sickle cell trait is a risk factor for early stroke. *Arch Neurol*, **62**, 1778–9.

Gringeri, A., and Mannucci, P. M. 2005. Italian guidelines for the diagnosis and treatment of patients with haemophilia and inhibitors. *Haemophilia*, **11**, 611–9.

Grundmann, K., Jaschonek, K., Kleine, B., Dichgans, J., and Topka, H. 2003. Aspirin non-responder status in patients with recurrent cerebral ischemic attacks. *J Neurol*, **250**, 63–6.

Gupta, R., Vora, N. A., Horowitz, M. B., *et al.* 2006. Multimodal reperfusion therapy for acute ischemic stroke: factors predicting vessel recanalization. *Stroke*, **37**, 986–90.

Hall, C., Richards, S., and Hillmen, P. 2003. Primary prophylaxis with warfarin prevents thrombosis in paroxysmal nocturnal hemoglobinuria (PNH). *Blood*, **102**, 3587–91.

Hankey, G. J., Eikelboom, J. W., van Bockxmeer, F. M., *et al.* 2001. Inherited thrombophilia in ischemic stroke and its pathogenic subtypes. *Stroke*, **32**, 1793–9.

Hara, H., Virmani, R., Ladich, E., *et al.* 2005. Patent foramen ovale: current pathology, pathophysiology, and clinical status. *J Am Coll Cardiol,* **46**, 1768–76.

Harrison, C. N. 2005. Platelets and thrombosis in myeloproliferative diseases. *Hematology Am Soc Hematol Educ Program,* 409–15.

Hart, R. G., Tonarelli, S. B., and Pearce, L. A. 2005. Avoiding central nervous system bleeding during antithrombotic therapy: recent data and ideas. *Stroke,* **36**, 1588–93.

Hartfield, D. S., Lowry, N. J., Keene, D. L., and Yager, J. Y. 1997. Iron deficiency: a cause of stroke in infants and children. *Pediatr Neurol,* **16**, 50–3.

Hassan, A. A., and Kroll, M. H. 2005. Acquired disorders of platelet function. *Hematology Am Soc Hematol Educ Program,* 403–8.

Haywood, S., Liesner, R., Pindora, S., and Ganesan, V. 2005. Thrombophilia and first arterial ischaemic stroke: a systematic review. *Arch Dis Child,* **90**, 402–5.

Hillmen, P., Lewis, S. M., Bessler, M., Luzzatto, L., and Dacie, J. V. 1995. Natural history of paroxysmal nocturnal hemoglobinuria. *N Engl J Med,* **333**, 1253–8.

Johansen, R. F., Sorensen, B., and Ingerslev, J. 2006. Acquired haemophilia: dynamic whole blood coagulation utilized to guide haemostatic therapy. *Haemophilia,* **12**, 190–7.

Juvela, S., and Kase, C. S. 2006. Advances in intracerebral hemorrhage management. *Stroke,* **37**, 301–4.

Kaplan, C. 2001. Immune thrombocytopenia in the foetus and the newborn: diagnosis and therapy. *Transfus Clin Biol,* **8**, 311–4.

Kaplan, C. 2005. [Fetal/neonatal allo-immune thrombocytopenias: the unsolved questions]. *Transfus Clin Biol,* **12**, 131–4.

Kenet, G., Sadetzki, S., Murad, H., *et al.* 2000. Factor V Leiden and antiphospholipid antibodies are significant risk factors for ischemic stroke in children. *Stroke,* **31**, 1283–8.

Kessler, C. M. 2005. New perspectives in hemophilia treatment. *Hematology Am Soc Hematol Educ Program,* 429–35.

Kizer, J. R., and Devereux, R. B. 2005. Clinical practice. Patent foramen ovale in young adults with unexplained stroke. *N Engl J Med,* **353**, 2361–72.

Koennecke, H. C., and Bernarding, J. 2001. Diffusion-weighted magnetic resonance imaging in two patients with polycythemia rubra vera and early ischemic stroke. *Eur J Neurol,* **8**, 273–7.

Kuo, K. H., and Kovacs, M. J. 2005. Fondaparinux: a potential new therapy for HIT. *Hematology,* **10**, 271–5.

Lalouschek, W., Schillinger, M., Hsieh, K., *et al.* 2005. Matched case-control study on factor V Leiden and the prothrombin G20210 A mutation in patients with ischemic stroke/transient ischemic attack up to the age of 60 years. *Stroke,* **36**, 1405–9.

Lanska, D. J., and Kryscio, R. J. 2000. Risk factors for peripartum and postpartum stroke and intracranial venous thrombosis. *Stroke,* **31**, 1274–82.

Lecumberri, R., Paramo, J. A., and Rocha, E. 2005. Anticoagulant treatment and survival in cancer patients. The evidence from clinical studies. *Haematologica,* **90**, 1258–66.

Lee, A. Y. 2006. Thrombosis and cancer: the role of screening for occult cancer and recognizing the underlying biological mechanisms. *Hematology Am Soc Hematol Educ Program,* 438–43.

Lee, J. H., Kim, S. W., and Sung Kim, J. 2000. Sagittal sinus thrombosis associated with transient free protein S deficiency after L-asparaginase treatment: case report and review of the literature. *Clin Neurol Neurosurg,* **102**, 33–6.

Leone, G., Sica, S., Chiusolo, P., Teofili, L., and De Stefano, V. 2001. Blood cells diseases and thrombosis. *Haematologica,* **86**, 1236–44.

Levi, M. 2005. Platelets. *Crit Care Med,* **33**, S523–S525.

Levine, S. R. 2005. Hypercoagulable states and stroke: a selective review. *CNS Spectr,* **10**, 567–78.

Lichy, C., Dong-Si, T., Reuner, K., *et al.* 2006. Risk of cerebral venous thrombosis and novel gene polymorphisms of the coagulation and fibrinolytic systems. *J Neurol,* **253**, 316–20.

Manno, C. S. 2005. Management of bleeding disorders in children. *Hematology Am Soc Hematol Educ Program,* 416–22.

Mannucci, P. M., Duga, S., and Peyvandi, F. 2004. Recessively inherited coagulation disorders. *Blood,* **104**, 1243–52.

Martinelli, I., Battaglioli, T., Pedotti, P., Cattaneo, M., and Mannucci, P. M. 2003. Hyperhomocysteinemia in cerebral vein thrombosis. *Blood,* **102**, 1363–6.

Martinowitz, U., and Michaelson, M. 2005. Guidelines for the use of recombinant activated factor VII (rFVIIa) in uncontrolled bleeding: a report by the Israeli Multidisciplinary rFVIIa Task Force. *J Thromb Haemost,* **3**, 640–8.

Masuhr, F., Mehraein, S., and Einhaupl, K. 2004. Cerebral venous and sinus thrombosis. *J Neurol,* **251**, 11–23.

Mayer, S. A., Brun, N. C., Begtrup, K., *et al.* 2008. Efficacy and safety of recombinant activated factor VII for acute intracerebral hemorrhage. *N Engl J Med,* **358**, 2127–37.

Mayer, S. A., and Rincon, F. 2006. Ultra-early hemostatic therapy for acute intracerebral hemorrhage. *Semin Hematol,* **43**, S70–6.

Meena, A. K., Naidu, K. S., and Murthy, J. M. 2000. Cortical sinovenous thrombosis in a child with nephrotic syndrome and iron deficiency anaemia. *Neurol India,* **48**, 292–4.

Menajovsky, L. B. 2005. Heparin-induced thrombocytopenia: clinical manifestations and management strategies. *Am J Med,* **118**, 21S–30S.

Miguez-Burbano, M. J., Jackson, J. Jr., and Hadrigan, S. 2005. Thrombocytopenia in HIV disease: clinical relevance, physiopathology and management. *Curr Med Chem Cardiovasc Hematol Agents,* **3**, 365–76.

Miller, S. T., Macklin, E. A., Pegelow, C. H., *et al.* 2001. Silent infarction as a risk factor for overt stroke in children with sickle cell anemia: a report from the Cooperative Study of Sickle Cell Disease. *J Pediatr,* **139**, 385–90.

Mohri, H., Yamazaki, E., Suzuki, Z., *et al.* 1997. Autoantibody selectively inhibits binding of von Willebrand factor to glycoprotein ib. Recognition site is located in the A1 loop of von Willebrand factor. *Thromb Haemost,* **77**, 760–6.

Muller, G. 1992. [Acquired antithrombin III deficiency]. *Z Gesamte Inn Med,* **47**, 74–7.

The National Institute of Neurological Disorders and Stroke rt-PA Stroke Study Group. 1995. Tissue plasminogen activator for acute ischemic stroke. *N Engl J Med,* **333**, 1581–7.

The National Institute of Neurological Disorders t-PA Stroke Study Group. 1997. Intracerebral hemorrhage after intravenous t-PA therapy for ischemic stroke. *Stroke,* **28**, 2109–18.

O'Connell, K. A., Wood, J. J., Wise, R. P., Lozier, J. N., and Braun, M. M. 2006. Thromboembolic adverse events after use of recombinant human coagulation factor VIIa. *JAMA,* **295**, 293–8.

Patrono, C. 2003. Aspirin resistance: definition, mechanisms and clinical readouts. *J Thromb Haemost,* **1**, 1710–3.

Petrides, P. E., and Siegel, F. 2006. Thrombotic complications in essential thrombocythemia (ET): clinical facts and biochemical riddles. *Blood Cells Mol Dis,* **36**, 379–84.

Pezzini, A., Del Zotto, E., Magoni, M., *et al.* 2003. Inherited thrombophilic disorders in young adults with ischemic stroke and patent foramen ovale. *Stroke,* **34**, 28–33.

Pohl, C., Harbrecht, U., Greinacher, A., *et al.* 2000. Neurologic complications in immune-mediated heparin-induced thrombocytopenia. *Neurology,* **54**, 1240–5.

Powars, D. R. 2000. Management of cerebral vasculopathy in children with sickle cell anaemia. *Br J Haematol,* **108**, 666–78.

Ries, M., Wolfel, D., and Maier-Brandt, B. 1995. Severe intracranial hemorrhage in a newborn infant with transplacental transfer of an acquired factor VII: C inhibitor. *J Pediatr,* **127**, 649–50.

Robetorye, R. S., and Rodgers, G. M. 2001. Update on selected inherited venous thrombotic disorders. *Am J Hematol,* **68**, 256–68.

Rosand, J., Eckman, M. H., Knudsen, K. A., Singer, D. E., and Greenberg, S. M. 2004. The effect of warfarin and intensity of anticoagulation on outcome of intracerebral hemorrhage. *Arch Intern Med,* **164**, 880–4.

Rosendaal, F. R. 2005. Venous thrombosis: the role of genes, environment, and behavior. *Hematology Am Soc Hematol Educ Program,* 1–12.

Rosse, W. F., Hillmen, P., and Schreiber, A. D. 2004. Immune-mediated hemolytic anemia. *Hematology Am Soc Hematol Educ Program,* 48–62.

Rossouw, J. E., Anderson, G. L., Prentice, R. L., *et al.* 2002. Risks and benefits of estrogen plus progestin in healthy postmenopausal women: principal results from the Women's Health Initiative randomized controlled trial. *JAMA,* **288**, 321–33.

Sacco, R. L., Adams, R., Albers, G., *et al.* 2006. Guidelines for prevention of stroke in patients with ischemic stroke or transient ischemic attack: a statement for healthcare professionals from the American Heart Association/American

Stroke Association Council on Stroke: co-sponsored by the Council on Cardiovascular Radiology and Intervention: the American Academy of Neurology affirms the value of this guideline. *Stroke*, **37**, 577–617.

Schafer, A. I. 2006. Molecular basis of the diagnosis and treatment of polycythemia vera and essential thrombocythemia. *Blood*, **107**, 4214–22.

Schror, K., Weber, A. A., and Hohlfeld, T. 2006. Aspirin "resistance." *Blood Cells Mol Dis*, **36**, 171–6.

Sebire, G., Tabarki, B., Saunders, D. E., *et al.* 2005. Cerebral venous sinus thrombosis in children: risk factors, presentation, diagnosis and outcome. *Brain*, **128(Pt 3)**, 477–89.

Shavit, L., and Grenader, T. 2005. Delayed diagnosis of HIV-associated thrombocytopenia in a man of 70. *J R Soc Med*, **98**, 515.

Siddiqi, F. A., Tepler, J., and Fantini, G. A. 1997. Acquired protein S and antithrombin III deficiency caused by nephrotic syndrome: an unusual cause of graft thrombosis. *J Vasc Surg*, **25**, 576–80.

Socie, G., Mary, J. Y., de Gramont, A., *et al.* 1996. Paroxysmal nocturnal haemoglobinuria: long-term follow-up and prognostic factors. French Society of Haematology. *Lancet*, **348**, 573–7.

Steiner, T., Rosand, J., and Diringer, M. 2006. Intracerebral hemorrhage associated with oral anticoagulant therapy: current practices and unresolved questions. *Stroke*, **37**, 256–62.

Sumner, M., and Williams, J. 2004. Type 3 von Willebrand disease: assessment of complications and approaches to treatment – results of a patient and Hemophilia Treatment Center Survey in the United States. *Haemophilia*, **10**, 360–6.

Szczeklik, A., Musial, J., Undas, A., and Sanak, M. 2005. Aspirin resistance. *J Thromb Haemost*, **3**, 1655–62.

Tefferi, A. 2006. Classification, diagnosis and management of myeloproliferative disorders in the JAK2V617F era. *Hematology Am Soc Hematol Educ Program*, 240–5.

Toole, J. F., Malinow, M. R., Chambless, L. E., *et al.* 2004. Lowering homocysteine in patients with ischemic stroke to prevent recurrent stroke, myocardial infarction, and death: the Vitamin Intervention for Stroke Prevention (VISP) randomized controlled trial. *JAMA*, **291**, 565–75.

Tosetto, A., Rodeghiero, F., Castaman, G., *et al.* 2006. A quantitative analysis of bleeding symptoms in type 1 von Willebrand disease: results from a multicenter European study (MCMDM-1 VWD). *J Thromb Haemost*, **4**, 766–73.

Tripodi, A., Valsecchi, C., Chantarangkul, V., Battaglioli, T., and Mannucci, P. M. 2003. Standardization of activated protein C resistance testing: effect of residual platelets in frozen plasmas assessed by commercial and homemade methods. *Br J Haematol*, **120**, 825–8.

Trouillas, P., and von Kummer, R. 2006. Classification and pathogenesis of cerebral hemorrhages after thrombolysis in ischemic stroke. *Stroke*, **37**, 556–61.

Vahdat, B., Canavy, I., Fourcade, L., *et al.* 2000. Fatal cerebral hemorrhage and severe thrombocytopenia during abciximab treatment. *Catheter Cardiovasc Interv*, **49**, 177–80.

Velat, G. J., Burry, M. V., Eskioglu, E., *et al.* 2006. The use of abciximab in the treatment of acute cerebral thromboembolic events during neuroendovascular procedures. *Surg Neurol*, **65**, 352–8.

Ventura, P., Cobelli, M., Marietta, M., *et al.* 2004. Hyperhomocysteinemia and other newly recognized inherited coagulation disorders (factor V Leiden and prothrombin gene mutation) in patients with idiopathic cerebral vein thrombosis. *Cerebrovasc Dis*, **17**, 153–9.

Viscoli, C. M., Brass, L. M., Kernan, W. N., *et al.* 2001. A clinical trial of estrogen-replacement therapy after ischemic stroke. *N Engl J Med*, **345**, 1243–9.

von Stuckrad-Barre, S., Berkefeld, J., Steckel, D., and Sitzer, M. 2003. Cerebral arterial thrombosis in paroxysmal nocturnal hemoglobinuria. *J Neurol*, **250**, 756–7.

Warkentin, T. E., and Bernstein, R. A. 2003. Delayed-onset heparin-induced thrombocytopenia and cerebral thrombosis after a single administration of unfractionated heparin. *N Engl J Med*, **348**, 1067–9.

Warkentin, T. E., and Greinacher, A. 2004. Heparin-induced thrombocytopenia: recognition, treatment, and prevention: the Seventh ACCP Conference on Antithrombotic and Thrombolytic Therapy. *Chest*, **126(3 Suppl)**, 311S–337S.

Weber, A. A., Przytulski, B., Schanz, A., Hohlfeld, T., and Schror, K. 2002. Towards a definition of aspirin resistance: a typological approach. *Platelets*, **13**, 37–40.

Williamson, L. M., Hackett, G., Rennie, J., *et al.* 1998. The natural history of feto-maternal alloimmunization to the platelet-specific antigen HPA-1a (PlA1, Zwa) as determined by antenatal screening. *Blood*, **92**, 2280–7.

Zandman-Goddard, G., and Shoenfeld, Y. 2002. HIV and autoimmunity. *Autoimmun Rev*, **1**, 329–37.

41

THROMBOTIC THROMBOCYTOPENIC PURPURA

Jorge Moncayo-Gaete

Introduction

Eighty years ago, Eli Moschkowitz first described thrombotic thrombocytopenic purpura (TTP) in a teenage girl who acutely developed fever, severe hemolytic anemia, thrombocytopenia, albuminuria, left-sided paralysis, and cardiac failure. She became comatose and died 2 weeks after onset of symptoms. The postmortem examination revealed widespread hyaline thrombi in the terminal arterioles of most organs, especially in those of the heart and kidneys (Moschkowitz, 1924). Singer et al. (1947) introduced the term "thrombotic thrombocytopenic purpura" to highlight the condition's principal histological lesion.

Since the initial description of this uncommon multisystem disorder, its pathogenesis has remained elusive. In the last two decades, however, important refinements in elucidating the pathophysiological basis of TTP have emerged. Considerable evidence now implicates the metabolic pathway of von Willebrand factor (vWF), particularly of its cleaving protease, as the key component in TTP pathogenesis.

Epidemiology

Historically, TTP has been considered an uncommon disorder. In fact, in a U.S. mortality data study conducted over a period of 30 years, the estimated annual incidence was 1.027 cases per million inhabitants (Petitt, 1980).

Several clinical variants of TTP, such as the hereditary form, however, may have been largely underestimated or misdiagnosed. In the last few years, the annual incidence of TTP has risen, with current estimates ranging from 3.8 to 6.5 cases per million (Miller et al., 2004; Terrel et al., 2005; Torok et al., 1995). The reasons for this apparent increase are uncertain, but may be related – at least in part – to an increasing awareness of the disease, less stringent diagnostic criteria, an increase in drug-induced and HIV-related events, or a true increase in incidence of idiopathic cases. Additionally, annual TTP incidence associated with severe ADAMTS-13 (von Willebrand cleaving protease) deficiency has recently been estimated to be 1.7 cases per million (Terrel et al., 2005).

TTP affects females more often than males, with a sex ratio of 3:1, and, based on the results of several recent studies, it may predominate in people of Afro-Caribbean origin (Coppo et al., 2004; Peyvandi et al., 2004; Sadler et al., 2004; Terrel et al., 2005; Zheng et al., 2004). It has been reported in all age groups, although onset usually occurs between the ages of 20 and 40 years (Gurkan et al., 2005; Kennedy et al., 1980; MacWhinney et al., 1962;

Peyvandi et al., 2004; Piastra et al., 2001; Sadler et al., 2004). Half of patients with familial TTP (Schulman-Upshaw syndrome) experience their first episode during childhood – some even very soon after birth – whereas the remainder are afflicted in adulthood, often as the result of infection, pregnancy, or some other triggering factor (Lämmle et al., 2005).

Pathophysiology

In the early 1980s, several lines of solid evidence found vWF to play a crucial role in TTP pathogenesis. First, extremely large vWF multimers were observed in plasma of patients with relapsing TTP. Later on, thrombi in the terminal arterioles and capillaries of distal organs involved in TTP were found to be composed mainly of vWF and degranulated platelets and nearly no fibrin (Asada et al., 1985; Moake et al., 1982).

Under physiological conditions, endothelial cells and megakaryocytes synthesize and secrete vWF multimers (approximately 20 000 kd in size). Under conditions of extreme shear stress, vWF mediates the initial adhesive link between platelets and the subendothelium of the damaged vessel walls (Kroll et al., 1996; Ruggeri et al., 1999). Immediately after its release in the circulation as highly adhesive, ultralarge multimers, vWF undergoes cleavage into two inactive fragments of 176 and 140 kd by a metal-containing proteolytic enzyme – metalloprotease (Sadler, 1998; Tsai, 2002). This metalloprotease cleaves the peptide bond between tyrosine at position 842 and methionine at position 843 within the central A2 domain of the mature vWF (Tsai, 1996). This protease was identified as the 13th member of the ADAMTS family of metalloproteases (ADAMTS-13 – a disentegrin and metalloprotease with thrombospondin type 1 motif) (Fujikawa et al., 2001; Zheng et al., 2001). Recently, ADAMTS-13 has been found to be deficient in the plasma of patients with acute TTP and those with chronic relapsing TTP (Furlan et al., 1997, 1998; Tsai and Lian, 1998). Thus, in TTP there is a failure of proteolysis of hyperadhesive and ultralarge vWF multimers, which then induces the adhesion and subsequent aggregation of platelets under high-flow, high-shear conditions that lead to platelet clumping with ensuing microvascular thrombosis in arterioles and capillaries, but not in venules (Kwaan, 1987; Moake, 2002; Tsai, 2002, 2003).

The underlying pathological mechanism of TTP is the presence of microvascular thrombi that partially occlude the vascular lumins with overlying proliferative endothelial cells. Widespread thrombi in microvessels results in ischemia that may involve any

Uncommon Causes of Stroke, 2nd edition, ed. Louis R. Caplan. Published by Cambridge University Press. © Cambridge University Press 2008.

Table 41.1 Characteristics of secondary TTP

Onset	Variable (very early or delayed, it depends on associated disorder)
Renal dysfunction	Variable (mild to renal failure)
CNS dysfunction	Prominent with ticlopidine
Pyrexia	Uncommon
Acute respiratory distress syndrome	Occasional
Peripheral digit ischemic syndrome	Occasional
Thrombocytopenia	Present
Hemolysis	Present
Schistocytosis	Mild
Prognosis	Variable (poor to high survival rates)
Relapse	Uncommon

CNS = central nervous system.

Table 41.2 Main clinical and hematological findings in TTP

Clinical findings	Prevalence % (range)
Thrombocytopenia	95–100
Microangiopathic hemolytic anemia	96–100
Neurological symptoms	72–92
Headache	39–60
Confusion	20–35
Focal deficits	22–30
Seizure	9
Renal impairment	10–70
Acute renal failure	5
Nausea, vomiting, diarrhea, abdominal pain	40–50
Generalized malaise	20
Fever	24–59
Hemorrhagic cutaneous lesions	20–30

organ, though it is most common in the brain, kidneys, pancreas, spleen, heart, and adrenal glands (Müller *et al.*, 2001).

Two types of TTP have been recognized: the autoimmune type caused by antibodies that inhibit ADAMTS-13 protease and the hereditary form caused by genetic mutations of ADAMTS-13. Most TTP cases in adults occur without a clear underlying cause or disease and are associated with either severe (<5% of activity in normal plasma) or moderate deficiency of vWF cleaving-protease activity, often due to the presence of ADAMTS-13-neutralizing immunoglobulin IgG or IgM antibodies (Furlan *et al.*, 1998; Rieger *et al.*, 2005; Tsai and Lian, 1998). Infectious agents, inflammation, drugs, or genetic factors may trigger or influence the production of these autoantibodies (Studt *et al.*, 2004). Secondary TTP may occur in association with drugs, pregnancy, organ transplantation, infections, autoimmune diseases, and cancer (Table 41.1).

The hereditary form of TTP (also called the Schulman-Upshaw syndrome) is extremely unusual. It is characterized by a constitutional ADAMTS-13 deficiency because of homozygous or compound heterozygous mutations of the ADAMTS-13 gene located at chromosome 9q34 (Assink *et al.*, 2003; Kokame and Miyata, 2004; Levy *et al.*, 2001; Tsai, 2003; Veyradier *et al.*, 2004). To date, more than 70 mutations of the ADAMTS-13 gene have been reported. The inheritance pattern is usually autosomal recessive. However, a complete deficiency of ADAMTS-13 is not sufficient to cause the clinical TTP syndrome, because patients with congenitally absent ADAMTS-13 activity may not have clinical symptoms until their 40s, suggesting that other cofactors may be needed to trigger onset (Furlan and Lämmle, 2001).

Clinical findings

TTP can manifest as one of the following three types: single episode with complete recovery and no recurrence; intermittent with infrequent relapses and normal hematology between attacks;

and chronic relapsing with persistent abnormalities (Moake and McPherson, 1989). The chronic and intermittent forms predominate in childhood (Piastra *et al.*, 2001).

Classically, TTP has been recognized by the pentad of microangiopathic hemolytic anemia, thrombocytopenia, neurological symptoms, fever, and renal involvement, though only 20%–40% of patients will manifest the classic pentad (Amorosi and Ultmann, 1966; Gurkan *et al.*, 2005; Meloni *et al.*, 2001). The usual presentation of TTP is quite diverse, making the initial diagnosis particularly difficult (Table 41.2). A triad consisting of microangiopathic hemolytic anemia, thrombocytopenia, and neurological symptoms is often seen in the early stages of the condition and currently constitutes the essential criteria for timely TTP diagnosis (Amorosi and Ultmann, 1966; Bukowski *et al.*, 1977; Ridolfi and Bell, 1981). Oligosymptomatic forms of presentation may also occur (Gurkan *et al.*, 2005).

Neurological involvement is a cornerstone of TTP diagnosis. Though one-third of all patients do not show neurological symptoms at onset, nearly all have neurological impairment during the course of the disease (Meloni *et al.*, 2001; Petz 1977; Peyvandi *et al.*, 2004; Ruggenenti and Remuzzi, 1996; Sadler *et al.*, 2004). Neurological involvement may be noticeable as a broad spectrum of generalized or focal neurological symptoms and signs, including headache, dizziness, abnormal behavior, and decreased level of consciousness, up to and including coma (Castellá *et al.*, 2004; Gurkan *et al.*, 2005; Kelly *et al.*, 1999; Park *et al.*, 2005; Peyvandi *et al.*, 2004; Soltes *et al.*, 2004; Veyradier *et al.*, 2004). Focal or generalized seizures have been reported mainly in the terminal phase of the illness, whereas convulsive and nonconvulsive status epilepticus are less common findings (Beydoun *et al.*, 2004; Blum and Drislane, 1996; Garrett *et al.*, 1996; Horton *et al.*, 2003; Kennedy *et al.*, 1980; Meloni *et al.*, 2001; Ridolfi and Bell, 1981; Silverstein, 1968).

TTP clinical manifestations may also include cortical blindness, homonymous hemianopsia, aphasia, dysarthria, bilateral ptosis, cranial nerve palsies, gaze-evoked nystagmus, ataxia, or paresis (Bornstein *et al.*, 1960; Bridgman and Witting, 1996; Castellá *et al.*,

2004; Kelly *et al.*, 1999; Park *et al.*, 2005; Petz, 1977; Meloni *et al.*, 2001; Rinkel and Wijdicks, 1991; Soltes *et al.*, 2004). Focal cerebral manifestations are often fluctuating or evanescent, suggesting in some instances transient ischemic attacks (TIAs), although permanent residual deficits have been reported even with small infarcts (Ben-Yehuda *et al.*, 1998; Kwaan and Boggio, 2005; Park *et al.*, 2005).

Thrombosis mainly affects the microvessels of gray or white matter, and cortical or small subcortical infarcts are found, as a result. Occasionally, large-vessel involvement may also occur, resulting from branch occlusion of the middle cerebral arteries (MCAs) or posterior cerebral arteries (PCAs) or, more rarely, of the entire MCA territory (Bakshi *et al.*, 1999; Kelly *et al.*, 1998; Rinkel and Wijdicks, 1991; Scheid *et al.*, 2004). Ischemia may be restricted to the brainstem or cerebellum, albeit very uncommonly (Bakshi *et al.*, 1999). Intracranial supratentorial or brainstem hemorrhages are both very rare forms of TTP presentation (Horton *et al.*, 2003; Piastra *et al.*, 2001).

Renal impairment is less frequent and severe than neurological involvement (Chang and Ikhlaque, 2004; George, 2000; Peyvandi *et al.*, 2004; Ridolfi and Bell, 1981; Rock *et al.*, 1998; Veyradier and Meyer, 2005). It may be present as gross hematuria or, less often, as oligoanuria or acute renal failure. Although rather uncommon, kidney-associated hypertension may also be present and is usually severe and refractory to standard measures (Remuzzi *et al.*, 1996).

Hemorrhagic cutaneous lesions (purpura, petechiae, and ecchymosis) are seen in one-third of patients. Retinal hemorrhages, epistaxis, and gingival, gastrointestinal, or vaginal bleeding may also occur, though overt bleeding is not typical (Castellá *et al.*, 2004; Gurkan *et al.*, 2005; Horton *et al.*, 2003).

Fever is usually low grade (Gurkan *et al.*, 2005; Rock *et al.*, 1998; Shepard *et al.*, 1991). Generalized malaise, fatigue, arthralgias, jaundice, abdominal pain, and a flu-like illness may also be present and may precede the main TTP clinical findings by several weeks (Amorosi and Ultmann, 1966; Ridolfi and Bell, 1981). Acute abdominal, pancreatic, and peripheral digit ischemic syndrome are atypical forms of TTP presentation (Bell *et al.*, 1990; Chang and Ikhlaque, 2004; Elias *et al.*, 1985; Muniz and Barbee, 2003). Acute respiratory distress, cardiac arrhythmias, and sudden death are very rare events in TTP (Kwaan and Boggio, 2005; Ridolfi and Bell, 1981).

Diagnosis

TTP is a clinical diagnosis with no pathognomonic laboratory test findings. Coombs-negative hemolytic anemia and severe thrombocytopenia owing to platelet clumping in the microcirculation are the most outstanding laboratory abnormalities. Platelet counts often drop to <20 000/mm^3 or even <10 000/mm^3 (Amorosi and Ultmann, 1966; Bukowski, 1982; Peyvandi *et al.*, 2004; Ridolfi and Bell, 1981; Rock *et al.*, 1998). Recently, the severity of thrombocytopenia was correlated with levels of ADAMTS-13 activity (Veyradier *et al.*, 2001).

Highly suggestive of TTP, but not pathognomonic, is red-blood-cell fragmentation on peripheral blood smear as a consequence of mechanical damage sustained when schistocytes attempt to traverse turbulent areas of the microcirculation that have been partially occluded by platelet clumps. The presence of schistocytes in pediatric patients is less prevalent than in adults; other red-cell abnormalities (anisocytes and poikilocytes) may also be found (Horton *et al.*, 2003). Reticulocyte count and indirect bilirubin level are high, whereas haptoglobin levels are low (Ruggenenti *et al.*, 2001). Coagulation tests and disseminated intravascular coagulation panel (fibrinogen, D-dimer) are usually normal (Rock, 2000; Rock *et al.*, 1998). At presentation, extremely high lactate dehydrogenase (LDH) serum levels are commonly found, resulting from ischemic or necrotic tissue leakage rather than intravascular red cell destruction (Brailey *et al.*, 1999; Ruggenenti *et al.*, 2001). Thrombocytopenia may precede schistocytosis and LDH elevation by several days.

Prompt diagnosis of TTP is crucial; therefore, it should be suspected on finding thrombocytopenia, schistocytosis, and significant elevations in LDH serum levels, without any other clinically apparent cause (Moake, 2002).

In approximately one-half of TTP patients, creatinine and blood urea nitrogen levels may be slightly elevated. Proteinuria, hemoglobinuria, and microscopic hematuria may also be observed (Peyvandi *et al.*, 2004; Rock *et al.*, 1998). Bone marrow or gingival biopsy may reveal diagnostic lesions (hyaline thrombi) in half of TTP cases, as well (Kennedy *et al.*, 1980; Kwaan, 1987).

The differential diagnosis between TTP and hemolytic uremic syndrome (HUS), both of which are thrombotic microangiopathic disorders, is often difficult because clinical and pathological findings may overlap. Severe renal dysfunction is not common in TTP, but is always found in HUS. The latter mainly occurs in children, manifesting as a single episode subsequent to a severe bloody diarrhea most often from enterohemorrhagic strains of *Escherichia coli* or *Shigella dysenteriae* that produce a Shiga toxin (Mead and Griffin, 1998; Ray and Liu, 2001). As in TTP, extrarenal manifestations can also occur in HUS.

One-fourth of all TTP patients show normal ADAMTS-13 activity levels (Bianchi *et al.*, 2002; Peyvandi *et al.*, 2004). When severe ADAMTS-13 deficiency (<5% of normal sensitivity threshold) is found, it is most often due to the presence of ADAMTS-13 neutralizing antibodies and will usually confirm an acquired TTP diagnosis (Tsai, 2003; Zheng *et al.*, 2004). In hereditary cases, however, the absence of ADAMTS-13 activity is not because of autoantibodies. Because of technical complexities, assay of the presence of ADAMTS-13 inhibitors and of ADAMTS-13 activity in plasma is not yet widely available in clinical practice (Veyradier and Meyer, 2005).

The correlation between the clinical course and ADAMTS-13 levels is not consistent. Long-lasting stable hematological remissions have been observed despite persistent undetectable ADAMTS-13 activity (Dong *et al.*, 2003).

Cerebral edema and infarction are the most common neuroimaging abnormalities observed during acute TTP. MRI is more sensitive than CT in revealing acute brain lesions, with figures around 80% and 50%, respectively (Bakshi *et al.*, 1999; Kay *et al.*, 1991). Abnormal brain CT and MRI may reveal multiple hypodense areas or multiple foci of high intensity in T2-weighted images, respectively (D'Aprile *et al.*, 1994; Tardy *et al.*, 1993). These lesions correspond to areas of cerebral edema, which predominantly affect white matter and, to a lesser extent, gray matter. When the occipito and/or parietal lobes are involved, radiological findings have an appearance similar to reversible posterior leukoencephalopathy (RPLS). In the TTP setting, RPLS-like findings may occur with or without hypertension and renal failure (Bakshi *et al.*, 1999; Hawley *et al.*, 2004). A noncontrast brain MRI may reveal increased signal intensity on both fluid-attenuated inversion recovery and T2-weighted images, whereas the signal is usually isointense on diffusion-weighted imaging and normal or increased in apparent diffusion coefficient map (Soltes *et al.*, 2004). Edema resolution usually occurs very soon after therapy is initiated; consequently, MRI may be normal during the convalescence phase (Bakshi *et al.*, 1999; Fiorani *et al.*, 1995; Soltes *et al.*, 2004). Large and small infarctions may also be found in neuroimaging studies, whether cerebral edema is present or not. Less often, petechial hemorrhages and supratentorial or brainstem hematomas are observed (Bakshi *et al.*, 1999; Meloni *et al.*, 2001; Piastra *et al.*, 2001). Electroencephalogram (EEG) is usually normal, even in TTP patients with evident neurological involvement. Less often, paroxysmal patterns may also be observed (Meloni *et al.*, 2001).

Treatment

TTP remains a life-threatening disease the mortality rate of which may be as high as 90% when untreated. Once TTP is suspected, therapy should be initiated as soon as possible. Fresh whole blood exchange, the first beneficial therapeutic intervention for TTP, reduced mortality rate to 50% (Rubinstein *et al.*, 1959). Subsequently, plasma exchange (PE) showed greater efficacy by reducing the mortality rate to 20% (Amorosi and Ultmann 1966; Bukowski *et al.*, 1977).

Since its widespread introduction in 1991, the first line of treatment in adults or older children with acute idiopathic acquired TTP continues to be PE. This procedure restores ADAMTS-13-deficient plasma and removes the pathogenic inhibitory antibodies and large vWF multimers (Cataland and Wu, 2005). The standard replacement fluid is usually fresh frozen plasma (FFP), although cryosupernatant plasma (CSP) and solvent-detergent-treated plasma – both lacking in the largest vWF multimers present in FFP – may be as efficacious as FFP (Brailey *et al.*, 1999).

The PE success rate in patients with acquired TTP has been estimated at approximately 90% (Bell *et al.*, 1991; Rock *et al.*, 1991). Lower titers of ADAMTS-13 autoantibodies have been associated with a better response to PE (Zheng *et al.*, 2004). Nevertheless, the optimal PE treatment schedule and the therapeutic targets continue to be a matter of debate. Early on, treatment is usually performed daily, and response is highly variable (Rock, 2000). Neurological symptoms and LDH serum levels will generally resolve soon after PE is initiated, whereas thrombocytopenia and anemia improve gradually (George, 2000). Clinical remission – an increase in platelet count $> 100–150 \times 10^9$/L and a drop in LDH levels for 2 or 3 days – is attained between 7 and 30 days after PE. Seventy-five percent of patients achieve remission by day 14 (Coppo *et al.*, 2003; Rock *et al.*, 1991; Willis and Bandarenko, 2005).

Incomplete response to daily PE or refractory TTP (lack of response within the first 7 days) may occur in 10%–20% of cases (Allford *et al.*, 2003). Delay in PE commencement is correlated with treatment failure, and lack of response to PE has been associated with either the secondary form of acquired TTP or high titers of ADAMTS-13 antibodies (Tsai, 2000). Corticosteroids have been used as an adjunct therapy to PE and in instances where PE has not been successful, but their role in TTP treatment remains to be properly established (Cataland and Wu, 2005; Gurkan *et al.*, 2005).

One-third of patients may relapse after 30 days of complete remission and discontinuation of PE (Bandarenko *et al.*, 1998; Onundarson *et al.*, 1992). ADAMTS-13 inhibitors may persist for a variable time – from months to years. When these inhibitors are found in high titers, relapses are more frequent (Sadler *et al.*, 2004; Zheng *et al.*, 2004). Relapses infrequently occur as acute strokes (Downes *et al.*, 2004).

In case reports and in smaller cohorts of patients, vincristine, rituximab, cyclosporine A, intravenous IgG, and splenectomy have proven to be successful in the treatment of refractory or relapsing TTP (Cataland and Wu, 2005; Rock, 2005). As with corticosteroids, controlled trials are needed to define the place of these adjunct therapies in relapsing TTP treatment.

Antiplatelet agents (aspirin or dipyridamole) are often added to PE, but hemorrhagic complications have been a main concern (Rock, 2000; Rock *et al.*, 1991). Aspirin (75 mg/day) may be used when the platelet count is $> 50 \times 10^9$/L (Allford *et al.*, 2003). Reluctance to use antiplatelet agents has also grown due to reported cases of TTP secondary to thienopyridine (ticlopidine and clopidogrel) use (Bennett *et al.*, 1998; Zakarija *et al.*, 2004).

Infusion of FFP, CSP, or solvent-detergent-treated plasma containing active ADAMTS-13 is sufficient for treatment of familial TTP patients. To avoid recurring episodes, the infusion should be repeated every 2 or 3 weeks (Furlan and Lämmle, 2001; Moake, 2002; Sadler *et al.*, 2004).

Prognosis

Prognosis for TTP patients has changed radically since the introduction of PE as standard therapy. However, the mortality rate for some subgroups remains unaffected, as in the case of patients with secondary TTP (mainly associated with bone marrow transplantation, cancer chemotherapy, or drugs), in whom mortality rates range from 86% to 100%, despite PE (Vesely *et al.*, 2003).

Normal neuroimaging studies or MRI demonstration of RPLS-like lesions may be associated with a favorable neurological outcome, whereas infarctions or hemorrhages may portend an unfavorable prognosis (Kay *et al.*, 1991). Most TTP patients with CNS involvement undergo minimal disability or have no long-term sequela (Kelly *et al.*, 1999; Meloni *et al.*, 2001).

Conclusion

TTP is a multisystem disorder that is being increasingly recognized. It may be described as a prothrombotic state in the microvasculature due to a perturbed metabolic pathway of vWF and its cleaving protease. Timely diagnosis and prompt initiation of therapy are essential for TTP patients. Diagnosis is mainly based on hematological findings and a broad variety of neurological abnormalities, including ischemic or, less often, hemorrhagic stroke. PE is currently the mainstay of treatment; however, rapid advances in the understanding of TTP pathophysiology may offer more specific and effective therapies in the near future.

REFERENCES

Allford, S. L., Hunt, B. J., Rose, P, and Machin, S. J. 2003. Guidelines on the diagnosis and management of the thrombotic microangiopathic haemolytic anaemias. *Br J Haematol*, **120**, 556–73.

Amorosi, E. L., and Ultmann, J. E. 1966. Thrombotic thrombocytopenic purpura: report of 16 cases and review of the literature. *Medicine (Baltimore)*, **45**, 139–59.

Asada, Y., Sumiyoshi, A., Hayashi, T., Suzumiya, J., and Kaketani, K. 1985. Immunohistochemistry of vascular lesion in thrombotic thrombocytopenic purpura, with special reference to factor VIII related antigen. *Thromb Res*, **8**, 469–79.

Assink, K., Schiphorst, R., Allford, S., *et al.* 2003. Mutations analysis and clinical implications of von Willebrand factor-cleaving protease deficiency. *Kidney Int*, **63**, 1995–9.

Bakshi, R., Shaikh, Z. A., Bates, V. E., and Kinkel, P. R. 1999. Thrombotic thrombocytopenic purpura: brain CT and MRI findings in 12 patients. *Neurology*, **52**, 1285–8.

Bandarenko, N., Brecher, M. E., and United States Thrombotic Thrombocytopenic Apheresis Study Group. 1998. Multicenter survey and retrospective analysis of current efficacy of therapeutic plasma exchange. *J Clin Apher*, **13**, 133–41.

Bell, M. D., Barnhart, J. S., and Martin, J. M. 1990. Thrombotic thrombocytopenic purpura causing sudden unexpected death – a series of 8 patients. *Am J Forensic Sci*, **35**, 601–13.

Bell, W. R., Braine, H. G., Ness, P. M., and Kickler, T. S. 1991. Improved survival in thrombotic thrombocytopenic purpura-hemolytic uremic syndrome: clinical experience in 108 patients. *N Engl J Med*, **325**, 398–403.

Bennett, C. L., Weinberg, P. D., Rozenberg-Ben-Dror, K., *et al.* 1998. Thrombotic thrombocytopenic purpura associated with ticlopidine. A review of 60 cases. *Ann Intern Med*, **128**, 541–4.

Ben-Yehuda, D., Rose, M., Michaeli, T., and Eldor, A. 1998. Permanent neurological complications in patients with thrombotic thrombocytopenic purpura. *Am J Hematol*, **29**, 74–8.

Beydoun, A., Vanderzant, C., Kutluay, E., and Drury, I. 2004. Full neurologic recovery after fulminant thrombotic thrombocytopenic purpura with status epilepticus. *Seizure*, **13**, 549–52.

Bianchi, V., Robles, R., Alberio, L., Furlan, M., and Lämmle, B. 2002. Von Willebrand factor-cleaving protease (ADAMTS 13) in thrombocytopenic disorders: a severely deficient activity is specific for thrombotic thrombocytopenic purpura. *Blood*, **100**, 710–3.

Blum, A. S., and Drislane, F. W. 1996. Nonconvulsive status epilepticus in thrombotic thrombocytopenic purpura. *Neurology*, **47**, 1079–81.

Bornstein, B., Boss, J. H., Casper, J., and Behar, M. 1960. Thrombotic thrombocytopenic purpura. Report of a case presenting as a chronic neurological disorder and characterized by unusual histological findings. *J Clin Pathol*, **13**, 124–32.

Brailey, L. L., Brecher, M. E., and Bandarenko, N. 1999. Apheresis and the thrombotic thrombocytopenic purpura syndrome: current advances in diagnosis, pathophysiology, and management. *Ther Apher*, **31**, 20–4.

Bridgman, J., and Witting, M. 1996. Thrombotic thrombocytopenic purpura presenting as a sudden headache with focal neurologic findings. *Ann Emerg Med*, **27**, 95–7.

Bukowski, R. 1982. Thrombotic thrombocytopenic purpura: a review. *Prog Hemost Thromb*, **6**, 287–337.

Bukowski, R. M., King, J. W., and Hewlett, J. S. 1977. Plasmapheresis in the treatment of thrombotic thrombocytopenic purpura. *Blood*, **50**, 413–7.

Castellá, M., Pujol, M., Julia, A., *et al.* 2004. Thrombotic thrombocytopenic purpura and pregnancy: a review of ten cases. *Vox Sang*, **87**, 287–90.

Cataland, S. R. and Wu, H. M. 2005. Immunotherapy for thrombotic thrombocytopenic purpura. *Curr Opin Hematol*, **12**, 359–63.

Chang, J. C., and Ikhlaque, N. 2004. Peripheral digit ischemic syndrome can be a manifestation of postoperative thrombotic thrombocytopenic purpura. *Ther Apher Dial*, **8**, 413–8.

Coppo, P., Bengoufa, D., Veyradier, A., *et al.* 2004. Severe ADAMTS-13 deficiency in adult idiopathic thrombotic microangiopathies defines a subset of patients characterized by various autoimmune manifestations, lower platelet count, and mild renal involvement. *Medicine*, **83**, 233–44.

Coppo, P., Bussel, A., Charrier, S., *et al.* 2003. High-dose plasma infusion versus plasma exchange as early treatment of thrombotic thrombocytopenic purpura/hemolytic-uremic syndrome. *Medicine (Baltimore)*, **82**, 27–38.

D'Aprile, P., Farchi, G., Pagliarulo, R., and Carella, A. 1994. Thrombotic thrombocytopenic purpura: MR demonstration of reversible brain abnormalities. *Am J Neuroradiol*, **15**, 19–20.

Dong, J. F., Moake, J. L., Bernardo, A., *et al.* 2003. ADAMTS-13 metalloprotease interacts with the endothelial cell-derived ultra-large von Willebrand factor. *J Biol Chem*, **278**, 29633–9.

Downes, K. A., Yomtovian, R., Tsai, H. M., *et al.* 2004. Relapsed thrombotic thrombocytopenic purpura presenting as an acute cerebrovascular accident. *J Clin Apher*, **19**, 86–9.

Elias, M., Flatau, E., and Bar-El, Y. 1985. Thrombotic thrombocytopenic purpura presenting as an acute abdomen. *Br J Surg*, **72**, 286.

Fiorani, L., Vianelli, N., Gugliotta, L., *et al.* 1995. Brain MRI and SPET in thrombotic thrombocytopenic purpura. *Ital J Neurol Sci*, **16**, 149–51.

Fujikawa, K., Suzuki, H., McMullen, B., and Chung, D. 2001. Purification of human von Willebrand factor-cleaving protease and its identification as a new member of the metalloproteinase family. *Blood*, **98**, 1662–6.

Furlan, M., and Lämmle, B. 2001. Aetiology and pathogenesis of thrombotic thrombocytopenic purpura and haemolytic uraemic syndrome: the role of von Willebrand factor-cleaving protease. *Best Pract Res Clin Haematol*, **14**, 437–54.

Furlan, M., Robles, R., Galbusera, M., *et al.* 1998. Von Willebrand factor-cleaving protease in thrombotic thrombocytopenic purpura and the hemolytic uremic syndrome. *N Engl J Med*, **339**, 1578–84.

Furlan, M., Robles, R., Solenthaler, M., *et al.* 1997. Deficient activity of von Willebrand-factor cleaving protease in chronic relapsing thrombotic thrombocytopenic purpura. *Blood*, **89**, 3097–103.

Garrett, W. T., Chang, C. W. J., and Bleck, T. P. 1996. Altered mental status in thrombotic thrombocytopenic purpura is secondary to nonconvulsive status epilepticus. *Ann Neurol*, **40**, 245–6.

George, J. N. 2000. How I treat patients with thrombotic thrombocytopenic purpura-hemolytic uremic syndrome. *Blood*, **96**, 1223–9.

Gurkan, E., Baslamisli, F., Guvenc, B., *et al.* 2005. Thrombotic thrombocytopenic purpura in southern Turkey: a single-center experience of 29 cases. *Clin Lab Haematol*, **27**, 121–5.

Hawley, J. S., Ney, J. P., and Swanberg, M. 2004. Thrombotic thrombocytopenic purpura-induced posterior leukoencephalopathy in a patient without significant renal or hypertensive complications. *J Postgrad Med*, **50**, 197–9.

Horton, T. M., Stone, J. D., Yee, D., *et al.* 2003. Case series of thrombotic thrombocytopenic purpura in children and adolescents. *J Pediatr Hematol Oncol*, **25**, 336–9.

Kay, A. C., Solberg, L. A., Nichols, D. A., and Pettit, R. M. 1991. Prognostic significance of computed tomography of the brain in thrombotic thrombocytopenic purpura. *Mayo Clin Proc*, **66**, 602–7.

Kelly, P. J., McDonald, C. T., O'Neill, G., *et al.* 1998. Middle cerebral artery main stem thrombosis in two siblings with familial thrombotic thrombocytopenic purpura. *Neurology*, **50**, 1157–60.

Kelly, F. E., Treacher, D. F., Williams, F. M., Hunt, B. J., and Howard, R. S. 1999. Coma in thrombotic thrombocytopenic purpura. *J Neurol Neurosurg Psychiatry*, **66**, 689–90.

Kennedy, S. S., Zacharski, L. R., and Beck, J. R. 1980. Thrombotic thrombocytopenic purpura: analysis of 48 unselected cases. *Semin Thromb Hemost*, **4**, 341–9.

Kokame, K., and Miyata, T. 2004. Genetic defects leading to hereditary thrombotic thrombocytopenic purpura. *Semin Hematol*, **41**, 34–40.

Kroll, M. H., Hellums, J. D., McIntire, L. V., Schafer, A. I., and Moake, J. L. 1996. Platelets and shear stress. *Blood*, **88**, 1525–41.

Kwaan, H. C. 1987. Clinicopathological features of thrombotic thrombocytopenic purpura. *Semin Hematol*, **24**, 74–81.

Kwaan, H. C., and Boggio, L. N. 2005. The clinical spectrum of thrombotic thrombocytopenic purpura. *Semin Thromb Hemost*, **31**, 673–80.

Lämmle, B., Kremer Hovinga, J. A., and Alberio, L. 2005. Thrombotic thrombocytopenic purpura. *J Thromb Haemost*, **3**, 1663–75.

Levy, G. A., Nichols, W. C., Lian, E. C., et al. 2001. Mutations in a member of the ADAMTS gene family cause thrombotic thrombocytopenic purpura. *Nature*, **413**, 488–94.

MacWhinney, J. B., Packer, J. T., Miller, G., and Greendyke, R. M. 1962. Thrombotic thrombocytopenic purpura in childhood. *Blood*, **19**, 181–99.

Mead, P. S., and Griffin, P. M. 1998. Coli 0157;H7. *Lancet*, **352**, 1207–12.

Meloni, G., Proia, A., Antonini, G., et al. 2001. Thrombotic thrombocytopenic purpura: prospective neurologic neuroimaging and neurophysiologic evaluation. *Haematologica*, **86**, 1194–9.

Miller, D. P., Kaye, J. A., Shea, K., et al. 2004. Incidence of thrombotic thrombocytopenic purpura/hemolytic uremic syndrome. *Epidemiology*, **15**, 208–15.

Moake, J. L. 2002. Thrombotic microangiopathies. *N Engl J Med*, **347**, 589–600.

Moake, J. L., and McPherson, P. D. 1989. Abnormalities of von Willebrand factor multimers in thrombotic thrombocytopenic purpura and the hemolytic-uremic syndrome. *Am J Med*, **87**, 9–15.

Moake, J. L., Rudy, C. K., Troll, J. H., et al. 1982. Unusually large plasma factor VIII: von Willebrand factor multimers in chronic relapsing thrombotic thrombocytopenic purpura. *N Engl J Med*, **307**, 1432–5.

Moschkowitz, E. 1924. Hyaline thrombosis of the terminal arterioles and capillaries: a hitherto undescribed disease. *Proc N Y Pathol Soc*, **24**, 21–4.

Müller, J., Czinyéri, J., Sasvári, I., Garami, M., and Kovács, G. 2001. Thrombotic thrombocytopenic purpura, Moschkowitz syndrome. *Int Pediatr*, **16**, 144–9.

Muniz, A. E., and Barbee, R. W. 2003. Thrombotic thrombocytopenic purpura (TTP) presenting as pancreatitis. *J Emerg Med*, **24**, 407–11.

Onundarson, P. T., Rowe, J. M., Heal, J. M., and Francis, C. W. 1992. Response to plasma exchange and splenectomy in thrombotic thrombocytopenic purpura. A 10-year experience at a single institution. *Arch Intern Med*, **152**, 791–6.

Park, S. A., Lee, T. K., Sung, K. B., and Park, S. K. 2005. Extensive brain stem lesions in thrombotic thrombocytopenic purpura: repeat magnetic resonance findings. *J Neuroimaging*, **15**, 79–81.

Petitt, R. M. 1980. Thrombotic thrombocytopenic purpura: a thirty-year review. *Semin Thromb Hemost*, **6**, 350–5.

Petz, L. D. 1977. Neurological manifestations of systemic lupus erythematosus and thrombotic thrombocytopenic purpura. *Stroke*, **8**, 719–22.

Peyvandi, F., Ferrari, S., Lavoretano, S., Canciani, M. T., and Mannucci, P. M. 2004. Von Willebrand factor cleaving protease (ADAMTS-13) and ADAMTS-13 neutralizing autoantibodies in 100 patients with thrombotic thrombocytopenic purpura. *Br J Hematol*, **127**, 433–9.

Piastra, M., Currò, V., Chiaretti, A., et al. 2001. Intracranial hemorrhage at the onset of thrombotic thrombocytopenic purpura in an infant: therapeutic approach and intensive care management. *Pediatr Emerg Care*, **17**, 42–5.

Ray, P. E., and Liu, X. H. 2001. Pathogenesis of Shiga toxin-induced hemolytic uremic syndrome. *Pediatr Nephrol*, **16**, 823–39.

Remuzzi, G., Galbusera, M., Salvadori, M., et al. 1996. Bilateral nephrectomy stopped disease progression in plasma-resistant hemolytic uremic syndrome with neurological signs and coma. *Kidney Int*, **49**, 282–6.

Ridolfi, R. L., and Bell, W. R. 1981. Thrombotic thrombocytopenic purpura: a report of 25 cases and a review of the literature. *Medicine (Baltimore)*, **60**, 413–28.

Rieger, M., Mannucci, P. M., Kremer Hovinga, J. A., et al. 2005. ADAMTS 13 autoantibodies in patients with thrombotic microangiopathies and other immunomediated diseases. *Blood*, **106**, 1262–7.

Rinkel, G. J. E., and Wijdicks, E. F. M. 1991. Stroke in relapsing thrombotic thrombocytopenic purpura. *Stroke*, **28**, 1087–9.

Rock, G. 2000. Management of thrombotic thrombocytopenic purpura. *Br J Haematol*, **109**, 496–507.

Rock, G. 2005. The management of thrombotic thrombocytopenic purpura in 2005. *Semin Thromb Hemost*, **31**, 709–16.

Rock, G. A., Shumak, K. H., Buskard, N. A., et al. 1991. Comparison of plasma exchange with plasma infusion in the treatment of thrombotic thrombocytopenic purpura. Canadian Apheresis Study Group. *N Engl J Med*, **325**, 393–7.

Rock, G., Kelton, J. G., Shumak, K. H., et al. 1998. Laboratory abnormalities in thrombotic thrombocytopenic purpura. Canadian Apheresis Group. *Br J Haematol*, **103**, 1031–6.

Rubinstein, M. A., Kagan, B. M., MacGillviray, M. H., Merliss, R., and Sacks, H. 1959. Unusual remission in a case of thrombotic thrombocytopenic purpura syndrome following fresh blood exchange transfusions. *Ann Intern Med*, **51**, 1409–19.

Ruggenenti, P., Noris, M., and Remuzzi, G. 2001. Thrombotic microangiopathy, hemolytic uremic syndrome, and thrombotic thrombocytopenic purpura. *Kidney Int*, **60**, 831–46.

Ruggenenti, P., and Remuzzi, G. 1996. The pathophysiology and management of thrombotic thrombocytopenic purpura. *Eur J Haematol*, **56**, 191–207.

Ruggeri, Z. M., Dent, J. A., and Saldívar, E. 1999. Contribution of distinct adhesive interactions to platelet aggregation in flowing blood. *Blood*, **94**, 172–8.

Sadler, J. E. 1998. Biochemistry and genetics of von Willebrand factor. *Annu Rev Biochem*, **67**, 395–424.

Sadler, J. E., Moake, J. L., Miyata, T., and George, J. M. 2004. Recent advances in thrombotic thrombocytopenic purpura. *Hematology Am Soc Hematol Educ Prog*, 407–23.

Scheid, R., Hegenbart, U., Ballaschke, O., and von Cramon, D. Y. 2004. Major stroke in thrombotic-thrombocytopenic purpura (Moschkowitz Syndrome). *Cerebrovasc Dis*, **18**, 83–5.

Shepard, K. V., Fishleder, A., Lucas, F. V., Goormastic, M., and Bukowski, R. 1991. Thrombotic thrombocytopenic purpura treated with plasma exchange or exchange transfusions. *West J Med*, **154**, 410–3.

Silverstein, A. 1968. Thrombotic thrombocytopenic purpura: initial neurologic manifestations. *Arch Neurol*, **18**, 358–62.

Singer, K., Bornstein, F. P., and Wiles, S. A. 1947. Thrombotic thrombocytopenic purpura. Hemorrhagic diathesis with generalized platelet thrombosis. *Blood*, **2**, 542–54.

Soltes, L., Schmalfuss, I. M., and Bhatti, T. M. 2004. Cortical blindness due to reversible posterior leukoencephalopathy syndrome in a patient with thrombotic thrombocytopenic purpura and preeclampsia. *Arch Ophthalmol*, **122**, 1885–7.

Studt, J. D., Hovinga, J. A., Radonic, R., et al. 2004. Familial acquired thrombotic thrombocytopenic purpura: ADAMTS 13 inhibitory autoantibodies in identical twins. *Blood*, **103**, 4195–7.

Tardy, B., Page, Y., Convers, P., et al. 1993. Thrombotic thrombocytopenic purpura: MR findings. *Am J Neuroradiol*, **14**, 489–90.

Terrel, D. R., Williams, L. A., Vesely, S. K., et al. 2005. The incidence of thrombotic thrombocytopenic purpura-hemolytic uremic syndrome: all patients, idiopathic patients, and patients with severe ADAMTS-13 deficiency. *J Thromb Haemost*, **3**, 1432–6.

Torok, T. J., Holman, R. C., and Chorba, T. I. 1995. Increasing mortality from thrombotic thrombocytopenic purpura in the United States: analysis of national mortality data, 1969–1991. *Am J Hematol*, **50**, 84–90.

Tsai, H. M. 1996. Physiologic cleavage of von Willebrand factor by a plasma protease is dependent on its conformation and requires calcium ion. *Blood*, **87**, 4235–44.

Tsai, H. M. 2000. High titers of inhibitors of von Willebrand factor-cleaving metalloproteinase in a fatal case of acute thrombotic thrombocytopenic purpura. *Am J Hematol*, **65**, 251–5.

Tsai, H. M. 2002. Von Willebrand factor, ADAMTS 13, and thrombotic thrombocytopenic purpura. *J Mol Med*, **80**, 639–47.

Tsai, H. M. 2003. Advances in the pathogenesis, diagnosis, and treatment of thrombotic thrombocytopenic purpura. *J Am Soc Nephrol*, **14**, 1072–81.

Tsai, H. M., and Lian, E. C. 1998. Antibodies to von Willebrand factor-cleaving protease in acute thrombotic thrombocytopenic purpura. *N Engl J Med*, **339**, 1585–94.

Vesely, S. K., George, J. N., Lämmle, B., et al. 2003. ADAMTS 13 activity in thrombotic thrombocytopenic purpura-hemolytic uremic syndrome: relation to presenting features and clinical outcomes in a prospective cohort of 142 patients. *Blood*, **102**, 60–8.

Veyradier, A., Lavergne, J. M., Ribba, A. S, *et al.* 2004. Ten candidate ADAMTS 13 mutations in six French families with congenital thrombotic thrombocytopenic purpura (Upshaw-Schulman syndrome). *J Thromb Haemost*, **2**, 424–9.

Veyradier, A., and Meyer, D. 2005. Thrombotic thrombocytopenic purpura and its diagnosis. *J Thromb Haemost*, **3**, 2420–7.

Veyradier, A., Obert, B., Houllier, A., Meyer, D., and Dima, J. P. 2001. Specific von Willebrand factor-cleaving protease in thrombotic microangiopathies: a study of 111 cases. *Blood*, **98**, 1765–72.

Willis, M. S., and Bandarenko, N. 2005. Relapse of thrombotic thrombocytopenic purpura: is it a continuum of disease? *Semin Thromb Hemost*, **31**, 700–8.

Zakarija, A., Bandarenko, N., Pandey, D. K., *et al.* 2004. Clopidogrel-associated TTP. An update of pharmacovigilance efforts conducted by independent researchers, pharmaceutical suppliers, and the Food and Drug Administration. *Stroke*, **35**, 533–8.

Zheng, X. L., Chung, D., Takayama, T. K., *et al.* 2001. Structure of von Willebrand factor-cleaving protease (ADAMTS13), a metalloprotease involved in thrombotic thrombocytopenic purpura. *J Biol Chem*, **276**, 41059–63.

Zheng, X. L., Kaufman, R. M., Goodnough, L. T., and Sadler, J. E. 2004. Effect of plasma exchange on plasma ADAMTS13 metalloprotease activity, inhibitor level, and clinical outcome in patients with idiopathic and nonidiopathic thrombotic thrombocytopenic purpura, *Blood*, **103**, 4043–9.

42

CEREBROVASCULAR COMPLICATIONS OF HENOCH-SCHÖNLEIN PURPURA

Sean I. Savitz and Louis R. Caplan

Henoch-Schönlein purpura (HSP), the most common vasculitis that affects children, is an acute, small-vessel leukocytoclastic process (Saulsbury, 2007). The frequency is about 10 cases per 100 000 persons per year (Calvino et al., 2001; Saulsbury, 1999, 2007). The condition also affects adults but much less often than children.

Historical background

The first case was probably reported by Heberden two centuries ago (Heberden, 1801; Saulsbury, 1999) who described a 5-year-old boy with abdominal pain, arthritic pain, melena, hematuria, and a purpuric rash. Schönlein (1837) described the association of purpura, arthritis, and precipitates in the urine, and Henoch (1874, 1899), a pupil of Schönlein, later elaborated on the gastrointestinal and renal findings in his patients. Sir William Osler (1914) published several reports on the condition emphasizing the renal involvement, and he provided some of the initial descriptions of the neurological complications of HSP: headache, behavioral alterations, and depressed consciousness (Osler 1914). Osler attributed the disease to anaphylaxis, and subsequent authors sometimes referred to the condition as "anaphylactoid purpura" (Saulsbury, 1999).

General clinical findings and pathogenesis

HSP is a systemic vasculitis involving vascular wall deposits of predominantly immunoglobulin (Ig) A within the small vessels of the gut, skin, joints, and kidneys, and in the mesangium of the renal glomeruli (Knight et al. 1988; Saulsbury, 1999, 2007). The disease is characterized by palpable purpura, arthralgias, abdominal pain, and renal abnormalities. Skin purpura is found in all patients and consists of palpable purpuric lesions that range in size from 2 to 10 mm in diameter (Saulsbury, 2007). Table 42.1 lists the most frequent clinical findings among a series of 100 patients (Saulsbury, 1999). Arthralgias, arthritis, and abdominal pain often precede the development of purpura. The onset of nephritis is often delayed by weeks (Saulsbury, 1999). Intussusception can develop and cause intestinal obstruction (Saulsbury, 1999; Trapani et al., 2005). Orchitis is also a problem in boys. Recurrences of disease after resolution of symptoms and signs develop in about one-third of patients (Saulsbury, 1999).

The most frequent laboratory abnormalities are high erythrocyte sedimentation rates, microscopic hematuria, proteinuria, and elevated levels of IgA (Saulsbury, 1999, 2007; Trapani et al.,

2005). Serum complement (C3 or C4 concentrations) is low in some patients (Calvino et al., 2001; Trapani et al., 2005). Biopsy of the skin in patients with HSP often shows neutrophilic infiltration in and around dermal blood vessels. Immunofluorescence analysis shows granular deposits of IgA and some quantity of complement (C3) and fibrin within the walls of the vessels (Giangiacomo and Tsai, 1977; Saulsbury, 1999; Stevenson et al., 1982). In the kidneys, focal or diffuse mesangial proliferation and glomerular crescents are sometimes found. Immunofluorescence shows that IgA is deposited diffusely within the renal mesangium (Giangiacomo and Tsai 1977; Levy et al., 1976; Saulsbury 1999).

A number of potential provoking agents have been posited. Group A β-hemolytic streptococcal infection has been the most extensively studied, but this agent has been cultured in only a minority of patients with HSP (Saulsbury, 1999). Other infections – bacterial, viral, and parasitic – have occasionally been reported in patients. Various drugs have also been implicated. Probably a wide variety of stimulants can provoke an immunological response that triggers the occurrence of HSP. Perhaps the relatively naïve immunological system found in childhood is more susceptible to an IgA response than in mature adults.

Neurological complications and strokes

HSP is known to cause neurological complications including seizure, chorea, encephalopathy, focal neurological signs, cortical blindness, as well as cranial and peripheral neuropathies and intracerebral hemorrhage (Chen et al., 2000; Eun et al., 2003; Ha and Cha, 1996; Saulsbury, 1999; Trapani et al., 2005). Although neurological symptoms and signs are common, few patients have been evaluated by neurologists who defined the mechanisms of the findings. Many of the cerebral manifestations have been attributed to central nervous system vasculitis. Although there are no reports detailing the neuropathological changes of patients with HSP, it is possible that IgA immune deposition might trigger arteriolar inflammation in the cerebral vasculature. There have been documented reports of neurological deficits in patients with HSP who have MRIs suggestive of cerebral vasculitis (Chen et al., 2000; Elinson et al., 1990; Eun et al., 2003; Ha and Cha, 1996).

Intracerebral hemorrhage has also been reported in the setting of possible vasculitis and is posited to develop secondary to a fulminant course of arterial inflammation (Wen et al., 2005). Intraparenchymal hemorrhages develop during a typical inflammatory attack but can occur before the onset of systemic symptoms

Uncommon Causes of Stroke, 2nd edition, ed. Louis R. Caplan. Published by Cambridge University Press. © Cambridge University Press 2008.

Table 42.1 Major findings among 100 children with HSP

Findings	Percentage of cases
Purpura	100
Arthritis	82
Abdominal pain	63
Nephritis	40
Gastrointestinal bleeding	33
Orchitis	5 (9% of boys)
Seizures	2

Note: Data from Saulsbury, 1999.

(Chiaretti *et al.*, 2002; Paolini *et al.*, 2003; Wen *et al.*, 2005). Ischemic infarction and strokes also occur in HSP. One case report described a 17-year-old girl who infarcted the left lenticular nucleus, caudate, and perioperculum. Evaluation showed that she had anti-phospholipid antibodies in serum and cerebrospinal fluid, suggesting that the latter may predispose HSP patients to develop ischemic stroke (Sokol *et al.*, 2000). Other potential mechanisms to explain neurological complications in patients with HSP include encephalopathy and reversible leukoencephalopathy from the acute nephropathy or corticosteroids.

Treatment

Pulse steroids have been shown to be effective, but sometimes plasmapheresis has been used to arrest disease progression (Eun *et al.*, 2003; Shin *et al.*, 2006; Wen *et al.*, 2005). Patients with severe nephritis, especially with the nephritic syndrome, have often been treated with corticosteroids and cyclophosphamide, cyclosporine, or azathioprine (Saulsbury, 2007).

REFERENCES

Calvino, M. C., Llorca, J., Garcia-Porrua, C., *et al.* 2001. Henoch-Schonlein purpura in children from northwest Spain: a 20 year epidemiologic and clinical study. *Medicine*, **80**, 279–90.

Chen, C. L., Chiou, Y. H., Wu, C. Y., Lai, P. H., and Chung, H. M. 2000. Cerebral vasculitis in Henoch-Schonlein purpura: a case report with sequential magnetic resonance imaging changes and treated with plasmapharesis alone. *Pediatr Nephrol*, **15**, 276–8.

Chiaretti, A., Caresta, E., Piastra, M., Pulitano, S., and Di Rocco, C. 2002. Cerebral hemorrhage in Henoch-Schoenlein syndrome. *Childs Nerv Syst*, **18**, 365–7.

Elinson, P., Foster, K. W., and Kaufman, D. B. 1990. Case report: magnetic resonance imaging of central system vasculitis. *Acta Paediatr Scand*, **70**, 710–3.

Eun, S. H., Kim, S. J., Cho, D. S., *et al.* 2003. Cerebral vasculitis in Henoch-Schonlein purpura: MRI and MRA findings, treated with plasmapheresis alone. *Pediatr Int*, **45**, 484–7.

Giangiacomo, J., and Tsai, C. C. 1977. Dermal and glomerular deposition of IgA in anaphylactoid purpura. *Am J Dis Child*, **131**, 981–3.

Ha, T. S., and Cha, S. H. 1996. Cerebral vasculitis in Henoch-Schonlein purpura: a case report with sequential magnetic resonance imaging. *Pediatr Nephrol*, **10**, 634–6.

Heberden, W. 1801. Commentari di morborium historia et curatione, London, Payne. Reprinted as "Commentaries on the history and cure of diseases" The Classics of Medicine Library, Division of Gryphon Editions Ltd, Birmingham Alabama, 1982, 395–7.

Henoch, E. H. 1874. Uber eine eigenthumliche form von purpura. Berlin: Klinische Wochenschrift **11**, 641–3.

Henoch, E. H. 1899. Vorlesungen uber kinderkrankheiten. In *Volhesunger uber Kinderkrankheiten*, A. Hirschward, ed. Berlin: Aufli, 839.

Knight, J. F., Harada, T., Thomas, M. A. B., *et al.* 1988. IgA rheumatoid factor and other autoantibodies in acute Henoch-Schonlein purpura. *Contrib Nephrol*, **67**, 117–20.

Levy, M., Broyer, M., Arsan, A., Levy-Bentolila, D., and Habib, R. 1976. Anaphylactoid purpura nephritis in childhood: natural history and immunopathology. *Adv Nephrol*, **6**, 183–228.

Osler, W. 1914. The visceral lesions of purpura and allied conditions. *Br Med J Clin Res*, **1**, 517–25.

Paolini, S., Ciappetta, P., Piattella, M. C., and Domenicucci, M. 2003. Henoch-Schonlein syndrome and cerebellar hemorrhage: report of an adolescent case and literature review. *Surg Neurol*, **60**, 339–42.

Saulsbury, F. T. 1999. Henoch-Schonlein purpura in children: report of 100 patients and review of the literature. *Medicine (Baltimore)*, **78**, 395–409.

Saulsbury, F. T. 2007. Clinical update: Henoch-Schonlein purpura. *Lancet*, **369**, 976–8.

Shin, J., Lee, J. S., Kim, H. D., and Lee, Y. M. 2006. Neurologic manifestations and treatment of Henoch-Schonlein purpura. *Brain Dev*, **28**, 547.

Sokol, D. K., McIntyre, J. A., Short, R. A., *et al.* 2000. Henoch-Schonlein purpura and stroke: antiphosphatidyl-ethanolamine antibody in CSF and serum. *Neurology*, **55**, 1379–81.

Stevenson, J. A., Leong, L. A., Cohen, A. H., and Border, W. A. 1982. Simultaneous demonstration of IgA deposits in involved skin, intestine, and kidney. *Arch Pathol Lab Med*, **106**, 192–5.

Trapani, S., Miceli, A., Grisolia, F., *et al.* 2005. Henoch Schonlein purpura in childhood: epidemiological and clinical analysis of 150 cases over a 5-year period and review of the literature. *Semin Arthritis Rheum*, **35**, 143–53.

Wen, Y.-K., Yang, Y., and Chang, C.-C. 2005. Cerebral vasculitis and intracerebral hemorrhage in Henoch-Schonlein purpura treated with plasmapheresis. *Pediatric Nephrology*, **20**, 223–5.

PART V: SYSTEMIC DISORDERS THAT ALSO INVOLVE THE CEREBROVASCULAR SYSTEM

43 MICROSCOPIC POLYANGIITIS AND POLYARTERITIS NODOSA

Marc D. Reichhart, Reto Meuli, and Julien Bogousslavsky

Introduction, nosology, diagnostic criteria of polyarteritis nodosa and microscopic polyangiitis

Kussmaul and Maier (1866) in Freiburg, Germany first reported a young patient with a fatal disease manifested by high fever, weight loss, abdominal pain, myalgias, muscle weakness, mononeuritis multiplex, and renal failure with proteinuria – symptoms that were previously described by Von Rokitansky in 1852 in Vienna (Brown and Swash, 1989; Tesar *et al.*, 2004). At autopsy, Kussmaul and Maier found abnormal segmental thickening (macroscopically discernable nodular lesions) and inflammation of small-to medium-sized arteries in many organs, and described the disease as "periarteritis nodosa." Since Ferrari (1903), it was renamed polyarteritis nodosa (PAN), and it remains the prototypic disorder of the group of systemic necrotizing arteritis, including also Churg-Strauss syndrome (see Chapter 44), microscopic polyangiitis (MPA), Kawasaki disease (see Chapter 13), and an overlap syndrome (Younger, 2004).

Zeek (1952) was the first to classify the various systemic vasculitides. The American College of Rheumatology's (ACR) classification of "classic" PAN was published nearly 50 years later (Lightfoot *et al.*, 1990). The 10 diagnostic criteria are summarized in Table 43.1. If a patient fullfils at least three of them, the diagnosis of PAN can be made with a sensitivity of 82.2% and a specificity of 86.6%. First recognized as a distinct microscopic form of PAN associated with crescentic glomerulonephritis (Davson *et al.*, 1948), Godman and Churg (1954) confirmed that Zeek's hypersensitivity angiitis was identical to "microscopic periarteritis" (Jennette and Falk, 2007; Segelmark and Selga, 2007), now called MPA since the Chapel Hill Conference Consensus on the nomenclature system of systemic vasculitis definitions (Jennette *et al.*, 1994). However, some have questioned whether these two entities should be separated because Kussmaul and Maier included glomerular lesions and small vessel involvement in their original description of PAN (Lie, 1994).

The association of positive hepatitis B virus serology with PAN was first recognized in 1970, whereas anti-neutrophil cytoplasmic antibodies (ANCAs) in the 1980s were more frequently detected in MPA (Jennette and Falk, 2007; Segelmark and Selga, 2007). Falk and Jennette (1988) first reported that perinuclear subtype ANCAs (p-ANCAs), directed against myeloperoxidase, were detectable in MPA. The combined detection of positive ANCA by indirect immunofluorescence and enzyme-linked immunosorbence assay

Table 43.1 1990 ACR criteria for the classification of PAN

Criterion	Definition
1. Weight loss $\geq$ 4 kg	Loss of $\geq$ 4 kg of body weight since illness began, not due to dieting or other factors
2. Livedo reticularis	Mottled reticular pattern over the skin (portions of the extremities or torso)
3. Testicular pain or tenderness	Pain or tenderness of the testicles, not due to infection, trauma, or other causes
4. Myalgias, weakness, or leg tenderness	Diffuse myalgias (excluding shoulder and hip girdle) or weakness of muscles or tenderness of leg muscles
5. Mononeuropathy or polyneuropathy	Development of mononeuropathy, multiple mononeuropathies, or polyneuropathy
6. Diastolic blood pressure > 90 mmHg	Development of hypertension with diastolic blood pressure > 90 mmHg
7. Elevated blood urea nitrogen (BUN) or creatinine	Elevation of BUN > 40 mg/dL or creatinine > 1.5 mg/dL, not due to dehydratation or obstruction
8. Hepatitis B virus	Presence of hepatitis B surface antigen or antibody in serum
9. Arteriographic abnormality	Arteriogram showing aneurysms or occlusions of the visceral arteries, not due to arteriosclerosis, fibromuscular dysplasia, or other noninflammatory causes
10. Biopsy of small or medium-sized artery containing polymorphonuclear neutrophils	Histologic changes showing the presence of granulocytes or granulocytes and mononuclear leukocytes in the artery wall

Source: Lightfoot *et al.*, 1990, with permission.

Uncommon Causes of Stroke, 2nd edition, ed. Louis R. Caplan. Published by Cambridge University Press. © Cambridge University Press 2008.

(ELISA) has a specificity of 73% and a sensitivity of 67% for the diagnosis of MPA (Bosch *et al.*, 2006). About 60% of patients with MPA show positive MPO-ANCA (p-ANCA), and 30% have proteinase 3 subtype ANCA (PR3-ANCA or c-ANCA) (Bosch *et al.*, 2006). Overall, more than 80% of MPA patients have ANCA (Jennette and Falk, 1997), but about 10% of them show negative assays for ANCA, so that ANCA negativity does not exclude this small-vessel vasculitis. Conversely, up to 20% of patients with "classic" PAN show positive ANCA (Guillevin and Lhote, 1995). Positive results for hepatitis B virus and p-ANCA may help to distinguish PAN from MPA (Guillevin *et al.*, 1995a; Jennette and Falk, 1997).

According to the Chapel Hill nomenclature (Jennette *et al.*, 1994), systemic vasculitis is characterized by the size and preferred type of vascular involvement: PAN, a medium-sized-vessel (main visceral arteries and their branches, such as renal, hepatic, coronary, and mesenteric arteries) vasculitis, is characterized by necrotizing inflammation of medium-sized or small arteries without glomerulonephritis or vasculitis in arterioles, capillaries, or venules, whereas MPA is defined as a necrotizing vasculitis with few or no immune deposits (pauci-immune) affecting small vessels (capillaries, venules, or arterioles), but necrotizing arteritis in the small and medium-sized arteries may be present; necrotizing glomerulonephritis is very common and pulmonary capillaritis occurs frequently. In a retrospective series of 99 British patients with primary systemic vasculitis from a single referral center (population, 415000 people) during 12 years (1988–2000), although initially 60 cases (60%) fulfilled the ACR criteria for the diagnosis of PAN, none of them could be confirmed according to the Chapel Hill criteria, including two patients with suspected PAN (2%) showing another type of vasculitis; overall, 24 (24%) had MPA (Lane, Watts, Shepstone, *et al.*, 2005). In a similar Swedish study (population, 1.5 million people), during 12 years (1990–2002), 10 patients fulfilled the Chapel Hill definition for PAN, giving an annual incidence of only 1.6 per million (Selga *et al.*, 2006), which is rarer than MPA (8.4–11.6 per million) (Watts *et al.*, 2001).

A more recent European consensus classification of the ANCA-associated vasculitides and PAN was validated (Watts *et al.*, 2007), using the ACR criteria and the Chapel Hill definitions with a stepwise algorithm. The following are used to separate MPA from classic PAN: surrogate markers for renal vasculitis, positive PR3- or MPO-ANCA testing, and histologically proven small-vessel vasculitis or glomerulonephritis. PAN is characterized by typical compatable histology or typical celiac axis angiographic abnormalities (see Figure 43.1B) (Das and Pangtey, 2006)) For recent data on the prevalence and incidence of MPA and classic PAN, see Lane, Watts, and Scott, 2005.

The largest reported series that included randomized clinical trial results focusing on treatment, and later pooled to obtain data on prognostic factors, outcome, and mortality in patients with PAN and MPA, came from the French Vasculitis Study Group, previously known as the Cooperative Study Group for Polyarteritis Nodosa (Agard *et al.*, 2003; Bourgarit *et al.*, 2005; Chanseaud *et al.*, 2005; Gayraud *et al.*, 2001; Guillevin *et al.*, 1995a, 1995b, 1999, 2005; Guillevin, Le Thi, Godeau, *et al.*, 1988; Guillevin and Lhote, 1995; Guillevin, Lhote, Amouroux, *et al.*, 1996; Guillevin, Lhote,

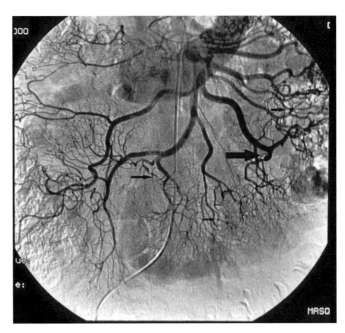

Figure 43.1 Visceral angiography of Patient 5, Lausanne, showing multiple microaneurysms (*arrow*).

Cohen, *et al.*, 1995b; Lhote *et al.*, 1996). The differential diagnosis of PAN and MPA is summarized in Table 43.2 (Guillevin *et al.*, 1997a; Guillevin and Lhote, 1995; Jennette *et al.*, 2001; Niles *et al.*, 1996). In a retrospective series of 72 patients with PAN and MPA (50% each), initial manifestations were similar in both vasculitides, except that peripheral neuropathy and gastrointestinal tract involvement were more frequent in PAN) and systemic symptoms alone (i.e. fever, weight loss, asthenia) were found only in MPA (Agard *et al.*, 2003).

MPA

Clinical features

MPA affects men more often than women (male-to-female ratio of 1–2:1) (Adu *et al.*, 1987; Gayraud *et al.*, 2001; Guillevin *et al.*, 1999; Hogan *et al.*, 1996; Lane, Watts, Shepstone, *et al.*, 2005; Nachman *et al.*, 1996; Savage *et al.*, 1985; Westman *et al.*, 1998). Most patients are older than 50 years (Adu *et al.*, 1987) (mean, 60; range, 50–70) (Agard *et al.*, 2003; Ara *et al.*, 1999; Gayraud *et al.*, 2001; Guillevin *et al.*, 1999; Hogan *et al.*, 1996; Lane, Watts, Shepstone, *et al.*, 2005; Nachman *et al.*, 1996; Pavone *et al.*, 2006; Rodgers *et al.*, 1989; Savage *et al.*, 1985; Westman *et al.*, 1998). MPA is a systemic necrotizing vasculitis that clinically and histologically involves capillaries, venules, or arterioles without granulomata, and is associated with necrotizing crescentic glomerulonephritis and hemorrhagic pulmonary capillaritis, which are the main causes of mortality and morbidity (Guillevin *et al.*, 1999; Jennette *et al.*, 2001; Lhote *et al.*, 1996, 1998; Lhote and Guillevin, 1995). Renal involvement is very common, found in 79%–92% of patients in recent series (Guillevin *et al.*, 1999; Lane, Watts, Shepstone, *et al.*, 2005; Pavone *et al.*, 2006). Kidney involvement requiring dialysis occurred in 16%–37% of cases (Guillevin *et al.*, 1999; Pavone *et al.*, 2006). Glomerulonephritis is found in 80%–100% of patients (Jennette *et al.*, 2001; Lhote

Table 43.2 Differential diagnosis of PAN and MPA,

Criteria	PAN	MPA
Histology		
Type of vasculitis	Necrotizing with mixed cells, rarely granulomatous	Necrotizing with mixed cells, not granulomatous
Type of vessels involved	Medium-sized and small muscle arteries, sometimes arterioles	Small vessels (i.e., capillaries, venules, or arterioles). Small- and medium-sized arteries may also be affected
Distribution and localization		
Kidney		
Renal vasculitis with renal infarcts and microaneurysms	Yes	No
Renovascular hypertension	Yes (10–33%)	No
Rapidly progressive glomerulonephritis	No	Yes (very common)
Lung		
Pulmonary hemorrhage	No	Yes
Pulmonary-renal syndrome Goodpasture' syndrome	No	Most frequent cause
Peripheral neuropathy	50–80%	10–20%
Relapses	Rare	Frequent
Laboratory data		
Perinuclear ANCA	Rare (<20% in frequency)	Frequent (50–80% of cases)
HBV infection	Yes (uncommon)	No
Abnormal angiography (microaneurysms, stenosis)	Yes (variable)	No (rare)

Adapted from Guillevin *et al.*, 1997a; Guillevin and Lhote, 1995; Jennette *et al.*, 2001; and Niles *et al.*, 1996.

et al., 1998). The other most frequent target of MPA is lung involvement, found in 22–63% of patients (Adu *et al.*, 1987; Agard *et al.*, 2003; Guillevin *et al.*, 1999; Hogan *et al.*, 1996; Lane, Watts, Shepstone, *et al.*, 2005; Nachman *et al.*, 1996; Pavone *et al.*, 2006; Rodgers *et al.*, 1989; Savage *et al.*, 1985; Westman *et al.*, 1998). Pulmonary hemorrhage or hemoptysis has been reported in 11%–38% of cases (Adu *et al.*, 1987; Agard *et al.*, 2003; Guillevin *et al.*, 1999; Lane, Watts, Shepstone, *et al.*, 2005; Pavone *et al.*, 2006; Rodgers *et al.*, 1989; Savage *et al.*, 1985). MPA is the most common

cause of the pulmonary-renal syndrome, so-called Goodpasture's syndrome (Jennette *et al.*, 2001; Jennette and Falk, 1997; Niles *et al.*, 1996). Other clinical features are: myalgias, arthralgias, and arthritis (50%–72%); purpura and splinter hemorrhages (44%–62%); abdominal pain (30%–58%); and gastrointestinal bleeding (29%) (Lhote *et al.*, 1998). Peripheral neuropathy (14%–58%) is less frequent than in PAN, whereas ear, nose, and throat lesions (5%–28%) are much more common (Adu *et al.*, 1987; Agard *et al.*, 2003; Guillevin *et al.*, 1999; Hogan *et al.*, 1996; Lane, Watts, Shepstone, *et al.*, 2005; Nachman *et al.*, 1996; Pavone *et al.*, 2006; Rodgers *et al.*, 1989; Savage *et al.*, 1985; Westman *et al.*, 1998).

Laboratory findings

Laboratory findings show nonspecific inflammation, with raised erythrocyte sedimentation rate (ESR) (>20 mm/hour) in 76%–100% of cases (Adu *et al.*, 1987; Guillevin *et al.*, 1999; Pavone *et al.*, 2006; Rodgers *et al.*, 1989; Savage *et al.*, 1985; Westman *et al.*, 1998), ranging from a mean of 74–88 mm/hour (Guillevin *et al.*, 1999; Pavone *et al.*, 2006; Westman *et al.*, 1998), increased C-reactive protein ranging from a mean of 56–69 mg/L (Ara *et al.*, 1999; Pavone *et al.*, 2006; Westman *et al.*, 1998), high white cell count (42%–90%) (Adu *et al.*, 1987; Rodgers *et al.*, 1989; Savage *et al.*, 1985), eosinophilia (3–6%) (Rodgers *et al.*, 1989; Savage *et al.*, 1985), low hemoglobin (75–100%) (Adu *et al.*, 1987; Rodgers *et al.*, 1989; Savage *et al.*, 1985; Westman *et al.*, 1998) and serum albumin (Savage *et al.*, 1985), elevated plasma creatinine level (25%–100%) (Agard *et al.*, 2003; Guillevin *et al.*, 1999; Hogan *et al.*, 1996; Pavone *et al.*, 2006; Rodgers *et al.*, 1989; Savage *et al.*, 1985; Westman *et al.*, 1998) ranging from a mean of 2.54–7.4 mg/dL (Guillevin *et al.*, 1999; Hogan *et al.*, 1996; Pavone *et al.*, 2006) or a median of 389 μmol/L (>115 μmol/L) (Westman *et al.*, 1998), microscopic hematuria (11%–100%) (Adu *et al.*, 1987; Guillevin *et al.*, 1999; Hogan *et al.*, 1996; Rodgers *et al.*, 1989; Savage *et al.*, 1985), and proteinuria (70%–100%) (Adu *et al.*, 1987; Guillevin *et al.*, 1999; Hogan *et al.*, 1996; Savage *et al.*, 1985). Concentrations of complement (C3,C4) are normal or high (19–68%) (Adu *et al.*, 1987; Rodgers *et al.*, 1989; Savage *et al.*, 1985). Rheumatoid factor (23%–50%) (Adu *et al.*, 1987; Guillevin *et al.*, 1999; Rodgers *et al.*, 1989; Savage *et al.*, 1985) and antinuclear antibodies (17%–33%) (Adu *et al.*, 1987; Guillevin *et al.*, 1999; Savage *et al.*, 1985) were detected in older series. Hepatitis B surface antigen (2.3%) (Guillevin *et al.*, 1999) is rarely positive in MPA, contrary to PAN, whereas anti-hepatitis B virus (2.4%) (Adu *et al.*, 1987), anti-hepatitis C virus (1%), and anti-HIV (1%) (Guillevin *et al.*, 1999) antibody detections were considered coincidental.

In three large old MPA series (Adu *et al.*, 1987; Savage *et al.*, 1985; Serra *et al.*, 1984) among 30 patients who underwent celiac axis/renal (visceral) angiography, only five showed microaneursyms (16.7%) (see Figure 43.1; 43.1A and B) (Das and Pangtey, 2006), including none in one series (Savage *et al.*, 1985). Small microaneurysms and stenosis in medium-sized vessels on visceral angiography are commonly present in PAN, and this invasive angiogram procedure still remains a useful diagnostic tool for discriminating PAN from MPA (Guillevin, Lhote, Amouroux, *et al.*, 1996; Lhote *et al.*, 1998).

Since the availability of non-invasive ANCA diagnostic testing, the most recently reported MPA series found increasing proportion of patients with positive ANCA, which has replaced visceral angiogram as the key investigation. Rogers et al. (1989) found that only 4/36 (11%) patients had positive ANCA. In later series, patients with MPA had positive serum ANCA in 85%–95% of cases (Bosch et al., 2006), but approximately 10% have negative ANCA assays (Jennette and Falk, 1997). Most patients with MPA and idiopathic necrotizing and crescentic glomerulonephritis display perinuclear pattern (indirect immunofluorescence) anti-neutrophil cytoplasmic antibodies (p-ANCA) directed to myeloperoxidase (MPO-ANCA), and increases in their levels precede or coincide with clinical relapses (Kallenberg et al., 2006, 2007). Moreover, detection of PR3- and/or MPO-ANCA by ELISA, in the clinical context, have a specificity of 98% for the diagnosis of ANCA-associated vasculitides, which includes Wegener's granulomatosis, MPA and its renal limited form, and the Churg-Strauss syndrome (see Chapter 44) (Kallenberg et al., 2006). The sensitivities of MPO-ANCA are 60% and 64% for MPA and idiopathic crescentic glomerulonephritis, respectively, whereas those of PR3-ANCA are 30% for each (Kallenberg et al., 2006). Indeed, p- and c-ANCA have been reported in 87%–93% and 7%–13% of cases in MPA series, respectively (Guillevin et al., 1999; Pavone et al., 2006), whereas MPO- and PR3-ANCA were found in 64%–89% and in 3.5%–25% of cases (Gibson et al., 2006; Hauer et al., 2002; Pavone et al., 2006; Weidner et al., 2004). About 60% of patients with MPA or renally limited necrotizing crescentic glomerulonephritis have MPO-ANCA, and 30% show PR3-ANCA (Wiik, 2002).

Pathology and pathogenesis

The pathological hallmark of acute vascular lesions in MPA is segmental vascular necrosis with infiltration of mainly neutrophils, and variable numbers of monocytes, lymphocytes, and eosinophils, often associated with fibrinoid necrosis and leukocytoclasia (i.e. transmural and perivascular leukocyte infiltration) of the media (Jennette et al., 2001; Lhote et al., 1996). The fibrinoid necrosis and inflammation may erode into perivascular tissue, resulting in pseudoaneurysm formation (Jennette et al., 2001). This produces various grades of hemorrhages resulting in purpura (dermal venulitis), pulmonary hemorrhage (alveolar capillaritis), and the hematuria of glomerulonephritis (Jennette et al., 2001). Thrombosis may occur, causing infarction only if arteries are involved. Arteritis is most frequently seen in nerve, skeletal muscle, heart, liver, pancreas, and digestive tract (Jennette et al., 2001). Another pathological feature of MPA is the coexistence of necrotizing vasculitis and healed lesions or normal artery in different parts of the same or in different tissues (Lhote et al., 1996). The vasculitic lesions involve (in order of decreasing frequency) the following organs: kidney (93%), spleen (33%), lung (27%), muscle (20%), and gastrointestinal tract, pericardium, central nervous system (CNS), testis, and uterus (7% each) (Lhote et al., 1996).

Clinical, in vitro, and in vivo experimental data support the pathological role of ANCA in MPA. ANCA can stimulate neutrophils to become adherent to endothelial cells, and primed neutrophils with cytokines such as tumor necrosis factor-α (TNF-α)

can lyse endothelial cells in vitro (Lhote et al., 1996). Cytokine-induced expression of adhesion molecules (lymphocyte function-associated antigen-1 [LFA-1], intercellular adhesion molecule 1 [ICAM-1], endothelial-leukocyte adhesion molecule 1 [ELAM-1]) enables contact between neutrophils and endothelial cells. The coexistence of primed neutrophils, endothelium, and circulating ANCA provokes the cascade of events leading to vasculitis (Lhote et al., 1996). Primed neutrophils with TNF-α express PR3 and MPO on their surface, and when incubated with PR3- or MPO-ANCA, they are further activated to produce lytic enzymes such as elastase and PR3. Neutrophil activation is even stronger in the presence of arachidonic acid, indicating a potential for additional activation in an already inflammatory state (Kallenberg et al., 2006). Fc-γ receptor (FcγR) interactions may play a role in ANCA-induced neutrophil activation, and in pathways other than those mediated by G proteins (Kallenberg et al., 2006). Increased numbers of neutrophils that express PR3 on their membrane have been found in Wegener's granulomatosis (associated with PR3-ANCA type contrary to MPA) and have been related to increased relapse frequency (Kallenberg et al., 2006).

MPO expression is also essential for MPO-ANCA-mediated neutrophil activation. ANCA can induce neutrophils and monocytes to adhere to the endothelial layer, where these cells become activated close to the vessel wall, resulting in small-vessel necrotizing vasculitis. Many in vivo studies showed the proinflammatory potential of MPO-ANCA in the development of MPA-like pulmonary vasculitis and glomerulonephritis. Presence of anti-MPO antibodies augments the inflammatory reaction, suggesting their potential neutrophil activation capacity. Priming of neutrophils and endothelial cells with lipopolysaccharide prepares neutrophils for the activating effects of MPO-ANCA. A case report described the first case of transplacental transfer of MPO-ANCA from a woman with a history of vasculitis (MPO-ANCA positive) resulting in pulmonary-renal syndrome in her newborn (Bansal and Tobin, 2004). The clinical presentation of MPO-ANCA-associated MPA lesions in humans is nearly identical to the lesions observed in experimental animals (Kallenberg et al., 2006). Finally, CD4-positive T cells may also play a role in the pathogenesis of MPO-ANCA-associated glomerulonephritis (Kallenberg, 2007).

Outcome

Another characteristic of MPA, contrary to PAN, is its tendency to relapse, ranging from 25.4% to 60% of cases and within a median time ranging from 12 to 88 months (Gayraud et al., 2001; Gordon et al., 1993; Guillevin et al., 1999; Hogan et al., 2005; Jayne et al., 1995; Nachman et al., 1996; Pavone et al., 2006; Westman et al., 1998). Relapse may be preceded and monitored by ANCA levels or positive seroconversion during therapy of patients with ANCA-associated vasculitis (Ara et al., 1999; Boomsma et al., 2000; Jayne et al., 1995; Kyndt et al., 1999; Nachman et al., 1996; Stegeman, 2002), but this strategy has been less well studied for MPA than for Wegener's granulomatosis. One Spanish series showed that positive-to-negative seroconversion p-ANCA directed against MPO (ELISA) was achieved in 75% (18/24 cases) of patients with MPA (14 cases), and so-called renal limited vasculitis (RLV) or rapidly progressive glomerulonephritis type III (10 cases) within 6 months following standard immunosuppressive therapy (Ara *et al.*, 1999). All relapses were associated with, or closely preceded by, seroconversion (negative-to-positive) or by an increase in the anti-MPO ANCA titers (Ara *et al.*, 1999). Another European series (Dutch) of patients with MPA/RLV found a trend of lower relapse-free survival at 5 years in PR3-ANCA (63%) compared with MPO-ANCA (84%) positive patients (Stegeman, 2002). In contrast, a large series from the southeastern United States including MPA (58%), RLV (25%), and Wegener's granulomatosis (17%) found that patients with anti-PR3 antibodies were 1.87 times more likely to relapse than were those who were anti-MPO seropositive, after achieving remission (Hogan *et al.*, 2005). A Swedish series including MPA and Wegener's granulomatosis found, in near half of the patients in each group, that very high PR3-ANCA level at time of diagnosis (>550 U), measured by the capture ELISA method (Westman *et al.*, 1998), was significantly associated with an increased risk of decreased patient survival (Westman *et al.*, 2003). These conflicting results may be explained by racial and geographical differences between Wegener's granulomatosis and MPA in the prevalence and association with PR3- or MPO-ANCA (Kallenberg, 2007).

The prognosis of MPA and Wegener's granulomatosis was only 18% at 1 year before the use of immunosuppressive therapy (Walton, 1958). Since the use of corticosteroids and cyclophosphamide, first reported by Fahey *et al.* (1954) and later by Fauci *et al.* (1971), patient survival improved to 80% at 5 years for Wegener's granulomatosis (Fauci *et al.*, 1983). As regards MPA, despite evolving modern immunosuppressive treatment over 20 years, the survival rates of patients still ranges as follows: at 1 year, 62%–93% (Adu *et al.*, 1987; Bourgarit *et al.*, 2005; Lane, Watts, Shepstone, *et al.*, 2005; Pavone *et al.*, 2006; Weidner *et al.*, 2004; Westman *et al.*, 2003), at 5 years, 45%–80% (mean, 74%) (Gayraud *et al.*, 2001; Guillevin *et al.*, 1999; Lane, Watts, Shepstone, *et al.*, 2005; Pavone *et al.*, 2006; Savage *et al.*, 1985; Weidner *et al.*, 2004; Westman *et al.*, 2003), and at 10 years, 52%–55% (Gordon *et al.*, 1993; Westman *et al.*, 2003).

Treatment

Early previous series highlighted the longer survival rate (i.e. 5.56 times better) (Hogan *et al.*, 1996) of patients treated with cyclophosphamide (3 mg/kg/day) and corticosteroids than of those receiving corticosteroids alone (Adu *et al.*, 1987; Hogan *et al.*, 1996; Rodgers *et al.*, 1989; Savage *et al.*, 1985). The dose and type of corticosteroid treatment depend on the severity of MPA and particularly the presence of renal involvement (methylprednisolone pulses intravenously 15 mg/kg over 60 minutes, at 24-hour intervals, for 3 days, or oral prednisone 1 mg/kg/day), which should be tapered as soon as possible, according to the European Vasculitis Study group (Guillevin and Lhote, 1998; Jayne, 2001). The gold standard regimen consisted 20 years ago in oral daily cyclophosphamide (2 mg/kg), accompanied by a tapering dose of oral prednisolone (Jayne, 2001). The European Vasculitis Study group designed prospective therapeutic trials for ANCA-associated vasculitis, comparing classic cyclophosphamide (with/without corticosteroids) with methotrexate, azathioprine, and plasma

exchange (Jayne, 2001) and their website (www.vasculitis.com, 2007). There was improved renal outcome in the plasma exchange/cyclophosphamide group versus the methylprednisolone/cyclophosphamide group in patients with severe renal involvement (creatinine > 500 μg/L) (Watts *et al.*, 2005). Plasmapheresis is effective in some patients with MPA and diffuse alveolar hemorrhage (Klemmer *et al.*, 2003). The largest prospective trial from the European Vasculitis Study group, which included 155 patients at randomization (Wegener's granulomatosis, 61%; MPA, 39%), investigated whether cyclophosphamide treatment could be reduced by substitution of azathioprine at remission (Jayne *et al.*, 2003). All patients received oral cyclophosphamide (2 mg/kg/day) and prednisolone (1 mg/kg/day) tapered at 3 months (0.25 mg/kg) before randomization. After randomization, patients received either cyclophosphamide (1.5 mg/kg/day) or azathioprine (2 mg/kg/day), together with prednisolone (10 mg/day). At 12 months, both groups received azathioprine (1.5 mg/kg/day) and prednisolone (7.5 mg/day). After randomization, 93% (144) entered remission and were assigned to azathioprine (71) or continued cyclophosphamide (73), with 15.5% and 13.7% relapsed, respectively ($p = .65$). Relapses were less frequent in patients with microscopic polgangiitis (8%) than in those with Wegener's granulomatosis (18%); $p = .03$) (Jayne *et al.*, 2003). Withdrawal of cyclophosphamide and substitution of azathioprine after remission did not increase the rate of relapse. These data suggest that the treatment of MPA should comprise initial high-dose corticosteroids with a cytotoxic agent, followed by transition to a less toxic maintenance agent after achieving remission (Molloy and Langford, 2006).

Intravenous immunoglobulin (IVIg) gave conflicting results. One placebo-controlled trial of relapsed ANCA-associated vasculitides included 17 patients treated with IVIg (0.4 g/kg/day for 5 days) versus 17 treated with placebo (Jayne *et al.*, 2000). Treatment responses were found in 14 (IVIg) versus 6 (placebo) patients per group, respectively ($p = .015$). Mild, reversible side effects were frequent in the IVIg group. A single course of IVIg reduced disease activity, but the effect was not maintained beyond 3 months (Jayne *et al.*, 2000). A French prospective study (2005) including patients with relapsed ANCA-associated systemic vasculitis received monthly infusions of IVIg for 6 months in addition to conventional treatment (Guillevin *et al.*, 2007). Complete remission was achieved in 59% of cases (13/22), without severe adverse effects. The therapeutic effects of IVIg are the following: modulation/regulation of FcγR expression in leukocytes and endothelial cells, interaction with complements, modulation of cytokine/chemokine synthesis/release, neutralization of circulating antibodies, and interaction with lymphocytes and monocytes (Guillevin *et al.*, 2007). Infliximab, an anti-TNF-α monoclonal antibody associated with conventional therapy, succeeded in remission in 88% of patients (32 cases) with active ANCA-associated vasculitis, including MPA (40%) and Wegener's granulomatosis (59%) (Booth *et al.*, 2004). Etanercept, another TNF-α blocker, has been tested only in Wegener's granulomatosis (The Wegener's granulomatosis etanercept trial (WGET) research group, 2005).

Rituximab is a chimeric monoclonal IgC1-κ immunoglobulin directed against the CD20 antigen of B lymphocytes. Rituximab

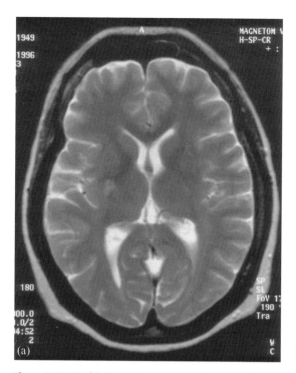 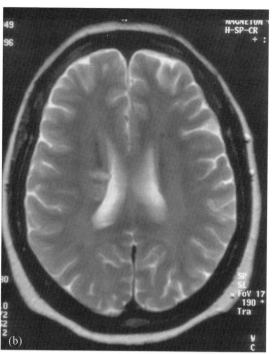

Figure 43.2 MRI of Patient 3, Lausanne, 1996; lacunar stroke involving the posterior limb of the right internal capsule (**A**) and adjacent corona radiate (**B**) on T2-weighted image (Reichhart *et al.*, 2000; patient 3).

has been proven an effective remission induction agent and is well tolerated for severe refractory Wegener's granulomatosis in 10 patients (Keogh *et al.*, 2006). A case series of nine patients with refractory ANCA-positive vasculitis (MPA, 2; Wegener's granulomatosis, 7) showed complete remission in all but one (partial remission) with rituximab therapy (Eriksson, 2005). Another similar series of 10 patients (MPA, 2; Wegener's granulomatosis, 8) also confirmed complete response in all but one (9 cases) including the two MPA-patients and partial remission in the remaining case at 6 month (Stasi *et al.*, 2006).

Neurological complications

Neurological complications of patients with MPA occur less frequently than in those with PAN, and were reported in 8%–16% of cases in early series (Hogan *et al.*, 1996; Nachman *et al.*, 1996; Westman *et al.*, 1998). Peripheral nerve involvement, including mononeuritis multiplex and polyneuropathy, occurs in 4%–58% of MPA patients (Adu *et al.*, 1987; Agard *et al.*, 2003; Ara *et al.*, 1999; Gordon *et al.*, 1993; Guillevin *et al.*, 1999; Jayne *et al.*, 1995; Lane, Watts, Shepstone, *et al.*, 2005; Pavone *et al.*, 2006; Rodgers *et al.*, 1989; Savage *et al.*, 1985; Weidner *et al.*, 2004). CNS involvement was reported in 8%–29% of cases in previous series (Agard *et al.*, 2003; Bourgarit *et al.*, 2005; Guillevin *et al.*, 1999; Lane, Watts, Shepstone, *et al.*, 2005; Pavone *et al.*, 2006; Rodgers *et al.*, 1989; Savage *et al.*, 1985; Weidner *et al.*, 2004). The type of CNS complication was specified as headache and seizure (Savage *et al.*, 1985), ischemic or hemorrhagic stroke in one case each (Agard *et al.*, 2003), and as seizure with monoplegia and alteration in consciousness level, optic atrophy and sensineural deafness, subarachnoid hemorrhage, and pseudo-bulbar palsy in one case each (Rodgers *et al.*, 1989).

MPA-associated strokes

Hemorrhagic (including secondary) strokes occur more frequently than ischemic infarction. Bleeding also occurs in other organs: hemoptysia/alveolar hemorrhage (lung) and hematuria (kidney). Among the six published MPA-associated strokes, three were ischemic with secondary hemorrhagic transformation (Honda *et al.*, 1996; Ito *et al.*, 2006; Sasaki *et al.*, 1998), one was purely hemorrhagic (Han *et al.*, 2006), and two were purely ischemic (Deshpande *et al.*, 2000; Reichhart *et al.*, 2000). One case report was excluded (Nakane *et al.*, 1997), because positive p-ANCA and antinuclear antibodies are known to occur in rheumatoid arthritis-associated vasculitis (Bosch *et al.*, 1995). Patient 3 (1996, Lausanne, reported below) with positive p-ANCA both in the serum and cerebrospinal fluid (CSF) (Reichhart *et al.*, 2000) represents a MPA-related stroke. She developed an ischemic infarct in the territory of the anterior choroidal artery (see Figure 43.2, A and B) (Reichhart *et al.*, 2000). The clinical and neuroradiological features, other organ involvement, laboratory results, treatment, and outcome of these five MPA-associated strokes are summarized in Table 43.3.

Patient 3, 1996 (Lausanne)

A 55-year-old Italian woman developed over 2 months asthenia, weight loss (5 kg), night fever (38.5°C), hypertension, large joint arthritis, myalgia, lower limb livedo reticularis, and Raynaud's phenomena. She was admitted for a bilateral asymmetric peroneal mononeuritis (confirmed electrophysiologically). There were biological signs of inflammation (ESR, 90 mm/h; white blood cell [WBC] count, 13.4 G/L; eosinophiles, 15%) and renal failure with nephrotic syndrome. The diagnosis of PAN was made by sural nerve and renal biopsy, although positive p-ANCAs were

Table 43.3 Clinical and neuroradiological features, other organ involvement, laboratory results, treatment, and outcome of six MPA-associated strokes

Author year	Age/ Sex	Clinical features	Neuroimaging	Organ involvement	Laboratory findings	Treatment	Outcome
Honda *et al.*, 1996	56/F	Seizures, L hemiparesis hypesthesia, R homonymous hemianopia	B occipital infarcts (1st MRI), L occipital + R temporal lobar hemorrhages (2nd MRI)	PNP, intestinal hemorrhage, NCGN	p-ANCA (MPO, 1000 EU/mL)	Pulsed MP, plasmapheresis, PSL	Favorable
Reichhart *et al.*, 2000 (Patient 3, 1996)	55/F	L sensorimotor syndrome	R lacunar infarct of the posterior limb of the internal capsule (MRI, Figure 43.2)	MM, renal failure + nephrotic syndrome, arthritis, myalgia, LR	p-ANCA (1/320 EIA), p-ANCA (CSF, 2 EIA)	Pulsed MP + CYC, P, ASA	Favorable
Sasaki *et al.*, 1998	78/M	L hemiparesis, homonymous hemianopia	R frontoparietal infarct (MRI), multiple hemorrhagic strokes(autopsy)	Renal failure (NCGN), digestive tract massive hemorrhage, alveolar hemorrhage	p-ANCA (637)	Unknown	Died
Deshpande *et al.*, 2000	15/F	Blurred vision, headache, seizures, probable visual agnosia	B occipital ischemic strokes, normalized at 2 mo (MRI)	NCGN, pulmonary edema, pleural effusion	p-ANCA (MPO, 26 EU/mL; N < 3)	Pulsed MP, CYC, P, 5 PE, pulsed CYC	Favorable
Ito *et al.*, 2006	56/M	R hemiparesis, dysarthria, coma	B corona radiata infarcts (MRI), cerebral + ventricular massive hemorrhage (CT)	PNP	p-ANCA (640 U)	Pulsed MP (2), PSL, heparin 10000 UI/day	Died
Han *et al.*, 2006	43/M	L amaurosis fugax, followed by L hemiparesis + homonymous hemianopia, coma	R ICA occlusion (1st MRI), R parietotemporal + ventricular hemorrhage (CT)	Myalgia, arthritis, deafness, NCGN, microinfarction of kidney, spleen, adrenals (no granuloma, necropsy)	c-ANCA (1:80), PR3 (40 U/ml)	Antibiotics, ASA, P, pulsed MP + CYC	Died

L = left; R = right; B = bilateral; MP = methylprednisolone; P = prednisone; PSL = prednisolone; LR = livedo reticularis; MM = mononeuritis multiplex; PNP = polyneuropathy; NCGN = necrotizing crescentic glomerulonephritis; mo = months; ASA = acetisylate acid; EIA= enzyme immuno assay; CYC = cyclophosphamide; PE = plasma exchange; ICA = internal carotid artery.

found in the serum (1/320 EIA). Corticosteroids were promptly initiated, but 8 hours later she developed a left-side sensorimotor syndrome without hemineglect (two adjacent right-side deep small infarcts, anterior choroidal artery territory; Figure 43.2, A and B). Echocardiography and Doppler studies of the carotids were normal, and tests for coagulation (including antithrombin III and anti-cardiolipin antibodies) were normal. CSF immunoelectrophoresis showed signs of blood-brain barrier rupture (p-ANCA could therefore also be detected in the CSF). Following treatment with intravenous corticosteroids then prednisone (1 mg/kg/d), together with antiplatelet drug (ASA, 200 mg), and intravenous pulsed cyclophosphamide therapy (750 mg/m^2/month), the clinical course improved. During a 3-year follow-up,

there was no stroke recurrence. Retrospectively, applying the Chapell Hill nomenclature, this patient represents the first published lacunar stroke syndrome associated with MPA rather than with PAN, as previously reported (Reichhart *et al.*, 2000).

PAN

Clinical features

Classic PAN is a rare disease, with an annual incidence of 0.7–1.8 and prevalence of 6.3 per 100 000 habitants (biopsy-proven study, 1983) (Brown and Swash, 1989; Guillevin *et al.*, 1997a; Lhote *et al.*, 1998). Applying the Chapel Hill definition for PAN, one series found an annual incidence of only 0.16 cases per 100 000 (Selga *et al.*, 2006). The PAN prevalence was estimated to be 2–9 per million using Chapel Hill criteria and 33 per million (ACR criteria; Table 43.1), respectively, whereas a recent French study estimated it at 30.7 per million, including about 30% of cases with hepatitis B virus (Mahr *et al.*, 2004). The annual incidence rate of PAN ranges from 4.6 (England), to 9.0 (Minnesota), to 77 per million in a hepatitis B virus hyperendemic Alaskan Eskimo population (Guillevin *et al.*, 1997a; Lhote *et al.*, 1998). The frequency of hepatitis B virus-associated PAN in developed countries has decreased from 36% in the 1970s to 7%–10% now (immunization, screening of blood donors) (Colmegna and Maldonado-Cocco, 2005; Guillevin *et al.*, 1997a; Lhote *et al.*, 1998).

The association between PAN and hepatitis B virus surface antigen (so-called Australia antigen) was first recognized by Trépo and Thivolet (1970) and Gocke *et al.* (1970). This etiology of PAN has been further confirmed in large hepatitis B virus-PAN series (Guillevin *et al.*, 2005; Guillevin, Lhote, Cohen, *et al.*, 1995b). The following viruses were found to be associated with PAN: hepatitis C virus, detected in <5% of PAN patients (Guillevin, 2004; Guillevin *et al.*, 1997b; Pagnoux *et al.*, 2006); HIV (Chetty, 2001; Gherardi *et al.*, 1993; Guillevin, 2004; Guillevin *et al.*, 1997b; Pagnoux *et al.*, 2006); erythrovirus B19 (Guillevin, 1999b; Guillevin and Lhote, 1998; Pagnoux *et al.*, 2006); cytomegalovirus (Pagnoux *et al.*, 2006); and Epstein-Barr virus (Caldeira *et al.*, 2007). However, except for hepatitis B virus, the role of these viruses in the pathogenesis of PAN remains controversial (Mandell and Calabrese, 1998; Stone, 2002). PAN may be secondary to hairy cell leukemia, Sjögren's syndrome, or rheumatoid arthritis (Colmegna and Maldonado-Cocco, 2005; Conn, 1990).

PAN affects equally men and women at any age and of all ethic groups, with a predominance between the ages of 40 and 60 years (Guillevin *et al.*, 1997a; Lhote *et al.*, 1998), and with a mean age of 52 years (Gayraud *et al.*, 2001; Guillevin, Lhote, Gayraud, *et al.*, 1996). A spectrum of systemic organ involvement exists in PAN, excepting the lung, which ranges from limited forms of PAN to multisystem disease (Colmegna and Maldonado-Cocco, 2005; Segelmark and Selga, 2007). Organ-limited varieties of PAN comprise the following: cutaneous form including nodules, ulcers, and livedo reticularis (Colmegna and Maldonado-Cocco, 2005; Segelmark and Selga, 2007); striated muscle form (Kamimura *et al.*, 2005; Segelmark and Selga, 2007); and primary angiitis of the CNS (see Chapter 1) form (MacLaren *et al.*, 2005; Segelmark and Selga, 2007). According to large series (Bonsib, 2001; Brown and Swash, 1989; Colmegna and Maldonado-Cocco, 2005; Conn, 1990; Guillevin *et al.*, 1997a), the frequency ranges of clinical features of PAN vary as follows, in decreasing order: general symptoms (76%–81%) including fever (31%–81%) and weight loss (54%–66%); peripheral neuropathy (50%–75%), renal involvement (35%–70%), musculoskeletal (25%–64%) including myalgias (30%–73%), arthralgia or arthritis (46%–53%), gastrointestinal tract (23%–60%) with abdominal pain (34%–43%) including acute surgical abdomen in one-third of cases, skin (25%–60%), hypertension (40%–54%), heart (20%–36%), genital tract (21%), CNS (10%–20%), and eye (20%). The clinical features of hepatitis B virus-associated PAN are roughly similar to classic PAN, with the exceptions of higher frequencies of malignant hypertension (29.6%), orchiepidymitis (26%), renal infarction (26%–28%), and abdominal manifestations (46.3%) (Guillevin *et al.*, 2005; Guillevin, Lhote, Cohen, *et al.*, 1995b; Guillevin, Lhote, Gayraud, *et al.*, 1996; Lhote *et al.*, 1998; Trepo and Guillevin, 2001). These differences were confirmed in a recent large hepatitis B virus-PAN series, which found no cases with positive ANCA or glomerulonephritis (Guillevin *et al.*, 2005). Contrary to MPA, no specific laboratory test or clinical findings confirms or excludes the diagnosis of PAN. The diagnosis requires the integration of clinical, angiographic, and biopsy findings. PAN should be suspected in patients with constitutional symptoms and multisystem involvement (Colmegna and Maldonado-Cocco, 2005). PAN must be highly considered in patients with systemic vasculitis, orchitis, abnormal angiographic findings, absence of glomerulonephritis, and ANCA negativity (Guillevin, Lhote, Amouroux, *et al.*, 1996).

Laboratory findings

An ESR > 60 mm/hour (78%–89%), increased C-reactive protein, high a2-globulin level, leukocytosis (45%–75%), normochromic anemia (34%–79%), and thrombocytosis are often found (Conn, 1990; Lhote *et al.*, 1998). Hypereosinophilia > 500/mm^3 (20%), diminished levels of serum albumin, and concentrations of serum whole complement and C3and C4 components (25%), presence of immune complexes, and positive rheumatoid factor (40%) are less common findings (Conn, 1990; Kirkland *et al.*, 1997; Lhote *et al.*, 1998). The presence of hepatitis B virus antigen was detected in 10%–54% of cases in the 1970s (Conn, 1990), in 36% of patients in the early 1980s (Guillevin, Le Thi, Godeau, *et al.*, 1988), in less than 10% of cases in 1990–92 (Guillevin, Lhote, Cohen, *et al.*, 1995b), and in 17.4% of cases in 1997–2002 (Guillevin *et al.*, 2005). Positive ANCAs were previously detected in 10%–27% of patients with PAN in the 1990s (Lhote *et al.*, 1998), but more recently in less than 10% of cases (Colmegna and Maldonado-Cocco, 2005), and were absent in the largest recent hepatitis B virus-PAN series (Guillevin *et al.*, 2005).

Biopsy and angiographic findings

The procedure of single biopsy followed by angiography has a diagnostic sensitivity of 85% and a specificity of 96% (Albert *et al.*, 1988). The "gold standard" for the diagnosis of PAN is a biopsy that shows focal, segmental, panmural necrotizing inflammation of medium-sized arteries (Colmegna and Maldonado-Cocco, 2005; Lhote *et al.*, 1998). Different stages of inflammation often co-exist: the acute stage shows fibrinoid necrosis of the media with neutrophils, monocytes, lymphocytes (CD8$^+$ T cells), and sometimes eosinophilic infiltration (see Figure 43.3, A–C), whereas the healing phase shows intimal and medial proliferation (i.e. with collagen deposition and fibrosis, so-called fibrotic endarteritis, see Figure 43.4) leading to arterial narrowing or occlusion, with secondary infarction (Bonsib, 2001; Colmegna and Maldonado-Cocco, 2005; Guillevin *et al.*, 1997a; Lhote and Guillevin, 1995). Aneurysms with either hemorrhage or thrombosis may be seen. No granulomas are present (Colmegna and Maldonado-Cocco, 2005).

(a)

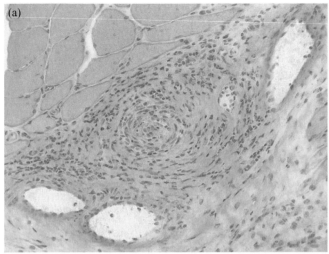

(b)

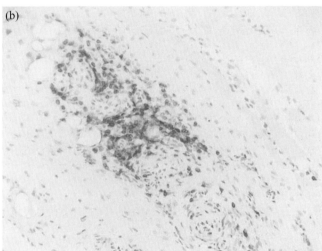

(c)

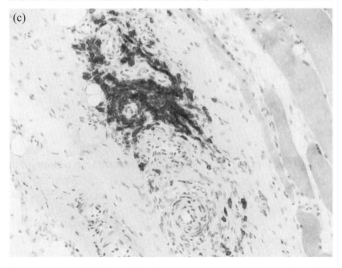

Figure 43.3 Muscular biopsy of Patient 6, 2004, Lausanne. Hematoxylin and eosin staining shows typical inflammation of a small-sized artery, with perivascular inflammation (**A**). Staining for CD3 confirms T lymphocytes infiltration (**B**). Staining for CD20 shows B lymphocyte infiltration (**C**). See color plate. Figures courtesy of Prof. R. Janzer, Department of Pathology, Lausanne.

A

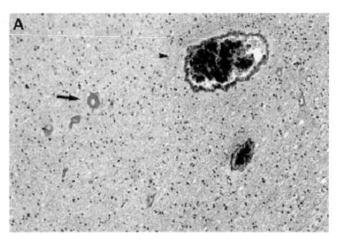

Figure 43.4 Microscopic examination of cerebral arteries of Patient 1, 1982, Lausanne (Van Gieson-Luxol), showing arterial wall fibrosis (*purple-red*) of arterioles and small arteries with fibrosis of the media and adventice (*full arrow*). Two small venules (*arrowhead*) are normal. See color plate. (Reichhart *et al.*, 2000).

The pathologic process affects medium- and small-sized arteries, less frequently arterioles, and rarely venules. Large elastic arteries such as the aorta and pulmonary arteries are rarely involved (Lhote *et al.*, 1998).

PAN has a predilection for arterial bifurcations and branch points (Bonsib, 2001), and the pattern of aneurysms was compared with "apples on a branching tree" by Kussmaul and Maier (1866). The most accessible symptomatic sites for biopsy are skeletal muscle (see Figure 43.3, A–C), sural nerve, kidney, testis, liver, and rectum (Lhote *et al.*, 1998). Biopsies of apparently unaffected muscles (see Figure 43.3, A–C) may show vasculitis in 30%–50% of cases (Conn, 1990; Lhote *et al.*, 1998). Kidney and liver biopsies are more invasive procedures, and visceral angiography should be performed prior to biopsy to demonstrate aneurysms, in order to avoid the hazard of visceral bleeding (Lhote *et al.*, 1998). Punch skin biopsies are easy to perform, but may show only nonspecific signs of small-vessel vasculitis (Lhote *et al.*, 1998).

First described by Bron *et al.* (1965), visceral angiography was only included near 30 years later as the gold standard radiologic procedure for the diagnosis of PAN in the ACR criteria (Lightfoot *et al.*, 1990). The hallmark of PAN is angiographic visualization of saccular or fusiform microaneurysms (1–5 mm) in medium-sized renal or visceral arteries (see Figure 43.1, A and B) (Das and Pangtey, 2006) (Colmegna and Maldonado-Cocco, 2005; Lhote *et al.*, 1998). In one large series, when other diagnostic tests were negative, angiography confirmed the diagnosis of PAN in one-fifth of cases (Guillevin *et al.*, 1992). Another hepatitis B-PAN series showed renal and/or celiomesenteric microaneurysms in 50% of patients with abdominal symptoms (Guillevin, Lhote, Cohen, *et al.*, 1995b). Finally, aneurysms were found in 61% (34) of 56 consecutive PAN patients with abnormal angiographic findings (Stanson *et al.*, 2001). Aneurysm demonstration by selective abdominal angiography has a sensitivity of 89% and a specificity of 90% for the diagnosis of PAN, with a positive predictive value of 55% and a negative predictive value of 98% (Hekali *et al.*, 1991).

Pathogenesis

The pathologic features of PAN are fully described (Bonsib, 2001). The pathogenesis of classic PAN is not as well established as for hepatitis B virus-PAN, particularly the role of immune complexes. In the setting of neurological complications, Moore and Cupps (1983) mentioned 20 years ago that "tissue ischemia is the common denominator of the vasculitides" and "even after the acute inflammation has resolved, ischemia may be sustained by fibrotic narrowing of the vessel wall." Ten years later, Moore (1995) and Conn (1990) postulated that endothelial cells play a prominent role in the vasculitic inflammatory process. First, a number of procoagulants and anticoagulants associated with the endothelium have an anticoagulant effect under normal physiological conditions, which balanced in favor of procoagulant effects (via interleukin-1 [IL-1] and TNF-α) on the endothelium during inflammation. Second, modulation of the vascular tone, which depends on the release of vasodilatators (i.e. prostacyclin; endothelium-derived relaxation factor, like nitric oxide, and vasoconstrictors, including endothelin), is also affected by inflammation with impaired endothelium-dependent relaxation and release of endothelin, which may further lead to vasoconstriction and thrombosis (Conn, 1990; Moore, 1995). As demonstrated in Kawasaki disease (see Chapter 13), circulating thromboxane B2 (derived from thromboxane A2) is increased, whereas prostacyclin is decreased, resulting in vasoconstriction and platelet aggregation (Conn, 1990). The analogy of these processes with those of atherosclerosis was first recognized by Conn (1990) Endothelial cell dysfunction, such as impaired endothelium-dependent (via nitrous oxide) vasodilatation is known to have a major role and is the earliest measurable physiological abnormality in atherosclerosis; impaired endothelium-derived vasodilatation was shown in PAN and other vasculitides (Filer *et al.*, 2003). The main issue is if direct (i.e. vasculitic process) mechanisms, indirect (cytokines or anti-endothelial antibodies) mechanisms, or both, promote endothelial cells dysfunction in PAN (and other vasculitides) (Colmegna and Maldonado-Cocco, 2005). A variety of anti-endothelial cell antibodies have been detected in ANCA-associated vasculitis but not in PAN (Chanseaud *et al.*, 2003). Conversely, increased serum levels of TNF-α, IFN-γ, IL-2, and more recently IL-8 (Freire *et al.*, 2004), a potent chemoattractant and activator of neutrophils, have been documented in PAN (Colmegna and Maldonado-Cocco, 2005). Moderated elevations of TNF-α and IL-1β also have been detected. Increased levels of circulating soluble adhesions molecules (ICAM-1, VCAM-1, E-selectin) have been found in PAN (Coll-Vinent *et al.*, 1997). The expression of class I and the inducing of major histocompability complex (MHC) class II antigens that lead to antigen presentation to T cells are increased by TNF-α and IFN-γ. Immunohistochemical studies from muscle and nerve biopsies showed that macrophages and T cells, mostly CD8+, are involved in the pathogenesis of PAN (Colmegna and Maldonado-Cocco, 2005).

In hepatitis B virus-PAN, as for virus-associated vasculitis pathogenesis, two mechanisms have been incriminated (Trepo and Guillevin, 2001). First, virus replication might induce direct injury of the vessel wall, like in equine viral arteritis (Trepo and Guillevin, 2001). Second, vascular damage might be the result of immune mechanisms, cellular and/or humoral, and include immune complex deposition and/or in situ formation (Trepo and Guillevin, 2001). These factors lead to activation of the complement cascade, whose products, in turn, attract and activate neutrophils (Colmegna and Maldonado-Cocco, 2005). In hepatitis B (HB) virus-PAN, glomerular deposits of HB s, c, and e antigens (together with immunoglobulins and C3) have been documented, together with low complement levels in the serum (CH50, C3, C4) (Trepo and Guillevin, 2001). The most likely responsible antigen is HB e antigen based on ultrastructural and immunostaining findings. Furthermore, HB e antigen measures 19 kd and complexes with Ig of 300 kd size, whereas HB s antigen alone is three million kd large. Experimental studies showed that only complexes of one million kilodaltons or less could induce serum sickness and glomerulonephritis. Finally, all cases of hepatitis B virus-PAN are associated with the wild-type hepatitis B virus and hepatitis B virus e antigenemia and high virus replication, supporting the hypothesis that lesions could result from viral antigen-antibody complexes soluble in antigen excess, possibly involving hepatitis B virus e antigen (Trepo and Guillevin, 2001). This hypothesis is challenged by recent observations of cases with PAN associated with precore mutation that abrogates hepatitis B e antigen formation (Wartelle-Bladou *et al.*, 2001). The immunologic process inducing PAN occurs within 6 months after hepatitis B virus infection. During active hepatitis B virus-PAN, serum levels of complements are low due to their consumption by immune complex deposition. Finally, no relationship between PAN and hepatitis B vaccination has been proven (Begier *et al.*, 2004).

Outcome and treatment

Classic PAN

In 1951, Bagenstoss *et al.* first reported two PAN patients treated with cortisone who had partial clinical improvement as well as complete vascular healing of all arterial lesions at autopsy, at 3 weeks and 3 months, respectively; they also noted "however, in the process of healing, that fibrous obliteration of the lumina of these vessels occurred and resulted in infarcts particularly in the kidneys, heart, and intestinal tract" (Bagenstoss *et al.*, 1951). Untreated patients with PAN had a 5-year survival rate of <15% (Frohnert and Sheps, 1967; Leib *et al.*, 1979). Corticosteroids were the first applied treatment and increased the 5-year survival to 48–57% (Cohen *et al.*, 1980; Frohnert and Sheps, 1967; Leib *et al.*, 1979; Sack *et al.*, 1975). The beneficial effects of corticosteroids are complex, acting both on the cell and humoral immune system, by inhibiting activated T and B cells, MHC class II antigen-presenting cell, leukocytes at inflammation sites, IFN-γ, induced class II expression, by interfering with macrophage differentiation, cytokine expression, complement activation, and immunomodulating cell adhesion molecules (Younger, 2004). Beneficial effects were also observed with combined therapy with cyclophosphamide and corticosteroids (Fauci *et al.*, 1979; Leib *et al.*, 1979), particularly in patients with advanced PAN (Fauci et al., 1978). Conversely, one series found no better improvement in outcome for patients treated with a combination of cyclophosphamide and corticosteroids as compared to those receiving corticosteroids alone (Cohen et al., 1980).

Most outcome and treatment data for the management of PAN have come from trials beginning in 1980 and performed by the French Vasculitis Study Group. In the first trial that included patients with PAN and Churg-Strauss syndrome, patients were randomized to receive prednisone plus plasma exchange, either alone or in combination with daily cyclophosphamide (Guillevin et al., 1991). The 3-year ad interim analysis (71 patients enrolled) showed a greater efficacy and fewer relapses in the cyclophosphamide group, but the cumulative 10-year survival rate showed no differences regarding patients initially treated with cyclophosphamide. Further studies also failed to confirm a difference in survival in the analysis of survival curves based on the initial use of cyclophosphamide (Guillevin, Lhote, Gayraud, et al., 1996). Although these trials showed the effectiveness of cyclophosphamide, questions were raised as to which treatment regimen might be more effective in patients with severe PAN and Churg-Strauss syndrome and poor outcome (Guillevin, Lhote, Gayraud, et al., 1996). The Five-Factors Score (FFS) was derived from the following items associated with increased mortality: serum creatinine > 1.58 mg/dL (≥140 μmol/L), proteinuria > 1 g/day, gastrointestinal tract involvement (bleeding, perforation, infarction, and pancreatitis), CNS involvement, and cardiomyopathy. A score of 0 is given when none of the five factors is present, 1 when 1 factor is present, and an FFS of ≥ 2 when ≥ 2 factors are present (Guillevin, Lhote, Gayraud, et al., 1996). Patients with an FFS of ≥ 2, 1, and 0 have had a 5-year survival rate of, respectively, 54%, 75%, and 88% (i.e. good prognosis PAN) (Guillevin, 1999a; Guillevin, Lhote, Gayraud, et al., 1996; Langford, 2001). In their largest trial, outcome was assessed by the FFS and the Birmingham Vasculitis Activity Score, and the entire cohort was reclassified according to the ACR, the Chapel Hill Consensus Conference, and their own criteria for discriminating PAN, hepatitis B virus-PAN, MPA, and Churg-Strauss syndrome (Gayraud et al., 2001). The results of this study showed that the initial treatment of patients with severe PAN (FFS of ≥ 2) should consist of corticosteroids together with cyclophosphamide (Gayraud et al., 2001). These findings were confirmed in a further prospective study that showed that the combination of corticosteroids plus cyclophosphamide improved prognosis for patients with FFS ≥ 2, and those with FFS = 0 could be initially treated with corticosteroids alone, with cyclophosphamide being added for unresponsive or worsening disease (Guillevin, 1999a; Guillevin et al., 2003; Langford, 2001). Cyclophosphamide remains the only cytotoxic drug that has been evaluated in such prospective trials in PAN. Regarding the route of administration, pulsed cyclophosphamide therapy (monthly intravenous pulses) is the recommended regimen for PAN (Colmegna and Maldonado-Cocco, 2005; Gayraud et al., 1997; Guillevin, 1999a; Guillevin, Lhote, Cohen, et al., 1995a). The aforementioned trial also studied the duration of cyclophosphamide pulse therapy (six over 4 months, 12 cases; 12 over 10 months, six cases) in 18 PAN patients with FFS ≥ 1, and found a

3-year event-free survival rate of 80% (12 cyclophosphamide pulses group) versus 71% (six cyclophosphamide pulses group) (Guillevin et al., 2003). The authors concluded that treating PAN patients with factors of poor prognosis with 12 rather than 6 cyclophosphamide pulses in combination with corticosteroids for 12 months significantly lowered the relapse rate and increased the probability of a good outcome (Guillevin et al., 2003).

Whether this regimen requires subsequent maintenance therapy needs further study. As regards TNF-α blockers, to date, only two case reports of patients with childhood PAN that was successfully treated with infliximab have been published (Brik et al., 2007; Keystone, 2004). In one of them (aged 20 months), presenting with CNS involvement (bilateral thalamic infarcts), the disease was resistant to standard intravenous corticosteroids and pulsed cyclophosphamide therapy, and marked clinical and neuroradiological improvement was observed after infliximab treatment over 10 months (Brik et al., 2007). However, anti-TNF-α antibody use should be restricted to patients with vasculitis refractory to corticosteroids and immunosuppressants who have relapsed (Guillevin and Mouthon, 2004).

Hepatitis B virus-related PAN

Whereas the clinical course of hepatitis B virus-PAN, occurring within 6 months after primary infection, is similar to those of classic PAN, the reported mortality rate is higher in the former (30%) than in the latter (15%) if the appropriate treatment is not promptly prescribed (Guillevin et al., 2005; Guillevin, Lhote, Cohen, et al., 1995b; Guillevin, Lhote, Gayraud, et al., 1996; Oyoo and Espinoza, 2005; Trepo and Guillevin, 2001). In the analysis of the largest French Vasculitis Study group cohort (595 patients), the first-year survival rate was 82% for hepatitis B virus-PAN, compared to 91% for classic PAN (Bourgarit et al., 2005). Factors associated with unfavorable outcome were severe gastrointestinal (50% vs. 27%) and renal involvements (36% vs. 27%). In the hepatitis B virus group, a trend toward better 1-year survival was observed in patients treated with antiviral agents compared to those who were not (86% vs. 74%) (Bourgarit et al., 2005). Guillevin and colleagues, based on the efficacy of antiviral agents in chronic hepatitis, and plasma exchange in immune complex-mediated diseases, combine both therapies to treat hepatitis B virus-PAN (Guillevin, 2004; Guillevin et al., 2007; Oyoo and Espinoza, 2005; Trepo and Guillevin, 2001). The rationale for this combination therapy was to obtain the following effects: (i) initial corticosteroids to control immediately the most severe life-threatening manifestations of PAN (first weeks); (ii) their abrupt stop to enhance immunological clearance of hepatitis B virus-infected hepatocytes and favor hepatitis B e antigen to anti-hepatitis B virus e antibody seroconversion; and (iii) plasma exchange combination to control the course of hepatitis B virus-PAN and clear immune complexes (Guillevin, 2004; Guillevin et al., 2007; Trepo and Guillevin, 2001).

The first results of this combined therapy in patients with hepatitis B virus-PAN were published in 1988 (Guillevin, Merrouche, Gayraud, et al., 1988). In a further prospective trial in 33 patients, using vidarabine as an antiviral agent, complete clinical recovery was achieved in three-quarters of cases, hepatitis B antigen to anti-hepatitis B e antibody seroconversion was obtained in about half of cases, whereas hepatitis B virus s to anti-hepatitis B s antigen to anti-hepatitis B s antibody seroconversion was observed only in 18% of cases (Guillevin *et al.*, 1993). This latter low seroconversion rate was attributed to the limited efficacy of vidarabine (Guillevin, 2004; Guillevin *et al.*, 1993). Other antiviral agents like IFN-α (Guillevin *et al.*, 1994), lamudivine (Guillevin *et al.*, 2004), and more recently adefovir (adefovir dipivoxil, 10 mg/day) (Farrell and Teoh, 2006; Guillevin *et al.*, 2007; Pagnoux *et al.*, 2006), give better results and should be preferred to vidarabine (Guillevin, 2004; Guillevin *et al.*, 2007). Adefovir has shown to be as effective and well-tolerated as lamudivine in the treatment of chronic hepatitis B, and can be effective against lamudivine-resistant virus strains, along or in combination with other new antiviral agents (entecavir, emtricitabine, clevudine); these drugs need further trials for the treatment of hepatitis B virus-PAN (Pagnoux *et al.*, 2006). The prescribed IFN-α dose is three million units, injected subcutaneously three times a week, for 4–6 months; if no seroconversion occurs, the dose can be increased to six million units (three times/week) (Guillevin, 2004; Pagnoux *et al.*, 2006). The prescribed dose of lamudivine is 100 mg/day, as for IFN-α, after a few days of corticosteroids, in combination with plasma exchange; in the case of seroconversion failure after 6 months, a combination with IFN-α or with newer antiviral agents should be proposed (Guillevin, 2004; Pagnoux *et al.*, 2006). The optimal schedule of plasma exchange is as follows: four sessions per week for 3 weeks, then three sessions per week for 2–3 weeks, followed by a tapering of frequency of sessions. One plasma volume (60 ml/kg) is usually exchanged using 4% albumin fluid (Guillevin, 2004; Guillevin *et al.*, 2007; Pagnoux *et al.*, 2006). With adequate therapy, the 7-year survival rate has improved to 83%, and relapses have been rare (Guillevin *et al.*, 2007).

As regards childhood vasculitis, hepatitis B virus–PAN and classic PAN are considered as completely separate entities (Ozen *et al.*, 2006).

Neurological complications

Neurological symptoms and signs are a major and common feature of PAN, occurring in nearly three-quarters of patients (Brown and Swash, 1989). The most frequent neurological complication and often inaugural manifestation of PAN is peripheral nervous system involvement, found in 50%–75% of cases (Bonsib, 2001; Brown and Swash, 1989; Cohen *et al.*, 1980; Cohen *et al.*, 1993; Colmegna and Maldonado-Cocco, 2005; Conn, 1990; Ford and Siekert, 1965; Guillevin *et al.*, 1997a; Lhote *et al.*, 1998; Moore and Cupps, 1983; Younger, 2004). The most common types of peripheral nervous system complications comprise polyneuropathy, mononeuritis, mononeuritis multiplex, and cutaneous sensory neuropathy, found in 50%–60% of cases (Moore and Cupps, 1983). Mononeuritis multiplex is the most frequent manifestation of PAN, found in 70% of cases in a large series of 182 PAN patients (Guillevin *et al.*, 1992), and more recently in 83.5% of 115 patients with hepatitis B virus-PAN (Guillevin *et al.*, 2005). Mononeuritis multiplex induces severe asymmetric distal

Table 43.4 Neurological manifestations of PAN	
Neurological manifestations	% frequency
Peripheral neuropathy	67
Headache	30
Retinopathy	29
Diffuse encephalopathy	16
Focal stroke or cerebral deficit	14
Cranial neuropathy	9
Seizure	7
Inflammatory myopathy	6
Retinal artery occlusion	3
Subarachnoid hemorrhage	<1

Source: Brown and Swash, 1989.

weakness and sensory loss due to sequential infarction of multiple individual peripheral nerves; the most vulnerable sites are the midthigh and midarm, which therefore predominantly affect the peroneal and tibial branches of the sciatic nerve, and less frequently the median and cubital nerves (Lhote *et al.*, 1998; Moore and Cupps, 1983). Peripheral neuropathy is typically mononeuropathy multiplex, but symmetric distal bilateral neuropathy may occur (Lhote *et al.*, 1998). The CSF analysis is usually normal (Lhote *et al.*, 1998). Less frequently, radiculopathy and plexopathy occur (Brown and Swash, 1989; Moore and Cupps, 1983). Cranial neuropathy, involving the II, III, IV, VI, VII, and VIII cranial nerves have been reported in 2%–9% of cases (Brown and Swash, 1989; Lhote *et al.*, 1998; Moore and Cupps, 1983).

CNS involvement, although reputed to be rare, occurred in 20%–40% of patients with PAN and developed 2–3 years after the initial diagnosis was made (Chin and Latov, 2005; Guillevin *et al.*, 1997a; Moore and Cupps, 1983). Two subgroups of CNS complications have been recognized: (i) a diffuse encephalopathy pattern with cognitive and behavioral abnormalities, stupor, and seizures (see case history, Patient 5, Lausanne, 2000), and (ii) a focal pattern that includes ischemic stroke of the cerebral hemisphere, cerebellum, brainstem, and spinal cord, intracranial or subarachnoid hemorrhage, and meningeal irritation (Brown and Swash, 1989; Guillevin *et al.*, 1997a; Moore and Cupps, 1983). Table 43.4 summarizes the frequency of neurological manifestations of PAN, according to a review of 215 patients (Brown and Swash, 1989).

PAN-associated strokes

Stroke occurs in 11%–14% of PAN patients (Brown and Swash, 1989). We found that stroke often occurs earlier than previously reported (i.e. within 8 months after the disease onset) (Reichhart *et al.*, 2000). In a recent series of 36 patients with PAN, stroke was the first clinical indication attributable to vasculitis in one patient (3%), with a median time to diagnosis of 6.6 months (Agard *et al.*, 2003). An ischemic stroke in the territory of the anterior choroidal artery was inaugural and revealed the diagnosis of PAN in an 81-year-old patient (Marignier *et al.*, 2002).

The mechanisms, i.e. corticosteroid- or hypertension-induced atherosclerosis versus arteritic occlusions, and patterns of PAN-associated strokes are less well known (Cohen *et al.*, 1980; Conn, 1990; Moore, 1995; Moore and Cupps, 1983; Moore and Fauci, 1981).

In 1965, Ford and Siekert described ischemic and hemorrhagic strokes as late CNS manifestations in 19% of patients (total 114 patients) with PAN. Among 14 patients with cerebral hemispheric infarcts, pure ischemic, ischemic and hemorrhagic, and pure hemorrhagic strokes occurred in near on-third of patients each, respectively. Five patients showed multiple deep small ischemic or petechial hemorrhagic infarcts involving the basal ganglia, internal capsule, or the thalamus. Clinical evidence (one necropsy) for brainstem strokes was found in seven patients.

A more recent series of 53 patients with PAN found cerebrovascular disease as the cause of death in five patients, with a mean latency after the onset of the vasculitis of 2 years (Cohen *et al.*, 1980). Because all strokes occurred while the vasculitis was controlled by immunosupressive therapy (corticosteroids with/without cyclophosphamide or azathioprine), it was hypothesized that atherosclerosis-like mechanisms (promoted by long-term use of corticosteroids) were the cause of arterial occlusion in PAN. Another series described five PAN patients with clinical evidence of focal deficits occurring at either the cerebral, brainstem, or cerebellum level (CT abnormalities in only three patients) (Moore and Fauci, 1981). Again, all strokes occurred on corticosteroid therapy (with a mean latency of 2 years). Three patients had hypertension. Thus, it was suggested that vascular scarring was responsible for those late CNS complications of PAN.

To study the relationship between PAN-associated strokes and the use of corticosteroids, and trying to delineate a specific stroke syndrome in PAN, we analyzed the reported data of 11 patients with PAN and stroke (de la Fuente Fernandez and Grana Gil, 1994; Harlé *et al.*, 1991; Hirohata *et al.*, 1993; Iaconetta *et al.*, 1994; Kasantikul *et al.*, 1991; Koppensteiner *et al.*, 1989; Long and Dolin, 1994; Mayo *et al.*, 1986; Squire *et al.*, 1993; Stahl *et al.*, 1995; Wildhagen *et al.*, 1989), together with four similar patients from Lausanne University Hospital (Neurology Department, 1982–98) (Reichhart *et al.*, 2000). The details of the source, patient age and sex, clinical and neuroradiological features, latencies (between the onset of PAN and the cerebrovascular insult), and current immuno-suppressive therapy at onset – i.e. methylprednisolone, corticosteroids, prednisone, prednisolone, with/without cyclophosphamide or azathioprine, for the 15 PAN-associated strokes are listed in Table 43.5. Since then, two additional patients with PAN were admitted in our department (Patient 5, 2000; Patient 6, 2004). Overall, from 1982 to 2007, six patients with PAN (ACR criteria, Table 43.1), including one with MPA (Patient 3, Lausanne) were admitted, confirming the rarity of PAN-associated strokes (450 stroke admissions per year).

Patient 5, 2000 (Lausanne)

A 53-year-old man was admitted with confirmed PAN (see visceral angiography, Figure 43.1). He developed oscillopsia and audi-tory loss, but examination showed a right internuclear ophthalmoplegia, bilateral corticospinal signs, and signs of bilateral VIII cranial nerve palsies and livedo reticularis 2.5 months after corticosteroid therapy (prednisolone 1 mg/kg/day). Electroneuromyography confirmed a sensorimotor polyneuropathy. The first MRI showed signs of pontine leukoaraiosis (Figure 43.5A). Positive anti-cardiolipin antibodies (IgM, 107.2 U/mL, IgG 10.9 U/mL, N < 10), repeated 2 months later (IgM, 43.5 U/mL), were found. A few days later, he developed an acute encephalopathy with delirium, visual hallucinations, and neurobehavioral and cognitive abnormalities. Electroencephalogram confirmed a diffuse encephalopathy pattern (tetha-delta waves diffuse slowing) whereas CSF analysis showed aseptic inflammation (15 WBC/mL; protein 1180 mg/L). Repeated MRI showed multiple abnormal fluid-attenuated inversion recovery (FLAIR) signals (see Figure 43.5B). Pulsed methylprednisolone and cyclophosphamide were initiated, together with aspirin (100 mg/day). At 1 year follow-up, a marked neuropsychology and neurological improvement was noted.

Patient 6, 2004 (Lausanne)

This 59-year-old woman was known to have PAN, confirmed by muscle biopsy (Figure 43.3, A–C) with mononeuritis multiplex, treated 2 years ago with corticosteroids (prednisone, 50 mg/day) and pulsed cyclophosphamide therapy (14, 1 per month), without treatment for 6 months. She was admitted for a sudden right-sided ataxic, hypesthetic hemiparesis with dysarthria, without oculomotor abnormalities. An MRI (Figure 43.6A) confirmed a left paramedian lacunar stroke, without stenosis of the basilar artery on magnetic resonance angiography (Figure 43.6B). The clinical course gradually improved, and the patient returned home 6 days later, on ASA 300 mg/d. At 3-year follow-up, no stroke recurrence occurred.

The present study of 15 PAN-associated strokes (Table 43.5) shows similar population characteristics as a previously published series (male-to-female ratio, 1.5:1; mean age, 49 years). Lacunar syndromes seem to be the specific and most frequent (73%, 11/15) stroke pattern associated with PAN. More than half of them (55%, 6/11) developed either pure (four patients) / sensory (one patient) – motor strokes or ataxic hemiparesis (one patient), which correlated with typical small deep infarcts (internal capsule, lenticulate and caudate nucleus, centrum semi-ovale or corona radiata). Pontine lacunes (together with asymptomatic small deep infarcts in one case) were found in three patients (27%, 3/11), and the remaining patients had leukoaraiosis (18%, 2/11). This distribution of lacunes is similar to that described by Fisher (1965) and confirms a predominantly small- and medium-sized artery involvement in PAN, inducing multiple, small penetrating artery occlusions at the subcortical or pontine level.

This preponderance of lacunar stroke may be partially explained by PAN-associated hypertension, seen in 40% (Lhote *et al.*, 1998) to more than half of the patients (Moore and Cupps, 1983). The short-time interval between disease onset and subsequent cerebrovascular complications in the present series allows hypertension to be considered only as a risk-factor for stroke in PAN, rather than the main etiology. In fact, stroke developed within 14 months in

Table 43.5 Clinical and neuroradiological features, latencies (disease-onset to stroke), and current corticosteroid (CS) therapy at stroke onset (latencies between stroke and corticosteroid initiation) for the 15 PAN-associated strokes

No., source	Age Y/Sex	Clinical features	CT	MRI	Latencies (Months)	CS (Latencies)
1, Reichhart et al., 2000	49/F	Blt blindness	Blt temporo-occipital infarcts	Not available	2 1/2	P (2 months)
2, Reichhart et al., 2000	44/M	R hemiparesis		Blt centrum semiovale lacurae	2	P (3 days)
3, Reichhart et al., 2000	55/F	L sensorimotor syndrome		R capsular lacune	2	MP (8 hours)
4, Reichhart et al., 2000	67/M	Wernicke's aphasia, R hemianopia	L temporo-parietal hematoma	R caudate petechial Infarct	1	None
5, Mayo et al., 1986	68/M	Parkinsonian syndrome	L striatum lacune		3 weeks	None
	(	R hemiparesis		L capsular lacune	11 days	MP, P + CY (11 days)
6, Wildhagen et al., 1989	55/M	R ataxic hemiparesis		Blt centrum semiovale lacunes	12	CS + AZA (6 months)
7, Koppensteiner et al., 1989	35/M	Seizures, R hemiparesis		Multiple white matter T2-weighted signals	5	None
8, Kasantikul et al., 1991	35/F	L hemiparesis, pseudo bulbar syndrome		R pontine lacune	Inaugural	None
9, Harlé et al., 1991	64/M	Dementia, incontinence Pyramidal tract signs	Leukoaraiosis	Multiple white matter T2-weighted signals	13	MP + CY (13 months)
10, Iaconetta et al., 1994	38/F	Dysarthria, L hemiparesis	R temporo-parietal hematoma		1	Unknown
11, Squire et al., 1993	43/M	Dysarthria, L hemiparesis	R basal ganglia lacune		14	None
		Hemiparesis deterioration	New R basal ganglia lacune		3 weeks later	P + CY
		Hemiparesis deterioration	R temporo-parietal infarct		5 days later	P + CY (5 days)
12, Hirohata et al., 1993	26/M	L sensorimotor syndrome		Pontine lacune	32 months	Prednisolone 32 months
13, Long and Dolin, 1994	23/F	Bilateral blindness		Blt parieto-occipital infarcts	2 months	P (10 days)
14, de la Fuente Fernandez and Grana Gil, 1994	58/F	L INO, L III, and R peripheral VII nerve palsies		T2-WI hypersignals in L pontomesesencephalic and R lower pontine Multiple old lacunes (pons, basal ganglia, thalamus)	8 months	P (6 months)
15, Stahl et al., 1995	70/M	R crural paresis	L caudate lacune		1 month	None

Notes: L = left; R = right; Blt = bilateral; P = prednisone; MP = methylprednisolone; CY = cyclophosphamide; AZA = azathioprine.

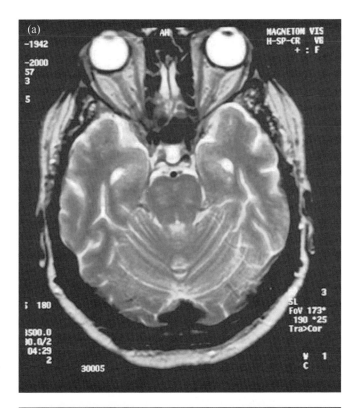

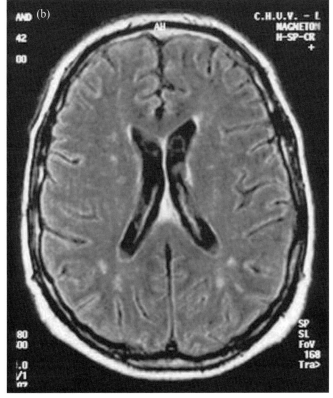

Figure 43.5 MRI of Patient 5, Lausanne, 2000. Leukoaraiosis of the pons is seen on T2-weighted images (**A**). Multiple abnormal signals of both hemispheres are seen on FLAIR (**B**).

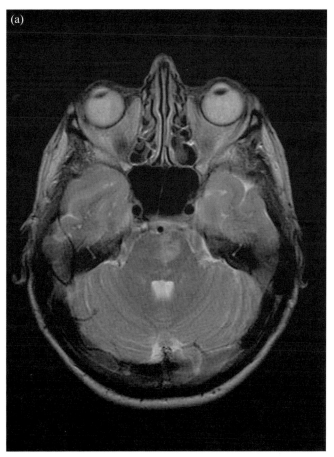

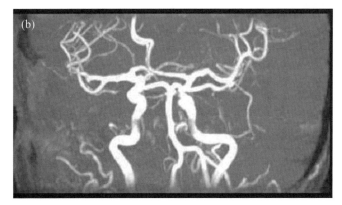

Figure 43.6 MRI of Patient 6, Lausanne, 2004. A left pontine lacunar infarct is seen on FLAIR (**A**). Basilar artery is normal (MRA, **B**).

all but one patient (mean latency, 6.5 months; range, 3 weeks to 32 months), within 8 months in 73% of patients (11/15), and was either inaugural or occurred within 1 month after the onset of PAN in one-third of patients (33%, 5/15). The earlier initiation and universal use of corticosteroid treatment in the recent cases of vasculitis probably explain the discrepancy between the previously late stroke occurrence (2–3 years) and the shorter latencies found in the present study. A close relationship between the use of corticosteroids and stroke exists in PAN. All strokes in the aforementioned series occurred while patients received adequate corticosteroid treatment. In the present study, most of the 77% of all first-time or recurrent ischemic strokes that developed despite corticosteroid therapy appeared within 6 months (80%) and 3 weeks (50%) of starting corticosteroid treatment (accompanied by other immunosuppressive therapy in only three patients). Although corticosteroids alone failed to prevent stroke (or recurrent stroke, see Patients 5 and 11) in PAN (concomitant immunosuppressive treatment being not yet active), the promoting effect of corticosteroids in the mechanisms of arterial occlusion seems to be confirmed in the present study. In fact, two of our patients (Patients 2 and 3) developed lacunar strokes within 8 hours and 3 days after corticosteroid therapy initiation, respectively, whereas two other patients (Patients 5 and 11) showed recurrent (two consecutive in Patient 11) new lacunes within 11 days and 3 weeks after the beginning of corticosteroid therapy.

Corticosteroids act on the primary inflammatory stage of PAN, without preventing the occurrence of later arteritic changes (intimal proliferation, granulation, and scarring) (Conn, 1990). Pathological studies of systemic arteries in two patients with PAN treated with corticosteroids showed no signs of active inflammation but multiple arterial occlusions (predominantly intimal fibrosis), within 3 weeks and 3 months, respectively, after initiation of cortisone acetate (Bagenstoss *et al.*, 1951). However, cerebral histological studies were normal, except in one patient (atheromatous small MCA aneurysm, medullar small infarct). In our study, four patients (one-fourth) with PAN and stroke were studied at autopsy. In one patient (Patient 8; inaugural pontine infarct) who died despite short-term corticosteroid therapy, although histological studies showed signs of necrotizing vasculitis of the medium- and small-sized arteries of the leptomeninges, there was only thrombosis of small pontine penetrating arteries. Among the three remaining patients who died despite a minimal 3-month corticosteroid therapy, no signs of active vasculitis were found. Cerebral histological studies of our Patient 1 performed 3 months after corticosteroid initiation showed arterial wall fibrosis of deep white matter arterioles (Figure 43.4; Reichhart *et al.*, 2000).

While corticosteroids should equally decrease production of both prostacyclin (vasodilator, platelet aggregation inhibitor) and thromboxane by inhibiting phospholipase A2 (Oates *et al.*, 1988a, 1988b), in vitro studies showed that the generation of prostacyclin was more depressed at pharmacological doses (Conn, 1990). Furthermore, thromboxane synthesis in platelets is corticosteroid-resistant due to the inability of platelets to induce lipocortin (phospholipase A2 inhibitor) because they are anucleated. Thromboxane may be increased in PAN (as in Kawasaki disease; see Chapter 13). Finally, one study showed cerebral medium-sized artery platelet fragment deposition in PAN by immunochemistry analysis (Ellison *et al.*, 1993). Penetrating medium-/small-sized arterial occlusions in PAN, producing deep small or pontine lacunar infarcts, are related to atherosclerosis-like mechanisms, which in turn may be promoted by both hypertension and corticosteroids, the latter promotting uncontrolled (thromboxane-mediated) platelet aggregation with further thrombus formation. From a therapeutic point of view, antiplatelet drugs, which also inhibit platelet thromboxane production, might reduce the risk of corticosteroid-induced arterial occlusion in PAN. The use of aspirin and corticosteroids prospectively prevented stroke

recurrence in four patients in the present study (Patients 3 and 14, Table 43.5; Patients 5 and 6). The promoting effect of corticosteroids on lacunar strokes in PAN is confirmed by the case histories of Patients 5 and 6, Lausanne.

Hemorrhagic strokes are unusual in PAN (20% of all patients). All patients with pure lobar hematoma (two cases) had no signs of microaneurysm on MRI/angiography. Because both hematomas involved the temporoparietal lobes, they could not be related to PAN-induced hypertension, but rather to rupture of the internal elastic lamina in the arterial wall (Bagenstoss *et al.*, 1951). The two other patterns of hemorrhagic strokes in PAN – i.e. hemorrhagic transformation of an ischemic infarct, and tiny petechial hemorrhage(s) (Ford and Siekert, 1965) – were found in only one case each. An extensive brain hemorrhage without aneurysm on conventional angiography in a child with PAN and Epstein-Barr virus infection has been reported (Caldeira *et al.*, 2007). Brain hemorrhages (Bouvard *et al.*, 2007; Oran *et al.*, 1999) and subarachnoidal hemorrhage (Rumboldt *et al.*, 2003) related to ruptured intracranial aneurysms in PAN have been reported.

Although echocardiographic studies were performed in only one-third of patients with PAN-associated ischemic strokes in this study, half of them showed signs consistent with a cardioembolic origin, which is similar to the frequency of cardiac involvement in PAN (40%) (Guillevin *et al.*, 1997a; Lhote *et al.*, 1998). However, only one patient had a large ischemic (bilateral parieto-occipital) stroke of cardioembolic origin (Patient 13), the only patient with an identified left intra-atrial thrombus had a lacunar stroke syndrome (Patient 15).

Livedo reticularis, common in PAN (Lhote *et al.*, 1998), was observed in near one-fourth of patients with PAN and stroke, but was only weakly correlated with positive anti-cardiolipin antibodies (one-fourth of patients with livedo reticularis). Among one-third of cases tested, 20% of patients with stroke had anti-cardiolipin antibodies. We found positive anti-cardiolipin antibodies in Patient 5. Multiple and recurrent strokes in patients with PAN and anti-phospholipid antibodies have been reported (Han *et al.*, 2004; Morelli *et al.*, 1998).

The role of anti-endothelial cell antibodies (not tested in any patients in this study), which have been reported in 28% of patients with active PAN without stroke and in 35% of patients with Sneddon's syndrome (strokes, anti-phospholipid antibodies, and livedo reticularis; see Chapter 56) (Frances *et al.*, 1995), requires further evaluation.

REFERENCES

Adu, D., Howie, A. J., Scott, D. G., *et al.* 1987. Polyarteritis and the kidney. *Q J Med*, **62**, 221–37.

Agard, C., Mouthon, L., Mahr, A., and Guillevin, L. 2003. Microscopic polyangiitis and polyarteritis nodosa: how and when do they start? *Arthritis Rheum*, **49**, 709–15.

Albert, D. A., Rimon, D., and Silverstein, M. D. 1988. The diagnosis of polyarteritis nodosa. I. A literature-based decision analysis approach. *Arthritis Rheum*, **31**, 1117–27.

Ara, J., Mirapeix, E., Rodriguez, R., Saurina, A., and Darnell, A. 1999. Relationship between ANCA and disease activity in small vessel vasculitis patients with anti-MPO ANCA. *Nephrol Dial Transplant*, **14**, 1667–72.

Bagenstoss, A. H., Shick, R. M., and Polley, H. F. 1951. The effect of cortisone on the lesions of periarteritis nodosa. *Am J Pathol*, **27**, 537–59.

Bansal, P. J., and Tobin, M. C. 2004. Neonatal microscopic polyangiitis secondary to transfer of maternal myeloperoxidase-antineutrophil cytoplasmic antibody resulting in neonatal pulmonary hemorrhage and renal involvement. *Ann Allergy Asthma Immunol*, **93**, 398–401.

Begier, E. M., Langford, C. A., Sneller, M. C., Wise, R. P., and Ball, R. 2004. Polyarteritis nodosa reports to the vaccine adverse event reporting system (VAERS): implications for assessment of suspected vaccine-provoked vasculitis. *J Rheumatol*, **31**, 2181–8.

Bonsib, S. M. 2001. Polyarteritis nodosa. *Semin Diagn Pathol*, **18**, 14–23.

Boomsma, M. M., Stegeman, C. A., van der Leij, M. J., *et al.* 2000. Prediction of relapses in Wegener's granulomatosis by measurement of antineutrophil cytoplasmic antibody levels: a prospective study. *Arthritis Rheum*, **43**, 2025–33.

Booth, A., Harper, L., Hammad, T., *et al.* 2004. Prospective study of TNFalpha blockade with infliximab in anti-neutrophil cytoplasmic antibody-associated systemic vasculitis. *J Am Soc Nephrol*, **15**, 717–21.

Bosch, X., Guilabert, A., and Font, J. 2006. Antineutrophil cytoplasmic antibodies. *Lancet*, **368**, 404–18.

Bosch, X., Llena, J., Collado, A., *et al.* 1995. Occurrence of antineutrophil cytoplasmic and antineutrophil (peri)nuclear antibodies in rheumatoid arthritis. *J Rheumatol*, **22**, 2038–45.

Bourgarit, A., le Toumelin P., Pagnoux, C., *et al.* 2005. Deaths occurring during the first year after treatment onset for polyarteritis nodosa, microscopic polyangiitis, and Churg-Strauss syndrome: a retrospective analysis of causes and factors predictive of mortality based on 595 patients. *Medicine (Baltimore)*, **84**, 323–30.

Bouvard, B., Lavigne, C., Marc, G., *et al.* 2007. [Two consecutive episodes of intracerebral hemorrhage as the presenting feature of polyarteritis nodosa.]. *Rev Med Interne*, **28**, 651–4.

Brik, R., Gepstein, V., Shahar, E., Goldsher, D., and Berkovitz, D. 2007. Tumor necrosis factor blockade in the management of children with orphan diseases. *Clin Rheumatol*, **26**, 1783–5.

Bron, K. M., Strott, C. A., and Shapiro, A. P. 1965. The diagnostic value of angiographic observations in polyarteritis nodosa. A case of multiple aneurysms in the visceral organs. *Arch Intern Med*, **116**, 450–4.

Brown, M. M., and Swash, M. 1989. Polyarteritis nodosa and other systemic vasculitides. In *Handbook of Clinical Neurology*, J. F. Toole, ed. 22 Vascular Diseases, Part III, Amsterdam: Elsevier Science Publishers, pp. 353–68.

Caldeira, T., Meireles, C., Cunha, F., *et al.* 2007. Systemic polyarteritis nodosa associated with acute Epstein-Barr virus infection. *Clin Rheumatol*, **26**, 1733–5.

Chanseaud, Y., de la Pena-Lefebvre, G., Guilpain, P., *et al.* 2003. IgM and IgG autoantibodies from microscopic polyangiitis patients but not those with other small- and medium-sized vessel vasculitides recognize multiple endothelial cell antigens. *Clin Immunol*, **109**, 165–78.

Chanseaud, Y., Tamby, M. C., Guilpain, P., *et al.* 2005. Analysis of autoantibody repertoires in small- and medium-sized vessels vasculitides. Evidence for specific perturbations in polyarteritis nodosa, microscopic polyangiitis, Churg-Strauss syndrome and Wegener's granulomatosis. *J Autoimmun*, **24**, 169–79.

Chetty, R. 2001. Vasculitides associated with HIV infection. *J Clin Pathol*, **54**, 275–8.

Chin, R. L., and Latov, N. 2005. Central nervous system manifestations of rheumatologic diseases. *Curr Opin Rheumatol*, **17**, 91–9.

Cohen, R. D., Conn, D. L., and Ilstrup, D. M. 1980. Clinical features, prognosis, and response to treatment in polyarteritis. *Mayo Clin Proc*, **55**, 146–55.

Cohen Tervaert, J. W., and Kallenberg, C. 1993. Neurologic manifestations of systemic vasculitides. *Rheum Dis Clin North Am*, **19**, 913–40.

Coll-Vinent, B., Grau, J. M., Lopez-Soto, A., *et al.* 1997. Circulating soluble adhesion molecules in patients with classical polyarteritis nodosa. *Br J Rheumatol*, **36**, 1178–83.

Colmegna, I., and Maldonado-Cocco, J. A. 2005. Polyarteritis nodosa revisited. *Curr Rheumatol Rep*, **7**, 288–96.

Conn, D. L. 1990. Polyarteritis. *Rheum Dis Clin North Am*, **16**, 341–62.

Das, C. J., and Pangtey, G. S. 2006. Images in clinical medicine. Arterial microaneurysms in polyarteritis nodosa. *N Engl J Med*, **355**, 2574.

Davson, J., Ball, J., and Platt, R. 1948. The kidney in periarteritis nodosa. *Q J Med*, **17**, 175–205.

de la Fuente Fernandez, R., and Grana Gil, J. 1994. Anticardiolipin antibodies and polyarteritis nodosa. *Lupus*, **3**, 523–4.

Deshpande, P. V., Gilbert, R., Alton, H., and Milford, D. V. 2000. Microscopic polyarteritis with renal and cerebral involvement. *Pediatr Nephrol*, **15**, 134–5.

Ellison, D., Gatter, K., Heryet, A., and Esiri, M. 1993. Intramural platelet deposition in cerebral vasculopathy of systemic lupus erythematosus. *J Clin Pathol*, **46**, 37–40.

Eriksson, P. 2005. Nine patients with anti-neutrophil cytoplasmic antibody-positive vasculitis successfully treated with rituximab. *J Intern Med*, **257**, 540–8.

Fahey, J. L., Leonard, E., Churg, J., and Godman, G. 1954. Wegener's granulomatosis. *Am J Med*, **17**, 168–79.

Falk, R. J., and Jennette, J. C. 1988. Anti-neutrophil cytoplasmic autoantibodies with specificity for myeloperoxidase in patients with systemic vasculitis and idiopathic necrotizing and crescentic glomerulonephritis. *N Engl J Med*, **318**, 1651–7.

Farrell, G. C., and Teoh, N. C. 2006. Management of chronic hepatitis B virus infection: a new era of disease control. *Intern Med J*, **36**, 100–13.

Fauci, A. S., Doppman, J. L., and Wolff, S. M. 1978. Cyclophosphamide-induced remissions in advanced polyarteritis nodosa. *Am J Med*, **64**, 890–4.

Fauci, A. S., Haynes, B. F., Katz, P., and Wolff, S. M. 1983. Wegener's granulomatosis: prospective clinical and therapeutic experience with 85 patients for 21 years. *Ann Intern Med*, **98**, 76–85.

Fauci, A. S., Katz, P., Haynes, B. F., and Wolff, S. M. 1979. Cyclophosphamide therapy of severe systemic necrotizing vasculitis. *N Engl J Med*, **301**, 235–8.

Fauci, A. S., Wolff, S. M., and Johnson, J. S. 1971. Effect of cyclophosphamide upon the immune response in Wegener's granulomatosis. *N Engl J Med*, **285**, 1493–6.

Ferrari, E. 1903. Ueber polyarteritis acuta nodosa (sogenannte periarteritis nodosa) und ihre Beziehungen zur polymyositis und polyneuritis acuta. *Beitr Pathol Anat*, **34**, 350–86.

Filer, A. D., Gardner-Medwin, J. M., Thambyrajah, J., *et al.* 2003. Diffuse endothelial dysfunction is common to ANCA associated systemic vasculitis and polyarteritis nodosa. *Ann Rheum Dis*, **62**, 162–7.

Fisher, C. M. 1965. Lacunes: small, deep cerebral infarcts. *Neurology*, **15**, 774–84.

Ford, R. G., and Siekert, R. G. 1965. Central nervous system manifestations of periarteritis nodosa. *Neurology*, **15**, 114–22.

Frances, C., Le Tonqueze, B. S., Salohzin, K. V., *et al.* 1995. Prevalence of anto-endothelial cell antibodies in patients with Sneddon's syndrome. *J Am Acad Dermatol*, **33**, 64–8.

Freire, A. L., Bertolo, M. B., de Pinho. A. J. Jr., Samara, A. M., and Fernandes, S. R. 2004. Increased serum levels of interleukin-8 in polyarteritis nodosa and Behcet's disease. *Clin Rheumatol*, **23**, 203–5.

Frohnert, P. P., and Sheps, S. G. 1967. Long-term follow-up study of periarteritis nodosa. *Am J Med*, **43**, 8–14.

Gayraud, M., Guillevin, L., Cohen, P., *et al.* 1997. Treatment of good-prognosis polyarteritis nodosa and Churg-Strauss syndrome: comparison of steroids and oral or pulse cyclophosphamide in 25 patients. French Cooperative Study Group for Vasculitides. *Br J Rheumatol*, **36**, 1290–7.

Gayraud, M., Guillevin, L., le Toumelin, P., *et al.* 2001. Long-term followup of polyarteritis nodosa, microscopic polyangiitis, and Churg-Strauss syndrome: analysis of four prospective trials including 278 patients. *Arthritis Rheum*, **44**, 666–75.

Gherardi, R., Belec, L., Mhiri, C., *et al.* 1993. The spectrum of vasculitis in human immunodeficiency virus-infected patients. A clinicopathologic evaluation. *Arthritis Rheum*, **36**, 1164–74.

Gibson, A., Stamp, L. K., Chapman, P. T., and O'Donnell, J. L. 2006. The epidemiology of Wegener's granulomatosis and microscopic polyangiitis in a Southern Hemisphere region. *Rheumatology (Oxford)*, **45**, 624–8.

Gocke, D. J., Hsu, K., Morgan, C., Bombardieri, S., Lockshin, M., and Christian, C. L. 1970. Association between polyarteritis and Australia antigen. *Lancet*, **2**, 1149–53.

Godman, G., and Churg, J. 1954. Wegener's granulomatosis. Pathology and review of the literature. *Arch Pathol Lab Med*, **58**, 533–53.

Gordon, M., Luqmani, R. A., Adu, D., *et al.* 1993. Relapses in patients with a systemic vasculitis. *Q J Med*, **86**, 779–89.

Guillevin, L. 1999a. Treatment of classic polyarteritis nodosa in 1999. *Nephrol Dial Transplant*, **14**, 2077–9.

Guillevin, L. 1999b. Virus-associated vasculitides. *Rheumatology (Oxford)*, **38**, 588–90.

Guillevin, L. 2004. Virus-induced systemic vasculitides: new therapeutic approaches. *Clin Dev Immunol*, **11**, 227–31.

Guillevin, L., Cohen, P., Mahr, A., et al. 2003. Treatment of polyarteritis nodosa and microscopic polyangiitis with poor prognosis factors: a prospective trial comparing glucocorticoids and six or twelve cyclophosphamide pulses in sixty-five patients. *Arthritis Rheum*, **49**, 93–100.

Guillevin, L., Durand-Gasselin, B., Cevallos, R., et al. 1999. Microscopic polyangiitis: clinical and laboratory findings in eighty-five patients. *Arthritis Rheum*, **42**, 421–30.

Guillevin, L., Jarrousse, B., Lok, C., et al. 1991. Longterm followup after treatment of polyarteritis nodosa and Churg-Strauss angiitis with comparison of steroids, plasma exchange and cyclophosphamide to steroids and plasma exchange. A prospective randomized trial of 71 patients. The Cooperative Study Group for Polyarteritis Nodosa. *J Rheumatol*, **18**, 567–74.

Guillevin, L., Le Thi, H. D., Godeau, P., Jais, P., and Wechsler, B. 1988. Clinical findings and prognosis of polyarteritis nodosa and Churg-Strauss angiitis: a study in 165 patients. *Br J Rheumatol*, **27**, 258–64.

Guillevin, L., and Lhote, F. 1995. Distinguishing polyarteritis nodosa from microscopic polyangiitis and implications for treatment. *Curr Opin Rheumatol*, **7**, 20–4.

Guillevin, L., and Lhote, F. 1998. Treatment of polyarteritis nodosa and microscopic polyangiitis. *Arthritis Rheum*, **41**, 2100–5.

Guillevin, L., Lhote, F., Amouroux, J., et al. 1996. Antineutrophil cytoplasmic antibodies, abnormal angiograms and pathological findings in polyarteritis nodosa and Churg-Strauss syndrome: indications for the classification of vasculitides of the polyarteritis Nodosa Group. *Br J Rheumatol*, **35**, 958–64.

Guillevin, L., Lhote, F., Brauner, M., and Casassus, P. 1995. Antineutrophil cytoplasmic antibodies (ANCA) and abnormal angiograms in polyarteritis nodosa and Churg-Strauss syndrome: indications for the diagnosis of microscopic polyangiitis. *Ann Med Interne (Paris)*, **146**, 548–50.

Guillevin, L., Lhote, F., Cohen, P., et al. 1995a. Corticosteroids plus pulse cyclophosphamide and plasma exchanges versus corticosteroids plus pulse cyclophosphamide alone in the treatment of polyarteritis nodosa and Churg-Strauss syndrome patients with factors predicting poor prognosis. A prospective, randomized trial in sixty-two patients. *Arthritis Rheum*, **38**, 1638–45.

Guillevin, L., Lhote, F., Cohen, P., et al. 1995b. Polyarteritis nodosa related to hepatitis B virus. A prospective study with long-term observation of 41 patients. *Medicine (Baltimore)*, **74**, 238–53.

Guillevin, L., Lhote, F., Gayraud, M., et al. 1996. Prognostic factors in polyarteritis nodosa and Churg-Strauss syndrome. A prospective study in 342 patients. *Medicine (Baltimore)*, **75**, 17–28.

Guillevin, L., Lhote, F., and Gherardi, R. 1997a. Polyarteritis nodosa, microscopic polyangiitis, and Churg-Strauss syndrome: clinical aspects, neurologic manifestations, and treatment. *Neurol Clin*, **15**, 865–86.

Guillevin, L., Lhote, F., and Gherardi, R. 1997b. The spectrum and treatment of virus-associated vasculitides. *Curr Opin Rheumatol*, **9**, 31–6.

Guillevin, L., Lhote, F., Jarrousse, B., and Fain, O. 1992. Treatment of polyarteritis nodosa and Churg-Strauss syndrome. A meta-analysis of 3 prospective controlled trials including 182 patients over 12 years. *Ann Med Interne (Paris)*, **143**, 405–16.

Guillevin, L., Lhote, F., Leon, A., et al. 1993. Treatment of polyarteritis nodosa related to hepatitis B virus with short term steroid therapy associated with antiviral agents and plasma exchanges. A prospective trial in 33 patients. *J Rheumatol*, **20**, 289–98.

Guillevin, L., Lhote, F., Sauvaget, F., et al. 1994. Treatment of polyarteritis nodosa related to hepatitis B virus with interferon-alpha and plasma exchanges. *Ann Rheum Dis*, **53**, 334–7.

Guillevin, L., Mahr, A., Callard, P., et al. 2005. Hepatitis B virus-associated polyarteritis nodosa: clinical characteristics, outcome, and impact of treatment in 115 patients. *Medicine (Baltimore)*, **84**, 313–22.

Guillevin, L., Mahr, A., Cohen, P., et al. 2004. Short-term corticosteroids then lamivudine and plasma exchanges to treat hepatitis B virus-related polyarteritis nodosa. *Arthritis Rheum*, **51**, 482–7.

Guillevin, L., Merrouche, Y., Gayraud, M., et al. 1988. [Periarteritis nodosa related to hepatitis B virus. Determination of a new therapeutic strategy: 13 cases]. *Presse Med*, **17**, 1522–6.

Guillevin, L., and Mouthon, L. 2004. Tumor necrosis factor-alpha blockade and the risk of vasculitis. *J Rheumatol*, **31**, 1885–7.

Guillevin, L., Pagnoux, C., Guilpain, P., et al. 2007. Indications for biotherapy in systemic vasculitides. *Clin Rev Allergy Immunol*, **32**, 85–96.

Han, B. K., Inaganti, K., Fahmi, S., and Reimold, A. 2004. Polyarteritis nodosa complicated by catastrophic antiphospholipid syndrome. *J Clin Rheumatol*, **10**, 210–3.

Han, S., Rehman, H. U., Jayaratne, P. S., and Carty, J. E. 2006. Microscopic polyangiitis complicated by cerebral haemorrhage. *Rheumatol Int*, **26**, 1057–60.

Harlé, J. R., Disdier, P., Ali Cherif, A., et al. 1991. Démence curable et panartérite noueuse. *Rev Neurol (Paris)*, **147**, 148–50.

Hauer, H. A., Bajema, I. M., Van Houwelingen, H. C., et al. 2002. Determinants of outcome in ANCA-associated glomerulonephritis: a prospective clinico-histopathological analysis of 96 patients. *Kidney Int*, **62**, 1732–42.

Hekali, P., Kajander, H., Pajari, R., Stenman, S., and Somer, T. 1991. Diagnostic significance of angiographically observed visceral aneurysms with regard to polyarteritis nodosa. *Acta Radiol*, **32**, 143–8.

Hirohata, S., Tanimoto, K., and Ito, K. 1993. Elevation of cerebrospinal fluid interleukin-6 activity in patients with vasculitides and central nervous involvement. *Clin Immunol Immunopathol*, **66**, 225–9.

Hogan, S. L., Falk, R. J., Chin, H., et al. 2005. Predictors of relapse and treatment resistance in antineutrophil cytoplasmic antibody-associated small-vessel vasculitis. *Ann Intern Med*, **143**, 621–31.

Hogan, S. L., Nachman, P. H., Wilkman, A. S., Jennette, J. C., and Falk, R. J. 1996. Prognostic markers in patients with antineutrophil cytoplasmic autoantibody-associated microscopic polyangiitis and glomerulonephritis. *J Am Soc Nephrol*, **7**, 23–32.

Honda, H., Hasegawa, T., Morokawa, N., Kato, N., and Inoue, K. 1996. [A case of MPO-ANCA related vasculitis with transient leukoencephalopathy and multiple cerebral hemorrhage]. *Rinsho Shinkeigaku*, **36**, 1089–94.

Iaconetta, G., Benvenuti, D., Lamaida, E., et al. 1994. Cerebral hemorrhagic complication in polyarteritis nodosa. *Acta Neurol (Napoli)*, **16**, 64–9.

Ito, Y., Suzuki, K., Yamazaki, T., et al. 2006. ANCA-associated vasculitis (AAV) causing bilateral cerebral infarction and subsequent intracerebral hemorrhage without renal and respiratory dysfunction. *J Neurol Sci*, **240**, 99–101.

Jayne, D. 2001. Update on the European Vasculitis Study Group trials. *Curr Opin Rheumatol*, **13**, 48–55.

Jayne, D., Rasmussen, N., Andrassy, K., et al. 2003. A randomized trial of maintenance therapy for vasculitis associated with antineutrophil cytoplasmic autoantibodies. *N Engl J Med*, **349**, 36–44.

Jayne, D. R., Chapel, H., Adu, D., et al. 2000. Intravenous immunoglobulin for ANCA-associated systemic vasculitis with persistent disease activity. *Q J Med*, **93**, 433–9.

Jayne, D. R., Gaskin, G., Pusey, C. D., and Lockwood, C. M. 1995. ANCA and predicting relapse in systemic vasculitis. *Q J Med*, **88**, 127–33.

Jennette, J. C., and Falk, R. J. 2007. Nosology of primary vasculitis. *Curr Opin Rheumatol*, **19**, 10–6.

Jennette, J. C., and Falk, R. J. 1997. Small-vessel vasculitis. *N Engl J Med*, **337**, 1512–23.

Jennette, J. C., Falk, R. J., Andrassy, K., et al. 1994. Nomenclature of systemic vasculitides. Proposal of an international consensus conference. *Arthritis Rheum*, **37**, 187–92.

Jennette, J. C., Thomas, D. B., and Falk, R. J. 2001. Microscopic polyangiitis (microscopic polyarteritis). *Semin Diagn Pathol*, **18**, 3–13.

Kallenberg, C. G. 2007. Antineutrophil cytoplasmic autoantibody-associated small-vessel vasculitis. *Curr Opin Rheumatol*, **19**, 17–24.

Kallenberg, C. G., Heeringa, P., and Stegeman, C. A. 2006. Mechanisms of disease: pathogenesis and treatment of ANCA-associated vasculitides. *Nat Clin Pract Rheumatol*, **2**, 661–70.

Kamimura, T., Hatakeyama, M., Torigoe, K., *et al.* 2005. Muscular polyarteritis nodosa as a cause of fever of undetermined origin: a case report and review of the literature. *Rheumatol Int*, **25**, 394–7.

Kasantikul, V., Suwanwela, N., and Pongsabutr, S. 1991. Magnetic resonance images of brain stem infarct in periarteritis nodosa. *Surg Neurol*, **36**, 133–6.

Keogh, K. A., Ytterberg, S. R., Fervenza, F. C., *et al.* 2006. Rituximab for refractory Wegener's granulomatosis: report of a prospective, open-label pilot trial. *Am J Respir Crit Care Med*, **173**, 180–7.

Keystone, E. C. 2004. The utility of tumour necrosis factor blockade in orphan diseases. *Ann Rheum Dis*, **63**(**Suppl 2**), ii79–83.

Kirkland, G. S., Savige, J., Wilson, D., *et al.* 1997. Classical polyarteritis nodosa and microscopic polyangiitis with medium vessel involvement–a comparison of the clinical and laboratory features. *Clin Nephrol*, **47**, 176–80.

Klemmer, P. J., Chalermskulrat, W., Reif, M. S., *et al.* 2003. Plasmapheresis therapy for diffuse alveolar hemorrhage in patients with small-vessel vasculitis. *Am J Kidney Dis*, **42**, 1149–53.

Koppensteiner, R., Base, W., Bognar, H., *et al.* 1989. Course of cerebral lesions in a patient with periarteritis nodosa studied by magnetic resonance imaging. *Klin Wochenschr*, **67**, 398–401.

Kussmaul, A., and Maier, R. 1866. Ueber eine bisher nicht beschriebene eigenthuemliche Arterienkrankung (Periarteritis nodosa), die mit Morbus Brightii und rapid fortschreitender allgemeiner Muskellaehmung einhergeht. *Deutsch Arch Klin Med*, **1**, 484–518.

Kyndt, X., Reumaux, D., Bridoux, F., *et al.* 1999. Serial measurements of antineutrophil cytoplasmic autoantibodies in patients with systemic vasculitis. *Am J Med*, **106**, 527–33.

Lane, S. E., Watts, R., and Scott, D. G. 2005. Epidemiology of systemic vasculitis. *Curr Rheumatol Rep*, **7**, 270–5.

Lane, S. E., Watts, R. A., Shepstone, L., and Scott, D. G. 2005. Primary systemic vasculitis: clinical features and mortality. *Q J Med*, **98**, 97–111.

Langford, C. A. 2001. Management of systemic vasculitis. *Best Pract Res Clin Rheumatol*, **15**, 281–97.

Leib, E. S., Restivo, C., and Paulus, H. E. 1979. Immunosuppressive and corticosteroid therapy of polyarteritis nodosa. *Am J Med*, **67**, 941–7.

Lhote, F., Cohen, P., Genereau, T., Gayraud, M., and Guillevin, L. 1996. Microscopic polyangiitis: clinical aspects and treatment. *Ann Med Interne (Paris)*, **147**, 165–77.

Lhote, F., Cohen, P., and Guillevin, L. 1998. Polyarteritis nodosa, microscopic polyangiitis and Churg-Strauss syndrome. *Lupus*, **7**, 238–58.

Lhote, F., and Guillevin, L. 1995. Polyarteritis nodosa, microscopic polyangiitis, and Churg- Strauss syndrome: clinical aspects and treatment. *Rheum Dis Clin North Am*, **21**, 911–47.

Lie, J. T. 1994. Nomenclature and classification of vasculitis: plus ca change, plus c'est la meme chose. *Arthritis Rheum*, **37**, 181–6.

Lightfoot, R. W. J., Michel, A. B., Bloch, D. A., *et al.* 1990. The American College of Rheumatology 1990 criteria for the classification of polyarteritis nodosa. *Arthritis Rheum*, **33**, 1088–93.

Long, S. M., and Dolin, P. 1994. Polyarteritis nodosa presenting as acute blindness. *Ann Emerg Med*, **24**, 523–5.

MacLaren, K., Gillespie, J., Shrestha, S., Neary, D., and Ballardie, F. W. 2005. Primary angiitis of the central nervous system: emerging variants. *Q J Med*, **98**, 643–54.

Mahr, A., Guillevin, L., Poissonnet, M., and Ayme, S. 2004. Prevalences of polyarteritis nodosa, microscopic polyangiitis, Wegener's granulomatosis, and Churg-Strauss syndrome in a French urban multiethnic population in 2000: a capture-recapture estimate. *Arthritis Rheum*, **51**, 92–9.

Mandell, B. F., and Calabrese, L. H. 1998. Infections and systemic vasculitis 1. *Curr Opin Rheumatol*, **10**, 51–7.

Marignier, R., Derex, L., Philippeau, F., *et al.* 2002. [Anterior choroidal artery infarction revealing polyarteritis nodosa]. *Rev Neurol (Paris)*, **158**, 221–4.

Mayo, J., Arias, M., Leno, C., and Berciano, J. 1986. Vascular parkinsonism and periarteritis nodosa. *Neurology*, **36**, 874–5.

Molloy, E. S., and Langford, C. A. 2006. Advances in the treatment of small vessel vasculitis. *Rheum Dis Clin North Am*, **32**, 157–72, x.

Moore, P. M. 1995. Neurological manifestations of vasculitis: update on immunopathogenic mechanisms and clinical features. *Ann Neurol*, **37**(**S1**), S131–S141.

Moore, P. M., and Cupps, T. R. 1983. Neurological complications of vasculitis. *Ann Neurol*, **14**, 155–67.

Moore, P. M., and Fauci, A. S. 1981. Neurologic manifestations of systemic vasculitis: a restrospective and prospective study of the clinicopathologic features and responses to therapy in 25 patients. *Am J Med*, **71**, 517–24.

Morelli, S., Perrone, C., and Paroli, M. 1998. Recurrent cerebral infarctions in polyarteritis nodosa with circulating antiphospholipid antibodies and mitral valve disease. *Lupus*, **7**, 51–2.

Nachman, P. H., Hogan, S. L., Jennette, J. C., and Falk, R. J. 1996. Treatment response and relapse in antineutrophil cytoplasmic autoantibody-associated microscopic polyangiitis and glomerulonephritis. *J Am Soc Nephrol*, **7**, 33–9.

Nakane, S., Tsujino, A., Shirabe, S., Nakamura, T., and Nagataki, S. 1997. [A case of malignant rheumatoid arthritis with transverse myelopathy and multiple lacunar infarction]. *Rinsho Shinkeigaku*, **37**, 685–9.

Niles, J. L., Bottinger, E. P., Saurina, G. R., *et al.* 1996. The syndrome of lung hemorrhage and nephritis is usually an ANCA-associated condition. *Arch Intern Med*, **156**, 440–5.

Oates, J. A., Fitzgerald, G. A., Branch, R. A., *et al.* 1988a. Clinical implications of prostaglandins and thromboxane A2 formation (part two). *N Engl J Med*, **319**, 761–7.

Oates, J. A., Fitzgerald, G. A., Branch, R. A., *et al.* 1988b. Clinical implications of prostaglandins and thromboxane A2 formation (part one). *N Engl J Med*, **319**, 689–98.

Oran, I., Memis, A., Parildar, M., and Yunten, N. 1999. Multiple intracranial aneurysms in polyarteritis nodosa: MRI and angiography. *Neuroradiology*, **41**, 436–9.

Oyoo, O., and Espinoza, L. R. 2005. Infection-related vasculitis. *Curr Rheumatol Rep*, **7**, 281–7.

Ozen, S., Ruperto, N., Dillon, M. J., *et al.* 2006. EULAR/PReS endorsed consensus criteria for the classification of childhood vasculitides. *Ann Rheum Dis*, **65**, 936–41.

Pagnoux, C., Cohen, P., and Guillevin, L. 2006. Vasculitides secondary to infections. *Clin Exp Rheumatol*, **24**, S71–S81.

Pavone, L., Grasselli, C., Chierici, E., *et al.* 2006. Outcome and prognostic factors during the course of primary small-vessel vasculitides. *J Rheumatol*, **33**, 1299–306.

Reichhart, M. D., Bogousslavsky, J., and Janzer, R. C. 2000. Early lacunar strokes complicating polyarteritis nodosa: thrombotic microangiopathy. *Neurology*, **54**, 883–9.

Rodgers, H., Guthrie, J. A., Brownjohn, A. M., and Turney, J. H. 1989. Microscopic polyangiitis: clinical features and treatment. *Postgrad Med J*, **65**, 515–8.

Rumboldt, Z., Beros, V., and Klanfar, Z. 2003. Multiple cerebral aneurysms and a dural arteriovenous fistula in a patient with polyarteritis nodosa. Case illustration. *J Neurosurg*, **98**, 434.

Sack, M., Cassidy, J. T., and Bole, G. G. 1975. Prognostic factors in polyarteritis. *J Rheumatol*, **2**, 411–20.

Sasaki, A., Hirato, J., Nakazato, Y., Tanaka, T., and Takeuchi, H. 1998. [An autopsy case of P-ANCA-positive microscopic polyangiitis with multiple cerebral hemorrhagic infarction]. *No To Shinkei*, **50**, 56–60.

Savage, C. O., Winearls, C. G., Evans, D. J., Rees, A. J., and Lockwood, C. M. 1985. Microscopic polyarteritis: presentation, pathology and prognosis. *Q J Med*, **56**, 467–83.

Segelmark, M., and Selga, D. 2007. The challenge of managing patients with polyarteritis nodosa. *Curr Opin Rheumatol*, **19**, 33–8.

Selga, D., Mohammad, A., Sturfelt, G., and Segelmark, M. 2006. Polyarteritis nodosa when applying the Chapel Hill nomenclature–a descriptive study on ten patients. *Rheumatology (Oxford)*, **45**, 1276–81.

Serra, A., Cameron, J. S., Turner, D. R., *et al.* 1984. Vasculitis affecting the kidney: presentation, histopathology and long-term outcome. *Q J Med*, **53**, 181–207.

Squire, I. B., Grosset, D. G., and Lees, K. R. 1993. Immunosupressive treatment in stroke and renal failure. *Ann Rheum Dis*, **52**, 165–8.

Stahl, H., Mihatsch, M. J., Orantes, M., and Lehmann, F. 1995. Pneumonia, biclonal gammopathy, paresis of the fibular nerve and cerebrovascular insult. *Schweiz Rund Med*, **84**, 1071–8.

Stanson, A. W., Friese, J. L., Johnson, C. M., *et al.* 2001. Polyarteritis nodosa: spectrum of angiographic findings. *Radiographics*, **21**, 151–9.

Stasi, R., Stipa, E., Del Poeta, G., *et al.* 2006. Long-term observation of patients with anti-neutrophil cytoplasmic antibody-associated vasculitis treated with rituximab. *Rheumatology (Oxford)*, **45**, 1432–6.

Stegeman, C. A. 2002. Anti-neutrophil cytoplasmic antibody (ANCA) levels directed against proteinase-3 and myeloperoxidase are helpful in predicting disease relapse in ANCA-associated small-vessel vasculitis. *Nephrol Dial Transplant*, **17**, 2077–80.

Stone, J. H. 2002. Polyarteritis nodosa. *JAMA*, **288**, 1632–9.

Tesar, V., Kazderova, M., and Hlavackova, L. 2004. Rokitansky and his first description of polyarteritis nodosa. *J Nephrol*, **17**, 172–4.

Trepo, C., and Guillevin, L. 2001. Polyarteritis nodosa and extrahepatic manifestations of HBV infection: the case against autoimmune intervention in pathogenesis. *J Autoimmun*, **16**, 269–74.

Trepo, C., and Thivolet, J. 1970. Hepatitis associated antigen and periarteritis nodosa (PAN). *Vox Sang*, **19**, 410–1.

Walton, E. W. 1958. Giant-cell granuloma of the respiratory tract (Wegener's granulomatosis). *Br Med J*, **2**, 265–70.

Wartelle-Bladou, C., Lafon, J., Trepo, C., *et al.* 2001. Successful combination therapy of polyarteritis nodosa associated with a pre-core promoter mutant hepatitis B virus infection. *J Hepatol*, **34**, 774–9.

Watts, R., Harper, L., Jayne, D., *et al.* 2005. Translational research in autoimmunity: aims of therapy in vasculitis. *Rheumatology (Oxford)*, **44**, 573–6.

Watts, R., Lane, S., Hanslik, T., *et al.* 2007. Development and validation of a consensus methodology for the classification of the ANCA-associated vasculitides and polyarteritis nodosa for epidemiological studies. *Ann Rheum Dis*, **66**, 222–7.

Watts, R. A., Gonzalez-Gay, M. A., Lane, S. E., *et al.* 2001. Geoepidemiology of systemic vasculitis: comparison of the incidence in two regions of Europe. *Ann Rheum Dis*, **60**, 170–2.

The Wegener's granulomatosis etanercept trial (WGET) research group. 2005. Etanercept plus standard therapy for Wegener's granulomatosis. *N Engl J Med*, **352**, 351–61.

Weidner, S., Geuss, S., Hafezi-Rachti, S., Wonka, A., and Rupprecht, H. D. 2004. ANCA-associated vasculitis with renal involvement: an outcome analysis. *Nephrol Dial Transplant*, **19**, 1403–11.

Westman, K. W., Bygren, P. G., Olsson, H., Ranstam, J., and Wieslander, J. 1998. Relapse rate, renal survival, and cancer morbidity in patients with Wegener's granulomatosis or microscopic polyangiitis with renal involvement. *J Am Soc Nephrol*, **9**, 842–52.

Westman, K. W., Selga, D., Isberg, P. E., Bladstrom, A., and Olsson, H. 2003. High proteinase 3-anti-neutrophil cytoplasmic antibody (ANCA) level measured by the capture enzyme-linked immunosorbent assay method is associated with decreased patient survival in ANCA-associated vasculitis with renal involvement. *J Am Soc Nephrol*, **14**, 2926–33.

Wiik, A. 2002. Rational use of ANCA in the diagnosis of vasculitis. *Rheumatology (Oxford)*, **41**, 481–3.

Wildhagen, K., Stoppe, G., Meyer, G. J., *et al.* 1989. Bildgebende diagnostik der zentralnervoesen beteiligung der panarteriitis nodosa. *Z Rheumatol*, **48**, 323–5.

www.vasculitis.com. 2007.

Younger, D. S. 2004. Vasculitis of the nervous system. *Curr Opin Neurol*, **17**, 317–36.

Zeek, P. M. 1952. Periarteritis nodosa: a critical review. *Am J Clin Pathol*, **22**, 777–90.

44 CHURG-STRAUSS SYNDROME

Manu Mehdiratta and Louis R. Caplan

The Churg-Strauss syndrome (CSS) is a type of small-vessel vasculitis that was originally described more than a half century ago (Churg and Strauss, 1951). The capillaries, arterioles, and venules are preferentially involved. In some patients, the larger vessels can be affected, but this is unusual. This condition tends to affect middle-age individuals and has a slight propensity for men. The incidence of CSS is approximately 1–3 per million, although among individuals with asthma, the incidence has been estimated to be as high as 6–7 per million. CSS represents only 20% of patients with the systemic necrotizing vasculitis of the polyarteritis nodosa group, making it relatively uncommon in comparison to the other vasculitides (Keogh and Specks, 2006).

Most patients have had asthma for years before developing systemic or neurological signs of CSS. In one series of 91 patients with CSS, the median time between the onset of asthma and other signs was 4 years (Keogh and Specks, 2003) In 13 patients, asthma and systemic signs occurred together, and in two patients systemic signs preceded the asthma (Keogh and Specks, 2003). The clinical findings are usually dominated by asthma and pulmonary disease. Livedo reticularis occured in some patients (7/112, 62%) in one large series (Sable-Fourtassou et al., 2005).

Pathologically, CSS consists of three classical features: necrotizing vasculitis, eosinophilic inflammation, and extravascular granulomas (Churg and Strauss, 1951). The triggering events and cause of CSS remain unclear. Some postulated mechanisms relate to antigen exposure (drugs, inhaled antigent, vaccines) resulting in activation of T lymphocytes, eosinophils, and neutrophils with resultant tissue injury.

In most patients with CSS there are associated anti-neutrophil cytoplasmic antibodies (ANCA) present which also have been shown to be pro-inflammatory (Keogh and Specks, 2006). French and Italian studies found that the clinical characteristics of patients with CSS differed according to their ANCA status (Sable-Fourtassou et al., 2005; Pagnoux et al., 2007). Cardiomyopathy predominated in ANCA-negative patients, whereas necrotizing glomerulonephritis, peripheral neuropathy, and biopsy-proven vasculitis were more often found in ANCA-positive patients (Sable-Fourtassou et al., 2005; Pagnoux et al., 2007). Recently, patients treated with leukotriene antagonists for asthma have been found to have a higher likelihood of developing CSS. A possible mechanism does exist as leukotriene antagonists were developed to act on leukotriene receptors in the lung, but these receptors also exist outside the lung in the vasculature. This mechanism continues to be investigated, and now it is not clear if there is a direct cause-and-effect relationship (Keogh and Specks, 2006).

Patients with CSS usually have a high level of eosinophils in their peripheral blood. The pathogenetic effects of eosinophils are linked to the release of their cytotoxic enzymes, which can result in tissue injury (Dorfman et al., 1983; Durack et al., 1979; Fauci, 1982; Pagnoux et al., 2007). Patients with CSS have high levels of eosinophilic toxic enzymes in their sera, urine, and bronchoalveolar lavage fluid (Pagnoux et al., 2007; Peen et al., 2000). (See also the discussion in Hypereosinophilic syndrome in Chapter 70.)

Like microscopic polyangiitis, the ANCA in CSS is associated with a perinuclear staining pattern (p-ANCA) on neutrophils. Up to 75% of patients with active CSS have associated p-ANCA present (Keogh and Specks, 2003). The presence of ANCA is associated with a "vasculitic" clinical picture, with central nervous system (CNS) involvement occurring much more often in those patients who are ANCA positive than in those who are ANCA negative. In patients who are ANCA positive, it is also more common to see evidence of mononeuritis multiplex, glomerulonephritis, alveolar hemorrhages, and purpuric lesions. ANCA-negative patients have been found to have a more "nonvasculitic" clinical presentation, with features such as eosinophilic myocarditis (Keogh and Specks, 2003).

There are different clinical and histopathological criteria for the diagnosis of CSS. The clinical criteria of Lanham et al. (1984) for the diagnosis of CSS is a triad consisting of asthma, peak eosinophilia $> 1.5 \times 10^9$/L, and systemic vasculitis involving two or more extrapulmonary organs. The most commonly effected extrapulmonary organs in CSS vasculitis are the gastrointestinal tract, skin, and heart. The skin lesions can take the form of purpura or nodules (which are found in up to two-thirds of patients). Cardiac involvement can manifest as congestive heart failure or pericardial effusions. The gastrointestinal involvement consists of diarrhea or abdominal pain, with bleeding present in some patients. According to Lanham and colleagues there are three clinical phases in CSS: (1) the prodromal phase consisting of asthma and, in some patients, allergic rhinitis and polyposis; (2) the second phase consisting of eosinophilia in the blood and possibly even eosinophilic tissue infiltration; and (3) the third (and most serious) phase consisting of a systemic vasculitis. However, the different phases do not always occur in order, and this makes the diagnosis more difficult, often leading to a delay in treatment (Chumbley et al., 1977; Keogh and Specks, 2003).

In order to effectively diagnose patients with CSS, the American College of Rheumatology developed clinical and histopathologic criteria for the diagnosis of CSS. Using these 1990 criteria, it is determined that a patient with vasculitis has CSS with a sensitivity

Uncommon Causes of Stroke, 2nd edition, ed. Louis R. Caplan. Published by Cambridge University Press. © Cambridge University Press 2008.

of 85% and a specificity of 99.7% if at least four of the following six criteria are met: asthma, eosinophilia (>10% of white blood cells [WBC]), mononeuropathy or polyneuropathy (including mononeuropathy multiplex), nonfixed pulmonary infiltrates, paranasal sinus abnormality, or a biopsy containing a blood vessel with eosinophils seen extravascularly (Masi *et al.*, 1990).

Cerebrovascular complications of CSS

Neurological involvement in CSS is relatively common with up to 76% of patients having evidence of a peripheral neuropathy, usually presenting as a mononeuritis multiplex. The CNS is much less often involved, but there is a higher prevalence of morbidity and mortality if CNS involvement is present (Keogh and Specks, 2006). In one series, among 91 patients, 69 (76%) had peripheral neuropathies, whereas only 10 (11%) had CNS involvement (Keogh and Specks, 2003). Among 112 patients with CSS in another series, 81 (72%) had peripheral nervous system signs, whereas 10 (9%) had CNS abnormalities (Sable-Fourtassou *et al.*, 2005).

Because many of the infarcts are small but widely disseminated, patients mostly present with confusion, decreased alertness, and diminished cognitive function. A rather diffuse encephalopathy is the typical finding. Occlusions of dural sinus and cerebral veins (Teresa Sartori *et al.*, 2006) and of arteries supplying the eye (Hoffman *et al.*, 2005; Udono *et al.*, 2003) indicate that a prothrombotic state develops in some patients with CSS. Thrombosis of systemic veins and arteries has also been reported (Ames *et al.*, 1996; Garcia *et al.*, 2005).

CSS brain infarcts

Large brain infarcts related to CSS are rare. In a case series by Sehgal *et al.* (1995), brain infarcts were seen in 3 of 47 patients with CSS. The three infarcts in this case series occurred in different vascular territories, in patients of both sexes, and in a range of ages. The first patient was a 62-year-old woman who had a left middle cerebral artery (MCA) infarct. The second patient was a 34-year-old man with a right MCA infarction related to a left ventricular thrombus in the presence of CSS. The third patient was a 62-year-old woman with a thalamic infarct. In all three patients, the diagnosis of CSS had been made at the time of the brain infarct. The time delay between the diagnosis of CSS and brain infarction ranged from 2 to 15 years (Sehgal *et al.*, 1995).

There are few other case reports of CSS presenting with focal neurological deficits related to brain infarction. Tsuda *et al.* (2005) reported a patient with CSS who presented with a third nerve palsy and midbrain infarction. Their patient was a 30-year-old man with a 20-year history of asthma. He developed horizontal diplopia and was found to have a partial left third nerve palsy and bilateral sural nerve hyperesthesia. MRI showed a midbrain infarction in the vascular territory supplied by the left superior median mesencephalic branch of the posterior cerebral artery. Complete blood count revealed a WBC count of 31 900/mm^3 with 66% eosinophils. Serum p-ANCA testing was positive. The patient was treated with pulsed methylprednisolone 1000 mg/day for 3 days followed by prednisolone 80 mg/day for 14 days with improvement

in symptoms. He was continued on prednisolone 15 mg/day and remained asymptomatic with no change in MRI (Tsuda *et al.*, 2005).

CSS-related hemorrhage

There have been several reports of CSS presenting with intracerebral hemorrhage. The mechanism has been thought to be related to uncontrolled hypertension in the setting of CSS (Liou *et al.*, 1997). However, there have also been reports in patients with CSS who do not have uncontrolled hypertension, suggesting a possible mechanism secondary to the underlying angiitis (Nishino *et al.*, 1999). In addition to intraparenchymal hemorrhage, there has also been a report of subarachnoid and intraventricular hemorrhage from a necrotizing vasculitis of the choroid plexus in CSS (Chang *et al.*, 1993).

Treatment of CSS

Glucocorticoids remain the mainstay of therapy in CSS. Initial therapy with prednisone is usually pulsed (15 mg/kg over 60 minutes repeated at 24-hour intervals for 1–3 days) followed by prednisone 1 mg/kg per day (Guillevin *et al.*, 1996).

Treatment must be optimized for each individual patient, and in some patients other immunosuppressant medications are added to the steroid regimen. Keogh and Specks (2006) recommended that cyclophosphamide be considered if the CSS is severe, as evidenced by cardiac, renal, or nervous system involvement (central or peripheral). The side effects of cyclophosphamide include hemorrhagic cystitis, bladder fibrosis, bone marrow suppression, ovarian failure, and neoplasms (bladder cancer and hematologic malignancies). Alternatively, methotrexate can be used in patients without life-threatening illness to induce remission. Methotrexate can also be used after cyclophosphamide therapy to maintain remission. Newer options for immunosuppression include azathioprine and mycophenolate-mofetil.

Prognosis

Guillevin *et al.* (1996) completed a prospective study of 342 patients (260 with polyarteritis nodosa and 82 with CSS) to determine prognosis. They established a five-factor prognostic score consisting of: renal insufficiency with serum Cr > 1.58 mg/dL, CNS involvement, cardiomyopathy, presence of proteinuria (>1 g/d) and gastrointestinal tract involvement. If none of these features was present, mortality at 5 years was 11.9%. If one feature was present, mortality increased to 25.9% compared to a mortality of 45.95% if three or more features were present. CNS involvement correlated with an RR of mortality of 1.76.

Conclusion

CSS is a rare and challenging disease process both to diagnose and manage. Nervous system involvement is usually peripheral but can also be central, presenting with cerebral infarction or hemorrhage. Involvement of the CNS is associated with an increased risk for mortality and requires aggressive treatment with steroids and immunosuppressants. The condition should be considered in any patient who has asthma and develops eosinophilia and peripheral and/or CNS signs.

REFERENCES

Ames, P. R., Roes, L., Lupoli, S., *et al.* 1996. Thrombosis in Churg-Strauss syndrome. Beyond vasculitis? *Br J Rheumatol*, **35**, 1181–3.

Chang, Y., Kargas, S. A., Goates, J. J., and Horoupian, D. S. 1993. Intraventricular and subarachnoid hemorrhage resulting from necrotizing vasculitis of the choroid plexus in a patient with Churg-Strauss syndrome. *Clin Neuropathol*, **12**, 84–7.

Chumbley, L. C., Harrison, E. G., and DeRemee, R. A. 1977. Allergic granulomatosis and angiitis (Churg-Strauss syndrome). *Mayo Clin Proc*, **52**, 477–84.

Churg, J. and Strauss, L. 1951. Allergic granulomatosis, allergic angiitis, and periarteritis nodosa. *Am J Pathol*, **27**, 277–301.

Dorfman, L. J., Ransom, B. R., Formo, L. S., and Klets, A. 1983. Neuropathy in the hypereosinophilic syndrome. *Muscle Nerve*, **6**, 291–8.

Durack, D. T., Sumi, S. M., and Klebanoff, S. J. 1979. Neurotoxicity of human eosinophils. *Proc Natl Acad Sci, U S A*, **76**, 1443–7.

Fauci, A. S. 1982. NIH conference: the idiopathic hypereosinophilic syndrome. *Ann Intern Med*, **97**, 78–92.

Garcia, G., Achouh, L., Cobarzan, D., Fichet, D., and Humbert, M. 2005. Severe venous thromboembolic disease in Churg-Strauss syndrome. *Allergy*, **60**, 409–10.

Guillevin, L., Lhote, F., Gayraud, M., *et al.* 1996. Prognostic factors in polyarteritis nodosa and Churg-Strauss syndrome. A prospective study in 342 patients. *Medicine (Baltimore)*, **75**, 17–28.

Hoffman, P. M., Godfrey, T., and Stawell, R. J. 2005. A case of Churg-Strauss syndrome with visual loss following central retinal artery occlusion. *Lupus*, **14**, 174–5.

Keogh, K. A., and Specks, U. 2003. Churg-Strauss syndrome. Clinical presentation, antineutrophil cytoplasmic antibodies and leukotriene receptor antagonists. *Am J Med*, **115**, 284–90.

Keogh, K. A., and Specks, U. 2006. Churg-Strauss syndrome: update on clinical, laboratory and therapeutic aspects. *Sarcoidosis Vasc Diffuse Lung Dis*, **23**, 3–12.

Lanham, J. G., Elkon, K. B., Pusey, C. D., and Hughes, C. R. 1984. Systemic vasculitis with asthma and eosinophilia: a clinical approach to the Churg-Strauss syndrome. *Medicine (Baltimore)*, **63**, 65–81.

Liou, H. H., Liu, H. M., Chiang, I. P., Yeh, T. S., and Chen, R. C. 1997. Churg-Strauss syndrome presented as multiple intracerebral hemorrhage. *Lupus*, **6**, 279–82.

Masi, A. T., Hunder, G. G., Lie, J. T., *et al.* 1990. The American College of Rheumatology 1990 criteria for the classification of Churg-Strauss syndrome (allergic granulomatosis and angiitis). *Arthritis Rheum*, **33**, 1094–100.

Nishino, R., Murata, Y., Oiwa, H., *et al.* 1999. A case of Churg-Strauss syndrome presented as right thalamic hemorrhage. *No To Shinkei*, **51**, 891–4.

Pagnoux, C., Guilpain, P., and Guillevin, L. 2007. Churg-Strauss syndrome. *Curr Opin Rheumatol*, **19**, 25–32.

Peen, E., Hahn, P., Lauwers, G., *et al.* 2000. Churg-Strauss syndrome: localization of eosinophil major basic protein in damaged tissues. *Arthritis Rheum*, **43**, 1897–900.

Sable-Fourtassou, R., Cohen, P., Mahr, A., *et al.* for the French Vasculitis Study Group. 2005. Antineutrophil cytoplasmic antibodies and the Churg-Strauss syndrome. *Ann Intern Med*, **143**, 632–8.

Sehgal, M., Swanson, J. W., Deremee, R. A., and Colby, T. V. 1995. Neurologic manifestations of Churg-Strauss syndrome. *Mayo Clin Proc*, **70**, 337–41.

Teresa Sartori, M., Briani, C., Munari, M., *et al.* 2006. Cerebral venous thrombosis as a rare onset of Churg-Strauss syndrome. *Thromb Haemost*, **96**, 90–2.

Tsuda, H., Ishikawa, H., Majima, T., *et al.* 2005. Isolated oculomotor nerve palsy in Churg-Strauss syndrome. *Intern Med*, **44**, 638–40.

Udono, T., Abe, T., Sato, H., and Tamai, M. 2003. Bilateral central retinal artery occlusion in Churg-Strauss syndrome. *Am J Ophthalmol*, **136**, 1181–3.

45

SYSTEMIC LUPUS ERYTHEMATOSUS

Nancy Futrell

Introduction

Patients with systemic lupus erythematosus (SLE) have an increased risk of stroke (Futrell and Millikan, 1989). As these patients are relatively young compared to other stroke patients, SLE is generally considered in the evaluation of stroke. SLE is actually a relatively uncommon etiology of stroke, even in young persons, being found in only 3.5% of patients presenting with stroke before the age of 45 (Adams *et al.*, 1995). The risk of recurrence of stroke in patients with SLE is much higher than in other stroke patients, and the preventative treatment is influenced by the underlying systemic disease. This, along with the need to determine when to order expensive diagnostic tests to rule out SLE in young stroke patients, makes an understanding of the systemic disease of SLE and many unique features of stroke in SLE an important part of the general knowledge base for the management and prevention of stroke.

Background

SLE was initially described as a skin disorder in the mid-nineteenth century, with recognition of the systemic, multiorgan involvement by Kaposi in 1872. Although Kaposi included descriptions of patients with brain dysfunction, including headache, delirium, and coma, the first description of focal neurological deficits was by Osler, who reported a patient with episodes of right hemiparesis and aphasia in 1904. The presence of systemic "thrombosis" (more likely cardiogenic emboli) was recognized as early as 1935, with a report of lupus patients with renal infarcts and endocarditis at autopsy (Baehr *et al.*, 1935). Multiple cerebral infarcts were described at autopsy in lupus patients with Libman-Sacks endocarditis in 1947 (von Albertini and Alb, 1947), and lupus presenting with stroke was reported in 1963 (Silverstein, 1963) and in 1971 (Jentsch *et al.*, 1971). Widespread recognition of stroke as a complication of SLE began in the early 1980s (Delaney, 1983; Haas, 1982; Harris *et al.*, 1984; Hart and Miller, 1983).

Diagnosis of SLE

A diagnosis of SLE includes documentation of 4 of 11 potential abnormalities (Tan *et al.*, 1982) (Table 45.1). In young stroke patients, an appropriate history should be taken to determine whether any clinical manifestations of SLE have been present, or whether there is a family history of SLE or other autoimmune

Table 45.1 Criteria for the diagnosis of SLE[a]

(i)	Malar rash
(ii)	Discoid rash
(iii)	Photosensitivity
(iv)	Oral ulcers (generally painless)
(v)	Arthritis (two or more joints, with swelling; arthralgias not sufficient)
(vi)	Serositis
	(a) Pleuritis (pleurisy, pleural effusion, pleural rub)
	(b) Pericarditis (pericardial effusion or rub, or typical EKG changes)
(vii)	Renal
	(a) 3+ proteinuria
	(b) Cellular casts
(viii)	Neurological
	(a) Seizures
	(b) Psychosis
(ix)	Hematological
	(a) Hemolytic anemia
	(b) Leukopenia (<4000/mm^3 on two or more occasions)
	(c) Lymphopenia (<1500/mm^3 on two or more occasions)
	(d) Thrombocytopenia (<100 000/mm^3)
(x)	Immunological
	(a) Positive LE prep (rarely performed now)
	(b) False-positive syphilis test
	(c) Anti-DNA antibody
(xi)	Anti-nuclear antibody (ANA) 1:320 or greater

Note: [a] The diagnosis of SLE requires positivity in 4 of the 11 categories. "Seronegative" lupus is described as lupus in patients without a positive ANA or anti-DNA. There is disagreement as to whether seronegative lupus is bona fide SLE.
Source: Tan *et al.*, 1982, reproduced with permission.

disorders. Review of systems should include questions about arthritis, skin rashes, photosensitivity, pleurisy, seizures, and psychotic episodes, which will screen for 6 of the 11 potential lupus criteria. The physical examination should include evaluation of the skin, mucous membranes, and joints, along with auscultation for pericardial or pleural rubs, screening for 5 of the 11 criteria. The usual admitting laboratory panel for stroke patients includes

Uncommon Causes of Stroke, 2nd edition, ed. Louis R. Caplan. Published by Cambridge University Press. © Cambridge University Press 2008.

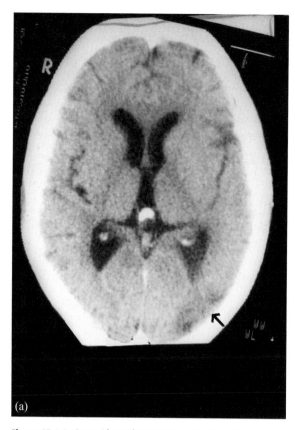

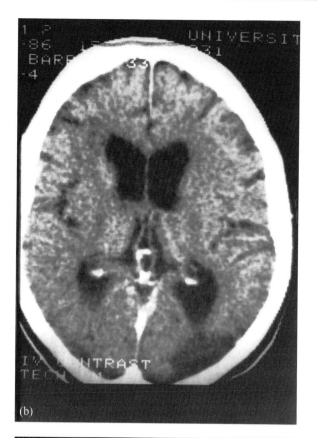

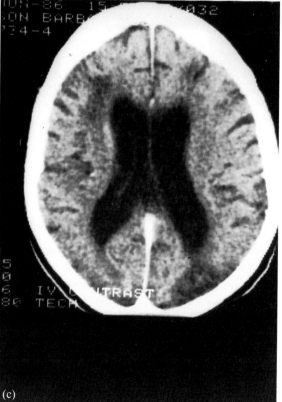

Figure 45.1 Patient with SLE, lupus anticoagulant, and 16 spontaneous abortions. (**a**) Head CT scan following a left parietal stroke (*arrow*). Major atrophy was not present at that time. Anticoagulant therapy was not initiated, as the patient was hospitalized for a major gastrointestinal (GI) bleed. (**b**) and (**c**) Head CT scan 2 years later, following multiple cerebral infarcts. Multiple areas of low density are present, along with significant interval enlargement of the ventricles. Anticoagulant was started because of a pulmonary embolus. The patient had no clinical strokes over the subsequent year.

a complete blood count, chemistry panel, prothrombin time, partial thromboplastin time (PTT), and urinalysis. This panel serves as a screen for the two additional lupus criteria, and also screens for the lupus anticoagulant (elevated PTT). An echocardiogram (standard portion of the stroke evaluation) would screen for a pericardial effusion if present.

If the admitting history, physical examination, and laboratory results do not suggest lupus, specific tests for SLE (ANA, double-stranded-DNA) or for lupus anticoagulant (Russell's Viper Venom Time) are not warranted.

Frequency

The exact frequency of stroke in lupus is not known. One report of consecutive patients in a university-based rheumatology clinic reports 4% of lupus patients having stroke, but some likely stroke patients with diplopia, gaze palsy, and/or vertigo were classed as having "brainstem syndrome" rather than stroke (Sibley *et al.*, 1992). Series selected from consecutive hospital admissions overestimate the frequency of stroke, as they are biased toward patients with more severe SLE. The San Antonio Lupus Study found ischemic stroke in 2% of patients, but the longitudinal portion of this study is now underway. The long-term risk of stroke in these patients has not yet been determined (Brey *et al.*, 2002).

The frequency of recurrent stroke in patients with SLE is better documented, with more than 50% of SLE patients who have a stroke going on to have multiple infarcts if preventative treatment is not instituted (Asherson *et al.*, 1987; Futrell and Millikan, 1989).

Microinfarcts and microhemorrhages (Hanly *et al.*, 1991; Johnson and Richardson, 1968) are seen frequently in autopsy specimens of SLE patients. Asymptomatic microinfarcts are common, and are now diagnosed due to the high sensitivity of MRI (Ishikawa *et al.*, 1994). Occlusions of large arteries (Trevor *et al.*, 1972) and major strokes also occur in lupus patients (Figure 45.1).

Etiology of stroke in patients with SLE

Vasculitis, an overestimated association

Lupus patients are known to have systemic vasculitis, most commonly in the kidney or the skin. This led Osler to postulate in 1903 that similar vascular lesions could be causing stereotyped transient ischemic attacks (TIAs) in one of his patients (Osler, 1904). Unfortunately, this concept has persisted in the absence of verification. "Cerebral vasculitis" has been reported as the etiology of stroke in series of patients who did not have neuropathological confirmation, but used indirect evidence such as concomitant vasculitis in the skin. Other errors in diagnosis come from series with an angiographic diagnosis of vasculitis, which has low specificity. Major autopsy studies have failed to provide evidence for cerebral vasculitis as the cause of stroke in SLE patients (Devinsky *et al.*, 1988; Hanly *et al.*, 1991; Johnson and Richardson, 1968). There are a few case reports in the literature of what appears to be a true vasculitis (Bertrand *et al.*, 1995), but the most common pathology is a vasculopathy, with perivascular inflammatory infiltrates (Johnson and Richardson, 1968), perivascular hemorrhages (Smith *et al.*, 1994), and proliferation of blood vessels (Lie, 1989), which includes vascular occlusion with multiple channels of recanalization (Futrell and Asherson, 1993) (Figure 45.2).

In spite of the lack of pathological evidence of central nervous system vasculitis in SLE, vasculitis is commonly a strong consideration in these patients. This may be because of widespread multifocal hyperintensity of white matter on T2-weighted MRI scans, as seen in a patient who presented with mild confusion and apraxia (Figure 45.3). This patient underwent biopsy, and tissue was sampled from four separate areas. One was normal, two were consistent with edema in otherwise normal brain tissue, and one showed subacute ischemia. There was no vasculitis. Apparently this patient had multifocal ischemic lesions with an unusually large amount of white matter edema. It is possible that cytokine abnormalities in patients with SLE could contribute to unusually severe white matter changes (Al-Janadi *et al.*, 1993; Gilad *et al.*, 1997).

In cases with inflammatory changes within brain tissue and brain blood vessels, infection rather than primary inflammatory vasculitis is an important consideration (Figure 45.4). Infections

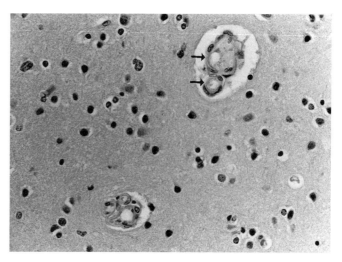

Figure 45.2 Typical vascular changes in the brain of an SLE patient with lupus anticoagulant who died of multiple organ involvement with SLE. She had multiple cerebral infarcts. Occluded vessels with recanalization are seen in this section (*small arrows*).

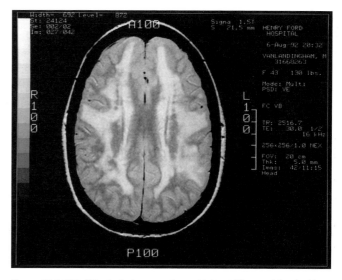

Figure 45.3 MRI of the brain from a patient with SLE. Diffuse multifocal white matter disease led to a presumptive diagnosis of vasculitis. Biopsy revealed subacute infarcts and normal tissue with edema. No vasculitis was present. The overdiagnosis of "vasculitis" based on multiple lesions on MRI is an important pitfall.

are common in patients with SLE, being a common cause of death. These can produce infected emboli. There can also be basilar meningitis from aspergillus (Futrell *et al.*, 1992), which is indeed a "vasculitis," but is a secondary rather than a primary inflammatory process. Appropriate treatment would emphasize antimicrobial therapy, as opposed to immunosuppression.

Without biopsy proof, cerebral vasculitis should not be considered the etiology of a stroke in a patient with SLE. Careful evaluation for cardiogenic emboli, hypercoagulable states, and atherosclerosis should be performed.

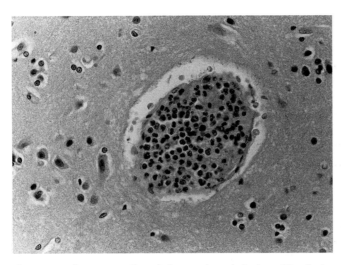

Figure 45.4 Inflammatory cells producing vascular occlusion in an SLE patient who died with pneumococcal pneumonia and positive blood cultures for pneumococcus. This is most likely an infected embolus.

Cardiogenic emboli

There are multiple cardiac abnormalities in patients with SLE. Libman-Sacks endocarditis is a verrucous endocarditis with deposition of hyalinized blood and platelet thrombus, not covered by endothelium (Libman and Sacks, 1924). These lesions can involve cardiac valves as well as the endocardium, and they can produce emboli. As many as 75% of SLE patients may have cardiac abnormalities on echocardiography, with valvular lesions in 37.5% (Ong et al., 1992). The most commonly diseased valve is the mitral valve. Cardiac valvular abnormalities are associated with anti-cardiolipin antibodies (Metz et al., 1994; Stein et al., 1994). Abnormalities of the mitral valve are the most common, and infective endocarditis is a frequent problem (Fluture et al., 2003). Based on autopsy material, cardiogenic sources of emboli appear to be the most common etiology in patients with stroke (Devinsky et al., 1988).

Hypercoagulable states

The lupus anticoagulant includes a heterogeneous group of antibodies that interfere with phospholipid coagulation tests in vitro (Espinoza and Hartmann, 1986). The lupus anticoagulant and anti-cardiolipin antibodies are partially overlapping autoantibodies (Branch et al., 1987) associated with venous thrombosis (Asherson et al., 1989), multiple spontaneous abortions (Branch et al., 1985), and stroke (Fields et al., 1990). They were initially described in patients with SLE, but the primary anti-phospholipid antibody syndrome in individuals without SLE was subsequently described (Asherson et al., 1989). The catastrophic anti-phospholipid antibody syndrome presents with life-threatening diffuse vascular occlusive events. In a cohort of 250 catastrophic anti-phospholipid antibody syndrome patients with multiple recurrent ischemic events, 100 of the patients also had lupus. Patients with lupus had significantly higher mortality than those with the primary anti-phospholipid antibody syndrome (59% vs.

39%, $p = .0003$), with stroke being the number one cause of death (Bucciarelli et al., 2006).

There is evidence that the lupus anticoagulant may convey a higher risk for thrombosis than anti-cardiolipin antibodies (Derksen et al., 1988). Those patients who are positive for beta(2)-glycoprotein I, a plasma cofactor that facilitates the binding of anti-phospholipid antibodies to phospholipids, may have an even higher risk of stroke (Fiallo et al., 2000). The thrombogenic tendency of both lupus anticoagulant and anti-cardiolipin antibody is multifactorial, with contributions from defects in protein C (Amer et al., 1990) and protein S (Amster et al., 1993). Both endogenous anticoagulants may contribute to this thrombogenic tendency, along with low functional levels of antithrombin III (Cosgriff and Martin, 1981).

Endothelial dysfunction (Byron et al., 1987) and fibrinolytic defects (Glas-Greenwalt et al., 1984) have also been reported in patients with SLE, with decreased endogenous tissue plasminogen activator (t-PA) activity and inhibition of plasminogen activation (Awada et al., 1988). Endothelial cell dysfunction has been correlated with the lupus anticoagulant (Byron et al., 1987), and specific antibodies against the endothelial cell are also reported (Vismara et al., 1988).

Atherosclerosis

Atherosclerosis may be more frequent in SLE patients than in the general population. Steroids, which are frequently administered to lupus patients, are associated with the development of a lipid profile that is atherogenic (MacGregor et al., 1992). This becomes even more important due to an atherogenic effect of low-density lipoprotein-containing immune complexes in lupus patients (Kabakov et al., 1992). The combination of increased triglycerides with anti-cardiolipin antibodies in these patients also has increased atherogenic potential (MacGregor et al., 1992). It is clear that atherosclerosis in lupus is more frequent than can be explained by the presence of standard vascular risk factors (Esdaile et al., 2001).

Thrombogenic cytokines

Multiple cytokine abnormalities are present in patients with SLE, with significant variability between patients (Al-Janadi et al., 1993). Tumor necrosis factor (TNF) is a thrombogenic cytokine (van der Poll et al., 1990). Baseline TNF levels are higher in patients with SLE, but levels may not elevate normally following stimulation (Malavé et al., 1989). The exact implications of abnormal cytokines in SLE are not yet clear, but presence of soluble interleukin-2 receptors in the spinal fluid, which is sometimes seen in lupus patients with brain involvement, may indicate immune mediated pathology in addition to vascular occlusion (Gilad et al., 1997).

Prevention of stroke in lupus patients

Warfarin

As the major causes of stroke in lupus are cardiogenic emboli and hypercoagulable (including hypofibrinolytic) states, the mainstay of stroke prevention is long-term warfarin, with an international normalized ratio (INR) of approximately 3.0 (Khamashta *et al.*, 1995). This is based on a study of 147 patients having a history of thrombosis who were positive for anti-phospholipid antibodies. SLE was present in 66 of these patients. More recent studies of stroke prevention in patients with anti-phospholipid antibodies suggest that there is no difference in efficacy between antiplatelet and anticoagulant therapy (Brey, 2005). These results should be interpreted with caution, as these patients had low positive anti-phospholipid antibody levels and they did not have lupus or other major systemic diseases. The risk-benefit ratio of long-term warfarin must be carefully weighed in patients with SLE. As many of them have serious underlying disorders, including anemia, GI bleeding (from vasculitic lesions or gastric irritation from steroids and nonsteroidal anti-inflammatory agents), seizures, and psychosis, anticoagulation may carry increased risk.

In patients with the catastrophic anti-phospholipid antibody syndrome, the only treatment to improve outcome was anticoagulation. The recovery rate increased by a factor of 3 in patients treated with anticoagulation versus those who did not receive anticoagulation. Corticosteroids, cyclophosphamide, plasma exchange, and intravenous immunoglobulin (IVIG) used alone did not improve the outcome. Combining anticoagulation with corticosteroids, plasma exchange, and IVIG improved recovery over that from anticoagulation alone. The addition of cyclophosphamide to anticoagulation, however, worsened outcome. By definition there is an active inflammatory process in patients who meet the definition of the catastrophic anti-phospholipid antibody syndrome. In patients with active lupus, perhaps the addition of anti-inflammatory or immunomodulating treatments might be a useful addition to anticoagulation. Importantly, strokes may occur in patients with lupus when the disease is not active (Futrell and Millikan, 1989), making improved outcome with immunomodulation unlikely.

Heparin

Even with an INR of 3.0–3.5, some lupus patients continue to have ischemic events. Also, during pregnancy, warfarin cannot be used as it crosses the placenta. In both of these situations, full dose subcutaneous heparin is a reasonable alternative. The 24-hour dose of heparin can be estimated from weight-based nomograms. Heparin can then be administered in three equal doses. As many of these patients are young women, the possibility of heparin-induced osteoporosis is important. Low-molecular-weight heparins are an excellent alternative, with less predisposition to osteoporosis.

Ancrod

Ancrod is extracted from the Malayan pit viper. It functions as an anticoagulant by decreasing fibrinogen levels, and there is also an indirect fibrinolytic effect (Reid *et al.*, 1963). It also may decrease blood viscosity (Hossmann *et al.*, 1983).

Ancrod has been used in patients with SLE and renal disease. Patients with fibrinolytic defects responded with improved

fibrinolysis, improved prostacyclin production, and improved renal function (Kant *et al.*, 1982). Those patients who did not respond had an α-2 antiplasmin (Kant *et al.*, 1985).

The use of ancrod at the present time may not be practical, as it is not widely available. The long-term role of ancrod in SLE requires further study, but theoretical considerations and preliminary data in patients with SLE are promising.

Platelet inhibition

The role of the platelet in thrombosis in SLE has not received as much attention as fibrin formation and lysis. It is clear that intramural platelet deposition is seen in occluded vessels in the brain (Ellison *et al.*, 1993), along with being present in the heart in patients with verrucous endocarditis (Libman and Sacks, 1924).

The matter of platelet inhibition is more complicated, as patients with lupus may have thrombocytopenia, and many of them are already on maximum doses of nonsteroidal anti-inflammatory medications, making aspirin therapy undesirable. Ticlopidine or clopidogrel are alternate medications, with the advantage of less direct GI irritation than aspirin. Both appear superior to aspirin in secondary stroke prevention in the general population, but there are increased expense and important side effects. Ticlopidine produces neutropenia and skin rashes that may complicate the management of the patient with SLE. Lupus patients seem to have more hematological and allergic reactions to anticonvulsant medications. There are no data on whether similar increased complications occur with clopedegril. An alternative possibility is clopidogrel, which does not have as many hematological complications but is associated with skin rash.

Steroid or immunosuppression

The failure of steroids alone to prevent stroke in lupus patients has been documented (Appan *et al.*, 1987). Steroids decrease lupus anticoagulant prothrombotic activity, but effects on anti-cardiolipin antibody levels are variable (Derksen *et al.*, 1986). Steroids have been successful in preventing recurrent spontaneous abortions in patients with SLE or the primary anti-phospholipid antibody syndrome. As SLE patients have a lifetime risk of stroke, and long-term steroids produce serious side effects, steroids should not be the first-line treatment for preventing stroke in patients with SLE. Steroids or immunosuppression are recommended only as a temporary measures, particularly if strokes or TIAs occur despite therapeutic anticoagulation. Combination therapy has been successful in patients with the catastrophic anti-phospholipid antibody syndrome, and may be applicable to patients with lupus (see the previous section on warfarin).

Conclusions

Lupus patients have a higher risk of stroke than the general population. Of greatest concern is the very high risk of multiple recurrent strokes if aggressive preventative treatment is not given. This must be balanced with the higher risk of treatments in this complicated, multisystem disease. As the major causes of stroke are cardiogenic emboli and hypercoagulable states, both of which are treated with warfarin, this is the mainstay for stroke prevention in lupus patients. Platelet inhibition may also be desirable. Steroids and immunomodulatory treatments should be reserved for patients with active systemic inflammatory processes or incomplete responses to anticoagulation and platelet inhibition. Previous dogma that stroke is caused by vasculitis and should be treated with steroids or immunosuppression cannot be validated by autopsy studies or biopsy data.

Although stroke is an important problem in lupus patients, leading to significant morbidity in young patients, SLE is relatively uncommon in young patients presenting with strokes or TIAs. Laboratory evaluation for SLE can be reserved for those patients with evidence of SLE by history, physical examination, or standard laboratory tests used in all stroke patients.

REFERENCES

Adams, H. P., Kappelle, L. J., Biller, J., *et al.* 1995. Ischemic stroke in young adults; experience in 329 patients enrolled in the Iowa registry of stroke in young adults. *Arch Neurol*, **52**, 491–5.

Al-Janadi, M., Al-Balla, S., Al-Dalaan, A., and Raziuddin, S. 1993. Cytokine profile in systemic lupus erythematosus, rheumatoid arthritis, and other rheumatic diseases. *J Clin Immunol*, **13**, 58–67.

Amer, L., Kisiel, W., Searles, R. P., and Williams, R. C. Jr. 1990. Impairment of the protein C anticoagulant pathway in a patient with systemic lupus erythematosus, anticardiolipin antibodies and thrombosis. *Thromb Res*, **57**, 247–58.

Amster, M. S., Conway, J., Zeid, M., and Pincus, S. 1993. Cutaneous necrosis resulting from protein S deficiency and increased antiphospholipid antibody in a patient with systemic lupus erythematosus. *J Am Acad Dermatol*, **29**, 853–7.

Appan, S., Boey, M. L., and Lim, K. W. 1987. Multiple thromboses in systemic lupus erythematosus. *Arch Dis Child*, **62**, 739–41.

Asherson, R. A., Khamashta, M. A., Gil, A., *et al.* 1987. Cerebrovascular disease and antiphospholipid antibodies in systematic lupus erythematosus, lupus-like disease, and the primary antiphospholipid syndrome. *Am J Med*, **86**, 391–9.

Asherson, R. A., Khamashta, M. A., Ordi-Ros, J., *et al.* 1989. The 'primary' antiphospholipid syndrome: major clinical and serological features. *Medicine (Baltimore)*, **68**, 366–74.

Asherson, R. A., Mercey, D., Phillips, G., *et al.* 1987. Recurrent stroke and multi-infarct dementia in systemic lupus erythematosus: association with antiphospholipid antibodies. *Ann Rheum Dis*, **46**, 605–11.

Awada, H., Barlowatz-Meimon, G., Dougados, M., *et al.*1988. Fibrinolysis abnormalities in systemic lupus erythematosus and their relation to vasculitis. *J Lab Clin Med*, **111**, 229–36.

Baehr, G., Klemperer, P. and Schifrin, A. 1935. A diffuse disease of the peripheral circulation (usually associated with lupus erythematosus and endocarditis). *Trans Assoc Am Physicians*, **50**, 139–55.

Bertrand, E., Kuczynska-Zardzewialy, A., Palasik, W., and Chorzelski, T. 1995. Rare vascular changes in the brain in a case of subacute cutaneous lupus erythematosus. *Folia Neuropathol*, **33**, 235–40.

Branch, D. W., Rote, N. S., Dostal, D. A., and Scott, J. R. 1987. Association of lupus anticoagulant with antibody against phosphatidylserine. *Clin Immunol Immunopathol*, **42**, 63–75.

Branch, D. W., Scott, J. R., Kochenour, N. K., and Hershgold, E. 1985. Obstetric complications associated with the lupus anticoagulant. *N Engl J Med*, **313**, 1322–6.

Brey, R. L. 2005. Antiphospholipid antibodies in young adults with stroke. *J Thomb Thrombolysis*, **20**, 105–12.

Brey, R. L., Holliday, S. L., Saklad, A. R., *et al.* 2002. Neuropsychiatric syndromes in lupus: prevalence using standardized definitions. *Neurology*, **58**, 1214–20.

Byron, M. A., Allington, M. J., Chapel, H. M., Mowat, A. G., and Cederholm-Williams, S. A. 1987. Indications of vascular endothelial cell dysfunction in systemic lupus erythematosus. *Ann Rheum Dis*, **46**, 741–5.

Cosgriff, T. M., and Martin, B. A. 1981. Low functional and high antigenic antithrombin III level in a patient with the lupus anticoagulant and recurrent thrombosis. *Arthritis Rheum*, **24**, 94–6.

Delaney, P. 1983. Neurologic complications of systemic erythematosus. *AFP*, **28**, 191–3.

Derksen, R. H., Beisma, D., Bouma, B. N., Gmelig Meyling, F. H., and Kater, L. 1986. Discordant effects of prednisone on anticardiolipin antibodies and the lupus anticoagulant [letter]. *Arthritis Rheum*, **29**, 1295–6.

Derksen, R. H., Hasselaar, P., Blokzijl, L., Gmelig-Meyling, F. H., and De Groot, P. G. 1988. Coagulation screen is more specific than the anticardiolipin antibody ELISA in evaluating a thrombotic subset of lupus patients. *Ann Rheum Dis*, **47**, 364–71.

Devinsky, O., Petito, C. K., and Alonso, D. R. 1988. Clinical and neuropathological findings in systemic lupus erythematosus: the role of vasculitis, heart emboli and thrombotic thrombocytopenic purpura. *Ann Neurol*, **23**, 380–4.

Ellison, D., Gatter, K., Heryet, A., and Esiri, M. 1993. Intramural platelet deposition in cerebral vasculopathy of systemic lupus erythematosus. *J Clin Pathol*, **46**, 37–40.

Esdaile, J. M., Abrahamowicz, M., Grodzicky, T., Li, Y. 2001. Traditional Framingham risk factors fail to fully account for accelerated atherosclerosis in systemic lupus erythematosus. *Arthritis Rheum*, **44**, 2331–7.

Espinoza, L. R., and Hartmann, R. C. 1986. Significance of the lupus anticoagulant. *Am J Hematol*, **22**, 331–7.

Fiallo, P., Tomasina, C., Clapasson, A., and Cardo, P. P. 2000. Antibodies to beta(2)-glycoprotein I in ischemic stroke. *Cerebrovasc Dis*, **10**, 293–7.

Fields, R. A., Sibbitt, W. L., Toubbeh, H., and Bankhurst, A. D. 1990. Neuropsychiatric lupus erythematosus, cerebral infarctions, and anticardiolipin antibodies. *Ann Rheum Dis*, **49**, 114–7.

Fluture, A., Chaudhari, S., and Frishman, W. H. 2003. Valvular heart disease and systemic lupus erythematosus: therapeutic implications. *Heart Dis*, **5**, 349–53.

Futrell, N., and Asherson, R. A. 1993. Probable antiphospholipid syndrome with recanalization of occluded blood vessels mimicking proliferative vasculopathy. *Clin Exp Rheumatol*, **11**, 230.

Futrell, N., and Millikan, C. 1989. Frequency, etiology, and prevention of stroke in patients with systemic lupus erythematosus. *Stroke*, **20**, 583–91.

Futrell, N., Schultz, L. R., and Millikan, C. 1992. Central nervous system disease in patients with systemic lupus erythematosus. *Neurology*, **42**, 1649–57.

Gilad, R., Lampl, Y., Eshel, Y., Barak, V., and Sarova-Pinhas, I. 1997. Cerebrospinal fluid soluble interleukin-2 receptor in cerebral lupus. *Br J Rheumatol*, **36**, 190–3.

Glas-Greenwalt, P., Kant, K. S., Allen, C., and Pollak, V. E. 1984. Fibrinolysis in health and disease: severe abnormalities in systemic lupus erythematosus. *J Lab Clin Med*, **104**, 962–76.

Haas, L. F. 1982. Stroke as an early manifestation of systemic lupus erythematosus. *J Neurol, Neurosurg, Psychiatry*, **45**, 554–6.

Hanly, J. G., Walsh, N. M. G., and Sangalang, V. 1991. Brain pathology in systemic lupus erythematosus. *J Rheumatol*, **71**, 416–22.

Harris, E. N., Gharavi, A. E., Asherson, R. A., Boey, M. L., and Hughes, G. R. V. 1984. Cerebral infarction in systemic lupus: association with anticardiolipin antibodies. *Clin Exp Rheumatol*, **2**, 47–51.

Hart, R. G., and Miller, V. T. 1983. Cerebral infarction in young adults: a practical approach. *Stroke*, **14**, 110–14.

Hossmann, V., Heiss, W. D., Bewermeyer, H., and Wiedemann, G. 1983. Controlled trial of ancrod in ischemic stroke. *Arch Neurol*, **40**, 803–8.

Ishikawa, O., Ohnishi, K., Miyachi, Y., and Ishizaka, H. 1994. Cerebral lesions in systemic lupus erythematosus detected by magnetic resonance imaging. Relationship to anticardiolipin antibody. *J Rheumatol*, **21**, 87–90.

Jentsch, H. J., Haas, H., Haffner, B., and Berger, H. 1971. Fokale Anfälle und hemiplegie als Erstmanifestation eine systemicher Lupus erythematodes. *Therapiewoche*, **29**, 1187–94.

Johnson, R. T., and Richardson, E. P. 1968. The neurological manifestations of systemic lupus erythematosus: a clinical-pathological study of 24 cases and review of the literature. *Medicine (Baltimore)*, **47**, 337–69.

Kabakov, A. E., Tertov, V. V., Saenko, V. A., Poverenny, A. M., and Orekhov, A. N. 1992. The atherogenic effect of lupus sera: systemic lupus erythematosus-derived immune complexes stimulate the accumulation of cholesterol in cultured smooth muscle cells from human aorta. *Clin Immunol Immunopathol*, **63**, 214–20.

Kant, K. S., Doeskun, A. K., Chandran, K. G. P., *et al.* 1982. Deficiency of a plasma factor stimulating vascular prostacyclin generation in patients with lupus nephritis and glomerular thrombi and its correction by ancrod: in-vivo and in-vitro observations. *Thromb Res*, **27**, 651–8.

Kant, K. S., Pollak, V. E., Dosekum, A., *et al.* 1985. Lupus nephritis with thrombosis and abnormal fibrinolysis: effect of ancrod. *J Lab Clin Med*, **105**, 77–88.

Kaposi, M. K. 1872. Neue Beiträge zur Kenntniss des Lupus erythematosus. *Arch Dermatitis Syphilis*, **4**, 36–78.

Khamashta, M. A., Cuadrado, M. J., Mujic, F., *et al.* 1995. The management of thrombosis in the antiphospholipid-antibody syndrome. *N Engl J Med*, **332**, 993–1027.

Libman, E., and Sacks, B. 1924. A hitherto undescribed form of valvular and mural endocarditis. *Arch Intern Med*, **33**, 701–37.

Lie, J. T. 1989. Vasculopathy in the antiphospholipid syndrome: thrombosis or vasculitis, or both? *J Rheumatol*, **16**, 713.

MacGregor, A. J., Dhillon, V. B., Binder, A., *et al.* 1992. Fasting lipids and anti-cardiolipin antibodies as risk factors for vascular disease in systemic lupus erythematosus. *Ann Rheum Dis*, **51**, 152–5.

Malavé, I., Searles, R. P., Montano, J., and Williams, R. C. Jr. 1989. Production of tumor necrosis factor/cachectin by peripheral blood mononuclear cells in patients with systemic lupus erythematosus. *Int Arch Allergy Appl Immunol*, **89**, 355–61.

Metz, D., Jolly, D., Graciet-Richard, J., *et al.* 1994. Prevalence of valvular involvement in systemic lupus erythematosus and association with antiphospholipid syndrome: a matched echocardiographic study. *Cardiology*, **85**, 129–36.

Ong, M. L., Veerapen, K., Chambers, J. B., *et al.* 1992. Cardiac abnormalities in systemic lupus erythematosus: prevalence and relationship to disease activity. *Int J Cardiol*, **34**, 69–74.

Osler, W. 1904. On the visceral manifestations of the erythema group of skin diseases. *Am J Med Sci*, **127**, 1–23.

Reid, H., Chan, K., and Thean, P. 1963. Prolonged coagulation defect (defibrination syndrome) in the Malayan viper bite. *Lancet*, **i**, 621–6.

Sibley, J. T., Olszynski, W. P., Decoteau, W. E., and Sundaram, M. B. 1992. The incidence and prognosis of central nervous system disease in systemic lupus erythematosus. *J Rheumatol*, **19**, 47–52.

Silverstein, A. 1963. Cerebrovascular accidents as the initial major manifestation of lupus erythematosus. *N Y State J Med*, **5**, 2942–8.

Smith, R., Ellison, D. W., Jenkind, E. A., Gallagher, P., and Cawley, M. I. D. 1994. Cerebellum and brainstem vasculopathy in systemic lupus erythematosus: two clinico-pathological cases. *Ann Rheum Dis*, **53**, 327–30.

Stein, P. D., Hull, R. D., and Raskob, G. 1994. Risks for major bleeding from thrombolytic therapy in patients with acute pulmonary embolism. *Ann Int Med*, **121**, 313–7.

Tan, E. M., Cohen, A. S., Fries, J. F., *et al.* 1982. The 1982 revised criteria for the classification of systemic lupus erythematosus. *Arthritis Rheum*, **25**, 1271–7.

Trevor, R. P., Sondheimer, F. K., Fessel, W. J., and Wolpert, S. M. 1972. Angiographic demonstration of major cerebral vessel occlusion in systemic lupus erythematosus. *Neuroradiology*, **4**, 202–7.

van der Poll, T., Büller, H. R., ten Cate, H. *et al.* 1990. Activation of coagulation after administration of tumor necrosis factor to normal subjects. *N Engl J Med*, **322**, 1622–7.

Vismara, A., Meroni, P. L., Tincani, A., *et al.* 1988. Relationship between anti-cardiolipin and anti-endothelial cell antibodies in systemic lupus erythematosus. *Clin Exp Immunol*, **74**, 247–53.

von Albertini, V. A., and Alb, O. 1947. Ueber die atypische verrucoese endocarditis Libman-Sacks und ihr beziehungen zum lupus erythematodes acutus. *Cardiologica*, **12**, 133–69.

46

RHEUMATOID ARTHRITIS AND CEREBROVASCULAR DISEASE

Elayna O. Rubens and Sean I. Savitz

Introduction

Rheumatoid arthritis (RA) is an autoimmune disease that is characterized by an inflammatory, symmetric polyarthritis. In addition to the intra-articular inflammation, the systemic disease leads to the well known, extra-articular manifestations including rheumatoid nodules, pericarditis, pleuritis, vasculitis, and Felty's syndrome. The most common neurological complications of RA are peripheral neuropathy and cervical myelopathy (Moore and Richardson, 1998). Although cerebrovascular complications are less common, there is a growing body of evidence that suggests that patients with RA are at increased risk for stroke and that this increased risk contributes significantly to the morbidity and mortality of RA (Sattar *et al.*, 2003).

Various epidemiological studies have shown an increased mortality and decreased life expectancy in patients with RA (Wolfe *et al.*, 1994). A follow-up of more than 300 RA patients showed the standardized mortality ratio (the ratio of observed to expected deaths) to be 1.65 (Chehata *et al.*, 2001). Much of the increased mortality has been attributed to an increased frequency of vascular disease. Noncardiac vascular disease is common among patients with RA; one patient cohort was found to have a 22% cumulative risk of cerebrovascular events during 30 years of follow-up (Liang *et al.*, 2005). The relative risk of stroke in patients with RA compared to the general population is less clear. A retrospective analysis of the Nurses' Health Study compared risk of myocardial infarction and stroke in women with and without RA. There was a clear increased risk of myocardial infarction in women with RA, but the relative risk of stroke (1.48) was not statistically significant (Solomon *et al.*, 2003). Similarly, Wolfe *et al.* (2003) compared cardiovascular and cerebrovascular disease prevalence between patients with RA and those with osteoarthritis. They found that patients with RA were 1.7 times more likely to have had a stroke in the preceding 6 months than were patients with osteoarthritis. There was also a trend toward increased lifetime risk of stroke among RA patients, although this was not statistically significant (Wolfe *et al.*, 2003).

The mechanisms by which RA patients are predisposed to stroke are varied. The most common of these causes is atherosclerotic disease, which seems to be accelerated by the underlying RA. Hypercoagulability, central nervous system (CNS) vasculitis, dural rheumatoid involvement, and vertebral artery occlusion are less common causes of strokes in patients with RA.

Accelerated atherosclerosis

An increased prevalence of a number of vascular risk factors has been demonstrated, all of which seem to accelerate atherosclerosis in patients with RA. The role of systemic inflammation in mediating atherosclerotic disease is becoming more clear and may be the underlying link between RA and vascular events. Destabilization of atherosclerotic plaques has been related to the activation of the inflammatory cascade where activated T cells seem to play a major role. In RA, these same activated T cells are present in inflamed synovium and other systemic sites of inflammation. Their presence and increased activity in RA patients may predispose to atherosclerotic plaque destabilization and rupture (Pasceri and Yeh, 1999).

Active RA is also characterized by release of cytokines from the inflamed synovia into the systemic circulation. Tumor necrosis factor-α (TNF-α), interleukin (IL)-1β, and IL-6 are present at high levels in the serum. These cytokines, particularly TNF-α and IL-6, contribute to the development of atherosclerotic disease by promoting insulin resistance, dyslipidemia, and endothelial dysfunction (Sattar *et al.*, 2003).

Patients with active and untreated RA also often have unfavorable lipid profiles. Compared to matched healthy controls, patients with RA have lower levels of high-density lipoprotein (HDL), higher HDL/low-density lipoprotein (LDL) ratios, and higher levels of lipoprotein-a. The low HDL seems to be inversely related to acute phase reactants, such as C-reactive protein, such that those patients with more inflammatory activity had more unfavorable lipid profiles (Park *et al.*, 1999).

The tendency for increased atherosclerosis and large-artery disease in RA has been further demonstrated by observations of carotid disease in this population. Studies examining carotid artery intima-media thickness with carotid ultrasound have shown an increased prevalence of carotid disease in patients with RA. One study showed that increased duration of disease (>1 year) was a risk-factor for asymptomatic carotid artery stenosis (Park *et al.*, 2002). Another study indicated prior steroid use as a potential risk factor for the development of carotid artery stenosis (Alkaabi *et al.*, 2003). These studies, however, were done on asymptomatic patients, and it is unclear if the increased prevalence of carotid atherosclerotic disease translates to increased rate of cerebrovascular events.

Hypercoagulability

There is evidence that patients with RA have an increased clotting tendency. RA patients have increased plasma levels of fibrinogen,

Uncommon Causes of Stroke, 2nd edition, ed. Louis R. Caplan. Published by Cambridge University Press. © Cambridge University Press 2008.

von Willebrand factor, tissue plasminogen activator antigen, and fibrin D-dimer (McEntegart *et al.*, 2001). Alterations in the hemostatic system in RA may be because of the subclinical vasculitis that is often present in the disease. Vasculitis and the resultant endothelial dysfunction may increase the level of circulating von Willebrand factor. Increased levels of von Willebrand factor and fibrinogen, in turn, promote thrombus formation by increasing platelet aggregation and adhesion. Elevated levels of tissue plasminogen activator and D-dimer, in contrast, indicate up-regulation of the fibrinolytic cascade, most likely in response to fibrin formation. When tissue plasminogen activator antigen patients were followed for 8 years in one study, those who developed a vascular event (myocardial infarction, stroke, or deep venous thrombosis/pulmonary embolism) were found to have significantly higher concentrations of von Willebrand factor and plasminogen activator inhibitor 1 activity than did RA patients who did not have vascular events in the follow-up period (Wallberg-Jonsson *et al.*, 2000).

Another factor that may contribute to the propensity to form clots in RA is the finding that this condition is associated with abnormal homocysteine metabolism. Fasting levels of homocysteine were 33% higher in RA patients than in the control subjects (Roubenoff *et al.*, 1997). Elevated homocysteine has been associated with thrombophilia and confers an increased risk of arterial disease. Whether lowering homocysteine levels in patients with RA would reduce risk of vascular events remains to be seen.

Vasculitis

Systemic vasculitis in RA often involves the vasa nervorum of the peripheral nervous system. CNS vasculitis, however, is an exceptionally rare complication of rheumatoid disease. In a review of the literature, 21 reported patients with RA had CNS involvement. Eleven of these had cerebral vasculitis with parenchymal involvement and subsequent infarction. Other CNS manifestations of RA include isolated meningeal vasculitis; dural, parenchymal, and choroid plexus rheumatoid nodules; and inflammatory encephalomyelitis (Kim, 1980; Tajima *et al.*, 2004). Extra-articular manifestations are most likely in patients with systemic symptoms and rheumatoid nodules. Nodules are most often found on extensor surfaces around the elbows.

Seven men and four women with cerebral vasculitis were identified in the literature. The mean age of these patients was 53 years, and mean duration of RA was 13 years. Clinical presentation varied with the site of neurological involvement. Involved areas of the CNS included basal ganglia, bilateral frontal cortex, visual cortex, splenium or the corpus callosum, fornix, pons, cerebellum, and spinal cord. Four patients had seizures, four developed a hemiparesis, six had impaired mentation, one had cortical blindness and Gerstmann syndrome, and two had ataxia and cranial nerve deficits (Beck and Corbett, 1983; Johnson *et al.*, 1959; Kemper *et al.*, 1957; Ouyang *et al.*, 1967; Pirani and Bennett, 1951; Ramos and Mandybur, 1975; Singleton *et al.*, 1995; Watson *et al.*, 1977). Cerebrospinal fluid findings available in five cases showed: 0–24 white bloods cells, 0–760 red blood cells, protein 30–133, and glucose 49–71 (Beck and Corbett, 1983; Ouyang *et al.*, 1967; Ramos and Mandybur, 1975; Singleton *et al.*, 1995; Watson *et al.*, 1977).

The pathologic features of the CNS vasculitis associated with RA are perivascular and transmural inflammatory infiltration, severe fibrinoid necrosis of the media, and perivascular nodule formation resembling polyarteritis nodosa (Ramos and Mandybur, 1975). Vasculitis without vessel necrosis has also been described mainly consisting of perivascular inflammatory infiltrates (lymphocytes and plasma cells) and vascular fibrosis of the vessels in the periventricular white matter (Singleton *et al.*, 1995). The vasculitis in RA can be isolated to the CNS or part of a generalized vascular involvement. In at least three of the reported cases, autopsy findings showed isolated cerebral vasculitis (Ouyang *et al.*, 1967; Steiner, 1959; Watson *et al.*, 1977).

Imaging studies are available for only two of the reported cases of RA-associated cerebral vasculitis. In one patient, a 52-year-old man who had had RA for 2 years presented with partial seizures involving both sides of his body on separate occasions. CT scan showed diffuse cortical enhancement of the anterior frontal lobes bilaterally. Brain and meningeal biopsy of the right frontal cortex confirmed meningeal and parenchymal perivascular inflammatory changes. He improved on prednisone and azathioprine and was reportedly asymptomatic after 2 years of follow-up (Beck and Corbett, 1983). Another reported patient, a 47-year-old woman with RA, presented with dysarthria and gait ataxia. MRI showed increased T2 signal in the pons with marked hyperintensity of the periventricular white matter with minimal extension to the gray-white junction. There was no enhancement nor was there involvement of the gray matter. Cerebral angiography showed no abnormalities. She was treated with prednisone and azathioprine with stabilization of her neurological deficits. A follow-up MRI 9 months later showed no interval change. She died unexpectedly 2 years after presentation, and postmortem examination of the brain showed perivascular inflammatory infiltrates in the periventricular white matter, pons, and right hippocampus (Singleton *et al.*, 1995).

Although MRI is a useful imaging study for detecting small-vessel vasculopathy, it should be noted that the findings are relatively nonspecific in rheumatoid vasculitis. Meningeal and brain biopsy therefore remains the gold standard in confirming a diagnosis of vasculitis in these patients. In RA, biopsy is particularly important given that the other CNS manifestations of the disease may produce similar abnormalities on imaging studies. Encephalomyelopathy, for example, has been reported in RA with similar brainstem and basal ganglia T2 hyperintensities on MRI in the absence of a diagnosis of vasculitis (Tajima *et al.*, 2004).

The underlying pathogenesis of CNS vasculitis associated with RA remains unclear. Possible causes include complications of disease-modifying therapy used in RA, immune complex deposition, or association of RA with other rheumatic diseases such as Sjögren's or polyarteritis nodosa (Ramos and Mandybur, 1975). Despite the rarity of the disease, CNS vasculitis should be considered in the differential diagnosis of any RA patient presenting with focal neurological signs and symptoms.

Venous sinus thrombosis

Rheumatoid involvement of the dura either by pachymeningitis or by dural rheumatoid nodules is an unusual occurrence (Kim, 1980). The inflammation of the meninges comprising the dural sinus or presence of rheumatoid nodules adjacent to the venous sinuses themselves could predispose to venous sinus thrombosis. A single case report described a woman with an 8-year history of RA who presented with paraparesis, dysarthria, and nystagmus. She was found to have sulcal effacement and edema of the bilateral frontal and parietal lobes associated with superior sagittal sinus thrombosis. She improved on heparin and was later found to have imaging evidence of pachymeningitis. An evaluation for other causes of hypercoagulability was negative (Cellerini *et al.*, 2001).

Vertebral arterial disease

Acquired as well as congenital lesions of the osseous and ligamentous structures at the craniocervical junction have also been posited to cause compression of the distal extracranial vertebral artery and posterior circulation ischemia. Although there is a theoretical risk of mechanical injury to the vertebral artery due to cervical arthritis and atlantoaxial subluxation in RA, this most often results in cervical myelopathy. Stroke due to vertebral dissection has been reported in RA, but the vertebral artery occlusion was sometimes associated with only minimal atlantoaxial subluxation (Loeb *et al.*, 1993).

A number of individual case reports do document compressive changes in vertebral arteries related to severe rheumatoid disease at the cervicocranial junction (Caplan 1996). Davis and Markley (1951) reported death from direct medullary compression by the odontoid process in a physician's wife who had severe RA. The dens had dislocated and herniated upward through the foramen magnum. No vascular compression was shown or sought in this patient. Robinson (1966) reviewed the clinical findings in 22 patients with RA who had atlantoaxial subluxation. Two of these patients had transient positional vertigo, one of whom also had transient visual blurring. Robinson (1966) reviewed the anatomical relationships of the vertebral artery, the odontoid process of C2, and the atlas and noted "while the neurological complaints are no doubt related to cord compression, it is possible that some of the manifestations such as vertigo and visual disturbance may be related to intermittent obstruction of the vertebral artery due to excessive mobility of C2."

Webb *et al.* (1968) reported the first well-documented patient with posterior circulation infarction related to RA of the upper cervical spine. A 53-year-old woman with severe RA had had occasional blackouts and occipital headaches. She became comatose, and autopsy showed severe atlantoaxial subluxation with protrusion of the dens into the foramen magnum adjacent to the medulla. The vertebral arteries were both thrombosed at "their upper ends where they followed a tortuous course along the disorganized collapsed remnants of the atlas and axis" (Webb *et al.*, 1968). Extensive cerebellar and brainstem infarction had caused her death.

Jones and Kaufman (1976) also reported a single autopsy-confirmed case of vertebral artery compression due to RA. A 74-year-old man had had intermittent spells of loss of consciousness, and then died after a period of "coma vigil." Autopsy showed extensive bilateral posterior cerebral artery territory infarction and brainstem and cerebellar infarcts. The odontoid was displaced to the right and herniated upwards for a distance of 1 cm through the foramen magnum. The right vertebral artery was markedly narrowed and constricted in an hourglass manner between the tip of the odontoid process and the lip of the foramen magnum. The left vertebral artery contained a recent thrombus at the site of 90% atheromatous stenosis (Jones and Kaufman, 1976).

Another rare, potential mechanism of vertebral artery occlusion in RA includes involvement of the vertebral artery by a spinal dural rheumatoid nodule (Steiner, 1959).

REFERENCES

Alkaabi, J. K., Ho, M., Levison, R., Pullar, T., and Belch, J. J. F. 2003. Rheumatoid arthritis and macrovascular disease. *Rheumatology*, **42**, 292–7.

Beck, D. O., and Corbett, J. J. 1983. Seizures due to central nervous system rheumatoid meningovasculitis. *Neurology*, **33**, 1058–61.

Caplan, L. R. 1996. *Posterior Circulation Disease: Clinical Findings, Diagnosis, and Management*. Cambridge, MA: Blackwell Science, pp. 235–7.

Cellerini, M., Gabbrielli, S., Maddali Bongi, S., and Cammelli, D. 2001. MRI of cerebral rheumatoid pachymeningitis: report of two cases with follow-up. *Neuroradiology*, **43**, 147–50.

Chehata, J. C., Hassel, A. B., Clarke, S. A., *et al.* 2001. Mortality in rheumatoid arthritis: relationship to single and composite measures of disease activity. *Rheumatology*, **40**, 447–52.

Davis, F. W., and Markley, H. E. 1951. Rheumatoid arthritis with death from medullary compression. *Ann Intern Med*, **35**, 451–4.

Johnson, R. L., Smyth, C. J., Holt, G. W., Lubchenko, A., and Valentine, E. 1959. Steroid therapy and vascular lesions is rheumatoid arthritis. *Arthritis Rheum*, **2**, 224–49.

Jones, M. W., and Kaufman, J. C. E. 1976. Vertebrobasilar insufficiency in rheumatoid atlanto-axial subluxation. *J Neurol Neurosurg Psychiatry*, **39**, 122–8.

Kemper, J. W., Baggenstoss, A. H., and Slocumb, C. H. 1957. The relationship of therapy with cortisone to the incidence of vascular lesions in rheumatoid arthritis. *Ann Intern Med*, **46**, 831–51.

Kim, R. C. 1980. Rheumatoid disease with encephalopathy. *Ann Neurol*, **7**, 86–91.

Liang, K. P., Liang, K. V., Matteson, E. L., *et al.* 2005. Incidence of non cardiac vascular disease in rheumatoid arthritis and relationship to extraarticular disease manifestations. *Arthritis Rheum*, **54**, 642–8.

Loeb, M., Bookman, A., and Mikulis, A. 1993. Rheumatoid arthritis and vertebral artery occlusion: a case report with angiographic and magnetic resonance demonstration. *J Rheumatol*, **20**, 1402–5.

McEntegart, A., Capell, H. A., Creran, D., *et al.* 2001. Cardiovascular risk factors, including thrombotic variables, in a population with rheumatoid arthritis. *Rheumatology*, **30**, 640–4.

Moore, P. M., and Richardson, B. 1998. Neurology of the vasculitides and connective tissue diseases. [Review]. *J Neurol Neurosurg Psychiatry*, **65**, 10–22.

Ouyang, R., Mitchell, D. M., and Rozdilsky, B. 1967. Central nervous system involvement in rheumatoid disease. Report of a case. *Neurology*, **17**, 1099–105.

Park, Y. B., Ahn, C. W., Choi, H. K., *et al.* 2002. Atherosclerosis in rheumatoid arthritis – morphologic evidence obtained by carotid ultrasound. *Arthritis Rheum*, **46**, 1714–9.

Park, Y. B., Lee, S. K., Lee, W. K., *et al.* 1999. Lipid profiles in untreated patients with rheumatoid arthritis. *J Rheumatol*, **26**, 1701–4.

Pasceri, V., and Yeh, E. T. 1999. A tale of two diseases-atherosclerosis and rheumatoid arthritis. *Circulation*, **100**, 2124–6.

Pirani, C. L., and Bennett, G. A. 1951. Rheumatoid arthritis: a report of three cases progressing from childhood and emphasizing certain systemic manifestations. *Bull Hosp Joint Dis*, **12**, 335–67.

Ramos, M., and Mandybur, T. I. 1975. Cerebral vasculitis in rheumatoid arthritis. *Arch Neurol*, **32**, 271–5.

Robinson, H. S. 1966. Rheumatoid arthritis-atlanto-axial subluxation and its clinical presentation. *Can Med Assoc J*, **94**, 470–7.

Roubenoff, R., Dellaripa, P., Nadeau, M. R., *et al.* 1997. Abnormal homocysteine metabolism in rheumatoid arthritis. *Arthritis Rheum*, **40**, 718–22.

Sattar, N., McCarey, D. W., Capell, H., and McInnes, I. B. 2003. Explaining how "high grade" systemic inflammation accelerates vascular risk in rheumatoid arthritis [Review]. *Circulation*, **108**, 2957–63.

Singleton, J. D., West, S. G., Reddy, V. V., and Rak, K. M. 1995. Cerebral vasculitis complicating rheumatoid arthritis. *South Med J*, **88**, 470–4.

Solomon, D. H., Karlson, E. W., Rimm, E. B., *et al.* 2003. Cardiovascular morbidity and mortality in women diagnosed with rheumatoid arthritis. *Arthritis Rheum*, **107**, 1303–7.

Tajima, Y., Kishimoto, R., Sudoh, K., and Matsumoto, A. 2004. Multiple central nervous system lesions associated with rheumatoid arthritis. *Arch Neurol*, **61**, 1794–5.

Wallberg-Jonsson, S., Cederfelt, M., and Dahlqvist, S. R. 2000. Hemostatic factors and cardiovascular disease in active rheumatoid arthritis: an 8 year followup study. *J Rheumatol*, **27**, 71–5.

Watson, P., Fekete, J., and Deck, J. 1977. Central nervous system vasculitis in rheumatoid arthritis. *Can J Neurol Sci*, **4**, 269–72.

Webb, F. W., Hickman, J. A., and Brew, D. 1968. Death from vertebral artery thrombosis in rheumatoid arthritis. *Br Med J*, **2**, 537–8.

Wolfe, F., Freundlich, B., and Straus, W. L. 2003. Increase in cardiovascular and cerebrovascular disease prevalence in rheumatoid arthritis. *J Rheumatol*, **30**, 36–40.

Wolfe, F., Mitchell, D. M., Sibley, J. T., *et al.* 1994. The mortality of rheumatoid arthritis. *Arthritis Rheum*, **37**, 481–94.

47

HYPERVISCOSITY AND STROKE

John F. Dashe

Introduction

The association of elevated hematocrit and fibrinogen levels with increased stroke risk has led to continued interest in hemorheologic factors and their role in the development of vascular disease and acute stroke. The neurological complications of the hyperviscosity syndromes are well described, but the relative importance of hemorheologic factors and viscosity in the more common ischemic stroke subtypes is still uncertain.

Basic principles of blood viscosity

Viscosity is the resistance to flow that arises from the friction between adjacent layers of a fluid in motion, and is defined as the ratio of shear stress to shear rate. Shear stress is the tangential force between flowing layers of fluid, and shear rate is the velocity gradient between the layers of flow (Wood and Kee, 1985). For Newtonian fluids such as water or plasma, viscosity is a fixed property, and is independent of flow rate. Whole blood is a non-Newtonian fluid, and has an apparent viscosity that varies as a function of its shear rate. Blood viscosity increases at low shear rates (low velocity) and decreases at high shear rates (high velocity). At very low flow velocities, blood viscosity may be from 100 to 10 000 times that of water; at high flow velocities, it may be of the order of 2–10 times that of water (Dintenfass, 1968).

Because of its non-Newtonian properties, blood viscosity is continuously changing in vivo as blood flows through vessels of different sizes and pressure gradients. In addition, shear rates cannot be measured directly, and their values are approximations for different parts of the circulation. For these reasons, a single in vitro measurement of blood viscosity has limited practical value (Thomas, 1982).

Blood viscosity is influenced by many factors including hematocrit, plasma protein and fibrinogen concentrations, cellular aggregation, red cell deformability and axial migration, vessel diameter, and flow rate. Leukocytes and platelets make a relatively minor contribution to whole-blood viscosity under normal conditions, but may be important in certain pathological conditions.

Effects of hyperviscosity in large and small vessels

Blood flow in the microcirculation (vessels with an internal diameter of ≤100 microns) is governed mainly by red cell deformability and plasma viscosity. Normal deformability allows erythrocytes with a diameter of 8 microns to squeeze through capillaries with diameters of 4–6 microns (Wood and Kee, 1985). Red cell deformability is determined by surface-to-volume area, cell morphology, mechanical properties of the membrane, and viscosity of the cell contents (Koenig and Ernst, 1992). Normal deformability requires sufficient adenosine triphosphate (ATP) levels to maintain cell shape and actively extrude calcium. Excess intracellular calcium can cause gelation of hemoglobin and contraction of the cell membrane (Grotta *et al.*, 1986). If intracellular ATP is depleted, as might occur in ischemic tissue, the red cell becomes more rigid, contributing to increased viscosity. Likewise, rigid erythrocytes in sickle cell blood cannot easily pass through the smaller vessels.

Because of the Fahraeus–Lindqvist effect (Fahraeus and Lindqvist, 1931), blood viscosity decreases as tube diameter decreases below 1 mm due to reduced contribution of normal red cells to viscous resistance ("Haemorheology, blood-flow and venous thrombosis," 1975). In these small vessels, blood viscosity approximates plasma viscosity, which becomes a direct determinant of capillary blood flow (Gaehtgens and Marx, 1987). Leukocytes may also play an important role at this level.

Red cell aggregation is a reversible process that causes most of the non-Newtonian flow behavior of whole blood. Large, electrically positive macromolecules in plasma, mainly fibrinogen and globulins, facilitate bridging and reduce the electronic repulsion between red blood cells. In large vessels, migration of red cells to the vessel axis increases blood fluidity and oxygen transport, and the higher velocities and shear rates tend to break up aggregations of red cells. Under low flow conditions, and accompanying lower shear rates, the process tilts toward formation of red cell aggregates (rouleau) that increase blood viscosity and may result in diminished perfusion (Koenig and Ernst, 1992). The width of capillaries precludes the passage of red cell aggregates unless a rouleau formation enters end on (Wells, 1964). Elevated fibrinogen and paraprotein levels cause an increase in erythrocyte aggregation.

Increased red cell aggregation also occurs with trauma, shock, burns, infection, complicated diabetes mellitus, malignancy, and rheumatic diseases. Red cell aggregation is increased in most conditions that are accompanied by an increased erythrocyte sedimentation rate (ESR) (Somer and Meiselman, 1993).

Viscosity increases logarithmically at the lowest shear rates (Somer and Meiselman, 1993), and this effect is magnified at higher hematocrit levels. Conditions that cause low flow, such as a high-grade arterial stenosis or systemic hypotension and hypovolemia, increase blood viscosity based on the associated low shear rates.

Uncommon Causes of Stroke, 2nd edition, ed. Louis R. Caplan. Published by Cambridge University Press.   © Cambridge University Press 2008.

The end result is a further reduction in flow, potentially leading to a "viscous, vicious circle" (Dintenfass, 1966; Thomas, 1982) consisting of reduced blood flow, aggregation of blood cells, and finally complete stasis favoring thrombus formation.

Acute ischemia also induces an acute-phase reaction and a further deterioration of blood fluidity, mainly by increasing fibrinogen. With stasis or zero shear rate, cell aggregation causes an increased structural viscosity, which must be overcome for flow to be re-established. The minimum force required to initiate flow in static blood is called the yield stress, and fibrinogen is the principle determinant of this property of blood (Wells, 1964).

Epidemiologic evidence

Patients with acute and chronic cerebrovascular disease may have abnormalities involving blood viscosity, plasma viscosity, hematocrit, red cell deformability, and fibrinogen (Coull *et al.*, 1991; Fisher and Meiselman, 1991; Ott *et al.*, 1974; Sakuta, 1981; Thomas, 1982).

Fibrinogen

Fibrinogen may play a causal role in ischemic stroke through several mechanisms (Lowe, 1995). The most prominent of these is its essential role in thrombosis, both as the substrate for fibrin clot formation and as a facilitator of platelet aggregation. Another is the contribution of fibrinogen to atherogenesis. Finally, and perhaps of least importance, is the effect of fibrinogen on whole-blood viscosity.

Perhaps the strongest evidence linking fibrinogen with stroke comes from a 2005 Fibrinogen Studies Collaboration meta-analysis of 31 prospective studies that included more than 150 000 healthy participants without stroke or coronary heart disease (CHD) (Danesh *et al.*, 2005). Within each age group (40–59, 60–69, and ≥70 years), there was an approximately log-linear association between fibrinogen level and the risk of any CHD, any stroke, and mortality due to other causes. The risk of stroke increased for each 1 g/L increase in fibrinogen level (age- and sex-adjusted hazard ratio [HR] 2.06, 95% confidence interval [CI], 1.83–2.33). After adjustment for several established vascular risk factors, the HR for stroke was reduced to about 1.8.

Analysis of pooled data from three prospective studies of patients with recent transient ischemic attack (TIA) or minor ischemic stroke also showed that fibrinogen levels above the median predicted subsequent ischemic stroke (HR 1.34, 95% CI, 1.13–1.60) (Rothwell *et al.*, 2004).

Despite the association of increased fibrinogen levels with stroke and CHD, it remains unclear whether fibrinogen plays a causal role in vascular disease, or is simply a marker of risk. Arguing against a causal role is the finding that fibrinogen is not specific for vascular disease but is also associated with the aggregate of all nonvascular mortality, mainly cancer, as demonstrated by the Fibrinogen Studies Collaboration meta-analysis (Danesh *et al.*, 2005; Lowe, 2006).

One alternative hypothesis is that the broad association of fibrinogen with vascular and nonvascular events and mortality may reflect an inflammatory response to cumulative lifetime environmental stressors (e.g. smoking, metabolic syndrome, infections, low socioeconomic status) that impacts the risk and progression of various chronic diseases (Lowe, 2005). The same hypothesis may explain why other markers of low-grade inflammation (e.g. plasma viscosity, white cell count, ESR, C-reactive protein, and low serum albumin) also appear to have associations with stroke, CHD, and nonvascular mortality, as shown in meta-analyses of prospective studies (Lowe, 2005).

Although fibrinogen is also an acute-phase reactant, a prospective epidemiological study found that hematocrit, fibrinogen, blood viscosity, and plasma viscosity are increased years before the onset of acute ischemic events, in addition to having an association with stroke risk (Lowe *et al.*, 1997). Furthermore, a prospective nested case-control study found that fibrinogen was associated with an increased risk of ischemic stroke after adjustment for C-reactive protein, a marker of inflammation, suggesting that the acute-phase behavior of fibrinogen was unlikely to be driving the association (Woodward *et al.*, 2005).

In patients with a history of stroke or risk factors for stroke, a prospective study found that a low albumin–globulin (A-G) ratio (≤1.45) was an independent risk-factor for the composite outcome of subsequent stroke, myocardial infarction, or vascular death (HR 2.4, 95% CI, 1.2–4.7) (Beamer *et al.*, 1993). A low A-G ratio in this study was inversely related to plasma fibrinogen concentration and appeared to reflect both higher fibrinogen and globulin levels and a lower concentration of albumin; the latter is a marker of inflammation.

Hematocrit

The Framingham study suggested an epidemiological link between elevated hematocrit and risk of stroke (Kannel *et al.*, 1972). A later report found that the risk of stroke increases progressively with fibrinogen level in men but not in women (Kannel *et al.*, 1987).

A year 2000 meta-analysis of 16 prospective population-based studies found that increased hematocrit (top third vs. bottom third of baseline hematocrit) was associated with a small but statistically significant risk of CHD (risk ratio [RR] 1.16, 95% CI, 1.05–1.29) (Danesh *et al.*, 2000). This study did not address stroke risk, and no comparable meta-analysis evaluating the relationship of hematocrit with stroke has been published to date.

Plasma viscosity

Plasma viscosity increases with age regardless of gender; is positively associated with untreated hypertension, hypercholesterolemia, and smoking in men; and is raised in hypertension and severe obesity in women (Koenig and Ernst, 1992).

Evidence regarding the association of plasma viscosity with stroke is conflicting. An earlier prospective study of 523 patients in stroke rehabilitation phase found that elevated blood viscosity, red cell aggregation, plasma and serum viscosity, fibrinogen, and cholesterol levels were associated with recurrent stroke (Ernst *et al.*, 1991). In addition, the prospective Edinburgh Artery Study

Table 47.1 Hematological hyperviscosity syndromes

Plasma abnormality	Increased cellularity	Decreased red cell deformability
Waldenstrom's macroglobulinemia	Polycythemia vera	Sickle cell anemia
Paraproteinemias	Erythrocytosis (secondary polycythemia)	Spherocytosis
Congenital hyperfibrinogenemia	Stress polycythemia (Gaisbock's syndrome)	Hemoglobinopathies
Hyperleukocytic leukemias		

Source: Modified from Dormandy *et al.*, 1981, with permission.

Table 47.2 Covert hyperviscosity states

Diabetes
Inflammation
Atherosclerosis
Systemic low flow states/hemoconcentration in:
Burn injury
Inappropriate red cell transfusion
Dehydration
Circulatory shock

found that mean levels of plasma viscosity, blood viscosity, hematocrit, and fibrinogen, adjusted for age, sex, and conventional risk-factors, were significantly higher in subjects who had first ischemic strokes than in subjects who did not (Lowe *et al.*, 1997). However, subsequent prospective studies have found no association between plasma viscosity and ischemic stroke (Baker *et al.*, 2002; Woodward *et al.*, 2005).

A 2000 meta-analysis of six prospective studies addressed the relationship of plasma viscosity and CHD and found that increased plasma viscosity (top third vs. bottom third of baseline values) was associated with a small but statistically significant risk of CHD (RR 1.57, 95% CI, 1.34–1.85) (Danesh *et al.*, 2000). In a combined analysis of two of the six studies that reported whole-blood viscosity measurements or calculations, blood viscosity (top third vs. bottom third of baseline values) was associated with a non-significantly increased risk of CHD (RR 1.24, 95% CI, 0.74–2.10). No comparable meta-analysis has addressed the relationship of plasma viscosity or blood viscosity with stroke.

Hyperviscosity syndromes

Diseases that cause hyperviscosity fall into three main categories: plasma abnormalities, increased cellularity, and decreased red cell deformability (Table 47.1). Each has a different rheological mechanism that leads to a hyperviscous state. A fourth category of "covert" hyperviscosity states is increasingly recognized (Table 47.2).

Plasma abnormalities

Plasma viscosity is determined mainly by the concentration of electrically neutral or slightly positively charged, nonspherical, high-molecular-weight proteins. These proteins, including fibrinogen, α-2 macroglobulins, and immunoglobulins, contribute to viscosity because of their physical characteristics as well as by their interactions with red cells. Fibrinogen is the principal determinant of plasma viscosity under normal conditions (Dormandy *et al.*, 1981; Wells, 1970). Although it makes up about 4% of normal plasma proteins by weight, fibrinogen is responsible for more

than one-fifth of the total plasma viscosity (Somer and Meiselman, 1993).

Increased production of high-molecular-weight globulins or macroglobulins is frequently found in patients with monoclonal and polyclonal immunoglobulinemias including lymphoma, Waldenstrom's macroglobulinemia, and less commonly in multiple myeloma (Fahey *et al.*, 1965). The plasma hyperviscosity syndrome is a clinical entity characterized by mucous membrane bleeding, blurred vision, visual loss, lethargy, headache, dizziness, vertigo, tinnitus, paresthesias, and occasionally seizures (Dintenfass, 1966; Fahey *et al.*, 1965; Pavy *et al.*, 1980; Wells, 1970). Funduscopic examination may show retinal hemorrhages and papilledema. Pathologically, this syndrome is explained by extremely elevated plasma viscosity and hypervolemia; intense red cell aggregation results from the elevated paraproteins (Somer and Meiselman, 1993).

Intravenous immunoglobulin (IVIG) can increase viscosity of plasma and whole blood both in vivo and in vitro, suggesting that IVIG therapy may impair blood flow and cause ischemic stroke, myocardial infarction, or venous thromboembolism (Reinhart and Berchtold, 1992). Other potential mechanisms for thromboembolism related to IVIG therapy include platelet activation and vasospasm (Emerson *et al.*, 2002).

The actual risk of stroke with IVIG therapy is unknown, but case reports and small case series suggest a possible association. In one report, a 70-year-old woman with stable polycythemia vera was treated with IVIG when she developed Guillain-Barré syndrome (Byrne *et al.*, 2002). Coma ensued 8 days later because of symmetric bilateral cerebral infarcts. Autopsy findings included infarction with necrotizing microangiopathy and intravascular aggregates of fibrin with immunoglobulin and platelets.

Another study reported 16 patients who developed ischemic stroke associated with IVIG infusions over a 4-year period at several regional centers in North Carolina (Caress *et al.*, 2003). The stroke rate among all hospitalized patients who received IVIG treatment during the 4-year study period was 0.6%. Stroke onset occurred within 24 hours of IVIG infusion in 14 patients, and multifocal infarctions were present in 9 patients. Eight of the 16 were receiving IVIG treatment for the first time. Stroke risk factors, including hypertension, diabetes mellitus, asymptomatic cerebrovascular disease or stroke, and hematologic disorders that may predispose to stroke, were present in 15 of the 16 patients.

While these reports suggest that each course of IVIG treatment is associated with a small risk of thromboembolic complications, particularly in patients with underlying risk factors (Vucic *et al.*, 2004), an alternative explanation is that ischemic stroke may be coincidental in patients with cardiovascular risk factors receiving IVIG therapy (Alexandrescu *et al.*, 2005).

Increased cellularity

Polycythemia vera is the most common cause of increased cellularity, and is characterized by overproduction of erythroid, myeloid, and megakaryocytic cell lines, leading to elevated peripheral blood cell counts and an increased red cell mass. Cerebral blood flow (CBF) is diminished with the high hematocrits found in polycythemia (Thomas *et al.*, 1977). The most common neurological symptoms related to polycythemia include headache, dizziness or vertigo, paresthesias, scotomata, blurred vision, and tinnitus (Silverstein *et al.*, 1962), similar to the symptoms reported in the plasma hyperviscosity syndrome.

The frequency of brain infarction due to hyperviscosity in polycythemia vera is unclear. Prospective controlled studies addressing this issue are lacking. Grotta *et al.* (1986) concluded that polycythemia rarely, if ever, plays a role in focal cerebral infarction, but other studies have reported an increased incidence of brain ischemia and thrombosis (Barabas *et al.*, 1973; Chievitz and Thiede, 1962; Millikan *et al.*, 1960; Silverstein *et al.*, 1962). The nature of the brain events themselves (whether focal or diffuse) is often difficult to ascertain from these studies, as they usually do not provide detailed clinical-pathological correlation or precise definitions of the cerebral thrombotic events.

The increased hematocrit in polycythemia may impede flow and increase coagulability in the presence of large artery occlusive disease, and contribute to decreased microvascular flow in patients with hypertensive small-vessel disease. Stroke could also be caused by the increased platelet counts and increased platelet reactivity found in myeloproliferative disorders such as polycythemia vera (Schafer, 1984). Pearson and Wetherley-Mein (1978) found that the incidence of vascular occlusive episodes correlated directly with the red cell mass; the same study showed an association between the frequency of thrombosis and thrombocytosis, but this association did not achieve statistical significance. Lacunar infarction (Pearce *et al.*, 1983), Binswanger's disease (Caplan, 1995), cerebral venous thrombosis (Melamed *et al.*, 1976), intracerebral hemorrhage, cerebral large-artery thrombosis, large-artery territorial infarction, and watershed infarction (Yazdi and Cote, 1986) have all been attributed to polycythemia (Barabas *et al.*, 1973).

Erythrocytosis from increased erythropoietin (so-called secondary polycythemia) causes elevated hematocrit and hyperviscosity. Increased erythropoietin production can be triggered by a physiologic response to chronic hypoxia in a number of conditions including cyanotic congenital heart disease, hypoxic lung disease, hypoventilation due to the Pickwickian syndrome, and high altitude. Nonphysiologically increased erythropoietin is associated with renal cysts, hydronephrosis, and a number of neoplasms (Grotta *et al.*, 1986). Stress polycythemia, or Gaisbock's syndrome, also causes elevated hematocrit. High altitude induces a physiologic erythrocytosis, but the limited epidemiological data in the United States suggest that stroke mortality actually declines with increasing altitude (Gordon *et al.*, 1977).

Evidence against an association of increased hematocrit with ischemic stroke comes from a study of 112 adults with cyanotic congenital heart disease that excluded those with independent stroke risk factors (Perloff *et al.*, 1993). At 1–12 years of follow-up, no patient with either compensated or decompensated erythrocytosis had clinical evidence brain infarction, irrespective of hematocrit level, iron stores, or the severity of hyperviscosity symptoms.

Children with congenital cyanotic heart disease do have an increased incidence of stroke, most frequently due to cerebral venous thrombosis (Cottrill and Kaplan, 1973; Phornphutkul *et al.*, 1973). Unlike adults, these children are likely to have a microcytic hypochromic red cell morphology consistent with iron deficiency, which has been shown to decrease red cell deformability (Cottrill and Kaplan, 1973; Phornphutkul *et al.*, 1973). Thus, hyperviscosity in children may be related more to decreased red cell deformability than to the level of hemoglobin or hematocrit.

Very high white blood cell counts in patients with leukemias are associated with hyperviscosity (Rampling, 2003). Normal white cells are by some estimates 1000-fold less deformable (and leukemic blast cells may be less deformable still) than normal red cells. The increased numbers of rigid leukemic cells tend to occlude small vessels and lead to global neurological dysfunction (Somer and Meiselman, 1993). Microinfarcts and petechial hemorrhages result. No strong evidence has emerged linking leukemic hyperviscosity to large-artery brain infarction.

Decreased red cell deformability

In sickle cell disease (SCD), the hemoglobin HbS structure is less soluble than normal hemoglobin, and has a tendency toward polymerization when exposed to hypoxia or low pH (Bunn, 1997). This causes the cell membrane to conform to a highly rigid sickle shape, and results in tremendously increased viscosity with abnormal flow and red blood cell sludging in the microcirculation and cerebral veins. Even oxygenated sickle blood from asymptomatic sickle patients has an elevated viscosity when compared to normal blood at the same hematocrit (Chien *et al.*, 1970).

Although the tissue damage is thought to occur in the microcirculation, large-artery occlusive disease involving the distal internal carotid artery and circle of Willis is a characteristic feature of SCD, occasionally developing into a moyamoya radiographic pattern (Stockman *et al.*, 1972). One potential mechanism for this large-vessel arteriopathy is repetitive flow-related injury to the endothelium (Jeffries *et al.*, 1980); sickle red cells may stimulate proliferation of the smooth muscle and fibrous components of arterial walls, leading to arterial stenoses. Another mechanism may be stasis and occlusion of the small vessels of the vaso vasorum that nourish the large arteries, leading to ischemia of the large artery walls, intimal proliferation, and gradual occlusion (Stockman *et al.*, 1972).

The risk of stroke in SCD varies according to genotype and is highest in patients with homozygous SS. In a series of 3647 patients with SCD, the likelihood of having a first stroke by age 20, 30, or 45 years was 11%, 15%, and 24%, respectively (Ohene-Frempong *et al.*, 1998). The same study found that the incidence of a first cerebral infarct was between ages 2 and 5 years, 6 and 9 years, 10 and 19 years, and 20 and 29 years was 0.7, 0.5, 0.24, and 0.04, respectively.

Patients with SCD are at risk for both cerebral infarction and intracerebral hemorrhage; the latter may develop from medial wall necrosis and rupture of cerebral arterioles (Stockman *et al.*, 1972). Cerebral infarctions occur in both deep and subcortical structures. Both neuropathologic (Rothman *et al.*, 1986) and neuroradiologic (Pavlakis *et al.*, 1988) evidence indicates that the majority of brain infarcts in patients with SCD involve the high cortical convexity border zone regions between the major arterial territories. Brainstem, spinal cord, and retinal infarctions also occur (Grotta *et al.*, 1986).

Other examples of decreased red cell deformability include hereditary spherocytosis, pyruvate kinase deficiency, and certain hemoglobinopathies; usually these disorders do not lead to major clinical symptoms or cerebrovascular involvement (Somer and Meiselman, 1993), although patients with brain infarction have been reported (van Hilten *et al.*, 1989).

Other conditions associated with hyperviscosity

Diabetes, inflammation, and atherosclerosis have been termed "covert" hyperviscosity syndromes (Somer and Meiselman, 1993), because their rheological manifestations are typically less pronounced than in the better known hematological hyperviscosity syndromes (Table 47.2). Diabetes is associated with a number of rheological abnormalities (McMillan 1985, 1989); the arteriolar hyalinization found in this disease may be mediated by a diabetes-specific impairment in red cell deformability, causing an increase in peak tangential arteriolar wall force (Juhan *et al.*, 1982; McMillan, 1997).

Increased viscosity may also occur in low-flow states that arise systemically from hemoconcentration with severe burns, inappropriate red cell transfusion, dehydration due to illness, and circulatory shock (Lowe, 1987).

In arterial hypertension, whole-blood viscosity, plasma viscosity, hematocrit, fibrinogen, and red cell aggregation and deformability are all increased (Hossmann *et al.*, 1985; Letcher *et al.*, 1981; Zannad *et al.*, 1988).

Lipoproteins have direct effects on blood rheology. Increases in triglycerides, chylomicrons (Seplowitz *et al.*, 1981), and low-density lipoprotein (LDL) and very low-density lipoprotein (VLDL) cholesterol fractions lead to a concentration-dependent increase in plasma viscosity (Leonhardt *et al.*, 1977; Rosenson and Lowe, 1998). Patients with hyperlipoproteinemia type II have elevated fibrinogen levels and increased blood viscosity, plasma viscosity, and hematocrit, as well as elevated levels of α-2 antiplasmin (Lowe *et al.*, 1982), an inhibitor of fibrinolysis. Elevated LDL causes increased viscosity by fostering red cell aggregation (Sloop, 1996), whereas high-density lipoprotein (HDL) has antiatherothrombotic properties that result in part from inhibition of platelet and erythrocyte aggregation and reduced blood viscosity (Rosenson and Lowe, 1998).

Cigarette smoking is associated with increased hemoglobin, fibrinogen levels, plasma viscosity, red cell aggregation, platelet aggregation, and leukocyte counts, resulting in a steep increase in whole-blood viscosity in smokers (Ernst, 1995). The effect of smoking is dose dependent and largely reversible (Lowe, 1998).

Role of hyperviscosity in ischemic stroke subtypes

Outside of the overt hematologic hyperviscosity syndromes, few studies have directly examined the role of rheological factors pertaining to ischemic stroke subtypes or vascular lesions. Tohgi *et al.* (1978) studied 432 consecutive patients with 'cerebral infarction' at autopsy and found that the risk of ischemic stroke rose dramatically for hematocrit values >46%; the increase occurred predominantly in deeper regions rather than in cortex, but this trend did not reach statistical significance. The proportion of large-versus small-vessel infarcts is not clear from their data.

The majority of studies have focused on the microcirculation. In a study of 40 patients with lacunar strokes confirmed by clinical and radiologic criteria, Schneider *et al.* (1985) found that erythrocyte aggregation, erythrocyte deformability, plasma viscosity, fibrinogen concentration, and shear stress were pathologic when compared to those of normal control patients, but hematocrit was not significantly different. A later study (Schneider *et al.*, 1987) found that fibrinogen levels were significantly higher in 40 patients with lacunar infarcts and 21 patients with Binswanger's disease compared to 275 healthy control subjects without vascular risk factors. The Binswanger patients alone had consistently elevated plasma viscosity.

Although most strongly associated with hypertension, Binswanger's disease may be associated with other conditions linked to hyperviscosity such as polycythemia, hyperglobulinemia, hyperlipidemia, and diabetes (Caplan, 1995). Kawamoto *et al.* (1991) found that asymptomatic patients with multiple lacunar infarcts by MRI criteria showed a higher predicted whole-blood viscosity and a lower HDL cholesterol than did hypertensive and normotensive controls. Taken together, these studies suggest that hyperviscosity and altered rheological factors may be involved in the pathophysiology of small-vessel ischemic disease.

Hyperviscosity appears to be associated with the pathogenesis and progression of atherosclerosis. There is evidence that atherosclerotic and thrombotic arterial lesions are promoted by altered rheological factors including fibrinogen, lipoproteins, plasma viscosity, hematocrit, red blood cell aggregation, and leukocyte activation (Koenig and Ernst, 1992). One hypothesis is that increased viscosity creates larger areas of decreased blood flow, thereby perpetuating the interaction of atherogenic elements with the endothelium (Sloop, 1996).

However, it remains unclear if increased viscosity is a primary cause or a secondary consequence of atherosclerosis (Stuart *et al.*, 1981). The issue is confounded by the relationship of whole-blood viscosity to its major determinants, including plasma viscosity and fibrinogen, which in turn are modified by the effects of inflammation, another factor thought to play an important role in atherogenesis. Shear stress is another confounding rheologic factor related to viscosity. Atherosclerotic lesions typically occur in regions of low shear stress, which appears to accelerate endothelial proliferation, shape change, and apoptosis, and to increase secretion of factors that promote vasoconstriction, coagulation, and platelet aggregation (Paszkowiak and Dardik, 2003).

In patients with angiographically confirmed carotid artery occlusion found after evaluation for TIA and minor stroke, infarct size on CT scans correlated significantly with increased hematocrit (Harrison *et al.*, 1981). Oder *et al.* (1998) reported significantly higher blood viscosity in patients with sonographic abnormalities of one vertebral artery compared to controls.

Hyperviscosity appears to be associated with carotid atherosclerosis. A longitudinal cohort study found that blood viscosity, plasma viscosity, fibrinogen, and hematocrit were all linearly related to carotid artery intima-media thickness in men (Lee *et al.*, 1998). Blood viscosity, plasma viscosity, and fibrinogen remained significantly associated on multivariate analysis. Furthermore, a cohort study of healthy subjects (246 men and 337 women) found that increased plasma viscosity (by 1 standard deviation) was associated with carotid atherosclerosis in men (odds ratio [OR] 2.27, 95% CI, 1.52–3.38) and women (OR 1.63, 95% CI, 1.17–2.26) (Levenson *et al.*, 2000). The association persisted with very little effect on these ORs after adjustment for age, waist-to-hip ratio, smoking, hypercholesterolemia, hypertension, diabetes, and fibrinogen.

Spontaneous echo contrast (SEC) seen in the left atrial cavity or appendage on echocardiographic examination has generated interest as a risk factor for cardioembolic stroke (Ansari and Maron, 1997; Daniel *et al.*, 1988). In vitro, static erythrocytes are highly echogenic. The swirling smoke-like appearance of SEC is present at low shear rates but disappears at high shear rates. Spontaneous echo contrast is associated with cardiac abnormalities that produce low-flow states within the left atrium, including atrial fibrillation, mitral stenosis, and left atrial enlargement (Black and Stewart, 1993). Most left atrial thrombi are accompanied by SEC (Black and Stewart, 1993).

Spontaneous echo contrast is likely a consequence of protein-mediated red blood cell aggregation in the setting of low shear forces (Merino *et al.*, 1992). Spontaneous echo contrast in patients with nonvalvular atrial fibrillation is independently related to hematocrit, fibrinogen concentration, and left atrial dimension (Black *et al.*, 1993). In a study of 185 patients with atrial fibrillation, 46% had SEC. The presence and severity of SEC was positively correlated with ESR, low-shear blood viscosity, and anti-cardiolipin antibody (Fatkin *et al.*, 1994). In 50 patients with acute or chronic cerebrovascular disease, Briley *et al.* (1994) found that the severity of SEC was related to elevated fibrinogen levels and concomitant increases in both plasma and serum viscosity; patients with severe SEC had double the prevalence of cardioembolic stroke compared to those with other causes of stroke.

Cerebral blood flow and oxygen delivery

Blood flow to an organ system is determined by the blood vessel size, the blood pressure, and the hemorheologic or flow properties of blood. In patients with polycythemia vera, CBF is low at high hematocrit levels; reducing hematocrit dramatically increases CBF

(Thomas *et al.*, 1977a, 1977b). Other studies have confirmed an inverse relationship between hematocrit and viscosity on the one hand, and CBF on the other (Grotta *et al.*, 1982; Thomas 1982). These observations have been interpreted as evidence that hyperviscosity causes a reduction in CBF, because hematocrit is the primary factor influencing blood viscosity. A similar inverse relationship between fibrinogen levels and viscosity, and between fibrinogen levels and CBF, has been shown (Grotta *et al.*, 1982, 1985).

However, other studies have found that the oxygen-carrying capacity of the blood is the critical factor in determining CBF, reflecting a homeostatic and physiological mechanism designed to maintain transport and delivery of oxygen to the brain despite falling hematocrit and arterial oxygen content (Harrison, 1989; Wade, 1983).

The rationale behind hemodilution and phlebotomy is that reducing the hematocrit lowers whole-blood viscosity, which in turn increases CBF to ischemic regions. To be useful, this increase in CBF must be sufficiently robust to overcome the diminished oxygen-carrying capacity of the blood that results from lowering the hematocrit. The optimal hematocrit for oxygen delivery to most tissues has been estimated at 30%–35% (Messmer *et al.*, 1973; Wood and Kee, 1985). It is unclear if this relationship is true for brain (Asplund, 1989); Gaehtgens and Marx (1987) place the optimal hematocrit for cerebral oxygen delivery at 42%. Lowering viscosity by reducing hematocrit runs the risk of worsening ischemia if the CBF is in fact regulated by homeostatic mechanisms designed to maintain oxygen-carrying capacity or oxygen delivery irrespective of viscosity. However, homeostatic regulation of CBF may be deranged in ischemic regions (Asplund, 1989), and the effect of hyperviscosity may take on greater importance as the physiological response to diminished oxygen delivery is blunted, or even exhausted as when vasodilation is maximal in an ischemic vascular bed (Grotta, 1987).

The studies examining oxygen delivery after hematocrit reduction are conflicting. Wade (1983) reported a small but significant increase in oxygen transport to the brain following phlebotomy to reduce hematocrit in 20 patients with polycythemia vera, and Yamauchi *et al.* (1993) found that CBF and oxygen transport were increased in the hemisphere ipsilateral to carotid occlusion in five patients after hemodilution. Henriksen *et al.* (1981) reported that oxygen delivery capacity did not change significantly from baseline following hemodilution in six patients with slightly elevated hematocrit.

Treatment

Plasma hyperviscosity syndromes are treated by plasmapheresis (plasma exchange) to remove the paraproteins and thereby reduce hyperviscosity and hypervolemia. Newer techniques of cell centrifugation, plasma separation, and filtration may also be useful.

For many years, phlebotomy has been the mainstay for treatment of polycythemia vera, with the goal of keeping the hematocrit <45% in men and <42% in women. However, phlebotomy increases the risk of thrombosis in the first 3–4 years of treatment, although it is associated with a better overall survival than is myelosuppression (Berk *et al.*, 1986).

Leukapheresis can be used to decrease levels of leukemic cells and blood viscosity in patients with leukocytic leukemias (Somer and Meiselman, 1993).

Treatment of SCD is aimed at maintaining the hemoglobin S concentration <30% by repeated exchange transfusion, which reduces the risk of stroke in SCD (Adams and Brambilla 2005; Adams et al., 1998; Pegelow et al., 1995). During acute crises, oxygen and intravenous fluids are used in an attempt to improve systemic blood flow and CBF.

Despite some promising results in a few human stroke trials (Strand et al., 1984; Wood and Fleischer, 1982), the majority of hemodilution studies failed to show significant benefit (Asplund, 1989; Grotta, 1987; Harrison, 1989). A 2002 systematic review of 18 trials evaluating hemodilution for acute ischemic stroke found no statistically significant benefits of any type of hemodiluting agents, but the statistical power to detect effects of hydroxyethyl starch and albumin was weak (Asplund, 2002). Many of the hemodilution trials may have been flawed by late initiation of therapy beyond the therapeutic time window to salvage brain cells within the ischemic penumbra.

Other methods of lowering viscosity in acute stroke or chronic cerebrovascular disease could theoretically improve blood flow and ameliorate ischemia. Pentoxifylline increases erythrocyte and leukocyte deformability, and decreases viscosity (Muller 1979; Schneider et al., 1983). Omega-3 fatty acids available in the form of fish oils decrease fibrinogen levels (Radack et al., 1989) and blood viscosity, and may increase erythrocyte deformability (Simopoulos, 1991). They also have lipid-lowering effects on triglycerides and total cholesterol (Haglund et al., 1990). However, the fibrinogen-lowering effects of omega-3 fish oil consumption may not be evident at typical intake levels consumed by the U.S. population (Archer et al., 1998).

Derivatives of fibric acid (fibrates), including clofibrate, gemfibrozil, fenofibrate, bezafibrate, and ciprofibrate, are most often used to treat elevations of VLDL cholesterol and plasma triglycerides (Miller and Spence, 1998). Fenofibrate and bezafibrate reduce plasma fibrinogen, whereas gemfibrozil does not (Durrington et al., 1998; Elisaf, 2002; Simpson et al., 1985). Koenig et al. (1992) found that lovastatin decreased plasma viscosity to the same extent as bezafibrate, but did not reduce fibrinogen. Heparin-induced extracorporeal LDL precipitation (HELP) is a last-resort method to rapidly reduce lipids for patients with medically refractory hypercholesterolemia; it also reduces fibrinogen and viscosity (Bosch and Wendler, 2004; Walzl et al., 1994).

Three fibrinolytic snake venoms – ancrod, batroxobin, and crotalase – act primarily by a proteolytic effect on circulating fibrinogen (Bell, 1997). Treatment with batroxobin or ancrod increases CBF and reduces blood viscosity (Grotta, 1987; Izumi et al., 1996). Ticlopidine directly reduced the mean fibrinogen level in a study of patients with polycythemia vera (Finelli et al., 1991); in another study, ticlopidine reduced fibrinogen levels of both healthy volunteers and patients with stable angina (de Maat et al., 1996).

The thrombolytic agents including streptokinase (Jan et al., 1990) and urokinase decrease fibrinogen, plasma viscosity, and red cell aggregation (Koenig and Ernst, 1992). Tissue plasminogen activator reduces fibrinogen and blood viscosity to a lesser degree than does streptokinase (Jan et al., 1990). Improved blood fluidity may be an additional beneficial effect of these agents beyond their primary role in thrombolysis (Moriarty et al., 1988).

Conclusions

Hyperviscosity remains an intriguing issue but appears to play a limited role in ischemic stroke risk. While the risk of focal brain infarction is increased in SCD, and probably in polycythemia, it is uncertain if hyperviscosity related to other conditions increases stroke risk. Stroke associated with IVIG treatment is rare and possibly coincidental in patients with underlying risk factors. The neurological symptoms that occur with the hematologic hyperviscosity syndromes are global, nonspecific for localization, and generally reversible with treatment.

Hyperviscosity, hyperfibrinogenemia, and altered rheological factors may increase the risk of ischemic stroke in certain conditions, including large-vessel stenosis, low flow, and hypertensive small-vessel disease. Hyperviscosity may also be important in the promotion of atherosclerosis and chronic cerebrovascular disease. However, a direct causative role for these rheologic factors in ischemic stroke remains speculative.

Many treatment options are available to decrease viscosity and potentially improve flow, but outside of the hematologic hyperviscosity syndromes there is no evidence that decreasing viscosity or its determinants is effective for treating or preventing acute ischemic stroke. Further study is needed to determine the precise role of hemorheology in the pathogenesis of cerebrovascular disease and ischemic stroke subtypes.

REFERENCES

Adams, R. J., and Brambilla, D. 2005. Discontinuing prophylactic transfusions used to prevent stroke in sickle cell disease. N Engl J Med, **353**(26), 2769–78.

Adams, R. J., McKie, V. C., et al. 1998. Stroke prevention trial in sickle cell anemia. Control Clin Trials, **19**, 110–29.

Alexandrescu, D. T., Dutcher, J. P., et al. (2005). Strokes after intravenous gamma globulin: thrombotic phenomenon in patients with risk factors or just coincidence? Am J Hematol, **78**, 216–20.

Ansari, A., and Maron, B. J. 1997. Spontaneous echo contrast and thromboembolism. Hosp Pract (Minneap), **32**, 109–11, 115–6.

Archer, S. L., Green, D., et al. 1998. Association of dietary fish and n-3 fatty acid intake with hemostatic factors in the coronary artery risk development in young adults (CARDIA) study. Arterioscler Thromb Vasc Biol, **18**, 1119–23.

Asplund, K. 1989. Randomized clinical trials of hemodilution in acute ischemic stroke. Acta Neurol Scand Suppl, **127**, 22–30.

Asplund, K. 2002. Haemodilution for acute ischaemic stroke. Cochrane Database Syst Rev, **4**, CD000103.

Baker, I. A., Pickering, J., et al. 2002. Fibrinogen, viscosity and white blood cell count predict myocardial, but not cerebral infarction: evidence from the Caerphilly and Speedwell cohort. Thromb Haemost, **87**, 421–5.

Barabas, A. P., Offen, D. N., et al. 1973. The arterial complications of polycythaemia vera. Br J Surg, **60**, 183–7.

Beamer, N., Coull, B. M., et al. 1993. Fibrinogen and the albumin-globulin ratio in recurrent stroke. Stroke, **24**, 1133–9.

Bell, W. R. Jr. 1997. Defibrinogenating enzymes. Drugs, **54**(**Suppl 3**), 18–30; discussion 30–1.

Berk, P. D., Goldberg, J. D., et al. 1986. Therapeutic recommendations in polycythemia vera based on Polycythemia Vera Study Group protocols. Semin Hematol, **23**, 132–43.

Black, I. W., Chesterman, C. N., *et al.* 1993. Hematologic correlates of left atrial spontaneous echo contrast and thromboembolism in nonvalvular atrial fibrillation. *J Am Coll Cardiol*, **21**, 451–7.

Black, I. W., and Stewart, W. J. 1993. The role of echocardiography in the evaluation of cardiac source of embolism: left atrial spontaneous echo contrast. *Echocardiography*, **10**, 429–39.

Bosch, T., and Wendler, T. 2004. State of the art of low-density lipoprotein apheresis in the year 2003. *Ther Apher Dial*, **8**, 76–9.

Briley, D. P., Giraud, G. D., *et al.* 1994. Spontaneous echo contrast and hemorheologic abnormalities in cerebrovascular disease. *Stroke*, **25**, 1564–9.

Bunn, H. F. 1997. Pathogenesis and treatment of sickle cell disease. *N Engl J Med*, **337**, 762–9.

Byrne, N. P., Henry, J. C., *et al.* 2002. Neuropathologic findings in a Guillain-Barre patient with strokes after IVIg therapy. *Neurology*, **59**, 458–61.

Caplan, L. R. 1995. Binswanger's disease–revisited. *Neurology*, **45**, 626–33.

Caress, J. B., Cartwright, M. S., *et al.* 2003. The clinical features of 16 cases of stroke associated with administration of IVIg. *Neurology*, **60**, 1822–4.

Chien, S., Usami, S., *et al.* 1970. Abnormal rheology of oxygenated blood in sickle cell anemia. *J Clin Invest*, **49**, 623–34.

Chievitz, E., and Thiede, T. 1962. Complications and causes of death in polycythaemia vera. *Acta Med Scand*, **172**, 513–23.

Cottrill, C. M., and Kaplan, S. 1973. Cerebral vascular accidents in cyanotic congenital heart disease. *Am J Dis Child*, **125**, 484–7.

Coull, B. M., Beamer, N., *et al.* 1991. Chronic blood hyperviscosity in subjects with acute stroke, transient ischemic attack, and risk factors for stroke. *Stroke*, **22**, 162–8.

Danesh, J., Collins, R., *et al.* 2000. Haematocrit, viscosity, erythrocyte sedimentation rate: meta-analyses of prospective studies of coronary heart disease. *Eur Heart J*, **21**, 515–20.

Danesh, J., Lewington, S., *et al.* 2005. Plasma fibrinogen level and the risk of major cardiovascular diseases and nonvascular mortality: an individual participant meta-analysis. *JAMA*, **294**, 1799–809.

Daniel, W. G., Nellessen, U., *et al.* 1988. Left atrial spontaneous echo contrast in mitral valve disease: an indicator for an increased thromboembolic risk. *J Am Coll Cardiol*, **11**, 1204–11.

de Maat, M. P., Arnold, A. E., *et al.* 1996. Modulation of plasma fibrinogen levels by ticlopidine in healthy volunteers and patients with stable angina pectoris. *Thromb Haemost*, **76**, 166–70.

Dintenfass, L. 1966. A preliminary outline of the blood high viscosity syndromes. *Arch Intern Med*, **118**, 427–35.

Dintenfass, L. 1968. Internal viscosity of the red cell and a blood viscosity equation. *Nature*, **219**, 956–8.

Dormandy, J. A., Yates, C. J., *et al.* 1981. Clinical relevance of blood viscosity and red cell deformability including newer therapeutic aspects. *Angiology*, **32**, 236–42.

Durrington, P. N., Mackness, M. I., *et al.* 1998. Effects of two different fibric acid derivatives on lipoproteins, cholesteryl ester transfer, fibrinogen, plasminogen activator inhibitor and paraoxonase activity in type IIb hyperlipoproteinaemia. *Atherosclerosis*, **138**, 217–25.

Elisaf, M. 2002. Effects of fibrates on serum metabolic parameters. *Curr Med Res Opin*, **18**, 269–76.

Emerson, G. G., Herndon, C. N., *et al.* 2002. Thrombotic complications after intravenous immunoglobulin therapy in two patients. *Pharmacotherapy*, **22**, 1638–41.

Ernst, E. 1995. Haemorheological consequences of chronic cigarette smoking. *J Cardiovasc Risk*, **2**, 435–9.

Ernst, E., Resch, K. L., *et al.* 1991. Impaired blood rheology: a risk factor after stroke? *J Intern Med*, **229**, 457–62.

Fahey, J. L., Barth, W. F., *et al.* 1965. Serum hyperviscosity syndrome. *JAMA*, **192**, 464–7.

Fahraeus, R., and Lindqvist, T. 1931. Viscosity of blood in narrow capillary tubes. *Am J Physiol*, **96**, 562–8.

Fatkin, D., Herbert, E., *et al.* 1994. Hematologic correlates of spontaneous echo contrast in patients with atrial fibrillation and implications for thromboembolic risk. *Am J Cardiol*, **73**, 672–6.

Finelli, C., Palareti, G., *et al.* 1991. Ticlopidine lowers plasma fibrinogen in patients with polycythaemia rubra vera and additional thrombotic risk factors. A double-blind controlled study. *Acta Haematol*, **85**, 113–8.

Fisher, M., and Meiselman, H. J. 1991. Hemorheological factors in cerebral ischemia. *Stroke*, **22**, 1164–9.

Gaehtgens, P., and Marx, P. 1987. Hemorheological aspects of the pathophysiology of cerebral ischemia. *J Cereb Blood Flow Metab*, **7**, 259–65.

Gordon, R. S. Jr., Kahn, H. A., *et al.* 1977. Altitude and CBVD death rates show apparent relationship. *Stroke*, **8**, 274.

Grotta, J., Ackerman, R., *et al.* 1982. Whole blood viscosity parameters and cerebral blood flow. *Stroke*, **13**, 296–301.

Grotta, J., Ostrow, P., *et al.* 1985. Fibrinogen, blood viscosity, and cerebral ischemia. *Stroke*, **16**, 192–8.

Grotta, J. C. 1987a. Can raising cerebral blood flow improve outcome after acute cerebral infarction? *Stroke*, **18**, 264–7.

Grotta, J. C. 1987b. Current status of hemodilution in acute cerebral ischemia. *Stroke*, **18**, 689–90.

Grotta, J. C., Manner, C., *et al.* 1986. Red blood cell disorders and stroke. *Stroke*, **17**, 811–7.

Haemorheology, blood-flow and venous thrombosis (editorial). 1975. *Lancet*, **2**, 113–4.

Haglund, O., Wallin, R., *et al.* 1990. Effects of a new fluid fish oil concentrate, ESKIMO-3, on triglycerides, cholesterol, fibrinogen and blood pressure. *J Intern Med*, **227**, 347–53.

Harrison, M. J. 1989. Influence of haematocrit in the cerebral circulation. *Cerebrovasc Brain Metab Rev*, **1**, 55–67.

Harrison, M. J., Pollock, S., *et al.* 1981. Effect of haematocrit on carotid stenosis and cerebral infarction. *Lancet*, **2**, 114–5.

Henriksen, L., Paulson, O. B., *et al.* 1981. Cerebral blood flow following normovolemic hemodilution in patients with high hematocrit. *Ann Neurol*, **9**, 454–7.

Hossmann, V., Auel, H., *et al.* 1985. Haemorheology in adolescent hypertensives. *J Hypertens*, **3**, S331–3.

Izumi, Y., Tsuda, Y., *et al.* 1996. Effects of defibrination on hemorheology, cerebral blood flow velocity, and CO2 reactivity during hypocapnia in normal subjects. *Stroke*, **27**, 1328–32.

Jan, K. M., Powers, E., *et al.* 1990. Altered rheological properties of blood following administrations of tissue plasminogen activator and streptokinase in patients with acute myocardial infarction. *Adv Exp Med Biol*, **281**, 409–17.

Jeffries, B. F., Lipper, M. H., *et al.* 1980. Major intracerebral arterial involvement in sickle cell disease. *Surg Neurol*, **14**, 291–5.

Juhan, I., Vague, P., *et al.* 1982. Abnormalities of erythrocyte deformability and platelet aggregation in insulin-dependent diabetics corrected by insulin in vivo and in vitro. *Lancet*, **1**, 535–7.

Kannel, W. B., Gordon, T., *et al.* 1972. Hemoglobin and the risk of cerebral infarction: the Framingham Study. *Stroke*, **3**, 409–20.

Kannel, W. B., Wolf, P. A., *et al.* 1987. Fibrinogen and risk of cardiovascular disease. The Framingham Study. *JAMA*, **258**, 1183–6.

Kawamoto, A., Shimada, K., *et al.* 1991. Factors associated with silent multiple lacunar lesions on magnetic resonance imaging in asymptomatic elderly hypertensive patients. *Clin Exp Pharmacol Physiol*, **18**, 605–10.

Koenig, W., and Ernst, E. 1992. The possible role of hemorheology in atherothrombogenesis. *Atherosclerosis*, **94**, 93–107.

Koenig, W., Hehr, R., *et al.* 1992. Lovastatin alters blood rheology in primary hyperlipoproteinemia: dependence on lipoprotein(a)? *J Clin Pharmacol*, **32**, 539–45.

Lee, A. J., Mowbray, P. I., *et al.* 1998. Blood viscosity and elevated carotid intima-media thickness in men and women: the Edinburgh Artery Study. *Circulation*, **97**, 1467–73.

Leonhardt, H., Arntz, H. R., *et al.* 1977. Studies of plasma viscosity in primary hyperlipoproteinaemia. *Atherosclerosis*, **28**, 29–40.

Letcher, R. L., Chien, S., *et al.* 1981. Direct relationship between blood pressure and blood viscosity in normal and hypertensive subjects. Role of fibrinogen and concentration. *Am J Med*, **70**, 1195–202.

Levenson, J., Gariepy, J., *et al.* 2000. Association of plasma viscosity and carotid thickening in a French working cohort. *Am J Hypertens*, **13**, 753–8.

Lowe, G. D. 1987. Blood rheology in general medicine and surgery. *Baillieres Clin Haematol*, **1**, 827–61.

Lowe, G. D. 1995. Fibrinogen and cardiovascular disease: historical introduction. *Eur Heart J*, **16**(**Suppl A**), 2–5.

Lowe, G. D. 1998. Etiopathogenesis of cardiovascular disease: hemostasis, thrombosis, and vascular medicine. *Ann Periodontol Am Acad Periodontol*, **3**, 121–6.

Lowe, G. D. 2005a. Circulating inflammatory markers and risks of cardiovascular and non-cardiovascular disease. *J Thromb Haemost*, **3**, 1618–27.

Lowe, G. D. 2005b. Fibrinogen measurement to assess the risk of arterial thrombosis in individual patients: not yet. *J Thromb Haemost*, **3**, 635–7.

Lowe, G. D. 2006. Can haematological tests predict cardiovascular risk? The 2005 Kettle Lecture. *Br J Haematol*, **133**, 232–50.

Lowe, G. D., Lee, A. J., *et al.* 1997. Blood viscosity and risk of cardiovascular events: the Edinburgh Artery Study. *Br J Haematol*, **96**, 168–73.

Lowe, G. D., McArdle, B. M., *et al.* 1982. Increased blood viscosity and fibrinolytic inhibitor in type II hyperlipoproteinaemia. *Lancet*, **1**, 472–5.

McMillan, D. E. 1985. Hemorheologic changes in diabetes and their role in increased atherogenesis. *Horm Metab Res*, **15**, 73–9.

McMillan, D. E. 1989. Increased levels of acute-phase serum proteins in diabetes. *Metab Clin Exp*, **38**, 1042–6.

McMillan, D. E. 1997. Development of vascular complications in diabetes. *Vasc Med (London, England)*, **2**, 132–42.

Melamed, E., Rachmilewitz, E. A., *et al.* 1976. Aseptic cavernous sinus thrombosis after internal carotid arterial occlusion in polycythaemia vera. *J Neurol Neurosurg Psychiatry*, **39**, 320–4.

Merino, A., Hauptman, P., *et al.* 1992. Echocardiographic "smoke" is produced by an interaction of erythrocytes and plasma proteins modulated by shear forces. *J Am Coll Cardiol*, **20**, 1661–8.

Messmer, K., Gornandt, L. *et al.* 1973. Oxygen transport and tissue oxygenation during hemodilution with dextran. *Adv Exp Med Biol*, **37**, 669–80.

Miller, D. B., and Spence, J. D. 1998. Clinical pharmacokinetics of fibric acid derivatives (fibrates). *Clin Pharmacokinet*, **34**, 155–62.

Millikan, C. H., Siekert, R. G., *et al.* 1960. Intermittent carotid and vertebral-basilar insufficiency associated with polycythemia. *Neurology*, **10**, 188–96.

Moriarty, A. J., Hughes, R., *et al.* 1988. Streptokinase and reduced plasma viscosity: a second benefit. *Eur J Haematol*, **41**, 25–36.

Muller, R. 1979. Pentoxifylline – a biomedical profile. *J Med*, **10**, 307–29.

Oder, B., Oder, W., *et al.* 1998. Hypoplasia, stenosis and other alterations of the vertebral artery: does impaired blood rheology manifest a hidden disease? *Acta Neurol Scand*, **97**, 398–403.

Ohene-Frempong, K., Weiner, S. J., *et al.* 1998. Cerebrovascular accidents in sickle cell disease: rates and risk factors. *Blood*, **91**, 288–94.

Ott, E. O., Lechner, H., *et al.* 1974. High blood viscosity syndrome in cerebral infarction. *Stroke*, **5**, 330–3.

Paszkowiak, J. J., and Dardik, A. 2003. Arterial wall shear stress: observations from the bench to the bedside. *Vasc Endovasc Surg*, **37**, 47–57.

Pavlakis, S. G., Bello, J., *et al.* 1988. Brain infarction in sickle cell anemia: magnetic resonance imaging correlates. *Ann Neurol*, **23**, 125–30.

Pavy, M. D., Murphy, P. L., *et al.* 1980. Paraprotein-induced hyperviscosity. A reversible cause of stroke. *Postgrad Med*, **68**, 109–12.

Pearce, J. M., Chandrasekera, C. P., *et al.* 1983. Lacunar infarcts in polycythaemia with raised packed cell volumes. *Br Med J*, **287**, 935–6.

Pearson, T. C., and Wetherley-Mein, G. 1978. Vascular occlusive episodes and venous haematocrit in primary proliferative polycythaemia. *Lancet*, **2**, 1219–22.

Pegelow, C. H., Adams, R. J., *et al.* 1995. Risk of recurrent stroke in patients with sickle cell disease treated with erythrocyte transfusions. *J Pediatr*, **126**, 896–9.

Perloff, J. K., Marelli, A. J., *et al.* 1993. Risk of stroke in adults with cyanotic congenital heart disease. *Circulation*, **87**, 1954–9.

Phornphutkul, C., Rosenthal, A., *et al.* 1973. Cerebrovascular accidents in infants and children with cyanotic congenital heart disease. *Am J Cardiol*, **32**, 329–34.

Radack, K., Deck, C., *et al.* 1989. Dietary supplementation with low-dose fish oils lowers fibrinogen levels: a randomized, double-blind controlled study. *Ann Intern Med*, **111**, 757–8.

Rampling, M. W. 2003. Hyperviscosity as a complication in a variety of disorders. *Semin Thromb Hemost*, **29**, 459–65.

Reinhart, W. H., and Berchtold, P. E. 1992. Effect of high-dose intravenous immunoglobulin therapy on blood rheology. *Lancet*, **339**, 662–4.

Rosenson, R. S., and Lowe, G. D. 1998. Effects of lipids and lipoproteins on thrombosis and rheology. *Atherosclerosis*, **140**, 271–80.

Rothman, S. M., Fulling, K. H., *et al.* 1986. Sickle cell anemia and central nervous system infarction: a neuropathological study. *Ann Neurol*, **20**, 684–90.

Rothwell, P. M., Howard, S. C. *et al.* 2004. Fibrinogen concentration and risk of ischemic stroke and acute coronary events in 5113 patients with transient ischemic attack and minor ischemic stroke. *Stroke*, **35**, 2300–5.

Sakuta, S. 1981. Blood filtrability in cerebrovascular disorders, with special reference to erythrocyte deformability and ATP content. *Stroke*, **12**, 824–8.

Schafer, A. I. 1984. Bleeding and thrombosis in the myeloproliferative disorders. *Blood*, **64**, 1–12.

Schneider, R., Korber, N. *et al.* 1985. The haemorheological features of lacunar strokes. *J Neurol*, **232**, 357–62.

Schneider, R., Ringelstein, E. B., *et al.* 1987. The role of plasma hyperviscosity in subcortical arteriosclerotic encephalopathy (Binswanger's disease). *J Neurol*, **234**, 67–73.

Schneider, R., Schmid-Schonbein, H., *et al.* 1983. The rheological efficiency of parenteral pentoxifylline (Trental) in patients with ischemic brain lesions. Preliminary results. *Eur Neurol*, **22**(**Suppl 1**), 98–104.

Seplowitz, A. H., Chien, S., *et al.* 1981. Effects of lipoproteins on plasma viscosity. *Atherosclerosis*, **38**, 89–95.

Silverstein, A., Gilbert, H., *et al.* 1962. Neurologic complications of polycythemia. *Ann Intern Med*, **57**, 909–16.

Simopoulos, A. P. 1991. Omega-3 fatty acids in health and disease and in growth and development. *Am J Clin Nutr*, **54**, 438–63.

Simpson, I. A., Lorimer, A. R., *et al.* 1985. Effect of Ciprofibrate on platelet aggregation and fibrinolysis in patients with hypercholesterolaemia. *Thromb Haemost*, **54**, 442–4.

Sloop, G. D. 1996. A unifying theory of atherogenesis. *Med Hypotheses*, **47**, 321–5.

Somer, T., and Meiselman, H. J. 1993. Disorders of blood viscosity. *Ann Med*, **25**, 31–9.

Stockman, J. A., Nigro, M. A., *et al.* 1972. Occlusion of large cerebral vessels in sickle-cell anemia. *N Engl J Med*, **287**, 846–9.

Strand, T., Asplund, K., *et al.* 1984. A randomized controlled trial of hemodilution therapy in acute ischemic stroke. *Stroke*, **15**, 980–9.

Stuart, J., George, A. J., *et al.* 1981. Haematological stress syndrome in atherosclerosis. *J Clin Pathol*, **34**, 464–7.

Thomas, D. J. 1982. Whole blood viscosity and cerebral blood flow. *Stroke*, **13**, 285–7.

Thomas, D. J., du Boulay, G. H., *et al.* 1977a. Cerebral blood-flow in polycythaemia. *Lancet*, **2**, 161–3.

Thomas, D. J., Marshall, J., *et al.* 1977b. Effect of haematocrit on cerebral blood-flow in man. *Lancet*, **2**, 941–3.

Tohgi, H., Yamanouchi, H., *et al.* 1978. Importance of the hematocrit as a risk factor in cerebral infarction. *Stroke*, **9**, 369–74.

van Hilten, J. J., Haan, J., *et al.* 1989. Cerebral infarction in hereditary spherocytosis. *Stroke*, **20**, 1755–6.

Vucic, S., Chong, P. S., *et al.* 2004. Thromboembolic complications of intravenous immunoglobulin treatment. *Eur Neurol*, **52**, 141–4.

Wade, J. P. 1983. Transport of oxygen to the brain in patients with elevated haematocrit values before and after venesection. *Brain*, **106**(**Pt 2**), 513–23.

Walzl, B., Walzl, M. *et al.* 1994. Extracorporeal fibrinogen and platelet precipitation as a new haemorheological treatment for acute stroke. *J Neurol Sci*, **126**, 25–9.

Wells, R. 1970. Syndromes of hyperviscosity. *N Engl J Med*, **283**, 183–6.

Wells, R. E., Jr. 1964. Rheology of blood in the microvasculature. *N Engl J Med*, **270**, 832–9.

Wood, J. H., and Fleischer, A. S. 1982. Observations during hypervolemic hemodilution of patients with acute focal cerebral ischemia. *JAMA*, **248**, 2999–304.

Wood, J. H., and Kee, D. B. Jr. 1985. Hemorheology of the cerebral circulation in stroke. *Stroke*, **16**, 765–72.

Woodward, M., Lowe, G. D. O., *et al.* 2005. Associations of inflammatory and hemostatic variables with the risk of recurrent stroke. *Stroke*, **36**, 2143–7.

Yamauchi, H., Fukuyama, H. *et al.* 1993. Hemodilution improves cerebral hemodynamics in internal carotid artery occlusion. *Stroke*, **24**, 1885–90.

Yazdi, R., and Cote, C. 1986. Watershed infarction in a case of polycythemia vera. *Clin Nucl Med*, **11**, 665–6.

Zannad, F., Voisin, P., *et al.* 1988. Haemorheological abnormalities in arterial hypertension and their relation to cardiac hypertrophy. *J Hypertens*, **6**, 293–7.

48

CALCIUM, HYPERCALCEMIA, MAGNESIUM, AND BRAIN ISCHEMIA

Philip B. Gorelick and Michael A. Sloan

Introduction

Calcium is an important constituent of many organs of the body, especially bones and teeth. Normal calcium and magnesium ion concentrations are crucial for the maintenance of homeostasis and cellular function. Calcium is an important mediator of striatal and smooth muscle contraction, and is integral in many coagulation and other blood reactions. The concentration of ionized calcium is normally much higher in the extracellular spaces than within cells. Excessive entry of calcium into cells promotes cell death (Choi, 1995; Lee et al., 1999; Orrenius et al., 1992; Siesjo, 1991; Siesjo and Bengtson, 1989). Hypercalcemia is a relatively common biochemical abnormality that is often caused by hyperparathyroidism but may also be related to a number of pathological entities that include cancer, bone metastases, sarcoidosis, and other conditions. Calcium has become recognized as a key mediator of cell death in cerebrovascular pathophysiology (Lee et al., 1999). As a result, calcium channel antagonists (CCAs) have been tested as neuroprotective agents for the treatment of acute stroke (Horn and Limburg, 2001; Mohr et al., 1994), as well as to mitigate vascular and neuronal effects of vasospasm after subarachnoid hemorrhage (Allen et al., 1983; Haley et al., 1994b; Rinkel et al., 2005; Shibuya et al., 1992). Reviews of the neurological manifestations of hypercalcemia rarely discuss stroke, although such has been reported (Gorelick and Caplan, 1985).

Magnesium is another important metallic ion that sometimes functions in a reciprocal way to calcium, a so-called natural calcium antagonist. Magnesium is one of the latest agents to be tested in acute ischemic stroke as a neuroprotectant as it may exert beneficial effects via multimodal mechanisms such as cerebral arterial vasodilation, noncompetitive N-methyl-D-aspartate (NMDA) receptor blockade, inhibition of presynaptic excitatory neurotransmitter release, potentiation of presynaptic adenosine, blockade of voltage-gated calcium channels, suppression of cortical spreading depression and anoxic depolarizations, and vascular smooth muscle relaxation (Gorelick and Ruland, 2004; Muir, 2000). Magnesium has been and is currently being tested for efficacy and safety in persons with acute ischemic stroke (Intravenous Magnesium Efficacy in Stroke [IMAGES] Investigators, 2004; Saver et al., 2004). In addition, systemic magnesium deficiency has been associated with delayed cerebral ischemia after aneurysmal subarachnoid hemorrhage (van den Bergh et al., 2003). As a result, magnesium infusions are being tested as a treatment for vasospasm after aneurysmal subarachnoid hemorrhage (van den Bergh, 2005; Wong et al., 2006).

This chapter reviews the role of calcium and magnesium in causing and ameliorating brain ischemia, respectively.

Calcium: theoretical considerations

Three different effects of hypercalcemia are posited to contribute to the development and severity of brain ischemia: (i) hypercalcemia stimulates vascular smooth muscle causing vasoconstriction; (ii) increased calcium concentrations enhance platelet aggregation and activate the body's intrinsic coagulation system; and (iii) calcium entry into cells, a process enhanced by an elevated extracellular-to-intracellular calcium ion gradient, causes cytotoxic effects that promote cell death and brain infarction. Another possible mechanism to explain stroke when there is a disturbance in calcium regulation relates to compensatory hyperparathyroidism (Sato et al., 2003).

Smooth muscle contraction

The role of calcium in smooth muscle contraction has been better understood since clarification of the relationship of calcium to magnesium. The roles of calcium and magnesium in relation to cerebral arterial vasoconstriction in diverse disease states have been reviewed previously (Sloan, 1995; Sloan et al., 1998). Calcium is an essential mediator of smooth muscle contraction. Contraction of the smooth muscle of blood vessels is often initiated by stimulation of α-adrenergic receptors, which in turn leads to a release of membrane-bound calcium. The increase in calcium ion concentration promotes entry of calcium ions through a voltage-sensitive calcium channel (VSCC) or receptor-operated calcium channel (ROC) into the cytosol of smooth muscle cells (Tymianski, 1996). Calcium ions bind with the protein calmodulin and activate myosin light-chain kinase, which in turn phosphorylates myosin heads. This reaction activates adenosine triphosphatase (ATPase), an enzyme that cleaves ATP, causing conformational change in myosin and stimulating smooth muscle contraction. When calcium is not present, ATPase activity in smooth muscle is extremely slight, ATP cannot be cleaved, and the contractile process does not occur. This process is slow, and other factors besides calcium ions can have large effects on the intensity of the contractile process (Guyton, 1986).

Two major types of CCAs have been used in diverse cerebrovascular disorders. The dihydropyridine VSCC agents, such as nimodipine and nicardipine, have differential effects on cerebral arterial tone. In the setting of aneurysmal subarachnoid hemorrhage, nimodipine has been shown to have weak cerebral vasodilatory effects (Allen *et al.*, 1983), whereas nicardipine has been shown to significantly reduce the proportion of patients with mean flow velocities >200 cm/s by transcranial Doppler ultrasonography and angiographic vasospasm (Haley *et al.*, 1994b). It is believed that nimodipine may either have a direct cytoprotective effect or dilate small collateral channels (Findlay *et al.*, 1991). AT877 (or fasudil hydrochloride) inhibits the action of free intracellular Ca$_2$+ ion, protein kinases A, G, and C, and myosin light-chain kinase, as well as antagonizing the actions of endothelin. AT877 has been shown to dilate vasospastic arteries in the setting of aneurysmal subarachnoid hemorrhage (Shibuya *et al.*, 1992).

Blood coagulation

Calcium is essential for blood clotting. It is required at multiple levels within the intrinsic and extrinsic pathways of coagulation to form activated blood coagulation factors and convert prothrombin to thrombin. Calcium also plays a role in adenosine diphosphate (ADP)-induced platelet aggregation and participates in platelet adhesion reactions to various surfaces. Various substances have been used to reduce the concentration of calcium ions in the blood. With potassium citrate, the citrate ion combines with calcium in the blood to cause an un-ionized calcium compound; the lack of ionic calcium prevents coagulation (Guyton, 1986). Severe hypercalcemia can trigger diffuse intravascular coagulation (Bauermeister *et al.*, 1967).

Calcium and cell death

Entry of calcium into cells is known to contribute to cell death. In neurons, the total intracellular calcium content is in the millimolar range, but its physiological intracellular concentration is very low, <0.1 mM. To maintain such a large gradient across the cell membrane, the movement of calcium is subject to strict and sensitive control, and multiple mechanisms are involved in its homeostasis (Blaustein, 1988; Miller, 1991; Siesjo and Bengtson, 1989). An increase in intracellular calcium can be brought about by one or more of three mechanisms: activation of influx, curtailment of efflux, and reduction in the intracellular calcium-buffering capacity, which includes release from internal stores. In hypoxia and ischemia, ATP production fails. The sodium-potassium channels fail, resulting in membrane depolarization. Brain hypoxia leads to a cascade of metabolic changes. Lactate, potassium, free radicals that contain active oxygen species, prostaglandins, leukotrienes, and thromboxane A$_2$ are all present in extracellular fluid in the hypoxic zone in much higher than normal levels. These biochemical changes alter cell membrane function and open voltage-dependent ion channels causing an increase in intracellular calcium (Siesjo and Bengtson, 1989). Other calcium-related damage includes changes in protein phosphorylation, enhanced proteolysis and microtubular disassembly, production of free radicals, and mitochondrial calcium overload. The combinations of these processes trigger apoptosis and necrotic cell death (Siesjo, 1991; Siesjo and Bengtson, 1989).

With the depolarization of ischemic neurons deprived of oxygen and glucose there is rapid build-up of synaptic-derived and depolarized-astrocytic origin glutamate (Lee *et al.*, 1999). The build-up of extracellular glutamate leads to overstimulation of the α-amino-3-hydroxy-5-methyl-4-isoxazoleproprionic acid (AMPA), kainate, and NMDA-type glutamate receptors with resultant influx of sodium and calcium ions via the channels gated by these cell receptors. The elevated intracellular calcium concentrations lead to lethal metabolic derangements. NMDA antagonists, however, reduce death of cultured neurons lacking oxygen and glucose. Although NMDA-antagonist drugs have shown promise in reducing ischemic damage in the laboratory, use of these drugs in clinical trials has not proved to be beneficial thus far (Gorelick, 2000). Similarly and experimentally, extracellular magnesium-dependent, NMDA-induced neuronal swelling may occur and increasing extracellular magnesium may reduce neuronal apoptosis by interfering with calcium entry through voltage- or agonist-gated channels (Lee *et al.*, 1999).

An alternate hypothesis

Atherosclerosis and osteoporosis may be related to one another by shared pathogenetic mechanisms (Sato *et al.*, 2003). Hyperparathyroidism may result from vitamin D deficiency, and osteoporosis occurs in elderly persons. A cycle occurs whereby hyperparathyroidism leads to bone resorption and calcium deposition in tissues (which include the vessel wall). Reduced bone mineral density and osteoporosis have been observed in elderly women with stroke. The vascular endothelium is a target of parathyroid hormone, and compensatory hyperparathyroidism may be characterized by endothelial vasodilatory dysfunction (Sato *et al.*, 2003). Therefore, endothelial dysfunction and calcium deposition could be mechanistically linked to stroke and other cardiovascular disease. This relationship, however, may be confounded by other cardiovascular risk factors such as hypertension, which may be associated with hyperparathyroidism.

Linking stroke to hypercalcemia – prior reports

An extensive analysis of the relationship between hypercalcemia and stroke was a report by Bostrom and Alveryd (1972) concerning their experience in Stockholm. Among 170 patients with hypercalcemia referred for parathyroid exploration, nine had well-defined strokes. The brain event consisted of a sudden or stepwise onset of severe focal deficits, usually hemiparesis or quadriparesis, without seizures. Although the patients were not evaluated with angiography or modern imaging technology, the events were likely to have been brain infarcts. Four of the nine stroke patients had autopsies that documented brain infarcts in three patients, occlusion of one vertebral and the basilar artery in one patient, and putaminal hemorrhage in one hypertensive patient. The average age of these nine patients was 71.6 years. Some patients also had hypertension, and two had atrial fibrillation. Bostrom and Alveryd (1972) screened 2268 consecutive internal medicine emergency patients for hypercalcemia and identified 12 with hyperparathyroidism, of whom three had had recent strokes. They also screened 86 consecutive stroke patients by repeated measurements of serum calcium and identified two patients with hyperparathyroidism among those patients with brain infarction. No patient with intracerebral hemorrhage was found to be hypercalcemic.

Gorelick and Caplan (1985) reviewed their experience with hypercalcemia and stroke at the Michael Reese Hospital in Chicago. During a 2-year period, among 502 patients seen by the stroke service, six stroke patients had hypercalcemia. The patients were black, and five of the six were women. All were hypertensive and elderly and all had hyperparathyroidism. A parathyroid adenoma and parathyroid hyperplasia were found in two patients; the others all had elevated parathyroid hormone levels. In four patients the hypercalcemia was found at the time of the strokes, whereas the other two patients were known to have hypercalcemia for 5 and 7 years, respectively. Three patients had single strokes with sudden onset of hemiplegia. The other patients had multiple instances of multiple focal neurological symptoms and signs that occurred during days, weeks, or months. Two patients had decreased consciousness, and two patients had seizures (Gorelick and Caplan, 1985). Angiography in three patients showed distal branch artery occlusions (two patients), and the third patient had severe large artery and distal branch narrowing probably caused by vasoconstriction. The patient with intracranial artery vasoconstriction was a psychotic woman with known longstanding hypercalcemia. She had refused treatment. She was lethargic, restless, and confused, and she often hallucinated. She had seizures and multifocal findings on examination. After parathyroidectomy and normalization of serum calcium levels, the patients improved (Gorelick and Caplan, 1985).

Focal seizures have been noted in hypercalcemic patients (Bauermeister et al., 1967; Gorelick and Caplan, 1985; Herishanu et al., 1970). One patient with parathyroid adenoma and acute pancreatitis died after developing focal seizures that led to stupor. Autopsy revealed multiple cerebral microthrombi, scattered microinfarcts, and small hemorrhages (Bauermeister et al., 1967).

Case reports have identified possible vasospasm as the mechanism for brain ischemia in some patients with hypercalcemia (Streeto, 1969; Walker et al., 1980; Yarnell and Caplan, 1986). For example, a 52-year-old woman with hypertension and severe hypercalcemia was evaluated for headache and polyuria (Walker et al., 1980). She developed a left hemiparesis, fluent aphasia, and bilateral Babinski signs. CT scan showed two separate right cerebral infarcts in the parasagittal parietal lobe in the anterior cerebral artery territory and in the occipital lobe in the posterior cerebral artery territory. Angiography showed intense spasm of the distal right internal carotid and proximal left anterior cerebral and middle cerebral arteries (MCAs). Localized areas of spasm were also identified in distal cortical branches, and transit of blood was slow through both cerebral hemispheres. After treatment of hypercalcemia, she improved clinically, and repeat angiography showed a marked decrease in cerebral vasospasm (Walker et al., 1980). The patient reported by Yarnell and Caplan (1986) was a 42-year-old hypertensive man who had a brainstem stroke that evolved during 1 week. Two angiograms (performed on days 8 and 20 of the stroke) showed an irregular constriction beginning at the midportion of the basilar artery extending from the anterior inferior cerebellar

artery origins to the superior cerebellar artery origins. Serum calcium and parathyroid hormone levels were persistently high. He had a parathyroidectomy. Repeat angiography 18 months after the stroke showed complete normalization of the basilar artery narrowing, identifying vasoconstriction related to hypercalcemia as the explanation for the findings on the initial angiograms (Yarnell and Caplan, 1986).

In some patients, stroke was accompanied by sleepiness, restlessness, confusion, stupor, muscle weakness, hallucination, altered intellectual function, and psychosis. In a single case report by Streeto (1969), a patient with hypercalcemia caused by vitamin D intoxication had visual hallucinations, ataxia, and hemianopia. The symptoms in this patient mimicked those often found in patients with vertebrobasilar arterial disease.

Hypercalcemia is most commonly found in older patients and is often accompanied by hypertension, which may confound the association. It may be difficult to determine how much of the cerebrovascular pathology in patients with ischemic stroke is related to the elevated serum calcium level and how much is better explained by coexisting hypertension and atherosclerosis.

Stroke treatment with calcium antagonists

Investigators have used CCAs to reduce neurological deficits and improve outcome from acute ischemic stroke. Nimodipine, a dihydropyridine compound that diminishes Ca_2+ flux through VSCCs, is the prototype agent in this class. One meta-analysis of nine trials suggested that a subgroup of patients treated within 12 hours might have better neurological recovery (odds ratio [OR] 0.62, 95% confidence interval [CI], 0.44–0.87) (Mohr, et al., 1994). A more recent meta-analysis of 29 clinical trials involving CCAs (Horn and Limburg, 2001) revealed no effect of nimodipine on poor outcome (relative risk [RR] 1.04, 95% CI, 0.98–1.09) or death (RR 1.07, 95% CI, 0.98–1.17). In trials of good methodological quality, a statistically significant negative effect of treatment was found (RR 1.09, 95% CI, 1.02–1.16). There were no differences in outcome by route of administration or time interval between stroke onset and onset of treatment.

Investigators have also actively explored the role of calcium and calcium channel blocking agents in contributing to intracranial arterial vasoconstriction related to subarachnoid hemorrhage. The rationale for the use of calcium antagonists in the prevention or treatment of secondary brain ischemia was based on the assumption that these drugs reduce the frequency of vasospasm by counteracting the influx of calcium into vascular smooth muscle cells. The antivasospastic effect of calcium antagonists was confirmed by many in vitro studies that used intracranial arteries and also by in vivo assessments of arterial lumen changes after experimental subarachnoid hemorrhage. Clinical trials have been undertaken with three calcium antagonists: nimodipine, AT877 (Asahi Chemical Industry Company, Japan), and nicardipine, of which nimodipine was the most extensively used and studied (Feigin et al., 1998). In a review of reported randomized controlled trials of calcium antagonists in patients with subarachnoid hemorrhage, pooled data from trials on all three calcium antagonists, totaling 2434 randomized patients, showed a significant reduction in the frequency of poor outcome, which resulted from a reduction in the frequency of secondary brain ischemia (Feigin *et al.*, 1998). When analyzed separately, the nimodipine trials showed a significant reduction in the frequency of a poor outcome, but the nicardipine and AT877 trials did not. These data suggest that the administration of nimodipine improves outcome in patients with subarachnoid hemorrhage, but it is uncertain whether nimodipine acts by reducing the frequency of vasospasm or through a neuroprotective mechanism, or both.

In the Nicardipine in Subarachnoid Hemorrhage Trial (Haley *et al.*, 1994a), the rates of favorable outcomes and mortality at 3 months were similar in the nicardipine- and placebo-treated groups. In the AT877 study (Shibuya *et al.*, 1992), vasospasm-associated low densities on CT scan and the number of patients with a poor outcome at 1 month after subarachnoid hemorrhage were lower in the AT877 group. These data indicate that while nicardipine and AT877 reduce the frequency of vasoconstriction, the effect on overall outcome remains uncertain.

In a more recent review of calcium antagonists in aneurysmal subarachnoid hemorrhage from the Cochrane Stroke Group Trials Register, it was concluded that calcium antagonists reduce risk of poor outcome and secondary ischemia after aneurysmal subarachnoid hemorrhage; however, the results for the poor outcome category were dependent largely on one trial with oral nimodipine (Rinkel *et al.*, 2005). Although not beyond doubt, oral nimodipine administered 60 mg every 4 hours is indicated for patients with aneurysmal subarachnoid hemorrhage given the background of this devastating disorder, whereas intravenous administration of calcium antagonists is not recommended. The evidence for nicardipine and AT877 therapies in aneurysmal subarachnoid hemorrhage is inconclusive (Rinkel *et al.*, 2005).

Calcium channel blockers have also been used to prophylactically treat common migraine and patients with classic and basilar artery migraine. The rationale behind the use of calcium channel blockers in migraine is to prevent vasoconstriction; however, the mechanism whereby migraine exerts its deleterious effect or may cause stroke is apparently complex (Goadsby *et al.*, 2002; Silberstein, 2004). Clues to deciphering migraine mechanisms, for example, have been linked to studies of familial hemiplegic migraine, an uncommon disorder (Ducros *et al.*, 2001; Moskowitz *et al.*, 2004). Mutations in CACNA1 A, an encoder for a neuronal calcium channel, have been identified in this condition.

In the course of our practice, we have described several other examples of stroke related to calcium. In one case, we described a 40-year-old man who had sudden onset of left-sided weakness, slurred speech, and bifrontal headache (Shanmugan *et al.*, 1997). He had a medical history of cigarette smoking and calcified bicuspid aortic valve. Cranial CT and brain MRI showed findings consistent with a right frontotemporal-parietal area infarction. On cranial CT there was a density consistent with calcium lodged in the horizontal portion (M1) of the right MCA, and magnetic resonance angiography showed diminished flow in this area. Echocardiography showed a heavily calcified bicuspid aortic valve and a significant gradient across the valve. Surgical replacement of the valve with a 27 St. Jude prosthesis revealed a severely stenotic, deformed, and heavily calcified bicuspid valve with a gap area suggesting the

site where a piece of calcium had broken off. Included in our report was a review of other cases of calcific embolism.

In another case, we reported a 26-year-old woman with end-stage renal disease, hyperparathyroidism with systemic calciphylaxis (CPX), and stroke (Katsamakis *et al.*, 1998). CPX is a rare complication of chronic renal failure and secondary hyperparathyroidism that manifests as diffuse calcification of the medial layer of small and intermediate arterial blood vessels and may manifest with skin necrosis and soft-tissue calcification of connective tissue in a variety of systemic organs. This patient presented with mitral annular calcification and a right MCA territory ischemic stroke. A high-density lesion was seen in the region of the right MCA on cranial CT that was thought to represent a calcified cerebral embolism originating from the mitral valve. In addition to disorders of calcium metabolism that might be associated with stroke in CPX, these patients might have protein S or C deficiencies that could lead to stroke. Our report emphasized the possibility of a cardiac source of calcific embolism causing ischemic stroke in CPX patients.

Dietary calcium and other electrolytes

Recently, there has been some interest in the role of dietary intake of calcium and its relationship to stroke. Iso *et al.* (1999) prospectively studied calcium, potassium, and magnesium intake and the risk of stroke among 85 746 women who filled out dietary questionnaires. After 1.6 million-years of follow-up, there were 690 strokes (129 subarachnoid hemorrhages, 74 intraparenchymal hemorrhages, 386 ischemic strokes, and 101 strokes of undetermined type). Women in the highest quintile of calcium intake had an adjusted RR of ischemic stroke of 0.69 compared with women in the lowest quintile (Iso *et al.*, 1999). These investigators concluded that low calcium intake and low potassium intake might contribute to the increased risk of ischemic stroke in middle-aged women. Due to the design of the study, it remains possible that women in the lowest quintile of calcium intake had unknown characteristics that may have made them susceptible to ischemic stroke.

Magnesium: theoretical considerations

Magnesium ions are involved in many essential biochemical reactions by acting as cofactors in protein and energy synthesis, as well as influencing many calcium-related processes (Muir, 2000). Active transport of magnesium across the blood-brain barrier maintains a concentration gradient between cerebrospinal fluid (CSF) and serum. In dietary magnesium deficiency, CSF magnesium is maintained preferentially. In the central nervous system, magnesium is predominantly intracellular, and approximately 80% is bound to ATP. Magnesium competes with calcium at VSCCs on both cell surface and intracellular membranes and is an antagonist at N-, P-, and (at high concentrations) L-type VSCCs. It may therefore impede calcium-dependent presynaptic glutamate release and VSCC-mediated calcium entry into ischemic neurons. At resting membrane potentials, opening of, affinity of, and current flow through the NMDA receptor is reduced or completely abolished by physiological extracellular magnesium concentrations.

Increasing extracellular magnesium concentrations to supraphysiologic levels noncompetitively antagonizes NMDA conductance. NMDA receptor activation causes a 20-fold increase in intracellular magnesium concentration, which may be large enough to block L-type VSCCs and sodium and potassium channels. Intracellular magnesium enhances mitochondrial buffering of intracellular free calcium and is required for uptake of calcium by endoplasmic reticulum (via membrane Mg_2+-Ca_2+ ATPase) in ischemic neurons. Brain intracellular magnesium concentrations can be measured with phosphorus (31P) magnetic resonance spectroscopy (Helpern et al., 1993). Ionized magnesium is believed to exert beneficial effects on cardiac contractility and vascular endothelial function.

Favorable vascular and neuronal effects with magnesium administration have been reported. Magnesium has direct vasodilatory effects on large, medium, and small cerebral vessels, either by antagonizing endothelin-1, neuropeptide Y, and angiotensin II in large vessels or as a direct calcium antagonist effect in medium-size vessels (Muir, 2000). In a rat model, administration of magnesium produces a dose-dependent inhibition (20%–85%) of cocaine-induced arteriolar spasms and attenuation (85%–95%) of venular vasospasm and microhemorrhages (Huang et al., 1990). In a rat model of subarachnoid hemorrhage (Ram et al., 1991), basilar artery vasospasm was reduced by intravenous magnesium sulfate at a mean plasma magnesium level of 4.32 mmol/L. Administration of magnesium sulfate, but not magnesium chloride, has been associated with neuroprotection in focal cerebral ischemia models. Use of magnesium chloride has been associated with hyperglycemia, which may exacerbate ischemic injury (Muir, 2000).

Linking stroke to disturbances of magnesium – prior reports

There are few reports evaluating the relationship between serum magnesium levels and stroke. In one study (Altura et al., 1997), 98 patients were admitted to three hospitals with a diagnosis of either ischemic or hemorrhagic stroke. The stroke patients had early and significant deficits in serum ionized magnesium, but not in total magnesium. Twenty-five percent had >65% reductions in the mean serum ionized magnesium level compared to controls. The stroke patients had significant elevation in the ratio of serum ionized calcium to ionized magnesium, a sign suggestive of increased vascular tone and vasoconstriction of intracranial arteries. Application of the low serum concentrations of ionized magnesium from stroke patients to cultured canine cerebral smooth muscle cells resulted in rapid and marked elevations in cytosolic free calcium ions. Coincident with the rise in intracellular calcium, many of the cerebral vascular smooth muscle cells contracted causing vasospasm. Reintroduction of normal extracellular magnesium ion concentrations failed to either lower the intracellular calcium overload or reverse the rounding-up of the cerebral vascular cells. These results suggested that changes in magnesium metabolism play an important role in stroke syndromes and in the etiology of intracranial artery vasoconstriction associated with subarachnoid hemorrhage.

In one magnetic resonance spectroscopy study (Helpern et al., 1993), compared with normal controls, ischemic stroke patients had a significant 45% increase in intracellular free magnesium concentration associated with acidotic brain pH, reduced phosphocreatine, and elevated inorganic phosphate. This pattern is consistent with disruption of the biochemical balance between ATP, hydrogen ions, and the release of bound magnesium. Because ATP has a greater binding affinity for hydrogen ions than for magnesium ions, the acidosis likely contributes to the increase in intracellular free magnesium concentration. These acute changes in intracellular magnesium may contribute to, or be a marker for, ischemic cell injury.

Recent data suggest that magnesium deficiency may promote the development and progression of atherosclerosis and symptomatic large-vessel cerebrovascular disease. In a cohort study of 323 patients with symptomatic peripheral artery occlusive disease and intermittent claudication followed for 20 months (Amighi et al., 2004), neurologic outcomes (ischemic stroke and carotid revascularization) occurred in 35 (11%) patients (15 stroke, 13 carotid revascularization, 7 stroke with subsequent revascularization). Compared with patients in the highest tertile of serum magnesium levels, patients with serum magnesium levels <0.76 mmol/L (lowest tertile) had a significantly increased risk for neurologic events after adjustment for diabetes mellitus, smoking, serum creatinine, history of myocardial infarction, history of stroke, use of diuretic therapy, and use of statin therapy (RR 3.29, 95% CI, 1.34–7.90, $p = .009$). Limitations of this study include a combined study endpoint that may reflect differing pathophysiologic entities, lack of data on other drugs that may affect magnesium levels, and a nonrepresentative study population.

Evidence is conflicting regarding the role of hypomagnesemia in the development of vasospasm after subarachnoid hemorrhage (Collignon et al., 2004; van den Bergh, et al., 2003). In one study of 107 consecutive patients with aneurysmal subarachnoid hemorrhage (van den Bergh et al., 2003), hypomagnesemia occurred in 50% of patients. Overall, hypomagnesemia (<0.70 mmol/L) on admission was univariately associated with the occurrence of delayed cerebral ischemia (crude hazard ratio 2.4, 95% CI, 1.0–5.6) and poor outcome (Glasgow Outcome Scale score 1–3; OR 2.5, 95% CI, 1.1–5.5), although not in multivariate analysis (delayed cerebral ischemia; hazard ratio 1.9, 95% CI, 0.7–4.7). However, in multivariate analysis, hypomagnesemia between days 2 and 12 after subarachnoid hemorrhage was associated with delayed cerebral ischemia (hazard ratio 3.2, 95% CI, 1.1–8.9). In another study of 128 consecutive patients with aneurysmal subarachnoid hemorrhage (Collignon et al., 2004), there was no difference in mean, minimal, or maximal serum magnesium level in the physiologic range between patients with or without delayed cerebral ischemia or between patients with severe, moderate, or no delayed cerebral ischemia.

Stroke treatment with magnesium

Muir (2000) reviewed five small pilot trials of intravenous magnesium in acute ischemic stroke. No adverse cardiovascular effects were reported.

The IMAGES Trial (IMAGES Investigators, 2004) enrolled 2386 patients within 12 hours of symptom onset to receive 16 mmol of magnesium sulfate intravenously over 15 minutes, followed by 65 mmol over 24 hours, or placebo. Primary outcome was a global endpoint statistic expressed as the common OR for death and disability at 90 days. Predefined subgroup analyses were for <6 hours versus >6 hours, ischemic versus nonischemic strokes, and cortical versus noncortical strokes. Median time to treatment was 7 hours, with only 3% treated within 3 hours of symptom onset. In the intention-to-treat analysis, the primary outcome was not improved by magnesium (OR 0.95, 95% CI, 0.80–1.13, $p = .59$). Mortality was slightly higher in the magnesium-treated group (hazard ratio 1.18, 95% CI, 0.97–1.42, $p = .098$). Surprisingly, subgroup analyses revealed that there was a significant reduction in poor outcomes in the noncortical stroke group (OR 0.75, 95% CI, 0.58–0.97, $p = .026$), with a significant interaction between this subgroup and treatment ($p = .011$). Study limitations include lack of a reliable measure of initial stroke severity, median time to treatment, and lack of demonstration of adequate drug concentration in the serum or in ischemic tissue (Goldstein, 2004).

The Field Administration of Stroke Therapy-Magnesium (FAST-MAG) pilot trial of 20 stroke patients (Saver et al., 2004) showed that field administration of magnesium can begin within a median of 100 minutes of symptom onset without occurrence of serious adverse events.

In the phase II Magnesium Sulfate in Aneurysmal Subarachnoid Hemorrhage (MASH) Trial (van den Bergh, 2005) 283 patients were randomized within 4 days of onset of aneurysmal subarachnoid hemorrhage to receive a continuous intravenous dose of 64 mmol/day or placebo until 14 days after occlusion of the aneurysm. The primary outcome, delayed cerebral ischemia (new hypodense lesion on CT compatible with clinical features of delayed cerebral ischemia), was analyzed by intention-to-treat methodology. Magnesium treatment reduced the risk of delayed cerebral ischemia (hazard ratio 0.66, 95% CI, 0.38–1.14) and poor outcome (hazard ratio 0.77, 95% CI, 0.54–1.09). A pilot study (Wong et al., 2006) randomized 60 patients to receive magnesium sulfate 80 mmol/day or saline for 14 days. Intravenous nimodipine was allowed as a concomitant therapy. The duration of sonographic vasospasm, defined as MCA mean flow velocities >120 cm/s or a Lindegaard index > 3, was shorter in the magnesium-treated group ($p <.01$). Symptomatic vasospasm was reduced from 43% (placebo) to 23% (magnesium), $p = .06$. However, there was no difference in functional recovery or Glasgow Outcome Scale score.

Conclusion

Case series suggest an association between hypercalcemia, ischemic stroke, and reversible cerebral vasoconstriction. The status of hypomagnesemia as a risk-factor for large-vessel ischemic stroke, or stroke in general, is not established. During acute cerebral ischemia, calcium overload of neurons and vascular smooth muscle cells is associated with ischemic cell injury and death. Administration of CCAs and magnesium has not yet been shown to improve outcome from acute ischemic stroke. However, there is

some benefit from the use of the dihydropyridine CCA nimodipine for improving outcome after aneurysmal subarachnoid hemorrhage. Ongoing studies of prehospital administration of magnesium for acute ischemic stroke and intravenous magnesium during the period of risk for vasospasm after aneurysmal subarachnoid hemorrhage will, it is hoped, prove to be efficacious and safe as treatments for these specific stroke types.

REFERENCES

Allen, G. S., Ahn, H. S., Preziosi, T. J., et al. 1983. Cerebral arterial spasm – a controlled trial of nimodipine in patients with subarachnoid hemorrhage. N Engl J Med, **308**, 619–24.

Altura, B. T., Memon, Z. I., Zang, A., et al. 1997. Low levels of serum ionized magnesium are found in patients early after stroke which result in rapid elevation in cytosolic free calcium and spasm in cerebral vascular muscle cells. Neurosci Lett, **230**, 37–40.

Amighi, J., Sabeti, S., Schlager, O., et al. 2004. Low serum magnesium predicts neurological events in patients with advanced atherosclerosis. Stroke, **35**, 22–7.

Bauermeister, D. E., Jennings, E. R., Cruse, D. R., and Sedgwick, V. D. 1967. Hypercalcemia with seizures, a clinical paradox. JAMA, **201**, 146–8.

Blaustein, M. P. 1988. Calcium transport and buffering in neurons. Trends Neurosci, **11**, 438–43.

Bostrom, H., and Alveryd, A. 1972. Stroke in hyperparathyroidism. Acta Med Scand, **192**, 299–308.

Choi, D. 1995. Calcium: still center-stage in hypoxic–ischemic neuronal death. Trends Neurosci, **18**, 58–60.

Collignon, F. P., Friedman, J. A., Piepgras, D. G., et al. 2004. Serum magnesium levels as related to symptomatic vasospasm and outcome following aneurysmal subarachnoid hemorrhage. Neurocrit Care, **1**, 441–8.

Ducros, A., Denier, C., Joutel, A., et al. 2001. The clinical spectrum of familial hemiplegic migraine associated with mutations in a neuronal calcium channel. N Engl J Med, **345**, 17–24.

Feigin, V. L., Rinkel, G. J., Algra, A., et al. 1998. Calcium antagonists in patients with subarachnoid hemorrhage: a systemic review. Neurology, **50**, 876–83.

Findlay, J. M., Macdonald, R. L., and Weir, B. K. 1991. Current concepts of pathophysiology and management of cerebral vasospasm following aneurysmal subarachnoid hemorrhage. Cerebrovasc Brain Metab Rev, **3**, 336–61.

Goadsby, P. G., Lipton, R. B., and Ferrari, M. D. 2002. Migraine – current understanding and treatment. N Engl J Med, **364**, 257–70.

Goldstein, L. B. 2004. Neuroprotective therapy for acute ischaemic stroke: down, but not out. Lancet, **363**, 414–5.

Gorelick, P. B. 2000. Neuroprotection in acute ischemic stroke: a tale of for whom the bell tolls? Lancet, **355**, 1925–6.

Gorelick, P. B., and Caplan, L. R. 1985. Calcium, hypercalcemia, and stroke. Current concepts of cerebrovascular disease. Stroke, **20**, 13–7.

Gorelick, P. B., and Ruland, S. 2004. IMAGES and FAST-MAG: magnesium for acute ischemic stroke. Lancet Neurol, **3**, 330.

Guyton, A. C. 1986. Textbook of Medical Physiology, 7th edn. W. B. Saunders Company.

Haley, E. C., Kassell, N. F., Torner, J. C., et al. 1994a. A randomized controlled trial of high-dose intravenous nicardipine in aneurysmal subarachnoid hemorrhage: a report of the Cooperative Aneurysm Study. J Neurosurg, **78**, 537–47.

Haley, E. C., Kassell, N. F., and Torner, J. C. 1994b. A randomized trial of nicardipine in subarachnoid hemorrhage: angiographic and transcranial Doppler results. A report of the Cooperative Aneurysm Study. J Neurosurg, **78**, 548–53.

Helpern, J. A., Vande Linde, A. M., Welch, K. M., et al. 1993. Acute elevation and recovery of intracellular [Mg2+] following human focal cerebral ischemia. Neurology, **43**, 1577–81.

Herishanu, U., Abramsky, O., and Lavy, S. 1970. Focal neurological manifestation in hypercalcemia. Eur Neurol, **4**, 283–8.

Horn, J., and Limburg, M. 2001. Calcium antagonists for ischemic stroke: a systematic review. *Stroke*, **32**, 570–6.

Huang, Q. F., Gebrewold, A., Altura, B. T., *et al.* 1990. Cocaine-induced cerebral vascular damage can be ameliorated by Mg2+ in rat brains. *Neurosci Lett*, **109**, 113–6.

Intravenous Magnesium Efficacy in Stroke (IMAGES) Study Investigators. 2004. Magnesium for acute stroke (intravenous magnesium in stroke trial: randomized controlled trial). *Lancet*, **363**, 439–45.

Iso, H., Stampfer, M. J., Manson, J. E., *et al.* 1999. Prospective study of calcium, potassium and magnesium intake and the risk of stroke in women. *Stroke*, **30**, 1772–9.

Katsamakis, G., Lukovits, T. G., and Gorelick, P. G. 1998. Calcific cerebral embolism in systemic calciphylaxis. *Neurology*, **51**, 295–7.

Lee, J.-M., Zipfel, G. J., and Choi, D. W. 1999. The changing landscape of ischemic brain injury mechanisms. *Nature*, **399(6738 Suppl)**, A7–14.

Miller, R. J. 1991. The control of neuronal Ca homeostasis. *Prog Neurobiol*, **37**, 255–85.

Mohr, J. P., Orgogozo, J. M., Harrison, M. J., *et al.* 1994. Meta-analysis of oral nimodipine trials in acute ischemic stroke. *Cerebrovasc Dis*, **4**, 197–203.

Moskowitz, M. A., Bolay, H., and Dalkara, T. 2004. Deciphering migraine mechanisms: clues from familial hemiplegic migraine genotypes. *Ann Neurol*, **55**, 276–80.

Muir, K. W. 2000. Therapeutic potential of magnesium in the treatment of acute stroke. *J Stroke Cerebrovasc Dis*, **9**, 257–67.

Orrenius, S., Burkitt, M. J., Kass, G. E. N., Dypbukt, J. M., and Nicotera, P. 1992. Calcium ions and oxidative cell injury. *Ann Neurol*, **32**, S33–42.

Ram, Z., Sadeh, M., Shacked, I., *et al.* 1991. Magnesium sulfate reverses experimental delayed cerebral vasospasm after subarachnoid hemorrhage in rats. *Stroke*, **22**, 922–7.

Rinkel, G. J. E., Feigin, V. L., Algra, A., *et al.* 2005. Calcium antagonists in aneurysmal subarachnoid hemorrhage. *Stroke*, **36**, 1816–7.

Sato, Y., Kaji, M., Metoki, N., *et al.* 2003. Does compensatory hyperparathyroidism predispose to ischemic stroke? *Neurology*, **60**, 626–9.

Saver, J. L., Kidwell C., Eckstein M., *et al.* 2004. Prehospital neuroprotective therapy for acute stroke: results of the Field Administration of Stroke Therapy-Magnesium (FAST-MAG) pilot trial. *Stroke*, **35**, 106–8.

Shanmugan, V., Chhablani, R., and Gorelick, P. B. 1997. Spontaneous calcific cerebral embolus. *Neurology*, **48**, 538–9.

Shibuya, M., Suzuki, Y., Takayasu, M., *et al.* 1992. Effect of AT877 on cerebral vasospasm after aneurysmal subarachnoid hemorrhage. Results of a prospective placebo-controlled double-blind trial. *J Neurosurg*, **76**, 571–7.

Siesjo, B. 1991. The role of calcium in cell death. In *Neurodegenerative Disorders: Mechanisms and Prospects for Therapy*, eds. D. Price, A. Aguayo, and H. Thoenen. Chichester, UK: Wiley, pp. 35–59.

Siesjo, B. K., and Bengtson, F. 1989. Calcium fluxes, calcium antagonists, and calcium related pathology in brain ischemia, hypoglycemia and spreading depression: a unifying hypothesis. *J Cereb Blood Flow Metab*, **9**, 127–40.

Silberstein, S. D. 2004. Migraine. *Lancet*, **363**, 381–91.

Sloan, M. A. 1995. Cerebral vasoconstriction: physiology, pathophysiology and occurrence in selected cerebrovascular disorders. In *Brain Ischemia: Basic Concepts and Their Clinical Relevance (Clinical Medicine and the Nervous System Series)*, ed. L. R. Caplan. London: Springer-Verlag, pp. 151–72.

Sloan, M. A., Kittner, S. J., and Price, T. R. 1998. Stroke and illicit drug use. In *Cerebrovascular Disease: Pathophysiology, Diagnosis and Management, Volume II*, eds. M. D. Ginsburg, J. Bogousslavsky. Cambridge, UK: Blackwell Science, Inc., pp. 1589–609.

Streeto, J. M. 1969. Acute hypercalcemia simulating basilar artery insufficiency. *N Engl J Med*, **280**, 427–9.

Tymianski, M. 1996. Cytosolic calcium concentrations and cell death in vitro. *Adv Neurol*, **71**, 85–105.

van den Bergh, W. M., Algra, A., van der Sprenkel, J. W. B., *et al.* 2003. Hypomagnesemia after aneurysmal subarachnoid hemorrhage. *Neurosurgery*, **52**, 276–82.

van den Bergh, W. M., on behalf of the MASH Study Group. 2005. Magnesium sulfate in aneurysmal subarachnoid hemorrhage: a randomized controlled trial. *Stroke*, **36**, 1011–5.

Walker, G. L., Williamson, P. M., Ravich, R. M. B., and Roche, J. 1980. Hypercalcemia associated with cerebral vasospasm causing infarction. *J Neurol Neurosurg Psychiatry*, **43**, 464–7.

Wong, G. K. C., Chan, M. T. V., Boet, M., Poon, W. S., and Gin, T. 2006. Intravenous magnesium sulfate after aneurysmal subarachnoid hemorrhage: a prospective randomized pilot study. *J Neurosurg Anesthesiol*, **18**, 142–8.

Yarnell, P., and Caplan, L. R. 1986. Basilar artery narrowing and hyperparathyroidism: illustrative case. *Stroke*, **17**, 1022–4.

49

STROKE AND SUBSTANCE ABUSE

John C. M. Brust

The term "substance abuse" refers to the nonmedical use of an agent in a manner perceived as harmful. The use may or may not produce psychological dependence (addiction) or physical dependence (resulting in physical symptoms and signs upon withdrawal), and the agent may be either illicit or legally available. When alcohol and tobacco are included, countless people worldwide are substance abusers, and many of them are at increased risk for ischemic or hemorrhagic stroke (Brust, 2004a,b).

Opiates

Opiate drugs include a large number of agonists (e.g. morphine), antagonists (e.g. naloxone), and mixed agonist/antagonists (e.g. pentazocine). The most widely abused opiate is the agonist heroin, which is injected intravenously or subcutaneously or, especially since the AIDS epidemic, sniffed or smoked. Among parenteral users infectious endocarditis is a major risk, especially with *Staphylococcus aureus* and *Candida*, and brain emboli are common. Strokes can be ischemic or hemorrhagic, the latter caused by rupture of either a septic "mycotic" aneurysm or nonaneurysmal infectious vasculitis. Unlike saccular "berry" aneurysms, septic aneurysmal rupture is often preceded by insidiously progressive neurological or systemic symptoms. Septic aneurysms may or may not disappear during appropriate antimicrobial therapy, and they can rupture during or following such treatment. It has been recommended, therefore, that septic aneurysms be angiographically sought in patients with endocarditis and suspicious neurological symptoms and that surgically accessible aneurysms be excised (Brust *et al.*, 1990).

Hemorrhagic stroke in heroin users may be a consequence of hepatitis with liver failure and deranged clotting or of heroin nephropathy with uremia or malignant hypertension. Ischemic stroke may be a complication of meningitis or AIDS (Brust, 1997a).

A number of reports describe ischemic stroke in young heroin users without evidence of endocarditis, additional drug use, or other risk factors (Brust and Richter, 1976). In some patients, cerebral infarction was associated with loss of consciousness after intravenous injection of heroin. In others, ischemic stroke occurred in active users but did not follow overdose or a recent injection. Angiography in some users suggested either large- or small-vessel arteritis (unconfirmed pathologically). Suggestive of hypersensitivity were eosinophilia, hypergammaglobulinemia, a positive direct Coombs test, and a positive latex fixation test. In one patient, hemiparesis was preceded by symptoms suggesting anaphylaxis (Woods and Strewler, 1972). Ischemic stroke has also followed heroin sniffing (Bartolomei *et al.*, 1992). A young woman had an intracerebral hemorrhage within minutes of intravenous heroin use (Knoblauch *et al.*, 1983).

Stroke in heroin users could have a number of different mechanisms. Overdose causes hypoventilation and hypotension, and bilateral globus pallidus infarction is often found at autopsies of heroin users. Direct toxic injury from heroin or an adulterant is another possibility. A variety of pharmacologically active and inactive ingredients find their way into heroin preparations (Caplan *et al.*, 1982a).

Embolization of foreign material has not been documented in heroin users but is well recognized in users of other agents, including opiates. During the 1970s, mixtures of pentazocine (Talwin) and tripelennamine (Pyribenzamine) – so-called "Ts and Blues" – became a popular form of drug abuse in the American Midwest. Oral tablets were crushed, suspended in water, and injected intravenously. Brain infarcts and hemorrhages were a frequent complication, and autopsies revealed talc and cellulose crystals in both pulmonary and brain arterioles. Cerebral angiography often showed arterial "beading," consistent with either multiple emboli or a vasoconstrictive or vasculitic reaction to the foreign material (Caplan *et al.*, 1982b).

Foreign body embolism was also suspected in cases of ischemic stroke associated with parenteral use of paregoric, oral meperidine, and hydromorphone (Dilaudid) suppository (Brust, 2004b).

Heroin myelopathy is probably ischemic in some cases. Several reports describe acute paraparesis, sensory loss, and urinary retention, occurring shortly after injection (and in one case sniffing) and often following a period of abstinence (McCreary *et al.*, 2000). Symptoms were sometimes present on awakening from coma, suggesting hypotension and border-zone infarction. In some patients, proprioception and vibratory sensation were spared, suggesting infarction in the territory of the anterior spinal artery (Pearson *et al.*, 1972). In one case, small-vessel arteritis was found histologically (Judice *et al.*, 1978).

Amphetamine and related agents

Amphetamine-like psychostimulants include dextroamphetamines, methamphetamines, methylphenidate (Ritalin), ephedrine, pseudoephedrine, phenylpropanolamine (PPA), and a large number of other agents marketed as decongestants or appetite suppressants. Ischemic or hemorrhagic stroke is a well-recognized complication of these drugs.

Uncommon Causes of Stroke, 2nd edition, ed. Louis R. Caplan. Published by Cambridge University Press. © Cambridge University Press 2008.

Dextroamphetamines and methamphetamine are taken orally, injected, sniffed, or smoked in a crystalline form ("ice," "crystal meth"). Strokes common to any parenteral drug use are encountered. Amphetamine overdose causes delirium, hypertension, malignant hyperthermia, vascular collapse, and death, and at autopsy there are cerebral edema and petechiae. Gross intracranial hemorrhage, however, has more often been associated with amphetamine use in the absence of other signs of overdose.

More than 50 such patients have been reported. Routes of administration were intravenous, oral, or by inhalation (Brust, 2004b). Most involved dextroamphetamines or methamphetamines, but single patients used pseudoephedrine or diethylpropion. Chronic use predominated. Severe headache usually occurred within minutes of drug use, and in most patients, blood pressure was elevated. CT showed either intracerebral or subarachnoid hemorrhage. In several patients, cerebral angiographic 'beading' was present, and cerebral vasculitic changes were occasionally found at autopsy. Some of these strokes were therefore probably secondary to acute hypertension, some to acute vasculitis, and some to both.

Amphetamine-induced cerebral vasculitis has also caused ischemic stroke. In one report, 14 polydrug abusers – all but two of whom used intravenous methamphetamines – developed a necrotizing arteritis that resembled polyarteritis nodosa, with systemic symptoms and signs and, in some, infarction or hemorrhage affecting the cerebrum, cerebellum, or brainstem (Citron et al., 1970). Such brain lesions have been found pathologically in other amphetamine and methamphetamine abusers (Bostwick, 1981; Brust, 2004a). In some reports, however, vasculitis was presumed on the basis of angiographic "beading," which could have other causes, including multiple emboli, vasospasm, and subarachnoid hemorrhage (Rothrock et al., 1988; Rumbaugh et al., 1971).

These reports are anecdotal. Epidemiological evidence for an association of amphetamine/methamphetamine with stroke is limited to a population-based case-control study of young women, in which the drugs were a risk factor for combined hemorrhagic and ischemic stroke (odds ratio 3.8) (Petitti et al., 1998).

Experimental studies with monkeys and rats confirmed that cerebral vasculitis – often involving vessels smaller than those affected by polyarteritis nodosa – can follow either single or repeated intravenous administration of either methamphetamine or methylphenidate (Rumbaugh et al., 1976). It is unclear if such lesions are the result of direct toxicity or hypersensitivity.

Numerous case reports described ischemic and hemorrhagic stroke in users of the decongestant and appetite suppressant PPA (Lake et al., 1990). A case-control study found that appetite suppressants containing PPA significantly increased the risk of hemorrhagic stroke in women (no men in the study used PPA-containing diet pills) and that there was a trend toward increased risk of hemorrhagic stroke in both women and men using PPA-containing decongestants (Kernan et al., 2000). Following this report, the U.S. Food and Drug Administration (FDA) ordered products containing PPA to be withdrawn from the market.

Anecdotally associated with ischemic or hemorrhagic stroke are the decongestants ephedrine and pseudoephedrine and the appetite suppressants phentermine, phendimetrazine, diethylpropion, and fenfluramine (Bruno et al., 1993; Derby et al., 1999; Harrington et al., 1983; Loizou et al., 1982). Fenfluramine and dexfenfluramine were removed from the market following reports of valvular heart disease in users (Jick et al., 1998).

"Food supplements" containing ephedra (Ma Huang) were banned by the FDA following a case-control study that found a trend toward an association of these products with hemorrhagic stroke (Morganstern et al., 2003).

MDMA (3,4-methylenedioxymethamphetamine, "ecstasy"), a drug with both psychostimulatory and hallucinogenic properties, became increasingly popular during the 1980s, especially on college campuses. Both ischemic and hemorrhagic strokes are described in users (Auer et al., 2002; Reneman et al., 2000; Schifano et al., 2003). Microembolization of talc to brain and retina was reported following intravenous (and inadvertent carotid artery) injection of crushed methylphenidate tablets (Chillar and Jackson, 1981; Mizutami et al., 1980).

Cocaine

Although cocaine's psychostimulatory effects are similar to those of amphetamine, its mode of action is different. Unlike amphetamine, cocaine blocks reuptake of monoamine neurotransmitters at synaptic nerve endings by binding to specific transporter proteins. Also unlike amphetamine, cocaine is a local anesthetic. Whether these different pharmacological properties confer different degrees of risk or different pathophysiological mechanisms for stroke is unclear.

The first report of stroke associated with cocaine use described cerebral infarction following intramuscular use (Brust and Richter, 1977). A handful of reports then described both ischemic and hemorrhagic stroke in intranasal users of cocaine hydrochloride. During the 1980s, cocaine production shifted to smokable alkaloidal "crack," which unlike cocaine hydrochloride can be administered in huge doses continuously over hours or even days. The resulting epidemic of use was accompanied by an upsurge in reports of cocaine-related stroke (Brust, 2004a,b; Kaku and Lowenstein, 1990; Levine et al., 1990, 1991). By 2003, more than 600 cases had been described, about half ischemic and half hemorrhagic.

Reports of brain ischemia include transient ischemic attacks (TIAs) and infarction of cerebrum, thalamus, brainstem, spinal cord, and retina. Infarction has occurred in pregnant women and in neonates whose mothers used cocaine shortly before delivery. As with amphetamine, cerebral vasculitis has sometimes been inferred on the basis of angiographic changes. In only five cases, however, was cerebral vasculitis confirmed pathologically, and in each case it was slight; most autopsies have shown histologically normal cerebral vessels, including cases with angiographic "beading."

Hemorrhagic strokes have been both intracerebral and subarachnoid, and of those patients receiving angiography, nearly half had vascular malformations or saccular aneurysms. Cocaine increases the likelihood of vasospasm after aneurysm rupture (Conway and Tamargo, 2001). Other hemorrhages include bleeding into embolic infarction or glioma. Intracerebral hemorrhages have occurred in postpartem women and their offspring.

Two case-control studies did not find any association between crack cocaine use and stroke. In one, information regarding acute crack use was missing in more than half the subjects and controls, and nearly half of the controls with information available had used crack (Qureshi *et al.*, 1997). In the other study the diagnosis of stroke was based on physician report, and "lifetime cocaine use" was based on patient report (Qureshi *et al.*, 2001). Two other case-control studies found that cocaine was a strong risk factor for stroke. One involved hemorrhagic and ischemic stroke in women aged 15–44 years (odds ratio 13:9) (Petitti *et al.*, 1998). The other involved aneurysmal subarachnoid hemorrhage in men and women aged 18–49 years (odds ratio 24:97) (Broderick *et al.*, 2003).

Cocaine causes vasoconstriction by blocking reuptake of norepinephrine at sympathetic nerve endings. Pharmacologically active metabolites perhaps account for ischemic strokes that occur hours or even days after cocaine use (Herning *et al.*, 1999). Coronary artery constriction causes myocardial infarction and with it the risk of cardioembolic stroke. (Cocaine also causes a cardiomyopathy probably independent of coronary artery constriction [Chokshi *et al.*, 1989].) Systemic artery constriction causes acute hypertension, predisposing to rupture of underlying vascular malformations or aneurysms. Cerebral artery constriction – a property verified angiographically in human volunteers (Kaufman *et al.*, 1998) – causes cerebral ischemia. Infarcts are sometimes multiple and carry a high risk of hemorrhagic transformation if cerebral vasoconstriction clears while systemic hypertension is still present (Green *et al.*, 1990). Animal studies, however, reveal greater complexity; cerebral vasodilatation as well as vasoconstriction occurs, depending on species and whether the drug is administered intravenously or applied topically (Diaz-Tejedor *et al.*, 1992).

In vitro studies have described both aggregation and deaggregation of platelets by cocaine (Jennings *et al.*, 1993). Other cocaine effects involve protein C, antithrombin III, nuclear factor-κB, activator protein-1, and von Willebrand factor. Synergism between cocaine and ethanol is also recognized; in the presence of ethanol, cocaine is metabolized to cocaethylene, which binds more powerfully than cocaine itself to monoamine transporter proteins (Brust, 2004a).

Relevant to cocaine and cerebrovascular disease are controversies over whether chronic cocaine use has long-term adverse effects on cognition, to what degree in utero exposure to cocaine affects psychomotor development, and whether such effects are vasculopathic rather than directly toxic (Brust, 2004a).

Phencyclidine

Phencyclidine (PCP, "angel dust") can be smoked, eaten, or injected. Low doses produce euphoria; higher doses produce psychosis. PCP's principal action is to block excitatory *N*-methyl-D-aspartate receptors. The basis of its circulatory effects is unclear but might involve specific receptors on blood vessels. Hypertension can appear either early or late during intoxication, and hemorrhagic stroke has either immediately followed use or occurred

after a delay of a few days. Temporally related hypertensive encephalopathy is also described (Boyko *et al.*, 1987; Eastman and Cohen, 1975). Transient monocular blindness occurred within a few hours of smoking phencyclidine (Ubogu, 2001).

LSD

The hallucinogenic drug D-lysergic acid diethylamide (LSD) is an ergot which in high doses causes severe hypertension and in vitro produces spasm of cerebral vessel strips. Ischemic stroke has occurred up to several days after LSD use, with cerebral angiography showing either (i) progressive narrowing and occlusion of the internal carotid artery or (ii) more widespread intracranial arterial "beading" (Sobel *et al.*, 1971).

Marijuana

Reports of ischemic stroke in marijuana users are mostly unconvincing as to causality (Alvaro *et al.*, 2002). Hypotension and cerebral vasospasm have been proposed as mechanisms, but neither has been documented in clinical reports. In humans, marijuana has unpredictable effects on cerebral blood flow (Mathew and Wilson, 1991).

Sedatives

Barbiturates, benzodiazepines, and other sedative drugs can cause cerebral infarction as a result of respiratory depression, hypotension, and decreased cerebral blood flow, but ischemic or hemorrhagic stroke has not otherwise been reported.

Inhalants

Inhaling the intoxicating vapors of household and industrial products is especially common among children. Death results from accidents, violence, suffocation, aspiration, and cardiac arrhythmia. Cerebral infarction occurred in a 12-year-old while sniffing glue containing trichloroethylene (Parker *et al.*, 1984). Aneurysmal rupture occurred during orgasm following amyl nitrite inhalation (Nudelman and Salcman, 1987).

Ethanol

The relationship between ethanol consumption and coronary artery disease follows a "J-shaped curve" – that is, mild-to-moderate drinking decreases risk whereas heavy drinking increases risk (Ahlawat and Siwach, 1994). Heavy drinkers are therefore indirectly at increased risk for cardioembolic stroke as an aftermath of myocardial infarction. Ethanol also directly precipitates cardiac arrhythmia ("holiday heart"), and thromboembolism is a prominent feature of alcoholic cardiomyopathy.

Stroke independent of ethanol's cardiac effects has been extensively studied. Finnish investigators reported a temporal association of heavy drinking and both ischemic and hemorrhagic stroke, but those studies were retrospective and the findings could not be duplicated by others (Gorelick *et al.*, 1989).

The relationship of chronic ethanol use and stroke has been addressed in many case-control and cohort studies. Contradictory findings are the result of differently selected endpoints, e.g. total stroke, ischemic stroke, hemorrhagic stroke, stroke mortality; amount and duration of ethanol consumption; correction for other risk factors, e. g. hypertension and tobacco; ethnicity and socioeconomics of populations being studied; and selection of controls. In 2003, a meta-analysis of 19 cohort studies and 16 case-control studies over a period of two decades revealed that, compared with abstention, consumption of 12–24 g of ethanol per day reduced the risk of ischemic stroke (relative risk 0.72) but not of hemorrhagic stroke. Consumption of more than 60 g/day increased the risk of both ischemic stroke (relative risk: 1.69) and hemorrhagic stroke (relative risk 2.18). Thus, as with myocardial infarction, a J-shaped association exists for ethanol consumption and risk for ischemic stroke, whereas a more linear association exists for ethanol consumption and risk for hemorrhagic stroke (Reynolds *et al.*, 2003).

The Northern Manhattan Stroke Study reported that drinking up to two drinks daily protected against ischemic stroke in whites, Hispanics, and African-Americans; higher doses increased risk. (A "standard drink" was defined as 120 mL of wine, 360 mL of beer, or 45 mL of liquor.) There was no difference in the effect of wine, beer, or liquor (Sacco *et al.*, 1999).

Studies with angiography and ultrasound parallel these clinical observations. Heavy ethanol consumption increases the risk of carotid artery atherosclerosis, whereas low ethanol consumption decreases it (Palomaki *et al.*, 1993).

Multiple mechanisms probably explain the complex association of ethanol and stroke. Ethanol acutely and chronically raises blood pressure (Beilin, 1995). It lowers blood levels of low-density lipoproteins and raises the levels of high-density lipoproteins. Ethanol acutely decreases fibrinolytic activity, increases factor VIII levels, and increases platelet reactivity to adenosine diphosphate. It also decreases plasma fibrinogen levels, increases levels of prostacyclin, decreases platelet function, and stimulates endothelial release of endothelin (Brust, 2004a). Alcoholic liver disease impairs clotting. During withdrawal, hemoconcentration and rebound platelet hyperaggregability occur. Acute ethanol intoxication causes cerebral vasodilatation, yet ethanol in vitro constricted cerebral artery segments, and in rats ethanol constricted cerebral arterioles (Gordon *et al.*, 1995).

Tobacco

Smoking is a major risk factor for coronary artery and peripheral vascular disease. Case-control and cohort studies show that, independent of these effects, tobacco increases the risk for both ischemic and hemorrhagic stroke (Hawkins *et al.*, 2002; Kurth *et al.*, 2003). Smokeless tobacco also carries risk (Asplund *et al.*, 2003). In women, the risk of ischemic and hemorrhagic stroke is greater in those also taking oral contraceptives. As with ethanol, multiple mechanisms probably contribute. Smoking aggravates atherosclerosis and reduces the blood's oxygen-carrying capacity. Nicotine damages endothelium, and acute smoking raises blood pressure. Smoking also increases platelet reactivity, inhibits prostacyclin formation, and raises blood fibrinogen levels. Smoking-induced polycythemia increases blood viscosity (Brust, 2004a).

REFERENCES

Ahlawat, S. K., and Siwach, S. B. 1994. Alcohol and coronary artery disease. *Int J Cardiol*, **44**, 157.

Alvaro, L. C., Iriondo, I., and Villaverde, F. J. 2002. Sexual headache and stroke in a heavy cannabis smoker. *Headache*, **42**, 224.

Asplund, K., Nasic, S., Janlert, V., *et al.* 2003. Smokeless tobacco as a possible risk factor for stroke in men. A nested case-control study. *Stroke*, **34**, 1754.

Auer, J., Berent, R., Weber, T., *et al.* 2002. Subarachnoid hemorrhage with "Ecstasy" abuse in a young adult. *Neurol Sci*, **23**, 199.

Bartolomei, F., Nicoli, F., Swiader, L., and Gastaut, J. L. 1992. Accident vasculaire cerebral ischemique apres prise nasale d'heroine. Une nouvelle observation. *Presse Medécin*, **21**, 983.

Beilin, L. J. 1995. Alcohol and hypertension. *Clin Exp Pharmacol Physiol*, **22**, 185.

Bostwick, D. G. 1981. Amphetamine induced cerebral vasculitis. *Hum Pathol*, **12**, 1031.

Boyko, O. B., Burger, P. C., and Heinz, E. R. 1987. Pathological and radiological correlation of subarachnoid hemorrhage in phencyclidine abuse: case report. *J Neurosurg*, **67**, 446.

Broderick, J. P., Viscoli, C. M., Brott, T., *et al.* 2003. Major risk factors for aneurysmal subarachnoid hemorrhage in the young are modifiable. *Stroke*, **34**, 1375.

Bruno, A., Nolte, K. B., and Chapin, J. 1993. Stroke associated with ephedrine use. *Neurology*, **43**, 1313.

Brust, J. C. M. 1997a. AIDS and stroke. In *Cerebrovascular Disease. A Primer*, K. M. A. Welch, L. R. Caplan, D. J. Reis, B. K. Siesjo, and B. Weir (eds.), San Diego: Academic Press, pp. 423–5.

Brust, J. C. M. 2004a. *Neurological Aspects of Substance Abuse*, 2nd edn. Boston: Butterworth-Heinemann.

Brust, J. C. M. 2004b. Stroke and substance abuse. In *Stroke: Pathophysiology, Diagnosis, and Treatment*, 4th edn, J. P. Mohr, D. W. Choi, J. C. Grotta, B. Weier, and P. A. Wolf (eds.), Philadelphia: Churchill Livingstone, pp. 725–46.

Brust, J. C. M., Dickinson, P. C. T., Hughes, J. E. O., and Holtzman, R. N. N. 1990. The diagnosis and treatment of cerebral mycotic aneurysms. *Ann Neurol*, **27**, 238.

Brust, J. C. M., and Richter, R. W. 1976. Stroke associated with addiction to heroin. *J Neurol Neurosurg Psychiatry*, **39**, 194.

Brust, J. C. M., and Richter, R. W. 1977. Stroke associated with cocaine abuse? *N Y State J Med*, **77**, 1473.

Caplan, L. R., Hier, D. B., and Banks, G. 1982a. Stroke and drug abuse. *Stroke*, **13**, 869.

Caplan, L. R., Thomas, C., and Banks, G. 1982b. Central nervous system complications of addiction to 'Ts and Blues.' *Neurology*, **32**, 623.

Chillar, R. K., and Jackson, A. L. 1981. Reversible hemiplegia after presumed intracarotid injection of Ritalin. *N Engl J Med*, **304**, 1305.

Chokshi, S. K., Moore, R., Pandian, N. G., and Isner, J. M. 1989. Reversible cardiomyopathy associated with cocaine intoxication. *Ann Intern Med*, **111**, 1039.

Citron, B. P., Halpern, M., McCarron, M., *et al.* 1970. Necrotizing angiitis associated with drug abuse. *N Engl J Med*, **283**, 1003.

Conway, J. E., and Tamargo, R. J. 2001. Cocaine use is an independent risk factor for cerebral vasospasm after aneurysmal subarachnoid hemorrhage. *Stroke*, **32**, 2338.

Derby, L. E., Myers, M. W., Jick, H., *et al.* 1999. Use of dexfenfluramine, fenfluramine and phentermine and the risk of stroke. *Br J Clin Pharmacol*, **47**, 565.

Diaz-Tejedor, E., Tejada, J., and Munoz, J. 1992. Cerebral arterial changes following cocaine IV administration: an angiographic study in rabbits. *J Neurol*, **239(Suppl. 2)**, 538.

Eastman, J. W., and Cohen, S. N. 1975. Hypertensive crisis and death associated with phencyclidine poisoning. *JAMA*, **231**, 1270.

Gordon, E. L., Nguyen, T. S., Ngai, A. C., and Winn, H. R. 1995. Differential effects of alcohols on intracerebral arterioles. Ethanol alone causes vasoconstriction. *J Cereb Blood Flow Metab*, **15**, 532.

Gorelick, P. B., Rodin, M. B., Langenberg, P. *et al.* 1989. Weekly alcohol consumption, cigarette smoking, and the risk of ischemic stroke: results of a case-control study at three urban medical centers in Chicago, Illinois. *Neurology*, **39**, 339.

Green, R., Kelly, K. M., Gabrielsen, T., *et al.* 1990. Multiple cerebral hemorrhages after smoking 'crack' cocaine. *Stroke*, **21**, 957.

Harrington, H., Heller, H. A., Dawson, D., *et al.* 1983. Intracerebral hemorrhage and oral amphetamine. *Arch Neurol*, **40**, 503.

Hawkins, B. T., Brown, R. C., and David, T. P. 2002. Smoking and ischemic stroke: a role for nicotine? *Trends Pharmacol Sci*, **23**, 8.

Herning, R. I., King, D. E., Better, W. C., and Cadet, J. L. 1999. Neurovascular deficits in cocaine users. *Neuropharmacology*, **21**, 110.

Jennings, L. K., White, M. M., Saver, C. M., *et al.* 1993. Cocaine induced platelet defects. *Stroke*, **24**, 1352.

Jick, H., Vasilakis, C., Weinrauch, L. A., *et al.* 1998. A population-based study of appetite-suppressant drugs and the risk of cardiac valve regurgitation. *N Engl J Med*, **339**, 719.

Judice, D. J., LeBlanc, H. J., and McGarry, P. A. 1978. Spinal cord vasculitis presenting as spinal cord tumor in a heroin addict. *J Neurosurg*, **48**, 131.

Kaku, D. A., and Lowenstein, D. H. 1990. Emergence of recreational drug abuse as a major risk factor for stroke in young adults. *Ann Intern Med*, **113**, 821.

Kaufman, M. J., Levin, J. M., Ross, M. H., *et al.* 1998. Cocaine-induced cerebral vasoconstriction detected in humans with magnetic resonance angiography. *JAMA*, **279**, 376.

Kernan, W. N., Viscoli, C. M., Brass, L. M., *et al.* 2000. Phenylpropanolamine and the risk of hemorrhagic stroke. *N Engl J Med*, **343**, 1826.

Knoblauch, A. L., Buchholz, M., Koller, M. G., and Kistler, H. 1983. Hemiplegie nach injektion von heroin. *Schweiz Medische Wochenschrift*, **113**, 402.

Kurth, T., Kase, C. S., Berger, K., *et al.* 2003. Smoking and the risk of hemorrhagic stroke in men. *Stroke*, **34**, 1151, 2792.

Lake, C. R., Gallant, S., Masson, E., and Miller, P. 1990. Adverse drug effects attributed to phenylpropanolamine: a review of 142 case reports. *Am J Med*, **89**, 195.

Levine, S. R., Brust, J. C. M., Futrell, N., *et al.* 1990. Cerebrovascular complications of the use of the 'crack' form of alkaloidal cocaine. *N Engl J Med*, **323**, 699.

Levine, S. R., Brust, J. C. M., Futrell, N., *et al.* 1991. A comparative study of the cerebrovascular complications of cocaine: alkaloidal versus hydrochloride – a review. *Neurology*, **41**, 1173.

Loizou, L. A., Hamilton, J. G., and Tsementzis, S. A. 1982. Intracranial hemorrhage in association with pseudoephedrine overdose. *J Neurol Neurosurg Psychiatry*, **45**, 471.

Mathew, R. J., and Wilson, W. H. 1991. Substance abuse and cerebral blood flow. *Am J Psychiatry*, **148**, 292.

McCreary, M., Emerman, C., Hanna, J., and Simon, J. 2000. Acute myelopathy following intranasal insufflation of heroin: case report. *Neurology*, **55**, 316.

Mizutami, T., Lewis, R., and Gonatas, N. 1980. Medial medullary syndrome in a drug abuser. *Arch Neurol*, **37**, 425.

Morganstern, M. D., Viscoli, C. M., Kernan, W. N., *et al.* 2003. Use of ephedra-containing products and risk for hemorrhagic stroke. *Neurology*, **60**, 132.

Nudelman, R. W., and Salcman, M. 1987. The birth of the blues. II. Blue movie. *JAMA*, **257**, 3230.

Palomaki, H., Kaste, M., Raininko, R. *et al.* 1993. Risk factors for cervical atherosclerosis in patients with transient ischemic attack or minor ischemic stroke. *Stroke*, **24**, 970.

Parker, M. J., Tarlow, M. J., and Milne-Anderson, J. 1984. Glue sniffing and cerebral infarction. *Arch Dis Child*, **59**, 675.

Pearson, J., Richter, R. W., Baden, M. M. *et al.* 1972. Transverse myelopathy as an illustration of the neurologic and neuropathologic features of heroin addiction. *Hum Pathol*, **3**, 109.

Petitti, D. B., Sidney S., Queensberry, C., and Bernstein, A. 1998. Stroke and cocaine or amphetamine use. *Epidemiology*, **9**, 596.

Qureshi, A. L., Akber, M. S., Czander, E. *et al.* 1997. Crack cocaine use and stroke in young patients. *Neurology*, **48**, 341.

Qureshi, A. L., Fareed, M., Suri, K., *et al.* 2001. Cocaine use and the likelihood of non-fatal myocardial infarction and stroke: data from the third National Health and Nutrition Examination Survey. *Circulation*, **103**, 502.

Reneman, L., Habraken, J. B., Majoie, C. B., *et al.* 2000. MDMA ("Ecstasy") and its association with cerebrovascular accidents: preliminary findings. *Am J Neuroradiol*, **21**, 1001.

Reynolds, K., Lewis, L. B., and Nolen, J. D. L. 2003. Alcohol consumption and risk of stroke. A meta-analysis. *JAMA*, **289**, 579.

Rothrock, J. F., Rubenstein, R., and Lyden, P. D. 1988. Ischemic stroke associated with methamphetamine inhalation. *Neurology*, **38**, 589.

Rumbaugh, C. L., Bergeron, R. T., Fang, H. C. H., and McCormick, R. 1971. Cerebral angiographic changes in the drug abuse patient. *Radiology*, **101**, 335.

Rumbaugh, C. L., Fang, H. C. H., Higgins, R. E., *et al.* 1976. Cerebral microvascular injury in experimental drug abuse. *Invest Radiol*, **11**, 282.

Sacco, R. L., Elkind, M., Boden-Albala, B., *et al.* 1999. The protective effect of moderate alcohol consumption on ischemic stroke. *JAMA*, **281**, 53.

Schifano, F., Oyefeso, A., Webb, L., *et al.* 2003. Review of deaths related to taking ecstasy, England and Wales, 1997–2000. *Br Med J*, **326**, 80.

Sobel, J., Espinas, O. E., and Friedman, S. A. 1971. Carotid artery obstruction following LSD capsule injection. *Arch Intern Med*, **127**, 290.

Ubogu, E. E. 2001. Amaurosis fugax associated with phencyclidine inhalation. *Eur Neurol*, **46**, 98.

Woods, B. T., and Strewler, G. J. 1972. Hemiparesis occurring six hours after intravenous heroin injection. *Neurology*, **22**, 863.

50

CANCER AND PARANEOPLASTIC STROKES

Rogelio Leira, Antonio Dávalos, and José Castillo

Introduction

Paraneoplastic syndromes are a variety of disorders that accompany the clinical evolution of tumors that are not produced directly by the primary neoplasm, by its metastasis, or as a result of diagnostic or therapeutic procedures. These syndromes may evolve in parallel with the development of the tumor, but may also be independent of it and even precede the initial diagnosis of neoplasm. Paraneoplastic syndromes are detected in about 7%–10% of patients at the time the tumor is diagnosed, although almost all patients with a malignant tumor develop a paraneoplastic syndrome during the course of its evolution (Nathanson and Hall, 1997).

Paraneoplastic syndromes can affect any part of the central nervous system (CNS). Occasionally, paraneoplastic syndromes arise from causal lesions in the CNS or peripheral nervous system, but neurological manifestations are more commonly due to lesions in organs outside of the CNS. The classic paraneoplastic neurological syndromes fall into the first group, whereas in the second group, the neurological manifestations are the result of blood vessel changes, blood-forming elements, hemostasis and coagulation disorders, metabolic changes, and infections (Table 50.1). Cerebrovascular paraneoplastic manifestations are included in the second group of neurological paraneoplastic syndromes.

Frequency

The association between neoplasm and atherothrombotic disease is recognized from the first clinical observations of Trosseau from more than 100 years ago (Rickles and Edwards, 1983). Cerebrovascular disease is the second most common cause of CNS disease found at autopsy of patients with cancer, and must be considered in any patient who has cerebral symptoms. Fifteen percent of patients with cancer present cerebrovascular disorders related to neoplastic disease, and half of these patients have clinical symptoms before dying. In some patients, the cerebrovascular manifestations are due to the tumor itself, its metastases, or to complications resulting from the diagnostic procedures or from treatment. However, in most cases, the paraneoplastic origin is the most common cause of strokes (Graus et al., 1985; Patchell and Posner, 1985).

Etiopathology

In all primary neurological paraneoplastic syndromes, the pathogenesis is autoimmune. Proteins normally expressed only in the CNS are expressed ectopically by the tumor. However, the immune system does not recognize these proteins as its own and produces antibodies against the proteins that destroy antigenically vulnerable neurons (Dalmau and Posner, 1997).

In the secondary neurological paraneoplastic syndromes, which are responsible for most cerebrovascular diseases that appear in patients with cancer, the pathogenesis has been linked to autoimmunity or to the release of procoagulant substances by the tumor. Some of them are associated with intracerebral hemorrhages, others with cerebral infarcts, and others with both (Table 50.2).

Microangiopathic hemolytic anemia, thrombocytopenia, von Willebrand's disease, antiphospholipid syndrome, and vasculitis all fall within the first group of etiopathological mechanisms. Microangiopathic hemolytic anemia, usually accompanied by thrombocytopenia, is an autoimmune disease that is sometimes associated with mucinous adenocarcinomas most often of the stomach, breast, and lung (Staszewski, 1997).

Thrombocytopenia of paraneoplastic origin may also be because of autoimmune thrombocytopenia accompanying chronic lymphocytic leukemia, B-cell lymphomas, and less commonly, in some solid tumors (lung and rectum), it may be because of thrombotic thrombocytopenic purpura (Steingart, 1988). In these cases, deposits of fibrin and platelet aggregates are found within the brain's microcirculation. These give rise to microinfarcts and subdural and intracerebral hemorrhages. An acquired form of von Willebrand's disease has been reported as a paraneoplastic manifestation in patients with lymphoproliferative and myeloproliferative neoplasms and with systemic hemorrhages (Mohri et al., 1987).

The association of high levels of anti-phospholipid antibodies with arterial and venous thrombosis is called the antiphospholipid syndrome, which may be primary or associated with other diseases such as neoplasms (Harris et al., 1985; McNeil et al., 1991). Even though the link between the presence of anti-phospholipid antibodies and thrombotic phenomena has clearly been established, we still do not know what the pathogenic mechanism is. One of the most widely accepted theories is based on the possible effects of the binding of anti-phospholipid antibodies with phospholipids that make up the cellular membranes of the endothelium and platelets. The inhibiting effect of I32-glycoprotein I on blood coagulation and platelet aggregation would be neutralized by antiphospholipid antibodies (Khamashta et al., 1990). Antiphospholipid syndrome might cause occlusion of the intracerebral arteries and of the large intracranial venous sinuses (Coull et al., 1992; Russell and Enevoldson, 1993).

Uncommon Causes of Stroke, 2nd edition, ed. Louis R. Caplan. Published by Cambridge University Press. © Cambridge University Press 2008.

Table 50.1 Classification of neurological paraneoplastic syndromes

Primary neurological paraneoplastic syndromes
Disorders of the brain and cranial nerves
Encephalomyelitis
Subacute cerebellar degeneration
Opsoclonus/myoclonus syndrome
Limbic encephalitis and other dementias
Brainstem encephalitis
Optic neuritis
Cancer-associated retinopathy
Disorders of the spinal cord
Necrotizing myelopathy
Subacute motor neuropathy
Stiff person (man) syndrome
Disorders of the peripheral nerve
Sensorimotor polyneuropathy
Subacute sensory neuronopathy
Guillain-Barré syndrome
Autonomic neuropathy
Disorders of the neuromuscular union
Lambert-Eaton myasthenic syndrome
Myasthenia gravis
Muscle disorders
Dermatomyositis, polymyositis
Carcinoid myopathies
Myotonia
Cachectic myopathy

Secondary neurological paraneoplastic syndromes
Disorder of the vessels
Vasculitis
Disorders of blood-forming elements
Thrombocytopenia
Thrombocytosis
Hemostasia and coagulation disorders
Disseminated intravascular coagulation
Nonbacterial thrombotic endocarditis
Acquired von Willebrand's disease
Hyperviscosity syndrome
Metabolic changes
Infections

Table 50.2 Etiopathology of paraneoplastic strokes

Intracerebral hemorrhage
Mediated by autoimmune mechanism
Autoimmune thrombocytopenia
Thrombotic thrombocytopenic purpura
Acquired von Willebrand's disease
Mediated by the release of procoagulant substances
Disseminated intravascular coagulation
Hyperviscosity due to myeloproliferative syndrome

Cerebral infarct
Mediated by autoimmune mechanism
Microangiopathic hemolytic anemia
Acquired von Willebrand's disease
Antiphospholipid syndrome
Vasculitis
Mediated by the release of procoagulant substances
States of hypercoagulability
Thrombocytosis
Bacterial thrombotic endocarditis
Disseminated intravascular coagulation
Hyperviscosity syndrome

Vasculitis is a heterogeneous group of multisystem processes characterized by inflammation of the arterial wall. These inflammatory arteriopathies may lead to ischemia of the CNS by two different mechanisms that are not mutually exclusive. First, arterial disease provides the right conditions for thrombosis to develop. Second, the change in the arterial wall can itself, though less commonly, cause stenosis of the vascular lumen to the point that it is destroyed. When vasculitis appears in association with malignant tumors, antigens deriving from the tumor itself play a part in the formation of immune complexes that are deposited on the vascular wall, causing inflammation. The clinical symptoms that arise from these arterial changes will depend on the vessel affected, its size and location, and the speed at which the obstruction develops. Even though they are rare, almost all forms of vasculities have been associated with neoplastic diseases, especially Hodgkin's disease, lymphomas, hairy cell leukemia, and lung cancer (Carsons, 1997; Kurzrock and Cohen, 1993; Lie, 1997). Approximately 5% of vasculities are paraneoplastic in origin (Sánchez-Guerrero *et al.*, 1990), but only a very small percentage cause brain infarction (Baumgartner *et al.*, 1998).

Granulomatous angiitis of the CNS has only been reported in 7% of patients with lymphoproliferative neoplasms, although 77% of these patients develop focal neurological manifestations (Younger *et al.*, 1997). In some cases, granulomatous angiitis affects the carotid artery, the middle cerebral artery, or the anterior cerebral artery, and appears weeks after herpes zoster infection of the contralateral ophthalmic branch (Hilt *et al.*, 1983).

The association between temporal arteritis, neoplastic disease, and stroke is difficult to quantify given that the patients are usually of an advanced age, when other diseases are also prevalent (Haga *et al.*, 1993). The association of neoplasia and temporal arteritis has been estimated at between 3.5% and 16% (Kurzrock and Cohen, 1993), and infarcts and transient ischemic attacks (TIAs) appear in 7% of these patients (Caselli and Hunder, 1997).

The second group of etiopathological mechanisms involved in paraneoplastic strokes is caused by the tumor-releasing procoagulant substances responsible for hypercoagulability.

Nonbacterial thrombotic endocarditis (often also called marantic endocarditis) is the most common cause of symptomatic cerebral infarcts in patients with cancer (Graus *et al.*, 1985; Patchell and Posner, 1985) and is produced by growths of fibrin and platelets in the cardiac valves, particularly on the left (Figure 50.1). The valvular lesions of nonbacterial thrombotic endocarditis usually affect

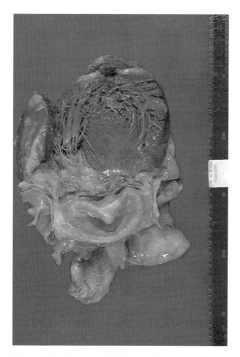

Figure 50.1 Nonbacterial thrombotic endocarditis in patients with adenocarcinoma of the lung. See color plate.

the mitral and aortic valves (Biller *et al.*, 1982; Lopez *et al.*, 1987) and can complicate any type of cancer except brain tumor, leading to a risk of brain embolism. This disorder is often associated with cerebral intravascular thrombosis. Both valvular deformation and a hypercoagulable state have been involved in the genesis of this paraneoplastic endocarditis. In autopsy studies of the general population, the prevalence of nonbacterial thrombotic endocarditis ranges from 0.3% to 9.3% (Chino *et al.*, 1975), whereas the postmortem prevalence among cancer patients has been reported to be up to 1–2% (Biller *et al.*, 1982; Graus *et al.*, 1985; Ondrias *et al.*, 1985); a third of these patients have emboli in the brain. The highest incidence of nonbacterial thrombotic endocarditis has been reported with lymphoma (Gallerini *et al.*, 2004; Glass, 2006), carcinomas of the gastrointestinal tract and lung (Edoute *et al.*, 1997; Ondrias *et al.*, 1985; Reisner *et al.*, 1992), medullary thyroid cancer (Lal *et al.*, 2003), and prostatic adenocarcinoma (Almela *et al.*, 2004), but it can complicate any kind of neoplasm and appear at any early or late stage (Rogers *et al.*, 1987).

More than 20% of patients with acute leukemia develop disseminated intravascular coagulation (Sletnes *et al.*, 1995), with increased fibrinogen degradation products, thrombocytosis, increased platelet adhesiveness, and hyperfibrinogenemia. The triggering of this process is because of the release of procoagulant material from the tumor cells into blood circulation (Staszewski, 1997). The chronic form of disseminated intravascular coagulation produces a state of hypercoagulability in which fibrin-platelet thrombi occlude small cerebral arteries and venules, large intracranial venous sinuses, or deposits on cardiac valves, leading to nonbacterial thrombotic endocarditis (Posner, 1995). This chronic form of disseminated intravascular coagulation is the second cause of symptomatic brain infarcts in patients with cancer

(Graus *et al.*, 1985; Patchell and Posner, 1985). The acute form of disseminated intravascular coagulation is associated with clinical hemorrhaging, consumption of coagulation factors and platelets, and an increase in fibrinolysis (Furui *et al.*, 1983; Rogers, 1991). Disseminated intravascular coagulation is common in gastric and pancreatic mucinous adenocarcinomas; cancers of the lung, ovary, and prostate; and in myeloproliferative syndromes (Cornuz *et al.*, 1988; Graus *et al.*, 1985; Posner, 1995). This process can complicate the evolution of the cancer at any stage but appears more frequently in the advanced phases and in the presence of sepsis (Posner, 1995).

The association of migratory thrombophlebitis and neoplasms (Trousseau's syndrome) was one of the first paraneoplastic syndromes described (Prandoni *et al.*, 1992). The mechanisms that affect hypercoagulability and thrombosis are complex and only partially elucidated. Fibrinopeptide A, a sensitive marker of thrombotic activity, appears in many developed neoplasms (Rickles and Edwards, 1983). Residues of sialic acid may be released by mucinous tumors and are responsible for the activation of the coagulation cascade. Autopsies in patients with mucinous adenocarcinomas, mostly pancreatic and gastrointestinal, may show mucin within small brain arteries and veins (Amico *et al.*, 1989). Mucin activates the body's coagulation system.

Other phospholipids and tissue factors, which activate hemostasis in normal situations following the disruption of the endothelium, may be released into the blood flow by the tumor itself or through abnormal vascularization arising from the growth of the tumor (Staszewski, 1997). Platelet hyperactivity can also contribute to the increased risk of thrombosis in these patients, presumably due to factors released by the tumor or induced by its presence (Staszewski, 1997). Acquired protein C and protein S deficiencies may be associated with a variety of diseases including malignancies (Coull *et al.*, 1998).

Many neoplasms are capable of releasing cytokines (interleukin [IL]-1, IL-6, IL-8, tumor necrosis factor [TNF], transforming growth factor [TGF], and intercellular adhesion molecule [ICAM]) that are responsible for the most common paraneoplastic syndromes, such as fever (Dinarello and Bunn, 1997), cachectic syndrome (Puccio and Nathanson, 1997), and hypercoagulability (Green and Silverstein, 1996). In addition, IL-6 is a powerful stimulant of thrombocytosis (Gastl *et al.*, 1993). Deep venous thrombosis, both in the limbs and in the brain, pulmonary thromboembolism, and systemic embolizations due to nonbacterial thrombotic endocarditis are all consequences of this state of hypercoagulability (Staszewski, 1997).

On rare occasions, some tumors release paraproteins and monoclonal immunoglobulins, leading to a hyperviscosity syndrome that interferes with the polymerization of fibrin and causes coagulation disorders and symptomatic hemorrhages (O'Kane *et al.*, 1994).

Clinical and diagnostic characteristics

Even though cerebrovascular manifestations in patients with cancer may be clinically similar and have the same etiopathology as the strokes that appear in the rest of the population (Chaturvedi

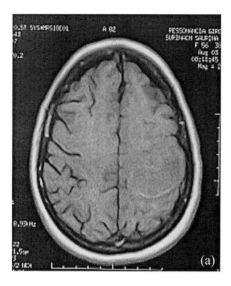

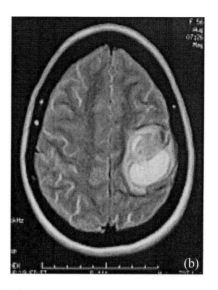

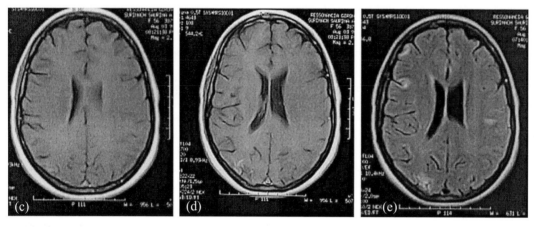

Figure 50.2 Woman (70 years old) admitted with intracerebral hemorrhage. She was admitted 1 month earlier with occipital infarct. During the current admission adenocarcinoma of the ovary was diagnosed. MRI carried out in acute phase, sectioned at the level of the corona radiata (*top*) and the semioval center (*bottom*). Lobar, Leith parietal intraparenchymatous hematoma, in amplified images in T1 (**a**) and T2 (**b**). At the level of the corona radiata no changes in signal were observed in amplified images in T1 (**c**); images in T1 with contrast (**d**) and fluid-attenuated inversion recovery (FLAIR) (**e**) show the presence of multiple ischemic cortical lesions, in the same stage and in different vascular areas.

et al., 1994), paraneoplastic strokes more commonly present with specific clinical manifestations (Baumgartner *et al.*, 1998; Patchell and Posner, 1985; Rogers, 1991, 1994). In contrast to non-neoplastic patients, among whom brain infarcts are more prevalent than hemorrhages, in patients with cancer the frequency of hemorrhages is almost the same as the frequency of infarcts (Graus *et al.*, 1985).

Symptomatic brain infarction is more common in patients with lymphoma and carcinoma than it is in those with leukemia, among whom brain hemorrhage predominates.

The classic ischemic stroke, preceded or not by TIAs, is a rare form of presentation in paraneoplastic strokes. The proportion of ischemic events in the vertebrobasilar territory and in the carotid artery is similar in patients with temporal arteritis, a fact that does not occur in arteriosclerotic disease. Neurological symptoms in these patients are usually the result of thrombotic obstruction of the vertebral and carotid arteries rather than of intracranial

arteritis (Caselli and Hunder, 1997). In other forms of vasculitis, the clinical pattern may also be focal, but cerebral manifestations appear just as often as spinal signs and isolated lesions in cranial nerves (Younger *et al.*, 1997). Brain infarcts with focal neurological manifestations also appear in nonbacterial thrombotic endocarditis, occasionally preceded by TIAs.

More often, paraneoplastic strokes show a clinical picture different from those observed in stroke patients without cancer. Diffuse and progressive encephalopathy, either isolated or accompanied by focal neurological manifestations, is usual in disseminated intravascular coagulation, nonbacterial thrombotic endocarditis, and paraneoplastic vasculitis. This is because brain infarcts in cancer patients are often multifocal, and the resulting multifocal manifestations are difficult to distinguish from those caused by encephalopathy. Many patients with paraneoplastic strokes progress towards stupor or coma (Rogers, 1991; Schwartzmann and Hill, 1982).

The clinical presentation of paraneoplastic cerebral venous thrombosis is very variable and includes severe, diffuse, and progressive headache due to intracranial hypertension, partial or generalized seizures, transient ischemia or cerebral infarct of venous origin, and progressive ischemic encephalopathy (Ameri and Bousser, 1992; Russell and Enevoldson, 1993). This clinical pattern is usually more serious than the one caused by metastatic cerebral venous thrombosis or by a thrombosis induced by treatment (Hickey et al., 1982).

The hemorrhagic presentation of paraneoplastic stroke is as common as ischemic forms (Figure 50.2). Brain hemorrhage occurs more often in patients with leukemia than in those with lymphomas or solid tumors, and is more frequent in acute than in chronic leukemias and in myelogenous than in lymphocytic leukemias. Intracerebral hemorrhaging may present itself with the usual clinical pattern, although hemorrhages are more often smaller and cause symptoms of diffuse encephalopathy (Posner, 1995). Subdural hemorrhaging may be acute, subacute, or chronic, with considerable clinical variability (Minette and Kimmel, 1989). Subarachnoid hemorrhaging is the rarest form of presentation of paraneoplastic hemorrhagic stroke (Graus et al., 1985).

In many cases the diagnostic process for paraneoplastic strokes is different from standard procedures for other types of stroke. Cerebral CT and MRI can be normal in ischemic events caused by disseminated intravascular coagulation (Schwartzman and Hill, 1982), or may show multiple images in several vascular territories in nonbacterial thrombotic endocarditis and vasculitis (Baumgartner et al., 1998).

Brain infarction due to disseminated intravascular coagulation should be diagnosed in patients with clinical manifestations coinciding with the characteristic hematological profile. Systemic thrombosis – including deep vein thrombosis, pulmonary embolism, and myocardial infarction – and systemic hemorrhages may occur together with the cerebral symptoms. Laboratory studies to confirm disseminated intravascular coagulation include determination of the number of platelets, prothrombin time, activated partial thromboplastin time, fibrinogen, fibrin split products, fibrinopeptide A, and D-dimer assay. Results of laboratory tests for coagulation function must be carefully interpreted in the clinical context, because abnormalities are not always clinically significant. Pleocytosis of cerebrospinal fluid helps in the diagnosis of vasculitis (Younger et al., 1997). Echocardiograms, including transesophageal echocardiograms, are usually normal in patients with nonbacterial thrombotic endocarditis, possibly because of the small size of the valve growths (Hofmann et al., 1990). The most useful test for diagnosing vasculitis and nonbacterial thrombotic endocarditis is the cerebral angiogram.

Treatment

Brain hemorrhages of paraneoplastic origin are difficult to treat. Surgical removal of hematomas during the course of coagulopathy is not indicated. Treatment with heparin and platelet concentrate or fresh plasma reverses the coagulopathy of consumption in some circumstances. Therapy with heparin and the administration of fresh plasma are usually more useful in preventing progression

of cerebral hemorrhaging in patients among whom hematological changes suggestive of disseminated intravascular coagulation are detected at an early stage (Rogers et al., 1987). Cytoreductive chemotherapy reduces the risk of cerebral hemorrhage in patients with chronic myeloproliferative processes (Wehmeier et al., 1991). However, in other patients, lysis of the primitive blood cells can exacerbate disseminated intravascular coagulation (Rogers, 1994).

Heparin may be effective in preventing cerebral infarction among patients with nonbacterial thrombotic endocarditis and does not increase the risk of hemorrhagic complications (Rogers et al., 1987). Vasculitis responds to treatment with steroids and cytostatic agents (Inwards et al., 1991). Administering aspirin and other antiplatelet agents has also been shown to be effective in preventing the recurrence of thrombotic complications in patients with essential thrombocythemia (Michiels et al., 1993).

REFERENCES

Almela, R., Aladro, Y., Munoz, C., Balda, I., and Mendoza, D. 2004. Recurrent ischemic strokes secondary to acquired hypercoagulability in a patient with prostatic adenocarcinoma. *Neurologia*, **19**, 69–73.

Ameri, A., and Bousser, M. G. 1992. Cerebral venous thrombosis. *Neurol Clin*, **10**, 87–109.

Amico, L., Caplan, L. R., and Thomas, C. 1989. Cerebrovascular complications of mucinous cancers. *Neurology*, **39**, 16–21.

Baumgartner, R. W., Mattle, H. P., and Cerny, T. 1998. Stroke and cancer. In *Cerebrovascular Disease: Pathophysiology, Diagnosis, and Management*, vol 2, M. D. Ginsberg and I. Bogousslavsky (eds.), Boston, MA: Blackwell Science, pp. 1727–36.

Biller, J., Challa, V. R., Toole, J. E., and Howard, V. I. 1982. Non-bacterial thrombotic endocarditis. A neurological perspective of clinicopathologic correlations of 99 patients. *Arch Neurol*, **39**, 95–8.

Carsons, S. 1997. The association of malignancy with rheumatic and connective tissue diseases. *Semin Oncol*, **24**, 360–72.

Caselli, R. J., and Hunder, G. G. 1997. Giant cell (temporal) arteritis. *Neurol Clin*, **15**, 893–902.

Chaturvedi, S., Ansell, J., and Recht, L. 1994. Should cerebral ischemic events in cancer patients be considered a manifestation of hypercoagulability? *Stroke*, **25**, 1215–8.

Chino, F., Kodama, A., Otake, M., and Docks, D. S. 1975. Non-bacterial thrombotic endocarditis in a Japanese autopsy sample. Review of eighty cases. *Am Heart J*, **90**, 190–8.

Cornuz, J., Bogousslavsky, J., Schapira, M., Regli, F., and Camenzind, E. 1988. Ischemic stroke as the presenting manifestation of localized systemic cancer. *Schweiz Arch Neurol Psychiatr*, **139**, 5–11.

Coull, B. M., DeLoughery, T. G., and Fenberg, W. M. 1998. Coagulation abnormalities in stroke. In *Stroke: Pathophysiology, Diagnosis, and Management*, 3rd edn., H. J. M. Barnett, J. P. Mohr, B. M. Stein, and F. D. Yatsu (eds.), Philadelphia: Churchill Livingstone, pp. 936–78.

Coull, B. M., Levine, S. R., and Brey, R. L. 1992. The role of antiphospholipid antibodies in stroke. *Neurol Clin*, **10**, 125–43.

Dalmau, J. O., and Posner, J. B. 1997. Paraneoplastic syndromes affecting the nervous system. *Semin Oncol*, **24**, 318–28.

Dinarello, C. A., and Bunn, P. A. 1997. Fever. *Semin Oncol*, **24**, 281–98.

Edoute, Y., Haim, N., Rinkevich, D., Brenner, B., and Reisner, S. A. 1997. Cardiac valvular vegetations in cancer patients: a prospective echographic study of 200 patients. *Am J Med*, **102**, 252–8.

Furui, T., Ichihara, K., and Ikeda, A. 1983. Subdural hematoma associated with disseminated intravascular coagulation in patients with advanced cancer. *J Neurosurg*, **58**, 398–401.

Gallerini, S., Fanucchi, S., Sonnoli, C., et al. 2004. Stroke in the young as a clinical onset of non-Hodgkin's lymphoma with paraneoplastic endocarditis. *Eur J Neurol*, **11**, 421–3.

Gastl, G., Plante, M., Finstad, C. L., *et al.* 1993. High IL-6 levels in ascitic fluid correlate with reactive thrombocytosis with epithelial ovarian cancer. *Br J Hematol*, **83**, 433–41.

Glass, J. 2006. Neurologic complications of lymphoma and leukaemia. *Semin Oncol*, **33**, 342–7.

Graus, E., Rogers, L. R., and Posner, J. B. 1985. Cerebrovascular complications in patients with cancer. *Medicine (Baltimore)*, **64**, 16–35.

Green, K. B., and Silverstein, R. L. 1996. Hypercoagulability in cancer. *Hematol Oncol Clin North Am*, **10**, 506–7.

Haga, H. L, Eide, G. E., Brun, J., Johansen, A., and Langmark, E. 1993. Cancer in association with polymyalgia rheumatica and temporal arteritis. *J Rheumatol*, **20**, 1335–9.

Harris, E. N., Gharavi, A. E., and Hughes, G. R. V. 1985. Antiphospholipid antibodies. *Clin Rheum Dis*, **11**, 591–608.

Hickey, W. E., Garnick, M. B., Henderson, L. C., and Dawson, D. M. 1982. Primary cerebral venous thrombosis in patients with cancer. A rarely diagnosed paraneoplastic syndrome. Report of three cases and review of the literature. *Am J Med*, **73**, 740–50.

Hilt, D., Buchholz, D., Krumholz, A., Weiss, H., and Wolinsky, J. S. 1983. Herpes zoster ophthalmicus and delayed contralateral hemiparesis caused by cerebral angiitis: diagnosis and management approaches. *Ann Neurol*, **14**, 543–53.

Hofmann, T., Kasper, W., Meinertz, T., Geibel, A., and Just, H. 1990. Echocardiographic evaluation of patients with clinically suspected arterial emboli. *Lancet*, **336**, 1421–4.

Inwards, D. J., Piepgras, D. G., Lie, J. T., *et al.* 1991. Granulomatous angiitis of the spinal cord associated with Hodgkin's disease. *Cancer*, **68**, 1318–22.

Khamashta, M. A., Cervera, R., Asherson, R. A., *et al.* 1990. Association of antibodies against phospholipids with heart valve disease in systemic lupus erythematosus. *Lancet*, **335**, 1541–4.

Kurzrock, R., and Cohen, P. R. 1993. Vasculitis and cancer. *Clin Dermatol*, **11**, 175–87.

Lal, G., Brennan, T. V., Hambleton, J., and Clarck, O. H. 2003. Coagulopathy, marantic endocarditis, and cerebrovascular accidents as paraneoplastic features in medullary thyroid cancer. Case report and review of the literature. *Thyroid*, **13**, 601–5.

Lie, L. T., 1997. Classification and histopathologic spectrum of central nervous system vasculitis. *Neurol Clin*, **15**, 805–19.

Lopez, J. A., Fishbeim, M. C., and Siegel, R. J. 1987. Echocardiographic features of nonbacterial thrombotic endocarditis. *Am J Cardiol*, **59**, 478–80.

McNeil, H. P, Chesterman, C. N., and Krilis, S. A. 1991. Immunology and clinical importance of antiphospholipid antibodies. *Adv Immunol*, **49**, 193–280.

Michiels, J. J., Koudstaal, P. J., Mulder, A. H., and van Vliet, H. H. 1993. Transient neurologic and ocular manifestations in primary thrombocythemia. *Neurology*, **43**, 1107–10.

Minette, S. E., and Kimmel, D. W. 1989. Subdural hematoma in patients with systemic cancer. *Mayo Clin Proc*, **64**, 637–42.

Mohri, H., Noguchi, T., Kodama, E., Itoh, A., and Ohkube, T. 1987. Acquired von Willebrand disease due to an inhibitor of human myeloma protein specific for von Willebrand factor. *Am J Clin Pathol*, **87**, 663–8.

Nathanson, L., and Hall, T. C. 1997. Paraneoplastic syndromes. *Semin Oncol*, **24**, 265–8.

O'Kane, M. J., Wisdom, G. B., Desai, Z. R., and Archbold, G. P. 1994. Inhibition of fibrin monomer polymerization by myeloma immunoglobulin. *J Clin Pathol*, **47**, 266–8.

Ondrias, F., Slugen, I., and Valach, A. 1985. Malignant tumors and embolizing paraneoplastic endocarditis. *Neoplasma*, **32**, 135–40.

Patchell, R. A., and Posner, J. B. 1985. Neurologic complications of systemic cancer. *Neurol Clin*, **3**, 729–50.

Posner, L. B. 1995. Neurologic complications of cancer. In *Contemporary Neurology*, vol 45, R. W. Reinhardt (ed.), Philadelphia: FA Davis, pp. 199–229.

Prandoni, P., Lensing, A. W. A., Buller, H. R., *et al.* 1992. Deep-vein thrombosis and the incidence of subsequent symptomatic cancer. *N Engl J Med*, **327**, 1128–38.

Puccio, M., and Nathanson, L. 1997. The cancer cachexia syndrome. *Semin Oncol*, **24**, 277–87.

Reisner, S. A., Rinkiewich, D., Markiewicz, W., Tatarsky, I., and Brenner, B. 1992. Cardiac involvement in patients with myeloproliferative disorders. *Am J Med*, **93**, 498–504.

Rickles, E. R., and Edwards, R. L. 1983. Activation of blood coagulation in cancer: Trousseau's syndrome revisited. *Blood*, **62**, 14–41.

Rogers, L. R. 1991. Cerebrovascular complications in cancer patients. *Neurol Clin*, **9**, 889–99.

Rogers, L. R. 1994. Cerebrovascular complications in cancer patients. *Oncology*, **8**, 23–30.

Rogers, L. R., Cho, E. S., Kempin, S., and Posner, J. B. 1987. Cerebral infarction from non-bacterial thrombotic endocarditis. *Am J Med*, **83**, 746–56.

Russell, R. W. R., and Enevoldson, T. P. 1993. Unusual types of ischemic stroke. In *Current Review of Cerebrovascular Disease*, M. Fisher and J. Bogousslavsky (eds.), Philadelphia: Current Medicine, pp. 63–77.

Sánchez-Guerrero, J., Gutiérrez-Urena, S., Vidaller, A., *et al.* 1990. Vasculitis as a paraneoplastic syndrome. Report of 11 cases and review of the literature. *J Rheumatol*, **17**, 1458–62.

Schwartzman, R. J., and Hill, J. B. 1982. Neurologic complications of disseminated intravascular coagulation. *Neurology*, **32**, 791–7.

Sletnes, K. E., Godal, H. C., and Wisloff, I. 1995. Disseminated intravascular coagulation (DIC) in adult patients with acute leukaemia. *Eur J Haematol*, **54**, 34–8.

Staszewski, H. 1997. Hematological paraneoplastic syndromes. *Semin Oncol*, **24**, 329–33.

Steingart, R. H. 1988. Coagulation disorders associated with neoplastic disease. *Recent Results Cancer Res*, **108**, 37–43.

Wehmeier, A., Daum, L., Jamin, H., and Schneider, W. 1991. Incidence and clinical risk factors for bleeding and thrombotic complications in myeloproliferative disorders. *Ann Hematol*, **63**, 101–6.

Younger, D. S., Calabrese, L. H., and Hays, A. P. 1997. Granulomatous angiitis of the nervous system. *Neurol Clin*, **15**, 821–34.

51 KOHLMEIER-DEGOS' DISEASE (MALIGNANT ATROPHIC PAPULOSIS)

Oriana Thompson and Daniel M. Rosenbaum

Introduction

Kohlmeier-Degos' disease (KDD) was initially described in 1941 by Kohlmeier (Kohlmeier, 1941a,b) and then in 1942 by Degos et al. Other synonyms for this disease are malignant atrophic papulosis, atrophic papulosquamous dermatitis, fatal cutaneous-intestinal syndrome, and thromboangiitis cutaneointestinalis disseminata (Magnnat et al., 1989). First described as a cutaneous disorder with a characteristic rash, two distinct forms are now recognized (Zamiri et al., 2005). The systemic or malignant variant is associated with a fatal outcome. Death is usually a consequence of involvement of the gastrointestinal tract or the central nervous system (Kocheril et al., 2004). The cutaneous or benign variant has characteristic cutaneous lesions with no evidence of systemic involvement, and these patients have a normal life expectancy. A number of these cases are familial (Habbema et al., 1986).

KDD is more common in white boys and men with age of onset ranging between 3 weeks of age to 67 years old, most commonly occurring in the second and third decades. The etiology and pathogenesis, although still unknown, is speculated to be immunologic dysfunction, coagulation or fibrinolysis abnormalities, or possible viral infections (Pallesen, 1979). Effective treatment also remains unknown.

Clinical findings

Cutaneous

Any organ system may be involved; the clinical manifestations are a result of multifocal infarctions. The cutaneous lesions, which usually precede the visceral symptoms (Figures 51.1 and 51.2), are usually asymptomatic but can cause slight burning or itching (Caviness et al., 2006). The skin lesions range in number from a few to hundreds, and typically involve the trunk and upper limbs. Other body regions are usually spared but there are reports of lesions involving more distal regions, including the penis (Aydogan et al., 2005). Initially, the lesions present as pink macules that soon become small, red, round, smooth, and firm (Ball et al., 2003). Within weeks they become umbilicated, with two distinct zones: a depressed porcelain white (necrotic) scaly center and an erythematous or telangiectatic border. In time, the reddish border disappears and the fully formed lesion measures <1 cm (Ball et al., 2003). The differential diagnosis includes: systemic lupus erythematous, dermatomyositis (Tsao et al., 1997), atrophic blanche, and allergic necrotizing vasculitis (Pallesen, 1979). The ocular conjuctiva is the most common site for mucosal involvement (Ball et al., 2003; Feuerman, 1966).

Gastrointestinal

Death is most often because of microvascular infarction of the intestines leading to perforation and peritonitis. Episodes of abdominal pain, nausea, diarrhea, and melena may occur weeks to years after the onset of the cutaneous lesions. These symptoms are often initially attributed to gastritis, peptic ulcer, ileus, dysentery, or pancreatitis (Degos, 1979; Muller and Landry, 1976). Laparoscopic examination, however, shows lesions similar in appearance to the skin lesions that may involve multiple areas of the small intestine. These lesions are secondary to infarction and have also been found in the esophagus, duodenum, stomach, colon, and rectum.

Neurological

Central nervous system involvement occurs in approximately 20% of patients as a consequence of brain and spinal cord infarction (Yoshikawa et al., 1996). A few patients with peripheral nervous system involvement have been reported (Horner et al., 1976; Label et al., 1983). Neurological involvement may precede the skin lesions by years. In the largest series of patients of KDD with neurological involvement who had a mean duration of follow-up to 13 years, 13 of 15 patients had skin lesions; only one had neurological findings as the first manifestation (Subbiah et al., 1996). The mean duration of signs and symptoms before diagnosis was 2 years (range: 1–16 years).

A variety of neurological signs were noted, depending on the site of involvement, including cognitive, motor, and sensory impairment, ophthalmoplegia, and other cranial neuropathies. Ophthalmic involvement has been reported in 35 of 105 published observations (Lee et al., 1984; Sotrel et al., 1983).

Other organs

Autopsy findings have included infarcts in the heart (Mauad et al., 1996), pericardium, kidneys (Bjorck et al., 1984), bladder, lungs, pleura, liver, and pancreas (Strole et al., 1967; Yoshikawa et al., 1996). These are usually asymptomatic.

Uncommon Causes of Stroke, 2nd edition, ed. Louis R. Caplan. Published by Cambridge University Press. © Cambridge University Press 2008.

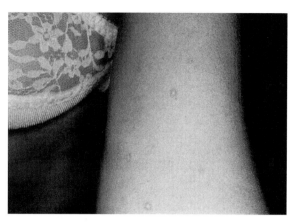

Figure 51.1 Cutaneous lesions of KDD on trunk and arm of a 35-year-old woman with KDD.

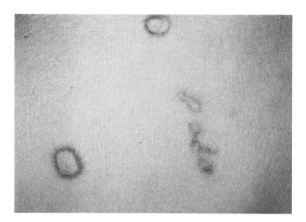

Figure 51.2 Papules with central atrophy showing porcelain appearance, surrounded by an erythematous peripheral circle, disseminated on the trunk.

Etiology/pathogenesis

The etiology and pathogenesis of KDD remain unknown. Ischemia and infarction are key pathophysiological mechanisms of the lesions seen, but there is still no consensus as to the nature of the injury. At least three major hypotheses have been proposed.

The first hypothesis is that KDD is a coagulopathy, with thrombus formation being the primary event (Magnnat *et al.*, 1989). Abnormalities in platelet function (Drucker, 1990; Stahl *et al.*, 1978; Vazquez-Doval *et al.*, 1993), increase in fibrinogen (Roegnik and Farmer, 1968; Vazquez-Doval *et al.*, 1993), decrease in plasminogen (Paramo *et al.*, 1985), as well as other alterations in the coagulation cascade (Yoshikawa *et al.*, 1996) have been reported to support this hypothesis. However, many patients with the disease do not have these abnormalities, either histopathologically or by laboratory studies. Moreover, therapies targeting these parameters have not been shown to be effective (see below).

The second hypothesis favors that KDD is a form of vasculitis, based on similarities between KDD and systemic lupus erythematous (Su *et al.*, 1985). The lack of response to immunosuppression argues against this theory (Ball *et al.*, 2003).

The third hypothesis is that KDD is a primary disorder of endothelial cells (Tribble *et al.*, 1986), which some investigators

have attributed to viral infection (Howard and Nishida, 1969). The nature of the endothelial defect that leads to thrombosis has not been elucidated.

Finally, there are those who postulate that KDD is not a specific disease but rather a distinctive pattern that expresses different pathological processes, primarily systemic lupus erythematosis, so that patients with manifestations of this disease should also be assessed for evidence of lupus and other collagen vascular disease (Ball *et al.*, 2003).

Pathology

The pathological findings in KDD are a noninflammatory occlusive endarteriopathy, mainly involving arterioles (Degos *et al.*, 1942; Kohlmeier, 1941). Increased intimal cellularity, secondary to endothelial cell proliferation, may be associated with superimposed thrombosis (Caviness *et al.*, 2006). The media is always spared (Demitsu *et al.*, 1992). The clinical manifestations are a consequence of ischemia and infarction that occurs secondary to the arteriolar occlusion. Three stages have been described: early, intermediate, and late. These findings are similar, regardless of the organ involved (Demitsu *et al.*, 1992; Molenaar *et al.*, 1987). Leptomeningeal involvement results in ischemia and infarction in the distribution of the affected arteries. In the parenchyma, foci of hemorrhagic necrosis may be seen. Cranial nerve and spinal root infarcts as well as myelomalacia of the posterolateral spinal cord have been described (Matsuura *et al.*, 2006; McFarland *et al.*, 1978).

Treatment

There is no known effective treatment for KDD (Caviness *et al.*, 2006). Therapies that have been used include antiplatelet (Stahl *et al.*, 1978; Tribble *et al.*, 1986), anticoagulant (Degos, 1979), immunosuppressive agents, plasma exchange (Burrow *et al.*, 1991; Caviness *et al.*, 2006), and nicotine patches (Kanekura *et al.*, 2003). Surgery is indicated in cases of intestinal perforation (Pallesen, 1979).

REFERENCES

Aydogan, L., Alkan, G., Karadogan, K. S., *et al.* 2005. Painful penile ulceration in a patient with malignant atrophic papulosis. *J Eur Acad Dermatol Venereol*, **5**, 612–6.

Ball, E., Newburger, A., and Ackerman, A. B. 2003. Degos' disease: a distinctive pattern of disease, chiefly of lupus erythematous, and not a specific disease per se. *Am J Dermatopathol*, **25**, 308–20.

Bjorck, S., Johansson, S. L., and Aurell, M. 1984. Acute renal failure caused by a rapidly progressive arterio-occlusive syndrome – Kohlmeier-Degos' disease? *Scand J Urol Nephrol*, **18**, 343–6.

Burrow, J. N., Blumbergs, P. C., Iyer, P. V., and Hallpike, J. F. 1991. Kohlmeier-Degos disease: a multisystem vasculopathy with progressive cerebral infarction. *Aust N Z J Med*, **21**, 49–51.

Caviness, V. S. Jr., Sagar, P., Israel, E. J., *et al.* 2006. Case 38–2006: a 5-year old boy with headache and abdominal pain. *N Engl J Med*, **355**, 2575–84.

Degos, R. 1979. Malignant atrophic papulosis. *Br J Dermatol*, **100**, 21–35.

Degos, R., Delort, J., and Tricot, R. 1942. Dermatite papulosquameuse atrophiante. *Bulletin Societe Francais Dermatologie et Syphilligraphie*, **49**, 148–50.

Demitsu, T., Nakajima, K., Okayuma, R., and Tadaki, T. 1992. Malignant atrophic papulosis (Degos' syndrome). *Int J Dermatol*, **31**, 99–102.

Drucker, C. R. 1990. Malignant atrophic papulosis: response to antiplatelet therapy. *Dermatologica*, **180**, 90–2.

Feuerman, E. J. 1966. Papulosis atrophicans maligna Degos with microaneurysms of the conjunctiva. *Arch Dermatol*, **94**, 440–5.

Habbema, L., Kisch, L. S., and Starink, T.,M. 1986. Familial malignant atrophic papulosis (Degos' disease) additional evidence for heredity and a benign course. *Br J Dermatol*, **114**, 134–5.

Horner, F. A., Myers, G. J., Stumpf, D. A., Oseroff, B. J., and Choi, B. H. 1976. Malignant atrophic papulosis (Kholmeier-Degos disease) in childhood. *Neurology*, **26**, 317–21.

Howard, R. O., and Nishida, S. 1969. A case of Degos' disease with electron microscopic findings. *Trans Am Acad Ophthalmol Otolaryngol*, **73**, 1097–112.

Kanekura, T., Uchino, Y., and Kanzaki, T. 2003. A case of malignant atrophic papulosis successfully treated with nicotine patches. *Br J Dermatol*, **149**, 655–80.

Kocheril, S. V., Blaivas, M., Appleton, B. E., McCune, W. J., and Ike, R. W. 2004. Degos' disease mimicking vasculitis. *Arthritis Rheum Arthritis Care Res*, **51**, 498–500.

Kohlmeier, W. 1941a. Multiple Hautnekrausen bei thrombangiitis obliterans. *Archiv Klinik Experimentale Dermatologie*, **181**, 783–92.

Kohlmeier, W. 1941b. Bulletin Société Francais. *Dermatologie et Syphiligraphie*, **49**, 148–50.

Label, L. S., Tandan, R., and Albers, J. W. 1983. Myelomalacia and hypoglycorrhachia in malignant atrophic papulosis. *Neurology*, **33**, 936–9.

Lee, D. A., Su, W. P., and Liesegant, T. J. 1984. Ophthalmic changes of Degos' disease (malignant atrophic papulosis). *Ophthalmology*, **91**, 295–9.

Magnnat, G., Kerwin, K. S., and Gabriel, D. A. 1989. The clinical manifestations of Degos syndrome. *Arch Pathol Lab Med*, **113**, 354–62.

Matsuura, F., Makino, K., Fukushima, T., *et al.* 2006. Optic nerve and spinal cord manifestations of malignant atrophic papulosis (Degos disease). *J Neurol Neurosurg Psychiatry*, **77**, 260–2.

Mauad, T., DeFatima Lopes Calvo Tiberio, I., Baba, E., *et al.* 1996. Malignant atrophic papulosis (Degos' disease) with extensive cardiopulmonary involvement. *Histopathology*, **28**, 84–6.

McFarland, H. R., Wood, W. G., Drowns, B. V., and Meneses, A. C. O. 1978. Papulosis atrophicans, maligna (Kohlmeier-Degos disease): a disseminated occlusive vasculopathy. *Ann Neurol*, **3**, 388–92.

Molenaar, W. M., Rosman, J. B., Donker, A. J., and Houthoff, H. J. 1987. The pathology and pathogenesis of malignant atrophic papulosis (Degos' disease). *Pathol Res Pract*, **182**, 98–106.

Muller, S. A., and Landry, M. 1976. Malignant atrophic papulosis (Degos' disease). *Arch Dermatol*, **112**, 357–63.

Pallesen, R. M. 1979. Malignant atrophic papulosis – Degos' syndrome. *Acta Chir Scand*, **145**, 279–83.

Paramo, J. A., Rocha, E., Cuesta, B., *et al.* 1985. Fibrinolysis in Degos' disease. *Thromb Haemost*, **54**, 730.

Roegnik, H. H., and Farmer, R. G. 1968. Degos' disease (malignant papulosis): report of three cases with clues to etiology. *J Am Acad Dermatol*, **206**, 1508–14.

Sotrel, A., Lacson, A. G., and Huff, K. 1983. Childhood Kohlmeier-Degos disease with atypica skin lesions. *Neurology*, **33**, 1146–51.

Stahl, D., Thomsen, K., and Hou-Jensen, K. 1978. Malignant atrophic papulosis. Treatment with aspirin and dipyridamole. *Arch Dermatol*, **114**, 1687–9.

Strole, W. E. Jr., Wallace, H., Clark, M. D. Jr., and Isselbacher, K. J. 1967. Progressive arterial occlusive disease (Kohlmeier-Degos). A frequently fatal cuteneosystemic disorder. *N Engl J Med*, **276**, 195–201.

Su, W. P., Schroeter, A. L., Lee, D. A., Hsu, T., and Muller, S. A. 1985. Clinical and histological findings in Degos' syndrome (malignant atrophic papulosis). *Cutis*, **35**, 131–8.

Subbiah, P., Wijdicks, E., Muenter, M., *et al.* 1996. Skin lesion with fatal neurological outcome (Degos' disease). *Neurology*, **46**, 636–40.

Tribble, K., Archer, M. E., Jorizzo, J. L., *et al.* 1986. Malignant atrophic papulosis: absence of circulating immune complexes or vasculitis. *J Am Acad Dermatol*, **15**, 365–9.

Tsao, H., Busam, K., Barnhill, R. L., and Haynes, H. A. 1997. Lesions resembling malignant atrophic papulosis in a patient with dermatomyositis. *J Am Acad Dermatol*, **36**, 317–9.

Vazquez-Doval, F. J., Ruiz de Erenchun, F., Paramo, J. A., and Quintanilla, E. 1993. Malignant atrophic papulosis. A report of two cases with altered fibrinolysis and platelet function. *Clin Exp Dermatol*, **5**, 441–4.

Yoshikawa, H., Maruta, T., Yokoji, H., *et al.* 1996. Degos' disease: radiological and immunological aspects. *Acta Neurol Scand*, **94**, 353–6.

Zamiri, M., Jarrett, P., and Snow, J. 2005. Benign cutaneous Degos disease. *Int J Dermatol*, **44**, 654–6.

52 STROKE IN PATIENTS WHO HAVE INFLAMMATORY BOWEL DISEASE

Michael A. De Georgia and David Z. Rose

Introduction

When reviewing the panoply of risk factors ascribed to ischemic stroke – diabetes, hypertension, hyperlipidemia, atrial fibrillation, and so on – gastrointestinal disorders rarely come to mind. However, a set of disorders collectively termed inflammatory bowel disease (IBD) also predisposes patients to thromboembolic events. Pelvic, peripheral, and pulmonary thromboemboli are among the better known extraintestinal complications of IBD, but ischemic stroke also occurs. This chapter highlights the clinical, pathophysiologic, and biochemical links between IBD and ischemic stroke.

IBD is the umbrella term for two disorders: Crohn's disease (CD) and ulcerative colitis (UC). Whereas CD and UC overlap in their clinical and histological features, they differ in pathogenesis. Whereas both diseases result from T-lymphocyte activation and humeral mechanisms, in general, CD involves mainly lymphocyte activation whereas UC is related mainly to humeral mechanisms. The unifying feature of CD and UC is chronic inflammation of intestinal mucosa. The diagnosis is based on a combined assessment of clinical, endoscopic, radiographic, and histological features. On histology, IBD is characterized by acute and chronic inflammation of the intestine. In UC, the inflammation is limited to the mucosa and superficial submucosa. In CD, there is architectural disruption of the intestinal wall (transmural inflammation and presence of noncaseating granulomatous infiltration).

Epidemiology and symptoms of IBD

An estimated four million people worldwide (including one million Americans) have IBD, with the incidence evenly divided between UC and CD. IBD can be accompanied by a markedly painful and debilitating course accounting for an estimated US$1 billion in missed workdays per year. The peak age of onset for IBD is 15–30 years. Both UC and CD have a bimodal age distribution, with a second, smaller peak occurring in individuals between 50 and 70 years old, yet IBD can appear at any age, and an estimated 10% of cases occur in children younger than 18 years. UC is slightly more common in men, whereas CD affects women more (Andres and Friedman, 1999). Breakdowns by racial and ethnic subgroups indicate higher rates of IBD in Caucasians and Ashkenazi Jews.

Severe, crampy abdominal pain and diarrhea (with or without rectal bleeding) are the chief complaints of patients with IBD. Fecal urgency, dramatic weight loss, skin and eye irritations, ulcers, fevers, and blood clots also are notorious complications of the disease. These symptoms are quite distressing and, in many cases, debilitating. Miserable intervals of active disease known as "flares" are relieved by periods of remission that can vary from weeks to years.

Pathogenesis of IBD

In CD, areas of normal bowel exist between areas of diseased bowel that disrupt parts of the entire digestive tract from mouth to anus. These "skip lesions" can evolve into devastating strictures, fissures, and fistulas by eventually tearing through all layers of the intestinal wall. CD is primarily a condition of chronic T-lymphocyte activation, and flares occur when secondary macrophage activation induces tissue damage. The exact etiology of the initial T-cell activation is unknown, but usual gastrointestinal microflora might be triggering the inappropriate inflammatory response. Normally, exposure to commensal bacteria downregulates inflammatory genes and blocks activation of an immune response. In CD, however, this tolerance is lost and luminal microflora can activate T cells. The amount of tissue damage – ranging from villous atrophy and crypt hyperplasia to total mucosal destruction – directly correlates with the degree of T-cell activation. Immunosuppression to inhibit T cells can reduce this damage. FK506, for example, in experimental models can completely inhibit mucosal damage (Lionetti *et al.*, 1993).

UC, in contrast, involves just the inner intestinal walls of only the colon and rectum. In UC, there is no strong evidence for T-cell activation, and humeral mechanisms seem to predominate. Activation of mucosal macrophages is seen with a dramatic increase of immunoglobulin G (IgG)-producing cells and complement activation. These antibodies try to remove antigens of the indigenous microbial flora and consequently become cytotoxic to the colonic walls (Brandtzaeg and Halstensen, 2006; MacDonald and Murch, 1994). Many patients with UC are positive for anti-neutrophil cytoplasmic antibodies (ANCAs), further corroborating a humoral stimulus.

Despite these differences in initial immune activations, both UC and CD share similar "downstream" inflammatory pathways – such as the production of cytokines and oxygen free radicals – that provoke intestinal vascular injury (MacDonald and Murch, 1994). Occlusive thromboses in intestinal arteries plague patients with CD, whereas submucosal thrombotic lesions have been reported in UC. This endothelial damage, vasospasm, and thrombosis might be secondary to vasculitis of the mesenteric circulation. Recent studies suggest that two principal macrophage cytokines – tumor necrosis factor-α (TNF-α) and interleukin (IL)-1 – embroil the inflammation, degrade the protective matrix, and induce focal vascular thrombosis (Araki *et al.*, 2003). Other cytokines like IL-6 contribute to the *systemic* effects of IBD, including growth suppression, anorexia, and chronic anemia as IL-6 suppresses erythropoietin production (Araki *et al.*, 2003; Breese *et al.*, 1994; Levine and Lukawski-Trubish, 1995; Murch, 1998). Higher levels of cytokines are seen in CD than in UC, probably due to the extensive T-cell activation in CD (Breese *et al.*, 1994).

The enhanced release of reactive oxygen species also plays a role in the pathogenesis of IBD. Certain reactive oxygen species such as nitrogen monoxide produced in high amounts by the enzyme inducible nitrogen oxide synthase (iNOS) may damage cellular DNA. Free-radical scavengers curb the destructive activity of reactive oxygen species, thereby reducing mucosal damage (Araki *et al.*, 2003).

Extraintestinal complications

Nonthrombotic

Non-neurologic

IBD is a *systemic* inflammatory disease; as many as 1 of 3 patients will have some form of extraintestinal manifestation. Perhaps the most disabling extraintestinal, nonthrombotic, non-neurologic complication of IBD is peripheral arthritis. Usually affecting large joints, peripheral arthritis in IBD is similar to reactive arthritis associated with enteric infections because the pathogenesis involves synovial exposure to arthritogenic bacterial antigens and inflammatory cell by-products.

Another nonthrombotic complication of IBD is primary sclerosing cholangitis. This disorder may arise from production of ANCAs that target antigens in both the biliary tract and bowel. More infrequent and poorly understood nonthrombotic complications include acute pancreatitis, gluten-sensitive enteropathy, and possibly even pulmonary bronchiectasis (Levine and Lukawski-Trubish, 1995). Similarities in the mucosal immune system of the lung and intestine may account for bronchial hyperreactivity in patients with active IBD.

Neurologic

Although neurologic sequelae of IBD can transpire at any time, most occur after a diagnosis of IBD already has been established (Manzino and Tomasina, 1996). There may be some correlation with activity of systemic disease, but neurologic symptoms can arise during an IBD flare or in periods of remission. To determine the frequency, spectrum, and clinical features of neurologic disorders associated with IBD, a team from Israel conducted a retrospective analysis of 638 IBD patients, looking for involvement of the nervous system (Lossos *et al.*, 1995). They identified 19 patients (10 CD and 9 UC) with neurologic involvement. In 14 (74%), the neurologic sequelae started about 6 years after the diagnosis of IBD, and in two (10%) it occurred during an IBD flare. The most common association was a peripheral neuropathy, which affected six patients, all of whom had UC. Ten others (nine of whom had CD) exhibited myelopathy, myopathy, and myasthenia gravis. Stroke occurred in two UC and two CD patients.

Thrombotic

Noncerebrovascular

Thromboembolic disease has had a longstanding association with IBD and ranks as the third leading cause of death in IBD patients. As early as 1936, the observation of extensive vascular thrombosis as a complication of UC was noted (Bargen and Barker, 1936). In 1966, Graef found 39 cases of thromboembolism in 100 patients with UC (Graef, 1966). Many IBD patients have subclinical thromboses; in the literature, when defined clinically, the incidence of thromboembolism in IBD patients varies from 1.2% to 7.1%, but this number increases to 39% when defined by autopsy. In one study of 1500 patients with UC, clinically significant thrombosis occurred in only 18 (1.2%); however, among 43 patients studied at autopsy, emboli and thrombi were found in 14 (33%) (Ricketts and Palmer, 1946).

Sometimes many clots develop in the same patient. In one study, multiple (two or more) thromboembolic events occurred in 13% of IBD patients (Jackson *et al.*, 1997). More than half of these patients were younger than 50 years; correlation with IBD flares was seen in 64%. Moreover, IBD patients have been found to develop thrombosis earlier in life than those without IBD who develop thrombosis (Grip *et al.*, 2000).

Deep venous thrombosis (DVT) and pulmonary embolism (PE) account for the overwhelming majority of thrombotic events in patients with IBD. Nevertheless, arterial thromboses also can and do occur, even in unusual locations. In IBD patients with either arterial or venous thromboembolic events, mesenteric microvascular changes have been noted; that some patients seem to benefit with anticoagulation supports a valid connection between this inflammation and systemic thrombosis. Specifically, a necrotizing, granulomatous vasculitis – mainly affecting small- and medium-sized vessels of the skin, lung, bowel, muscle, retina, and central nervous system (CNS) – has been reported to cause systemic thrombosis in IBD patients.

Coagulation abnormalities are common in patients with IBD (Schneiderman *et al.*, 1979). These include genetic deficiencies of protein C, protein S, and antithrombin; factor V Leiden (fVL) and prothrombin 20210A mutations; activated protein C (APC) resistance; and high concentrations of fibrinogen, platelets, factor VIII, and homocysteine. Laboratory irregularities may normalize after medical and surgical control of intestinal inflammation. Acquired risk factors for thrombosis include immobilization, surgery, trauma, pregnancy, puerperium, lupus anticoagulant, malignancy, and female hormones (Koutroubakis, 2001). Patients may have a combination of these conditions which, when combined with oral contraceptive use, may increase the risk for thrombosis (Breckwoldt *et al.*, 1990; Fraser, 1993).

Cerebrovascular

Cerebrovascular thrombosis in IBD is well recognized with an incidence ranging from 0.1% to 4.2% (Mayeux and Fahn, 1978). The actual incidence and prevalence of IBD and stroke remain unknown and probably underestimated. In one study, among 52 IBD patients who developed thrombosis requiring hospitalization, thrombus occurred in the deep leg veins in 52%, in the pulmonary vasculature in 37%, intracranially in 9%, and intracardiac in 2% (Jackson et al., 1997). In this same study, multiple thromboses occurred in 13% and 60% of all episodes occurred in patients younger than 50 years.

In a review of patients from the New England Medical Center and the Cleveland Clinic, 38 patients were identified with both IBD and stroke including 23 with CD and 15 with UC. Overall, the average age was 52 ±19 years. Most patients (86%) had ischemic stroke, including 19 of 23 patients with CD and 12 of 15 with UC. Most patients (72%) also had other vascular risk factors for stroke: carotid atherosclerotic disease in 45% and hypertension in 35%. Atrial fibrillation was found in three patients, and one patient had a vertebral artery dissection. Three patients had lacunar strokes.

While disease activity may promote a stroke, a minority of patients had active disease immediately before their event. When flares were present during a stroke, they were more frequent in patients with CD than in those with UC (39% vs. 16.7%, respectively). In another study, evidence for inflammatory disease activity was found in 89% of patients with CD at the time of their thromboembolic event, in contrast to 45% of those with UC. A less clear relationship to duration or activity of IBD has been reported in other studies (Johns, 1991).

Cerebral venous thrombosis (CVT) is not uncommon in patients with IBD; several cases of CVT with IBD appear in the literature (Calderon et al., 1998). Seven of our patients had cerebral venous occlusion, including 4 of 23 (17.3%) patients with CD and 3 of 15 (20%) patients with UC. These patients were much younger with an average age of 33 ±13.6 years. Typical vascular risk factors were not present, and most (all four with CD and one with UC) had active disease before their event.

The literature consists of numerous case reports of stroke in IBD patients. One account describes a 39-year-old woman with a past medical history of CD and hypertension who presented with an ischemic stroke of the left internal carotid artery (ICA) territory (Schneiderman et al., 1979). Evaluation revealed bilateral high-grade ICA stenosis. She also had increased levels of fibrinogen and factor IX, and a marked hyperhomocysteinemia. Vitamin B_1 and B_6 levels were decreased, and heterozygous C677 T methylenetetrahydrofolate reductase (MTHFR) gene mutation was present.

Another case, a 35-year-old man with refractory CD in his terminal ileum, complained of headaches and blurred vision and suddenly developed tonic-clonic seizures (Mayeux and Fahn, 1978). CT-scan revealed an ischemic stroke in the left cerebral hemisphere. Laboratory studies were significant for elevated factor VIII and platelet counts.

Likewise, a 30-year-old woman with a UC exacerbation developed both a CVT and a lower extremity DVT. Her laboratory data uncovered a functional APC resistance, yet after colectomy, her APC ratio normalized (Manzino and Tomasina, 1996).

Table 52.1 summarizes the literature of thrombosis in the setting of IBD.

Vasculitis

In most reported cases of IBD and stroke, full neurologic and laboratory evaluations have been incomplete, thus it is difficult to establish the exact underlying causal mechanism of the strokes. Systemic vasculitis is associated with a variety of thromboses in patients with IBD and thus may affect the CNS and has been posited to cause ischemic stroke (Karacostas et al., 1991). Studies with vascular brain imaging mostly have reported occlusions of the carotids and middle cerebral artery (or its branches). Occasionally, the central retinal artery and posterior ciliary central arteries also are involved.

A case of IBD-related CNS vasculitis involves a young man with UC who developed seizures, became comatose, and was found to have multiple low-density enhancing cerebral lesions on brain MRI. Anti-nuclear antibodies (ANA) and rheumatoid factor (RF) were negative, and skin and muscle biopsies revealed a mild perivascular infiltrate with inflammation. Brain biopsy showed necrotizing vasculitis involving meningeal and cortical vessels. Treatment with prednisone and cyclophosphamide (Cytoxan) was complicated by systemic thrombosis and sepsis before full recovery was made.

Other descriptions of IBD-associated CNS vasculitis are based on angiography showing segmental narrowing in the small to medium-sized arteries. This is a nonspecific finding and is more often related to vasoconstriction than to true arteritis (Schmidely, 2000). One patient with UC so far has been reported among 25 with biopsy-proven giant cell arteritis (Dare and Byrne, 1980).

Hypercoagulability

Several abnormalities in the coagulation cascade may cause thromboses in IBD patients. Of the many IBD-related hypercoagulable state manifestations, an estimated 10% are ischemic strokes. An extensive search for a single unifying coagulation defect explaining the hypercoagulability in IBD patients is currently underway. Such a single defect – genetic or otherwise – has not yet been elucidated, but many distinct defects have been reported in the literature. Regardless of the number of defects, though, it is believed that the severity of a patient's IBD correlates with the magnitude and timing of that patient's hypercoagulable state. Secondary or nonspecific inflammatory responses comprise the majority of hypercoagulable changes seen in these patients; such changes may stabilize during IBD remission. Even if transient, it is likely that these hypercoagulable changes play a key role in inducing clinical, overt thrombosis. Hypercoaguable abnormalities that persist in these patients (those that are not transient and do not normalize during remissions) probably reflect on-going disease and manifest as thromboses subclinically or upon autopsy.

Plasma fibrinopeptide A levels have been strongly linked with the level of disease activity in CD as measured by the Crohn's Disease Activity Index. Patients with active CD who undergo medical or surgical treatment usually have a reduction of fibrinopeptide A levels; a failure of fibrinopeptide A levels to normalize often heralds a relapse. Fibrinopeptide A levels also correlate with monocyte

Table 52.1 Main case series of systemic thrombosis and cerebrovascular disorders in IBD

Study	Number	IBD	Total number of cases Thrombosis (%)	Number (%)	Cerebrovascular disorders Diagnosis
Autopsy					
Bargen and Barker, 1936	43	UC	14 (33%)	NS	
Sloan *et al.*, 1950	99	UC	33 (33%)	2 (2%)	1 Hemorrhagic encephalitis
					1 NS
Graef, 1966	100	UC	39 (39%)	2 (2%)	2 CVT
Clinical					
Bargen and Barker, 1936	1500	UC	18 (1.2%)	NS	
Edwards and Truelove, 1964	624	UC	50 (8%)	NS	
Talbot *et al.*, 1986	7199	UC and CD	92 (1.3%)	9 (0.1%)	1 Cerebral arterial thrombosis
					1 Retinal venous thrombosis
					2 Transient ischemic attacks
					5 NS
Lloyd-Still and Tomasi, 1989	180	UC and CD	6 (3.3%)	6 (3.3%)	1 Retinal artery thrombosis
					1 CVT
					1 Cerebral arteritis
					1 Hypertensive encephalopathy
					2 NS
Elsebety and Bertorini, 1991	263	CD	NS	11 (4.2%)	11 NS
Lossos *et al.*, 1995	638	UC and CD	NS	4 (0.6%)	1 Cerebral arterial thrombosis
					1 Transient ischemic attacks
					2 CVT
Jackson *et al.*, 1997	NS	UC and CD	52	4	NS

Notes: NS = not specified.

tissue factor generation, which may contribute to hypercoagulability as well (Edwards *et al.*, 1987).

IBD exacerbations also tend to correlate with a rise in platelet counts. Thrombocytosis and increased platelet activation and aggregation are well documented in patients with IBD. Increased platelet number and activity may be directly responsible for microvascular thrombosis in the intestinal wall and may mediate initial mucosal injury. Many of the cytokines involved in the pathogenesis of IBD are released by activated platelets.

APC resistance because of a fVL mutation is now known to be the most common genetic cause of venous thrombosis worldwide. As expected, fVL mutations and APC resistance have been incriminated in patients with stroke. A retrospective analysis of 11 patients with IBD plus arterial or venous thrombosis and 51 IBD patients without thrombosis found the presence of fVL mutations in 4 of 11 (36%) thrombotic patients compared with only 2 of the 51 controls (4%) (Liebman *et al.*, 1998). Of note, APC resistance can be transient. For example, a 30-year-old woman was described with both a CVT and a DVT of her leg during a flare of her UC. Laboratory investigations revealed a functional APC resistance, without fVL mutation, and slight hyperhomocysteinemia. After colectomy, her APC ratio returned to normal limits. These findings may help explain the probable increased thrombophilia during active IBD flares (Gonera *et al.*, 1997). A study from France revealed that 14% of thrombotic patients with IBD had fVL mutation versus 0%

of control patients with IBD without thrombosis. About 16% of thrombotic patients without IBD had fVL, but this was not significant when compared to the thrombotic IBD patients with fVL (Guedon *et al.*, 2001).

The prothrombin gene 20210A mutation has been associated with thrombosis in patients with IBD. The aforementioned French study also found that 14% of thrombotic patients with IBD and 12% of thrombotic patients without IBD carried the prothrombin 20210A mutation, compared to 1.7% of control patients with IBD without thrombosis; however, this difference was just below statistical significance (Guedon *et al.*, 2001).

Protein S deficiency has also been reported in IBD. One case was of a 29-year-old woman with UC and thrombosis of the veins of Galen and straight sinus. A transient protein S deficiency was discovered (Vaezi *et al.*, 1995). The role of protein S and many other hypercoagulable factors was evaluated in a Turkish study that enlisted 27 patients with active IBD flares. Specifically, international normalized ratio, activated partial thromboplastin time, lupus anticoagulant, anticardiolipin IgG, IgM antibodies, protein C, protein S, antithrombin-III, factor V, and factor II mutation all were measured in the 27 IBD patients and in a group of sex-matched, age-matched, non-IBD controls. Every factor was comparable between the two groups except for antithrombin-III, which was significantly lower in the IBD group compared with the healthy controls (Yuerlki *et al.*, 2006).

Anti-cardiolipin (aCL) antibodies have been reported in patients with IBD and stroke. In one report, a 44-year-old woman with CD for 25 years developed a left temporal stroke associated with aCL antibodies and lupus anticoagulant, suggesting antiphospholipid syndrome (Mevorach *et al.*, 1996). In another study, antibodies against the aCL cofactor, β2-glycoprotein I, which has a higher specificity for thrombosis, were found in several IBD patients. Comparing 128 patients with IBD (83 with UC and 45 with CD) with 100 controls, the prevalence of aCL positivity was 18.1% for UC patients, 15.6% for CD patients, and a mere 3% for controls (Koutroubakis *et al.*, 1998).

Hyperhomocysteinemia has recently emerged as an independent risk factor for stroke; homocysteine is a sulfur-containing amino acid formed during the demethylation of the amino acid methionine. It may be elevated in the blood and urine if a genetic C677 T MTHFR enzyme polymorphism is present. Patients with IBD appear to have elevated plasma levels of homocysteine most likely from vitamin B12 and B6 deficiencies, not necessarily from a MTHFR enzyme polymorphism. Vitamin B12 and B6 deficiency can be because of malnutrition or malabsorption (not an uncommon phenomenon in IBD patients) and can result in high levels of homocysteine in the blood and urine. A study from Canada involving 65 IBD patients found high levels of plasma homocysteine (8.7 μmol/L) compared with healthy control subjects (6.6 μmol/L). In another study, homocysteine levels in 138 healthy control subjects were compared with those in the IBD cohort, and adjustments for age and sex were made using logistic regression. Hyperhomocysteinemia was significantly more common in patients with IBD compared with healthy controls, and is associated with lower (but not necessarily deficient) vitamin B12 levels (Romagnuolo *et al.*, 2001).

Increased homocysteine levels have also been associated with progressive atherosclerosis. In one case report, a 39-year-old woman with CD presented with an ischemic stroke. Evaluation revealed bilateral high-grade internal carotid stenosis and atheroma of the subclavian and vertebral arteries. The patient was found to have hyperhomocysteinemia in addition to increased levels of fibrinogen and factor IX (Younes-Mhenni *et al.*, 2004).

In another case report, a 45-year-old woman had two ischemic strokes a full 16 years after ileal resection for CD. Blood tests revealed an elevated random serum homocysteine level and a low serum vitamin B12 level. Intramuscular vitamin B12 injections normalized her homocysteine level (Penix, 1998).

Conclusion

Patients with IBD are at risk for a host of thromboembolic events, up to 10% of which are ischemic strokes. When compared to the general population, the exact incremental stroke risk that IBD patients face remains unknown, yet it appears higher for younger patients. The mechanism for ischemic strokes in IBD patients is multifactorial, but likely secondary to an abnormal coagulability profile and, in rare situations, cerebral vasculitis. A search for a unifying coagulation defect has not been discovered. An IBD patient's current hypercoagulable state seems to correlate with the magnitude and timing of IBD flares. Serious extraintestinal complications – including the more common pelvic, peripheral, and pulmonary thromboemboli, as well as the less common ischemic stroke – likely occur with greater frequency during flares.

Microvascular injury, endothelial damage, vasospasm, and coagulation diatheses all curtail mesenteric blood flow and harm the walls lining the intestines and other organs. An increased cytokine milieu develops and becomes a nexus for extraintestinal micro- and macrovascular thromboses. Elevated factors V, VIII, fibrinogen, homocysteine, platelets, and aCL antibodies as well as a decline in the B vitamins, folate, and antithrombin III levels all predispose IBD patients to ischemic attacks. Some abnormalities appear inherited whereas others may be reactive from an IBD flare. Subpopulations of IBD patients who have certain hemostatic, thrombophilic abnormalities may wind up with a higher incidence of IBD manifestations, thrombotic complications, or both.

Better management of IBD flares, improved compliance with newer IBD medications, and quicker surgical interventions might lead to better outcomes and stroke risk reduction. It is reasonable to believe that the addition of low-dose anticoagulation or antiplatelet therapy to an IBD regimen would lessen ischemic stroke risk. However, this must be weighed against each individual's bleeding risk, which can be significant in patients with recurrent hematochezia.

REFERENCES

Andres, P. G., and Friedman, L. S. 1999. Epidemiology and the natural course of inflammatory bowel disease. *Gastroenterol Clin North Am*, **28**, 255–81.

Araki, Y., Andoh, A., and Fujiyama, Y. 2003. The free radical scavenger edaravone suppresses experimental dextran sulfate sodium-induced colitis in rats. *Int J Mol Med*, **12**, 125–9.

Bargen, J. A., and Barker, N. W. 1936. Extensive arterial and venous thrombosis complicating chronic ulcerative colitis. *Arch Intern Med*, **58**, 17–31.

Brandtzaeg, P. C. H., and Halstensen, T. S. 2006. The B-cell system in inflammatory bowel disease. *Adv Exp Med Biol*, **579**, 149–67.

Breckwoldt, M., Wieacker, P., and Geisthovel, F. 1990. Oral contraception in disease states. *Am J Obstet Gynecol*, **163**, 2213–6.

Breese, E. J., Michie, C. A., Nicholls, S. W., *et al.* 1994. Tumor necrosis factor alpha-producing cells in the intestinal mucosa of children with inflammatory bowel disease. *Gastroenterology*, **106**, 1455–66.

Calderon, R., Cruz-Correa, M. R., and Torres, E. A. 1998. Cerebral thrombosis associated with active Crohn's disease. *P R Health Sci J*, **17**, 293–5.

Dare, B., and Byrne, E. 1980. Giant cell arteritis. A five-year review of biopsy-proven cases in a teaching hospital. *Med J Aust*, **1**, 372–3.

Edwards, R. L., Levine, J. B., Green, R., *et al.* 1987. Activation of blood coagulation in Crohn's disease. Increased plasma fibrinopeptide A levels and enhanced generation of monocyte tissue factor activity. *Gastroenterology*, **92**, 329–37.

Edwards, F. C., and Truelove, S. C. 1964. The course and prognosis of ulcerative colitis. III. Complications. *Gut*, **5**, 1–22.

Elsehety, A., and Bertorini, T. E. 1997. Neurologic and neuropsychiatric complications of Crohn's disease. *Southern Medical Journal*, **90(6)**, 606–10.

Fraser, I. S. 1993. Contraceptive choice for women with 'risk factors'. *Drug Saf*, **8**, 271–9.

Gonera, R. K., Timmerhuis, T. P., Leyten, A. C., and van der Heul, C. 1997. Two thrombotic complications in a patient with active ulcerative colitis. *Neth J Med*, **50**, 88–91.

Graef, V. 1966. Venous thrombosis occurring in nonspecific ulcerative colitis. *Arch Intern Med*, **117**, 377–82.

Grip, O., Svensson, P. J., and Lindgren, S. 2000. Inflammatory bowel disease promotes venous thrombosis earlier in life. *Scand J Gastroenterol*, **35**, 619–23.

Guedon, C., Le Cam-Duchez, V., Lalaude, O., *et al.* 2001. Prothrombotic inherited abnormalities other than factor V Leiden mutation do not play a role in venous thrombosis in inflammatory bowel disease. *Am J Gastroenterol*, **96**, 1448–54.

Jackson, L. M., O'Gorman, P. J., O'Connell, J., *et al.* 1997. Thrombosis in inflammatory bowel disease: clinical setting, procoagulant profile and factor V Leiden. *Q J M*, **90**, 183–8.

Johns, D. R. 1991. Cerebrovascular complications of inflammatory bowel disease. *Am J Gastroenterol*, **86**, 367–70.

Karacostas, D., Mavromatis, J., Artemis, K., and Milonas, I. 1991. Hemorrhagic cerebral infarct and ulcerative colitis. A case report. *Funct Neurol*, **6**, 181–4.

Koutroubakis, I. E. 2001. Unraveling the mechanisms of thrombosis in inflammatory bowel disease [comment]. *Am J Gastroenterol*, **96**, 1325–7.

Koutroubakis, I. E., Petinaki, E., Anagnostopoulou, E., *et al.* 1998. Anti-cardiolipin and anti-beta2-glycoprotein I antibodies in patients with inflammatory bowel disease. *Dig Dis Sci*, **43**, 2507–12.

Levine, J. B., and Lukawski-Trubish, D. 1995. Extraintestinal considerations in inflammatory bowel disease. *Gastroenterol Clin North Am*, **24**, 633–46.

Liebman, H. A., Kashani, N., Sutherland, D., McGehee, W., and Kam, A. L. 1998. The factor V Leiden mutation increases the risk of venous thrombosis in patients with inflammatory bowel disease. *Gastroenterology*, **115**, 830–4.

Lionetti, P., Breese, E., Braegger, C. P., *et al.* 1993. T-cell activation can induce either mucosal destruction or adaptation in cultured human fetal small intestine. *Gastroenterology*, **105**, 373–81.

Lloyd-Still, J. D., and Tomasi, L. 1989. Neurovascular and thromboembolic complications of inflammatory bowel disease in childhood. *Journal of Pediatric Gastroenterology & Nutrition*, **9(4)**, 461–6.

Lossos, A., River, Y., Eliakim, A., and Steiner, I. 1995. Neurologic aspects of inflammatory bowel disease. *Neurology*, **45**, 416–21.

MacDonald, T. T., and Murch, S. H. 1994. Aetiology and pathogenesis of chronic inflammatory bowel disease. *Baillieres Clin Gastroenterol*, **8**, 1–34.

Manzino, M., and Tomasina, C. 1996. Infarti cerebrali multipli in corso di morbo di Crohn. Descrizione di un caso. *Minerva Med*, **87**, 253–5.

Mayeux, R., and Fahn, S. 1978. Strokes and ulcerative colitis. *Neurology*, **28**, 571–4.

Mevorach, D., Goldberg, Y., Gomori, J. M., and Rachmilewitz, D. 1996. Antiphospholipid syndrome manifested by ischemic stroke in a patient with Crohn's disease. *J Clin Gastroenterol*, **22**, 141–3.

Murch, S. H. 1998. Local and systemic effects of macrophage cytokines in intestinal inflammation. *Nutrition*, **14**, 780–3.

Penix, L. P. 1998. Ischemic strokes secondary to vitamin B12 deficiency-induced hyperhomocystinemia. *Neurology*, **51**, 622–4.

Ricketts, W. E., and Palmer, W. L. 1946. Complications of chronic non-specific ulcerative colitis. *Gastroenterology*, 25–38.

Romagnuolo, J., Fedorak, R. N., Dias, V. C., Bamforth, F., and Teltscher, M. 2001. Hyperhomocysteinemia and inflammatory bowel disease: prevalence and predictors in a cross-sectional study [see comment]. *Am J Gastroenterology*, **96**, 2143–9.

Schmidely, J. W. 2000. *Central Nervous System. Angiitis*. Boston: Butterworth-Heinemann.

Schneiderman, J. H., Sharpe, J. A., and Sutton, D. M. 1979. Cerebral and retinal vascular complications of inflammatory bowel disease. *Ann Neurol*, **5**, 331–7.

Sloan, W. P. Jr., Bargen, J. A., and Gage, R. P. 1950. Life histories of patients with chronic ulcerative colitis: a review of 2,000 cases. *Gastroenterology*, **16(1)**, 25–38.

Vaezi, M. F., Rustagi, P. K., and Elson, C. O. 1995. Transient protein S deficiency associated with cerebral venous thrombosis in active ulcerative colitis. *Am J Gastroenterol*, **90**, 313–5.

Younes-Mhenni, S., Derex, L., Berruyer, M., *et al.* 2004. Large-artery stroke in a young patient with Crohn's disease. Role of vitamin B6 deficiency-induced hyperhomocysteinemia. *J Neurol Sci*, **221**, 113–5.

Yuerlki, B., Aksoy, D., Aybar, M., *et al.* 2006. The search for a common thrombophilic state during the active state of inflammatory bowel disease. *J Clin Gastroenterol*, **40**, 809–13.

53 SWEET'S SYNDROME (ACUTE FEBRILE NEUTROPHILIC DERMATOSIS)

Bernhard Neundörfer

Introduction

Sweet's syndrome (SS), also referred to as acute febrile neutrophilic dermatosis, is characterized by a constellation of symptoms and findings: fever, neutrophilia, erythematous and tender skin lesions that typically show an upper dermal infiltrate of mature neutrophils, and prompt improvement of both symptoms and lesions after the initiation of treatment with systemic corticosteroids (Sweet, 1964, 1979). Crow *et al.* (1969) were the first authors to call this disease "Sweet's syndrome." Hundreds of patients with this dermatosis have been reported. The manifestations of SS in these individuals have not only confirmed those originally described by Dr Robert Douglas Sweet in 1964, but have also introduced new features that have expanded the clinical and pathologic concepts of this condition (Cohen and Kurzrock, 1993, 2003).

History

The condition was originally described by Dr Robert Douglas Sweet in 1964 in the *British Journal of Dermatology* (Sweet, 1964). He summarized the cardinal features of a distinctive and severe illness that he had encountered in eight women during the period from 1949 through 1964.

Epidemiology and classification

SS has a worldwide distribution and no racial predilection. An annual incidence of 2:1 000 000 was estimated in Scotland (Kemmett and Hunter, 1990). Prevalences of 1:250 (Gunawardena *et al.*, 1975) to 1:1 200 (von den Driesch, 1994) were found in dermatology outpatient departments. The disease occurs in patients of any age. The female sex predominates with a ratio of 2.3:1 to 3.7:1 (von den Driesch, 1994). However, this predilection of one sex cannot be discerned in childhood. Women between the ages of 30 and 50 years are the individuals in whom SS most often occurs. However SS may also involve younger patients. Classical or idiopathic SS may be associated with infection (upper respiratory or gastrointestinal tract), inflammatory bowel disease, and/or pregnancy (Cohen and Kurzrock, 1993, 2003).

As many cases of SS are cancer related, several authors distinguish between the classical form and the malignancy-associated form of the disease (Cohen *et al.*, 1988, 1993; Cohen and Kurzrock 1993; Cooper *et al.*, 1983). Several patients with a drug-related variant of the dermatosis have been recently described (Walker and Cohen, 1996). Many drugs (trans retinoic acid, carbamazepine,

diazepam, hydralazine, diclofenac, minocycline, nitrofurantoine, propylthiouracil, levonorgestrel, ethinyl estradiol) have been associated with the occurrence of the dermatosis (Sitjas *et al.*, 1993; Walker and Cohen, 1996); however, the administration of granulocyte-colony stimulating factor is considered to be responsible for the majority of drug-induced SS (Shimizu *et al.*, 1996).

SS may recur following either therapy induced or spontaneous remission (Cohen *et al.*, 1989). The duration of remission is variable between recurrent episodes of the dermatosis. In cancer patients, SS recurrences are more common; often the reappearance of dermatosis-associated symptoms and lesions represents the initial manifestation of recurrent malignancy (Cohen and Kurzrock, 1987).

Symptoms

Fever and leukocytosis usually accompany the skin eruption. The fever can precede the skin disease by several days or weeks or be present concurrently during the entire episode of the dermatosis. Other symptoms include arthralgia, general malaise, headache, and myalgia. The eyes are involved in about two-thirds of patients; these ophthalmological conditions are mainly conjunctivitis and episcleritis (Cohen and Kurzrock, 2000; Hisanaga *et al.*, 2005).

Skin lesions

The skin lesions typically appear as tender and red or purplered. They most often occur on the upper extremities, face, and/or neck. The lesions may have a transparent, vesicle-like appearance secondary to pronounced edema. The lesions enlarge over a period of days to weeks. The painful lesions resolve spontaneously or after treatment, without scarring (Gunawardena *et al.*, 1975). Less commonly, the lesions can present as a pustular dermatosis. This clinical variant of SS includes patients with neutrophilic dermatosis of the dorsal hands (DiCaudo and Connolly, 2002; Sommer *et al.*, 2000).

Concomitant diseases

A malignancy may be found in about one-third of SS patients. Many instances are related to lymphoproliferative disorders such as acute and chronic leukemia, acute and chronic lymphatic leukemia, hairy cell leukemia, polycythemia vera, non-Hodgkin's lymphoma, Hodgkin's lymphoma, and other diseases of the hematopoietic system (von den Driesch, 1994). Some patients

Uncommon Causes of Stroke, 2nd edition, ed. Louis R. Caplan. Published by Cambridge University Press. © Cambridge University Press 2008.

with solid tumors have been repeatedly described in association with SS (Cohen *et al.*, 1993; Geelkerken *et al.*, 1994; von den Driesch, 1994), including mainly breast, uterine, prostate, colon, and rectal cancers. All other organs may also be affected. An infection is sometimes found simultaneously with SS and is caused by the most diverse pathogens such as yersinias, salmonellae, *Helicobacter pylori*, *Mycobacteria leprae*, HIV, mycobacteria, and cytomegalovirus (further references in von den Driesch, 1994). Autoimmune diseases such as Behçet's disease (Cho *et al.*, 1989; Mizoguchi *et al.*, 1988), Crohn's disease (Ly *et al.*, 1995; Perales *et al.*, 1997), ulcerative colitis (Hommel *et al.*, 1993; Kemmett and Hunter, 1990; Sitjas *et al.*, 1993; Sweet, 1964; von den Driesch, 1994), Sjögren syndrome (Bianconcini *et al.*, 1991; Levenstein *et al.*, 1991; Vatan *et al.*, 1997), lupus erythematosus (Goette, 1985; Sequeira *et al.*, 1986), thyroiditis (Alcalay *et al.*, 1987; von den Driesch, 1994), and rheumatoid arthritis (Delaporte *et al.*, 1989; Kemmett and Hunter, 1990; von den Driesch, 1994) may also be associated with SS. SS has also been frequently described in pregnancy (see references in von den Driesch, 1994).

Pathology

The pathologic features of SS characteristically involve the dermis. There is an infiltrate of mature neutrophils in the superficial dermis (Jordaan, 1989; Su *et al.*, 1995; Sweet, 1964; von den Driesch, 1994). Swelling of the endothelial cells, dilatation of the small blood vessels, and fragmentation of the neutrophil nuclei (which is referred to as leukocytoclasia) are also often present. The composition and location of the inflammatory infiltrate can vary. The mature neutrophil is the typical and most frequent inflammatory cell in SS lesions, yet occasional lymphocytes or histiocytes may be present in the inflammatory infiltrate. In addition, eosinophils have been noted in the cutaneous lesions of some patients with drug-induced SS (Going *et al.*, 1987; Matsuda *et al.*, 1994).

Laboratory findings

An elevated erythrocyte sedimentation rate (ESR) and peripheral leukocytosis with neutrophilia are the most consistent laboratory findings in SS (Cohen and Kurzrock, 2000). Specifically in patients with malignancy-associated SS, anemia, a normal or low neutrophil count, and/or abnormal platelet count may be observed (Cohen and Kurzrock, 1993).

Diagnosis and clinical differential diagnosis

For the diagnosis of SS, two obligatory (major) and two of the four facultative (minor) criteria must be fulfilled (Table 53.1). The morphology of SS skin lesions can mimic that of several other mucocutaneous and systemic conditions. The differential diagnosis of SS includes infectious and inflammatory disorders such as bacterial sepsis, cellulitis, erysipelas, herpes simplex virus infection, leprosy, lymphangitis, panniculitis, pyoderma gangrenosum, syphilis, systemic mycosis, thrombophlebitis, tuberculosis, and varicella-zoster virus infection; neoplastic conditions such as chloroma, leukemia cutis, lymphoma, and metastatic tumor;

Table 53.1 Diagnostic criteria for SS

Major criteria

Abrupt onset of tender, painful erythematous or violaceous plaques or nodules

Predominantly neutrophilic infiltration in dermis without leukocytoclastic vasculitis

Minor criteria

Prodromal symptoms of fever or infection

Concurrent association with fever, arthralgia, conjunctivitis, or underlying malignancy

Laboratory finding or leukocytosis or ESR >50 mm/1 h

Good response to therapy with systemic steroids

Both major criteria and at least two of the minor criteria must be fulfilled to justify a diagnosis of SS.

Source: Su *et al.*, 1995, with permission from Elsevier © 1995.

reactive erythemas such as vasculitis (leukocytoclastic vasculitis; other cutaneous conditions such as acne vulgaris and granuloma faciale; and other systemic diseases such as Behçet's disease, bowel bypass syndrome, dermatomyositis, familial Mediterranean fever, and lupus erythematosus (Cohen and Kurzrock, 2003).

SS and the central nervous system

Hisanaga *et al.* (2005) reported 27 cases of probable neuro-Sweet disease. Both sexes were almost equally affected. Encephalitis and meningitis were the most common neurological manifestations. Any region of the central nervous system (CNS) may be involved resulting in a variety of neurological symptoms (Table 53.2). Furthermore, a high frequency of human leukocyte antigen (HLA) B54 is reported in particular in Japanese patients with SS. Systemic corticosteroids were effective for most of the neurological symptoms. Other patients with involvement of the CNS have been reported in the literature. In 1983, Chiba described a 46-year-old man with SS who had convulsions and showed slowing on electroencephalograms (EEGs) as well as cerebral atrophy on cranial CT scans. The patient later developed myoclonus resistant to treatment as well as depression. The cerebrospinal fluid (CSF) was normal. In 1992, Dunn *et al.* reported a 7-week-old boy with SS and aseptic meningitis that developed following otitis media and an infection of the upper airways. Furukawa *et al.* (1992) as well as Martínez *et al.* (1995) each described a patient with slight meningitis (cell count 29/mm^3 [Furukawa *et al.*, 1992] and 31/mm^3 [Martínez *et al.*, 1995]) without neurological deficits in connection with SS.

Only two patients with brain ischemia with focal neurological deficits have been reported to date. The first patient was reported by Druschky *et al.* in 1996. This was a 69-year-old man who developed bronchitis 14 days before inpatient admission. He received antibiotic treatment for suspected meningitis. On inpatient admission, he showed the typical skin changes of SS, meningism, and a slight to moderately severe right hemiparesis. The ESR was very high (100 m/h). Leukocytosis of 26 600/mL with 87.2% granulocytes and 7.7% lymphocytes was found with

Table 53.2 Neurological signs and symptoms in patients with neuro-Sweet ($n = 27$)

Signs and symptoms	n	%
Headache	14	50
Consciousness disturbance	11	41
Epilepsy	8	29
Hemiparesis	8	29
Memory disturbance	5	19
Psychiatric disorder	5	19
Involuntary movement	4	15
Ocular movement disorder	4	15
Dysarthria	4	15
Sensory disturbance	4	15
Ataxia	3	11

Source: Hisanaga *et al.*, 2005, with permission.

pleocytosis of 51 cells/mm^3 in the CSF. Polymerase chain reaction for *Borrelia burgdorferi* and herpesvirus were negative. MRI and Doppler sonography were normal. A broad-scale antibiotic treatment (ceftriaxone, fosfomycin, penicillin) administered for 2 weeks remained unsuccessful. After confirmation of the diagnosis by the dermatological consultant on the basis of the typical histological finding, 100-mg methylprednisolone treatment was begun. The patient then initially developed slight paresis of the left arm and the left leg. Assuming that the patient had cerebral vasculitis, 250 mg of prednisolone was then administered intravenously. The skin changes regressed quickly under this treatment, and the cell count in the CSF fell to 8/mm^3 after 13 days. After 4 weeks, the motor deficit had markedly improved. A CT scan and cerebral angiography did not show any indications of vasculitis.

The second patient was reported by Ohori *et al.* (1999). A 54-year-old woman visited the emergency service complaining of a severe language disturbance. She spoke fluently, but most of the words were merely meaningless syllables. This jargon state lasted only 4 hours, then her abnormal speech rapidly and completely recovered within 24 hours. She had also developed painful oral ulcers, fever, and erythema-like eruptions on her face for about 3 weeks. Skin biopsy of a facial lesion showed a dense infiltrate of neutrophils in the dermis and minimal features of vasculitis, which, with other typical clinical findings, led us to the diagnosis of SS. Although head CT scans, MRIs, magnetic resonance angiography (MRA), or single photon emission computed tomography (SPECT) could not detect any brain lesions, a CSF examination showed a slight pleocytosis of 38/mm^3 with 47% polymorphonuclear cells. It was speculated that the transient aphasia was due to a focal lesion in the CNS attributable to SS.

Treatment

The standard therapy is administration of prednisone or prednisolone at an initial dose of 0.5–1.5 mg/kg body weight with a subsequent slow reduction over 2–4 weeks. Fever and arthralgias mostly subside within 2 days and the skin eruptions within 7 days

(Su *et al.*, 1995; von den Driesch, 1994). Twenty to thirty percent of patients have recurrences (Kemmett and Hunter, 1990; Sitjas *et al.*, 1993). Potassium iodide, colchicine, dapsone, doxycycline, clofazimine, and nonsteroid anti-inflammatory drugs (indomethacin, naproxen) are recommended as alternatives (especially in the context of recurrences).

REFERENCES

Alcalay, J., Filhaber, A., David, M., *et al.* 1987. Sweet's syndrome and subacute thyroiditis. *Dermatologica*, **174**, 28–9.

Bianconcini, G., Mazzali, F., Gardini, G., *et al.* 1991. Sindrome di Sweet (dermatosi neutrofila acuta febbrile) associata a sindrome di Sjögren. Un caso clinico. *Minerva Med*, **82**, 869–76.

Chiba, S. 1983. Sweet's syndrome with neurologic signs and psychiatric symptoms. *Arch Neurol*, **40**, 829.

Cho, K. H., Shin, K. S., Sohn, S. J., *et al.* 1989. Behçet's disease with Sweet's syndrome-like presentation: a report of six cases. *Clin Exp Dermatol*, **14**, 20–4.

Cohen P. R., Almeida, L., and Kurzrock, R. 1989. Acute febrile neutrophilic dermatosis. *Am Fam Physician*, **39**, 199–204.

Cohen, P. R., Holder, W. R., Tucker, S. B., *et al.* 1993. Sweet syndrome in patients with solid tumors. *Cancer*, **72**, 2723–31.

Cohen P. R., and Kurzrock, R. 1987. Sweet's syndrome and malignancy. *Am J Med*, **82**, 1220–6.

Cohen, P. R., and Kurzrock, R. 1993. Sweet's syndrome and cancer. *Clin Dermatol*, **11**, 149–57.

Cohen P. R., and Kurzrock, R. 2000. Sweet's syndrome: a neutrophilic dermatosis classically associated with acute onset and fever. *Clin Dermatol*, **18**, 265–82.

Cohen, P. R., and Kurzrock, R. 2003. Sweet's syndrome revisited: a review of disease concepts. *Int J Dermatol*, **42**, 761–78.

Cohen, P. R., Talpaz, M., and Kurzrock, R. 1988. Malignancy-associated Sweet's syndrome: review of the world literature. *J Clin Oncol*, **6**, 1887–97.

Cooper, P. H., Innes, D. J. J., and Greer, K. E. 1983. Acute febrile neutrophilic dermatosis (Sweet's syndrome) and myeloproliferative disorders. *Cancer*, **51**, 1518–26.

Crow, K. D., Kerdel-Vergas, F., and Rook, A. 1969. Acute febrile neutrophilic dermatosis: Sweet's syndrome. *Dermatologica*, **139**, 123–34.

Delaporte, E., Gaveau, D. J., Piette, F. A., *et al.* 1989. Acute febrile neutrophilic dermatosis (Sweet's syndrome): association with rheumatoid vasculitis. *Arch Dermatol*, **125**, 1101–4.

DiCaudo D. J., and Connolly, S. M. 2002. Neutrophilic dermatosis (pustular vasculitis) of the dorsal hands: a report of seven cases and review of the literature. *Arch Dermatol*, **138**, 361–5.

Druschky, A., von den Driesch, P., Anders, M., *et al.* 1996. Sweet's syndrome (acute febrile neutrophilic dermatosis) affecting the central nervous system. *J Neurol*, **243**, 556–7.

Dunn, T. R., Saperstein, H. W., Biederman, A., *et al.* 1992. Sweet syndrome in a neonate with aseptic meningitis. *Pediatr Dermatol*, **9**, 288–92.

Furukawa, F., Toriyama, R., and Kawanishi, T. 1992. Neutrophils in cerebrospinal fluid of a patient with acute febrile neutrophilic dermatosis (Sweet's syndrome). *Int J Dermatol*, **31**, 670–1.

Geelkerken, R. H., Lagaay, M. B., van Deijk, W. A., *et al.* 1994. Sweet syndrome associated with liposarcoma: a case report. *Neth J Med*, **45**, 107–9.

Goette, D. K. 1985. Sweet's syndrome in subacute cutaneous lupus erythematodes. *Arch Dermatol*, **121**, 789–91.

Going, J. J., Going, S. M., Myskov, M. W., *et al.* 1987. Sweet's syndrome: histological and immunohistochemical study of 15 cases. *J Clin Pathol*, **40**, 175–9.

Gunawardena, D. A., Gunarwardena, K. A., Ratnayaka, M. R. S., *et al.* 1975. The clinical spectrum of Sweet's syndrome (acute febrile neutrophilic dermatosis): a report of eighteen cases. *Br J Dermatol*, **92**, 363–73.

Hisanaga, K., Iwasaki, Y., and Itoyama, Y. 2005. Neuro-Sweet disease: clinical manifestations and criteria for diagnosis. *Neurology*, **64**, 1756–61.

Hommel, L., Harms, M., and Saurat, J.-H. 1993. The incidence of Sweet's syndrome in Geneva: a retrospective study of 29 cases. *Dermatology*, **187**, 303–5.

Jordaan, H. F. 1989. Acute febrile neutrophilic dermatosis: a histopathological study of 37 patients and a review of the literature. *Am J Dermatopathol*, **11**, 99–111.

Kemmett, D., and Hunter, J. A. A. 1990. Sweet's syndrome: a clinico-pathologic review of twenty-nine cases. *J Am Acad Dermatol*, **23**, 503–7.

Levenstein, M. M., Fisher, B. K., Fisher, L. O. L., *et al.* 1991. Simultaneous occurrence of subacute cutaneous lupus erythematosus and Sweet syndrome. A marker of Sjögren syndrome? *Int J Dermatol*, **30**, 640–3.

Ly, S., Beylot-Barry, M., Beyssac, R., *et al.* 1995. Syndrome de Sweet associé à une maladie de Crohn. *La Revue de Medecine Interne*, **16**, 931–3.

Martínez, E., Fernández, A., Mayo, J., *et al.* 1995. Sweet's syndrome associated with cerebrospinal fluid neutrophilic pleocytosis. *Int J Dermatol*, **34**, 73–4.

Matsuda, T., Abe, Y., Arata, J., *et al.* 1994. Acute febrile neutrophilic dermatosis (Sweet's syndrome) associated with extreme infiltration of eosinophils. *J Dermatol*, **21**, 341–6.

Mizoguchi, M., Matsuki, M., Mochizuki, M., *et al.* 1988. Human leukocyte antigen in Sweet's syndrome and its relationship to Behçet's syndrome. *Arch Dermatol*, **124**, 1069–73.

Ohori, N., Kinoshita, T., Toda, K., *et al.* 1999. A case of Sweet's syndrome (acute febrile neutrophilic dermatosis) showing transient jargon aphasia. *Rinsho Shinkeigaku*, **39**, 1156.

Perales, J. L. G., Ortí, R. T., Fayos, J. B., *et al.* 1997. Un caso de síndrome de Sweet Asociado a enfermedad de Crohn. *Gastroenterologia y Hepatologia*, **20**, 134–7.

Sequeira, W., Polisky, R. B., and Alrenga, B. P. 1986. Neutrophilic dermatosis (Sweet's syndrome): association with a hydralazine-induced lupus syndrome. *Am J Med*, **81**, 558–61.

Shimizu, T., Yoshida, I., Eguchi, H., *et al.* 1996. Sweet syndrome in a child with aplastic anemia receiving recombinant granulocyte colony-stimulating factor. *J Pediatr Hematol Oncol*, **18**, 282–4.

Sitjas, D., Puig, L., Cuatrecasas, M., *et al.* 1993. Acute febrile neutrophilic dermatosis (Sweet's syndrome). *Int J Dermatol*, **32**, 261–8.

Sommer, S., Wilkinson, S. M., Merchant, W. J., *et al.* 2000. Sweet's syndrome presenting as palmoplantar pustulosis. *J Am Acad Dermatol*, **42**, 332–4.

Su, W. P. D., Fett, D. L., Gibson, L. E., *et al.* 1995. Sweet syndrome: acute febrile neutrophilic dermatosis. *Semin Dermatol*, **14**, 173–8.

Sweet, R. D. 1964. An acute febrile neutrophilic dermatosis. *Br J Dermatol*, **74**, 349–56.

Sweet, R. D. 1979. Acute febrile neutrophilic dermatosis. *Br J Dermatol*, **100**, 93–9.

Vatan, R., Sire, S., Constans, J., *et al.* 1997. Association syndrome de Goujerot-Sjögren primitif et syndrome de Sweet. À propos d'un cas. *La Revue de Medecine Interne*, **18**, 734–5.

von den Driesch, P. 1994. Sweet's syndrome (acute febrile neutrophilic dermatosis). *J Am Acad Dermatol*, **31**, 535–56.

Walker, D. C., and Cohen, P. R. 1996. Trimethoprim-sulfamethoxazole-associated acute febrile neutrophilic dermatosis: case report and review of drug-induced Sweet's syndrome. *J Am Acad Dermatol*, **34**, 918–23.

54 NEPHROTIC SYNDROME AND OTHER RENAL DISEASES AND STROKE

Rima M. Dafer, José Biller, and Alfredo M. Lopez-Yunez

Introduction

Nephrotic syndrome is defined as proteinuria exceeding 3.5 grams per day, hypoalbuminemia, hyperlipidemia, and edema. (Arneil, 1971; Orth and Ritz, 1998) Nephrotic syndrome, first described by Volhard and Fahr in 1914, is common in both children and adults. Idiopathic nephrotic syndrome accounts for 85% of children and 25% of adults with the disorder. Secondary systemic disorders, which may affect the renal glomeruli, could also contribute to the syndrome.

Minimal change disease (MCD) is the most common cause of nephrotic syndrome in children, although it is not uncommon among adults. The cause of minimal change nephrotic syndrome is unknown; the disease may be preceded by viral infection, allergic reactions, or recent immunizations. Membranous glomerulonephropathy (MGN) accounts for most of the cases of nephrotic syndrome in adults older than 40 years. MGN may be idiopathic or may result secondary to systemic conditions, which may affect the renal glomeruli such as diabetes mellitus or amyloidosis (Orth and Ritz, 1998). Others causes include malignancies (e.g. solid tumors, lymphoma, leukemia, multiple myeloma, pheochromocytoma), systemic infections (e.g. group A β-hemolytic streptococci, hepatitis B, hepatitis C, human immunodeficiency virus, malaria, varicella, infectious mononucleosis, tuberculosis, syphilis), noninfectious inflammatory systemic vasculopathies (e.g. systemic lupus erythematosus [SLE], polyarteritis nodosa, Wegener granulomatosis, Takayasu's, Sjögrens' disease, rheumatoid arthritis), hypersensitivity vasculitides (e.g. Henoch-Schönlein purpura, mixed cryoglobulimemia), and Fabry's disease. Other potential causes include medications such as gold, penicillamine, nonsteroidal anti-inflammatory drugs, trimethadione, probenecid, captopril, lithium, warfarin, penicillamine, mercury, paramethadione), toxins (e.g. mercury, bee sting, poison ivy and oak, snake venom (Olson and Schwartz, 1998).

Thromboembolic events are rare but known complications of renal diseases. Nephrotic syndrome, particularly when associated with idiopathic MGN, and less frequently with diabetic nephropathy and MCD carries a high risk of thrombotic complications with a cumulative incidence of approximating 50% (Andrassy et al., 1983; Cameron, 1987). Most thrombotic complications occur outside the central nervous system, most commonly renal vein thrombosis with an incidence of 10–20% (Harris and Ismail, 1994). The incidence of extrarenal venous thrombosis is 20%; deep venous thrombosis and pulmonary embolism are the most common venoocclusive manifestations in children (8%–28%) (Bernard, 1988; Llach, 1984).

Cerebral thrombo-occlusive complications have been well-recognized complications of the nephrotic syndrome in both children and adults. Such complications usually correlate with the severity of hypoalbuminemia and hypercholesterolemia. Other contributing factors include poor response to steroids, hypovolemia, and degree of hyperviscosity.

Pathophysiology

The pathogenesis of thromboembolic complications in patients with nephrotic syndrome remains unclear. Several factors have been implicated in the development of venous and arterial thromboembolism. Endothelial cell injury (Cosson et al., 2006; Malyszko et al., 2004), platelet hyperreactivity and hyperaggregability secondary to increased activity of adenosine biphosphate (Kanfer, 1990; Orth and Ritz, 1998, lead to thrombosis. Other mechanisms of thrombosis include hyperviscosity and disturbance of the coagulation cascade secondary to excessive urinary excretion of physiological coagulation proteins such as antithrombin (AT), free protein S, and protein C, hypoalbuminemia, and increased levels of several procoagulant coagulation factors such as V, VII, VIII, and X (Table 54.1) (Cameron, 1984; Citak et al., 2000; Molino et al., 2004; Vaziri, 1983).

Microalbuminuria and vascular complications

Microalbuminuria is an index of generalized vascular endothelial dysfunction, especially in hypertension and diabetes (Cao et al., 2006; Jager et al., 1999) and a well-recognized risk factor for stroke in men and women, independent of other vascular risk factors and regardless of stroke mechanism (Beamer et al., 1999; Romundstad et al., 2003).

Microalbuminuria is defined as a urinary albumin-creatinine ratio of 30–299 μg/mg per hour period; it is prevalent in 6.1% of men and 9.7% of women in the general population in the United States (Jones et al., 2002). In normal urine, the biggest excreted protein fraction consists of Tamm-Horsfall protein, originating from renal tubular cells. Low-molecular-weight plasma proteins such as insulin and parathormone are filtered through the glomerular basement membrane and then reabsorbed by the tubular cells. The appearance of any of these proteins in urine is indicative of tubular damage. Conversely, medium-sized (40–150 kd) plasma

Uncommon Causes of Stroke, 2nd edition, ed. Louis R. Caplan. Published by Cambridge University Press. © Cambridge University Press 2008.

Table 54.1 Potential contributing factors for hypercoagulability in nephrotic syndrome

Platelet disorders

Thrombocytosis

Increased thromboglobulin levels

Increased platelet hyperaggregability

Increased platelet activity and function

Increased von Willebrand factor levels

Release of b-thrombomodulin

Elevated Platelet factor 4

Abnormal sialoglycoprotein and other negative-charge sites

Increased procoagulant activity

a2–macroglobulin

C4b-binding protein

Anti-cardiolipin antibodies

Lupus anticoagulant

Factor V Leiden mutation

Fibrinogen level

Factor V, VII, VIII, X

α 2 antiplasmin

Hypoalbuminemia

tPA and PAI-1

Hyperhomocysteinemia

Lipoprotein (a)

Decreased physiological proteins

AT

Free protein-S

Protein C activity

Decreased fibrinolysis

Decreased factor IX, XI, XII

Decreased plasminogen

Hemoconcentration and hyperviscosity

Volume depletion

Hypertension

Pregnancy

Malignancy

Immune complex deposition

Infections

Dyslipidemia

Altered endothelial function

Increased thrombomodulin

Increased intracellular adhesion molecules

Increased vascular cell adhesion molecules

Increased TAFI

Increased vascular endothelial growth factor

Drugs

Steroids

Diuretics

Oral contraceptives

tPA = tissue plasminogen activator; PAI-1 = plasminogen activator inhibitor type I; TAFI = thrombin activatable fibrinolysis inhibitor; AT = antithonbin.

proteins (albumin, transferrin, and high-density lipoprotein particles among others) are not filtered in the glomerulus; therefore, the appearance of these proteins in the urine indicates alteration of the glomerular barrier (Schnaper and Robson, 1996).

In patients with arterial hypertension, the presence of low renal plasma flow and increased renal vascular resistance may lead to higher filtration fraction and increased albumin transmembrane escape. Microalbuminuria occurs in 11%–40% of persons with essential hypertension, the prevalence increasing with age and the duration of hypertension. Hypertensive patients with microalbuminuria have shown higher glomerular filtration rates and higher plasma renin activity when compared with patients without microalbuminuria. Several studies in general unselected populations and in nondiabetic populations have also shown positive correlations between increased urinary albumin excretion and systolic and diastolic blood pressures (Bianchi *et al.*, 1999; Jensen *et al.*, 2000; Karalliedde and Viberti, 2004).

Microalbuminuria is a predictor of all-cause mortality in the general population, with a higher risk of death from coronary artery disease, mainly among type 2 diabetics. (Bloch and Basile, 2005) In a study by Hillege *et al.* (2002), a twofold increase in urine albumin excretion was associated with a relative risk of 1.29 for cardiovascular mortality (95% confidence interval [CI], 1.18–1.40) and 1.12 (95% CI, 1.04–1.21) for other causes of death.

Microalbuminuria is independently associated with approximately 50% increased risk of stroke in the general population (Beamer *et al.*, 1999; Ravera *et al.*, 2002; Turaj *et al.*, 2001; Yuyun *et al.*, 2004). In a prospective study of 23 630 individuals aged 40–79 years, microalbuminuria was independently associated with a 50% increased risk of stroke in the general population, with a hazard ratio (95% CI) of 2.01 (1.29–3.31). Bigazzi *et al.* (1995) reported an increased intima-media thickening in patients with essential hypertension, which significantly correlated with microalbuminuria, blood pressure, and hyperlipidemia (Bigazzi *et al.*, 1995; Mykkanen *et al.*, 1997).

Microalbuminuria is also associated with proliferative diabetic retinopathy (Manaviat *et al.*, 2004; Singh *et al.*, 2001). In a cross-sectional study of 590 patients with type 2 diabetes, the prevalence of microalbuminuria and macroalbuminuria was 25.9% and 14.5%, respectively ($p = .001$). (Manaviat *et al.*, 2004). Patients with diabetic retinopathy and microalbuminuria represent a group with incipient diabetic nephropathy with higher risk for progression to overt proteinuria (Kim *et al.*, 2004).

Microalbuminuria is considered to be a marker of overt nephropathy in diabetic patients, with evident widespread angiopathy (Jensen *et al.*, 2000). The risk of progression from subclinical to overt clinic disease within 10 years is as high as 80% (Mogensen and Christianson, 1994).

Hyperlipidemia

Hyperlipidemia may also contribute to the increased risk for thrombosis seen in nephrotic syndrome. Several abnormalities in lipid metabolism are observed, including elevations in total cholesterol, very low-density lipoprotein, intermediate-density lipoprotein, low-density lipoprotein, and hepatic overproduction

Table 54.2 Mechanisms of cerebral infarction in nephrotic syndrome

Hypercoagulability

Hypovolemia

Large-vessel atherosclerotic occlusive disease

Non-atherosclerotic noninfectious inflammatory vasculopathies

Non-atherosclerotic infectious inflammatory vasculopathies

of lipoprotein (a) (Kronenberg, 2005). These abnormalities may lead to the development of atherosclerosis, endothelial dysfunction, or exacerbation of glomerular injury. Lipoprotein (a), an atherogenic and thrombogenic lipoprotein, inhibits fibrinolysis by competing with the binding of plasminogen to fibrin and to the plasminogen receptor (Kronenberg, 2005). Lipoprotein (a) has been associated with increased risk for atherosclerotic coronary and cerebrovascular disease (Kronenberg et al., 1996; Kuge et al., 2004).

Cerebrovascular disorders and nephrotic syndrome

Brain infarction due to arterial pathology

Arterial complications are relatively less common than venous thrombosis. Nephrotic syndrome carries a risk for coronary artery disease and arterial cerebrovascular disease, predominantly in diabetics (Cameron, 1987; Crew et al., 2004; Ordonez et al., 1993).

Cerebral arterial infarction is an uncommon yet treatable cause of stroke in patients with nephrotic syndrome, predominantly in patients with MGN followed by focal segmental glomerulosclerosis and immunoglobulin A (IgA) nephropathy, and rarely minimal change nephropathy.

The association between arterial ischemic strokes and nephrotic syndrome is well recognized but not well understood. Potential mechanisms of arterial strokes in patients with nephrotic syndrome are summarized in Table 54.2.

Miller et al. (1969) first reported the association of stroke and nephrotic syndrome, but the information was insufficient to exclude other causes of cerebral infarction. Fewer than 20 reports of artery-related brain infarction with nephrotic syndrome in both adults and children have been published in the English literature since this early observation, with fatal outcome in four patients. In 1990, Parag et al. evaluated a young man with nephrotic syndrome associated with left hemiparesis secondary to middle cerebral artery (MCA) thrombosis. On examination he also had anasarca and a superficial abdominal cellulitis. He had a serum albumin of 0.7 g/dL, a 24-hour urinary protein of 10 g, hypercholesterolemia, elevated fibrinogen of 1440 mg/dL, and a decreased AT level of 36%. Clinical course was complicated by a left femoral artery thrombosis. Treatment included embolectomy and heparin, but he eventually died from pulmonary edema. On autopsy, the kidney showed MCD with fusion of podocytes on electron microscopy.

Marsh et al. (1991) reported two young patients with MCA distribution stroke and nephrotic syndrome. The first patient, a 36-year-old man, had a left MCA occlusion in the absence of vascular risk factors or family history of hypercoagulable disorder. There was no evidence of deep venous thrombosis, cardioembolic sources, or large-vessel disease. He had severe hypoalbuminemia and proteinuria, hypocomplementemia, elevated fibrinogen levels, and low free protein S, with otherwise negative prothrombotic and rheumatologic evaluation. Renal biopsy was not obtained. He showed partial improvement after warfarin treatment. The second patient, a 34-year-old man, had a right MCA territory infarction. He had a history of pulmonary embolism and cigarette smoking and a remote history of polysubstance abuse. Family history suggested arterial thrombotic events. Ancillary tests excluded cardioembolic and large-vessel occlusive sources. He had an elevated erythrocyte sedimentation rate, hypoalbuminemia, marked proteinuria, elevated fibrinogen levels, and normal rheumatologic and prothrombotic evaluation. Free protein S was not obtained. Renal biopsy showed membranous glomerulonephritis. He received prednisone and aspirin, but 4 months later, following recurrent pulmonary embolism, he received anticoagulant therapy.

Fritz and Braune (1992) reported a 51-year-old man with a right MCA territory infarction. Aside from cigarette smoking, no other vascular risk factors were found. The patient had all the cardinal manifestations of nephrotic syndrome, including hyperlipidemia. Serum fibrinogen level was elevated, and AT and plasminogen levels were decreased. No renal biopsy was obtained. A diagnosis of associated hypercoagulable disorder was made, but no information was given regarding treatment (Fritz and Braune, 1992). Fuh et al. (1992) found evidence of similar hemostatic abnormalities in seven patients with stroke associated with nephrotic syndrome.

Chaturvedi (1993) reported a fatal case of bilateral cerebral infarctions associated with membranous nephropathy in a 37-year-old woman with a history of arterial hypertension and cigarette smoking. She presented with a left MCA territory infarction and also had occlusion of both the right axillary and radial arteries. Ancillary investigations showed elevated erythrocyte sedimentation rate, raised fibrinogen levels, and findings consistent with nephrotic syndrome. Treatment included intravenous heparin and thrombectomy of the right arm thrombi. Her course was complicated by bilateral cerebellar infarctions progressing rapidly to brain death, despite a suboccipital decompression. Autopsy disclosed left ventricular hypertrophy with no cardiac embolic source and early membranous nephropathy with subepithelial intramembranous deposits on electron microscopy. No evidence for malignancy or cerebral vasculitis was found (Chaturvedi, 1993).

Song et al. (1994) described a 39-year-old woman with a history of membranoproliferative glomerulonephritis who had dysarthria and a left hemiparesis. She had a slight anemia, hypoalbuminemia, and a 24-hour proteinuria of 3.4 g. Platelet count and serum fibrinogen level were normal. Protein C activity was elevated, and plasma antigen level of total protein S and free protein S content were decreased. CT scan of the brain showed multiple subcortical hypodensities involving the right frontal lobe. The patient received warfarin and showed partial improvement (Song *et al.*, 1994).

Another cause of stroke among patients with nephrotic syndrome is cardioembolism. Huang and Chau (1995) evaluated a diabetic patient with nephrotic syndrome without significant carotid atherosclerosis or cardiac disease who developed biventricular thrombi complicated by cerebral infarction. Two-dimensional echocardiography showed a left ventricular thrombus, an intramural right ventricular thrombus, normal chamber size and septum wall thickness, and no regional wall motion abnormalities. He received warfarin, and eventually attained full neurological recovery. The authors concluded that, in the absence of overt cardiac pathology, a hypercoagulable state associated with nephrotic syndrome was the likely cause of biventricular thrombi.

De Gauna *et al.* (1996) evaluated a 45-year-old man with MGN and nephrotic syndrome complicated by occlusion of the posterior inferior cerebellar artery resulting in a Wallenberg syndrome; he also had elevated fibrinogen levels.

Ahmed and Saeed (1995) described a 42-year-old man who presented with chest pain, hemoptysis, and dyspnea. He was found to have disseminated venous thrombosis in the pulmonary artery, deep veins of the lower extremities, renal veins, and inferior vena cava. He had thrombocytopenia, hypoalbuminemia, decreased AT levels, hypercholesterolemia, and elevated fibrinogen. He received anticoagulants and prednisone, but 2 years later developed a right MCA territory infarction. Prothrombin time was 12.4 s (international normalized ratio [INR] was not reported), and 24-h urine protein was 18 g. The authors reported no additional ancillary studies from the second admission, and they attributed his cerebral infarction to an underlying hypercoagulable disorder and subtherapeutic anticoagulation; the possibility of paradoxical embolism was apparently not entertained.

Leno *et al.* (1992) evaluated a 30-year-old hypertensive man who had a fatal basilar artery thrombosis 10 months following the diagnosis of MGN and hypercholesterolemia of 857 mg/dL. Aside from hyperlipidemia and an elevated erythrocyte sedimentation rate, there was no laboratory evidence to support the diagnosis of thrombophilia.

Lee *et al.* (2000) described a 35-year-old woman with brain infarction and concurrent femoral artery thrombosis. She received a thrombectomy of the femoral artery and achieved full recovery on anticoagulation and immunosuppressive therapy.

Pandian *et al.* (2000) reported a patient with nephrotic syndrome secondary to minimal-change disease in a 42-year-old man with history of hypertension, hyperlipidemia, and cigarette smoking, complicated by deep vein thrombosis, and fulminant infarction secondary to thrombosis of the right internal carotid artery extending to the anterior cerebral arteries and MCAs. Albumin level was 1.5 g/dL; protein C, protein S, AT, fibrinogen, and plasminogen tests were not performed.

More recently, Yun *et al.* (2004) described a 53-year-old man with a longstanding history of cigarette smoking who presented with left-sided weakness, dysarthria, and headache 3 weeks following the diagnosis of nephrotic syndrome secondary to focal glomerular sclerosis. Patient was on diuretics, angiotensin-converting enzyme inhibitors (ACEIs), prednisolone, and lamivudine for viral

hepatitis prevention. Magnetic resonance angiography (MRA) showed a right MCA distribution infarction. Free protein S level was 35%. AT and fibrinogen levels were normal. He received anticoagulation and had no recurrent neurological symptoms at 1-year follow up (Yun *et al.*, 2004).

Kotani and Kawano (2005) evaluated a 28-year-old woman with right hemiparesis. She had a personal history of cigarette smoking and a family history of stroke and coronary artery disease. Hematological studies including coagulation and fibrinolysis were normal. Cholesterol level was 294 mg/dL, and albumin was 2.6 g/dL. Serum lipoprotein (a) was 266 mg/dL. CT scan showed a subcortical white matter infarction. The patient was subsequently diagnosed with nephrotic syndrome. She declined renal biopsy. She was treated with ACEIs, platelet antiaggregants, and corticosteroids. At 3 months follow up, lipoprotein (a) remained elevated (Kotani and Kawano, 2005).

Other reported causes of cerebral infarction and myocardial infarction associated with hyperlipoproteinemia and nephrotic syndrome have been reported in patients with SLE (Haba *et al.*, 1988; Takegoshi *et al.*, 1990).

Reports of brain artery-related infarctions in adults with nephrotic syndrome are summarized in Table 54.3.

Brain infarction may also complicate the course of children with nephrotic syndrome. Thrombosis may be either venous or arterial, occurring anywhere from <2% (Egli *et al.*, 1973) to one-third of patients (Hoyer *et al.*, 1986). In 1984, the International Study of Kidney Disease in Children studied the mortality of children with nephrotic syndrome and minimal change on renal biopsy (Report of the International Study of Kidney Disease in Children, 1984). Of 389 patients with minimal changes on renal biopsy, 10 patients died, one had cerebral venous thrombosis (CVT), and none had a cerebral infarction. Although these data stress the low frequency of these complications, it should be remembered that cerebrovascular events might be asymptomatic, overlooked, or (not uncommonly) misinterpreted.

Thrombi involving the large vessels have been found on autopsy in 20% of patients affected by the congenital nephrotic syndrome of the Finnish type (Huttunen, 1976). Many cases of cerebral infarctions secondary to arterial thrombosis have been reported in children, with fulminant outcome (Chou and Chen, 1991; Raghu *et al.*, 1981). While some reports provide insufficient information to allow further analysis of stroke mechanisms, others suggest hemodynamic rather than thromboembolic mechanisms (Huemer *et al.*, 1998; Raghu *et al.*, 1981).

Congenital nephrotic syndrome may also follow focal segmental glomerulosclerosis in association with dysmorphic features and systemic involvement (Ehrich *et al.*, 1995). Ehrich *et al.* described five patients with steroid-resistant nephrotic syndrome associated with spondyloepiphyseal dysplasia, growth failure, and lymphopenia. They also had episodic neurologic deficits including ataxia, dysarthria, hemiparesis, and amaurosis fugax. The authors hypothesized that these transient ischemic attacks are secondary to a generalized vascular defect involving the glomerular capillaries and the cerebral arteries. However, in the absence of definitive ancillary studies to allow exclusion of other causes of cerebral ischemia in these children, a sensible conclusion

Table 54.3 Arterial cerebral thrombosis in adults with nephrotic syndrome

Author (Year)	Age/Gender	Disease	Arterial distribution	Hematological abnormalities				Rx	Neurological Outcome
				Albg/dL	Free PS%	AT%	Other		
Levine et al., 1989	40/F	N/A	Bilateral PCA and SCA	N/A					Partial R
Parag et al., 1990	23/M	MCD	Left MCA	0.7		Low		AC	Died
Takegoshi et al., 1990	18/M	N/A	N/A				Lipoprotein (a)	Apheresis	
Marsh et al., 1991	36/M	N/A	Left MCA	2.4	Low	NL		AC	Partial R
Marsh et al., 1991	34/M	MGN	Right MCA	2.7		NL		ASA + P; AC	
Fritz and Braune, 1992	51/M	NA	MCA	2.0		Low			
Fuh et al., 1992	28/M	MGN	Right MCA	1.6		Low		AC	Partial R
Fuh et al., 1992	21/M	MCD	Right MCA	1.5		Low	Low PC	AC	Partial R
Leno et al., 1992	30/M	MGN	VB	2.9	NL	NL			Died
Chatuvedi, 1993	37/F	MGN	Bilateral MCA	2.6	Low			AC	Died
Kanazawa et al., 1994	78/F	N/A	Left MCA						
Song et al., 1994	39/F	MPGN	Right MCA		Low			AC	Partial R
Huang and Chau, 1995	M	N/A	N/A				Cardiac thrombi	AC	Full R
de Gauna et al., 1996	45/M	MGN	PICA						
Ahmed and Saeed, 1995	42/M	N/A	Right MCA			Low		AC	
Ogawa et al., 1999	59/M	MGN	Bilateral PCA	1.7	NL				
Lee et al., 2000	35/F	IGA	Left MCA	1.1	NL			AC	Partial R
Pandian et al., 2000	42/M	MCD	Right MCA Right ACA	1.5					Died
Naganuma et al., 2003	47/M	N/A	Left MCA					AC	Partial R
Kotani and Kawano, 2005	28/F	N/A	White matter	2.6	NL	NL	Lipoprotein (a)	ASA + P	Partial R
Yun et al., 2004	53/M	FSG	MCA	1.2	Low	NL		AC	Partial R

FSG = focal glomerular sclerosis; P = prednisone; ASA = aspirin; AC = anticoagulation; PE = pulmonary embolism; PCA = posterior cerebral artery; PICA = posterior inferior cerebellar artery; SCA = superior cerebellar artery; ACA = anterior cerebral artery; PS = protein S; PC = protein C; NL = normal; N/A = not available; Rx = treatment; Alb = albumin; IGA = immunoglobulin A; MGN = membranous glomerulonephritis; MCD = minimal change disease; MPGN = membranoproliferative glomerulonephritis; R = recovery.

is that stroke mechanisms remain undetermined among these patients.

Igarashi et al. (1988) reported two children with brain infarction, one with congenital nephrotic syndrome, and one with minimal change nephrotic syndrome. The first patient, born at 34 weeks gestational age, required 4 weeks of hospitalization in an intensive care setting because of respiratory distress syndrome. He had motor and language developmental delay. At 9 months of age, congenital nephrotic syndrome resistant to prednisone and cyclophosphamide was diagnosed on the basis of severe proteinuria, hypoalbuminemia, and focal glomerulosclerosis with mesangial proliferation on renal biopsy. At age 3 years, he had partial seizures with secondary generalization prompting phenytoin treatment. Six months later, he developed right hemiparesis, lethargy, and a head tilt. Ancillary studies disclosed anemia, thrombocytosis, hypoalbuminemia of 1.5 g/dL, total proteinuria of 3.4 g/dL, borderline low AT levels of 22.5 (normal 24.8–30.0), and multiple bilateral hypodensities on brain CT. His course was complicated by brain edema leading to death 6 days later. Autopsy showed multiple, bilateral hemispheric infarctions and thrombosis of the small cerebral arteries. The second patient, an 11-year-old boy with a 9-year history of nephrotic syndrome had

Table 54.4 CVT in adults with nephrotic syndrome

Author (Year)	Age/Gender	Disease	Clinical Picture	Site	Hematologic abnormalities	Rx	Outcome
Barthélémy et al., 1980	50/M	MCD	Headache, papilledema	SSS, LS		AC	Complete R
Levine et al., 1989	32/M	N/A	Headache, papilledema, superior oblique palsy	SSS, SS	LA		Complete R
Purvin et al., 1987	34/M	N/A	Headache, loss of vision, papilledema	LS			
Tovi et al., 1988	46/M	N/A	Superior vena cava syndrome	LS			Complete R
Burns et al., 1995	20/M	MCD	Seizures, personality changes	SSS	Low AT		Fatal
Burns et al., 1995	35/M	MCD	Headache, oculomotor nerve	ISS	High fibrinogen		Partial R
Laversuch et al., 1995	42/F	MGN	Headache, seizure	LS	Low protein S	AC	Complete R
Urch and Pusey, 1996	41/F	MCD	Headache aphasia, hemiparesis	SSS			Complete R
Urch and Pusey, 1996	?/M	MCD	Headache, aphasia	SSS, LS			Complete R
Akatsu et al., 1997	65/F		Headache hemiparesis	SSS	AT		Complete R
Hirata et al., 1999	46/M	MCD	Headache, papilledema	SSS, LS		AC	Complete R
Philips et al., 1999	29/M		Seizures, cranial nerve palsies	SSS, LS, SiS IJV		Lysis	Complete R
Sung et al., 1999	45/F		Hemiparesis, hemiparesthesia	SSS	Low protein S		Complete R
Nishi et al., 2006	79/F	Amyl.	Altered mental status	LS, SiS			Fatal

SSS = superior sagittal sinus; SS = straight sinus; LS = lateral sinus; SiS = sigmoid sinus; IJV = internal jugular vein; N/A = not available; LA = lupus anticoagulant; Rx = treatment; AC = anticoagulation; Amyl. = amyloidosis; R = recovery.

dysarthria and bifrontal headaches that progressed to aphasia and right-sided hemiparesis. Laboratory data showed thrombocytosis of 658 000/mm^3, albumin of 1.7, and AT levels of 58%. He received prednisone and warfarin until nephrotic syndrome remitted, but was left with a moderate right-sided hemiparesis and aphasia requiring special education classes.

An unusual case of Capgras syndrome has been described in association with nephrotic syndrome in a 31-year-old eclamptic woman who became agitated and disoriented. Capgras syndrome is a rare misidentification phenomenon whereby a patient believes that someone, usually a loved one, has been replaced by an identical looking impostor. She had the delusion that her husband had been replaced by an impostor. Brain CT scan was normal. Renal biopsy showed IgA nephropathy. Symptoms subsided within 3 days. This observation raises the possibility of a probable reversible ischemic leukoencephalopathy in the context of hypertensive encephalopathy and nephrotic syndrome (Collins et al., 1990).

Diffuse cerebral hypoperfusion has been reported on single photon emission computed tomography (SPECT) in a boy with steroid-resistant nephrotic syndrome who developed speech, motor, and developmental delay. The findings on SPECT resolved as the nephrotic syndrome remitted, with remarkable clinical improvement (Ito et al., 2002).

Several vasculitides may also result in nephrotic syndrome, usually associated with membranoproliferative and cresentric glomerulonephritis. These include SLE, Wegener's granulomatosis, Goodpasture syndrome, polyarteritis nodosa, and Takayasu's disease (Arita et al., 1988; Garcia et al., 2004; Haba et al., 1988; Levine et al., 1989; Takegoshi et al., 1990). Finally, noninflammatory vasculopathies may play a pathogenic role as in the patient with Sneddon's syndrome, mesangial glomerulonephritis with segmental IgA deposition, and lacunar infarctions reported by Ohtani et al. (1995).

CVT

CVT is a well-recognized complication of nephrotic syndrome. Both dural sinuses and cerebral veins can be involved, most commonly the superior sagittal sinus. Unlike arterial thrombosis, which is predominantly seen in MGN, venous thrombosis is common in minimal-change disease (Burns et al., 1995; Cameron, 1987; Lin et al., 2002).

Table 54.5 CVT in children with nephrotic syndrome

Author (Year)	Age (yr)/Gender	Disease	CP	Venous Occlusion	Hematologic abnormalities	Rx	Outcome
Egli et al., 1973	12/M		Headache	SS			Complete R
Lau et al., 1980	2H/M		Seizure, hemiparesis	SSS	Low factor XII; high factor V		Complete R
Parchoux et al., 1981	4m/M		Hydrocephalus	Bilateral LS			Complete R
Purvin et al., 1987	4/F		Coma, headache, papilledema	SSS, SS			Partial R
Negrier et al., 1991	2/M		Seizure, vomiting	SSS, CV	Low factor XII		Fatal
Freycon et al., 1992	3/M		Vomiting, papilledema	SSS			Complete R
Burns et al., 1995	17/M	MCD	Headaches, seizures	CV	High vWF		Complete R
Divekar et al., 1996	3/M		Seizures, papilledema	SSS, LS	Low AT		Complete R
de Saint-Martin, 1997	3/?		Drowsiness, hemiparesis	SSS		AC	Complete R
Fofah and Roth, 1997	Newborn/F		Seizure	SSS, SS, LS	Low protein S and protein C		Partial R
Mandai et al., 1997	12/M		Altered consciousness, hemiparesis, convulsions	SSS			
Pillekamp et al., 1997	5/M		Vomiting, headache, seizure	SSS	Low AT		Complete R
Tullu et al., 1999	2.5/M	MCD	Fever, irritability	SSS			Complete R
Sung et al., 1999	15/M		Headache, seizure, hemiparesis	SSS	Low protein S ACL		Partial R
Meena et al., 2000	4/M	MCD	Headache, vomiting, papilledema, seizures	SSS	Thrombocytosis	AC	Complete R
Lin et al., 2002	7/M		Status epilepticus, papilledema, coma	SS		AC	Partial R
Rodrigues et al., 2003	9/M		Headache, vomiting, papilledema	SSS, LS		AC	Complete R
Papachristou et al., 2005	8.5/F		Vomiting, headache, impaired consciousness	SSS		AC	Complete R
Gangakhedkar et al., 2005	9/M		Dehydration, seizure		Low AT	AC	Partial R

SSS = superior sagittal sinus; SS = straight sinus; LS = lateral sinus; SiS = sigmoid sinus; IJV = internal jugular vein; CV = cerebral vein; N/A = not available; ACL = anti-cardiolipin antibodies; Rx = treatment; AC = anticoagulation; vWF = von Willebrand Factor; R = recovery.

Since first described by Barthélémy et al. in 1980, CVT as a complication of nephrotic syndrome has been well reported. The majority of cases of CVT may go unnoticed. When symptomatic, patients usually present with headaches, vomiting, seizures, papilledema, and focal neurological deficit. The risk is increased with the severity of hypoalbuminemia. The risk is increased in patients with associated thrombotic tendencies such as cigarette smoking and/or estrogen supplementation.

Contrasted CT scan or MRI examinations usually demonstrate hyperdense areas along the dural sinuses. MR venogram may show filling defects in the involved sinus or cerebral vein, and may eliminate the need for conventional cerebral angiogram. Patients with SLE are particularly at risk of CVT. At least one-third of the reported cases of CVT associated with SLE had nephrotic syndrome (Vidailhet et al., 1990), with an increased risk in the presence of anti-cardiolipin antibodies and lupus anticoagulant. Tables 54.3 and 54.4 summarize reported CVT in adults and children with nephrotic syndrome.

Intracranial hemorrhage

Intracranial hemorrhage is not a direct complication of nephrotic syndrome. When present, a clear cause such as hemorrhagic transformation in CVT (Mandai et al., 1997), thrombocytopenia (Leung et al., 1998), or coexistent intracranial aneurysms (Nagayasu et al., 1986) is implicated.

Management

A high suspicion for stroke should be raised in patients with nephrotic syndrome, especially in children and young adults when other well-recognized risk factors of stroke are absent. MRA and MR venography are helpful to confirm the diagnosis, and dye-contrast catheter cerebral angiography is rarely necessary. Maintenance of a normovolemic state, management of plasma lipid abnormalities, proteinuria, blood pressure control, and treatment of underlying infection are keys in the prevention of thrombotic complications. Caution should be taken in patients on prednisone, because steroids may contribute to decreased fibrinolytic activity by incomplete breakdown of thrombus, and may therefore potentiate the risk of thrombotic complications. In contrast, diuretics may lead to volume depletion and thereby contribute to plasma hemoconcentration and hyperviscosity (Cameron, 1987; Orth and Ritz, 1998).

Despite the high risk of thrombotic complications in nephrotic syndrome, prophylactic therapy with platelet antiaggregants remains controversial. Neurologists have empirically used prophylactic anticoagulation in patients with severe hypoalbuminemia and marked coagulation abnormalities, especially in patients with MGN, in the absence of prospective randomized trials evaluating the efficacy of such treatment.

Anticoagulation should be initiated in all patients with documented symptomatic thromboembolic events (Crew *et al.*, 2004; Orth and Ritz, 1998). Caution should be taken when starting patients on oral anticoagulation, because of the relatively decreased AT levels of a short course of heparin is recommended initially, followed by warfarin (Singhal and Brimble, 2006). The dose of warfarin must be adjusted as necessary with changes in serum albumin levels. In patients with CVT presenting with seizures, concomitant use of anticonvulsants should be cautiously monitored because of the potential interaction with warfarin, and fluctuation of the INR. Thrombolytic therapies with urokinase or streptokinase may be considered in patients with rapidly progressing symptoms and in patients with acute pulmonary emboli (Beaufils *et al.*, 1985; Philips *et al.*, 1999). Low-density lipoprotein apheresis is an alternative therapy in symptomatic patients with veno-occlusive complications and drug-resistant hyperlipidemia, especially in diabetics and in patients with recurrent focal glomerulosclerosis resistant to steroids (Stenvinkel *et al.*, 2000; Takegoshi *et al.*, 1990).

Conclusion

Neurologists should remain attentive to the potential danger associated with arterial and venous pathology in patients with nephrotic syndrome, specifically when membranous glomerulonephritis is the culprit. Nephrotic syndrome should be considered in any patient with ischemic stroke and pre-existing renal disease, especially in young patients without other defined predisposing conditions for cerebrovascular disease. While no consensus exists about the need for prophylactic anticoagulation, antiplatelet therapy could be beneficial in high-risk patients and in those with severe hypoalbuminemia. Once the diagnosis of thrombotic or occlusive cerebral event is established, anticoagulation should be immediately initiated.

REFERENCES

Ahmed, K., and Saeed, E. 1995. Nephrotic syndrome and pulmonary artery thrombosis. *Am J Nephrol*, **15**, 274–6.

Akatsu, H., Vaysburd, M., *et al.* 1997. Cerebral venous thrombosis in nephrotic syndrome. *Clin Nephrol*, **48**, 317–20.

Andrassy, K., Poertel, P. J., *et al.* 1983. Thromboembolic complications and haemostasis in the nephrotic syndrome – is there a difference between children and adults? *Proc Eur Dial Transplant Assoc*, **19**, 597–601.

Arita, M., Iwane, M., Nakamura, Y., Nishio, I. 1998. Anticoagulants in Takayasu's arteritis associated with crescentic glomerulonephritis and nephrotic syndrome: a case report. *Angiology*, **49**, 75–8.

Arneil, G. C. 1971. The nephrotic syndrome. *Pediatr Clin North Am*, **18**, 547–59.

Barthélémy, M., Bousser, M. G., *et al.* 1980. Cerebral venous thrombosis, complication of the nephrotic syndrome (author's transl). *Nouv Presse Med*, **9**, 367–9.

Beamer, N. B., Coull, B. M., *et al.* 1999. Microalbuminuria in ischemic stroke. *Arch Neurol*, **56**, 699–702.

Beaufils, F., Schlegel, N., *et al.* 1985. Urokinase treatment of pulmonary artery thrombosis complicating the pediatric nephrotic syndrome. *Crit Care Med*, **13**, 132–4.

Bernard, D. B. 1988. Extrarenal complications of the nephrotic syndrome. *Kidney Int*, **33**, 1184–202.

Bianchi, S., Bigazzi, R., *et al.* 1999. Microalbuminuria in essential hypertension: significance, pathophysiology, and therapeutic implications. *Am J Kidney Dis*, **34**, 973–95.

Bigazzi, R., Bianchi, S., *et al.* 1995. Increased thickness of the carotid artery in patients with essential hypertension and microalbuminuria. *J Hum Hypertens*, **9**, 827–33.

Bloch, M. J., and Basile, J. 2005. Lower levels of microalbuminuria are associated with an increased risk of coronary heart disease and death in hypertensive subjects. *J Clin Hypertens (Greenwich)*, **7**, 555–7.

Burns, A., Wilson, E., *et al.* 1995. Cerebral venous sinus thrombosis in minimal change nephrotic syndrome. *Nephrol Dial Transplant*, **10**, 30–4.

Cameron, J. S. 1984. Coagulation and thromboembolic complications in the nephrotic syndrome. *Adv Nephrol Necker Hosp*, **13**, 75–114.

Cameron, J. S. 1987. The nephrotic syndrome and its complications. *Am J Kidney Dis*, **10**, 157–71.

Cao, J. J., Barzilay, J. I., *et al.* 2006. The association of microalbuminuria with clinical cardiovascular disease and subclinical atherosclerosis in the elderly: the Cardiovascular Health Study. *Atherosclerosis*, **187**, 372–7. Epub 2005 Oct 20.

Chaturvedi, S. 1993. Fulminant cerebral infarctions with membranous nephropathy. *Stroke*, **24**, 473–5.

Chou, K. S., and Chen, J. Y. 1991. [Nephrotic syndrome complicated with cerebral infarction: report of one case]. *Zhonghua Min Guo Xiao Er Ke Yi Xue Hui Za Zhi*, **32**, 396–402.

Citak, A., Emre, S., *et al.* 2000. Hemostatic problems and thromboembolic complications in nephrotic children. *Pediatr Nephrol*, **14**, 138–42.

Collins, M. N., Hawthorne, M. E., *et al.* 1990. Capgras syndrome with organic disorders. *Postgrad Med J*, **66**, 1064–7.

Cosson, E., Pham, I., *et al.* 2006. Impaired coronary endothelium-dependent vasodilation is associated with microalbuminuria in patients with type 2 diabetes and angiographically normal coronary arteries. *Diabetes Care*, **29**, 107–12.

Crew, R. J., Radhakrishnan, J., *et al.* 2004. Complications of the nephrotic syndrome and their treatment. *Clin Nephrol*, **62**, 245–59.

de Gauna, R. R., Alcelay, L. G., *et al.* 1996. Thrombosis of the posterior inferior cerebellar artery secondary to nephrotic syndrome. *Nephron*, **72**, 123.

de Saint-Martin, A., Terzic, J., *et al.* 1997. Superior sagittal sinus thrombosis and nephrotic syndrome: favorable outcome with low molecular weight heparin. *Arch Pediatr*, **4**, 849–52.

Divekar, A. A., Ali, U. S., et al. 1996. Superior sagittal sinus thrombosis in a child with nephrotic syndrome. Pediatr Nephrol, 10, 206–7.

Egli, F., Elmiger, P., et al. 1973. Thrombosis as a complication of nephrotic syndrome. Helv Paediatr Acta, 30(Suppl), 20–1.

Ehrich, J. H., Burchert, W., Schirg, E., et al. 1995. Steroid resistant nephrotic syndrome associated with spondyloepiphyseal dysplasia, transient ischemic attacks and lymphopenia. Clin Nephrol, 43, 89–95.

Fofah, O., and Roth, P. 1997. Congenital nephrotic syndrome presenting with cerebral venous thrombosis, hypocalcemia, and seizures in the neonatal period. J Perinatol, 17, 492–4.

Freycon, M. T., Richard, O., et al. 1992. Intracranial venous sinus thrombosis in nephrotic syndrome. Pediatrie, 47, 513–6.

Fritz, C., and Braune, H. J. 1992. Cerebral infarction and nephrotic syndrome. Stroke, 23, 1380–1.

Fuh, J. L., Teng, M. M., et al. 1992. Cerebral infarction in young men with nephrotic syndrome. Stroke, 23, 295–7.

Gangakhedkar, A., Wong, W., et al. 2005. Cerebral thrombosis in childhood nephrosis. J Paediatr Child Health, 41, 221–4.

Garcia, C., Renard, C., et al. 2004. A "pulseless" woman with proteinuria! Ann Biol Clin (Paris), 62, 441–5.

Haba, T., Hirai, J., et al. 1988. Myocardial and cerebral infarction in a 17-year-old man with hyper-lp (a) lipoproteinemia and hypercholesterolemia associated with nephrotic syndrome due to systemic lupus erythematosus. Nippon Naika Gakkai Zasshi, 77, 591–2.

Harris, R. C., and Ismail, N. 1994. Extrarenal complications of the nephrotic syndrome. Am J Kidney Dis, 23, 477–97.

Hillege, H. L., Fidler, V., et al. 2002. Urinary albumin excretion predicts cardiovascular and noncardiovascular mortality in general population. Circulation, 106, 1777–82.

Hirata, M., Kuroda, M., et al. 1999. [Cerebral venous thrombosis in minimal change nephrotic syndrome]. Nippon Jinzo Gakkai Shi, 41, 464–8.

Hoyer, P. F., Gonda, S., et al. 1986. Thromboembolic complications in children with nephrotic syndrome. Risk and incidence. Acta Paediatr Scand, 75, 804–10.

Huang, T. Y., and Chau, K. M. 1995. Biventricular thrombi in diabetic nephrotic syndrome complicated by cerebral embolism. Int J Cardiol, 50, 193–6.

Huemer, M., Emminger, W., et al. 1998. Kinking and stenosis of the carotid artery associated with homolateral ischaemic brain infarction in a patient treated with cyclosporin A. Eur J Pediatr, 157, 599–601.

Huttunen, N. P. 1976. Congenital nephrotic syndrome of Finnish type. Study of 75 patients. Arch Dis Child, 51, 344–8.

Igarashi, M., Roy, S. 3rd, et al. 1988. Cerebrovascular complications in children with nephrotic syndrome. Pediatr Neurol, 4, 362–5.

Ito, S., Nezu, A., et al. 2002. Latent cerebral hypoperfusion in a boy with persistent nephrotic syndrome. Brain Dev, 24, 780–3.

Jager, A., Kostense, P. J., et al. 1999. Microalbuminuria and peripheral arterial disease are independent predictors of cardiovascular and all-cause mortality, especially among hypertensive subjects: five-year follow-up of the Hoorn Study. Arterioscler Thromb Vasc Biol, 19, 617–24.

Jensen, J. S., Feldt-Rasmussen, B., et al. 2000. Arterial hypertension, microalbuminuria, and risk of ischemic heart disease. Hypertension, 35, 898–903.

Jones, C. A., Francis, M. E., et al. 2002. Microalbuminuria in the US population: third National Health and Nutrition Examination Survey. Am J Kidney Dis, 39, 445–59.

Kanazawa, A., Hattori, Y., et al. 1994. [A 78-year-old woman with rheumatoid arthritis, right hemiparesis, and renal failure]. No To Shinkei, 46, 1191–200.

Kanfer, A. 1990. Coagulation factors in nephrotic syndrome. Am J Nephrol, 10(Suppl 1), 63–8.

Karalliedde, J., and Viberti, G. 2004. Microalbuminuria and cardiovascular risk. Am J Hypertens, 17, 986–93.

Kim, K. S., Koh, J. M., et al. 2004. Incidence of overt proteinuria and coronary artery disease in patients with type 2 diabetes mellitus: the role of microalbuminuria and retinopathy. Diabetes Res Clin Pract, 65, 159–65.

Kotani, K., and Kawano, M. 2005. A young female with marked hyperlipoprotein(a)emia associated with nephrotic syndrome and stroke. J Atheroscler Thromb, 12, 234.

Kronenberg, F. 2005. Dyslipidemia and nephrotic syndrome: recent advances. J Ren Nutr, 15, 195–203.

Kronenberg, F., Utermann, G., et al. 1996. Lipoprotein(a) in renal disease. Am J Kidney Dis, 27, 1–25.

Kuge, Y., Nozaki, S., et al. 2004. A case of marked hyperlipoprotein(a)emia associated with nephrotic syndrome and advanced atherosclerosis. J Atheroscler Thromb, 11, 293–8.

Lau, S. O., Bock, G. H., et al. 1980. Sagittal sinus thrombosis in the nephrotic syndrome. J Pediatr, 97, 948–50.

Laversuch, C. J., Brown, M. M., et al. 1995. Cerebral venous thrombosis and acquired protein S deficiency: an uncommon cause of headache in systemic lupus erythematosus. Br J Rheumatol, 34, 572–5.

Lee, C. H., Chen, K. S., et al. 2000. Concurrent thrombosis of cerebral and femoral arteries in a patient with nephrotic syndrome. Am J Nephrol, 20, 483–6.

Leno, C., Pascual, J., et al. 1992. Nephrotic syndrome, accelerated atherosclerosis, and stroke. Stroke, 23, 921–2.

Leung, T. F., Tsoi, W. C., Li, C. K., et al. 1998. A Chinese adolescent girl with Fechtner-like syndrome. Acta Paediatr, 87, 705–7.

Levine, S. R., Quint, D. J., et al. 1989. Intraluminal clot in the vertebrobasilar circulation: clinical and radiologic features. Neurology, 39, 515–22.

Lin, C. C., Lui, C. C., et al. 2002. Thalamic stroke secondary to straight sinus thrombosis in a nephrotic child. Pediatr Nephrol, 17, 184–6.

Llach, F. 1984. Thromboembolic complications in nephrotic syndrome. Coagulation abnormalities, renal vein thrombosis, and other conditions. Postgrad Med J, 76, 111–4, 116–8, 121–3.

Malyszko, J., Malyszko, J. S., et al. 2004. Endothelial cell injury markers in chronic renal failure on conservative treatment and continuous ambulatory peritoneal dialysis. Kidney Blood Press Res, 27, 71–7.

Manaviat, M. R., Afkhami, M., et al. 2004. Retinopathy and microalbuminuria in type II diabetic patients. BMC Ophthalmol, 4, 9.

Mandai, K., Tamaki, N., et al. 1997. [A case of intracranial hemorrhage following superior sagittal sinus thrombosis associated with nephrotic syndrome]. No Shinkei Geka, 25, 1101–3.

Marsh, E. E. 3rd, Biller, J., et al. 1991. Cerebral infarction in patients with nephrotic syndrome. Stroke, 22, 90–3.

Meena, A. K., Naidu, K. S., Murthy, J., M. 2000, Cortical sinovenous thrombosis in a child with nephrotic syndrome and iron deficiency anaemia. Neurol India. 48, 292–4.

Mogensen, C. E., and Christianson, C. K. 1994. Predicting diabetic nephropathy in insulin-dependent patients. N Engl J Med, 311, 89–93.

Molino, D., De Santo, N. G., et al. 2004. Plasma levels of plasminogen activator inhibitor type 1, factor VIII, prothrombin activation fragment 1+2, anticardiolipin, and antiprothrombin antibodies are risk factors for thrombosis in hemodialysis patients. Semin Nephrol, 24, 495–501.

Mykkanen, L., Zaccaro, D. J., et al. 1997. Microalbuminuria and carotid artery intima-media thickness in nondiabetic and NIDDM subjects. The Insulin Resistance Atherosclerosis Study (IRAS). Stroke, 28, 1710–6.

Naganuma, M., Sugimoto, R., et al. 2003. [A case of brain infarction with nephrotic syndrome]. Rinsho Shinkeigaku, 43, 126–9.

Nagayasu, S., Hanakita, J., Miyake, H., Suzuki, T., and Nishi, S. 1986. A case of systemic lupus erythematosus associated with multiple intracranial aneurysms. No Shinkei Geka, 14, 1251–5.

Negrier, C., Delmas, M. C., et al. 1991. Decreased factor XII activity in a child with nephrotic syndrome and thromboembolic complications. Thromb Haemost, 66, 512–3.

Nishi, H., Abe, A., Kita, A., et al. 2006. Cerebral venous thrombosis in adult nephrotic syndrome due to systemic amyloidosis. Clin Nephrol, 65, 61–4.

Ogawa, M., Tsukahara, T., et al. 1999. Nephrotic syndrome with acute renal failure and cerebral infarction in a patient with myasthenia gravis. Am J Nephrol, 19, 622–3.

Ohtani, H., Imai, H., Yasuda, T. et al. 1995. A combination of livedo racemosa, occlusion of cerebral blood vessels, and nephropathy: kidney involvement in Sneddon's syndrome. Am J Kidney Dis, 26, 511–5.

Olson, J. L., and Schwartz, M. 1998. The nephrotic syndrome: minimal change disease, focal segmental glomerulosclerosis, and miscellaneous causes. In Heptinstall's Pathology of the Kidney, 5th edn, C. Jenette, J. Olson, M. Schwartz, and F. Silva (eds.). Boston: Lippincott-Raven, pp. 196–9.

Ordonez, J. D., Hiatt, R. A., *et al.* 1993. The increased risk of coronary heart disease associated with nephrotic syndrome. *Kidney Int*, **44**, 638–42.

Orth, S. R., and Ritz, E. 1998. The nephrotic syndrome. *N Engl J Med*, **338**, 1202–11.

Pandian, J. D., Sarada, C., *et al.* 2000. Fulminant cerebral infarction in a patient with nephrotic syndrome. *Neurol India*, **48**, 179–81.

Papachristou, F. T., Petridou, S. H., *et al.* 2005. Superior sagittal sinus thrombosis in steroid-resistant nephrotic syndrome. *Pediatr Neurol*, **32**, 282–4.

Parag, K. B., Somers, S. R., *et al.* 1990. Arterial thrombosis in nephrotic syndrome. *Am J Kidney Dis*, **15**, 176–7.

Parchoux, B., Cotton, J. B., *et al.* 1981. [Congenital nephrotic syndrome, thrombosis of a renal vein and hydrocephalus. Apropos of a case]. *Pediatrie*, **36**, 55–9.

Philips, M. F., Bagley, L. J., *et al.* 1999. Endovascular thrombolysis for symptomatic cerebral venous thrombosis. *J Neurosurg*, **90**, 65–71.

Pillekamp, F., Hoppe, B., *et al.* 1997. Vomiting, headache and seizures in a child with idiopathic nephrotic syndrome. *Nephrol Dial Transplant*, **12**, 1280–1.

Purvin, V., Dunn, D. W., *et al.* 1987. MRI and cerebral venous thrombosis. *Comput Radiol*, **11**, 75–9.

Raghu, K., Malik, A. K., *et al.* 1981. Focal glomerulosclerosis with cerebral infarction in a young nephrotic patient. *Indian Pediatr*, **18**, 754–6.

Ravera, M., Ratto, E., *et al.* 2002. Microalbuminuria and subclinical cerebrovascular damage in essential hypertension. *J Nephrol*, **15**, 519–24.

Report of the International Study of Kidney Disease in Children. 1984. Minimal change nephrotic syndrome in children: deaths during the first 5 to 15 years' observation. *Pediatrics*, **73**, 497–501.

Rodrigues, M. M., Zardini, L. R., *et al.* 2003. Cerebral sinovenous thrombosis in a nephrotic child. *Arq Neuropsiquiatr*, **61**, 1026–9.

Romundstad, S., Holmen, J., *et al.* 2003. Microalbuminuria and all-cause mortality in 2089 apparently healthy individuals: a 4.4-year follow-up study. The Nord-Trondelag Health Study (HUNT), Norway. *Am J Kidney Dis*, **42**, 466–73.

Schnaper, H. W., and Robson, A. M. 1996. Nephrotic syndrome: minimal change disease, focal glomerulosclerosis, and related disorders. In *Diseases of the Kidney*, 6th edn, R. Schrier, and C. Gottschalk (eds.). Boston: Little, Brown & Co., pp. 1747–9.

Singh, S. K., Behre, A., *et al.* 2001. Diabetic retinopathy and microalbuminuria in lean type 2 diabetes mellitus. *J Assoc Physicians India*, **49**, 439–41.

Singhal, R., and Brimble, K. S. 2006. Thromboembolic complications in the nephrotic syndrome: pathophysiology and clinical management. *Thromb Res*, **118**, 397–407. Epub 2005 Jun 28.

Song, K. S., Won, D. I., *et al.* 1994. A case of nephrotic syndrome associated with protein S deficiency and cerebral thrombosis. *J Korean Med Sci*, **9**, 347–50.

Stenvinkel, P., Alvestrand, A., *et al.* 2000. LDL-apheresis in patients with nephrotic syndrome: effects on serum albumin and urinary albumin excretion. *Eur J Clin Invest*, **30**, 866–70.

Sung, S. F., Jeng, J. S., *et al.* 1999. Cerebral venous thrombosis in patients with nephrotic syndrome – case reports. *Angiology*, **50**, 427–32.

Takegoshi, T., Haba, T., *et al.* 1990. A case of hyperLp(a)aemia, associated with systemic lupus erythematosus, suffering from myocardial infarction and cerebral infarction. *Jpn J Med*, **29**, 77–84.

Tovi, F., Hirsch, M., *et al.* 1988. Superior vena cava syndrome: presenting symptom of silent otitis media. *J Laryngol Otol*, **102**, 623–5.

Tullu, M. S., Deshmukh, C. T., *et al.* 1999. Superior sagittal sinus thrombosis: a rare complication of nephrotic syndrome. *J Postgrad Med*, **45**, 120–2.

Turaj, W., Slowik, A., *et al.* 2001. The prognostic significance of microalbuminuria in non-diabetic acute stroke patients. *Med Sci Monit*, **7**, 989–94.

Urch, C., and Pusey, C. D. 1996. Sagittal sinus thrombosis in adult minimal change nephrotic syndrome. *Clin Nephrol*, **45**, 131–2.

Vaziri, N. D. 1983. Nephrotic syndrome and coagulation and fibrinolytic abnormalities. *Am J Nephrol*, **3**, 1–6.

Volhard, F., and Fahr, T. H. 1914. *Die Brightsche Nierenkrankheit: Klinik, Pathlogie und Atlas*. Vol. 2. Springer Verlag, Berlin, Germany, 247–265.

Vidailhet, M., Piette, J.-C., Wechsler, B., Bousser, M., and Brunet, P. 1990. Cerebral venous thrombosis in systemic lupus erythematosus. *Stroke*, **21**, 1226–31.

Yun, Y. W., Chung, S., *et al.* 2004. Cerebral infarction as a complication of nephrotic syndrome: a case report with a review of the literature. *J Korean Med Sci*, **19**, 315–9.

Yuyun, M. F., Khaw, K. T., *et al.* 2004. Microalbuminuria and stroke in a British population: the European Prospective Investigation into Cancer in Norfolk (EPIC-Norfolk) population study. *J Intern Med*, **255**, 247–56.

Epidermal nevus

A nevus is a hamartoma or malformation of skin in its broadest sense. An epidermal nevus is a benign hamartoma of the epidermis that may often involve the papillary dermis. Epidermal nevi arise primarily from the embryonic ectoderm, although mesoderm may also be involved (Rogers *et al.*, 1996). The nevi are usually present at birth. Rogers *et al.* (1989) reported that 60% of the nevi were present at birth, 81% by 1 year, and 96% were evident by 7 years of age. The nevus may enlarge with age in proportion to, or in excess of, body growth. Disproportionate extension of nevi with age is rare when the nevus is present on the head and neck. Also, nevi present at birth enlarge much less often, irrespective of their location. There is no racial or gender predilection, and the nevi occur with equal frequency in males and females. Although most epidermal nevi are sporadic, autosomal dominant transmission has been described (Meschia *et al.*, 1992; Rogers *et al.*, 1996).

Solomon *et al.* (1968) and Solomon and Esterly (1975) used the term epidermal nevus in a generic sense to encompass lesions such as nevus verrucosus, epithelial nevi, systematized nevi, linear nevus comedonicus, acanthosis nigricans, ichthyosis hystrix, ichthyosis cornea, ichthyosis linearis neuropathica, linear sebaceous nevus, nevus sebaceous of Jadassohn, and nevus unius lateris. Nevus verrucosus is often a solitary lesion, gray to yellow-brown in color, and velvety, granular, warty, or papillomatous in appearance. Nevus unius lateris is a single linear or spiral lesion, limited to one side of the body. This lesion may be in a continuous or interrupted pattern and may affect multiple sites. The nevus follows the long axis on the extremities and is in groups or spiral streaks when present on the trunk. The term systematized epidermal nevus is used when this lesion is present on large parts of the body and is called ichthyosis hystrix when the histology of the lesion shows epidermolytic hyperkeratosis (Hurwitz, 1983). The most common clinical variant of epidermal nevi is nevus unius lateris occurring frequently as a unilateral linear verrucous lesion. Next in frequency are whorled ichthyosis hystrix, acanthosis nigricans, and linear sebaceous nevi. Almost one-third of patients may have a combination of these nevi (Hurwitz, 1983; Solomon and Esterly, 1975). Hyperplasia of both epidermis and dermis is present in all types of epidermal nevi, whereas involvement of skin appendages may vary. The nevus may be composed primarily of keratinocytes, hair follicle elements, sweat glands, or sebaceous glands. Skin biopsy may show a variety of histologic patterns in a given patient, although most often one pattern predominates. Interaction of the dermis with epidermis and the role of dermal induction in epidermal nevi are not understood, although the nevus tends to recur if only the epidermal component is removed (Solomon and Esterly, 1975).

Epidermal nevus syndrome

The epidermal nevus syndrome refers to the association of any epidermal nevus with extracutaneous abnormalities. The most common extracutaneous abnormalities are neurologic, skeletal, and ocular, although other organs may also be involved. In general, head and neck nevi are associated with neurologic abnormality, and skeletal abnormalities are seen more commonly when nevi are present on the trunk or limbs (Grebe *et al.*, 1993; Solomon and Esterly, 1975). This association of an epidermal nevus with nervous system abnormalities constitutes the neurologic type of epidermal nevus syndrome. A wide variety of abnormalities have been described in the neurologic type of epidermal nevus syndrome. These include mental retardation; early-onset seizures, including infantile spasms; hemiparesis; cerebral vascular abnormalities; cranial nerve disorders, especially involving nerves VI, VII, and VIII; hemimegalencephaly; cerebral gyral malformations; and epilepsy (Solomon and Esterly, 1975).

Skeletal abnormalities may be seen in 60%–70% of patients with epidermal nevus syndrome. These are most often associated with nevi on the trunk and limbs and include vertebral anomalies, kyphosis, scoliosis, short limbs, syndactyly, and other bony deformities, as well as hemihypertrophy, bone cysts, and spina bifida. Kyphoscoliosis is the most common abnormality, often becoming manifest in adolescence. Other limb deformities besides syndactyly include genu valgum, equinovarus, and bone hypoplasia. Vitamin D-resistant rickets has also been reported (Aschinberg *et al.*, 1977; Besser, 1976; Golitz and Weston, 1979; Marden and Venters, 1966; Mollica *et al.*, 1974; Olivares *et al.*, 1999; Paller, 1987; Rogers *et al.*, 1989; Solomon and Esterly, 1975; Sugarman and Reed, 1969).

Up to one-half of the patients with epidermal nevus syndrome have ocular abnormalities such as micro-ophthalmia; macroophthalmia; coloboma of the lid, iris, and retina; and conjunctival lipodermoids. Nystagmus and congenital blindness have been described (Alfonso *et al.*, 1987; Brodsky *et al.*, 1997; Diven *et al.*, 1987). Cardiac and vascular abnormalities including ventricular septal defect, coarctation of the aorta, patent ductus arteriosus, aneurysms, and arteriovenous malformations have been reported (Eichler *et al.*, 1989; Grebe *et al.*, 1993; Rogers *et al.*, 1989).

Uncommon Causes of Stroke, 2nd edition, ed. Louis R. Caplan. Published by CAMBRIDGE UNIVERSITY PRESS. © Cambridge University Press 2008.

Other cutaneous abnormalities also may be seen in patients with epidermal nevus syndrome and include café-au-lait spots, congenital hypopigmented macules, capillary hemangiomas, and melanocytic nevi (Eichler *et al.*, 1989; Rogers *et al.*, 1989; Solomon and Esterly, 1975). Happle (1987) proposed that mosaicism may explain the varied cutaneous manifestations. The observation that most epidermal nevi follow the lines of Blaschko, which probably represent migration tracks of clones of genetically identical cells, is in favor of this hypothesis.

Nevus sebaceous

Of the epidermal nevi, nevus sebaceous described by Jadassohn in 1895 is probably the most common nevus associated with the neurologic type of epidermal nevus syndrome (Holden and Dekaban, 1972). The sebaceous nevus is often present on the face and scalp. It reportedly occurs in 0.3% of births (Wagner and Hansen, 1995), although the estimate of Solomon and Esterly (1975) of the overall incidence of epidermal nevi at 1:1000 live births is probably more accurate. The nevus sebaceous (sometimes called the linear sebaceous nevus) occurs sporadically with no racial or gender predilection. Familial occurrence is rare (Benedetto, 1990; Sahl, 1990). Nevus sebaceous is usually congenital; rarely late appearance in childhood has been reported. Rogers (1992) reviewed 233 patients who had epidermal nevi and found 104 of the patients had nevus sebaceous. In 103 of these 104 cases of nevus sebaceous, the lesion was noted at birth, and in 102 of them the nevus involved the head. The nevus was on the scalp in 58 instances, on the face in 38, and ear in 1 case. The nevus itself is most often isolated, slightly raised, and yellowish orange, with a waxy appearance of the skin. The nevus is often linear or oval in shape. There is alopecia when the lesion is in the scalp (Figure 55.1). The nevus evolves with age, and three stages may be recognized (Lantis *et al.*, 1968; Mehregan and Pinkus, 1965). In the first stage in infancy, the lesion is characterized by a localized yellowish-orange patch of alopecia. The surface of the skin is most often smooth but may be rough, depressed, or verrucous. At this stage, histological examination shows multiple small underdeveloped sebaceous glands and immature hair follicles; apocrine glands are rare. By puberty (second stage), the sebaceous glands mature and become hyperplastic. Androgenic stimulation may have a role in this enlargement. The hair follicles continue to remain immature and rudimentary while apocrine glands (usually present in axilla and groin, and a few on the breast and eyelids, but seen in almost half of the sebaceous nevi) begin to mature and occasionally may be cystic or hyperplastic. The third stage is characterized by onset of neoplastic transformation in puberty or adulthood. Benign or malignant tumors may arise in 10%–31% of nevi. A nodular nonaggressive type of basal cell epithelioma or a syringocystadenoma papilliferum is most common. Other tumor types include squamous cell carcinoma, apocrine carcinoma, adnexal carcinoma, syringoma, keratocanthoma, apocrine cystadenoma, and osteoma. Metastatic spread usually does not occur in the pediatric age group but rarely may be seen in adults. Neoplasms probably develop more often in sebaceous nevus than in other epidermal nevi. Local excision of the nevus before puberty is therefore recommended (Hurwitz, 1983;

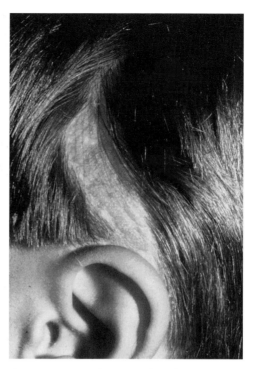

Figure 55.1 Nevus sebaceous on the scalp just above the ear. Note alopecia in the area of the nevus. (Photograph courtesy of Patricia Treadwell, MD, Department of Dermatology, Indiana University School of Medicine, Indianapolis.)

Mostafa and Satti, 1991; Rogers *et al.*, 1996; Solomon and Esterly, 1975).

Neurologic abnormalities

The epidermal nevus syndrome, characterized by the presence of an epidermal nevus and malformation in at least one extracutaneous organ system, was found in 65% of 300 patients with epidermal nevus. In this study by Solomon, one-third of the patients with the epidermal nevus syndrome had central nervous system (CNS) involvement (Micali *et al.*, 1995). In another study, 40% of patients with epidermal nevus syndrome had neurologic involvement. The most common neurologic abnormality in this study was epilepsy, present in 33.3%, followed by mental retardation of varying severity in 30.8% of patients (Holden and Dekaban, 1972). Others have found a much higher incidence of CNS involvement (Baker *et al.*, 1987; Barth *et al.*, 1977; Clancy *et al.*, 1985; Eichler *et al.*, 1989; Solomon and Esterly, 1975; Zaremba, 1978). Skin lesions on the face and scalp seem to correlate more strongly with CNS involvement in comparison to lesions limited to the trunk and limbs (Grebe *et al.*, 1993). Baker and colleagues (1987) found that cerebral hemiatrophy and hemimegalencephaly were present in 7% each, whereas gyral malformation was seen in 3% of patients. Gurecki *et al.* (1996) studied 23 patients with epidermal nevus syndrome who had biopsy-proven epidermal nevus and adequate data on neurologic and anatomical studies. Seizures were present in 50% of patients and mental retardation in 50% of patients for whom information was available. Only 9 of the 19 patients for whom data were available had normal cognition in this study. Five of the 23 patients had hemiparesis, nine had cranial nerve abnormalities, six patients each had hemiatrophy and vascular anomalies, and five patients each had hemimegalencephaly and gyral abnormalities. Widespread use of MRI has resulted in an increasing appreciation of the role of cortical malformations in patients with neurological symptoms. Studies prior to the general availability of MRI probably underestimated the prevalence of gyral and other cortical malformations in the neurologic type of epidermal nevus syndrome.

We reviewed data on 63 patients with epidermal nevus syndrome with severe neurologic abnormalities (Pavone *et al.*, 1991). From this group, 17 patients in whom adequate data were available and who had hemimegalencephaly were studied further. Nevus was ipsilateral to the hemimegalencephaly in all. Macrocephaly was present in four and microcephaly in one patient. Mental retardation and seizures of various types were common. Morphological and microscopic studies revealed pachygyria, polymicrogyria, irregularly thickened cortex, heterotopic nodules in the white matter, giant neurons, giant astrocytes, and areas of astrocytic proliferation. Sakuta *et al.* (1989, 1991) reported clinical and neuropathologic findings in a 5-year-old boy. In addition to the hemimegalencephaly and increased white matter volume, there was cerebral polymicrogyria with pachygyria, heterotopic neurons, and prominent astrogliosis. Hypertrophic neurons with increased dendrites and spines were seen on Golgi staining. Hemimegalencephaly limited to the temporal lobe has also been described (Kwa *et al.*, 1995). This clinical syndrome may be called the hemimegalencephalic variant of the neurologic type of epidermal nevus syndrome.

Vascular abnormalities

Strokes and vascular abnormalities have been reported in patients with the epidermal nevus syndrome. We reported one patient in whom cranial CT showed an infarct in the distribution of the right middle cerebral artery (Dobyns and Garg, 1991). There was ipsilateral atrophy and ventriculomegaly. We reviewed data on our patient and on three additional patients in whom the neurologic manifestations were because of vascular abnormalities. Two of the four patients had a clinically recognizable stroke. In the other two patients cerebral angiograms showed vascular dysplasia. In all four patients the facial or scalp epidermal nevus was ipsilateral to the vascular and brain abnormalities. The neurologic abnormalities could best be explained on the basis of either hemorrhage or ischemia of the underlying brain.

Arteriovenous malformations and leptomeningeal angiomas have been found in some patients with the epidermal nevus syndrome (Chatkupt *et al.*, 1993; Mollica *et al.*, 1974; Solomon and Esterly, 1975). Patients with absent dural sinuses and with dysplastic and partially thrombosed left carotid artery and branches have been reported. Patients with other venous anomalies and carotid artery malformation have been reported (Chalhub *et al.*, 1975; David *et al.*, 1990; Seawright *et al.*, 1996). Coarctation of the aorta has been found in some patients. Renal artery stenosis has been reported in one patient (Aizawa *et al.*, 2000). Vascular

abnormalities may also be the underlying mechanism in some patients with epidermal nevus syndrome reported to have cerebral atrophy, hypoplasia, or hemiatrophy although adequate information is often lacking.

We believe that an underlying vascular dysplasia may be the cause of neurologic abnormalities in patients with the neurologic type of the epidermal nevus syndrome who do not have the hemimegalencephalic variant. Others have disputed this hypothesis, although there are no documented reports implicating other mechanisms. Differences in the extent and location of the vascular dysplasia (which may predispose to occlusion, ischemia, and infarcts ipsilateral to the nevus) may be an adequate explanation for the wide variety of neurologic manifestation seen in these patients (Dobyns and Garg, 1991).

Clinical investigations

Generally, the diagnosis of an epidermal nevus is not in doubt. If there are any doubts, a skin biopsy should be obtained. The biopsy may also help in further characterizing the nevus type although as mentioned earlier there is considerable variability in the histologic patterns. In all children who have an epidermal nevus, a thorough physical examination must be carried out to discover any associated abnormality in other organ systems. The organs most commonly involved are the CNS, eyes, and the skeletal system, although others may also be involved. In children with involvement of the CNS, an imaging study such as CT or MRI should be considered. MRI is usually the study of choice. Cerebral angiographic evaluation may be necessary in selected patients. Neuropsychiatric testing may be helpful in the management of children with mental retardation or learning disabilities.

Genetics

The epidermal nevus syndrome, sometimes also referred to as the Schimmelpenning-Feuerstein-Mims syndrome, is a sporadic condition. Autosomal dominant cases have been described (Meschia *et al.*, 1992; Sahl, 1990). It should be distinguished from other phacomatoses, Proteus syndrome, and encephalocraniocutaneous lipomatosis. Parents should be counseled accordingly. Treatment of the nevus with dermabrasion, diathermy, laser treatment, and cryotherapy is associated with a fairly high risk of recurrence of the nevus. Focal resection of the epidermal nevus before puberty is advised because of the increased risk of tumor development. Resection must be complete as the nevus tends to recur if only the epidermal component is removed.

REFERENCES

Aizawa, K., Nakamura, T., Ohyama, Y., *et al.* 2000. Renal artery stenosis associated with epidermal nevus syndrome. *Nephron*, **84**, 67–70.

Alfonso, I., Howard, C., Lopez, P., Palomino, J., and Gonzalez, C. 1987. Linear nevus sebaceous syndrome: a review. *J Clin Neuroophthalmol*, **7**, 170–7.

Aschinberg, L., Solomon, L., Zeis, P., Justice, P., and Rosenthal, I. 1977. Vitamin D-resistant rickets associated with epidermal nevus syndrome: demonstration of a phosphaturic substance in the dermal lesions. *J Pediatr*, **91**, 56–60.

Baker, R., Ross, P., and Baumann, R. 1987. Neurologic complications of the epidermal nevus syndrome. *Arch Neurol*, **44**, 227–32.

Barth, P., Valk, J., Kalsbeck, G., and Blom, A. 1977. Organoid nevus syndrome linear nevus sebaceous of Jadassohn): clinical and radiological study of a case. *Neuropädiatrie*, **8**, 418–28.

Benedetto, L. 1990. Familial nevus sebaceous. *J Am Acad Dermatol*, **23**, 130–2.

Besser, F. 1976. Linear sebaceous nevi with convulsions and mental retardation (Feuerstein-Mims' syndrome), vitamin-D-resistant rickets. *Proc Roy Soc Med*, **69**, 518–20.

Brodsky, M., Kincannon, J., Nelson-Adesokan, P., and Brown, H. 1997. Oculocerebral dysgenesis in the linear nevus sebaceous syndrome. *Ophthalmology*, **104**, 497–503.

Chalhub, E. G., Volpe, J. J., and Gado, M. H. 1975. Linear sebaceous syndrome associated with porencephaly and nonfunctioning major cerebral venous sinuses. *Neurology*, **25**, 857–60.

Chatkupt, S., Ruzicka, P. O., and Lastra, C. R. 1993. Myelomeningocele, spinal arteriovenous malformations and epidermal nevi syndrome: a possible rare association. *Dev Med Child Neurol*, **35**, 727–41.

Clancy, R., Kurtz, M., Baker, D., *et al.* 1985. Neurologic manifestations of the organoid nevus syndrome. *Arch Neurol*, **42**, 236–40.

David, P., Elia, M., Garcovich, A., *et al.* 1990. A case of epidermal nevus syndrome with carotid malformation. *Ital J Neurol Sci*, **11**, 293–6.

Diven, D., Solomon, A., McNeely, M., and Font, R. 1987. Nevus sebaceous associated with major ophthalmologic abnormalities. *Arch Dermatol*, **123**, 383–6.

Dobyns, W., and Garg, B. 1991. Vascular abnormalities in epidermal nevus syndrome. *Neurology*, **41**, 276–8.

Eichler, C., Flowers, F., and Ross, J. 1989. Epidermal nevus syndrome: case report and review of clinical manifestations. *Pediatr Dermatol*, **6**, 316–20.

Golitz, L., and Weston, W. 1979. Inflammatory linear verrucous epidermal nevus. Association with epidermal nevus syndrome. *Arch Dermatol*, **115**, 1208–9.

Grebe, T., Rimsza, M., Richter, S. Hansen, R., and Hoyme, E. 1993. Further delineation of the epidermal nevus syndrome: two cases with new findings and literature review. *Am J Med Genet*, **47**, 24–30.

Gurecki, P., Holden, K., Sahn, E., Dyer, D., and Cure, J. 1996. Developmental neural abnormalities and seizures in epidermal nevus syndrome. *Dev Med Child Neurol*, **38**, 716–23.

Happle, R. 1987. Lethal genes surviving by mosaicism: a possible explanation for sporadic birth defects involving the skin. *J Am Acad Dermatol*, **16**, 899–906.

Holden, K., and Dekaban, A. 1972. Neurological involvement in nevus unius lateris and nevus linearis sebaceous. *Neurology*, **22**, 879–87.

Hurwitz, S. 1983. Epidermal nevi and tumors of epidermal origin. *Pediatr Clin North Am*, **30**, 483–94.

Kwa, V., Smitt, J., Verbeeten, B., and Barth, P. 1995. Epidermal nevus syndrome with isolated enlargement of one temporal lobe: a case report. *Brain Dev*, **17**, 122–5.

Lantis, S., Thew, M., and Heaton, C. 1968. Nevus sebaceous of Jadassohn: part of a new neurocutaneous syndrome? *Arch Dermatol*, **98**, 117–23.

Marden, P., and Venters, H. 1966. A new neurocutaneous syndrome. *Am J Dis Child*, **112**, 79–81.

Mehregan, A., and Pinkus, H. 1965. Clinical studies: life history of organoid nevi: special reference to nevus sebaceous of Jadassohn. *Arch Dermatol*, **91**, 574–88.

Meschia, J., Junkins, E., and Hofman, K. 1992. Brief clinical report. Familial systematized epidermal nevus syndrome. *Am J Med Genet*, **44**, 664–7.

Micali, G., Bene-Bain, M., Guitart, J., and Solomon, L. 1995. Genodermatoses. In *Pediatric Dermatology*, 2nd edn, L. Schachner, and R. Hansen (eds.), New York: Churchill Livingston, p. 397.

Mollica, F., Pavone, L., and Nuciforo, G. 1974. Linear sebaceous nevus syndrome in a newborn. *Am J Dis Child*, **128**, 868–71.

Mostafa, W., and Satti, M. 1991. Epidermal nevus syndrome: a clinicopathologic study with six-year follow-up. *Pediatr Dermatol*, **8**, 228–30.

Olivares, J. L., Ramos, F. J., Carapeto, F. J., and Bueno, M. 1999. Epidermal naevus syndrome and hypophosphataemic rickets: description of a new patient with central nervous system anomalies and review of the literature. *Eur J Pediatr*, **158**, 103–7.

Paller, A. 1987. Epidermal nevus syndrome. *Neurol Clin*, **5**, 451–7.

Pavone, L., Curatolo, P., Rizzo, R., *et al.* 1991. Epidermal nevus syndrome: a neurological variant with hemimegalencephaly, gyral malformation, mental retardation, seizures, and facial hemihypertrophy. *Neurology*, **41**, 266–71.

Rogers, M. 1992. Epidermal nevi and the epidermal nevus syndromes: a review of 233 cases. *Pediatr Dermatol*, **9**, 342–4.

Rogers, M., Fischer, G., and Hogan, P. 1996. Nevoid conditions of epidermis, dermis, and subcutaneous tissue. In *Cutaneous Medicine and Surgery. An Integrated Program*, K. Arndt, P. LeBoit, J. Robinson, and B. Wintroub (eds.), Philadelphia: W. B. Saunders Company, p. 1787.

Rogers, M., McCrossin, I., and Commens, C. 1989. Epidermal nevi and the epidermal nevus syndrome. *J Am Acad Dermatol*, **20**, 476–88.

Sahl, S. Jr. 1990. Familial nevus sebaceous of Jadassohn: occurrence in three generations. *J Am Acad Dermatol*, **22**, 853–4.

Sakuta, R., Aikawa, H., Takashima, S., and Ryo, S. 1991. Epidermal nevus syndrome with hemimegalencephaly: neuropathological study. *Brain Dev*, **13**, 260–5.

Sakuta, R., Aikawa, H., Takashima, S., Yoza, A., and Ryo, S. 1989. Epidermal nevus syndrome with hemimegalencephaly: a clinical report of a case with acanthosis nigricans-like nevi on the face and neck, hemimegalencephaly, and hemihypertrophy of the body. *Brain Dev*, **11**, 191–4.

Seawright, A. A., Sullivan, T. J., Pelekanos, J. T., and Masel, J. 1996. Coexistent orbital and cerebellar venous anomalies in sebaceous naevus syndrome. *Aust N Z J Ophthalmol*, **24**, 373–6.

Solomon, L., and Esterly, N. 1975. Epidermal and other congenital organoid nevi. *Curr Probl Pediatr*, **6**, 1–56.

Solomon, L., Fretzin, D., and Dewald, R. 1968. The epidermal nevus syndrome. *Arch Dermatol*, **97**, 273–85.

Sugarman, G., and Reed, W. 1969. Two unusual neurocutaneous disorders with facial cutaneous signs. *Arch Neurol*, **21**, 242–7.

Wagner, A., and Hansen, R. 1995 Neonatal skin and skin disorders. In *Pediatric Dermatology*, 2nd edn, L. Schachner, and R. Hansen (eds.), New York: Churchill Livingstone, p. 288.

Zaremba, J. 1978. Jadassohn's naevus phakomatosis: 2. A study based on a review of thirty-seven cases. *J Ment Defic Res*, **22**, 103–23.

SNEDDON'S SYNDROME

Jacques L. De Reuck and Jan L. De Bleecker

Introduction

Sneddon's syndrome (SS) refers to an infrequent disorder combining skin and ischemic cerebral lesions in patients without a recognizable connective tissue or inflammatory or chronic infectious disease. The skin lesions consist of a purplish mottling of the skin (livedo racemosa, mostly used synonymously with livedo reticularis in English usage), and central nervous system (CNS) manifestations ranging from transient ischemic attacks to multiple strokes. The first description dates back to Ehrmann (1906), who described a syphilitic patient with an ischemic stroke and the typical skin lesions. Champion and Rook (1960) described a typical patient in 1960. In 1965, the dermatologist Sneddon was the first to recognize the syndrome as a separate clinical entity (Sneddon, 1965). He was struck by the severe and generalized bluish discoloration of the skin, involving the limbs and often the trunk (Sneddon used the term livedo reticularis), and the multiple strokes "often leaving little residual disability" in five young women and one young man. All of those patients had arterial hypertension. Skin biopsies and clinical evaluations showed no known etiology of livedo racemosa such as polyarteritis nodosa, systemic lupus erythematosus (SLE), or essential thrombocytopenia. Sneddon suggested endarteritis obliterans or an unknown type of arteriopathy causing venous dilatation and stasis of the skin as the underlying pathology.

A similar syndrome combining livedo racemosa and multiple strokes had been reported by Divry and van Bogaert (1946) as a familial disease leading to dementia, pseudobulbar palsy, and epilepsy. Further sporadic and familial cases of this syndrome have been reported under various eponyms: diffuse meningocerebral angiomatosis and leukoencephalopathy, corticomeningeal angiomatosis, venous capillary angiomatosis, Divry-van Bogaert syndrome, etc. (Baro, 1964; Bussone et al., 1984; Divry and van Bogaert, 1946; Ellie et al., 1987; Pellat et al., 1976). These patients cannot be distinguished from SS patients on clinical grounds. Therefore, they can be considered as part of it until the underlying genetic or pathophysiological abnormalities are better defined (Ellie et al., 1987).

SS, which originally was a clinical diagnosis, is now regarded as a common clinical manifestation of different disease entities. It has been divided into idiopathic, autoimmune, and thromboembolic subsets or into SLE-associated, antiphospholipid syndrome-associated, and primary forms (Szmyrka-Kaczmarek et al., 2005).

Epidemiology

Following Sneddon's description, a number of cases or small series were reported, initially mainly in Europe. Although most reported patients were Caucasians, there is no definite evidence of ethnic differences in incidence. Some authors claim an incidence of four cases per 1 000 000 per year (Zelger et al., 1993). In hospital-based series of stroke patients, the frequency of SS is between 0.25% and 0.50% (Berciano, 1988; De Reuck et al., 1987).

At least in sporadic cases, there is a marked female preponderance. Of 200 literature cases reviewed by us, 80% are women. The average age at onset of the neurological symptoms is around 40 years, with a range of 10–65 years. In more than two-thirds of the patients, the disorder occurs sporadically, whereas in the others there is familial occurrence (Mascarenhas et al., 2003; Pettee et al., 1994; Rehany et al., 1998; Szmyrka-Kaczmarek et al., 2005). In apparently familial cases, no single pattern of inheritance is identified, but autosomal dominant inheritance has been most frequently reported (Berciano, 1988; Rebollo et al., 1983; Scott and Boyle, 1986).

Clinical expression

Cutaneous manifestations

Livedo racemosa is usually the first manifestation of the disease, and tends to precede the neurological symptoms by 10 years on average (Quimby and Perry, 1980; Rebollo et al., 1983; Sneddon, 1965; Thomas et al., 1982; Zelger et al., 1993). In some patients, the livedo is first detected at the time of stroke occurrence, and rarely it develops years after the first neurological symptoms (Thomas et al., 1982). Livedo racemosa is defined as a dusky erythematous-to-violaceous, irregular, net-like pattern in the skin (Burton, 1988; Daoud et al., 1995). The lesions are typically distributed over the lower trunk, the buttocks, and proximal region of the thighs. The lesions occasionally become more generalized and extend to the upper back, the distal extremities, and volar parts of the lower arms (Figure 56.1). The livedo is increased in the cold, in conjunction with exacerbations of neurological symptoms, and sometimes during pregnancy (Gibson et al., 1997). In the European literature, the term livedo reticularis refers to a regular, deep-bluish net-like pattern that disappears after the skin is warmed. In the American literature, livedo reticularis is used interchangeably with livedo racemosa, whereas the reticular changes that

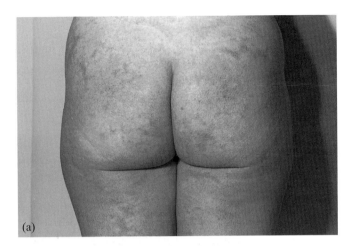

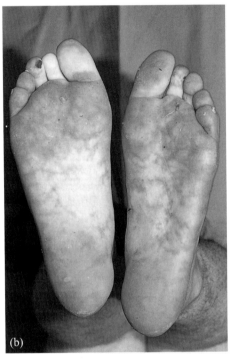

Figure 56.1 (a and b) Livedo racemosa involving the buttocks, feet, and lower legs in two SS patients. See color plate. (Courtesy of Prof. J.-M. Naeyaert, Ghent University Hospital.)

disappear after warming are sometimes referred to as "cutis marmorata." Livedo reticularis and livedo racemosa are caused by different pathophysiologic mechanisms (Daoud *et al.*, 1995). Livedo reticularis is caused by temporary vasoconstriction, whereas livedo racemosa results from persistent impairment of peripheral blood flow caused by occlusion of small or medium-sized arteries. However, there is a broad spectrum of transition between livedo reticularis (especially cutis marmorata and amantadine-induced livedo reticularis) and livedo racemosa (especially SS, Divry-van Bogaert syndrome, SLE, anti-phospholipid antibody syndrome, polyarteritis nodosa, cholesterol embolization syndrome, livedoid vasculopathy, and hematological diseases) (Kraemer *et al.*, 2005). Some patients also have acrocyanosis of the

distal extremities or typical Raynaud phenomenon (Daoud *et al.*, 1995).

Neurological manifestations

Virtually all syndromes caused by transient or permanent cerebral ischemia have been described (Toubi *et al.*, 2005). In a prospective 6-year clinical and neuroradiological follow-up study, headache occurred in 62% of the patients, vertigo in 54%, and transient ischemic attacks (TIAs) in 54%. Although not demented, 77% of the patients reported loss of concentration ability, memory disturbances, or emotional impairment. None of the patients developed a stroke during that period (Boesch *et al.*, 2003).

The frequency of headache is not significantly higher in persons with positive anti-phospholipid antibodies compared to an anti-phospholipid antibody-negative cohort (Tietjen *et al.*, 2006). However, those with anti-phospholipid antibodies have a significantly higher incidence of seizures, mitral regurgitation, and thrombocytopenia (Frances *et al.*, 1999, 2000).

As a rule, the transient ischemic attacks and strokes are multiple and recurrent in the same or different vascular territories (Stephens and Ferguson, 1982). Both cortical and subcortical areas in the anterior and posterior circulation can be affected, but the most common lesions leading to progressive clinical disability are white matter abnormalities and lacunar infarcts (Boesch *et al.*, 2003; Fetoni *et al.*, 2000). Aphasia, hemiparesis, hemisensory deficit, and visual field defects are the most common clinical signs. However, most of the strokes are minor with good recovery. Recurrent transient global amnesia has sometimes been the initial clinical presentation (Rumpl and Rumpl, 1979). Tremor as the first neurological manifestation has occasionally been described (Da Silva *et al.*, 2005). Spinal cord ischemia is rare (Baleva *et al.*, 1995).

In later stages, mild to severe cognitive impairment can occur in many patients, with symptoms varying from inability to concentrate, slight memory loss, frontal lobe type behavioral and emotional disturbances, to severe multi-infarct dementia. Dementia without precedent focal deficits has been the clinical presentation in some patients (Adair *et al.*, 2001; Antoine *et al.*, 1994; Baleva *et al.*, 1995; Bruyn *et al.*, 1987; Cosnes *et al.*, 1986; Devuyst *et al.*, 1996; Scott and Boyle, 1986).

Subarachnoid or intracerebral hemorrhage has been reported (Aquino Gondim *et al.*, 2003; Diez-Tejedor *et al.*, 1990; Dupont *et al.*, 1996; Serrano-Pozo *et al.*, 2004; Uitdehaag *et al.*, 1992), but an increased incidence of bleedings in SS patients is not supported by larger series.

Focal or secondary generalized seizures are more common in SS than in a general stroke population. Of 109 randomly selected SS patients from the neurological literature, seizures are mentioned in 26 (24%) (De Reus *et al.*, 1985; Ellie *et al.*, 1987; Frances *et al.*, 1999; Menzel *et al.*, 1994; Rebollo *et al.*, 1983; Rumpl and Rumpl, 1979; Sneddon, 1965; Stockhammer *et al.*, 1993), which is far more than the 8.6% observed in a prospective multicenter study of ischemic stroke patients (Bladin *et al.*, 2000). The explanation for the high frequency of seizures in SS patients is unknown, but irregular cortical infarcts and repeated strokes with good recovery are predisposing for the appearance of late-onset seizures (De Reuck et al., 2005, 2006).

Other manifestations

Slight to moderate arterial hypertension occurs in a significant proportion (60%–80%) of SS patients. The pathophysiological basis for the hypertension is not well understood. Very few hypertensive SS patients have renal vascular disease (Antoine et al., 1994; Macario et al., 1997).

Valvular heart disease, mostly mitral valve thickening, was found in 36% in one series (Lubach et al., 1992) and in up to 61% of patients in another series (Tourbah et al., 1997). The valvular disease sometimes was recognized before the onset of neurological symptoms and was considered rheumatic in some patients (Antoine et al., 1994; Tourbah et al., 1997; Vaillant et al., 1990). Valve disease is a common finding in patients with the anti-phospholipid antibody syndrome (Barbut et al., 1992; Brenner et al., 1991; Caplan and Manning, 2006). Thrombosis of peripheral arteries and pulmonary embolus can also occur (Alegre et al., 1990), as well as symptomatic involvement of mesenteric arteries (Khoo and Belli, 1999).

Ophthalmologic manifestations include transient monocular or binocular blindness, hypertensive vascular changes, retinal artery or vein thrombosis, and microaneurysms (Donders et al., 1998; Gobert, 1994; Jonas et al., 1986), in addition to CNS visual symptoms such as homonymous visual field defects, internuclear ophthalmoplegia, diplopia, and pupillary defects (Narbay, 1997; Rehany et al., 1998).

Those patients with anti-phospholipid antibodies may present the full clinical spectrum of the primary anti-phospholipid antibody syndrome (Hess, 1992; Levine and Welch, 1987; Lockshin, 1992; see also Chapter 38).

Pathology

Dermatopathology

For obvious reasons, skin biopsies have been studied more frequently than brain tissue. The most informative skin biopsies are those taken in the central normal areas within the bordering of the livedo (Copeman, 1975; Daoud et al., 1995; Zelger et al., 1992). The main abnormalities involve medium-sized arteries in the deep dermal or subcutaneous tissue and progress over time. The early stage is characterized by arteriolar endothelitis and a mixed inflammatory cellular infiltrate and is then followed by occlusion of the arteriolar lumen by a fibrotic plug and dilatation of neighboring arterioles and venules (Beurey et al., 1984; Lewandowska et al., 2005; Marsch and Muckelmann, 1985; Stockhammer et al., 1993; Zelger et al., 1992). Later, subendothelial cell proliferation with collapse of the lamina elastica and recanalization follows. Finally, the arteriole becomes completely involuted and occluded. The sensitivity to detect the diagnostic vascular lesions increases from 27% with one biopsy, to 53% with two biopsies, and to 80% with three biopsies taken from the white skin areas in all cases (Wohlrab et al., 2001).

Digital artery biopsies have been performed by Rebollo et al. (1983). They found segmental intimal hyperplasia, adventitial fibrosis, thrombosis, and narrowing of the lumen. Temporal artery biopsies are usually normal (Pauranik et al., 1987; Rumpl et al., 1985) or show nonspecific subintimal hyperplasia and medial fibrosis (De Reuck et al., 1987; De Reus et al., 1985; Kalashnikova et al., 1990).

Neuropathology

Few autopsies or brain biopsies have been reported. Nonspecific signs of cortical and subcortical infarction and gliosis, without vascular or perivascular inflammation or fibrinoid necrosis, are observed (Devuyst et al., 1996; Geschwind et al., 1995; Rumpl et al., 1985; Scott and Boyle, 1986). Boortz-Marx et al. (1995) found granulomatous inflammation of the leptomeninges without vessel involvement in one patient. Noninflammatory thrombosis of leptomeningeal arteries was a rare finding in one autopsy case (Pinol-Aguade et al., 1999). However, in a more recently described postmortem case, multiple small cortical infarcts associated with occlusion of medium-sized arteries and prominent focal smooth muscle hyperplasia of smaller arterial vessels were observed (Hilton and Footitt, 2003).

Pathogenesis

SS is unlikely to reflect a single, specific etiology. Two main hypotheses emerge: (i) a hypercoagulable state, itself of variable origin, and (ii) an intrinsic small-vessel vasculopathy.

Hypercoagulable state

The notion that anti-phospholipid antibody or the lupus anticoagulant are frequently present in SS patients has greatly supported the theory that SS is part of the clinical spectrum of the primary anti-phospholipid antibody syndrome (Alegre et al., 1990; Jonas et al., 1986; Kalashnikova et al., 1990; Levine et al., 1988; Moral et al., 1991). The proportion of anti-phospholipid antibody-positive patients is widely different in various cohorts of SS patients, e.g. 0/17 (Stockhammer et al., 1993), 1/5 (Burton, 1988), 3/13 (Sitzer et al., 1995), 6/17 (Kalashnikova et al., 1990), and 19/33 (Farronay et al., 1992). Natural or treatment-induced fluctuation of anti-phospholipid antibody levels, methods for assay determination, and criteria for positive results may partly explain the different incidences (Tanne et al., 1998). Rare familial SS cases with anti-phospholipid antibodies have also been documented (Pettee et al., 1994; Vargas et al., 1989).

Anti-prothrombin antibodies, a new serologic marker of anti-phospholipid antibody syndrome, were elevated in 57% of patients with SS. The addition of anti-prothrombin antibody data increases the proportion of SS with at least one type of anti-phospholipid antibody syndrome marker from 65% to 78% (Kalashnikova et al., 1999).

Less frequently, SS occurs in patients with anti-nuclear antibodies, some of whom turn out to have SLE (Antoine et al., 1994;

McHugh *et al.*, 1988). Rarely reported coagulation or platelet aggregation deficits include antithrombin-III deficiency (Bolayir *et al*, 1999; Donnet *et al.*, 1992; Matsumura *et al.*, 2001; Sauter and Rudin, 1992) and essential thrombocythemia (Michel *et al.*, 1996). Protein Z, a down-regulator of coagulation and linked to an increased risk of arterial thrombosis, is found to be deficient in 31% of patients with antiphospholipid-negative SS (Ayoub *et al.*, 2004). Factor V Leiden mutation is only found in 11.3% of SS cases (Besnier *et al.*, 2003).

Up to about 60% of SS patients have a cardiac valvulopathy (Antoine *et al.*, 1994; Lubach *et al.*, 1992; Tourbah *et al.*, 1997). The incidence of valvular disease is unexpectedly high in the young population. It is unclear whether the valvulopathies per se are the direct cause of embolic strokes or become symptomatic because of a coexistent hypercoagulable state (Geschwind *et al.*, 1995). In patients with the anti-phospholipid antibody syndrome, the valvular abnormalities consist of fibrinous and fibrous deposits on heart valves. The lesions are identical to those found in patients with SLE (Libman-Sacks endocarditis) and in nonbacterial thrombotic endocarditis (NBTE) often associated with cancer or other debilitating condition (Caplan and Manning, 2006). Frank vegetations may be visible on echocardiography.

Primary vasculopathy

In many patients, no anti-phospholipid antibody or primary coagulation deficits are detected (Martinez-Menendez *et al.*, 1990; Stockhammer *et al.*, 1993). Mainly based on observations in skin biopsies, it is assumed that a nonvasculitic small and medium-sized vessel arteriopathy causes both brain and skin symptoms. The common clinical observation of exacerbation of the livedo racemosa at times that new cerebrovascular symptoms develop is suggestive of a common factor causing skin and CNS symptoms. The type and origin of the arteriopathy is unknown. In some cases, heritable factors play a role. In others, endothelial dysfunction may be secondary to acquired autoimmune or other factors that circulate in the serum. Circulating proteins, presumably immunoglobulins, could cause both the hypercoagulable state and an endotheliopathy, thus linking both hypothesized mechanisms underlying the SS (Moral *et al.*, 1991). Signaling pathways specific to certain parts of the vascular bed, i.e. brain and skin, may explain why systemic congenital or acquired hypercoagulable states or endotheliopathies produce focal deficits of hemostasis (Rosenberg and Aird, 1999).

Diagnostic work-up

Any patient suspected of SS should undergo extensive blood tests, spinal tap, thorough cardiovascular evaluation including cardiac monitoring and transesophageal echo-Doppler, cerebral MRI, four-vessel intra-arterial angiography, and skin biopsy. A meningocortical brain biopsy is warranted only when clinical, angiographic, cerebrospinal fluid, or skin biopsy findings suggest a possible CNS vasculitis or a vasculopathy of other origin.

Blood tests should screen for the lupus anticoagulant, immunoglobulin (Ig)G and possibly IgM anti-cardiolipin antibodies, anti-nuclear and anti-double-stranded DNA autoantibodies, decreased complement factors, thrombocytopenia, leukopenia, and other indications for SLE, VDRL assay, cryoglobulins, and circulating immune complexes. Heritable causes of hypercoagulable states such as deficiency of antithrombin-III, protein C, or protein S should be sought.

The cerebrospinal fluid is usually normal. Mild increase of protein content or slight pleocytosis may reflect infarction, but marked lymphocytic pleocytosis suggests other causes of stroke including intracranial vasculitides or chronic CNS infections such as tertiary syphilis or tuberculosis.

MRI scan is more informative than CT scan (Ruscalleda *et al.*, 1991). Multiple, mainly subcortical infarcts and white matter changes in various vascular territories are usually present at the time of diagnosis (Figure 56.2). Mild to moderate cortical and subcortical atrophy with ventricular enlargement is common. Angiography is mandatory to exclude other types of cerebral vasculopathy. Many SS patients have normal angiograms, but a subset of patients have multiple distal arterial occlusions or narrowings, combined with a moyamoya type collateral network in a smaller proportion of the patients (Antoine *et al.*, 1994; Blom, 1989; Pettee *et al.*, 1994). The "beading type" segmental narrowing and dilation of large and medium-sized vessels typical of CNS vasculitis is not reported in SS.

Mitral and other cardiac valvulopathies are more commonly observed on transesophageal echocardiography in SS patients than predicted from observations in age-matched controls (Donnet *et al.*, 1992; Vaillant *et al.*, 1990). Selection bias alone is unlikely to explain the difference. Some authors claim that the cardiac emboli resulting from these mitral valve abnormalities are the main cause of the brain infarcts (Geschwind *et al.*, 1995). Alternatively, the mitral valve proliferations could be the consequence of a systemic hypercoagulable state.

Cervical Doppler sonography shows no significant atherosclerotic changes in most patients. Clinically silent cerebral microembolism was detected in one-third of the patients by transcranial duplex sonography of the middle cerebral artery in one study. The microemboli may be a marker of disease activity (Sitzer *et al.*, 1995).

Menzel *et al.* (1994) reported decreased cerebral blood flow as adjudged by technetium-99m-HMPAO-single photon emission computed tomography (SPECT) scan, even in patients without MRI abnormalities. Transcranial duplex sonography was normal in the same patients. These authors suggested that SPECT scan may allow presymptomatic detection of impaired cerebral blood flow in patients with livedo racemosa.

A skin biopsy including the deep dermis should be taken in the central normal areas within the bordering of the livedo (Daoud *et al.*, 1995; Zelger *et al.*, 1992). Three biopsies taken from the central normal white skin areas have a sensitivity of 80% (Wohlrab *et al.*, 2001). The pathologic changes in the various stages of the disease process have been detailed in the dermatopathology paragraph. The differential diagnosis of livedo racemosa should include leukocytoclastic and livedoid vasculitis, polyarteritis nodosa, SLE, cryoglobulinemia, macroglobulinemia, polycythemia, thrombotic thrombocytopenic purpura, essential thrombocythemia, atheromatous or cholesterol emboli,

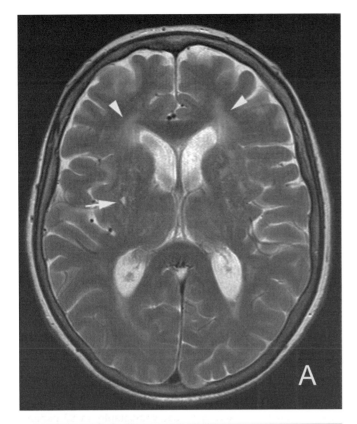

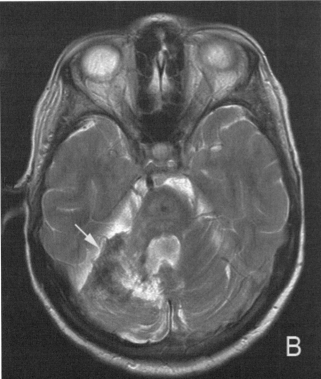

Figure 56.2 T2-weighted MRIs: (**a**) widespread frontal white matter abnormalities (*triangles*) and a right putaminal lacune (*arrow*). (**b**) large old hemorrhagic infarct in the right cerebellar hemisphere (*arrow*), partly involving the middle cerebellar peduncle and the pons in a 56-year-old woman with SS.

disseminated intravascular coagulation, infectious diseases such as syphilis and tuberculosis, and drug toxicity (Daoud *et al.*, 1995; Gibson *et al.*, 1997).

Treatment

No prospective studies are available (Hachulla *et al.*, 2000), but individual case reports suggest that warfarin sodium is probably more effective than aspirin for stroke recurrence (Krnic-Barrie *et al.*, 1997). By analogy with the anti-phospholipid antibody syndrome and based on the presumed pathogenesis of SS, most clinicians advocate warfarin anticoagulation for the treatment of SS patients (Dupont *et al.*, 1996). A large retrospective study on the anti-phospholipid antibody syndrome demonstrated that treatment with high-intensity warfarin (producing an international normalized ratio [INR] of >3) with or without low-dose aspirin (75 mg/day) is significantly more effective than treatment with low-intensity warfarin (producing an INR of <3) with or without treatment with low-dose aspirin or treatment with aspirin alone in preventing further thrombotic events. The risk of bleeding compared favorably with the risk of bleeding associated with long-term oral anticoagulation therapy in other conditions (Khamashta *et al.*, 1995).

Immunosuppression with steroids, azathioprine, and cyclophosphamide have been reported to be ineffective in SS (Floel *et al.*, 2002).

Conclusion

SS is a clinically well-delineated syndrome that probably stems from a number of acquired or congenital hemostatic abnormalities that preferentially involve the cerebral and cutaneous vascular beds. Further pathophysiological studies will undoubtedly continue to identify more etiological subgroups. Pending future therapeutic trials that may identify different treatment modalities for different etiological subgroups, the general concept of "Sneddon's syndrome" is currently still a valid and workable diagnosis in daily neurological clinical practice.

REFERENCES

Adair, J. C., Digre, K. B., Swanda, R. M., *et al.* 2001. Sneddon's syndrome: a cause of cognitive decline in young adults. *Neuropsychiatry Neuropsychol Behav Neurol*, **14**, 197–204.

Alegre, V. A., Winkelmann, R. K., and Gastineau, D. A. 1990. Cutaneous thrombosis, cerebrovascular thrombosis, and lupus anticoagulant – the Sneddon syndrome. *Int J Dermatol*, **29**, 45–9.

Antoine, J. C., Michel, D., Garnnier, P., *et al.* 1994. Syndrome de Sneddon: 9 cas. *Rev Neurol*, **150**, 435–43.

Aquino Gondim, F. A., Leacock, R. O., Subrammanian, T. A., and Cruz-Flores, S. 2003. Intracerebral hemorrhage associated with Sneddon's syndrome: is ischemia-related angiogenesis the cause? Case report and review of the literature. *Neuroradiology*, **45**, 368–72.

Ayoub, N., Esposito, G., Barete, S., *et al.* 2004. Protein Z deficiency in antiphospholipid-negative Sneddon's syndrome. *Stroke*, **35**, 1329–32.

Baleva, M., Chauchev, A., Dikova, C., *et al.* 1995. Sneddon's syndrome: echocardiographic, neurological, and immunological findings. *Stroke*, **26**, 1303–4.

Barbut, D., Borer, J., Gharavi, A., *et al.* 1992. Prevalence of anticardiolipin antibody in isolated mitral or aortic regurgitation, or both, and possible relation to cerebral ischemic events. *Am J Cardiol*, **70**, 901–5.

Baro, F. 1964. Angiomatose méningée non calcifiante, état granulaire de l' écorce, sclérose diffuse axiale et cutis marmorata congenita. Nouvelle observation clinique sporadique du syndrome décrit par Divry et van Bogaert. *Acta Neurol Psychiatr Belg*, **64**, 1042–63.

Berciano, J. 1988. Sneddon syndrome: another Mendelian etiology of stroke. *Ann Neurol*, **24**, 586–7.

Besnier, R., Frances, C., Ankri, A., Aiach, M., and Piette, J. C. 2003. Factor V Leiden mutation in Sneddon syndrome. *Lupus*, **12**, 406–8.

Beurey, J., Weber, M., Edelson, F., Thomas, I., and Eich, D. 1984. Livédo reticularis et accidents vasculaires cérébraux. *Ann Dermatol Venereol*, **111**, 25–9.

Bladin, C., Alexandrov, A., Bellevance, A., *et al.*, for the Seizures After Stroke Study Group. 2000. Seizures after stroke. A prospective multicenter study. *Arch Neurol*, **57**, 1617–22.

Blom, R. J. 1989. Sneddon syndrome: CT, arteriography, and MR imaging. *J Comput Assist Tomogr*, **13**, 119–22.

Boesch, S. M., Plorer, A. L., Auer, A. J., *et al.* 2003. The natural course of Sneddon syndrome: clinical and magnetic resonance imaging findings in a prospective six year observation study. *J Neurol Neurosurg Psychiatry*, **74**, 542–4.

Bolayir, E., Kecceci, H., Akyol, M., Tas, A., and Polat, M., 1999. Sneddon's syndrome and antithrombin III. *J Dermatol*, **26**, 532–4.

Boortz-Marx, R. L., Clark, H. B., Taylor, S., Wesa, K. M., and Anderson, D. C. 1995. Sneddon's syndrome with granulomatous leptomeningeal infiltration. *Stroke*, **26**, 492–5.

Brenner, B., Blumenfeld, Z., Markiewicz, W., and Reisner, S. A. 1991. Cardiac involvement in patients with primary antiphospholipid syndrome. *J Am Coll Cardiol*, **18**, 931–6.

Bruyn, R., Van Der Veen, J., Donker, A., Valk, J., and Wolters, E. C. 1987. Sneddon's syndrome. Case report and review of the literature. *J Neurol Sci*, **79**, 243–53.

Burton, J. L. 1988. Livedo reticularis, porcelain-white scars, and cerebral thromboses. *Lancet*, **2**, 1263–4.

Bussone, G., Parati, E. A., Boiardi, A., *et al.* 1984. Divry-Van Bogaert syndrome. Clinical and ultrastructural findings. *Arch Neurol*, **41**, 560–2.

Caplan, L. R., and Manning, W. J. 2006. Cardiac sources of embolism: the usual suspects. In *Brain Embolism*, L. R. Caplan and W. J. Manning (eds.), New York: Informa Healthcare, pp. 129–59.

Champion, R. H., and Rook, A. J. 1960. Livedo reticularis. *Proc Roy Soc Med*, **53**, 961–2.

Copeman, P. W. M. 1975. Livedo reticularis: signs in the skin of disturbance of blood viscosity and of blood flow. *Br J Dermatol*, **93**, 519–29.

Cosnes, A., Perroud, A. M., Mathieu, A., Jourdain, C., and Touraine, R. 1986. Livedo reticularis et accidents vasculaires cérébraux. *Ann Dermatol Venereol*, **113**, 137–41.

Daoud, M. S., Wilmoth, G. J., Su, W. P. D., and Pittelkow, M. R. 1995. Sneddon syndrome. *Semin Dermatol*, **14**, 166–72.

Da Silva, A. M., Rocha, N., Pinto, M., *et al.* 2005. Tremor as the first neurological manifestation of Sneddon's syndrome. *Mov Dis*, **20**, 248–51.

De Reuck, J., De Groote, L., and Van Maele, G. 2006. Delayed transient worsening of neurological deficits after ischaemic stroke. *Cerebrovasc Dis*, **22**, 27–32.

De Reuck, J., De Reus, R., and De Koninck, J. 1987. Sneddon's syndrome. A not unusual cause of stroke in young women. In *Cerebral Vascular Disease 6. Proceedings of the World Federation of Neurology 13th International Salzburg Conference*, J. S. Meyer, H. Lechner, M. Reivich, and E. O. Ott (eds.), Amsterdam: Excerpta Medica, pp. 171–4.

De Reuck, J., Goethals, M., Vonck, K., and Van Maele, G. 2005. Clinical predictors of late-onset seizures and epilepsy in patients with cerebrovascular disease. *Eur Neurol*, **54**, 68–72.

De Reus, R., De Reuck, J., Vermander, F., Kint, A., and Van de Velde, E. 1985. Livedo racemosa generalisata and stroke. *Clin Neurol Neurosurg*, **87**, 143–8.

Devuyst, G., Sindic, C., Laterre, E.-C., and Brucher, J.-M. 1996. Neuropathological findings of a Sneddon's syndrome presenting with dementia not preceded by clinical cerebrovascular events. *Stroke*, **27**, 1008–10.

Diez-Tejedor, E., Lara, M., Frank, A., Gutierrez, M., and Barreiro, P. 1990. Cerebral haemorrhage in Sneddon's syndrome. *J Neurol*, **237**(**Suppl**), 78–9.

Divry, P., and van Bogaert, L. 1946. Une maladie familiale caractérisée par une angiomatose diffuse cortico-meningée non calcifiante et une démyélinisation progressive de la substance blanche. *J Neurol Neurosurg Psychiatr*, **9**, 41–54.

Donders, R., Kappelle, L. J., Derksen, R., *et al.* 1998. Transient monocular blindness and antiphospholipid antibodies in systemic lupus erythematosus. *Neurology*, **51**, 535–40.

Donnet, A., Khalil, R., Terrier, G., *et al.* 1992. Cerebral infarction, livedo reticularis, and familial deficiency in antithrombin-III. *Stroke*, **23**, 611–2.

Dupont, S., Fénelon, G., Saiag, P., and Sirmai, J. 1996. Warfarin in Sneddon's syndrome. *Neurology*, **46**, 1781–2.

Ehrmann, S. 1906. Ein neues Gefassymptom bei Lues. *Wien Med Wochenschr*, **16**, 777–82.

Ellie, E., Julien, J., Henry, P., Vital, C., and Ferrer, X. 1987. Angiomatose cortico-méningée de Divry-van Bogaert et syndrome de Sneddon. Etude nosologique. A propos de quatre cas. *Rev Neurol*, **143**, 798–805.

Farronay, O. W., Kalashnikova, L. A., Vereschaguin, N. V., *et al.* 1992. Cerebrovascular and immunological studies in Sneddon's syndrome. *Ann Neurol*, **32**, 266.

Fetoni, V., Grisoli, M., Salmaggi, A., Carrieiro, R., and Girotti, F. 2000. Clinical and neuroradiological aspects of Sneddon's syndrome and primary antiphospholipid antibody syndrome. A follow-up study. *Neurol Sci*, **21**, 157–64.

Floel, A., Imai, T., Lohmann, H., *et al.* 2002. Therapy of Sneddon syndrome. *Eur Neurol*, **48**, 126–32.

Frances, C., Papo, T., Wechsler, B., *et al.* 1999. Sneddon syndrome with or without antiphospholipid antibodies. A comparative study of 46 patients. *Medicine (Baltimore)*, **78**, 209–19.

Frances, C., and Piette, J. C. 2000. The mystery of Sneddon syndrome: relationship with antiphospholipid syndrome and systemic lupus erythematosus. *J Autoimmunol*, **15**, 139–43.

Geschwind, D., FitzPatrick, M., Mischel, P., and Cummings, J. 1995. Sneddon's syndrome is a thrombotic vasculopathy: neuropathologic and neuroradiologic evidence. *Neurology*, **45**, 557–60.

Gibson, G. E., Su, W. P., and Pittelkow, M. R. 1997. Antiphospholipid syndrome and the skin. *J Am Acad Dermatol*, **36**, 970–82.

Gobert, A. 1994. Sneddon's syndrome with bilateral peripheral retinal neovascularization. *Bull Soc Belge Ophtalmol*, **255**, 85–90.

Hachulla, E., Piette, A. M., Hatron, P. Y., and Blétry, O. 2000. Aspirin and antiphospholipid syndrome. *Rev Med Interne*, **21**(**Suppl 1**), 83s–88s.

Hess, D. C. 1992. Stroke associated with antiphospholipid antibodies. *Stroke*, **23**(**Suppl**), 23–8.

Hilton, D. A., and Footitt, D. 2003. Neuropathological findings in Sneddon's syndrome. *Neurology*, **60**, 1181–2.

Jonas, J., Koelble, K., Voelcker, H. E., and Kalden, J. R. 1986. Central retinal artery occlusion in Sneddon's disease associated with antiphospholipid antibodies. *Am J Opthalmol*, **102**, 37–40.

Kalashnikova, L. A., Korczyn, A. D., Shavit, S., *et al.* 1999. Antibodies to protrombin in patients with Sneddon's syndrome. *Neurology*, **53**, 223–5.

Kalashnikova, L. A., Nasonov, E. L., Kushekbaeva, A. E., and Gracheva, L. A. 1990. Anticardiolipin antibodies in Sneddon's syndrome. *Neurology*, **40**, 464–7.

Khamashta, M. A., Cuadrado, M. J., Mujic, F., *et al.* 1995. The management of thrombosis in the antiphospholipid syndrome. *N Engl J Med*, **332**, 993–7.

Khoo, L. A., and Belli, A. M. 1999. Superior mesenteric artery stenting for mesenteric ischaemia in Sneddon's syndrome. *Br J Radiol*, **72**, 607–9.

Kraemer, M., Linden, D., and Berlit, P. 2005. The spectrum of differential diagnosis in neurological patients with livedo reticularis and livedo racemosa. A literature review. *J Neurol*, **252**, 1155–66.

Krnic-Barrie, S., O'Connor, C. R., Looney, S. W., Pierangeli, S. S., and Harris, E. N. 1997. A retrospective review of 61 patients with antiphospholipid syndrome. Analysis of factors influencing recurrent thrombosis. *Arch Intern Med*, **157**, 2101–8.

Levine, S. R., Langer, S. L., Albers, J. W., and Welch, K. M. A. 1988. Sneddon's syndrome: an antiphospholipid antibody syndrome? *Neurology*, **38**, 798–800.

Levine, S. R., and Welch, K. M. A. 1987. The spectrum of neurologic disease associated with antiphospholipid antibodies. *Arch Neurol*, **44**, 876–83.

Lewandowska, E., Wierzba-Bobrowicz, T., Wagner, T., *et al.* 2005. Sneddon's syndrome as a disorder of small arteries with endothelial cells proliferation: ultrastructural and neuroimaging study. *Folia Neuropathol*, **43**, 345–54.

Lockshin, M. D. 1992. Antiphospholipid antibody syndrome. *JAMA*, **268**, 1451–3.

Lubach, D., Schwabe, C., Weissenborn, K., *et al.* 1992. Livedo racemosa generalisata: an evaluation of thirty-four cases. *Stroke*, **23**, 1182–3.

Macario, F., Macario, M. C., Ferro, A., *et al.* 1997. Sneddon's syndrome: a vascular systemic disease with kidney involvement? *Nephron*, **75**, 94–7.

Marsch, W. C. L., and Muckelmann, R. 1985. Generalized racemose livedo with cerebrovascular lesions (Sneddon syndrome): an occlusive arteriolopathy due to proliferation and migration of medial smooth muscle cells. *Br J Dermatol*, **112**, 703–8.

Martinez-Menendez, B., Perez-Sempere, A., Gonzalez-Rubio, M., Villaverde-Amundarain, F. J., and Bermejo-Pareja, F. 1990. Sneddon's syndrome with negative antiphospholipid antibodies. *Stroke*, **21**, 1510–1.

Mascarenhas, R., Santo, G., Goncola, M., *et al.* 2003. Familial Sneddon's syndrome. *Eur J Dermatol*, **13**, 283–7.

Matsumura, Y., Tomimoto, H., Yamamoto, M., Imamura, S., and Miyachi, Y. 2001. Sneddon syndrome with multiple cerebral infarctions 12 years after the onset of livedo vasculitis: a possible involvement of platelet activation. *J Dermatol*, **28**, 508–10.

McHugh, N. J., Mayamo, J., Skinner, R. P., James, I., and Maddison, P. J. 1988. Anticardiolipin antibodies, livedo reticularis and major cerebrovascular and renal disease in systemic lupus erythematosus. *Ann Rheum Dis*, **47**, 110–5.

Menzel, C., Reinhold, U., Grunwald, F., *et al.* 1994. Cerebral blood flow in Sneddon syndrome. *J Nucl Med*, **35**, 461–4.

Michel, M., Bourquelot, P., and Hermine, O. 1996. Essential thrombocythaemia: a cause of Sneddon's syndrome. *Lancet*, **347**, 395.

Moral, A., Vidal, J. M., Moreau, I., Olhaberriague, L., and Montalban, J. 1991. Sneddon's syndrome with antiphospholipid antibodies and arteriopathy. *Stroke*, **22**, 1327–8.

Narbay, G. 1997. Sneddon's syndrome in a patient with homonymous hemianopia with macular sparing. *Bull Soc Belge Ophtalmol*, **263**, 103–7.

Pauranik, A., Parwani, S., and Jain, S. 1987. Simultaneous bilateral central retinal artery occlusion in a patient with Sneddon syndrome: case history. *J Vasc Dis*, **12**, 158–63.

Pellat, J., Perret, J., Pasquier, B., *et al.* 1976. Etude anatomoclinique et angiographie d'une observation de thromboangiose disséminée à manifestations cérébrales prédominantes. *Rev Neurol*, **132**, 517–35.

Pettee, A. D., Wasserman, B. A., Adams, N. L., *et al.* 1994. Familial Sneddon's syndrome. Clinical, hematological, and radiographic findings in two brothers. *Neurology*, **44**, 399–405.

Pinol-Aguade, J., Ferrandiz, C., Ferrer-Roca, O., and Ingelmo, M. 1999. Livedo reticularis y accidentes cerebrovasculares. *Med Cutan Ibero Lat Am*, **3**, 257–65.

Quimby, S. R., and Perry, H. O. 1980. Livedo reticularis and cerebrovascular accidents. *J Am Acad Dermatol*, **3**, 377–83.

Rebollo, M., Val, J. F., Garijo, F., Quintana, F., and Berg, E. L. 1983. Livedo reticularis and cerebrovascular lesions (Sneddon's syndrome). *Brain*, **106**, 965–79.

Rehany, U., Kassif, Y., and Rumelt, S. 1998. Sneddon's syndrome: neuro-ophthalmologic manifestations in a possible autosomal recessive pattern. *Neurology*, **51**, 1185–7.

Rosenberg, R. D., and Aird, W. C. 1999. Vascular-bed-specific hemostasis and hypercoagulable states. *N Engl J Med*, **340**, 1555–64.

Rumpl, E., Neuhofer, J., Pallua, A., *et al.* 1985. Cerebrovascular lesions and livedo reticularis (Sneddon's syndrome): a progressive cerebrovascular disorder? *J Neurol*, **231**, 324–30.

Rumpl, E., and Rumpl, H. 1979. Recurrent transient global amnesia in a case with cerebrovascular lesions and livedo reticularis (Sneddon syndrome). *J Neurol*, **221**, 127–31.

Ruscalleda, J., Coscojuela, P., Guardia, E., and De Juan, M. 1991. General case of the day. *Radiographics*, **11**, 929–31.

Sauter, A., and Rudin, M. 1992. Cerebral infarction, livedo reticularis, and familial deficiency in antithrombin-III. *Stroke*, **23**, 611–2.

Scott, I. A., and Boyle, R. S. 1986. Sneddon's syndrome. *Aust N Z Med*, **16**, 799–802.

Serrano-Pozo, A., Gomez-Aranda, F., Franco-Macias, E., and Serrano-Cabrera, A. 2004. Cerebral haemorrhage in Sneddon's syndrome: case report and literature review. *Rev Neurol*, **39**, 731–3.

Sitzer, M., Sohngen, D., Siebler, M., *et al.* 1995. Cerebral microembolism in patients with Sneddon's syndrome. *Arch Neurol*, **52**, 271–5.

Sneddon, I. B. 1965. Cerebro-vascular lesions and livedo reticularis. *Br J Dermatol*, **77**, 777–82.

Stephens, W. P., and Ferguson, I. T. 1982. Livedo reticularis and cerebro-vascular disease. *Postgrad Med J*, **58**, 70–3.

Stockhammer, G., Felber, S. R., Zelger, B., *et al.* 1993. Sneddon's syndrome: diagnosis by skin biopsy and MRI in 17 patients. *Stroke*, **24**, 685–90.

Szmyrka-Kaczmarek, M., Daikeler, T., Benz, D., and Koetter, I. 2005. Familial inflammatory Sneddon's syndrome-case report and review of the literature. *Clin Rheumatol*, **24**, 79–82.

Tanne, D., Triplett, D. A., and Levine, S. R. 1998. Antiphospholipid-protein antibodies and ischemic stroke. Not just cardiolipin anymore. *Stroke*, **29**, 1755–8.

Thomas, D. J., Kirby, J. D. T., Britton, K. E., and Galton, D. J. 1982. Livedo reticularis and neurological lesions. *Br J Dermatol*, **106**, 711–2.

Tietjen, G., Al-Qasmi, M., Gunda, P., and Herial, N. 2006. Sneddon's syndrome: another migraine-stroke association? *Cephalgia*, **26**, 225–32.

Toubi, E., Krause, I., Fraser, A., Lev, S., *et al.* 2005. Livedo reticularis is a marker for predicting multi-system thrombosis in antiphospholipid syndrome. *Clin Exp Rheumatol*, **23**, 499–504.

Tourbah, A., Piette, J., Iba-Zizen, M. T., *et al.* 1997. The natural course of cerebral lesions in Sneddon's syndrome. *Arch Neurol*, **54**, 53–60.

Uitdehaag, B. M. J., Scheltens, P., Bertelsmann, F. W., and Bruyn, R. P. M. 1992. Intracerebral hemorrhage and Sneddon's syndrome. *J Neurol Sci*, **111**, 227–8.

Vaillant, L., Larmande, P., Arbeille, B., *et al.* 1990. Livedo reticularis, accidents vasculaires cérébraux et maladie mitrale: une nouvelle cause du syndrome de Sneddon. *Ann Dermatol Venereol*, **117**, 925–30.

Vargas, J. A., Yerba, M., Pascual, M. L., Manzano, L., and Durantez, A. 1989. Antiphospholipid antibodies and Sneddon's syndrome. *Am J Med*, **87**, 597.

Wohlrab, J., Fischer, M., Wolter, M., and Marsch, W. C. 2001. Diagnostic impact and sensitivity of skin biopsies in Sneddon's syndrome. A report of 15 cases. *Br J Dermatol*, **145**, 285–8.

Zelger, B., Sepp, N., Schmid, K. W., *et al.* 1992. Life history of cutaneous vascular lesions in Sneddon's syndrome. *Hum Pathol*, **23**, 668–75.

Zelger, B., Sepp, N., Stockhammer, G., *et al.* 1993. Sneddon's syndrome. A long-term follow-up of 21 patients. *Arch Neurol*, **129**, 437–47.

Genetic and metabolic etiologies of stroke are considered in the differential diagnosis of stroke in children and young adults presenting with acute focal neurologic deficits. The incidence of stroke secondary to a metabolic disorder is unknown, and mortality data in the general population are lacking. In this chapter, we review mitochondrial and other selective metabolic causes of stroke (Schapira, 2006).

Mitochondrial disorders

Mitochondrial cytopathies are heterogeneous groups of disorders with a wide range of clinical features, preferentially affecting the muscles and the nervous system. The concept of mitochondrial disease was first described by Luft *et al.* (1962) in a young Swedish woman with severe hypermetabolism of nonthyroid origin. Abnormal deposits of mitochondria defined as "ragged-red fibers" were described by Engel and Cunningham (1963), and defects of mitochondrial metabolism causing a wide range of human diseases have been subsequently reported in the literature since the 1970s (Spiro *et al.*, 1970; Willems *et al.*, 1977). In 1988, Holt *et al.* described a pathogenic mutation of mitochondrial DNA (mtDNA) in a patient with mitochondrial myopathy (Holt *et al.*, 1988; Johns, 1995). Mitochondrial myopathies are caused either by mutations in the maternally inherited mitochondrial genome, or by nuclear DNA mutations, with defects in the respiratory chain complexes.

MELAS (mitochondrial encephalomyopathy, lactic acidosis, and stroke-like episodes)

Mitochondrial diseases are far more common than previously anticipated, with a prevalence of 5.7 per 100 000 in the population older than 14 years (Arpa *et al.*, 2003; Schapira, 2006). The acronym MELAS – describing a clinical syndrome with mitochondrial encephalopathy, myopathy, lactic acidosis, and stroke-like episodes – was introduced by Pavlakis *et al.* (1984), and is the most frequently occurring maternally inherited mitochondrial disorder. MELAS is a multiorgan syndrome, predominantly involving the central nervous system (CNS). There is considerable variability in the clinical presentation of MELAS. Neurological findings range from asymptomatic, to progressive muscle weakness, migraine-like headaches, cognitive impairment, recurrent seizures, ataxia, to stroke-like episodes during adolescence, and encephalopathy. Most patients present with migraine-like headache and seizures, in the setting of recurrent stroke-like episodes (Ohno *et al.*, 1997; Schapira, 2006). Brain imaging abnormalities in patients with

MELAS usually involve the posterior parietal and occipital lobes, and usually do not follow a specific vascular arterial distribution (Figure 57.1) (Coelho-Miranda *et al.*, 2000; Matsumoto *et al.*, 2005; Noguchi *et al.*, 2005; Ohno *et al.*, 1997; Schapira, 2006). Cardiac involvement includes valvulopathy, conduction defects, and progressive hypertrophic or dilated cardiomyopathies, resulting in congestive heart failure or end-stage heart disease (Hirano and Pavlakis, 1994; Hoffmann *et al.*, 1994; Johns, 1995; Momiyama *et al.*, 2001; Noer *et al.*, 1988; Pavlakis *et al.*, 1984; van den Berg *et al.*, 2000). Brain embolization in patients with cardiac involvement may occur. Full expression of the disease may result in gradual cognitive decline secondary to recurrent strokes, and death may follow. Other clinical features may include deafness (Mikol *et al.*, 2005; Takeshima and Nakashima, 2005; Tawankanjanachot *et al.*, 2005) and ocular manifestations such as bilateral eyelid ptosis, chronic external ophthalmoplegia, posterior subcapsular cataracts, atypical pigmentary retinopathy, and optic nerve atrophy (Bene *et al.*, 2003; Isashiki *et al.*, 1998; Rummelt *et al.*, 1993). Endocrinopathies are common including diabetes mellitus, hypothyroidism, and hypogonadism (Drouet *et al.*, 2000; Mikol *et al.*, 2005; Momiyama *et al.*, 2001; Murakami *et al.*, 2002; Schmiedel *et al.*, 2003; Topaloglu *et al.*, 1998).

MELAS is associated with a number of pathogenic point mutations in mtDNA (Schmiedel *et al.*, 2003), with more than 80% of the heteroplasmic A-to-G point mutations occurring in the dihydrouridine loop of the mitochondrial leucine transfer RNA of the mtDNA gene at base pair 3243 (A3243G mutation). Eighty to ninety percent of cases are associated with a point mutation (Goto, 2005; Goto *et al.*, 1991; Mamourian and du Plessis, 1991). The frequency of the A3243G mutation approximates 16.3 per 100 000 in adult populations (Majamaa *et al.*, 1997, 1998). Because mtDNA is maternally inherited, the majority of patients with mitochondrial disorders have a maternal pattern of inheritance; however, sporadic cases have also been described.

The pathophysiology of MELAS is not completely understood. Several mechanisms are proposed to contribute to this disease. These include decreased aminoacylation of mitochondrial transfer RNA (tRNA), resulting in decreased mitochondrial protein synthesis, changes in calcium homeostasis, and alterations in nitric oxide metabolism.

The pathogenesis of stroke-like episodes in MELAS remains unclear. Despite the microangiopathic findings in the brain and muscles (Iizuka and Sakai, 2005), the stroke-like episodes are more likely attributed to mitochondrial and metabolic dysfunction in neural tissue and glia rather than to ischemic vascular pathology

Uncommon Causes of Stroke, 2nd edition, ed. Louis R. Caplan. Published by Cambridge University Press. © Cambridge University Press 2008.

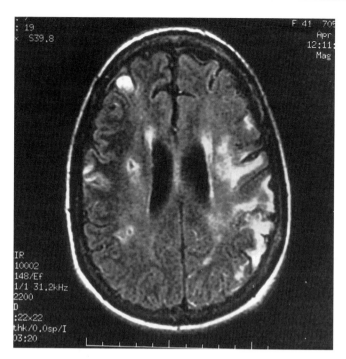

Figure 57.1 Hyperintense lesions on fluid-attenuated inversion recovery (FLAIR) in patients with MELAS.

(Michelson and Ashwal, 2004; Molnar *et al.*, 2000; Nariai *et al.*, 2000; Takahashi *et al.*, 1998).

The diagnosis of MELAS requires incorporating clinical, neuroimaging, histochemical, and molecular investigations. Hirano *et al.* (1992) proposed clinical criteria for establishing a diagnosis of MELAS. The main criteria are: (a) stroke-like episodes before age 40; (b) encephalopathy characterized by seizures, dementia, or both; and (c) lactic acidosis, ragged red fibers, or both. Additional criteria are: (d) normal early development, (e) recurrent headaches, and (f) recurrent vomiting. Elevated serum and cerebrospinal fluid (CSF) lactate, with the characteristic findings on neuroradiological testing, raise suspicion of the condition. A muscle biopsy with the characteristic ragged-red fibers confirms the diagnosis (Scaglia and Northrop, 2006; Schapira, 2006; Thambisetty and Newman, 2004). MRI with abnormal and normal-to-increased apparent diffusion coefficient in young patients presenting with acute stroke should raise the suspicion of metabolic causes of stroke (Abe *et al.*, 2004; Oppenheim *et al.*, 2000; Wang *et al.*, 2003; Yoneda *et al.*, 1999). Genetic mutation analysis may be performed on peripheral blood leukocytes, skeletal muscle, or both.

Characteristically, patients with MELAS have a slowly progressive course, with recurrent neurological deficits (with relapses and remissions) and gradual progression to dementia. A considerable number of patients succumb to the disease in the third decade of life.

To date, there is no consensus on the treatment of MELAS. Treatment is mainly supportive, directed toward the management of multisystem complications. Antioxidants, respiratory chain substrates and cofactors, and multivitamins have been suggested (Scaglia and Northrop, 2006). The use of L-arginine and free-radical scavengers such as edaravone has been reported to reduce cerebral edema in a patient with MELAS after acute cerebral infarction (Kubota *et al.*, 2004; Maeda *et al.*, 2005).

MERFF (myoclonic epilepsy with ragged-red fibers)/MELAS overlap syndrome

A rare point mutation at nucleotide position 8356 in the tRNA gene in mtDNA has been described in Japanese, American, and Italian families (Campos *et al.*, 1996; Zeviani *et al.*, 1993). Like MELAS, patients present with migraine, stroke-like episodes associated with lactic acidosis and dementia in addition to myoclonic epilepsy with ataxia and ragged-red fibers in a muscle biopsy specimen consistent with the clinical characteristics of MERRF. Sporadic mutation has also been reported (Campos *et al.*, 1996).

Kearns Sayre syndrome

Kearns Sayre syndrome (KSS) is a mitochondrial disorder caused by large heteroplasmic deletions in mtDNA. It is characterized by myopathy, chronic progressive external ophthalmoplegia, pigmentary retinopathy (salt-pepper like appearance), endocrinopathies, and cardiac abnormalities (Laloi-Michelin *et al.*, 2006; Park *et al.*, 2004). Brain infarction, presumably secondary to cardioembolic sources, may occur (Chabrol and Paquis, 1997; Kosinski *et al.*, 1995; Muller *et al.*, 2003; Provenzale and VanLandingham, 1996). Muscle biopsy shows ragged-red fibers under Gomori-trichrome staining. Insertion of pacemaker devices may prolong survival in patients with cardiac abnormalities and may decrease the risk of cardioembolic stroke (Provenzale and VanLandingham, 1996).

Subacute necrotizing encephalomyelopathy (Leigh syndrome)

The first case of subacute necrotizing encephalomyelopathy was described by Denis Leigh at autopsy in a 7-month-old infant with symmetrical lesions involving the thalamus, midbrain, pons, medulla, and posterior column of the spinal cord and resembling Wernicke's encephalopathy (Leigh, 1951).

Leigh's syndrome is a genetically heterogeneous, neurodegenerative disorder of infancy and childhood caused by mutation of the nuclear or mtDNA genome. The pathogenesis of Leigh's syndrome appears to represent the neuropathologic endpoint of disordered cerebral mitochondrial energy production (Holt *et al.*, 1990). The commonest biochemical abnormalities involve the cytochrome *c* oxidase (COX) complex I/II (Morris *et al.*, 1996; Moslemi *et al.*, 2003; Tay *et al.*, 2005; Taylor *et al.*, 2002; Ugalde *et al.*, 2003), and the pyruvate dehydrogenase complex (Chabrol *et al.*, 1994; Naito *et al.*, 1997).

The clinical presentation is highly variable. The classical presentation includes developmental delay, ataxia, hypotonia, brainstem dysfunction, respiratory abnormalities, and hypertrophic cardiomyopathy. Atypical presentation with progressive limb weakness, demyelinating neuropathy, progressive diplegia, blindness, bull's-eye maculopathy-like fundus abnormality, and tonic seizures have been reported (Huntsman *et al.*, 2005). The infantile form progresses very rapidly and results in death within 2 years (Montpetit *et al.*, 1971). The juvenile form has a subacute or acute

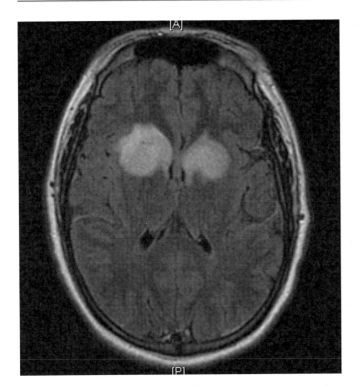

Figure 57.2 Bilateral symmetric putaminal hyperdensities on FLAIR in a patient with juvenile Leigh disease.

course. Mild spastic paraparesis, visual impairment, and movement disorders have been reported. Juvenile-onset Leigh's syndrome may present with an acute polyneuropathy (Stickler *et al.*, 2003); chronic sensory motor neuropathy, ataxia, deafness and retinitis pigmentosa (NARP); or myopathy and cardiomyopathy resulting in marked respiratory depression and coma (Grunnet *et al.*, 1991).

The condition is usually suspected in infants and children with developmental delay, elevated serum, and CSF lactate. Muscle and skin biopsies are usually helpful.

MRI examination of brain typically shows symmetrical hypointense lesions on T1/hyperintense on T2 in the basal ganglia, mainly in the putamen, and brainstem, with sparing of the mamillary bodies and red nuclei (Kissel *et al.*, 1987; Medina *et al.*, 1990) (Figure 57.2). White matter involvement is also common (Lerman-Sagie *et al.*, 2005).

Pathologically, there is gray matter degeneration and focal brainstem and spinal cord necrosis with marked spongiosis, endothelial proliferation, and extensive demyelination.

Treatment is symptomatic. Administration of coenzyme Q10 (Van Maldergem *et al.*, 2002), thiamine (Di Rocco *et al.*, 2000), sodium dichloroacetate (Craigen, 1996; Takanashi *et al.*, 1997), and a ketogenic diet (Wijburg *et al.*, 1992) has been found helpful.

COX deficiency (Saguenay-Lac St-Jean)

Saguenay-Lac St-Jean is a rare autosomal recessive disorder characterized by congenital systemic deficiency of COX (Lee *et al.*, 2001). It is clinically heterogeneous, ranging from isolated myopathy to severe multisystem disease, with onset from infancy to

adulthood. Lactic acidosis, developmental delay, and hypotonia are common features. Stroke-like episodes have been reported (Morin *et al.*, 1999). .

Tangier disease

Tangier disease is an autosomal recessive disorder characterized by deficiency or absence of high-density lipoprotein (HDL) cholesterol and apolipoprotein (apo) A-I levels (both <10 mg/dL), decreased low-density lipoprotein (LDL) cholesterol levels (about 40% of normal), and mild hypertriglyceridemia (Nofer and Remaley, 2005). The disorder is caused by mutations in the adenosine triphosphate (ATP)-binding cassette transporter A1 (ABCA1), leading to impairment of HDL-mediated cholesterol transport, and deposition of cholesteryl esters in reticuloendothelial tissues (Bared *et al.*, 2004; Neufeld *et al.*, 2004; Zuchner *et al.*, 2003). Enlarged lobulated tonsils (yellow-orange tonsils) and hepatosplenomegaly are common. Neurological symptoms are also common (Kocen, 2004). A predominantly proximal asymmetric sensorimotor peripheral neuropathy, which is usually slowly progressive, is the presenting feature in 30% of cases (Pietrini *et al.*, 1985). Facial diplegia and mononeuritis multiplex may occur. Children are predisposed to premature atherosclerosis (Mautner *et al.*, 1992); cardiac involvement (Pressly *et al.*, 1987) and brain infarction have been reported (Serfaty-Lacrosniere *et al.*, 1994).

The diagnosis is usually made when laboratory evaluation shows hypocholesterolemia with severely reduced HDL in the presence of a suggestive clinical picture.

There is currently no treatment for Tangier disease. ABCA1 is a promising therapeutic target for preventing atherosclerotic disease because of its ability to deplete cells of cholesterol and to raise plasma HDL levels (Nofer and Remaley, 2005).

Menkes disease

Menkes disease (kinky hair disease, steely hair disease, trichopoliodystrophy) is an X-linked neurodegenerative disease caused by a defective gene that regulates the metabolism of copper transport, with accumulation of copper at abnormally low levels in the liver and brain, but at higher-than-normal levels in the kidney and intestinal lining (George *et al.*, 2005). The mutant gene is located on the long arm of the X chromosome at Xq13.3. The incidence of the disease is 1 in 50 000–250 000. The disease occurs in infancy, and the clinical manifestations usually begin within the first 1–2 months. Affected patients may present with seizures, failure to thrive, subnormal body temperature, and strikingly peculiar kinky, light, abnormally pigmented, and easily broken hair.

Pathologically, there is extensive neurodegeneration in the gray matter. Intracranial and extracranial vascular pathology may occur, including arterial tortuosity, stenosis, or arterial rupture (Hsich *et al.*, 2000; Seay *et al.*, 1979; Takahashi *et al.*, 1993). If untreated, the disease is progressive, and death usually occurs by 3 years of age.

Early diagnosis is difficult in the absence of a suggestive clinical picture. The disease should be suspected in infants with developmental delay and clinical characteristics. The diagnosis is confirmed by low serum copper and ceruloplasmin levels, and by copper uptake studies on fibroblast cultures. The urine homovanillic acid/vanillylmandelic acid ratio is also a useful screening method for the disorder. Gene analysis may be useful and is often reliable when a mutation in ATP7A is present, and may help in prenatal diagnosis (Liu *et al.*, 2002; Poulsen *et al.*, 2004). Oral copper treatment is not effective. Early treatment, if started within 1 month of life with subcutaneous parenteral copper-histidine, may prevent neurological disturbance and may prolong survival rate (Kirodian *et al.*, 2002).

Hyperhomocysteinemia and homocystinuria

Hyperhomocysteinemia is a clinical syndrome caused by several enzyme deficiencies in methionine metabolism. Homocysteine is a sulfhydryl-containing amino acid produced during the metabolism of methionine. Its intracellular metabolism is controlled by two pathways: transsulfuration to cysteine and remethylation to methionine. The majority of homocysteine is catabolized via pyridoxine (B6)-dependent condensation with serine to form cystathionine. Cystathionine β-synthase catalyzes the first committed step of transsulfuration and is the most common enzyme deficient in classical homocystinuria (Kraus *et al.*, 1998). This defect is associated with disorders of the connective tissue, muscles, CNS, and cardiovascular system. A second pathway is remethylation of homocysteine back to methionine by methionine synthase, which requires methylenetetrahydrofolate and methylcobalamin as cofactors.

A number of hereditary defects in the enzymes involved in homocysteine metabolism and various acquired deficiencies in the vitamin cofactors of these enzymes are associated with the development of hyperhomocysteinemia. Deficiency of three enzymes – cystathionine β-synthetase, methylenetetrahydrofolate reductase (MTHFR), and methionine synthase – leads to hyperhomocysteinemia. High plasma levels of homocysteine are also observed with advanced age, in smokers, and in certain nutritional disorders associated with vitamin B12 (cobalamin), pyridoxine (vitamin B6), or folic acid deficiencies. Additionally, elevated homocysteine levels are seen following exposure to various drugs, including fibrates, statins, niacin, antihypertensive agents, metformin, methotrexate, sulfasalazine, anticonvulsants, levodopa, and theophylline (Apeland *et al.*, 2001; Dierkes and Westphal, 2005; Sener *et al.*, 2006; Siniscalchi *et al.*, 2005; Ueland and Refsum, 1989); The estimated incidence of homocystinuria is more common than previously reported, approximately 1:83 000 live births (Sokolova *et al.*, 2001).

The most common enzyme deficiency is cystathionine β-synthetase deficiency (Mudd *et al.*, 1964). The genetic defect in cystathionine β-synthetase is located on chromosome 21 (Kraus *et al.*, 1993). The homozygous trait of congenital homocystinuria is rare. Approximately 0.3–1.5% of the population is heterozygous for cystathionine β-synthetase deficiency. At least 24 mutations have been identified for the heterozygosity for cystathionine β-synthetase. Plasma homocysteine concentrations are slightly elevated (two to four times more than normal) in heterozygotes. Thromboembolism is a major cause of mortality and morbidity

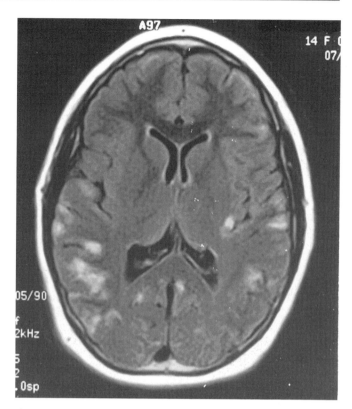

Figure 57.3 Cortical infarctions and white matter lesions in patients with MTHFR deficiency.

in patients with homocystinuria (Mudd *et al.*, 1972; Uhlemann *et al.*, 1976).

MTHFR mutation is an autosomal recessive disorder affecting folate metabolism. The gene is localized to chromosome 1p. MTHFR is a critical enzyme in the metabolism of folate and methionine. It is also prevalent in the population; about 50% of North Americans are heterozygous, and 11% are homozygous for a thermolabile mutation of MTHFR (Rozen, 1996). Unlike the A1298C mutation, MTHFR C677T homozygous polymorphism contributes to hyperhomocysteinemia and increases the risk factor for ischemic stroke (Figure 57.3) (Dikmen *et al.*, 2006; Li *et al.*, 2003; Rook *et al.*, 2005).

Homocystinuria promotes premature atherosclerosis and arterial dilatation. Mechanisms involved in homocysteine-induced atherosclerosis include increased tissue factor expression, attenuated anticoagulant processes, enhanced platelet reactivity, increased thrombin generation, augmented factor V activity, impaired fibrinolytic potential, endothelial dysfunction with smooth muscle cell proliferation, and increased monocyte recruitment into developing atherosclerotic lesions by upregulating monocyte chemotactic protein-1 (MCP-1) and interleukin (IL)-8 expression in vascular smooth muscle cells (Desai *et al.*, 2001; Undas *et al.*, 2005). Fibrous intimal plaques, medial fibrosis, and disruption of the internal elastic lamina are typical features (McCully, 1969; Tsai *et al.*, 1996). Homocysteine suppresses expression of thrombomodulin and heparin sulfate, resulting in a prothrombotic state (Lentz and Sadler, 1991). Neuropathologic changes are widespread and include microgyria and perivascular changes such as demyelination, macrophage infiltration, and gliosis.

Patients with homocystinuria have markedly elevated plasma homocysteine concentrations. Most patients present with peripheral venous thrombosis, including pulmonary embolism. Stroke, peripheral arterial occlusions, or myocardial infarction can be the initial presentation (Clarke and Lewington, 2002; Sacco *et al.*, 1998). The increased tendency for thrombosis usually presents as an ischemic stroke. There is also an increased risk of Alzheimer disease and vascular dementia in patients with homocystinuria. Other manifestations may include dystonia (Kempster *et al.*, 1988; Zupanc *et al.*, 1991) or osteoporosis (Sato *et al.*, 2005).

Hyperhomocysteinemia is accepted as an independent risk factor for cardiovascular disease and stroke (Graham *et al.*, 1997; McIlroy *et al.*, 2002). Stroke may occur secondary to artery-to-artery embolism or arterial dissection (Kelly *et al.*, 2003). While the Framingham Heart Study showed a strong relationship between elevated homocysteine levels and carotid artery disease (Selhub *et al.*, 1995), B-mode ultrasound imaging did not show evidence of increased intima-media thickness of carotid arteries in patients with homocystinuria because of homozygosis for cystathionine β-synthetase deficiency, suggesting arterial dilatations with resultant medial damage as the cause of thrombosis rather than typical atherosclerotic lesions in these patients (Rubba *et al.*, 1994).

The classic early childhood homocystinuria is associated with early atherosclerosis, marfanoid features, mental retardation, and ectopia lentis (Mudd *et al.*, 1985). Malar flush, livedo reticularis, myopia, glaucoma, and (rarely) optic atrophy may be present. The multiple clinical presentations that are possible relate to the genetic heterogeneity involved with this deficiency state. Approximately 50% of these patients will have a thromboembolic event before age 30 (Mudd *et al.*, 1985).

MTHFR deficiency is the most common inherited disorder of folate metabolism. A typical presentation is infantile global delay and failure to thrive, with associated seizures and progressive neurological deterioration. With infantile onset, cerebrovascular manifestations tend to be more striking than in cystathionine β-synthetase deficiency. MTHFR deficiency is associated with a possible increase in myocardial infarctions and adverse cardiac events after myocardial revascularization in patients with coronary artery disease (Botto *et al.*, 2004; Kluijtmans *et al.*, 1996). Adult-onset cerebrovascular disease is also possible, but currently data are lacking to support this mutation as an independent risk factor for stroke.

All young patients and adults with unexplained ischemic or retinal vascular occlusive disease, and coronary atherosclerosis should be considered for plasma homocysteine testing. The range of normal plasma homocysteine levels is still debatable. Plasma homocysteine levels 10.2 mmol/L or higher, were associated with an increase in vascular events (Graham *et al.*, 1997). Infants with cystathionine β-synthetase deficiency may be identified with neonatal screening for methionine. The cyanide nitroprusside test may be used for neonatal screening of infants with cystathionine β-synthetase. Prenatal diagnosis can be possible by amniocentesis and enzymatic essay of cultured amniocytes. MTHFR deficiency is also characterized by low CSF folate levels and low plasma

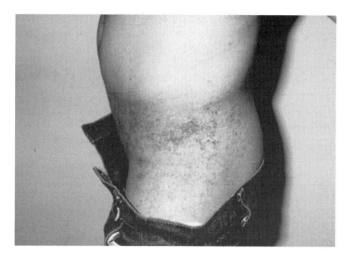

Figure 57.4 Angiokeratomas in a patient with Fabry disease.

methionine without megaloblastic anemia. Prenatal diagnosis is possible.

Although various observational studies have shown some benefit of vitamin supplementation with folic acid, pyridoxine, and vitamin B12 in reducing the risk of coronary heart disease and stroke, the strength of association of homocysteine with risk of vascular diseases remain weak (B-Vitamin Treatment Trialists' Collaboration, 2006). Despite moderate reduction of total homocysteine after nondisabling cerebral infarction, the Vitamin Intervention in Stroke Prevention (VISP) study failed to prove the potential benefit of high-dose vitamin supplementation in reducing the risk of recurrent stroke or myocardial infarction at 2 years (Furie and Kelly, 2006; Toole *et al.*, 2004). Similarly, both the Heart Outcomes Prevention Evaluation (HOPE)-2 and the Norwegian Vitamin Trial (NORVIT) studies did not show a reduction in the risk of major cardiovascular events in vascular disease patients receiving vitamin supplementation with folic acid, B6, and B12 (Bonaa *et al.*, 2006; Lonn *et al.*, 2006). An ongoing large-scale randomized, double-blinded, placebo-controlled trial based in Australia is currently in progress to test whether lowering blood homocysteine levels can reduce the risks of vascular sequelae following recent stroke or transient ischemic attack (VITATOPS Trial Study Group, 2002).

Anderson–Fabry disease

Anderson–Fabry disease is a rare X-linked disorder, caused by a deficient activity of the lysosomal enzyme α-galactosidase A resulting in progressive deposition of neutral glycosphingolipid (predominantly globotriaosylceramide trihexoside) in multivisceral organs, including the skin, eyes, kidney, heart, vascular system, and nervous system. (Brady and Schiffmann, 2000). Male hemizygotes are generally more severely affected than are female heterozygotes.

Clinical disease in women is thought to be due to unequal X chromosome inactivation. Children and adolescents usually present with angiokeratomas corporis diffusum (Figure 57.4), acroparesthesias, severe crisis of pain in the extremities, anhidrosis, gastrointestinal disturbances, corneal dystrophy (corneal verticillata), vascular lesions in the conjunctiva and retina, kidney disease,

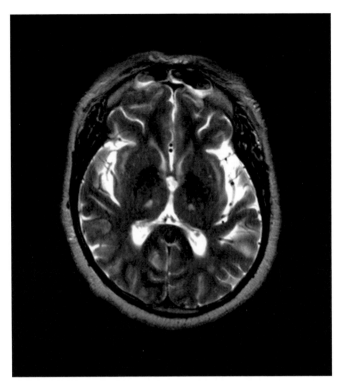

Figure 57.5 Bilateral thalamic hyperdensities on T2-weighted MRI in an adult patient with Fabry disease and history of renal transplantation.

cardiovascular complications, and vestibular, autonomic peripheral neuropathic symptoms. Seizures, aseptic meningitis, and pulvinar calcification may also occur. Deposition of glycosphingolipids in the vascular endothelium can lead to ischemia, predominantly in the deep white matter, brainstem, and basal ganglia, because of thrombosis or stenosis of small perforating vessels (Figure 57.5) (Clavelou et al., 2006; Giacomini et al., 2004; Grewal, 1994; Tanaka et al., 2005). Central retinal artery occlusion, cerebral aneurysm, and intraparenchymal hemorrhage may also occur (Andersen et al., 1994; Callegaro and Kaimen-Maciel, 2006; Schiffmann and Ries, 2005). Patients may present with stroke at a young age in the absence of other typical clinical features of Fabry disease.

Histologically, lysosomal aggregates are usually present in the organs affected or in the endothelium. Biochemical and histological findings on muscle biopsy may assist in the diagnosis (Giacomini et al., 2004; Grewal, 1994; Grewal and Barton, 1992; Schiffmann and Ries, 2005).

Beneficial effects of intravenous enzyme replacement therapy with algalsidase β (Fabrazyme) have been reported (del Toro et al., 2004; Spinelli et al., 2004). Fabry disease is the topic of Chapter 19.

Organic acidemias

Propionic acidemia

Propionic acidemia is a rare metabolic disorder in which a defective enzyme, propionyl-coenzyme A (CoA) carboxylase, results in an accumulation of propionic acid. Patients may present with vomiting, dehydration, lethargy, encephalopathy, and rapidly fatal symmetric necrosis of the caudate, globus pallidus, and putamen (Haas et al., 1995). Diagnosis is made by organic acid analysis in urine.

Methylmalonic acidemia

Methylmalonic acidemia (MMA) is an inborn disorder of amino acid metabolism characterized by accumulation of toxic organic methylmalonic acid and its by-products in biological fluids. The disorder is identified in 1:250 000 newborns screened. It commonly presents with neurologic deficits, including retinopathy, hydrocephalus, and microcephaly. Metabolic stroke due to hypoxemia and vascular insufficiency may occur. Gas chromatography-mass spectrometry (GC-MS) demonstrates large amounts of methylmalonic acid and its metabolite in the urine (Chakrapani et al., 2002; Heidenreich et al., 1988; Thompson et al., 1989). Proton magnetic resonance spectroscopy and diffusion-weighted imaging of the brain in two patients with methylmalonic acidemia showed restricted diffusion and elevated lactate in the globi pallidi, compatible with acute infarctions and metabolic acidosis (Michel et al., 2004; Trinh et al., 2001; Yesildag et al., 2005).

Glutaric aciduria

Glutaric aciduria is an inborn error of metabolism that results from a deficiency of glutaryl-CoA dehydrogenase. The disorder is characterized by macrocephaly, seizures, spasticity, and extrapyramidal dysfunction. Frontotemporal atrophy, basal ganglia infarctions, and bilateral subdural collections may be seen on neuroimaging studies (Hoffmann et al., 1994; Kohler and Hoffmann, 1998; Osaka et al., 1993).

Glutaric aciduria type I

Typical features are macrocephaly and attacks of fever of unknown origin and sweating. Acute cerebral infarctions, seizures, and coma may occur (Hoffmann et al., 1994; Strauss and Morton, 2003; Strauss et al., 2003; Vallee et al., 1994). Spasticity, dystonia, intellectual impairment, and choreoathetosis may be seen (Goodman et al., 1975). This condition may resemble Leigh's disease or nonaccidental head trauma in infants (shaken baby syndrome), with retinal hemorrhages and intracranial (subdural/subarachnoid) bleeding (Stutchfield et al., 1985). Neuroimaging studies may show frontotemporal atrophy and signal changes in putamen and caudate nuclei (Altman et al., 1991; Strauss and Morton, 2003) Glutaryl-CoA dehydrogenase is the deficient enzyme in this condition, with the gene located on the short arm of chromosome 19. Organic acid analysis of urine or culture of fibroblasts and leukocytes is useful in the diagnosis.

Treatment includes a low-protein diet and a combination of riboflavin (Brandt et al., 1979) and carnitine (Seccombe et al., 1986). Baclofen (Awaad et al., 1996) and vigabatrin (Francois et al., 1990) may be useful.

Glutaric aciduria type II

In glutaric aciduria type II, there is impairment of various acyl-CoA dehydrogenases. This condition is also referred to as multiple acyl-CoA dehydrogenase deficiency. Three different forms have been described: neonatal, infantile, and later onset. All forms are characterized by vomiting, hypoglycemia, metabolic acidosis, a strong "sweaty-feet" odor, stroke-like episode, seizures, aphasia, ataxia, and myoclonus (Vallee *et al.*, 1994). Cardiomyopathy and renal cysts may also present. Pathologically there is fatty degeneration of multiple organs. Diagnosis is made by detection of large amounts of urinary organic acids.

Sulfatide oxidase deficiency

Sulfatide oxidase deficiency is a rare autosomal recessive disorder usually presenting in early infancy. Clinical features include seizures, developmental delay, microcephaly, ectopia lentis, and acute infantile hemiplegia (Shih *et al.*, 1977). Cerebral atrophy and cystic encephalomalacia have been reported (Dublin *et al.*, 2002; Tan *et al.*, 2005). Biochemical assay for specific urinary and plasma metabolites is diagnostic. Prenatal diagnosis of sulfite oxidase deficiency is possible by measuring S-sulfocysteine in amniotic fluid (Shih *et al.*, 1977). There is no current treatment for the disorder. A diet restricted in cysteine and methionine has not shown benefit in improving neurological outcome.

Ornithine transcarbamylase deficiency

Ornithine transcarbamylase deficiency is an X-linked recessive disorder and the most common inherited cause of hyperammonemia secondary to urea cycle deficiency. The disorder is characterized by recurrent neonatal hyperammonemia, hyperglutaminemia, encephalopathy, coma, and death (Amir *et al.*, 1982). Female patients are usually asymptomatic. Late-onset presentation is infrequent, but has been reported in patients receiving valproic acid therapy (Oechsner *et al.*, 1998; Thakur *et al.*, 2006; Tokatli *et al.*, 1991) and in women heterozygous for the mutations in the postpartum period (Gilchrist and Coleman, 1987). Seizures, autistic-like symptoms, hyperactivity, ataxia, and dysarthria have been reported (Christodoulou *et al.*, 1993; Gorker and Tuzun, 2005; Keegan *et al.*, 2003). Recurrent stroke-like episodes, cerebral infarction, or intracranial hemorrhage are rare. Neurodiagnostic imaging findings may resemble infarctions (Amir *et al.*, 1982; de Grauw *et al.*, 1990).

The disorder should be suspected in children and adults with unexplained hyperammonemia (Rimbaux *et al.*, 2004). Therapies include protein restriction, ketoacid derivative administration, and branched chain amino acid supplementation (Rowe *et al.*, 1986; Scaglia *et al.*, 2004).

Purine nucleoside phosphorylase deficiency

Purine nucleoside phosphorylase (PNP) deficiency is an autosomal recessive disorder characterized by combined cellular humoral and immunodeficiency, recurrent infection, and neurologic dysfunction. Neurological manifestations include developmental delay, hypotonia, ataxia, and spasticity. Tam and Leshner (1995) reported the first case of stroke in a 13-year-old girl with purine nucleoside phosphorylase deficiency who presented with hemiparesis secondary to a capsular infarction (Tam and Leshner, 1995). Various mutations have been identified, with R234P being the most common mutation reported to date in this disease (Grunebaum *et al.*, 2004; Markert *et al.*, 1997). Umbilical cord blood transplantation has been reported to correct the immunodeficiency disorder (Myers *et al.*, 2004).

In conclusion, metabolic causes of stroke are quite heterogeneous. Genetic and metabolic disorders should be included in the work-up of unexplained acute focal neurologic deficit predominantly in the pediatric population. Accurate diagnosis is of the utmost importance for genetic counseling, prevention, and potential treatment.

REFERENCES

Abe, K., Yoshimura, H., Tanaka, H., *et al.* 2004. Comparison of conventional and diffusion-weighted MRI and proton MR spectroscopy in patients with mitochondrial encephalomyopathy, lactic acidosis, and stroke-like events. *Neuroradiology*, **46**, 113–7.

Altman, N. R., Rovira, M. J., and Bauer, M. 1991. Glutaric aciduria type 1: MR findings in two cases. *Am J Neuroradiol*, **12**, 966–8.

Amir, J., Alpert, G., Statter, M., Gurman, A., and Reisner, S. H. 1982. Intracranial haemorrhage in siblings and ornithine transcarbamylase deficiency. *Acta Paediatr Scand*, **71**, 671–3.

Andersen, M. V., Dahl, H., Fledelius, H., and Nielsen, N. V. 1994. Central retinal artery occlusion in a patient with Fabry's disease documented by scanning laser ophthalmoscopy. *Acta Ophthalmol (Copenh)*, **72**, 635–8.

Apeland, T., Mansoor, M. A., and Strandjord, R. E. 2001. Antiepileptic drugs as independent predictors of plasma total homocysteine levels. *Epilepsy Res*, **47**, 27–35.

Arpa, J., Cruz-Martínez, A., Campos, Y., *et al.* 2003. Prevalence and progression of mitochondrial diseases: a study of 50 patients. *Muscle Nerve*, **28**, 690–5.

Awaad, Y., Shamato, H., and Chugani, H. 1996. Hemidystonia improved by baclofen and PET scan findings in a patient with glutaric aciduria type I. *J Child Neurol*, **11**, 167–9.

Bared, S. M., Buechler, C., Boettcher, A., *et al.* 2004. Association of ABCA1 with syntaxin 13 and flotillin-1 and enhanced phagocytosis in tangier cells. *Mol Biol Cell*, **15**, 5399–407.

Bene, J., *et al.* 2003. Congenital cataract as the first symptom of a neuromuscular disease caused by a novel single large-scale mitochondrial DNA deletion. *Eur J Hum Genet*, **11**, 375–9.

Bonaa, K. H., *et al.* 2006. Homocysteine lowering and cardiovascular events after acute myocardial infarction. *N Engl J Med*, **354**, 1578–88.

Botto, N., *et al.* 2004. C677T polymorphism of the methylenetetrahydrofolate reductase gene is a risk factor of adverse events after coronary revascularization. *Int J Cardiol*, **96**, 341–5.

Brady, R. O., and Schiffmann, R. 2000. Clinical features of and recent advances in therapy for Fabry disease. *JAMA*, **284**, 2771–5.

Brandt, N. J., *et al.* 1979. Treatment of glutaryl-CoA dehydrogenase deficiency (glutaric aciduria). Experience with diet, riboflavin, and GABA analogue. *J Pediatr*, **94**, 669–73.

B-Vitamin Treatment Trialists' Collaboration. 2006. Homocysteine-lowering trials for prevention of cardiovascular events: a review of the design and power of the large randomized trials. *Am Heart J*, **151(2)**, 282–7.

Callegaro, D., and Kaimen-Maciel, D. R. 2006. Fabry's disease as a differential diagnosis of MS. *Int MS J*, **13**, 27–30.

Campos, Y., *et al.* 1996. Sporadic MERRF/MELAS overlap syndrome associated with the 3243 tRNA(Leu(UUR)) mutation of mitochondrial DNA. *Muscle Nerve*, **19**, 187–90.

Chabrol, B., *et al.* 1994. Leigh syndrome: pyruvate dehydrogenase defect. A case with peripheral neuropathy. *J Child Neurol*, **9**, 52–5.

Chabrol, B., and Paquis, V. 1997. Cerebral infarction associated with Kearns-Sayre syndrome. *Neurology*, **49**, 308.

Chakrapani, A., *et al.* 2002. Metabolic stroke in methylmalonic acidemia five years after liver transplantation. *J Pediatr*, **140**, 261–3.

Christodoulou, J., *et al.* 1993. Ornithine transcarbamylase deficiency presenting with strokelike episodes. *J Pediatr*, **122**, 423–5.

Clarke, R., and Lewington, S. 2002. Homocysteine and coronary heart disease. *Semin Vasc Med*, **2**, 391–9.

Clavelou, P., *et al.* 2006. [Neurological aspects of Fabry's disease]. *Rev Neurol (Paris)*, **162**, 569–80.

Coelho-Miranda, L., *et al.* 2000. [Mitochondrial encephalomyelitis, lactic acidosis and cerebrovascular accidents (MELAS) in pediatric age with the A3243G mutation in the tRNALeu(UUR) gene of mitochondrial DNA]. *Rev Neurol*, **31**, 804–11.

Craigen, W. J. 1996. Leigh disease with deficiency of lipoamide dehydrogenase: treatment failure with dichloroacetate. *Pediatr Neurol*, **14**, 69–71.

de Grauw, T.J., *et al.* 1990. Acute hemiparesis as the presenting sign in a heterozygote for ornithine transcarbamylase deficiency. *Neuropediatrics*, **21**, 133–5.

del Toro, N., Milan, J. A., and Palma, A. 2004. Enzyme replacement in the treatment of Fabry's disease. Is there a point-of-no-return? *Nephrol Dial Transplant*, **19**, 1018.

Desai, A., Lankford, H. A., and Warren, J. S. 2001. Homocysteine augments cytokine-induced chemokine expression in human vascular smooth muscle cells: implications for atherogenesis. *Inflammation*, **25**, 179–86.

Dierkes, J., and Westphal, S. 2005. Effect of drugs on homocysteine concentrations. *Semin Vasc Med*, **5**, 124–39.

Dikmen, M., *et al.* 2006. Acute stroke in relation to homocysteine and methylenetetrahydrofolate reductase gene polymorphisms. *Acta Neurol Scand*, **113**, 307–14.

Di Rocco, M., *et al.* 2000. Outcome of thiamine treatment in a child with Leigh disease due to thiamine-responsive pyruvate dehydrogenase deficiency. *Eur J Paediatr Neurol*, **4**, 115–7.

Drouet, A., *et al.* 2000. [Mitochondrial diabetes complicated by or associated with "MELAS" syndrome?]. *Rev Neurol (Paris)*, **156**, 892–5.

Dublin, A. B., Hald, J. K., and Wootton-Gorges, S. L. 2002. Isolated sulfite oxidase deficiency: MR imaging features. *AJNR Am J Neuroradiol*, **23**, 484–5.

Engel, W. K., and Cunningham, G. G. 1963. Rapid examination of muscle tissue. An improved trichrome method for fresh-frozen biopsy sections. *Neurology*, **13**, 919–23.

Francois, B., Jaeken, J., and Gillis, P. 1990. Vigabatrin in the treatment of glutaric aciduria type I. *J Inherit Metab Dis*, **13**, 352–4.

Furie, K. L., and Kelly, P. J. 2006. Homocyst(e)ine and stroke. *Semin Neurol*, **26**, 24–32.

George, S., *et al.* 2005. Menkes' kinky hair syndrome. *Indian J Pediatr*, **72**, 891–2.

Giacomini, P. S., *et al.* 2004. Fabry's disease presenting as stroke in a young female. *Can J Neurol Sci*, **31**, 112–4.

Gilchrist, J. M., and Coleman, R. A. 1987. Ornithine transcarbamylase deficiency: adult onset of severe symptoms. *Ann Intern Med*, **106**, 556–8.

Goodman, S. I., *et al.* 1975, Glutaric aciduria; a "new" disorder of amino acid metabolism. *Biochem Med*, **12**, 12–21.

Gorker, I., and Tuzun, U. 2005. Autistic-like findings associated with a urea cycle disorder in a 4-year-old girl. *J Psychiatry Neurosci*, **30**, 133–5.

Goto, Y. 2005. [Pathogenic mutations in human mtDNA and their phenotypes]. *Tanpakushitsu Kakusan Koso*, **50(14 Suppl)**, 1760–4.

Goto, Y., Nonaka, I., and Horai, S. 1991. A new mtDNA mutation associated with mitochondrial myopathy, encephalopathy, lactic acidosis and stroke-like episodes (MELAS). *Biochim Biophys Acta*, **1097**, 238–40.

Graham, I. M., *et al.* 1997. Plasma homocysteine as a risk factor for vascular disease. The European Concerted Action Project. *JAMA*, **277**, 1775–81.

Grewal, R. P. 1994. Stroke in Fabry's disease. *J Neurol*, **241**, 153–6.

Grewal, R. P., and Barton, N. W. 1992. Fabry's disease presenting with stroke. *Clin Neurol Neurosurg*, **94**, 177–9.

Grunebaum, E., Zhang, J., and Roifman, C. M. 2004. Novel mutations and hotspots in patients with purine nucleoside phosphorylase deficiency. *Nucleosides Nucleotides Nucleic Acids*, **23**, 1411–5.

Grunnet, M. L., *et al.* 1991. Juvenile Leigh's encephalomyelopathy with peripheral neuropathy, myopathy, and cardiomyopathy. *J Child Neurol*, **6**, 159–63.

Haas, R. H., *et al.* 1995. Acute basal ganglia infarction in propionic acidemia. *J Child Neurol*, **10**, 18–22.

Heidenreich, R., *et al.* 1988. Acute extrapyramidal syndrome in methylmalonic acidemia: "metabolic stroke" involving the globus pallidus. *J Pediatr*, **113**, 1022–7.

Hirano, M., *et al.* 1992. Melas: an original case and clinical criteria for diagnosis. *Neuromuscul Disord*, **2**, 125–35.

Hirano, M., and Pavlakis, S. G. 1994. Mitochondrial myopathy, encephalopathy, lactic acidosis, and strokelike episodes (MELAS): current concepts. *J Child Neurol*, **9**, 4–13.

Hoffmann, G. F., *et al.* 1994. Neurological manifestations of organic acid disorders. *Eur J Pediatr*, **153(7 Suppl 1)**, S94–100.

Holt, I. J., *et al.* 1990. A new mitochondrial disease associated with mitochondrial DNA heteroplasmy. *Am J Hum Genet*, **46**, 428–33.

Holt, I. J., Harding, A. E., and Morgan-Hughes, J. A. 1988. Deletions of muscle mitochondrial DNA in patients with mitochondrial myopathies. *Nature*, **331**, 717–9.

Hsich, G. E., *et al.* 2000. Cerebral infarction in Menkes' disease. *Pediatr Neurol*, **23**, 425–8.

Huntsman, R. J., *et al.* 2005. Atypical presentations of Leigh syndrome: a case series and review. *Pediatr Neurol*, **32**, 334–40.

Iizuka, T., and Sakai, F. 2005. Pathogenesis of stroke-like episodes in MELAS: analysis of neurovascular cellular mechanisms. *Curr Neurovasc Res*, **2**, 29–45.

Isashiki, Y., *et al.* 1998. Retinal manifestations in mitochondrial diseases associated with mitochondrial DNA mutation. *Acta Ophthalmol Scand*, **76**, 6–13.

Johns, D. R. 1995. Seminars in medicine of the Beth Israel Hospital, Boston. Mitochondrial DNA and disease. *N Engl J Med*, **333**, 638–44.

Keegan, C. E., *et al.* 2003. Acute extrapyramidal syndrome in mild ornithine transcarbamylase deficiency: metabolic stroke involving the caudate and putamen without metabolic decompensation. *Eur J Pediatr*, **162**, 259–63.

Kelly, P. J., *et al.* 2003. Stroke in young patients with hyperhomocysteinemia due to cystathionine beta-synthase deficiency. *Neurology*, **60**, 275–9.

Kempster, P.A., *et al.* 1988. Dystonia in homocystinuria. *J Neurol Neurosurg Psychiatr*, **51**, 859–62.

Kirodian, B. G., *et al.* 2002. Treatment of Menkes disease with parenteral copper histidine. *Indian Pediatr*, **39**, 183–5.

Kissel, J. T., *et al.* 1987. Magnetic resonance imaging in a case of autopsy-proved adult subacute necrotizing encephalomyelopathy (Leigh's disease). *Arch Neurol*, **44**, 563–6.

Kluijtmans, L.A., *et al.* 1996. Molecular genetic analysis in mild hyperhomocysteinemia: a common mutation in the methylenetetrahydrofolate reductase gene is a genetic risk factor for cardiovascular disease. *Am J Hum Genet*, **58**, 35–41.

Kocen, R. S. 2004. Tangier disease. *J Neurol Neurosurg Psychiatr*, **75**, 1368.

Kohler, M., and Hoffmann, G. F. 1998. Subdural haematoma in a child with glutaric aciduria type I. *Pediatr Radiol*, **28**, 582.

Kosinski, C., *et al.* 1995. Evidence for cardioembolic stroke in a case of Kearns-Sayre syndrome. *Stroke*, **26**, 1950–2.

Kraus, J. P., *et al.* 1998. The human cystathionine beta-synthase (CBS) gene: complete sequence, alternative splicing, and polymorphisms. *Genomics*, **52**, 312–24.

Kraus, J. P., *et al.* 1993. Human cystathionine beta-synthase cDNA: sequence, alternative splicing and expression in cultured cells. *Hum Mol Genet*, **2**, 1633–8.

Kubota, M., *et al.* 2004. Beneficial effect of L-arginine for stroke-like episode in MELAS. *Brain Dev*, **26**, 481–3; discussion 480.

Laloi-Michelin, M., *et al.* 2006. Kearns Sayre syndrome: an unusual form of mitochondrial diabetes. *Diabetes Metab*, **32**, 182–6.

Lee, N., *et al.* 2001. A genomewide linkage-disequilibrium scan localizes the Saguenay-Lac-Saint-Jean cytochrome oxidase deficiency to 2p16. *Am J Hum Genet*, **68**, 397–409.

Leigh, D. 1951. Subacute necrotizing encephalomyelopathy in an infant. *J Neurol Neurosurg Psychiatr*, **14**, 216–21.

Lentz, S. R., and Sadler, J. E. 1991. Inhibition of thrombomodulin surface expression and protein C activation by the thrombogenic agent homocysteine. *J Clin Invest*, **88**, 1906–14.

Lerman-Sagie, T., *et al.* 2005. White matter involvement in mitochondrial diseases. *Mol Genet Metab*, **84**, 127–36.

Li, Z., *et al.* 2003. Elevated plasma homocysteine was associated with hemorrhagic and ischemic stroke, but methylenetetrahydrofolate reductase gene C677T polymorphism was a risk factor for thrombotic stroke: a multicenter case-control study in China. *Stroke*, **34**, 2085–90.

Liu, P.,C., McAndrew, P. E., and Kaler, S. G. 2002. Rapid and robust screening of the Menkes disease/occipital horn syndrome gene. *Genet Test*, **6**, 255–60.

Lonn, E., *et al.* 2006. Homocysteine lowering with folic acid and B vitamins in vascular disease. *N Engl J Med*, **354**, 1567–77.

Luft, R., *et al.* 1962. A case of severe hypermetabolism of nonthyroid origin with a defect in the maintenance of mitochondrial respiratory control: a correlated clinical, biochemical, and morphological study. *J Clin Invest*, **41**, 1776–804.

Maeda, K., *et al.* 2005. [A case of stroke-like episode of MELAS of which progressive spread would be prevented by edaravone]. *Rinsho Shinkeigaku*, **45**, 416–21.

Majamaa, K., *et al.* 1998. Epidemiology of A3243G, the mutation for mitochondrial encephalomyopathy, lactic acidosis, and strokelike episodes: prevalence of the mutation in an adult population. *Am J Hum Genet*, **63**, 447–54.

Majamaa, K., *et al.* 1997. The common MELAS mutation A3243G in mitochondrial DNA among young patients with an occipital brain infarct. *Neurology*, **49**, 1331–4.

Mamourian, A. C., and du Plessis, A. 1991. Urea cycle defect: a case with MR and CT findings resembling infarct. *Pediatr Radiol*, **21**, 594–5.

Markert, M. L., *et al.* 1997. Mutations in purine nucleoside phosphorylase deficiency. *Hum Mutat*, **9**, 118–21.

Matsumoto, J., *et al.* 2005. Mitochondrial encephalomyopathy with lactic acidosis and stroke (MELAS). *Rev Neurol Dis*, **2**, 30–4.

Mautner, S. L., *et al.* 1992. The heart in Tangier disease. Severe coronary atherosclerosis with near absence of high-density lipoprotein cholesterol. *Am J Clin Pathol*, **98**, 191–8.

McCully, K. S. 1969. Vascular pathology of homocysteinemia: implications for the pathogenesis of arteriosclerosis. *Am J Pathol*, **56**, 111–28.

McIlroy, S. P., *et al.*, 2002. Moderately elevated plasma homocysteine, methylenetetrahydrofolate reductase genotype, and risk for stroke, vascular dementia, and Alzheimer disease in Northern Ireland. *Stroke*, **33**, 2351–6.

Medina, L., *et al.* 1990. MR findings in patients with subacute necrotizing encephalomyelopathy (Leigh syndrome): correlation with biochemical defect. *AJR Am J Roentgenol*, **154**, 1269–74.

Michel, S. J., Given, C. A. 2nd, and Robertson, W. C. Jr. 2004. Imaging of the brain, including diffusion-weighted imaging in methylmalonic acidemia. *Pediatr Radiol*, **34**, 580–2.

Michelson, D. J., and Ashwal, S. 2004. The pathophysiology of stroke in mitochondrial disorders. *Mitochondrion*, **4**, 665–74.

Mikol, J., Guillausseau, P. J., and Massin, P. 2005. [Diabetes and mitochondrial cytopathies: pathological studies]. *Ann Pathol*, **25**, 292–8.

Molnar, M. J., *et al.* 2000. Cerebral blood flow and glucose metabolism in mitochondrial disorders. *Neurology*, **55**, 544–8.

Momiyama, Y., *et al.* 2001. Left ventricular hypertrophy and diastolic dysfunction in mitochondrial diabetes. *Diabetes Care*, **24**, 604–5.

Montpetit, V. J., *et al.* 1971. Subacute necrotizing encephalomyelopathy. A review and a study of two families. *Brain*, **94**, 1–30.

Morin, C., *et al.* 1999. Stroke-like episodes in autosomal recessive cytochrome oxidase deficiency. *Ann Neurol*, **45**, 389–92.

Morris, A. A., *et al.* 1996. Deficiency of respiratory chain complex I is a common cause of Leigh disease. *Ann Neurol*, **40**, 25–30.

Moslemi, A. R., *et al.* 2003. SURF1 gene mutations in three cases with Leigh syndrome and cytochrome c oxidase deficiency. *Neurology*, **61**, 991–3.

Mudd, S. H., *et al.* 1985. The natural history of homocystinuria due to cystathionine beta-synthase deficiency. *Am J Hum Genet*, **37**, 1–31.

Mudd, S. H., *et al.* 1972. Homocystinuria associated with decreased methylenetetrahydrofolate reductase activity. *Biochem Biophys Res Commun*, **46**, 905–12.

Mudd, S. H., *et al.* 1964. Homocystinuria: an enzymatic defect. *Science*, **143**, 1443–5.

Muller, W., *et al.* 2003. Is there a final common pathway in mitochondrial encephalomyopathies? Considerations based on an autopsy case of Kearns-Sayre syndrome. *Clin Neuropathol*, **22**, 240–5.

Murakami, C., Nunomura, J., and Baba, M. 2002. [MELAS syndrome associated with Klinefelter syndrome]. *Nippon Rinsho*, **60(Suppl 4)**, 625–8.

Myers, L.A., *et al.* 2004. Purine nucleoside phosphorylase deficiency (PNP-def) presenting with lymphopenia and developmental delay: successful correction with umbilical cord blood transplantation. *J Pediatr*, **145**, 710–2.

Naito, E., *et al.* 1997. Biochemical and molecular analysis of an X-linked case of Leigh syndrome associated with thiamin-responsive pyruvate dehydrogenase deficiency. *J Inherit Metab Dis*, **20**, 539–48.

Nariai, T., *et al.* 2000. Cerebral blood flow, vascular response and metabolism in patients with MELAS syndrome – xenon CT and PET study. *Keio J Med*, **49(Suppl 1)**, A68–70.

Neufeld, E. B., *et al.* 2004. The ABCA1 transporter modulates late endocytic trafficking: insights from the correction of the genetic defect in Tangier disease. *J Biol Chem*, **279**, 15571–8.

Noer, A. S., *et al.* 1988. Mitochondrial DNA deletion in encephalomyopathy. *Lancet*, **2**, 1253–4.

Nofer, J. R., and Remaley, A. T. 2005. Tangier disease: still more questions than answers. *Cell Mol Life Sci*, **62**, 2150–60.

Noguchi, A., *et al.* 2005. Stroke-like episode involving a cerebral artery in a patient with MELAS. *Pediatr Neurol*, **33**, 70–1.

Oechsner, M., *et al.* 1998. Hyperammonaemic encephalopathy after initiation of valproate therapy in unrecognised ornithine transcarbamylase deficiency. *J Neurol Neurosurg Psychiatr*, **64**, 680–2.

Ohno, K., Isotani, E., and Hirakawa, K. 1997. MELAS presenting as migraine complicated by stroke: case report. *Neuroradiology*, **39**, 781–4.

Oppenheim, C., *et al.* 2000. Can diffusion weighted magnetic resonance imaging help differentiate stroke from stroke-like events in MELAS? *J Neurol Neurosurg Psychiatr*, **69**, 248–50.

Osaka, H., *et al.* 1993. Chronic subdural hematoma, as an initial manifestation of glutaric aciduria type-1. *Brain Dev*, **15**, 125–7.

Park, S. B., *et al.* 2004. Kearns-Sayre syndrome –3 case reports and review of clinical feature. *Yonsei Med J*, **45**, 727–35.

Pavlakis, S. G., *et al.* 1984. Mitochondrial myopathy, encephalopathy, lactic acidosis, and strokelike episodes: a distinctive clinical syndrome. *Ann Neurol*, **16**, 481–8.

Pietrini, V., *et al.* 1985. Neuropathy in Tangier disease: a clinicopathologic study and a review of the literature. *Acta Neurol Scand*, **72**, 495–505.

Poulsen, L., *et al.* 2004. X-linked Menkes disease: first documented report of germ-line mosaicism. *Genet Test*, **8**, 286–91.

Pressly, T. A., *et al.* 1987. Cardiac valvular involvement in Tangier disease. *Am Heart J*, **113**, 200–2.

Provenzale, J. M., and VanLandingham, K. 1996. Cerebral infarction associated with Kearns-Sayre syndrome-related cardiomyopathy. *Neurology*, **46**, 826–8.

Rimbaux, S., *et al.* 2004. Adult onset ornithine transcarbamylase deficiency: an unusual cause of semantic disorders. *J Neurol Neurosurg Psychiatr*, **75**, 1073–5.

Rook, J. L., Nugent, D. J., and Young, G. 2005. Pediatric stroke and methylenetetrahydrofolate reductase polymorphisms: an examination of C677T and A1298C mutations. *J Pediatr Hematol Oncol*, **27**, 590–3.

Rowe, P. C., Newman, S. L., and Brusilow, S. W. 1986. Natural history of symptomatic partial ornithine transcarbamylase deficiency. *N Engl J Med*, **314**, 541–7.

Rozen, R. 1996. Molecular genetic aspects of hyperhomocysteinemia and its relation to folic acid. *Clin Invest Med*, **19**, 171–8.

Rubba, P., *et al.* 1994. Premature carotid atherosclerosis: does it occur in both familial hypercholesterolemia and homocystinuria? Ultrasound assessment of arterial intima-media thickness and blood flow velocity. *Stroke*, **25**, 943–50.

Rummelt, V., *et al.* 1993. Ocular pathology of MELAS syndrome with mitochondrial DNA nucleotide 3243 point mutation. *Ophthalmology*, **100**, 1757–66.

Sacco, R. L., Roberts, J. K., and Jacobs, B. S. 1998. Homocysteine as a risk factor for ischemic stroke: an epidemiological story in evolution. *Neuroepidemiology*, **17**, 167–73.

Sato, Y., *et al.* 2005. Homocysteine as a predictive factor for hip fracture in elderly women with Parkinson's disease. *Am J Med*, **118**, 1250–5.

Scaglia, F., *et al.* 2004. Effect of alternative pathway therapy on branched chain amino acid metabolism in urea cycle disorder patients. *Mol Genet Metab*, **81 (Suppl 1)**, S79–85.

Scaglia, F., and Northrop, J. L. 2006. The mitochondrial myopathy encephalopathy, lactic acidosis with stroke-like episodes (MELAS) syndrome: a review of treatment options. *CNS Drugs*, **20**, 443–64.

Schapira, A. H. 2006. Mitochondrial disease. *Lancet*, **368**, 70–82.

Schiffmann, R., and Ries, M. 2005. Fabry's disease – an important risk factor for stroke. *Lancet*, **366**, 1754–6.

Schmiedel, J., *et al.* 2003. Mitochondrial cytopathies. *J Neurol*, **250**, 267–77.

Seay, A. R., *et al.* 1979. CT scans in Menkes disease. *Neurology*, **29**, 304–12.

Seccombe, D. W., James, L., and Booth, F. 1986. L-carnitine treatment in glutaric aciduria type I. *Neurology*, **36**, 264–7.

Selhub, J., *et al.* 1995. Association between plasma homocysteine concentrations and extracranial carotid-artery stenosis. *N Engl J Med*, **332**, 286–91.

Sener, U., *et al.* 2006. Effects of common anti-epileptic drug monotherapy on serum levels of homocysteine, vitamin B12, folic acid and vitamin B6. *Seizure*, **15**, 79–85.

Serfaty-Lacrosniere, C., *et al.* 1994. Homozygous Tangier disease and cardiovascular disease. *Atherosclerosis*, **107**, 85–98.

Shih, V. E., *et al.* 1977. Sulfite oxidase deficiency. Biochemical and clinical investigations of a hereditary metabolic disorder in sulfur metabolism. *N Engl J Med*, **297**, 1022–8.

Siniscalchi, A., *et al.* 2005. Increase in plasma homocysteine levels induced by drug treatments in neurologic patients. *Pharmacol Res*, **52**, 367–75.

Sokolova, J., *et al.* 2001. Cystathionine beta-synthase deficiency in Central Europe: discrepancy between biochemical and molecular genetic screening for homocystinuric alleles. *Hum Mutat*, **18**, 548–9.

Spinelli, L., *et al.* 2004. Enzyme replacement therapy with agalsidase beta improves cardiac involvement in Fabry's disease. *Clin Genet*, **66**, 158–65.

Spiro, A.J., *et al.* 1970. A cytochrome-related inherited disorder of the nervous system and muscle. *Arch Neurol*, **23**, 103–12.

Stickler, D. E., Carney, P. R., and Valenstein, E. R. 2003. Juvenile-onset Leigh syndrome with an acute polyneuropathy at presentation. *J Child Neurol*, **18**, 574–6.

Strauss, K.A., *et al.* 2003. Type I glutaric aciduria, part 1: natural history of 77 patients. *Am J Med Genet C Semin Med Genet*, **121**, 38–52.

Strauss, K. A., and Morton, D. H. 2003. Type I glutaric aciduria, part 2: a model of acute striatal necrosis. *Am J Med Genet C Semin Med Genet*, **121**, 53–70.

Stutchfield, P., *et al.* 1985. Glutaric aciduria type I misdiagnosed as Leigh's encephalopathy and cerebral palsy. *Dev Med Child Neurol*, **27**, 514–8.

Takanashi, J., *et al.* 1997. Dichloroacetate treatment in Leigh syndrome caused by mitochondrial DNA mutation. *J Neurol Sci*, **145**, 83–6.

Takahashi, S., *et al.* 1998. Cerebral blood flow and oxygen metabolism before and after a stroke-like episode in patients with mitochondrial myopathy, encephalopathy, lactic acidosis and stroke-like episodes (MELAS). *J Neurol Sci*, **158**, 58–64.

Takahashi, S., *et al.* 1993. Cranial MRI and MR angiography in Menkes' syndrome. *Neuroradiology*, **35**, 556–8.

Takeshima, T., and Nakashima, K. 2005. MIDD and MELAS: a clinical spectrum. *Intern Med*, **44**, 276–7.

Tam, D. A. Jr., and Leshner, R. T. 1995. Stroke in purine nucleoside phosphorylase deficiency. *Pediatr Neurol*, **12**, 146–8.

Tan, W. H., *et al.* 2005. Isolated sulfite oxidase deficiency: a case report with a novel mutation and review of the literature. *Pediatrics*, **116**, 757–66.

Tanaka, N., *et al.* 2005. Recurrent strokes in a young adult patient with Fabry's disease. *Eur J Neurol*, **12**, 486–7.

Tawankanjanachot, I., Channarong, N. S., and Phanthumchinda, K. 2005. Auditory symptoms: a critical clue for diagnosis of MELAS. *J Med Assoc Thai*, **88**, 1715–20.

Tay, S. K., *et al.* 2005. Unusual clinical presentations in four cases of Leigh disease, cytochrome C oxidase deficiency, and SURF1 gene mutations. *J Child Neurol*, **20**, 670–4.

Taylor, R. W., *et al.* 2002. Leigh disease associated with a novel mitochondrial DNA ND5 mutation. *Eur J Hum Genet*, **10**, 141–4.

Thakur, V., *et al.* 2006. Fatal cerebral edema from late-onset ornithine transcarbamylase deficiency in a juvenile male patient receiving valproic acid. *Pediatr Crit Care Med*, **7**, 273–6.

Thambisetty, M., and Newman, N. J. 2004. Diagnosis and management of MELAS. *Expert Rev Mol Diagn*, **4**, 631–44.

Thompson, G. N., Christodoulou, J., and Danks, D. M. 1989. Metabolic stroke in methylmalonic acidemia. *J Pediatr*, **115**, 499–500.

Tokatli, A., *et al.* 1991. Valproate-induced lethal hyperammonaemic coma in a carrier of ornithine carbamoyltransferase deficiency. *J Inherit Metab Dis*, **14**, 836–7.

Toole, J. F., *et al.* 2004. Lowering homocysteine in patients with ischemic stroke to prevent recurrent stroke, myocardial infarction, and death: the Vitamin Intervention for Stroke Prevention (VISP) randomized controlled trial. *JAMA*, **291**, 565–75.

Topaloglu, H., *et al.* 1998. mtDNA nt3243 mutation, external ophthalmoplegia, and hypogonadism in an adolescent girl. *Pediatr Neurol*, **18**, 429–31.

Trinh, B. C., Melhem, E. R., and Barker, P. B. 2001. Multi-slice proton MR spectroscopy and diffusion-weighted imaging in methylmalonic acidemia: report of two cases and review of the literature. *AJNR Am J Neuroradiol*, **22**, 831–3.

Tsai, J. C., *et al.* 1996. Induction of cyclin A gene expression by homocysteine in vascular smooth muscle cells. *J Clin Invest*, **97**, 146–53.

Ueland, P. M., and Refsum, H. 1989. Plasma homocysteine, a risk factor for vascular disease: plasma levels in health, disease, and drug therapy. *J Lab Clin Med*, **114**, 473–501.

Ugalde, C., *et al.* 2003. Impaired complex I assembly in a Leigh syndrome patient with a novel missense mutation in the ND6 gene. *Ann Neurol*, **54**, 665–9.

Uhlemann, E. R., *et al.* 1976. Platelet survival and morphology in homocystinuria due to cystathionine synthase deficiency. *N Engl J Med*, **295**, 1283–6.

Undas, A., Brozek, J., and Szczeklik, A. 2005. Homocysteine and thrombosis: from basic science to clinical evidence. *Thromb Haemost*, **94**, 907–15.

Vallee, L., *et al.* 1994. Stroke, hemiparesis and deficient mitochondrial beta-oxidation. *Eur J Pediatr*, **153**, 598–603.

van den Berg, J. S., *et al.* 2000. Prevalence of symptomatic intracranial aneurysm and ischaemic stroke in pseudoxanthoma elasticum. *Cerebrovasc Dis*, **10**, 315–9.

Van Maldergem, L., *et al.* 2002. Coenzyme Q-responsive Leigh's encephalopathy in two sisters. *Ann Neurol*, **52**, 750–4.

VITATOPS Trial Study Group. 2002. The VITATOPS (Vitamins to Prevent Stroke) Trial: rationale and design of an international, large, simple, randomised trial of homocysteine-lowering multivitamin therapy in patients with recent transient ischaemic attack or stroke. *Cerebrovasc Dis*, **13**, 120–6.

Wang, X. Y., *et al.* 2003. Serial diffusion-weighted imaging in a patient with MELAS and presumed cytotoxic oedema. *Neuroradiology*, **45**, 640–3.

Wijburg, F. A., *et al.* 1992. Leigh syndrome associated with a deficiency of the pyruvate dehydrogenase complex: results of treatment with a ketogenic diet. *Neuropediatrics*, **23**, 147–52.

Willems, J. L., *et al.* 1977. Leigh's encephalomyelopathy in a patient with cytochrome c oxidase deficiency in muscle tissue. *Pediatrics*, **60**, 850–7.

Yesildag, A., *et al.* 2005. Magnetic resonance imaging and diffusion-weighted imaging in methylmalonic acidemia. *Acta Radiol*, **46**, 101–3.

Yoneda, M., *et al.* 1999. Vasogenic edema on MELAS: a serial study with diffusion-weighted MR imaging. *Neurology*, **53**, 2182–4.

Zeviani, M., *et al.* 1993. A MERRF/MELAS overlap syndrome associated with a new point mutation in the mitochondrial DNA tRNA(Lys) gene. *Eur J Hum Genet*, **1**, 80–7.

Zuchner, S., *et al.* 2003. A novel nonsense mutation in the ABC1 gene causes a severe syringomyelia-like phenotype of Tangier disease. *Brain*, **126(Pt 4)**, 920–7.

Zupanc, M. L., *et al.* 1991. Deletion of mitochondrial DNA in patients with combined features of Kearns-Sayre and MELAS syndromes. *Ann Neurol*, **29**, 680–3.

58 BONE DISORDERS AND CEREBROVASCULAR DISEASES

Natan M. Bornstein and Alexander Y. Gur

Bone disorders are among the most uncommon causes of stroke. The publications on rare stroke occurrences associated with specific bone disorders will be reviewed in this chapter. For the sake of clarity, these disorders have been divided into subgroups based on body bone pathology, specific skull diseases, and periodontal diseases.

Body bone pathology

There are possible links between bone mineral density (BMD) and stroke, because both conditions may be related to estrogen deficiency, diabetes, hypertension, a low level of physical activity, and smoking. A more difficult question is whether there is a causal relationship between low BMD and high risk of stroke, or whether low BMD is a marker of poor general health and aging. Trivedi and Khaw (2001) published the results of a prospective follow-up of men aged 65–76 years after compiling measurements of their BMD at the hip. BMD was significantly inversely related to mortality from all causes including cardiovascular disease. The association remained significant after adjusting for age; body mass index; cigarette smoking status; serum cholesterol; systolic blood pressure; past history of heart attack, stroke, or cancer; and other lifestyle factors that included the use of alcohol, physical activity, and general health status. Based on these data, the authors concluded that low BMD at the hip is a strong and independent predictor of all-cause and cardiovascular mortality in older men. The relationship between BMD and cerebrovascular disorders can be shown not only after stroke occurrence but before the stroke event as well. Browner *et al.* (1993) showed that low BMD is significantly related to stroke mortality and stroke incidence in women.

Jørgensen *et al.* (2001) examined the relationship between BMD and acute stroke in a case-control study among noninstitutionalized men and women aged 60 years. BMD was measured by using dual-energy x-ray absorptiometry at both proximal femurs. The BMD at the femoral neck in the female stroke patients was significantly (8%) lower than in the control subjects, whereas there was no difference in BMD between the male stroke patients and their controls. Women with BMD values in the lowest quartile had a higher risk of stroke than did women with BMD values in the highest quartile, and the probability value for linear trend over the quartiles was statistically significant. The BMD in the patients had been measured 6 days after stroke onset, and the authors considered that this short gap was not sufficient to reflect BMD changes after stroke. In an earlier longitudinal study, the same authors showed

that patients who were completely wheelchair-bound had a significant (3%) BMD loss in the femoral neck on the paretic side and a nonsignificant (1%) loss on the nonparetic side 2 months after stroke (Jørgensen *et al.*, 2000). Regardless of possible biases, the authors suggested that there was a lower BMD in women who had stroke, but not in men, and that a low BMD value might predict stroke in women. This assumption was not confirmed in a large national study, the first National Health and Nutrition Examination Survey, which covered a nationally representative sample of noninstitutionalized persons (Mussolino *et al.*, 2003). This survey was done on a cohort of 3402 white and black subjects who were 45–74 years of age at baseline (1971–1975) and observed through 1992. Hospital records and death certificates were used to identify a total of 416 new stroke cases. The results were evaluated to determine the relative risk for stroke per decrease in BMD, after controlling for age at baseline, smoking status, alcohol consumption, history of diabetes, history of heart disease, education, body mass index, recreational physical activity, and blood pressure medication. Cox proportional-hazards analyses revealed that the incidence of stroke was not associated with a decrease in BMD in any of the three race-sex groups (i.e. white men, white women, or blacks). Furthermore, there was no association between BMD and stroke mortality. Therefore, the long-term predictive usefulness of BMD for stroke incidence and mortality remains unresolved.

In 2001, Browner *et al.* presented the results of a study aimed at evaluating the association of osteoprotegerin (OPG) with stroke, mortality, and cardiovascular risk factors, including diabetes mellitus, BMD, and fractures. OPG and its ligand are cytokines that regulate osteoclastogenesis and may be involved in the regulation of vascular calcification. A cohort of 490 white female participants who were at least 65 years old were studied prospectively. Although the authors found that OPG levels, which had been assayed blinded from serum obtained at baseline, were about 30% greater in the women with diabetes and were significantly correlated with all-cause mortality, the OPG levels were not associated with baseline BMD or with subsequent strokes or fractures. As such, osteogenesis-related markers were also not found to be associated with stroke.

Fibrocartilaginous emboli

The phenomenon of fibrocartilaginous embolism (FE) is well documented in the veterinary literature (Cook, 1988; Jeffrey and Weels, 1986; Johnson *et al.*, 1988; Kon and de Visser, 1981; Neer, 1992;

Ryan *et al.*, 1981; Schubert, 1980; Uhthoff and Rahn, 1981). However, FE is a rare cause of brain ischemia, and its pathogenesis remains poorly understood. Only one case of FE has been reported in humans (Toro-Gonzalez *et al.*, 1993). A previously healthy 17-year-old girl fell while playing basketball. Left hemiparesis and unresponsiveness developed, followed by signs of right uncal herniation over a period of 3 days and then by death. She had no evidence of neck, head, or spine trauma, and the cardiac evaluation was normal. The neuropathologic examination showed an extensive ischemic infarction of the right middle cerebral artery territory due to complete embolic occlusion by fibrocartilaginous material, consistent with nucleus pulposus. Small, terminal coronary artery branches also showed embolism by the same material in addition to limited areas of myocardial infarction.

FE from the ruptured nucleus pulposus was described in the spinal cord in only 17 cases (Bots *et al.*, 1981). In 1994, Toro *et al.* reported another 32 cases of nucleus pulposus embolism. Women were more frequently affected (69%), and age distribution was bimodal, with peaks at ages 22 and 60 years (median 38.5). Embolization was either arterial and venous (50%) or purely arterial (50%). Ischemic myelopathy occurred more commonly in the cervical (69%) and lumbosacral (22%) regions. Schmorl's nodes, larger volume, and vascularization of the nucleus pulposus in younger patients, and spinal arteriovenous communications, trauma, and degenerative changes in older patients, are potentially important pathogenetic factors. Han *et al.* (2004) reported a case report and reviewed the literature on this issue.

Multifocal ischemic encephalomyelopathy associated with fibrocartilaginous emboli was first described in a lamb by Jeffrey and Weels (1986). The emboli contained mucosubstances that were identified by the Alcian blue critical electrolyte concentration method as mainly keratin sulfate. This composition indicates that the probable origin of the emboli was the nucleus pulposus of intervertebral disks.

Skull disorders

Osteopetrosis (OP) is a rare, hereditary metabolic disorder of unknown etiology, characterized by an abnormal accumulation of bone mass, probably caused by diminished bone resorption (Bollerslev, 1987). This disorder has been given various names in the literature, among them marble disease, "marble bone" disease, marble brain disease, and Albers-Schonberg disease (a malignant adult form of OP). Although some neurological complications have been described in patients with OP, cerebrovascular involvement is very rare (Allen *et al.*, 1982; Lerman-Sagie *et al.*, 1987; Miyamoto *et al.*, 1980). Wilms *et al.* (1990) reported a 16-year-old patient with OP who had transient sensory and motor disturbances in the left upper limb and dizziness upon changing the position of his head. Selective angiography of the cerebral vessels showed severe narrowing of the internal carotid artery within the petrous carotid canal and in its supraclinoid portion. The cervical vertebral arteries showed multiple stenoses within the vertebral canal. These findings are explained by a mechanical narrowing of the basal foramina by the osteopetrotic bone. Stroke associated with OP is rare

and probably due to compression of the arteries by osteopetrotic bones.

Paget disease, a relatively common bone pathology, is a chronic osteodystrophy of unknown etiology that usually occurs in individuals 50 years of age or older (Farre and Declambre, 1989). This disorder is characterized by the progressive and extensive replacement of normal bone tissue by a rough and irregular structure (Renier, 1989). Some authors prefer the term *osteitis deformans* for this condition. Neurological manifestations are diverse and are due to anatomic alterations vascular steal syndromes (Farre and Declambre, 1989). Cerebrovascular disorders of these patients have a mainly mechanical origin (Fournie *et al.*, 1989).

Craniosynostosis

Premature fusion of multiple cranial sutures has been associated with increased intracranial pressure and the potential for mental impairment. Isolated craniosynostosis, however, has been thought to be a benign condition (David *et al.*, 1996). Craniosynostosis may be associated with decreased cerebral blood flow as a result of the constriction of the brain because of the prematurely fused sutures. Single positron emission computed tomography (SPECT) was used to assess differences in cerebral perfusion in the areas that were compressed secondary to the fused cranial suture before and after cranial reconstructive surgery in patients with simple craniostenosis (David *et al.*, 1996). These authors prospectively studied seven children with craniostenosis, six boys and one girl (3–28 months old). Six of the seven had cranial asymmetry on preoperative cranial CT scans, and one had a symmetric defect and served as a control. Each patient had a preoperative SPECT scan approximately 3–5 days before the cranial reconstructive procedure and a follow-up scan 6–10 weeks postoperatively. Preoperative asymmetries in cerebral perfusion ranged from 0% to 30% (mean, 13%) and were found in the areas that were compressed secondary to the premature suture fusion. In five patients, cerebral blood flow, which was asymmetric before surgery, became symmetric after craniofacial reconstruction, and no new perfusion defects were documented. The control patient and one other patient had symmetric perfusion both pre- and postoperatively. This difference in blood flow supports a policy of early surgical intervention to prevent any potential central nervous system compromise secondary to abnormal blood flow in these patients.

Spondyloepiphyseal dysplasia

Immuno-osseous dysplasia is an autosomal recessive spondyloepiphyseal dysplasia that was first described by Schimke *et al.* (1971). It is associated with premature arteriosclerosis and cerebral ischemia. Boerkoel *et al.* (1998) described two girls with immuno-osseous dysplasia and cerebral ischemia associated with the moyamoya phenomenon. This was the first presentation of the cerebral vascular abnormality found in spondyloepiphyseal dysplasia, and it was based on magnetic resonance angiography and magnetic resonance venography. Three other children who had a transient ischemic attack associated with focal segmental glomerulosclerosis, nephrotic syndrome, chronic renal failure, spondyloepiphyseal dysplasia, growth failure, and lymphopenia were reported (1995). Positron emission tomography revealed perfusion defects of both cerebral and cerebellar arteries. Two boys and one girl developed the full syndrome at age 5, 6, and 10 years.

Camurati-Engelmann disease

Camurati-Engelmann disease (CED) is an autosomal dominant disorder, characterized by a progressive diaphyseal dysplasia with cortical sclerosis of the diaphyses and the metaphyses of the long bones and cranial hyperostosis, particularly involving the skull base (Sparkes and Graham, 1972). Clinical features include diffuse bony deformities, exophthalmia, waddling gait, leg pain, muscular weakness, and generalized fatigue. Neurological complications consist of cranial nerve palsy because of restriction of the foramina at the skull base. Most CED patients carry a mutation in a gene located in chromosome 19q13.2, coding for the transforming growth factor-β1 (TGF-β1), an important mediator of bone remodeling, expressed in both osteoblasts and osteoclasts of the developing bone (Janssens et al., 2000; Massagué, 1990). The disease shows variable expressivity and, occasionally, incomplete penetrance (Campos-Xavier et al., 2001). Cerrato et al. (2005) reported a 39-year-old man with apparently sporadic CED who was admitted because of the recurrence of four transient episodes of vestibular symptoms associated with visual disturbances (diplopia on two occasions and blurred vision with hemianopsia to the left on another occasion) and lasting for 2–3 hours. The patient complained of an almost continuous cranial pain involving the occipital area often radiating to the frontal region. The family history did not show features suggestive of CED, nor was there a history of early stroke. Neurological examination at admission revealed gait ataxia and moderate hearing impairment. A marked hyperostosis with bone deformities in the skull, arms, and legs was evident. No vascular risk factors were present. Laboratory investigations were normal except for raised alkaline phosphatase. The diagnosis of CED was confirmed by denaturing high-performance liquid chromatography screening of the TGF-β1 gene that highlighted a missense mutation (652C1T; Arg 218Cys) in exon 4 (coding the TGF-β1 latency-associated peptide). Immunological and coagulation tests (namely, proteins C and S, homocysteine plasma levels, activated protein C resistance, prothrombin polymorphism, lupus anticoagulant, anti-cardiolipin antibodies) were unremarkable. Cranial CT showed a dramatic increase in the thickness of the skull bones, particularly in the lower half. Brain MRI revealed multiple small ischemic lesions involving the cerebellar hemispheres, the left thalamus, and the right occipital region and a T1 hyperintensity on the course of the intracranial right vertebral artery. Duplex sonography showed increased carotid wall thickness and reduced flow in both vertebral arteries. Digital subtraction angiography showed that the right vertebral artery was occluded immediately after the origin of the posteroinferior cerebellar artery, and the left vertebral artery had a reduced lumen between the origin of the posteroinferior cerebellar artery and the vertebrobasilar junction and furnished a normal basilar artery. Cranial CT revealed patent intravertebral foramina despite the huge thickness of the skull base bone. Transthoracic and transesophageal echocardiography

revealed only a slight increase in thickness of the endocardium and in the aortic valve. The patient was treated with low-molecular-weight heparin for 2 weeks followed by ticlopidine. No further ischemic events occurred. This was the first report of a cerebrovascular event related to CED. Several mechanisms were hypothesized for its etiopathogenesis. One, an extrinsic compression of the vertebral artery caused by a hyperostosis of the vertebral foramina, seems unlikely because the vertebral foramina were patent on cranial CT scan. An alternative hypothesis is atherothrombosis, dissection of the intracranial vertebral arteries, and a nonatheromatous vasculopathy due to a thickening of the blood vessel wall. Dissection of the right vertebral artery is plausible considering the clinical features of persistent cervicocephalic pain preceding the ischemic events. Moreover, the lack of angiographic evidence of the typical narrowing of the vertebral artery lumen and the apparent absence of the intramural hematoma on the axial MRI scan do not exclude this hypothesis. Intrigued by the recent experimental evidence of the enhanced TGF-β1 signaling associated with CED mutations (including R218C), the authors suggested that a constitutive excess of the active form of TGF-β1 might have a role in the premature onset of arteriopathy, either directly causing vertebral atherothrombosis or indirectly favoring a disorder of the vessel wall, which becomes predisposed to dissection. Moreover, TGF-β1 is involved in inflammation and atherosclerosis even if the role of TGF-β1-dependent vascular remodeling is controversial (Metcalfe and Grainger, 1995). TGF-β1 inhibits both proliferation and migration of endothelial and smooth muscle cells, and this inhibition is associated with an increase in the extracellular matrix and proteoglycan synthesis, leading to thickening of the intima and media (Chamberlain, 2001). Thus, a relationship between premature arteriopathy with stroke and CED is reasonable.

Periodontal disorders

Periodontal diseases are highly prevalent and can affect up to 90% of the worldwide population. Gingivitis, the mildest form of periodontal disease, is caused by the bacterial biofilm (dental plaque) that accumulates on teeth adjacent to the gingiva. Gingivitis does not, however, affect the underlying supporting structures of the teeth, and it is reversible. Periodontitis, in contrast, results in loss of connective tissue and bone support, and is a major cause of tooth loss in adults (Pihlstrom et al., 2005). Markers of acute inflammation and chronic infectious diseases were proposed as indicators of increased stroke risk (Grau et al., 1997). It was concluded from retrospective analyses of two longitudinal cohort studies and two smaller case-control studies that periodontitis could be an independent risk factor for cardiovascular disease and ischemic stroke (Beck et al., 1996; Syrjänen et al., 1989; Wu et al., 2000). These associations were questioned in the case of cardiovascular disease, and were rather explained away by inadequate corrections for confounding variables, such as smoking (Armitage, 2000; Hujoel et al., 2002). The association of gingivitis and periodontitis with ischemic stroke, however, remained significant after adjustment for several demographic variables and well-established cardiovascular risk factors. Dörfer et al. (2004) assessed the associations of different periodontal conditions with cerebral ischemia. Patients were examined on an average of 3 days after an ischemic event. The individual mean clinical attachment loss measured at four sites per tooth was used as an indicator variable for periodontitis. The results showed that patients with ischemic stroke had higher clinical attachment loss than the general population and, after adjustment for age, gender, number of teeth, vascular risk factors and diseases, childhood and adult socioeconomic conditions, and lifestyle factors, subjects with a mean clinical attachment loss >6 mm, a gingival index >1.2, and a radiographic bone loss had a 7.4-fold, an 18.3-fold, and a 3.6-fold higher risk of cerebral ischemia, respectively, than did subjects without periodontitis or gingivitis. The authors concluded that periodontitis is an independent risk factor for stroke and that acute exacerbation of inflammatory processes in the periodontium might be a trigger for the advent of stroke.

The association between periodontal disease and stroke has several possible pathophysiologic links. Periodontitis represents a systemic burden of bacteria, endotoxin, and other bacterial products (Carroll and Sebor, 1980; Solver et al., 1977). Several periodontal pathogens can induce platelet aggregation and may thus be thrombogenic when entering the systemic circulation, as in periodontitis (Herzberg and Meyer, 1996). Periodontal bacteria have been found in the atheromatous plaques of stroke patients and also can influence well-established cardiovascular risk factors, such as lipids, fibrinogen, and C-reactive protein, modifying those factors toward a profile that is more atherogenic (Haraszthy et al., 1998; Wu et al., 2000). Scannapieco et al. (2003) attempted to summarize all published data on the association between periodontal disease and atherosclerosis, cardiovascular disease, stroke, and peripheral vascular disease from 1966 through 2002. They included randomized controlled clinical trials and longitudinal, cohort, and case-control studies. Because the studies used different methods for oral assessment, it was not possible to perform a meta-analysis of the combined data. Taken together, most of the literature supports a modest association between periodontal disease and atherosclerosis, although several studies fail to show such an association. The absence of a standard definition and measures for periodontal disease complicates the interpretation of results. Additional large-scale longitudinal epidemiologic and intervention studies are necessary to validate this association.

Summary

Although the association of bone disorders with cerebrovascular diseases is frequently indirect and accidental, it is worthwhile to draw attention to the body bones and skull status of stroke patients in order to determine possible causality and preventive measures.

REFERENCES

Allen, H. A., Haney, P., and Rao, K. C. 1982. Vascular involvement in cranial hyperostosis. *AJNR Am J Neuroradiol*, **3**, 193–5.

Armitage, G. C. 2000. Periodontal infections and cardiovascular disease – how strong is the association? *Oral Dis*, **6**, 335–50.

Beck, J., Garcia, R., Heiss, G., Vokonas, P. S., and Offenbacher, S. 1996. Periodontal disease and cardiovascular disease. *J Periodontol*, **67**, 1123–37.

Boerkoel, C. F., Nowaczyk, M. J., Blaser, S. I., Meschino, W. S., and Weksberg, R. 1998. Schimke immunoosseous dysplasia complicated by moyamoya phenomen. *Am J Med Genet*, **78**, 118–22.

Bollerslev, J. 1987. Osteopetrosis. A genetic and epidemiological study. *Clin Genet*, **31**, 86–90.

Bots, G. T., Wattendorff, A. R., Buruma, O. J., Roos, R. A., and Endtz, L. J. 1981. Acute myelopathy caused by fibrocartilaginous emboli. *Neurology*, **31**, 1250–6.

Browner, W. S., Lui, L. Y., and Cummings, S. R. 2001. Associations of serum osteoprotegerin levels with diabetes, stroke, bone density, fractures, and mortality in elderly women. *J Clin Endocrinol Metab*, **86**, 631–7.

Browner, W. S., Pressman, A. R., Nevitt, M. C., Cauley, J. A., and Cummings, S. R. 1993. Association between low bone density and stroke in elderly women. The study of osteoporotic fractures. *Stroke*, **24**, 940–6.

Campos-Xavier, A. B., Saraiva, J. M., Savarirayan, R., et al. 2001. Phenotypic variability at the TGF-β1 locus in Camurati-Engelmann disease. *Hum Genet*, **109**, 653–8.

Carroll, G. C., and Sebor, R. J. 1980. Flossing and its relationship to transient bacteremia. *J Periodontol*, **51**, 691–2.

Cerrato, P., Baima, C., Bergui, M., et al. 2005. Juvenile vertebrobasilar ischaemic stroke in a patient with Camurati-Engelmann disease. *Cerebrovasc Dis*, **20**, 283–4.

Chamberlain, J. 2001. Transforming growth factor-β: a promising target for antistenosis therapy. *Cardiovasc Drug Rev*, **19**, 329–44.

Cook, J. R. 1988. Fibrocartilaginous embolism. *Vet Clin North Am Small Anim Pract*, **18**, 581–92.

David, L. R, Wilson, J. A, Watson, N. E, and Argenta, L. C. 1996. Cerebral perfusion defects secondary to simple craniosynostosis. *J Craniofac Surg*, **7**, 177–85.

Dörfer, C. E., Becher, H., Ziegler, C. M., et al. 2004. The association of gingivitis and periodontitis with ischemic stroke. *J Clin Periodontol*, **31**, 396–401.

Farre, J. M., and Declambre, B. 1989. Functional consequences and complications of Paget's disease. *Rev Prat*, **39**, 1129–36.

Fournie, A., Fournie, B., and Lassoued, S. 1989. Paget's disease: errors to be avoided. *Rev Prat*, **39**, 1143–6.

Grau, A. J., Buggle, F., Ziegler, C., et al. 1997. Association between acute cerebrovascular ischemia and chronic and recurrent infection. *Stroke*, **28**, 1724–9.

Han, J. J., Massagli, T. L., and Jaffe, K. M. 2004. Fibrocartilaginous embolism-an uncommon cause of spinal cord infarction: a case report and review of the literature. *Arch Phys Med Rehabil*, 85, 153–7.

Haraszthy, V. I., Zambon, J. J., Trevisan, M., Zeid, M., and Genco, R. J. 1998. Identification of pathogens in atheromatous plaques [abstract]. *J Dent Res*, **77**(**special issue B**), abstract 273.

Herzberg, M. C., and Meyer, M. W. 1996. Effects of oral flora on platelets: possible consequence in cardiovascular disease. *J Periodontol*, **67**(**suppl 10**), 1138–42.

Hujoel, P. P., Drangsholt, M., Spiekerman, C., and DeRouen, T. A. 2002. Pre-existing cardiovascular disease and periodontitis: a follow-up study. *J Dent Res*, **81**, 186–91.

Janssens, K., Gershoni-Baruch, R., Guanabens, N., et al. 2000. Mutations in the gene encoding the latency-associated peptide of TGFB1 cause Camurati-Engelmann disease. *Nat Genet*, **26**, 273–5.

Jeffrey, M., and Weels, G. A. 1986. Multifocal ischemic encephalomyelopathy associated with fibrocartilaginous emboli in the lamb. *Neuropathol Appl Neurobiol*, **12**, 415–24.

Johnson, R. C., Anderson W. I., and King J. M. 1988. Acute pelvic limb paralysis induced by a lumbar fibrocartilaginous embolism in a sow. *Cornell Vet*, **78**, 231–4.

Jørgensen, L., Engstad, T., and Jacobsen, B. K. 2001. Bone mineral density in acute stroke patients. Low bone mineral density may predict first stroke in women. *Stroke*, **32**, 47–51.

Jørgensen, L., Jacobsen, B. K., Wilsgaard, T., and Magnus, J. H. 2000. Walking after stroke: does it matter? Changes in bone mineral density within the first 12 months after stroke. A longitudinal study. *Osteoporos Int*, **11**, 381–7.

Kon, M., and de Visser, A. C. 1981. A poly (HEMA) sponge for restoration of articular cartilage defects. *Plast Reconstr Surg*, **63**, 288–94.

Lerman-Sagie, T., Levi, Y., Kidron, D., Grunebaum, M., and Nitzan, M. 1987. Syndrome of osteopetrosis and muscular degeneration associated with cerebro-oculo-facio-skeletal changes. *Am J Med Genet*, **28**, 137–142.

Massagué, J. 1990. The transforming growth factor-beta family. *Annu Rev Cell Biol*, **6**, 597–641.

Metcalfe, J. C., and Grainger, D. J. 1995. Transforming growth factor-beta and the protection from cardiovascular injury hypothesis. *Biochem Soc Trans*, **23**, 403–6.

Miyamoto, R. T., House, W. F., and Brackmann, D. E. 1980. Neurotologic manifestations of the osteopetroses. *Arch Otolaryngol*, **106**, 210–4.

Mussolino, M. E., Madans, J. H., and Gillum, R. F. 2003. Bone mineral density and stroke. *Stroke*, **34**, e20–2.

Neer, T. M. 1992. Fibrocartilaginous emboli. *Vet Clin North Am Small Anim Pract*, **22**, 1017–26.

Pihlstrom, B. L., Michalowicz, B. S., and Johnson, N. W. 2005. Periodontal diseases. *Lancet*, **366**, 1809–20.

Renier, J. C. 1989. What is Paget's disease? *Rev Prat*, **39**, 1104–8.

Ryan, L. M., Cheung, H. S., and McCarty, D. J. 1981. Release of pyrophosphate by normal mammalian articular hyaline and fibrocartilage in organ culture. *Arthritis Rheum*, **24**, 1522–7.

Scannapieco, F. A., Bush, R. B., and Paju, S. 2003. Associations between periodontal disease and risk for atherosclerosis, cardiovascular disease, and stroke. A systematic review. *Ann Periodontol*, **8**, 38–53.

Schimke, R. N., Horton, W. A., and King, C. R. 1971. Chondroitin-6-sulphaturia, defective cellular immunity, and nephrotic syndrome. *Lancet*, **13**, 1088–9.

Schubert, T. A. 1980. Fibrocartilaginous infarct in a German Shepherd dog. *Vet Clin North Am Small Anim Pract*, **75**, 839–42.

Solver, J. G., Martin, A. W., and McBride, B. C. 1977. Experimental transient bacteremias in human subjects with varying degrees of plaque accumulation and gingival inflammation. *J Clin Periodontol*, **4**, 92–9.

Sparkes, R. S., and Graham, C. B. 1972. Camurati-Engelmann disease. Genetics and clinical manifestations with a review of the literature. *J Med Genet*, **9**, 73–85.

Syrjänen, J., Peltola, J., Valtonen, V., *et al.* 1989. Dental infections in association with cerebral infarction in young and middle-aged men. *J Intern Med*, **225**, 179–84.

Toro, G., Roman, G. C., Navarro-Roman, L., *et al.* 1994. Natural history of spinal cord infarction caused by nucleus pulposus embolism. *Spine*, **19**, 360–6.

Toro-Gonzalez, G., Havarro-Roman, L., Roman, G. C., *et al.* 1993. Acute ischemic stroke from fibrocartilaginous embolism to the middle cerebral artery. *Stroke*, **24**, 738–40.

Trivedi, D. P., and Khaw, K. T. 2001. Bone mineral density at the hip predicts mortality in elderly men. *Osteoporos Int*, **12**, 259–65.

Uhthoff, H. K., and Rahn, B. A, 1981. Healing patterns of metaphyseal fractures. *Clin Orthop Relat Res*, **160**, 295–303.

Wilms, G., Casaer, P., Alliet, P., *et al.* 1990. Cerebrovascular occlusive complications in osteopetrosis major. *Neuroradiology*, **32**, 511–3.

Wu, T., Trevisan, M., Genco, R. J., *et al.* 2000. Periodontal disease and risk of cerebrovascular disease: the first national health and nutrition examination survey and its follow-up study. *Arch Intern Med*, **160**, 2749–55.

59 SCLERODERMA

Elayna O. Rubens

Introduction

Scleroderma (progressive systemic sclerosis) is a multisystem connective tissue disorder characterized by inflammation, fibrosis, and vasculopathy of affected tissues. Involvement of the nervous system is uncommon, but may manifest as either peripheral nervous system or central nervous system (CNS) dysfunction. Reports of neurological manifestations of progressive systemic sclerosis have emphasized the peripheral pathology including myopathy and peripheral neuropathy (Clements *et al.*, 1978; Lee *et al.*, 1984). Although rare, CNS involvement in scleroderma has been retrospectively identified in case series and described in several case reports. Hietaharju *et al.* (1993) investigated CNS and neuropsychiatric signs and symptoms among patients with systemic sclerosis and found that 16% of patients had prominent CNS or psychiatric symptoms and 6% had cerebrovascular symptoms. Another retrospective study of fifty scleroderma patients found that 6% of patients had transient ischemic attacks (TIAs) or minor strokes during the course of the disease (Averbuch-Heller *et al.*, 1992).

The etiology of brain ischemia in patients with scleroderma is varied and poorly understood. Confounding factors such as malignant hypertension and renal failure make determination of additional cerebrovascular pathology difficult. Information available from reported cases, however, suggests that CNS vasculitis, segmental vasospasm, and cerebrovascular calcifications may all play a role in causing strokes in patients with scleroderma.

CNS vasculitis

CNS vasculitis has been diagnosed in several patients with scleroderma and has been posited to cause strokes. However, pathological confirmation of a vasculitic process (in this case involving the internal carotid artery) was available in only one reported patient (Lee and Haynes, 1967). Otherwise, the diagnoses of vasculitis were largely based on angiographic findings and/or response to immunosuppressive therapy. Other ancillary tests reported were nondiagnostic. Markers of inflammation such as C-reactive protein and erythrocyte sedimentation rate (ESR) were normal to modestly elevated (ESR 20–60 mm/h). Cerebrospinal fluid (CSF) studies were often normal or associated with nonspecific elevations in protein content (70–100 mg%) (Das *et al.*, 2002; Estey *et al.*, 1979; Ishida *et al.*, 1993; Pathak and Gabor, 1991). In one patient the CSF did show a mild pleocytosis (8 white blood cells:

4 polymorphonucleocytes and 4 lymphocytes) (Estey *et al.*, 1979). Review of these putative examples of vasculitis highlights the variable nature of their presentations, involved cerebral vascular territories, and associated symptoms.

Pathak and Gabor (1991) reported a 45-year-old woman who presented with throbbing headaches and was found to have a small subarachnoid hemorrhage. She developed acute confusion, fluctuating blood pressure, and a seizure followed by intermittent episodes of numbness on her right side associated with expressive aphasia. Angiography revealed narrowing of several distal, medium, and small branches of the anterior and middle cerebral arteries and an occluded medium-sized branch of the middle cerebral artery on the right. There were also multiple, long segments of smooth and symmetric narrowing in the large- and medium-sized vessels within the posterior circulation, particularly the superior cerebellar arteries at their origins. Skin as well as leptomeningeal and brain biopsies were performed and showed no evidence of vasculitis. She was started on high dose oral prednisone and improved dramatically. Tapering of the steroid dose was followed by recurrent transient neurological symptoms including numbness and aphasia. She was later successfully treated with cyclophosphamide therapy (Pathak and Gabor, 1991). Although the angiographic findings and negative biopsy could suggest vasoconstriction alone as a cause for her transient cerebrovascular symptoms, her complete response to immunosuppressive therapy does support an underlying vasculitic process.

A 43-year-old woman who also presented with throbbing headaches (with associated visual symptoms), followed by seizures, transient hemiparesis, and confusion was described by Estey *et al.* (1979). In contrast to the case of Pathak and Gabor, this patient had evidence of malignant hypertension (papilledema and flame hemorrhages) and renal scleroderma, although recorded blood pressures in the hospital were not consistent with hypertensive encephalopathy. A CT scan was unrevealing, and cerebral angiography showed diffuse attenuation of the right and left middle cerebral opercular branches. No biopsy was performed, but the patient recovered quickly after the initiation of high dose intravenous methylprednisolone suggesting a focal arteritis due to her underlying scleroderma (Estey *et al.*, 1979).

A 67-year-old woman with scleroderma and no other identifiable vascular risk-factors was found to have right occipital, right middle cerebellar peduncle, and pontine infarcts associated with the angiographic finding of localized stenosis and poststenotic dilatation ("string of beads" appearance) involving the distal right

Uncommon Causes of Stroke, 2nd edition, ed. Louis R. Caplan. Published by Cambridge University Press. © Cambridge University Press 2008.

vertebral and proximal basilar arteries. Skin biopsy was negative for vasculitis. She was started on cyclosporin A to treat presumed CNS vasculitis. Her neurological signs remained stable whereas her Raynaud's phenomenon, skin changes, and respiratory symptoms improved (Ishida *et al.*, 1993).

Das *et al.* (2002) reported a 19-year-old woman with a 2-year history of scleroderma who presented with right hemiparesis and speech difficulty and was found on MRI to have multifocal parieto-occipital, left frontal, and right temporal infarcts. Magnetic resonance angiography showed poor flow through both carotids with prominent collateral circulation from the vertebral and basilar arteries. Skin biopsy was negative for vasculitis. Her course was complicated by bilateral optic neuropathies that may have been because of vasculitis as well as gangrene and ulcerations of her fingertips. She had no other vascular risk factors and responded to prednisone and intravenous cyclophosphamide therapy (Das *et al.*, 2002).

Despite the lack of pathological evidence of vasculitis in these case reports, the angiographic evidence combined with the overall clinical courses and responses to therapy favors the occurrence of a vasculitis of the CNS among patients with scleroderma. Certainly, cerebral infarction in scleroderma patients in the absence of other plausible, causative factors should prompt an aggressive work-up for vasculitis including angiography and, when appropriate, brain and/or meningeal biopsy. Negative results, however, do not obviate the use of immunosuppressive therapy as shown by these reported cases.

Segmental vasoconstriction

An alternative explanation for the narrowing of cerebral blood vessels seen in some patients with scleroderma is localized cerebrovascular spasm. Focal or multifocal constrictions of the cerebral blood vessels can induce transient ischemia and subsequent infarction of brain tissue. In scleroderma, changes in the endothelial cells and basal lamina cause vascular abnormalities that may predispose cerebral vessels to vasospasm. Evaluation for transient focal neurological symptoms reported in scleroderma patients is often entirely unrevealing with no definable cause of vascular pathology (Averbuch-Heller *et al.*, 1992). Intermittent vessel spasm may be the explanation for the transient ischemic symptoms seen in such patients.

A scleroderma patient seen in our hospital had a lifelong history of migraine. She developed her typical migraine aura after treatment for an epidural infection. The aura persisted intermittently for days and was associated with a hemianopia and hemisensory loss. MRI showed abnormalities involving the almost entire right cerebral hemisphere. The symptoms, signs, and MRI abnormalities all remitted after treatment with calcium channel blockers indicating that vasoconstriction was the likely cause of her CNS findings.

Results of cerebral angiography in several patients thought to have vasculitis are consistent with the diagnosis of vasoconstriction. Arteriography revealed segmental, often smoothly contoured, narrowing of arteries of multiple sizes (small, medium, and large) in both the anterior and posterior circulations. In one

reported patient, this was associated with subarachnoid hemorrhage which, by itself, can cause vasospasm and subsequent stroke (Pathak and Gabor, 1991).

Several reported patients with arterial narrowing on angiography presented with a unilateral, vascular type headache as well as transient neurological symptoms including positive visual phenomena, episodic paresthesias, and weakness reminiscent of complicated migraine (Estey *et al.*, 1979; Pathak and Gabor, 1991). Migraine may be more common in patients with scleroderma with a reported prevalence of 31% in one study population (Hietaharju *et al.*, 1993). Medical therapy to prevent vasospasm (with calcium channel blockers, for instance) may help to prevent recurrent cerebrovascular symptoms.

Cerebrovascular calcification

Although pathological information about the brains of scleroderma patients is extremely scant, one report described advanced cerebrovascular calcifications in two autopsy cases of patients with scleroderma and cerebrovascular symptoms (Heron *et al.*, 1998). A 41-year-old woman who had systemic sclerosis (calcinosis, Raynaud's phenomenon, esophageal dysmotility, sclerodactyly, telangiectasia [CREST] variant) became encephalopathic and died of septic shock several months later. At autopsy, small areas of ischemic necrosis were found accompanied by mineral deposits in the walls of small arteries and arterioles, especially in the basal ganglia, hippocampus, and dentate nucleus. The mineralized vessels could not be accounted for by patient age, hypoparathyroidism, or other hereditary or metabolic diseases. Some arteries were thickened by intimal hyperplasia (Heron *et al.*, 1998).

Another patient who also had the CREST variant of systemic sclerosis had a history of TIAs consisting of episodes of expressive aphasia and, later, nonspecific balance problems. No discernable cause of her cerebrovascular symptoms was found, and head CT showed only moderate atrophy and basal ganglia calcifications. She died of complications of a gastrointestinal infection. Like the first patient, she too had small areas of ischemic necrosis with vascular calcium deposits in the basal ganglia, hippocampus, and dentate nucleus as well as the frontal lobes, cerebellar cortex, and mamillary bodies (Heron *et al.*, 1998).

Whether these vascular calcium deposits were responsible for the patients' cerebrovascular symptoms is speculative. Whether the mineralization itself directly causes ischemia or serves as a marker for another pathologic process is unknown.

Conclusion

Further information regarding the clinical-pathological correlation between stroke and scleroderma is needed to more accurately assess the etiology of strokes and transient ischemic symptoms in these patients. For now, our approach to patient management is based on speculation from limited case reports and small case series. As such, work-up of scleroderma patients with cerebrovascular disease must take into consideration the potential causes of stroke we have discussed here, but also keeping in mind the potential for discovery of new, yet unreported disease mechanisms in this patient population.

REFERENCES

Averbuch-Heller, L., Steiner, I., and Abramsky, O. 1992. Neurologic manifestations of progressive systemic sclerosis. *Arch Neurol*, **49**, 1292–5.

Clements, P. J., Furst, D. E., Campion, D. S., *et al.* 1978. Muscle disease in progressive systemic sclerosis: diagnostic and therapeutic considerations. *Arthritis Rheum*, **21**, 62–71.

Das, C. P., Prabhakar, S., Lal, V., and Kharbanda, P. S. 2002. Scleroderma, stroke and optic neuropathy: a rare association. *Neurol India*, **50**, 504–7.

Estey, E., Lieberman, A., Pinto, R., Meltzer, M., and Ransohoff, J. 1979. Cerebral arteritis in scleroderma. *Stroke*, **10**, 595–7.

Heron, E., Fornes, P., Rance, A., *et al.* 1998. Brain involvement in scleroderma-two autopsy cases. *Stroke*, **29**, 719–21.

Hietaharju, A., Jääskeläinen, S., Hietarinta, M., and Frey, H. 1993. Central nervous system involvement and psychiatric manifestations in systemic sclerosis (scleroderma): clinical and neurophysiological evaluation. *Acta Neurol Scand*, **87**, 382–7.

Ishida, K., Kamata, T., Tsukagoshi, H., and Tanizaki, Y. 1993. Progressive systemic sclerosis with CNS vasculitis and cyclosporin A therapy. *J Neurol Neurosurg Psychiatry*, **56**, 720.

Lee, J. E., and Haynes, J. M. 1967. Carotid arteritis and cerebral infarction due to scleroderma. *Neurology*, **17**, 18–22.

Lee, P., Bruni, J., and Sukenik, S. 1984. Neurological manifestations in systemic sclerosis (scleroderma). *J Rheumatol*, **11**, 480–3.

Pathak, R., and Gabor, A. 1991. Scleroderma and central nervous system vasculitis. *Stroke*, **22**, 410–3.

PART VI: NONINFLAMMATORY DISORDERS OF THE ARTERIAL WALL

60 CERVICO-CEPHALIC ARTERIAL DISSECTIONS

Marcel Arnold and Mathias Sturzenegger

General considerations

The term cervico-cephalic arterial dissection (CAD) encompasses a group of arteriopathies not necessarily with an identical pathogenesis but that have in common an intramural hemorrhage (Hart and Easton, 1983; Schievink, 2001) (Figure 60.1). This most frequently affects the extracranial arterial segments (88%), predominantly the internal carotid artery (ICA) (58%–75%), the vertebral artery (VA) (19–30%), or multiple arteries (16%–28%) in typical locations. Intracranial dissections are rare (12%), affecting the vertebral arteries, carotid branches, or basilar artery and branches in that order of frequency (Mokri *et al.*, 1986; Vilela and Goulao, 2003).

In the case of carotid dissection, the mural hematoma usually causes local symptoms such as pain or Horner's syndrome and lower cranial nerve compression. It may or may not lead to vessel lumen stenoses with artery-to-artery embolic or (rarely) hemodynamic consequences to the brain (Figure 60.1).

Depending on the imaging aspect, three forms of dissection are recognized: stenotic (45%–66%), occlusive (21%–42%), and aneurysmal (12%–49%); stenosis and dissecting aneurysm may be combined, and multiple vessel dissections are more frequent in women (Arnold *et al.*, 2006; Lee *et al.*, 2006; Ozdoba *et al.*, 1996; Pelkonen *et al.*, 2003; Touze *et al.*, 2003). With increasing availability and use of noninvasive neuroimaging techniques such as ultrasound, MRI, magnetic resonance angiography (MRA), CT, and CT angiography, the attributable clinical spectrum of the disease is getting broader; more monosymptomatic, minimally symptomatic, and even asymptomatic cases have been detected. In the past, many such cases would have gone undiagnosed or wrongly diagnosed as the symptoms would not have warranted subjecting the patients to invasive angiographic studies. The sensitivity of these noninvasive methods, however, critically depends on the quality of the images (Shah *et al.*, 2004; Yang *et al.*, 2005) and on the examination of the correct vessel segments. MRI, therefore, can be considered as the diagnostic gold standard only under certain prerequisites (Nassenstein *et al.*, 2005; Ozdoba *et al.*, 1996). The increasing number of publications on this topic and the recognized significance of dissections as cause of strokes in young patients – frequently preventable if readily recognized (Nassenstein *et al.*, 2005; Sturzenegger, 1995; Sturzenegger *et al.*, 1995) – have fortunately increased familiarity of clinicians and radiologists with the clinical and radiological features of this disorder.

The most feared consequence of CAD is stroke. While dissections are the cause of 2.5% of all strokes in the general population, they are among the major causes of strokes in young and middle-aged

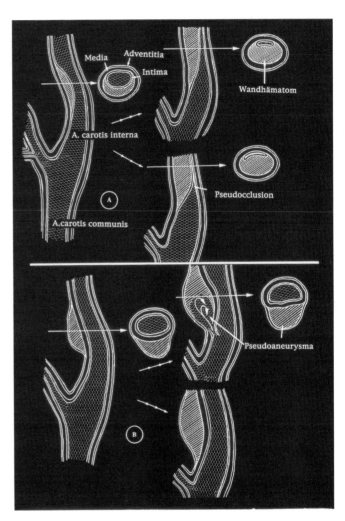

Figure 60.1 Mural hematoma and its local consequences.

persons (<45 years): 10%–20% (Bogousslavsky *et al.*, 1987; Giroud *et al.*, 1994; Schievink, 2001).

Usually dissections are called "traumatic" when there is history of major penetrating or blunt trauma (Bok and Peter, 1996). Otherwise, dissections are called "spontaneous." However, many patients with "spontaneous dissections" have a history of "minor" or so-called "trivial" trauma, which may or may not be of clinical significance. Spontaneous cervico-cephalic arterial dissections (sCAD) have typical predilection sites in the different arteries affected, which in part may be explained by mechanical influences: high cervical segment of extracranial ICA or V2 and V3 segments of VA (Arnold *et al.*, 2006). Other factors influencing the dissection site may be different vessel wall structures.

Incidence

Two population-based incidence studies of spontaneous internal carotid artery dissection (sICAD) from Rochester, Minnesota (Schievink *et al.*, 1993), and Dijon, France (Giroud *et al.*, 1994), reported an annual incidence rate of 2.6 and 2.9 per 100 000, mainly based on patients presenting with strokes. Because many patients with CAD never develop strokes, these studies do not reflect the true incidence of dissections. In a population-based case series, the frequency of spontaneous vertebral artery dissections (sVAD) is about one-third that of sICAD (Lee *et al.*, 2006). Furthermore, an unknown number of dissections occur asymptomatically. There is little doubt that, nowadays with more accurate noninvasive imaging and wider awareness, more cases of these dissections are diagnosed. No studies report the true incidence of traumatic CAD (tCAD), but these are likely less common than spontaneous ones. A 0.08% incidence of tCAD has been reported in blunt trauma patients (Davis *et al.*, 1990) but is more frequent in head injuries (Hughes *et al.*, 2000). VA abnormalities were detected in 50% of a prospective angiographic study in patients with cervical spine trauma (Willis *et al.*, 1994). tCAD is certainly underrecognized in the setting of polytrauma or craniocervical trauma because symptoms may be masked by the underlying head or spine injury (Bok and Peter, 1996; Schellinger *et al.*, 2001; Yang *et al.*, 2006). There are no incidence data for the pediatric age group.

Pathology

Histopathological studies of affected arteries are rare and result from two sources: (i) single case reports with autopsies of patients who died following severe stroke (Blanco Pampin *et al.*, 2002); and (ii) surgery specimens at times when patients with pseudo-occlusions or pseudoaneurysms were operated on, because the nature and prognosis of the disease were not yet known (Muller *et al.*, 2000).

The major finding is a blood clot either between the tunica intima and media (subintimal dissection) or between the tunica media and adventitia (subadventitial dissection) (Figure 60.1). It is not known whether the hematoma location gives any clue regarding etiology or risk factors. Subintimal dissection is said to cause predominantly stenosis, whereas subadventitial dissection should cause more frequently dissecting aneurysms (pseudoaneurysms) and local symptoms such as Horner's syndrome or cranial nerve palsy. Such a correlation seems logical, however; because no imaging method is able to delineate exact hematoma location within the vessel wall layers, they are not really proven.

In a histological analysis of the specimens of 50 surgically treated internal carotid artery dissections (ICAD), signs of traumatic alteration were observed in 18% and of fibromuscular dysplasia (FMD) in 12% (Muller *et al.*, 2000).

Direct evidence for an arteriopathy from histological analyses of an affected vessel is almost nonexistent and indirectly comes from skin biopsies or from biopsies of remote superficial vessels

Table 60.1 Pathogenetic factors in CAD

Environmental

Trauma

Definite trauma– "traumatic dissections"

  Cervical spine fracture

  blunt neck trauma

  penetrating neck injury

"Trivial" or "minor" trauma– many cases of "spontaneous dissections"

Every day activities	(e.g. coughing, sneezing, shaving, falls, car parking, bending over, coitus, hit to the head)
Sports	(e.g. basket, volley, tennis, polo, squash, soccer, bowling, diving, Yoga, aerobics, skiing, hockey, weight-lifting, bungee jumping, roller coaster)
Medical manoeuvres	(Intubation, delivery, reanimation, manipulation)

Contraceptives, Drugs (sympathomimetics)

Recent infection

Constitutional

Arterial disease

Direct evidence

Arterial redundancy: Vessel tortuousity (kinking, coiling) (~30%)

Fibromuscular dysplasia (10–20%)

Cystic medial necrosis (Erdheim-Gsell)

Known heritable connective tissue disorders [Marfan's syndrome, Type IV Ehlers–Danlos syndrome, Osteogenesis imperfecta, Pseudoxanthoma elasticum, Adult polycystic kidney disease (ADPKD)]

Dilated aortic root diameter (>34 mm)

Abnormal CCA elastance in sonographic tests

Indirect evidence

Abnormal or deficient elastin or fibrillin in cultured dermal fibroblasts

Multivessel dissections

Higher incidence of intracranial aneurysms in patients with ICAD

High prevalence of ICADs and cerebral aneurysms in siblings of patients with ICADs

Vasculitis (Syphilis, Polyarteriitis nodosa)

Endothelial dysfunctions in different tests

Familial occurrence of	ICA dissections
	ICA dissections and intracranial aneurysms bicuspid aortic valve and arterial dissections arterial dissections with lentiginosis

α1-Antitrypsin deficiency

Hyperhomocysteinemia

Migraine

Hypertension

in patients with dissections (Brandt and Grond-Ginsbach, 2002; Grond-Ginsbach *et al.*, 2002; Volker *et al.*, 2005).

Pathogenesis of dissections

In most patients with CAD, the exact pathogenesis of the dissection remains undetermined. Table 60.1 gives a list of potential risk factors with varying degree of evidence. Essentially, two major groups are presumed: (i) constitutional, best summarized as arterial disease and (ii) environmental, such as trauma (Rubinstein *et al.*, 2005).

In the case of a severe head and/or neck trauma, such as e.g. cervical spine fracture, the pathogenesis is straightforward; these dissections are called *traumatic*. Otherwise, dissections are called *spontaneous*. Some kind of predisposing arterial disease, together with a triggering event, such as e.g., an infection or trivial (may be unrecognized) trauma, seems the most logical pathogenetic chain. Yet, most patients with sCAD have no evidence for an arteriopathy or connective tissue disorder in their family history, personal history, or at clinical examination.

Trauma

Major trauma

The role of major trauma to the head or neck in the production of CAD is well recognized. In case of ICAD, hyperextension and rotation of the neck forces traction on the ICA as it crosses the transverse processes of C2 and C3 vertebrae. The intima (the least elastic layer of the arterial wall) may tear, and arterial dissection results. Abrupt full neck flexion may directly crush the ICA between the angle of the mandible and the upper cervical spine (Figure 60.2). Further causes are direct trauma to the anterior neck (blunt such as e.g. a punch or strangling) or penetrating trauma such as e.g. a knife thrust; a prominent styloid process may also injure the ICA during abrupt or steady and severe rotations of the neck. Such injuries are not infrequent with motor vehicle accidents, which seem to be the leading cause of traumatic ICAD (Mokri *et al.*, 1988) (Blanco Pampin *et al.*, 2002).

Traumatic dissections of the VA are primarily related to injuries associated with rotations of the neck (Bok and Peter, 1996). With

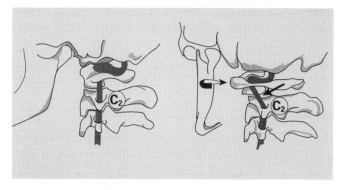

Figure 60.3 Potential mechanisms causing traumatic vertebral artery dissections (tVAD).

forceful, sudden, or extreme rotations, the artery is most intensively distorted and stretched in the V3 segment at the C2/C1 and less at the C3/C2 level (Figure 60.3); it may also be distorted by muscles and fascial bends at the junction of the V1 and V2 segment or by adjacent osteophytes as the artery travels upward in the transverse foramina (V2 segment).

Chiropractic manipulations, therefore, tend to cause more vertebral artery dissections (VAD) than ICAD. tVAD usually occur at the C1/C2 level (Hart, 1988; Smith *et al.*, 2003; Sturzenegger, 1993). A pathogenetic effect of a chiropractic maneuver could be proven only in a minority of cases (Rothwell *et al.*, 2001). Also, few histological examinations have shown evidence of a primary arterial disease in cases of tCAD.

Trivial or minor trauma

Many patients with CAD give a history of minimal or trivial trauma, especially if asked for it. A variety of traumas such as forceful coughing, sports activities, blowing the nose, sexual activity, sustained head turning, sleeping with head in an awkward position, prolonged neck extension, and so forth, have been reported (Hart and Easton, 1983) (see Table 60.1). Some of the reported events may be of no clinical significance, whereas others might have played an etiologic role. There is, however, no study suggesting that any neck movement or trivial neck trauma poses an independent risk factor for CAD (Rubinstein *et al.*, 2005).

Arterial disease

The relationship between sCAD and various constitutional as well as environmental risk factors is complex (Brandt and Grond-Ginsbach, 2002; Grond-Ginsbach *et al.*, 2002). According to the actual knowledge, CAD is regarded as an endpoint of a heterogeneous group of vasculopathies – permanent, transient, or both combined – developing under the influence of various genetic and environmental factors. The actual prevailing hypothesis for a vasculopathy is an extracellular matrix defect that may have various (genetic) origins (Guillon *et al.*, 2000).

Direct evidence of arterial disease

Redundancy of ICAs with the presence of coils, loops, or kinks is overrepresented in patients with ICAD (up to 30%) (Barbour *et al.*, 1994; Sturzenegger, 1995) and is probably the most frequent associated vessel anomaly (Figure 60.4). It may frequently

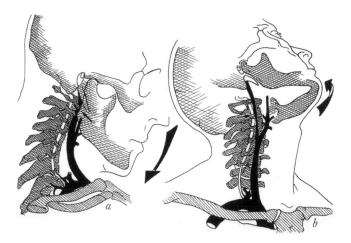

Figure 60.2 Mechanisms of traumatic ICA dissections.

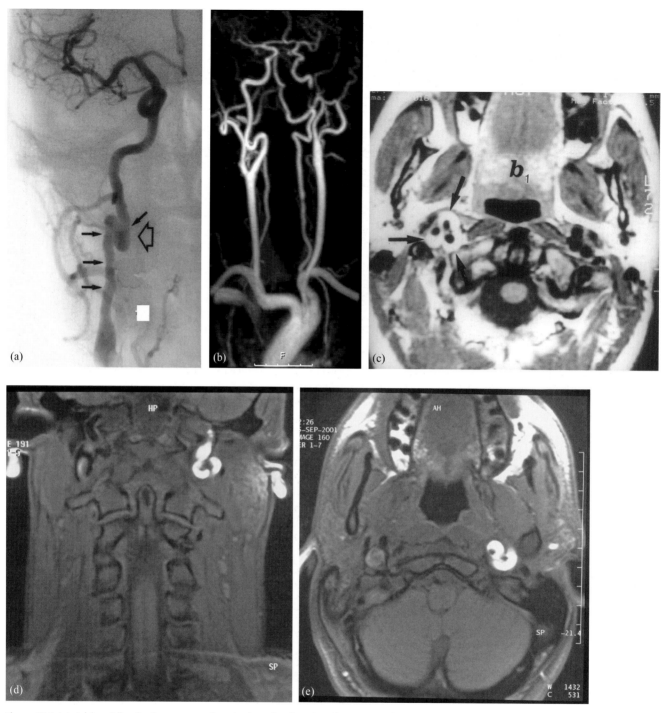

Figure 60.4 Arterial (carotid) redundancy as a predisposing factor for dissection. a) conventional angiography showing irregular stenosis (arrows) and a kinking of right ICA; b) MR-bolus contrast enhanced angiography showing kinking of right ICA and string sign (long distance tight stenosis) of left ICA; c) axial T1 showing the coiled right ICA with surrounding hemorrhage cut three times in the same plane; d) coronal T1, fat suppressed; e) axial T1 fat suppressed MR scans; d) and e) again show mural hematoma (hyperintense) around the coiled prepetrosal ICA segment.

go undetected in the case of vessel occlusion (Sturzenegger, 1995).

Angiographic evidence of FMD (Figure 60.5) or histological evidence of cystic medial necrosis has been noted in some patients with CAD (Thapedi *et al.*, 1970). Up to 15% of patients with ICAD have angiographic changes suggesting FMD in carotid, vertebral, or renal arteries (Table 60.1).

Hereditary connective tissue disorders, in particular the Type IV Ehlers-Danlos syndrome, but also Marfan's syndrome, osteogenesis imperfecta (mutations in one of the two genes [Col 1A1 and Col 1A2] encoding collagen type I), pseudoxanthoma elasticum, and adult polycystic kidney disease (ADPKD), are likely to be risk factors for sCAD (Brandt and Grond-Ginsbach, 2002; Grond-Ginsbach *et al.*, 2002). However, such underlying genetic disease

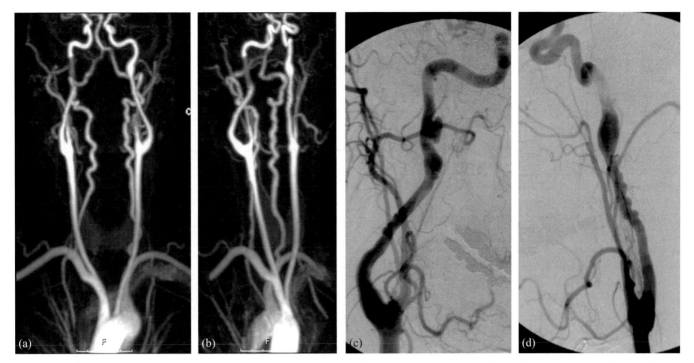

Figure 60.5 Fibromuscular dysplasia (FMD) probably more frequently underlies CAD than assumed since it is not well detected using MRI and may be masked by mural hemorrhage. a) and b): MR-bolus contrast enhanced angiography showing string sign of the right and irregular lumen of the left ICA. c) and d): conventional angiograms (frontal and lateral view) showing typical "string of beads" sign of the ICA with a dissecting aneurysm.

is found in a minority of sCAD patients. One group found connective tissue aberrations (abnormalities of collagen fibrils and elastic fibers) in skin biopsies in about half of examined CAD patients and their relatives (Brandt *et al.*, 1998, 2001). Another group found microbleeds at the tunica media-adventitia junction and altered smooth muscle cells in superior temporal artery branch biopsy in a small sample of sCAD patients (Volker *et al.*, 2005). The evaluation of CAD family members with connective tissue alterations in skin biopsy by linkage analysis suggested locus heterogeneity (Wiest *et al.*, 2006).

In a case-control study, aortic root diameter >34 mm as well as mitral valve dystrophy and prolapse were found to be associated with increased risk for sCAD (Tzourio *et al.*, 1997). Aortic and valvular abnormalities are considered markers of an extracellular matrix defect and are also a hallmark of Marfan's syndrome (Brandt *et al.*, 2001).

Functional tests using ultrasound in case-control studies showed evidence of impaired endothelium-dependent flow-mediated vasodilatation (Lucas *et al.*, 2004), increased common carotid artery diameter change (distensibility) during cardiac cycle (Guillon *et al.*, 2000), and higher circumferential wall stress of the carotids indicating abnormal elastic properties (Calvet *et al.*, 2004) in patients with sCAD in nondissected vessels as compared to controls or peripheral arterial segments.

The relatively young age of affected patients, the involvement of arterial segments usually not affected by atherosclerosis, and the absence of signs of atherosclerosis on imaging are additional arguments for a nonatherosclerotic vasculopathy.

Indirect evidence of arterial disease

The occurrence of multivessel dissections (unilateral or bilateral ICAD plus unilateral or bilateral VAD with renal artery or other visceral artery dissections), the higher incidence of intracranial aneurysms in patients with ICAD (Schievink *et al.*, 1992), the familial occurrence of spontaneous ICAD and congenitally bicuspid aortic valve (Schievink *et al.*, 1996), the occurrence of a familial syndrome of arterial dissections and lentiginosis, the familial association of intracranial aneurysms and CAD, and the familial occurrence of spontaneous ICAD all point to the possibility of an underlying arterial disease that, at least in some cases, may be familial (Table 60.1).

Whereas α1-antitrypsin plays a crucial role in maintaining the integrity of connective tissues and also arterial wall structure, the role of a deficiency of this enzyme with CAD is debated. One study found low levels of α1-antitrypsin in sCAD patients compared with controls (Vila *et al.*, 2003). In a recent case-control study, there was no difference in α1-antitrypsin deficiency alleles (Grond-Ginsbach *et al.*, 2004).

The role of hypertension and of cigarette smoking remains unsettled: these two vascular risk factors were found only rarely to be associated with CAD (Konrad *et al.*, 2004) but not so in most studies (Rubinstein *et al.*, 2005). A recent multicenter, prospective, hospital based, case-control study found a trend towards an increased risk of sCAD in hypertensive patients (adjusted odds ratio [OR] 1.79) (Pezzini *et al.*, 2006).

Oral contraceptive use was associated with CAD in three studies, significantly in only one (D'Anglejan-Chatillon *et al.*, 1989; Grau *et al.*, 1999; Tzourio *et al.*, 2002). Atherosclerosis does not seem to be a risk factor. Indeed, CAD seems to be less common in older atherosclerotic patients (Rubinstein *et al.*, 2005).

The role of hyperhomocysteinemia is controversial (Rubinstein *et al.*, 2005). It has been shown to cause endothelial dysfunction; however, CAD is not the result of endothelial disease. Two studies reporting a weak association are flawed by selection biases, above all in the controls (Caso and Gallai, 2003; Gallai *et al.*, 2001; Pezzini *et al.*, 2002).

Infection

Recent infection has been found to be an independent risk factor for CAD in two case-control studies (Grau *et al.*, 1999; Guillon *et al.*, 2003). Such an association may explain both a triggering role of an acute infection and a seasonal pattern of CAD occurrence, or it may stress the role of blood pressure because blood pressure is known to be higher in winter (Paciaroni *et al.*, 2006; Schievink *et al.*, 1998). The association of CAD with thyroid autoimmunity generates the hypothesis of genetically determined susceptibility to inflammatory stimuli as a predisposing factor for CAD (Pezzini *et al.*, 2006).

Age and sex

Spontaneous ICAD and VAD occur most frequently in the middle-aged or younger persons. The overall mean age for sICAD is around 45 years (with a wide range from <10 to >70 years) and for sVAD around 43 years (range >20 to 70) (Arnold *et al.*, 2006; Baumgartner *et al.*, 2001; Schievink, 2001). Overall, approximately 70% of the patients are reported to be younger than 50 years, and less than 10% of the patients are younger than 30 years. However, the age may change with the population studied: in one prospective study of stroke patients, 32% of those with an underlying dissection were older than 60 years (Ahl *et al.*, 2004). Older patients are less frequently referred to stroke centers and investigated using MRI, which may lead to underestimation of CAD in this age group.

The largest study to date including 696 patients with first-ever CAD reported a slight male predominance (57%). Women were younger than men (42.5 vs. 47.5 years). In men, there was a higher frequency of hypertension; in women, of migraine (Arnold *et al.*, 2006).

In children, dissection shows a clear male preponderance whether traumatic or not, and is predominantly extracranial in traumatic but intracranial in spontaneous cases (Fullerton *et al.*, 2001; Schievink *et al.*, 1994). sCAD in the pediatric age group (18 years or younger) seems to be rare; in the Mayo Clinic series, this accounted for less than 5% of the group (Schievink *et al.*, 1994). However, in a recent consecutive stroke series in children, dissection accounted for 20% of all causes, as in adults (Chabrier *et al.*, 2003). Almost all children with CAD diagnosed had a stroke, and only half had pain as a warning symptom (Fullerton *et al.*, 2001), which may, however, reflect a selection bias due to low index of suspicion in children, and poor assessment of warning symptoms.

The mean age of patients with traumatic dissections reported is around 30 years, and two-thirds are men (Hicks *et al.*, 1994).

Migraine and ICAD

Several case-control studies found an association between migraine and CAD (D'Anglejan-Chatillon *et al.*, 1989; Tzourio *et al.*, 2002). Dissections, in contrast, may have transient or even recurrent symptoms such as pain and neurological disturbances mimicking migraine with or without aura (Silverman and Wityk, 1998). Finally, CAD may trigger the trigeminovascular system and thus migraine; we have seen patients with pre-existing migraine in whom the dissection only caused either more frequent typical migraine attacks or prolonged migraine-like headache.

Clinical presentation

ICAD

The clinical manifestations of ICAD are highly variable. There are no clear differences in the clinical presentation of spontaneous versus traumatic ICAD.

Headache, neck and facial pain, pulsatile tinnitus, Horner's syndrome, cranial nerve palsies, anterior circulation stroke, transient ischemic attack (TIA), amaurosis fugax, and retinal infarction may be present in isolation or in various combinations (Table 60.2).

Symptoms caused by ICAD may be classified into two groups: (i) local symptoms, present in at least 75%, caused by intramural hemorrhage with vessel wall stenosis and/or distension or local space-occupying effect (Baumgartner *et al.*, 2001; Sturzenegger, 1995; Sturzenegger and Huber, 1993); and (ii) remote, as a consequence of ocular or cerebral ischemia, presenting as TIA in 10–20% or stroke in 60% (30–80%) (Baumgartner *et al.*, 2001; Biousse *et al.*, 1998; Dziewas *et al.*, 2003; Nassenstein *et al.*, 2005; Touze *et al.*, 2003) (Figure 60.6).

Ischemic symptoms are often preceded by local warning symptoms or signs such as head, facial, or neck pain; tinnitus; Horner's syndrome; or cranial nerve palsies. The knowledge and recognition of these symptoms and often subtle signs are the key to an early diagnosis and treatment of ICAD before ischemic complications occur (Biousse *et al.*, 1995; Sturzenegger, 1995).

Table 60.2 Clinical manifestations of ICAD

Local symptoms or signs	Remote symptoms or signs (ischemia)
Headache, facial and neck pain (fronto-temporal, orbital, periorbital, anterior neck); 64–90%	Stroke (mainly in the MCA territory); 41%–64%
Horner's syndrome; 25%–58%	TIA; 15%–29%
Pulsatile tinnitus; 16%–27%	Amaurosis fugax; 3%–28%
Cranial nerve palsies (mainly cranial nerves IX to XII, less frequently VII, VI, V, IV, III); 5%–16%	Ischemic optic neuropathy; <5%
	Retinal infarction; <5%

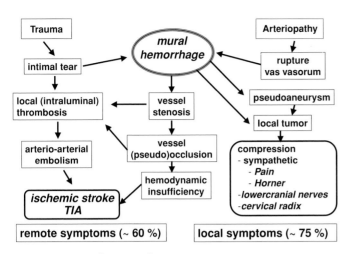

Figure 60.6 CAD. Pathogenesis of symptoms.

Local symptoms of ICAD

The most common symptom of ICAD is pain. Pain is the inaugural symptom in more than 50% and finally is reported by 64%–90% of ICAD patients (Baumgartner *et al.*, 2001; Biousse *et al.*, 1994; Dziewas *et al.*, 2003; Vilela and Goulao, 2003). Pain usually is an acute and early manifestation; however, it may also develop progressively and later in the disease course (Biousse *et al.*, 1994; Silbert *et al.*, 1995). Patients may present with headache, facial pain, or neck pain. Headache is present in 66%–68%, facial pain in 34%–53%, and neck pain in 9%–26%. In 17% of the patients, headache, facial pain, and neck pain occur simultaneously (Biousse *et al.*, 1994).

Pain can occur simultaneously with retinal or cerebral ischemia but more often precedes the ischemic symptoms by hours to several weeks, and then is an important warning symptom (Sturzenegger, 1995; Sturzenegger and Steinke, 1996). Location of pain is variable but usually unilateral, i.e. ipsilateral to the ICAD. The most frequent locations involve the frontotemporal, periorbital face and head, and/or upper anterolateral cervical region (Figure 60.7). (Biousse *et al.*, 1994; Silbert *et al.*, 1995; Sturzenegger, 1995). Less frequently, patients may complain of bilateral pain, occipital headache, or entire hemicrania.

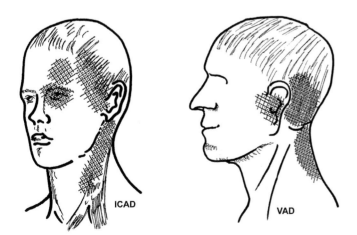

Figure 60.7 Pain location in CAD.

Pain is severe in more than 70% of patients and is often described as unique or unusual (Sturzenegger, 1995). Its character can be throbbing, constrictive, or pulsatile. Patients may even complain about extremely severe and sudden headache, like a thunderclap (Evans and Mokri, 2002). Pain following ICAD can also mimic cluster headache or migraine (Frigerio *et al.*, 2003). Pain as the only manifestation of sICAD has been reported in up to 5% (Arnold *et al.*, 2006).

Pulsatile tinnitus may occur in stenotic dissection, but only 16%–27% of patients describe a pulsatile tinnitus (Silbert *et al.*, 1995). In one large study, women more often than men (16% vs. 8%) reported the presence of a pulsatile tinnitus (Arnold *et al.*, 2006). Clinical examination may reveal a carotid bruit in these patients.

Local signs of ICAD

ICAD patients may present with Horner's syndrome if the ipsilateral cervical sympathetic fibers are affected by ischemia or compression or stretching due to mural hematoma (Hart and Easton, 1983; Sturzenegger and Huber, 1993). It may occur isolated or in combination with other local and ischemic symptoms. It may be detected at the onset of pain as a heralding sign, or with a delay of several days, when stroke has already occurred (Sturzenegger and Huber, 1993). In total, Horner's syndrome is reported in 25%–58% of patients with ICAD (Biousse, Touboul, D'Anglejan-Chatillon, *et al.*, 1998; Arnold, Kappeler, Georgiadis, *et al.*, 2006). However, the so-called classical triad of ICAD (including ipsilateral pain, Horner's syndrome, and anterior circulation cerebral ischemia) is present in less than 30% of ICAD (Schievink, 2001).

Single or multiple cranial nerve palsies in various combinations are found in 5%–16% of patients with extracranial ICAD (Arnold *et al.*, 2006; Mokri *et al.*, 1986, 1996; Sturzenegger and Huber, 1993). The most frequently involved nerve is the hypoglossal nerve followed by the other lower cranial nerves including the accessory, vagal, and glossopharyngeal nerves. The facial, trigeminal, and oculomotor nerves also may be affected in rare cases. Dysgeusia, probably due to affection of the chorda tympani nerve, has been described.

Possible pathomechanisms leading to cranial nerve palsies include direct compression or stretching of the nerves by the expanded carotid artery or the compromise of their vasa nervorum (Sturzenegger and Huber, 1993). Isolated local signs, without remote ischemic events, are reported in up to 25% (Touze *et al.*, 2003).

Ischemic manifestations of ICAD

Cerebral and ocular ischemic manifestations are the most feared symptoms of ICAD. The frequency of cerebral ischemia mainly depends on the delay to diagnosis and on patient selection, and varies between 50% and 90% (Baumgartner *et al.*, 2001; Biousse *et al.*, 1998; Touze *et al.*, 2003).

Patients with ICAD with ischemic manifestations more often have severe carotid stenoses or occlusion or intracranial obstruction, and their ICAD are less frequently accompanied by cranial nerve palsy and Horner's syndrome compared with ICAD without ischemia (Baumgartner *et al.*, 2001).

Anterior circulation TIA occurs in 15%–29% of patients with ICAD (Treiman *et al.*, 1996). It was the inaugural symptom of

ICAD in 8 of 80 patients (Biousse *et al.*, 1995). Most TIAs occurred within the first few days of symptom onset, and recurrent TIAs have been observed in several patients. Among 42 patients who had suffered a cerebral infarction, it was preceded by TIAs in 7 (Biousse *et al.*, 1995).

Most ischemic strokes (82%) occur within the first week of symptom onset. Late infarcts more than a month after symptom onset and a single case with a disabling stroke arising 5 months after ICAD have been reported (Biousse *et al.*, 1995; Martin and Humphrey, 1998). More than two-thirds of ischemic strokes are preceded by local warning symptoms, amaurosis fugax, and/or TIA (Biousse *et al.*, 1995; Sturzenegger, 1995).

Artery-to-artery embolism (and not hemodynamic impairment) seems to be the main stroke mechanism as assessed by stroke pattern analysis (Benninger *et al.*, 2006; Bounds, 1999; Lucas *et al.*, 1998; Pelkonen *et al.*, 2003; Steinke *et al.*, 1996). In a recent study, all patients had territorial infarcts, 130 of 131 in the middle cerebral artery (MCA) territory and 1 in the anterior cerebral artery (ACA) territory. In six patients, additional border zone infarcts were visualized. Rarely, patients with MCA infarcts had additional ACA (4%) or posterior cerebral artery (PCA) infarcts (2%) (Benninger, Georgiadis, Gandjour, *et al.*, 2006). Watershed infarcts are reported in 3%–15% of CAD-associated strokes (Dreier *et al.*, 2004; Lucas *et al.*, 1998; Steinke *et al.*, 1996).

Single or multiple episodes of transient monocular visual loss (amaurosis fugax) is a frequent symptom of ICAD and occurs in up to 28% of patients. Patients sometimes describe positive monocular visual phenomena such as monocular scintillations or flashing lights (Biousse *et al.*, 1998). These symptoms may be caused by transient emboli or more likely hemodynamic impairment of the retina, choroidea, or optic nerve. In a large series, none of 41 patients with transient monocular visual symptoms following ICAD had retinal emboli on fundus examination.

Many patients with amaurosis fugax ignore these warning symptoms and subsequently develop a stroke. Persisting visual loss due to retinal infarction is a rare event in ICAD (Rao *et al.*, 1994). Only 10 of 533 patients with ICAD suffered a retinal infarction (our unpublished observations).

Rarely, anterior or posterior ischemic optic neuropathy may occur as an early sign of ICAD with severe stenosis or occlusion. Patients may present with monocular visual impairment without retinal artery occlusion on fundus examination. An ipsilateral mydriasis with absent or poor reactivity to light stimulation may be present in these patients, probably because ischemia of the ciliary ganglion or the iris.

Asymptomatic ICAD

Asymptomatic ICADs have been reported to occur simultaneously with symptomatic VAD or contralateral ICAD, or have been detected incidentally during routine follow-up examinations on ultrasound or MRI.

VAD

The clinical picture of VAD again is broad and variable (Arnold *et al.*, 2006; Mokri *et al.*, 1988) (Table 60.3). Occipital headache,

Table 60.3 Clinical manifestations of VAD

Local symptoms or signs	Remote symptoms or signs (Ischemia, subarachnoid hemorrhage)
History of head or neck trauma: 16%–44%	Posterior circulation stroke (often Wallenberg's syndrome): 67%–83%
Posterior headache or neck pain: 81%–88%	Posterior circulation TIA (e.g., diplopia, visual blurring, gait disturbance, vertigo, dysphagia, dysarthria, hemisensory symptoms, motor symptoms): 11%–23%
Cervical root affection mostly at the C5-C6 level: <1%	Subarachnoid hemorrhage (in intracranial VAD): 4%–13%
Lower brainstem compression (in intracranial VAD) : <1%	Rostral or mid-cervical spinal cord ischemia: <1%

neck pain (sometimes preceded by a major or minor head or neck trauma), and posterior circulation ischemia are the main clinical features. Rarer clinical manifestations include cervical root impairment and spinal cord ischemia. In patients with intracranial VAD, subarachnoid hemorrhage (SAH) or in single cases lower brainstem compression (in intracranial VAD) may occur (Garnier *et al.*, 2004; Hosoya *et al.*, 1999).

Local symptoms and signs of VAD

Posterior headache or neck pain occurs in up to 88% of patients with VAD (Figure 60.7; Arnold *et al.*, 2006; Mokri *et al.*, 1988; Sturzenegger, 1994). The posterior location of headache may be explained by the innervation of the occipital region by the upper cervical nerves. The pain is ipsilateral to the dissected VAD in the majority of patients, but bilateral pain is not rare (Sturzenegger, 1994). Rarely generalized or frontal headache has been described. The character of headache was steady in 56% and pulsatile in 44% (Evans and Mokri, 2002; Silbert *et al.*, 1995). About one-fourth of patients reported abrupt onset of pain, and three-fourths gradual onset. Only about 50% of patients described the pain to be unique and different than previously experienced (Silbert *et al.*, 1995). Isolated headache or neck pain may be the only symptom in VAD, even when multiple arteries are dissected. Because of the heterogeneity of pain topographics, dynamics, quality, and intensity, it is difficult to establish an early diagnosis. Therefore, we recommend immediate imaging studies of the cervical arteries in patients with new-onset unexplained headache or neck pain (Arnold *et al.*, 2006).

In the case of intracranial extension of extracranial VAD or primarily intracranial VAD, SAH may occur when the dissection tears the adventitia (Garnier *et al.*, 2004; Yamaura *et al.*, 1990). Patients present with headache of severe intensity and sudden onset. In a study of 24 patients with SAH following intracranial VAD, 15 patients had a grade III to grade V on the Hunt and Kosnik scale and 9 a grade I or II. A severe neurological deficit on admission, rebleeding, and a pearl-and-string-like aspect on angiography were predictors of an unfavorable outcome (Hosoya et al., 1999). Rare cases of spinal SAH because of VAD have been reported (Crum et al., 2000).

Cervical root irritation, mainly affecting the C5–C6 level, is a very rare local symptom of VAD (Crum et al., 2000).

Single cases of lower brainstem compression by a dissecting aneurysm of the intracranial VA without SAH have been described (Caplan et al., 1988; Miyazaki et al., 1984).

Ischemic manifestations of VAD

The majority of patients present with symptoms and signs of posterior circulation ischemia, consisting mainly of stroke (67%–83%). Ischemia may be caused by artery-to-artery embolism or by hemodynamic impairment of the territory supplied by the VA.

Lateral medullar infarction leading to Wallenberg syndrome is a frequent manifestation of VAD. Other locations include medial medullar, cerebellar, pontine, thalamic, and PCA infarcts (Mokri et al., 1988). In the case of basilar artery occlusion because of embolism, devastating brainstem infarct leading to "locked-in" state or death may occur (Hicks et al., 1994). In a large series of 169 patients with VAD, ischemia occurred in 131 patients (77%). Among these patients, 114 suffered an ischemic stroke (67%). Fifteen (13%) of them had at least one TIA before stroke, with a median time interval from the first TIA to stroke onset of 1 day (range, 1 hour to 17 days). A total of 17 patients (10%) presented with TIA without a subsequent stroke. Three patients with ischemic stroke also showed signs of SAH (Arnold et al., 2006). Posterior and anterior radicular branches of the VA supply the rostral and middle cervical spinal cord. Therefore, spinal cord ischemia in the territory of the anterior or posterior spinal artery or both is a potential complication of VAD. Bilateral spinal cord infarction may occur if spinal radicular arteries arise from only one VA (Crum et al., 2000).

Asymptomatic patients with VAD

Some patients with VAD may be asymptomatic, with the VAD being detected during the diagnostic procedures in patients with ICAD (Pelkonen et al., 2003; Shah et al., 2004; Touze et al., 2001).

Intracranial dissections

Dissections of the intracranial segments of ICA and VA seem to be rare and usually present with severe headache, ischemic symptoms, or SAH (Chaves et al., 2002; Hosoda et al., 1991; Yamaura et al., 1990). Affected subjects are mostly young with a mean age less than 30 years. Intracranial dissections seem to occur most frequently in the V4 segment of the VA (Garnier et al., 2004; Hosoya et al., 1999; Yamaura et al., 1990). In the anterior circulation, the supraclinoid ICA segment is most frequently involved (Chaves et al., 2002). Brain ischemia is almost the rule and usually follows immediately after headache onset (Chaves et al., 2002). However, diagnosis is difficult because the clinical spectrum is broad and may be severe at presentation. Extensive diagnostic work-up (usually with conventional angiography) is necessary so as not to miss correct diagnosis (Garnier et al., 2004; Hosoda et al., 1991;

Hosoya et al., 1999). Clinical manifestations of intracranial VAD include headache, neck pain, SAH, (rarely) rostral cervical spinal cord ischemia, or brainstem compression. These symptoms have been discussed previously.

The visualization of a mural hematoma in intracranial arteries is difficult, and imaging of intracranial arteries is not systematically performed in some stroke centers (Hosoya et al., 1999). Therefore, the incidence of intracranial dissections is likely to be underestimated. Prognosis is thought to be poorer than in patients with extracranial CAD (Chaves et al., 2002; Garnier et al., 2004). However, the seriousness of the disease may be overestimated because of a publication bias in favor of autopsy cases due to the difficulty of the intra vitam diagnosis (Chaves et al., 2002).

Diagnostic evaluation

The wide spectrum of clinical manifestations only allows for diagnostic suspicion without the use of imaging methods, especially before ischemic events have occurred. More than 90% of all cerebral ischemic events are of (artery-to-artery) embolic origin (Benninger et al., 2004; Lucas et al., 1998). Because anticoagulant treatment is accepted to prevent the latter, early and reliable confirmation is mandatory (Lee et al., 2006; Sturzenegger and Steinke, 1996; Treiman et al., 1996). During the last years, MRI and MRA have replaced intra-arterial digital subtraction angiography (DSA) as the diagnostic gold standard (Charbonneau et al., 2005; Levy et al., 1994). The crucial advantage of MRI is its ability to show the intramural hematoma proving dissection (Figures 60.8, 60.9, and 60.13). Combined with cervical vessel MRA, luminal compromise is shown as well (Figures 60.8–60.10 and 60.12), and cerebral MRI may show (also subclinical) ischemic complications. Meanwhile, sophisticated protocols exist that allow noninvasive imaging of vessel wall, vessel lumen, and brain within a 30-minute examination time (Nassenstein et al., 2005). Older studies report brain ischemia in 60%–80% of patients with dissection (Baumgartner et al., 2001; Biousse et al., 1995; Dziewas et al., 2003; Sturzenegger, 1995); however, a delay between first symptoms (local, such as pain, Horner's syndrome, or pulsatile tinnitus) and stroke is well known and may last hours to days (Sturzenegger, 1994, 1995). A high degree of suspicion and an early active search for CAD with noninvasive imaging methods (especially MRI) in patients at risk can reduce the stroke rate in CAD dramatically to less than 30% (Nassenstein et al., 2005; Sturzenegger, 1995).

Angiography

Compared to MRI, the main shortcoming of conventional catheter angiography is its inability to image pathology of the vessels wall (mural hematoma) and its invasiveness.

ICAD

Common angiographic abnormalities in ICAD include luminal stenosis, which frequently has a typical appearance: irregular, elongated ("string sign"), and tapered stenosis (Figure 60.11); rapid luminal reconstitution at skull base; association with vessel tortuosity, dissecting aneurysms (pseudoaneurysm), intimal flaps, and slow ICA-MCA flow; occlusion (usually beginning about 1–2 cm

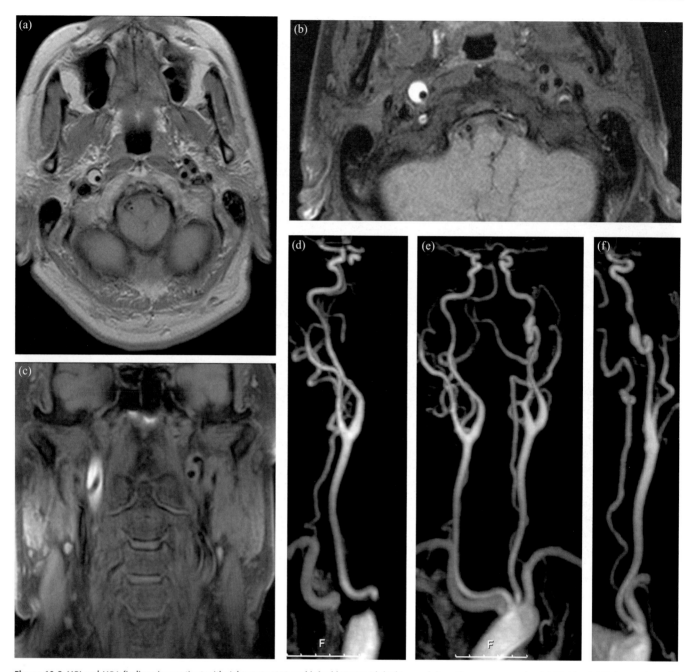

Figure 60.8 MRI and MRA findings in a patient with right acute ICAD and left old ICAD with kinking and dissecting aneurysm. a) axial PD; b) axial T1 fat suppressed; c) coronal T1 fat suppressed MR images showing (hyperintense) mural hematoma asymmetrically surrounding narrowed vessel lumen (flow void, black); d, e, f) MR bolus contrast enhanced angiography.

above the bifurcation and tapering to a complete occlusion with a flame-like or radish-tail appearance) ("flame sign") (see also Figure 60.1); and distal branch occlusions (a sign of distal embolization) (Fisher *et al.*, 1978; Houser *et al.*, 1984). In traumatic ICAD, aneurysms and occlusions are more frequent.

VAD

The most common angiographic features of VAD again include stenosis (elongated, irregular, and sometimes tapered), dissecting aneurysms, occlusion, and intimal flaps (Figure 60.12). Because of the smaller vessel dimensions and the curvilinear course of the VA,

MRI and MRA are less sensitive and have more confusing artifacts than in the carotid artery and therefore are less specific.

Basilar artery and other intracranial artery dissections

On angiography they may appear as an elongated stenosis, double lumen, dissecting aneurysm, or occlusion (Alexander *et al.*, 1979; Berger and Wilson, 1984; Berkovic *et al.*, 1983; Hosoda *et al.*, 1991; Pozzati *et al.*, 1995) (Figure 60.12). Dissections of the smaller intracranial vessels such as PCAs or MCAs have a much less specific angiographic appearance: nonspecific segment of stenosis or occlusion; stenosis may show luminal irregularities or be

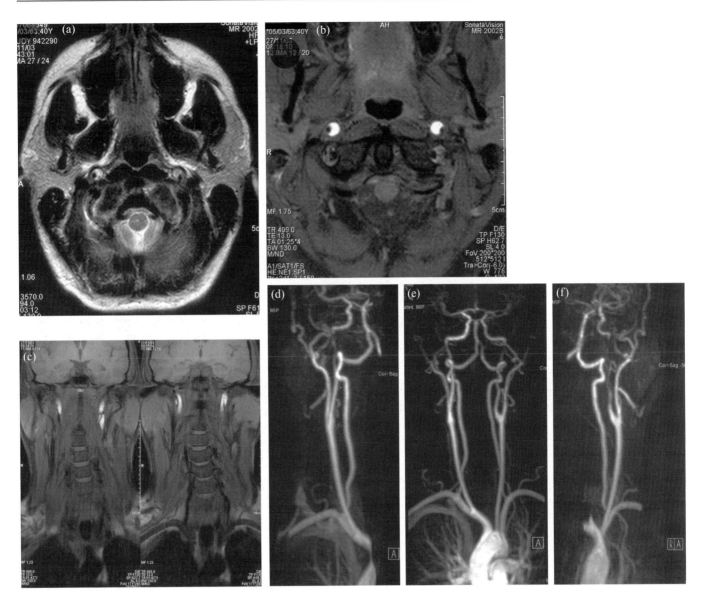

Figure 60.9 (a–f) MR and MRA in a patient with bilateral ICAD.

associated with luminal expansion or dilatation (Grosman *et al.*, 1980; Maillo *et al.*, 1991; Sasaki *et al.*, 1991). It is not unusual that entities such as "vasculitis" or meningeal infection or inflammation enter into the differential diagnosis. Overall, in most cases it becomes visually impossible to make an angiographic diagnosis of dissection with certainty in these small vessels.

MRI and MRA

MRI and MRA have replaced angiography as the gold standard, at least in the extracranial segments of ICA and VA. Special imaging protocols of MRI and contrast-enhanced MRA should be combined to get the highest diagnostic yield (Phan *et al.*, 2001; Shah *et al.*, 2004). With contrast-enhanced MRA techniques (such as bolus gadolinium injection), stenoses, some of the luminal irregularities, and many of the aneurysms can be seen (Figures 60.8–10, 60.12) (Auer *et al.*, 1998; Levy *et al.*, 1994; Ozdoba *et al.*, 1996;

Yang *et al.*, 2005). For the quality of MRA examination, a correct technique is crucial (Okumura *et al.*, 2001; Phan *et al.*, 2001). More subtle luminal irregularities (such as e.g. in FMD) and small aneurysmal dilatations could be missed with MRA when sensitivity is compared with that of high-quality conventional catheter arteriograms. Cross-sectional MR images at the level of dissection frequently reveal specific MRI abnormalities consisting of a dark small circle of flow void (which is smaller than the normal caliber of the original lumen as compared with the contralateral flow void area and best depicted on axial T2-weighted sequences) representing the narrowed lumen. This is surrounded by a bright hyperintense crescent- or donut-shaped zone that represents the intramural hematoma, best visualized with fat-suppressed axial or coronal T1-weighted sequences (Figures 60.8–60.10, 60.13). Double lumen is a rarer finding. These MRI abnormalities, which are quite specific, can be seen in ICA, VA, and basilar artery dissections. However, for the smaller intracranial vessels,

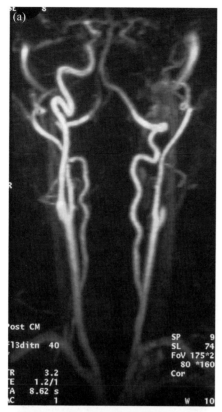

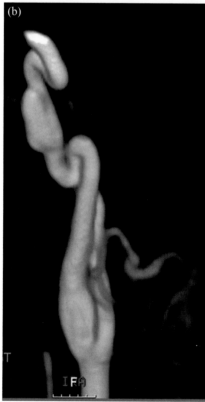

Figure 60.10 Bolus contrast enhanced MRA (a) and CT angiography (b) in ICAD showing kinking (a right and b), flame shaped occlusion (a, left), and dissecting aneurysm (a and b) in various combinations.

the diagnostic role of MRI and MRA remains limited, and the diagnosis of these dissections still remains a challenge. In vessel segments with a more tortuous course, such as the V3 and intracranial segments, flow-related artifacts may imitate mural hematoma (Mascalchi *et al.*, 1997). Furthermore, the mural hematoma may be isointense to the surrounding tissue in the very early phase of CAD.

Also in tCAD MRI is the method of choice; however, new CT-angiographic techniques may well allow detection of vessel compromise in trauma patients (Bok and Peter, 1996).

CT and CT angiography

High resolution, multichannel thin slice CT and CT angiography have shown promising results in visualization of vessel stenoses or occlusion and vessel diameter extension (Figures 60.10 and 60.14) as well as associated vessel tortuosities (Nunez *et al.*, 2004). However, direct imaging of mural hematoma is limited. The examination times are shorter than those of MRI; however, CT uses radiation and potentially nephrotoxic contrast agents (Yang *et al.*, 2005).

Ultrasound

Doppler combined with color duplex imaging is a simple, widely available, and noninvasive technique; however, it needs substantial experience of the examiner. Morphologic and hemodynamic sonographic criteria should be assessed in combination. In skilled hands, sensitivity is high (96%) for ICAD diagnosis in patients with arterial stenoses and/or carotid territory ischemia (Benninger *et al.*, 2006; Steinke *et al.*, 1994; Sturzenegger, 1991; Sturzenegger *et al.*, 1995). Typical findings are high resistance flow profile in the proximal ICA (because of distal stenoses or pseudo-occlusion), tapering stenoses distal to the bifurcation, stenoses in the high cervical retromandibular ICA segment, double lumen, intimal flap, low-density intramural hematoma (2–6 cm distal above the bifurcation), and absence of atherosclerotic wall changes (Figure 60.15). There are, however, pitfalls (especially in FMD patients), and sensitivity is only 71% in sCAD with only local symptoms (Baumgartner *et al.*, 2001). Therefore, confirmation with MRI/MRA is also considered mandatory regarding treatment and secondary prophylaxis. Sensitivity of ultrasound is much lower because of much less specific findings in cases of VAD (Sturzenegger *et al.*, 1993) or intracranial dissections.

Ultrasound is useful in monitoring the evolution and resolution of ICAD, e.g. to guide duration of anticoagulant therapy (Sturzenegger, 1995; Sturzenegger *et al.*, 1995; Treiman *et al.*, 1996).

Genetic testing

Although many aspects point to a genetically based anomaly of extracellular matrix components as a potential underlying cause (Table 60.1), despite many efforts, the candidate gene approach has not yet led to the identification of genes that are involved in the pathogenesis of CAD (Wiest *et al.*, 2006). Pedigree studies indicate locus heterogeneity for the connective tissue phenotype of CAD patients.

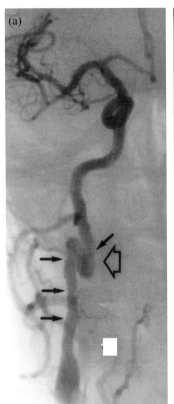

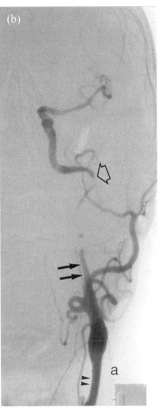

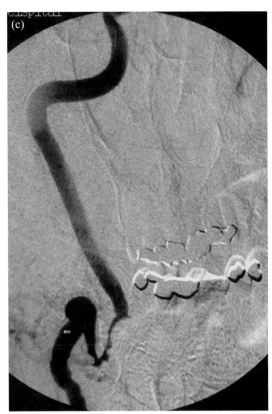

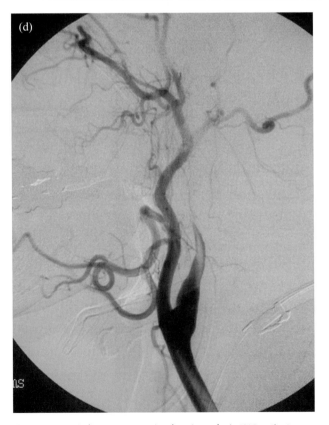

Figure 60.11 Findings on conventional angiography in ICAD patients: a) irregular luminal narrowing and kinking; b) pseudo-oclusion with abrupt luminal reconstitution at skull base; c) irregular high grade stenosis; d) flame-shaped occlusion.

Tissue biopsies

Two studies have provided some evidence for underlying and/or predisposing systemic connective tissue disorder or arteriopathy in sCAD:

1. Connective tissue abnormalities in dermal biopsies found on electron microscopy in 36 of 65 CAD patients and also in family members without CAD showed abnormalities of collagen fibrils and elastic fibers (fragmentation, calcification) (Brandt *et al.*, 1998, 2001)
2. So-called segmental mediolytic arteriopathy (microbleeds at the tunica media-adventitia junction) and altered smooth muscle cells (vacuolated, synthetic phenotype) were found in nine patients with sCAD in a superior temporal artery branch biopsy (Volker *et al.*, 2005)

These findings are, however, not specific and have not yet been reproduced by other groups.

Neither genetic testing nor tissue biopsies are part of the routine evaluation of CAD patients.

Treatment of cervico-cephalic dissections

Acute treatment

Thrombolysis

In acute CAD with severe cerebral ischemia, thrombolysis is a therapeutic option. CAD was not a contraindication in the large randomized intravenous thrombolysis trials (National Institute of Neurological Disorders and Stroke [NINDS], Second European-Australasian Acute Stroke Study [ECASS II]). However, the number

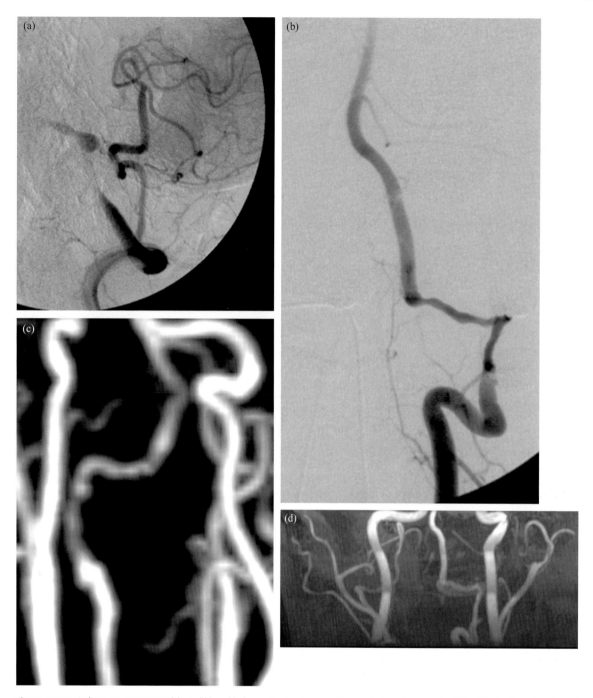

Figure 60.12 Findings on conventional (a and b) and bolus contrast enhanced MR (c and d) angiography in VAD patients. There is an irregular usually long distance vessel stenosis (a to d). There may also be a pseudo-aneurysm (a).

of CAD patients included in these trials is unknown. Recent case series of CAD patients treated with intravenous or intra-arterial thrombolysis suggest that efficacy and complication rates may be similar to those in other stroke patients, and a rupture of the dissected vessel because of thrombolysis has not been reported to date (Arnold *et al.*, 2002; Derex *et al.*, 2001; Georgiadis *et al.*, 2006). However, it remains unclear whether thrombolysis might enlarge the wall hematoma because such cases have not been described so far.

Vasoactive drugs and endovascular treatment

When hemodynamic ischemia is suspected based on perfusion MRI or transcranial ultrasound, patients are left recumbent (Biousse *et al.*, 1995). Rarely, hemodynamic impairment leads to clinical deterioration that may be prevented by the administration of vasoactive drugs or endovascular treatment. Balloon dilatation and stenting has been successfully used in such patients with progressive stoke symptoms despite an optimal conventional treatment (Cohen *et al.*, 2003, 2005).

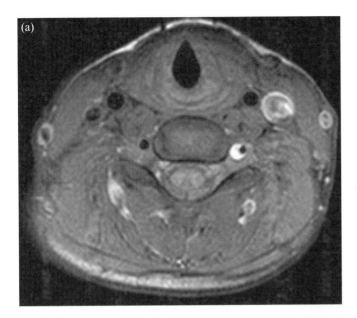

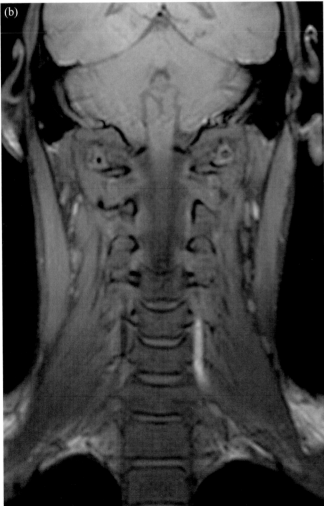

Figure 60.13 (**a** and **b**) MRI findings in VAD.

Secondary prevention

Antithrombotic treatment

To date, there are no randomized controlled trials comparing anticoagulant drugs with aspirin for the prevention of stroke in patients with CAD. Several attempts to perform such a study failed because most physicians familiar with CAD would not agree to have their patients randomized to the aspirin arm and because a very large study would be necessary to show a difference given the low rate of stroke recurrence under both treatments (Beletsky et al., 2003; Bounds, 1999). There is a general consensus in the stroke community that either heparin followed by warfarin or aspirin should be administered for at least 3–6 months following extracranial CAD (Bounds, 1999; Lee et al., 2006). A recent meta-analysis showed no difference in death or disability between anti-coagulant and antiplatelet therapy (Lyrer and Engelter, 2004). This meta-analysis is limited by its small sample size (n = 178 for the analysis of death or disability), inclusion of several very small case series, different diagnostic criteria, variable follow-up periods, and by the fact that many data (including baseline National Institutes of Health Stroke Scale [NIHSS] score, as well as causes of death) were not available. For these reasons, it remains under debate whether anticoagulants or aspirin should be used as first-line agents, and a prospective randomized trial is suggested (Beletsky et al., 2003; Bounds, 1999).

The usual treatment of extracranial CAD without intracranial extension at our stroke center consists of intravenous heparin followed by oral warfarin (target international normalized ratio [INR] 2.0–3.0) for a period of 3–6 months. This preference for anti-coagulation in the early phase of extracranial CAD is based on pathophysiological arguments and clinical experience. Transcranial ultrasound studies showed frequent microemboli in the MCA in up to 59% of patients with ICAD (Droste et al., 2001; Koennecke et al., 1997; Molina et al., 2000). These microembolic signals were reduced by the administration of intravenous heparin (Srinivasan et al., 1996). In addition, analyzing the stroke pattern on brain MRI and CT, several studies showed that most of the infarcts are attributable to embolism (Benninger et al., 2004; Lucas et al., 1998; Pelkonen et al., 2003; Steinke et al., 1996). Furthermore, it is rare to see a patient with CAD have a stroke after anticoagulant treatment has been started. However, increased risk of intracranial bleeding or potential extension of the mural hematoma theoretically may offset the benefits of the anticoagulant treatment. Therefore, we do not anticoagulate patients with large brain infarcts or with intracranial extension of CAD. An extension of mural hematoma under anticoagulant treatment has been assumed to be the cause of delayed ICA occlusion in rare cases and was associated with higher activated partial thromboplastin time (aPPT) ratios (over-anticoagulation) (Dreier et al., 2004).

In the case of intracranial vessel dissection or extension of the dissection to the intracranial vessel segments, which mainly occurs in VAD, we avoid anticoagulant agents because of the danger of SAH (Garnier et al., 2004). Curiously, SAH as a consequence of VAD has been reported predominantly from Asian medical centers and only rarely from Europe or the United States.

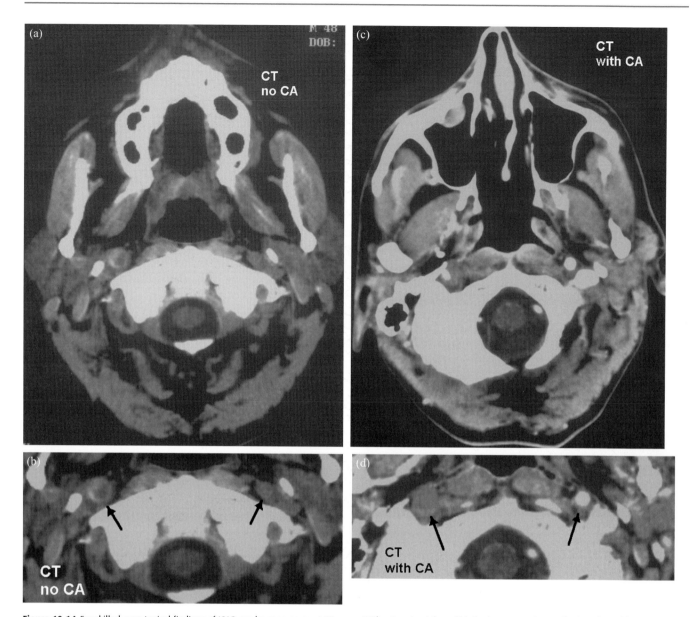

Figure 60.14 For skilled eyes typical findings of ICAD can be seen on most CT scans. Without contrast (a and b) the hematoma is usually ring-shaped hyperintense; with contrast (c and d) there is absent luminal contrast filling or a stenosis. Compare with the contra-lateral side. b) and d) are magnifications of a) and c).

After 6 months, we either stop antithrombotic treatment (if the artery has completely normalized on ultrasound or MRA) or we switch to aspirin 100 mg daily for long-term prevention (when there is persistent residual stenosis, occlusion or aneurysm, or an underlying arterial disease such as FMD).

Endovascular treatment and surgery

ICAD have a favorable long-term prognosis with low rates of recurrent dissection or recurrent stroke. The stroke recurrence rate is less than 1% per year irrespective of the persistence of severe stenoses or occlusion of the dissected artery (Baumgartner *et al.*, 2001). Aneurysms following ICAD have a favorable long-term prognosis with a very low risk of ischemic stroke or rupture (Guillon, 2001; Guillon *et al.*, 1999). These results suggest that endovascular or surgical treatment of a persisting stenosis or aneurysm should only be considered in the rare cases with recurrent ischemic

symptoms in the vascular territory supplied by the dissected artery despite antithrombotic treatment.

Prognosis

Outcome

For extracranial ICAD and VAD, the prognosis is typically good and is essentially defined by the occurrence, extent, and location of stroke. CAD causing severe stenosis or occlusion are more likely to lead to brain ischemia than are those without luminal narrowing (Baumgartner *et al.*, 2001). CAD patients with an occlusion have more severe large MCA territory infarcts with a definitely worse outcome, probably because of poor functioning collateral pathways (Milhaud *et al.*, 2002). Tertiary referral series report a higher frequency of serious outcomes (16%–37%

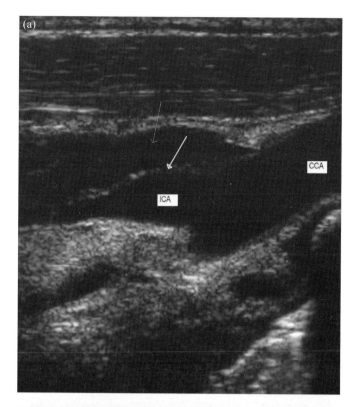

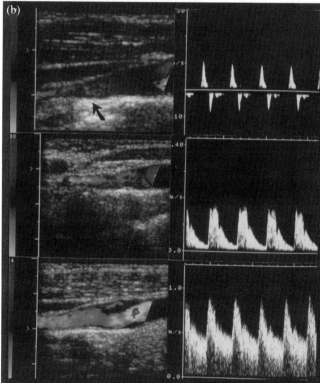

Figure 60.15 Ultrasound in ICAD. Usually there are no signs of atherosclerosis. There may be an intimal flap (a), a hypodense mural hematoma (a), a tapering stenosis with a high resistance flow profile (b, upper row), or a stenosis in the upper cervical ICA segment (b lower row). See color plate.

severe persisting deficits) (Stapf *et al.*, 2000), whereas in a population-based study of 48 CAD patients, good outcome (defined as modified Rankin score of 0–2) was seen in 92% (Lee *et al.*, 2006). Considering the broad spectrum of clinical presentation, including asymptomatic and monosymptomatic or minimally symptomatic cases, the overall mortality rate is less than 5%. Around three-fourths of the patients have complete or excellent recoveries, and less than 5% are left with marked neurological deficits (Biousse *et al.*, 1995; Hart and Easton, 1983; Leys and Debette, 2006). Considering ICAD patients presenting with stroke, after 1 year mean Rankin Scale score is 0.9 ± 1.2, with about 20% having disabling strokes (Rankin Scale score 3–5) (Kremer *et al.*, 2003). Angiographically on follow-up, 75%–90% of the stenoses either improve or completely resolve (Steinke *et al.*, 1994; Treiman *et al.*, 1996), most dissecting aneurysms decrease in size or resolve (Djouhri *et al.*, 2000; Guillon *et al.*, 1999), and 10%–70% of (pseudo)occlusions recanalize (Kremer *et al.*, 2003; Pelkonen *et al.*, 2003).

Outcome was favorable in 88 of 107 (82%) patients with VAD and ischemic stroke, and mortality was 2%. Low baseline NIHSS score and younger age were independent predictors of a favorable outcome (Arnold *et al.*, 2006).

The outcome for tCAD is usually less favorable than for the spontaneous ones: stroke is almost the rule, and cerebral deficits are usually more severe; pseudoaneurysm are more frequent, and fewer aneurysms resolve or become smaller; and fewer stenoses resolve or improve whereas more stenoses tend to progress to occlusion. Traumatic internal carotid artery dissection (tICAD) and also tVAD have higher mortality rates and are more likely to leave patients with neurological deficits (Martin *et al.*, 1991; Mokri, 1990; Schellinger *et al.*, 2001).

According to certainly biased data from the literature, intracranial dissections carry a significantly less favorable prognosis than do extracranial dissections, with higher rates of mortality and morbidity (Chaves *et al.*, 2002). It seems that intracranial dissections carry a high risk of developing pseudoaneurysms and of SAH. Mortality of intracranial dissections in a pediatric age group (predominantly affected by this location) was 51% (Fullerton *et al.*, 2001). This may, however, reflect a bias towards reporting cases with histopathologic diagnosis and the known difficulties making an antemortem diagnosis.

Recurrence

Dissection

Recurrence of dissection is a rare phenomenon, is reported in tertiary referral series (Schievink *et al.*, 1994; Touze *et al.*, 2003), but is not found in a population-based study during an 8-year follow-up (Lee *et al.*, 2006). Redissection usually does not occur in a previously dissected and healed cervical artery but rather in another cervical artery or in the renal arteries of the same patient (Bassetti *et al.*, 1996; Lee *et al.*, 2006).

For vertebral and extracranial ICAD, the rate of recurrence has been studied (Schievink *et al.*, 1994; Touze *et al.*, 2003). The risk of recurrence was small and maximal for the first month (2%), and subsequently much lower (1% per year for all age groups) (Schievink *et al.*, 1994). The 10-year rate of recurrence for all age groups was 12%; for patients younger than 45 years (the mean age of the cohort) the rate was 17%, and for those older than 45 years it was only 6%. In a multicenter French study, among 432 CAD patients there was a 0.9% recurrence rate during a mean follow-up of 31 months (Touze *et al.*, 2003). Recurrent dissections are likely more frequent in patients who have underlying arterial disease (Schievink *et al.*, 1996).

Stroke

The risk of having a (recurrent) stroke or TIA after having suffered a CAD in general is very low (Kremer *et al.*, 2003; Touze *et al.*, 2003). In a 1 year follow-up, annual rates for recurrent ischemic stroke in the territory of the dissected ICA and for any stroke were similarly low in patients with permanent (0.7% and 1.4%) and transient (0.3% and 0.6%) stenosis or occlusion of ICA (Kremer *et al.*, 2003). Thus, stroke recurrence rate was not significantly associated with persistence of ICA stenosis or occlusion (Kremer *et al.*, 2003). In another retrospective series, among 432 survivors of CAD, 0.9% had a recurrent stroke and 1.8% a TIA during a mean follow-up of 31 months, giving an incidence for stroke of 0.3% per year and of TIA of 0.6% per year (Touze *et al.*, 2003). Low stroke recurrence rates are confirmed by other studies (Bassetti *et al.*, 1996; Treiman *et al.*, 1996), and only one study reported an unexpectedly high event rate of 10.4% in 105 CAD patients followed for 10 months (Beletsky *et al.*, 2003).

Persistent aneurysm

Dissecting aneurysms due to CAD are reported in 12%–49% (Lee *et al.*, 2006; Ozdoba *et al.*, 1996; Pelkonen *et al.*, 2003; Touze *et al.*, 2001, 2003). Several studies show that these aneurysms frequently persist but that the patients carry a very low risk of stroke or any other complication (Mokri, 1990). Among 55 patients with 68 aneurysms and a clinical and radiological follow-up of >3 years, no patient had signs of cerebral ischemia, local compression, or rupture. Fifty-eight percent of the aneurysms were unchanged, 25% had disappeared, 17% had decreased in size, and none had increased (Djouhri *et al.*, 2000; Touze *et al.*, 2001). Surgical treatment has a high local and remote complication rate (Muller *et al.*, 2000). In the acute stage of traumatic and spontaneous CAD, stenting may restore a hemodynamically critical brain perfusion in selected cases (Cohen *et al.*, 2003; Cohen *et al.*, 2003). However, in patients with persistent pseudoaneurysm after tICAD, stent placement bears an increased risk of local and remote complications compared to antiplatelet treatment alone (Cothren *et al.*, 2005). Therefore, medical management with antiplatelet therapy is sufficient in most patients, and surgical or endovascular management is not indicated (Guillon *et al.*, 1999).

REFERENCES

Ahl, B., Bokemeyer, M., Ennen, J. C., *et al.* 2004. Dissection of the brain supplying arteries over the life span. *J Neurol Neurosurg Psychiatry*, **75**, 1194–6.

Alexander, C. B., Burger, P. C., and Goree, J. A. 1979. Dissecting aneurysms of the basilar artery in 2 patients. *Stroke*, **10**, 294–9.

Arnold, M., Bousser, M. G., Fahrni, G., *et al.* 2006. Vertebral artery dissection. Presenting findings and predictors of outcome. *Stroke*, **37**, 2499–503. Epub 2006 Sep 7. Erratum in: *Stroke*, 2007, **38**, 208.

Arnold, M., Cumurciuc, R., Stapf, C., *et al.* 2006. Pain as the only symptom of cervical artery dissection. *J Neurol Neurosurg Psychiatry*, **77**, 1021–4.

Arnold, M., Kappeler, L., Georgiadis, D., *et al.* 2006. Gender differences in spontaneous cervical artery dissection. *Neurology*, **67**, 1050–2.

Arnold, M., Nedeltchev, K., Sturzenegger, M., *et al.* 2002. Thrombolysis in patients with acute stroke caused by cervical artery dissection: analysis of 9 patients and review of the literature. *Arch Neurol*, **59**, 549–53.

Auer, A., Felber, S., Schmidauer, C., Waldenberger, P., and Aichner, F. 1998. Magnetic resonance angiographic and clinical features of extracranial vertebral artery dissection. *J Neurol Neurosurg Psychiatry*, **64**, 474–81.

Barbour, P. J., Castaldo, J. E., Rae-Grant, A. D., *et al.* 1994. Internal carotid artery redundancy is significantly associated with dissection. *Stroke*, 25, 1201–6.

Bassetti, C., Carruzzo, A., Sturzenegger, M., and Tuncdogan, E. 1996. Recurrence of cervical artery dissection. A prospective study of 81 patients. *Stroke*, **27**, 1804–7.

Baumgartner, R. W., Arnold, M., Baumgartner, I., *et al.* 2001. Carotid dissection with and without ischemic events: local symptoms and cerebral artery findings. *Neurology*, **57**, 827–32.

Beletsky, V., Nadareishvili, Z., Lynch, J., *et al.* 2003. Cervical arterial dissection: time for a therapeutic trial? *Stroke*, **34**, 2856–60.

Benninger, D. H., Georgiadis, D., Gandjour, J., and Baumgartner, R. W. 2006. Accuracy of color duplex ultrasound diagnosis of spontaneous carotid dissection causing ischemia. *Stroke*, **37**, 377–81.

Benninger, D. H., Georgiadis, D., Kremer, C., *et al.* 2004. Mechanism of ischemic infarct in spontaneous carotid dissection. *Stroke*, **35**, 482–5.

Berger, M. S., and Wilson, C. B. 1984. Intracranial dissecting aneurysms of the posterior circulation. Report of six cases and review of the literature. *J Neurosurg*, **61**, 882–94.

Berkovic, S. F., Spokes, R. L., Anderson, R. M., and Bladin, P. F. 1983. Basilar artery dissection. *J Neurol Neurosurg Psychiatry*, **46**, 126–9.

Biousse, V., D'Anglejan-Chatillon, J., Massiou, H., and Bousser, M. G. 1994. Head pain in non-traumatic carotid artery dissection: a series of 65 patients. *Cephalalgia*, **14**, 33–6.

Biousse, V., D'Anglejan-Chatillon, J., Touboul, P. J., Amarenco, P., and Bousser, M. G. 1995. Time course of symptoms in extracranial carotid artery dissections. A series of 80 patients. *Stroke*, **26**, 235–9.

Biousse, V., Schaison, M., Touboul, P. J., D'Anglejan-Chatillon, J., and Bousser, M. G. 1998. Ischemic optic neuropathy associated with internal carotid artery dissection. *Arch Neurol*, **55**, 715–9.

Biousse, V., Touboul, P., J., and D'Anglejan-Chatillon, J., 1998. Ophthalmologic manifestations of internal carotid artery dissection. *Am J Ophthalmol*, **126**, 565–77.

Blanco Pampin, J., Morte Tamayo, N., Hinojal Fonseca, R., Payne-James, J. J., and Jerreat, P. 2002. Delayed presentation of carotid dissection, cerebral ischemia, and infarction following blunt trauma: two cases. *J Clin Forensic Med*, **9**, 136–40.

Bogousslavsky, J., Despland, P. A., and Regli, F. 1987. Spontaneous carotid dissection with acute stroke. *Arch Neurol*, **44**, 137–40.

Bok, A. P., and Peter, J. C. 1996. Carotid and vertebral artery occlusion after blunt cervical injury: the role of MR angiography in early diagnosis. *J Trauma*, **40**, 968–72.

Bounds, J. A. 1999. Carotid dissection: pathophysiology of stroke and treatment implications. *Stroke*, **30**, 1149–50.

Brandt, T., and Grond-Ginsbach, C. 2002. Spontaneous cervical artery dissection: from risk factors toward pathogenesis. *Stroke*, **33**, 657–8.

Brandt, T., Hausser, I., Orberk, E., *et al.* 1998. Ultrastructural connective tissue abnormalities in patients with spontaneous cervicocerebral artery dissections. *Ann Neurol*, **44**, 281–5.

Brandt, T., Orberk, E., Weber, R., *et al.* 2001. Pathogenesis of cervical artery dissections: association with connective tissue abnormalities. *Neurology*, **57**, 24–30.

Calvet, D., Boutouyrie, P., Touze, E., et al. 2004. Increased stiffness of the carotid wall material in patients with spontaneous cervical artery dissection. Stroke, 35, 2078–82.

Caplan, L. R., Baquis, G. D., Pessin, M. S., et al. 1988. Dissection of the intracranial vertebral artery. Neurology, 38, 868–77.

Caso, V., and Gallai, V. 2003. Why should mild hyperhomocysteinemia be responsible for CAD? Stroke, 34, e209.

Chabrier, S., Lasjaunias, P., Husson, B., Landrieu, P., and Tardieu, M. 2003. Ischaemic stroke from dissection of the craniocervical arteries in childhood: report of 12 patients. Eur J Paediatr Neurol, 7, 39–42.

Charbonneau, F., Gauvrit, J. Y., Touze, E., et al. 2005. [Diagnosis and follow-up of cervical arterial dissections–results of the SFNV-SFNR study]. J Neuroradiol, 32, 255–7.

Chaves, C., Estol, C., Esnaola, M. M., et al. 2002. Spontaneous intracranial internal carotid artery dissection: report of 10 patients. Arch Neurol, 59, 977–81.

Cohen, J. E., Ben-Hur, T., Rajz, G., Umansky, F., and Gomori, J. M. 2005. Endovascular stent-assisted angioplasty in the management of traumatic internal carotid artery dissections. Stroke, 36, e45–7.

Cohen, J. E., Gomori, J. M., and Umansky, F. 2003. Endovascular management of symptomatic vertebral artery dissection achieved using stent angioplasty and emboli protection device. Neurol Res, 25, 418–22.

Cohen, J. E., Leker, R. R., Gotkine, M., Gomori, M., and Ben-Hur, T. 2003. Emergent stenting to treat patients with carotid artery dissection: clinically and radiologically directed therapeutic decision making. Stroke, 34, e254–7.

Cothren, C. C., Moore, E. E., Ray, C. E. Jr., et al. 2005. Carotid artery stents for blunt cerebrovascular injury: risks exceed benefits. Arch Surg, 140, 480–5; discussion 485–6.

Crum, B., Mokri, B., and Fulgham, J. 2000. Spinal manifestations of vertebral artery dissection. Neurology, 55, 304–6.

D'Anglejan-Chatillon, J., Ribeiro, V., Mas, J. L., Youl, B. D., and Bousser, M. G. 1989, Migraine – a risk factor for dissection of cervical arteries. Headache, 29, 560–1.

Davis, J. W., Holbrook, T. L., Hoyt, D. B., et al. 1990. Blunt carotid artery dissection: incidence, associated injuries, screening, and treatment. J Trauma, 30, 1514–7.

Derex, L., Tomsick, T. A., Brott, T. G., et al. 2001. Outcome of stroke patients without angiographically revealed arterial occlusion within four hours of symptom onset. AJNR Am J Neuroradiol, 22, 685–90.

Djouhri, H., Guillon, B., Brunereau, L., et al. 2000. MR angiography for the long-term follow-up of dissecting aneurysms of the extracranial internal carotid artery. AJR Am J Roentgenol, 174, 1137–40.

Dreier, J. P., Lurtzing, F., Kappmeier, M., et al. 2004. Delayed occlusion after internal carotid artery dissection under heparin. Cerebrovasc Dis, 18, 296–303.

Droste, D. W., Junker, K., Stogbauer, F., et al. 2001. Clinically silent circulating microemboli in 20 patients with carotid or vertebral artery dissection. Cerebrovasc Dis, 12, 181–5.

Dziewas, R., Konrad, C., Drager, B., et al. 2003. Cervical artery dissection–clinical features, risk factors, therapy and outcome in 126 patients. J Neurol, 250, 1179–84.

Evans, R. W., and Mokri, B. 2002. Headache in cervical artery dissections. Headache, 42, 1061–3.

Fisher, C. M., Ojemann, R. G., and Roberson, G. H. 1978. Spontaneous dissection of cervico-cerebral arteries. Can J Neurol Sci, 5, 9–19.

Frigerio, S., Buhler, R., Hess, C. W., and Sturzenegger, M. 2003. Symptomatic cluster headache in internal carotid artery dissection–consider anhidrosis. Headache, 43, 896–900.

Fullerton, H. J., Johnston, S. C., and Smith, W. S. 2001. Arterial dissection and stroke in children. Neurology, 57, 1155–60.

Gallai, V., Caso, V., Paciaroni, M., et al. 2001. Mild hyperhomocyst(e)inemia: a possible risk factor for cervical artery dissection. Stroke, 32, 714–8.

Garnier, P., Demasles, S., Januel, A. C., and Michel, D. 2004. [Intracranial extension of extracranial vertebral artery dissections. A review of 16 cases]. Rev Neurol (Paris), 160, 679–84.

Georgiadis, D., Caso, V., and Baumgartner, R. W. 2006. Acute therapy and prevention of stroke in spontaneous carotid dissection. Clin Exp Hypertens, 28, 365–70.

Giroud, M., Fayolle, H., Andre, N., et al. 1994. Incidence of internal carotid artery dissection in the community of Dijon. J Neurol Neurosurg Psychiatry, 57, 1443.

Grau, A. J., Brandt, T., Buggle, F., et al. 1999. Association of cervical artery dissection with recent infection. Arch Neurol, 56, 851–6.

Grond-Ginsbach, C., Engelter, S., Werner, I., et al. 2004. Alpha-1-antitrypsin deficiency alleles are not associated with cervical artery dissections. Neurology, 62, 1190–2.

Grond-Ginsbach, C., Schnippering, H., Hausser, I., et al. 2002. Ultrastructural connective tissue aberrations in patients with intracranial aneurysms. Stroke, 33, 2192–6.

Grosman, H., Fornasier, V. L., Bonder, D., Livingston, K. E., and Platts, M. E. 1980. Dissecting aneurysm of the cerebral arteries. Case report. J Neurosurg, 53, 693–7.

Guillon, B. 2001. [Is it necessary to treat persistent aneurysms after dissection of the cervical arteries?]. Rev Neurol (Paris), 157, 1304–8.

Guillon, B., Berthet, K., Benslamia, L., et al. 2003. Infection and the risk of spontaneous cervical artery dissection: a case-control study. Stroke, 34, e79–81.

Guillon, B., Brunereau, L., Biousse, V., et al. 1999. Long-term follow-up of aneurysms developed during extracranial internal carotid artery dissection. Neurology, 53, 117–22.

Guillon, B., Tzourio, C., Biousse, V., et al. 2000. Arterial wall properties in carotid artery dissection: an ultrasound study. Neurology, 55, 663–6.

Hart, R. G. 1988. Vertebral artery dissection. Neurology, 38, 987–9.

Hart, R. G., and Easton, J. D. 1983. Dissections of cervical and cerebral arteries. Neurol Clin, 1, 155–82.

Hicks, P. A., Leavitt, J. A., and Mokri, B. 1994. Ophthalmic manifestations of vertebral artery dissection. Patients seen at the Mayo Clinic from 1976 to 1992. Ophthalmology, 101, 1786–92.

Hosoda, K., Fujita, S., Kawaguchi, T., et al. 1991. Spontaneous dissecting aneurysms of the basilar artery presenting with a subarachnoid hemorrhage. Report of two cases. J Neurosurg, 75, 628–33.

Hosoya, T., Adachi, M., Yamaguchi, K., et al. 1999. Clinical and neuroradiological features of intracranial vertebrobasilar artery dissection. Stroke, 30, 1083–90.

Houser, O. W., Mokri, B., Sundt, T. M. Jr., Baker, H. L. Jr., and Reese D. F. 1984. Spontaneous cervical cephalic arterial dissection and its residuum: angiographic spectrum. AJNR Am J Neuroradiol, 5, 27–34.

Hughes, K. M., Collier, B., Greene, K. A., and Kurek, S. 2000. Traumatic carotid artery dissection: a significant incidental finding. Am Surg, 66, 1023–7.

Koennecke, H. C., Trocio, S. H. Jr., Mast, H., and Mohr, J. P. 1997. Microemboli on transcranial Doppler in patients with spontaneous carotid artery dissection. J Neuroimaging, 7, 217–20.

Konrad, C., Muller, G. A., Langer, C., et al. 2004. Plasma homocysteine, MTHFR C677 T, CBS 844ins68bp, and MTHFD1 G1958 A polymorphisms in spontaneous cervical artery dissections. J Neurol, 251, 1242–8.

Kremer, C., Mosso, M., Georgiadis, D., et al. 2003. Carotid dissection with permanent and transient occlusion or severe stenosis: long-term outcome. Neurology, 60, 271–5.

Lee, V. H., Brown, R. D. Jr., Mandrekar, J. N., and Mokri, B. 2006. Incidence and outcome of cervical artery dissection: a population-based study. Neurology, 67, 1809–12.

Levy, C., Laissy, J. P., Raveau, V., et al. 1994. Carotid and vertebral artery dissections: three-dimensional time-of-flight MR angiography and MR imaging versus conventional angiography. Radiology, 190, 97–103.

Leys, D., and Debette, S. 2006. Long-term outcome in patients with cervical-artery dissections: there is still a lot to know. Cerebrovasc Dis, 22, 215.

Lucas, C., Lecroart, J. L., Gautier, C., et al. 2004. Impairment of endothelial function in patients with spontaneous cervical artery dissection: evidence for a general arterial wall disease. Cerebrovasc Dis, 17, 170–4.

Lucas, C., Moulin, T., Deplanque, D., Tatu, L., and Chavot, D. 1998. Stroke patterns of internal carotid artery dissection in 40 patients. Stroke, 29, 2646–8.

Lyrer, P., and Engelter, S. 2004. Antithrombotic drugs for carotid artery dissection. *Stroke*, **35**, 613–4.

Maillo, A., Diaz, P., and Morales, F. 1991. Dissecting aneurysm of the posterior cerebral artery: spontaneous resolution. *Neurosurgery*, **29**, 291–4.

Martin, P. J., and Humphrey, P. R. 1998. Disabling stroke arising five months after internal carotid artery dissection. *J Neurol Neurosurg Psychiatry*, **65**, 136–7.

Martin, R. F., Eldrup-Jorgensen, J., Clark, D. E., and Bredenberg, C. E. 1991. Blunt trauma to the carotid arteries. *J Vasc Surg*, **14**, 789–93; discussion 793–5.

Mascalchi, M., Bianchi, M. C., Mangiafico, S., *et al.* 1997. MRI and MR angiography of vertebral artery dissection. *Neuroradiology*, **39**, 329–40.

Milhaud, D., de Freitas, G. R., van Melle, G., and Bogousslavsky, J. 2002. Occlusion due to carotid artery dissection: a more severe disease than previously suggested. *Arch Neurol*, **59**, 557–61.

Miyazaki, S., Yamaura, A., Kamata, K., and Fukushima, H. 1984. A dissecting aneurysm of the vertebral artery. *Surg Neurol*, **21**, 171–4.

Mokri, B. 1990. Traumatic and spontaneous extracranial internal carotid artery dissections. *J Neurol*, **237**, 356–61.

Mokri, B., Houser, O. W., Sandok, B. A., and Piepgras, D. G. 1988. Spontaneous dissections of the vertebral arteries. *Neurology*, **38**, 880–5.

Mokri, B., Piepgras, D. G., and Houser, O. W. 1988. Traumatic dissections of the extracranial internal carotid artery. *J Neurosurg*, **68**, 189–97.

Mokri, B., Silbert, P. L., Schievink, W. I., and Piepgras, D. G. 1996. Cranial nerve palsy in spontaneous dissection of the extracranial internal carotid artery. *Neurology*, **46**, 356–9.

Mokri, B., Sundt, T. M. Jr., Houser, O. W., and Piepgras, D. G. 1986. Spontaneous dissection of the cervical internal carotid artery. *Ann Neurol*, **19**, 126–38.

Molina, C. A., Alvarez-Sabin, J., Schonewille, W., *et al.* 2000. Cerebral microembolism in acute spontaneous internal carotid artery dissection. *Neurology*, **55**, 1738–40.

Muller, B. T., Luther, B., Hort, W., *et al.* 2000. Surgical treatment of 50 carotid dissections: indications and results. *J Vasc Surg*, **31**, 980–8.

Nassenstein, I., Kramer, S. C., Niederstadt, T., *et al.* 2005. [Incidence of cerebral ischemia in patients with suspected cervical artery dissection: first results of a prospective study]. *Rofo*, **177**, 1532–9.

Nunez, D. B. Jr., Torres-Leon, M., and Munera, F. 2004. Vascular injuries of the neck and thoracic inlet: helical CT-angiographic correlation. *Radiographics*, **24**, 1087–98; discussion 1099–100.

Okumura, A., Araki, Y., Nishimura, Y., *et al.* 2001. The clinical utility of contrast-enhanced 3D MR angiography for cerebrovascular disease. *Neurol Res*, **23**, 767–71.

Ozdoba, C., Sturzenegger, M., and Schroth, G. 1996. Internal carotid artery dissection: MR imaging features and clinical-radiologic correlation. *Radiology*, **199**, 191–8.

Paciaroni, M., Georgiadis, D., Arnold, M., *et al.* 2006. Seasonal variability in spontaneous cervical artery dissection. *J Neurol Neurosurg Psychiatry*, **77**, 677–9.

Pelkonen, O., Tikkakoski, T., Leinonen, S., *et al.* 2003. Extracranial internal carotid and vertebral artery dissections: angiographic spectrum, course and prognosis. *Neuroradiology*, **45**, 71–7.

Pezzini, A., Caso, V., Zanferrari, C., *et al.* 2006. Arterial hypertension as risk factor for spontaneous cervical artery dissection. A case-control study. *J Neurol Neurosurg Psychiatry*, **77**, 95–7.

Pezzini, A., Del Zotto, E., Archetti, S., *et al.* 2002. Plasma homocysteine concentration, C677 T MTHFR genotype, and 844ins68bp CBS genotype in young adults with spontaneous cervical artery dissection and atherothrombotic stroke. *Stroke*, **33**, 664–9.

Pezzini, A., Del Zotto, E., Mazziotti, G., *et al.* 2006. Thyroid autoimmunity and spontaneous cervical artery dissection. *Stroke*, **37**, 2375–7.

Phan, T., Huston J. 3rd, Bernstein, M. A., Riederer, S. J., and Brown, R. D. Jr. 2001. Contrast-enhanced magnetic resonance angiography of the cervical vessels: experience with 422 patients. *Stroke*, **32**, 2282–6.

Pozzati, E., Andreoli, A., Padovani, R., and Nuzzo, G. 1995. Dissecting aneurysms of the basilar artery. *Neurosurgery*, **36**, 254–8.

Rao, T. H., Schneider, L. B., Patel, M., and Libman, R. B. 1994. Central retinal artery occlusion from carotid dissection diagnosed by cervical computed tomography. *Stroke*, **25**, 1271–2.

Rothwell, D. M., Bondy, S. J., and Williams, J. I. 2001. Chiropractic manipulation and stroke: a population-based case-control study. *Stroke*, **32**, 1054–60.

Rubinstein, S. M., Peerdeman, S. M., van Tulder, M. W., Riphagen, I., and Haldeman, S. 2005. A systematic review of the risk factors for cervical artery dissection. *Stroke*, **36**, 1575–80.

Sasaki, O., Ogawa, H., Koike, T., Koizumi, T., and Tanaka, R. 1991. A clinicopathological study of dissecting aneurysms of the intracranial vertebral artery. *J Neurosurg*, **75**, 874–82.

Schellinger, P. D., Schwab, S., Krieger, D., *et al.* 2001. Masking of vertebral artery dissection by severe trauma to the cervical spine. *Spine*, **26**, 314–9.

Schievink, W. I. 2001. Spontaneous dissection of the carotid and vertebral arteries. *N Engl J Med*, **344**, 898–906.

Schievink, W. I., Mokri, B., and O'Fallon, W. M. 1994. Recurrent spontaneous cervical-artery dissection. *N Engl J Med*, **330**, 393–7.

Schievink, W. I., Mokri, B., and Piepgras, D. G. 1992. Angiographic frequency of saccular intracranial aneurysms in patients with spontaneous cervical artery dissection. *J Neurosurg*, **76**, 62–6.

Schievink, W. I., Mokri, B., and Piepgras, D. G. 1994. Spontaneous dissections of cervicocephalic arteries in childhood and adolescence. *Neurology*, **44**, 1607–12.

Schievink, W. I., Mokri, B., Piepgras, D. G., and Gittenberger-de Groot, A. C. 1996. Intracranial aneurysms and cervicocephalic arterial dissections associated with congenital heart disease. *Neurosurgery*, **39**, 685–9; discussion 689–90.

Schievink, W. I., Mokri, B., Piepgras, D. G., and Kuiper, J. D. 1996. Recurrent spontaneous arterial dissections: risk in familial versus nonfamilial disease. *Stroke*, **27**, 622–4.

Schievink, W. I., Mokri, B., and Whisnant, J. P. 1993. Internal carotid artery dissection in a community. Rochester, Minnesota, 1987–1992. *Stroke*, **24**, 1678–80.

Schievink, W. I., Wijdicks, E. F., and Kuiper, J. D. 1998. Seasonal pattern of spontaneous cervical artery dissection. *J Neurosurg*, **89**, 101–3.

Shah, G. V., Quint, D. J., and Trobe, J. D. 2004. Magnetic resonance imaging of suspected cervicocranial arterial dissections. *J Neuroophthalmol*, **24**, 315–8.

Silbert, P. L., Mokri, B., and Schievink, W. I. 1995. Headache and neck pain in spontaneous internal carotid and vertebral artery dissections. *Neurology*, **45**, 1517–22.

Silverman, I. E., and Wityk, R. J. 1998. Transient migraine-like symptoms with internal carotid artery dissection. *Clin Neurol Neurosurg*, **100**, 116–20.

Smith, W. S., Johnston, S. C., Skalabrin, E. J., *et al.* 2003. Spinal manipulative therapy is an independent risk factor for vertebral artery dissection. *Neurology*, **60**, 1424–8.

Srinivasan, J., Newell, D. W., Sturzenegger, M., Mayberg, M. R., and Winn, H. R. 1996. Transcranial Doppler in the evaluation of internal carotid artery dissection. *Stroke*, **27**, 1226–30.

Stapf, C., Elkind, M. S., and Mohr, J. P. 2000. Carotid artery dissection. *Annu Rev Med*, **51**, 329–47.

Steinke, W., Rautenberg, W., Schwartz, A., and Hennerici, M. 1994. Noninvasive monitoring of internal carotid artery dissection. *Stroke*, **25**, 998–1005.

Steinke, W., Schwartz, A., and Hennerici, M. 1996. Topography of cerebral infarction associated with carotid artery dissection. *J Neurol*, **243**, 323–8.

Sturzenegger, M. 1991. Ultrasound findings in spontaneous carotid artery dissection. The value of duplex sonography. *Arch Neurol*, **48**, 1057–63.

Sturzenegger, M. 1993. [Vertebral artery dissection following manipulation of the cervical vertebrae]. *Schweiz Med Wochenschr*, **123**, 1389–99.

Sturzenegger, M. 1994. Headache and neck pain: the warning symptoms of vertebral artery dissection. *Headache*, **34**, 187–93.

Sturzenegger, M. 1995. Spontaneous internal carotid artery dissection: early diagnosis and management in 44 patients. *J Neurol*, **242**, 231–8.

Sturzenegger, M., and Huber, P. 1993. Cranial nerve palsies in spontaneous carotid artery dissection. *J Neurol Neurosurg Psychiatry*, **56**, 1191–9.

Sturzenegger, M., Mattle, H. P., Rivoir, A., and Baumgartner, R. W. 1995. Ultrasound findings in carotid artery dissection: analysis of 43 patients. *Neurology*, **45**, 691–8.

Sturzenegger, M., Mattle, H. P., Rivoir, A., Rihs, F., and Schmid, C. 1993. Ultrasound findings in spontaneous extracranial vertebral artery dissection. *Stroke*, **24**, 1910–21.

Sturzenegger, M., and Steinke, W. 1996. [Cerebral artery dissection]. *Ther Umsch*, **53**, 544–51.

Thapedi, I. M., Ashenhurst, E. M., and Rozdilsky, B. 1970. Spontaneous dissecting aneurysm of the internal carotid artery in the neck. Report of a case and review of the literature. *Arch Neurol*, **23**, 549–54.

Touze, E., Gauvrit, J. Y., Moulin, T., *et al.* 2003. Risk of stroke and recurrent dissection after a cervical artery dissection: a multicenter study. *Neurology*, **61**, 1347–51.

Touze, E., Randoux, B., Meary, E., *et al.* 2001. Aneurysmal forms of cervical artery dissection: associated factors and outcome. *Stroke*, **32**, 418–23.

Treiman, G. S., Treiman, R. L., Foran, R. F., *et al.* 1996. Spontaneous dissection of the internal carotid artery: a nineteen-year clinical experience. *J Vasc Surg*, **24**, 597–605; discussion 605–7.

Tzourio, C., Benslamia, L., Guillon, B., *et al.* 2002. Migraine and the risk of cervical artery dissection: a case-control study. *Neurology*, **59**, 435–7.

Tzourio, C., Cohen, A., Lamisse, N., Biousse, V., and Bousser, M. G. 1997. Aortic root dilatation in patients with spontaneous cervical artery dissection. *Circulation*, **95**, 2351–3.

Vila, N., Millan, M., Ferrer, X., Riutort, N., and Escudero, D. 2003. Levels of alpha1-antitrypsin in plasma and risk of spontaneous cervical artery dissections: a case-control study. *Stroke*, **34**, E168–9.

Vilela, P., and Goulao, A. 2003. [Cervical and intracranial arterial dissection: review of the acute clinical presentation and imaging of 48 cases]. *Acta Med Port*, **16**, 155–64.

Volker, W., Besselmann, M., Dittrich, R., *et al.* 2005. Generalized arteriopathy in patients with cervical artery dissection. *Neurology*, **64**, 1508–13.

Wiest, T., Hyrenbach, S., Bambul, P., *et al.* 2006. Genetic analysis of familial connective tissue alterations associated with cervical artery dissections suggests locus heterogeneity. *Stroke*, **37**, 1697–702.

Willis, B. K., Greiner, F., Orrison, W. W., and Benzel, E. C. 1994. The incidence of vertebral artery injury after midcervical spine fracture or subluxation. *Neurosurgery*, **34**, 435–41; discussion 441–2.

Yamaura, A., Watanabe, Y., and Saeki, N. 1990. Dissecting aneurysms of the intracranial vertebral artery. *J Neurosurg*, **72**, 183–8.

Yang, C. W., Carr, J. C., Futterer, S. F., *et al.* 2005. Contrast-enhanced MR angiography of the carotid and vertebrobasilar circulations. *AJNR Am J Neuroradiol*, **26**, 2095–101.

Yang, S. T., Huang, Y. C., Chuang, C. C., and Hsu, P. W. 2006. Traumatic internal carotid artery dissection. *J Clin Neurosci*, **13**, 123–8.

61

CEREBRAL AMYLOID ANGIOPATHIES

Charlotte Cordonnier and Didier Leys

The term "amyloid" describes deposits of proteins sharing specific physical characteristics: -pleated sheet configuration, apple green birefringence under polarized light after Congo red staining, fibrillary structure, and insolubility in water (Castano and Frangione, 1988; Glenner, 1980a, b). Amyloid proteins are fluorescent under ultraviolet light after thioflavin S or T stains (Stokes and Trickey, 1973). The amyloid properties, depending on the physical configuration of the protein and the biochemical characteristics (Glenner, 1980a, b), are used to classify cerebral amyloid angiopathies (CAA) (Table 61.1).

In this chapter, we will not consider amyloid deposition associated with vascular malformations, radiation necrosis, angiitis, plasmocytomas, and pseudotumoral amyloid lesions called amyloidomas.

Common features in CAA

CAA are defined by the deposition of amyloid proteins in the wall of the cerebral vessels (Glenner, 1980a, b). The clinical presentation ranges from asymptomatic deposition in normal vessels, to a severe involvement of the wall of cerebral vessels leading to intracerebral hemorrhages (ICHs) or brain ischemia (Mandybur, 1986; Vonsattel et al., 1991). CAA are frequent but underdiagnosed causes of lobar ICH. They also contribute to the pathogenesis of leukoencephalopathies (Greenberg et al., 1993), but often remain undiagnosed in the absence of a neuropathological examination (Greenberg, 1998). Dementia is frequent in patients with CAA because of the association of brain infarcts and hemorrhages, leukoencephalopathies, and sometimes Alzheimer's pathology (Pasquier and Leys, 1997).

An overproduction or an abnormal degradation of circulating precursor proteins causes most CAA. A genetic abnormality leading to the production of variant precursor proteins is possible (Stone, 1990). A tissue or organ affinity often exists for each amyloid protein. Immunocytochemical studies are crucial to characterize the type of amyloid. The two types of cerebral amyloid deposition most frequently associated with CAA are amyloid-β (Aβ) and cystatin C.

Hereditary cases of CAA have a dominant autosomal transmission and have been reported in very few families. However, they play a crucial role in our knowledge of sporadic cases, and they may serve as a model for diagnostic and therapeutic purposes.

Classification of CAA

Aβ CAA

Aβ is responsible for the most frequent type of CAA (Glenner and Wong, 1984). The peptide deposited in the arterial wall was formerly called amyloid peptide, then A-4 or βA4, and finally Aβ. Aβ is the 40- to 43-amino-acid proteolysis product of a large precursor, the amyloid β-protein precursor (APP), with features of a cell surface receptor (Kang et al., 1987). APP has several isoforms generated by alternative splicing from a single gene located on chromosome 21. The prominent transcripts are APP695, APP751, and APP770. They differ in that APP751 and APP770 contain exon 7, which encodes a Kunitz serine protease inhibitor domain. APP695 is the prominent form in neuronal tissue, whereas APP751 is the prominent variant in other tissues. Protease nexin-II, a protease inhibitor synthesized and secreted by various cultured extravascular cells, is identical to APP751 (Van Nostrand et al., 1989). This angiopathy is limited to the cerebral vessels and has been reported in various clinical conditions. Aβ deposits are found in the walls of cerebral vessels of patients with sporadic CAA (the most frequent type of CAA), hereditary ICH with amyloidosis Dutch type (HCHWA-D) or other hereditary conditions, Alzheimer's disease (AD), and Down syndrome. Despite similarities between the vascular amyloid and the Aβ in the cerebral extracellular amyloid deposits (senile plaques) of AD, some features distinguish Aβ in CAA, especially the prominence of the Aβ species ending at amino acid position 39–40 (Alonzo et al., 1998; Suzuki et al., 1994) and the tendency of particular mutant forms of Aβ to accumulate preferentially in vessels (Hendriks et al., 1992). Cystatin C colocalizes with Aβ in the wall of cerebral vessels of patients with AD, HCHWA-D, and sporadic CAA, but not in senile plaques (Nagai et al., 1998).

Sporadic Aβ CAA

Epidemiology Most Aβ° CAA are sporadic, and are found at autopsy in normal elderly subjects, or in patients with AD or Down syndrome (Vinters, 1992). They have also been reported in dementia pugilistica, and postanoxic encephalopathies (Salama et al., 1986).

Depending on selection criteria of patients, and on staining methods, the prevalence of sporadic CAA largely varies between studies, but all studies suggest that CAA is common in the elderly. In population-based studies, the annual incidence rate of lobar

Uncommon Causes of Stroke, 2nd edition, ed. Louis R. Caplan. Published by Cambridge University Press. © Cambridge University Press 2008.

Table 61.1 Classification of CAA

Aβ CAA

Sporadic Aβ CAA

Hereditary Aβ CAA

Hereditary cerebral hemorrhages with amyloidosis (Dutch type; HCHWA-D)

Flemish type

Italian type

Iowa type

Other familial CAA with APP-gene mutations

Familial AD with CAA

Hereditary cystatin C CAA (Icelandic type; HCAAA-I)

Gelsolin-related amyloidosis (familial amyloidosis, Finnish type; AGel amyloidosis)

Transthyretin CAA (familial oculoleptomeningeal amyloidosis)

PrP CAA

Amyloid angiopathies of undetermined biochemical nature with mutation of the gene BRI

British type (so-called "Worster-Drought type")

Danish type

Amyloid angiopathies of undetermined biochemical nature without mutation of the gene BRI

APP = amyloid protein precursor; AD = Alzheimer's disease; AGel amyloidosis = Gelsolin amyloidosis; PRP = prion protein.

hemorrhages range from 30 to 40 per 100 000 persons older than 70 years (Broderick et al., 1993; Schutz et al., 1990). CAA accounts for approximately one-third of them (Broderick et al., 1993; Schutz et al., 1990). The question of the clinical impact of CAA and the risk of bleeding in patients under antithrombotic therapies remains unsettled. In a general hospital, 30% of autopsied patients older than 80 years had amyloid deposits in their cerebral vessels. The prevalence of Aβ CAA is higher in women (Wildi and Dago-Akribi, 1968), and increases with age: 2.3% between 65 and 74 years old (Greenberg and Hyman, 1997), 12.1% older than 85 years (Greenberg and Hyman, 1997), and up to 75% older than 90 years (Yamada et al., 1987). In AD patients, the prevalence of CAA at autopsy ranges from 25% to 100% (Glenner et al., 1981; Greenberg and Hyman, 1997; Vonsattel et al., 1991), 5.1% of AD patients having CAA-related ICH (Greenberg and Hyman, 1997). In Down syndrome, CAA is rare before 40 years of age.

In an autopsy sample of 211 Japanese-American men from the population-based Honolulu-Asia Aging Study, 44.1% had CAA in at least one neocortical area (Pfeifer et al., 2002). The presence of CAA was associated with higher mean neurofibrillary tangles and neuritic plaques counts and having at least one apolipoprotein E (APOE) ε4 allele (Pfeifer et al., 2002).

Neuropathology Aβ CAA involve small- and medium-sized arteries and veins of the cortex, leptomeninges, and (in severe cases) cortical capillaries. The deposits involve the external layers of the vessels. Progressively, the arterial walls appear eosinophilic and thickened, whereas muscle cells disappear. The lumen may be reduced or occluded. All cerebral vessels can be affected, but spinal cord vessels are spared. Surprisingly, the hippocampal vessels are rarely involved. Cystatin C is sometimes found to colocalize with Aβ, and immunoreactivity can be present in white matter vessels (Wang et al., 1997) and to indicate a higher risk of CAA-associated ICH (Izumihara et al., 2001).

Besides amyloid deposits, nonspecific changes are associated in two-thirds of patients (Vonsattel et al., 1991). They are similar to vascular changes seen in chronic arterial hypertension, including fibrinoid necrosis and microaneurysms. The severity of the amyloid deposition and the presence of fibrinoid necrosis are consistently related to ICH (Vonsattel et al., 1991). Another possibly associated vessel lesion is vasculitis (Masson et al., 1998). Their cause remains unsettled, but a chronic inflammatory process leading to amyloid deposition is plausible. Conversely, amyloid may also be the causative agent of vasculitis (Yamada et al., 1996). CAA may be associated with brain lesions such as senile plaques, dystrophic neurites, and neurofibrillary tangles, i.e. abnormalities of the phosphorylation of τ proteins (Buee et al., 1994). These vascular amyloid deposits may play a role in the constitution of senile plaques. Whether a continuum exists between CAA and AD remains unsettled.

Clinical features We know only the clinical presentation of patients who were autopsied or operated on for an ICH. If a biological marker of CAA becomes available in routine medical practice, the clinical spectrum of CAA will probably change.

1. Most sporadic CAA are silent and are just coincidental findings at autopsy
2. Recurrent ICH is the most frequent feature of CAA. Although no reliable statistics are available, CAA may account for 4–17% of all ICH and even more in very old patients. Because of the possible coexistence of arterial hypertension, ICH cannot always be attributed with certainty to CAA. ICHs associated with sporadic CAA do not occur before 55 years. They are lobar in location and more frequent in temporal and occipital lobes areas. Cerebellar and pontine hemorrhages are rare. The clinical presentation is not specific, but headache, seizures, and recurrences (Cosgrove et al., 1985) are frequent. In a few autopsied patients, the primary hemorrhage caused by CAA occurred in the subarachnoid space and then spread to the brain parenchyma (Takeda et al., 2003). CAA may play a major role in the pathogenesis of ICH even in patients with more obvious risk factors (Ritter et al., 2005)
3. Cerebral ischemia may be more frequent than ICH. It usually consists of multiple, nonhemorrhagic, small, cortical infarcts, that are sometimes silent or revealed by transient neurological deficits (Greenberg et al., 1993). However, transient episodes may also be because of epileptic seizures in patients with small hemorrhages.
4. Dementia is frequent in CAA. Three types of dementia may occur (Pasquier and Leys, 1997): (i) vascular dementia because of the coexistence of multiple infarcts and hemorrhages and leukoencephalopathy; (ii) AD; and (iii) dementia because of the coexistence of stroke, AD, and leukoencephalopathy. Cases of dementia of rapid onset and course have been reported, either

isolated (Probst and Ulrich, 1985) or in association with angiitis of the nervous system (Masson *et al.*, 1998; Probst and Ulrich, 1985; Scolding *et al.*, 2005). The presence of CAA significantly influences the neuropsychological status (Pfeifer *et al.*, 2002). CAA may, therefore, contribute to the clinical presentation of dementia by interacting with other neuronal pathologies, leading to more severe cognitive impairment in men with both CAA and AD compared with men with only AD or CAA (Pfeifer *et al.*, 2002)

5. Reversible acute leukoencephalopathies associated with CAA have been reported (Masson *et al.*, 1998; Oh *et al.*, 2004; Probst and Ulrich, 1985; Sarazin *et al.*, 2002; Scolding *et al.*, 2005): they are characterized by a rapid progression of neurologic symptoms followed by dramatic clinical and radiological improvement. Pathologically, CAA is associated with varying degrees of inflammation (Oh *et al.*, 2004). In the appropriate clinical context, the MRI findings of lobar white matter edema with evidence of prior hemosiderin deposition may indicate the presence of a reversible CAA leukoencephalopathy (Oh *et al.*, 2004)

Genetics While the ε4 allele of APOE has been identified as a risk factor for AD by promoting the aggregation and deposition of Aβ amyloid within the cerebral cortex (Strittmatter *et al.*, 1993), APOE ε2 might play a major role in facilitating the deposition of Aβ amyloid in cerebral blood vessels. This may lead to amyloid angiopathy and ICH (Greenberg and Hyman, 1997). A study conducted in 33 patients with sporadic Aβ CAA did not identify any mutation in the cystatin C gene (McCarron *et al.*, 2000). However, it has been shown that the cystatin C gene is associated with an increased risk of late-onset AD, and is the first gene with a recessive expression found as predisposing to AD (Finckh *et al.*, 2000). Several gene polymorphisms have been reported to be associated with sporadic CAA or CAA-related ICH, including APOE, presenilin 1 (PS1), and α1-antichymotrypsin (ACT). Yamada (2004) investigated whether gene polymorphisms of neprilysin (NEP), an Aβ-degrading enzyme, and the transforming growth factor β1 (TGF-β1), a multifunctional cytokine implicated in Aβ deposition, are associated with sporadic CAA: concerning a GT repeat polymorphism in the enhancer/promoter region of NEP, the shorter repeat alleles were associated with CAA severity; the T/C polymorphism at codon 10 in exon 1 of TGF-β1 was also associated with the severity of CAA (Hamaguchi *et al.*, 2005; Yamada, 2004), especially in non-AD patients and in APOE non-ε4 carriers (Hamaguchi *et al.*, 2005). These data suggest that multiple gene polymorphisms could be associated with the risk of sporadic CAA (Yamada, 2004).

Diagnosis

- Radiological findings have no specificity. The most useful radiological technique to approach a diagnosis of CAA is MRI with gradient-echo sequences that are sensitive to hemorrhages. The major arguments supporting the diagnosis of CAA are:
  - Lobar location of the ICH, sparing the basal ganglia, thalamus, and pons;
  - Presence of one or more previous ICH, as reported in three-quarters of CAA-related ICH (Greenberg, 1998). In addition, gradient-echo MRI may show the disease's progression with

new ICH (Hendriks *et al.*, 1992). In patients with probable CAA-related ICH, hemorrhagic lesions are located preferentially in the temporal and occipital lobes, and within individuals, ICH tend to cluster, regardless of lobe (Rosand *et al.*, 2005). Among subjects followed prospectively for recurrence, clustering of new symptomatic and asymptomatic hemorrhages was observed (Rosand *et al.*, 2005). These data suggest that regional differences within the brain play a role in the development of CAA-related ICH (Rosand *et al.*, 2005).

- Presence of leukoencephalopathies: they may be isolated, or associated with ICH or cerebral infarcts. Most leukoencephalopathies are not severe (Gray *et al.*, 1985). They have no specificity. They may occur in the absence of arterial hypertension. Hypoperfusion of the white matter supplied by long perforating arteries originating in leptomeningeal arteries involved by the CAA is the most likely mechanism (Gray *et al.*, 1985). In rare cases, leukoencephalopathies may have a clinical and a radiological presentation suggesting a tumor: such cases may require a brain biopsy and may improve under corticosteroid therapy (Greenberg *et al.*, 1993). Recent studies suggest a role for circulating Aβ peptides in leukoencephalopathies (van Dijk *et al.*, 2004): although soluble Aβ is present in blood and cerebrospinal fluid (CSF) of normal subjects, its toxicity on the blood vessels wall has been found in vitro (Thomas *et al.*, 1996). Gurol *et al.* (2006) performed a cross-sectional study of clinical, biochemical, and genetic factors associated with leukoencephalopathy in patients with either AD or mild cognitive impairment (AD/MCI) and in an independent group of patients with CAA. Biochemical measurements included plasma concentrations of the 40- and 42-amino-acid species of Aβ (Aβ40 and Aβ42). Plasma Aβ40 concentrations were associated with leukoencephalopathies in both groups after adjustment for age, hypertension, diabetes, homocysteine, creatinine, folate, vitamin B12, and APOE genotype (Gurol *et al.*, 2006). The presence of lacunar infarctions was also associated with increased Aβ40, but not Aβ42, in both groups (Gurol *et al.*, 2006). If these data are confirmed by longitudinal cohort studies, this would mean that circulating Aβ40 peptide is either a biomarker or a risk factor for microvascular damage in AD/MCI patients and in CAA patients. How Aβ40 relates to leukoencephalopathy is not clear. The main hypotheses are that: (i) serum Aβ40 levels reflect the severity of CAA, and therefore of leukoencephalopathy; and (ii) Aβ40 has a direct effect on the vasoreactivity of deep perforating arteries (Lee and Markus, 2006). Other studies are needed to determine whether Aβ40 is the cause of leukoencephalopathy.

- Presence of microbleeds described as small, rounded areas of marked and homogeneous signal loss on gradient-echo sequences (Koennecke, 2006). Their size is usually defined as smaller than 5 or 10 mm (according to criteria used), and they can be found throughout the brain. Whereas the prevalence in healthy populations is around 5% (Horita *et al.*, 2003; Jeerakathil *et al.*, 2004; Roob *et al.*, 1999; Tsushima *et al.*, 2002), it is 69% in the HCHWA-D type (Van Den Boom *et al.*, 2005). It has also been studied in patients older than 55 years with

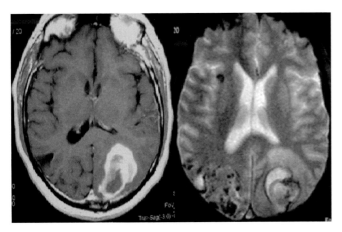

Figure 61.1 Patient with recurrent cortical ICH (*left*) and multiple microbleeds (*right*) in a case of sporadic Aβ amyloid angiopathy.

primary lobar ICH (Greenberg *et al.*, 1996, 1999, 2004; Walker *et al.*, 2004). In a group of 15 patients older than 60 years who had a lobar ICH, 12 (80%) had microbleeds, and 9 of these 12 microbleeds (60%) were restricted to the cortico-subcortical region, suggestive of probable CAA (Greenberg *et al.*, 1996). To date, microbleeds are not validated as diagnostic criteria for CAA. The Boston criteria (Knudsen *et al.*, 2001) for probable CAA do not mention microbleeds. Although some data suggest that, in CAA, microbleeds are more likely to be cortical, there is not enough evidence to conclude that patients with cortical microbleeds are likely to have CAA. Walker *et al.* (2004) studied 97 patients older than 70 years who underwent MRI for various clinical reasons. Fifteen patients presented with microbleeds, defined as small lesions of 2–5 mm restricted to lobar-cortical distributions. Among those 15 patients, only two patients (one of whom had biopsy proven CAA) had a history of suspected CAA, even though four did have dementia. Greenberg *et al.* (2004) tried to determine whether hemorrhages detected at the time of lobar ICH predict the major clinical complications of CAA: recurrent ICH or decline in cognition and function. New microbleeds appeared in 17 of 34 patients older than 55 years followed-up after a primary lobar ICH, and predicted increased risk of subsequent symptomatic ICH (3-year cumulative risks 19%, 42%, and 67% for subjects with 0, 1–3, or ≥4 new microbleeds; $p =.02$) but not subsequent clinical decline. Microbleeds may reflect the same underlying pathological process as symptomatic ICH. Therefore, if confirmed, the presence of microbleeds could be used as a surrogate marker to study the impact of treatment on the progression of the disease. An example of microbleeds is provided in Figure 61.1.
- CSF abnormalities are not specific. A decreased level in the CSF of protease nexin-II (the secreted form of APP751), APOE, and cystatin C have been reported in some patients (Vinters *et al.*, 1994). The contribution of CSF abnormalities to the diagnosis of CAA in patients with ICH has not been determined and CSF abnormalities cannot be regarded as useful diagnostic tools.
- Genetic mutations reported in familial cases of CAA are not present in patients with sporadic CAA. Therefore, genetics is

not useful for diagnostic purposes in the absence of a familial history.
- Neuropathological examination in patients operated on for ICH is the only way to make a diagnosis of CAA (Masson *et al.*, 1998; Probst and Ulrich, 1985), but it cannot be considered as a routine procedure. The frequency of ICH because of brain biopsy in patients with sporadic CAA reduces the number of indications to a very small number of patients. A biopsy is, however, useful in pseudotumoral leukoencephalopathies and in patients in whom an associated angiitis is suggested by the clinical and laboratory findings (Masson *et al.*, 1998).

Hereditary Aβ CAA HCHWA-D HCHWA-D is an autosomal dominant disease characterized by recurrent ICH occurring during the 4th and 5th decades (Haan *et al.*, 1989; Luyendijk *et al.*, 1988; Wattendorff *et al.*, 1982).

Epidemiology This rare disorder has been reported in four unrelated Dutch families originating from Schewingen (Wattendorff *et al.*, 1982) and Katwijk (Luyendijk *et al.*, 1988), two cities located in the western part of The Netherlands, close to Rotterdam. Another family has been identified in Western Australia, with similar neuropathological and genetic findings (Panegyres *et al.*, 2005).

Neuropathology Neuropathological findings are similar to those of sporadic AD, with the following differences (Durlinger *et al.*, 1993; Haan *et al.*, 1990; Haan and Roos, 1990; Luyendijk *et al.*, 1988; Maat-Schieman *et al.*, 1992; Timmers *et al.*, 1990; Wattendorff *et al.*, 1982): (i) AD lesions are frequent, with senile plaques but only few neurofibrillary tangles; (ii) white matter abnormalities occur early in the time course of the disease; (iii) ICHs occur more often in posterior areas; and (iv) a severe reduction of the lumen of small arteries due to severe hyalinosis and sclerosis of the arterial walls is frequent. Dementia appears to be associated with CAA and to be independent of the presence of plaques and tangles (Natte *et al.*, 2001). Protease nexin-II (the APP751 isoform) may have a local anticoagulant effect that may contribute to the pathogenesis of spontaneous ICH in HCHWA-D patients (Schmaier *et al.*, 1993), and it accumulates in cerebral blood vessels (Schmaier *et al.*, 1993).

Clinical features HCHWA-D is characterized by recurrent ICH occurring between 40 and 60 years of age (Haan *et al.*, 1989; Luyendijk *et al.*, 1988; Wattendorff *et al.*, 1982). Patients who survive several ICH usually develop a stepwise dementia (Haan *et al.*, 1990). Progressive dementia without stroke, suggestive of AD, is also possible (Haan *et al.*, 1992; Wattendorff *et al.*, 1982). Migraine, transient neurological deficits, and epileptic seizures are also frequent. The diagnosis may be difficult in the absence of a clear family history.

Genetics The underlying genetic defect is a point mutation in the APP gene located on chromosome 21, leading to an abnormal APP (Van Broeckhoven *et al.*, 1990). The gene mutation leads to an amino acid modification at codon 693 (glutamic acid to glutamine change) (Bakker *et al.*, 1991; Levy *et al.*, 1990). The APOE ε4 and ε2 alleles (Haan *et al.*, 1995) do not influence the clinical expression of the codon 693 mutation (Hendriks *et al.*, 1992). The penetrance of the gene is almost complete (Luyendijk *et al.*, 1988). Other types of mutations, which differ between families, have been identified in the same gene in other disorders leading to dementia, ICH, or familial cases of AD. However, most familial AD cases are associated with mutations located in the APP gene (located on chromosome 21) on chromosomes 1 and 14 in the PS1 gene (where more than 70 mutations have been identified), or on the PS2 gene (where 4 mutations are known) (Tandon *et al.*, 2000). The clinical characteristics of familial AD associated with PS1 or PS2 gene mutations are not influenced by the presence of CAA (Nochlin *et al.*, 1998; Yasuda *et al.*, 1997).

Diagnosis Direct evidence of the gene mutation by molecular methods is possible (Bakker *et al.*, 1991).

Flemish type The disease has been described in a single family from The Netherlands, but as the mutation was identified in the Belgian city of Antwerp, it was called "Flemish type." Amyloid consists of Aβ, and the disease is the consequence of a mutation in the APP gene at codon 692 (Hendriks *et al.*, 1992). This particular family – formerly called "Family 1302" – with hereditary CAA, was followed-up for 4 generations (Hendriks *et al.*, 1992). Most patients had early-onset AD, but several patients also had ICH at around 40 years of age. The cerebral Aβ CAA was identified in a patient who underwent surgery for an ICH. This patient also had diffuse Aβ deposits with only a few senile plaques, and no neurofibrillary tangles (Hendriks *et al.*, 1992). The clinical expression differs considerably from that of HCHWA-D. The reason why the prominent lesions involve the brain vessels in HCHWA-D and the brain tissue in Family 1302 remains unknown. However, De Jonghe *et al.* (1998) provided evidence that APP692 and APP693 have a different effect on Aβ secretion as determined by complementary DNA (cDNA) transfection experiments. While APP692 upregulates both Aβ-40 and Aβ-42 secretion, APP693 does not. These data corroborate the previous findings that increased Aβ secretion, and particularly increased secretion of Aβ-42, is specific for AD pathology and extracellular amyloid deposits. Thus, these data further support that the Flemish type of CAA is closer to familial AD than is HCHWA-D.

Italian type Patients have lobar ICH and dementia. HCHWA-It has been reported in two Italian families, as abstracts. Amyloid consists of Aβ, and, as seen in HCHWA-D, the disease is caused by an APP-gene mutation at codon 693, but of a different type.

Iowa type The most prominent feature is the absence of ICH. The clinical presentation consists of a progressive aphasia during the sixth and seventh decades, followed by dementia, and on imaging, occipital calcifications, infarcts, and white matter changes. The mutation is located at APP position 694 (Grabowski *et al.*, 2001).

Other familial CAA with APP-gene mutation A new mutation (L705 V) in the APP gene has been identified in a family with autosomal dominant recurrent ICH and neither plaques nor tangles (Obici *et al.*, 2005).

Familial cases of AD with CAA Most autosomal dominant AD families have a mutation in the PS1 gene on chromosome 14, where more than 100 mutations have been reported (Larner and Doran, 2006). A few families have a PS2 mutation on chromosome 1 (Tandon *et al.*, 2000). A duplication of the APP locus on chromosome 21 has also been identified in five families with early onset AD and CAA (Rovelet-Lecrux *et al.*, 2006). These mutations lead to progressive dementia associated with parenchymal Aβ amyloid deposits. The clinical features of patients from these CAA-families" are not distinguishable from those of PS1 or PS2 families without CAA. Cases reported in Volga German families are associated with PS2 mutation (Nochlin *et al.*, 1998). A Finnish family with dementia in four generations and with frequent co-occurrence of dementia and ICH was identified (Remes *et al.*, 2004). Neuropathologic examination revealed AD changes. In addition to cognitive decline, five patients had had lobar ICH and one was diagnosed with cerebral microbleeds. No causative mutations were identified in candidate genes associated with amyloid diseases, but linkage to APP region could not be entirely excluded. The AD in this Finnish family shares similarities with the Italian, Flemish, and Iowa types of AD, but no amyloidogenic mutations were identified.

Hereditary cystatin C CAA (Icelandic type)

Hereditary cystatin C amyloid angiopathy (HCAAA-I), previously called "hereditary ICH with amyloidosis, Icelandic type," is a rare autosomal dominant disorder. It has been reported in only eight Icelandic families (Jensson *et al.*, 1987), and is caused by a point mutation (leucine [L] to glutamine [Q]) change at codon 68 on the cystatin gene located on chromosome 20, consisting of a L68Q substitution (Palsdottir *et al.*, 1988). Cystatin C is a potent inhibitor of various cysteine proteases.

Abrahamson and Grubb (1994) produced normal cystatin C and L68Q cystatin C in an *Escherichia coli* expression system. Normal cystatin C and L68Q cystatin C differ considerably in their tendency to dimerize and form aggregates. Whereas wild-type cystatin C was monomeric and functionally active even after prolonged storage at elevated temperatures, L68Q cystatin C started to dimerize and lose biologic activity immediately after transfer to a nondenaturing buffer. The aggregation at physiologic concentrations was increased by 60% at 40°C compared to 37°C (Abrahamson and Grubb, 1994).

The first clinical symptoms occur between 20 and 30 years of age, and consist of ICH that may involve the corticomedullary junction and the basal ganglia (Blondal *et al.*, 1989). Infarcts are rare. Vascular dementia is possible in survivors (Blondal *et al.*, 1989; Jensson *et al.*, 1987). Patients may remain stable for several years (Jensson *et al.*, 1987). In the family reported by Gudmundsson *et al.* (1972), the mean age at death was 44 years in the first two generations, decreasing to 29.6 and 22.5 years in the third and fourth generations. Death usually occurs before the age of 50.

An example of sporadic CAA with ICH was reported in an elderly Croatian man who had a mutation in cystatin C similar to that of HCAAA-I (Graffagnino *et al.*, 1995).

Autopsy findings consist of multiple and extensive ICH of different ages and extensive amyloid depositions in the arterial walls of the cerebral and leptomeningeal vessels. The involvement of the most distal microcirculation (including capillaries) is usual. Areas of demyelination can also be observed (Blondal *et al.*, 1989; Gudmundsson *et al.*, 1972), but there are no AD changes (Gudmundsson *et al.*, 1972). Cystatin C deposits may also be found in lymph nodes, spleen, salivary glands, seminal vesicles, testes, and skin (Benedikz *et al.*, 1990; Lofberg *et al.*, 1987), but they remain silent.

Reduction to one-third of the normal level of cystatin C in CSF can be used as a diagnostic test (Jensson *et al.*, 1987). A specific diagnosis by polymerase chain reaction-based analysis is also available (Abrahamson *et al.*, 1992).

AGel amyloidosis (familial amyloidosis, Finnish type)

This is an autosomal dominant type of systemic amyloidosis where two mutations of the gelsolin gene have been described on chromosome 9 at codon 654 (aspartic acid 187 to asparagine change or aspartic acid 187 to tyrosine change) (de la Chapelle *et al.*, 1992; Kiuru *et al.*, 1994; Levy *et al.*, 1990). As demonstrated by cDNA transfection, both mutant forms of gelsolin are abnormally processed and secreted as an aberrant 68 kd gelsolin fragment in cell culture. This fragment contains the suggested amyloid-forming sequence (Paunio *et al.*, 1998). AGel is deposited in both the gray and white matter vessels of the brain and spinal cord. Clinical symptoms, such as dementia or mood disorders, and white matter lesions on MRI may be related to the gelsolin-related CAA (Kiuru *et al.*, 1994).

Transthyretin CAA (familial oculoleptomeningeal amyloidosis)

Familial oculoleptomeningeal amyloidosis (transthyretin CAA) is an autosomal dominant disorder with hemiplegic migraine, dementia, seizures, strokes, and visual deterioration (Goren *et al.*, 1980; Uitti *et al.*, 1988). Amyloid deposition can be found in leptomeningeal and retinal vessels. The cerebral vessels are usually spared, but superficial ICH can occur when vessels of the superficial neocortex are involved. Transthyretin CAA may also be seen in type I familial amyloid neuropathy, but usually remains asymptomatic. Two French patients were reported (Ellie *et al.*, 2001) with recurrent subarachnoid hemorrhages associated with amyloid deposits in the leptomeningeal vessels and a new mutation (Gly53Glu) in codon 53.

Prion protein CAA

Hereditary disorders because of prion protein (PrP) gene mutations in chromosome 20 are: familial Creutzfeldt-Jakob disease, Gerstmann-Straussler-Scheinker disease, and fatal familial insomnia. In a family with progressive dementia close to AD and a PrP gene mutation at codon 145, a severe amyloid angiopathy because of PrP has been reported (Ghetti *et al.*, 1996).

Amyloid angiopathies of undetermined biochemical nature with mutation of the gene BRI

British type (so-called "Worster-Drought type")

The Worster-Drought type CAA (Griffiths *et al.*, 1982; Plant *et al.*, 1990; Worster-Drought *et al.*, 1940), also called Familial British Dementia (FBD) is a rare autosomal dominant disorder characterized by progressive dementia, spasticity, and ataxia, with diffuse white matter changes (Plant *et al.*, 1990). The clinical onset occurs in the fifth decade, and death usually occurs less than 10 years after onset. Clinically obvious strokes are not frequent. Three families, two of them sharing a common ancestor, have been identified. At autopsy, patients have multiple ICH and lacunes, amyloid angiopathy, and senile plaques in the hippocampus and cerebellum. The biochemical nature of the amyloid deposits is unknown, but a genetic mutation has been identified in the BRI gene located on chromosome 13 (Kim *et al.*, 2000; Mead *et al.*, 2000). The mutant BRI codes for an abnormal protein dubbed ABri, a major component of plaques in FBD. The structure of ABri suggested that it was cleaved by the prohormone convertase furin (Kim *et al.*, 1999). Furin constitutively processes both ABRi and the normal protein product of BRI, with subsequent secretion of carboxyl terminal peptides that encompass all or part of ABRi. More significantly, furin generates more peptide product in the presence of the mutant BRI protein coded by chromosome 13, and the peptides thus produced assemble into irregular, short fibrils. Although the role of BRI peptides in the genesis of FBD is not known, it seems likely that the elucidation of this process can shed light on the role of abnormal protein aggregation in other neurodegenerative diseases such as AD. The disease is caused by a stop-codon mutation in the BRI gene on chromosome 13.

Danish type

Familial Danish dementia is also known as heredopathia ophthalmo-oto-encephalica, and is characterized by cataracts, deafness, progressive ataxia, and dementia. The disease causing mutation is a decamer duplication in the BRI gene on chromosome 13 (Vidal *et al.*, 2000).

Amyloid angiopathies of undetermined biochemical nature without mutation of the gene BRI

Other familial disorders with amyloid deposits of unknown origin have been identified (Haan and Roos, 1990).

The future

Improvement in diagnostic tools

The diagnosis of definite CAA requires neuropathological examination of autopsic or surgical material. However, there are clinical circumstances in which the diagnosis should be suspected (Table 61.2). In the Dutch type, there is an important heterogeneity in the age at onset and clinical presentation between and within families. Diagnostic criteria have therefore been established for CAA (Table 61.3).

Table 61.2 Possible clinical presentation of patients with CAA

Recurrent lobar ICH

Multiple lobar ICH

Lobar ICH with leukoencephalopathy

Unexplained leukoencephalopathy

Dementia + lobar ICH (with or without leukoencephalopathy)

Lobar ICH during anticoagulation or thrombolytic therapy

Any neurological symptom in a patient from a family with hereditary CAA

Association of ataxia, spasticity, and progressive dementia in at least two persons from the same family

Source: Haan *et al.*, 2001.

Table 61.3 Diagnostic criteria of CAA

1. Definite CAA

Full postmortem examination demonstrating:

  Lobar, cortical, or cortico-subcortical hemorrhage

  Severe CAA with vasculopathy (Vonsattel *et al.*, 1991)

  Absence of other diagnostic lesion

2. Probable CAA with supporting pathology

Clinical data and pathologic tissue (evacuated hematoma or cortical biopsy) demonstrating:

  Lobar, cortical, or cortico-subcortical hemorrhage

  Some degree of CAA in specimen

  Absence of other diagnostic lesion

3. Probable CAA

Clinical data and MRI or CT demonstrating:

  Multiple hemorrhages restricted to lobar, cortical, or

  cortico-subcortical regions (cerebellar hemorrhage allowed)

  Age $\geq$ 55 years

  Absence of other cause of hemorrhage*

4. Possible CAA

Clinical data and MRI or CT demonstrating:

  Single lobar, cortical, or cortico-subcortical hemorrhage

  Age $\geq$ 55 years

  Absence of other cause of hemorrhage*

*Other causes of ICH: excessive warfarin (international normalized ratio [INR] > 3.0); antecedent of head trauma or ischemic stroke; central nervous system tumor; vascular malformation, or vasculitis; and blood dyscrasia or coagulopathy. (INR > 3.0 or other nonspecific laboratory abnormalities permitted for diagnosis of possible CAA).
Source: Knudsen *et al.*, 2001 with permission.

Genetic counseling in hereditary CAA should aim at giving adequate information specific for the type of CAA. DNA diagnosis, possibly even prenatal, should be offered, accompanied by psychological support to cope with the DNA test result. In the Dutch type, there are important ethical issues for the prenatal test as the natural history of the disease is not completely known, and many patients may have a normal life for 40 or more years.

CAA can only be diagnosed with certainty by means of histological investigation. Therefore, attempts should be made to improve the diagnostic possibilities in vivo, for example, by means of new MRI techniques or radioactive labeled compounds.

Biochemical analysis of the amyloid vessels, genetic studies of so-called "sporadic cases," and determination of risk factors for amyloid deposition are the main research activities that will help to achieve this goal.

Treatment of ICH

There is no reason to treat CAA-related ICH differently than other varieties of ICH. However, when a patient is expected to have CAA, surgery should be avoided if at all possible because of a high risk of rebleeding and a good spontaneous recovery.

Prevention of ICH

CAA is the only major type of stroke without any effective prevention. Aspirin and anticoagulants should be avoided as much as possible in these patients. Early treatment of febrile periods might reduce amyloid formation as suggested in HCAAA-I where it might slow down the in vivo formation of L68Q cystatin C aggregates (Abrahamson and Grubb, 1994). In transthyretin amyloidosis, liver transplantation appears to reduce the amount of amyloid deposition, but it is very unlikely to be an option for CAA as well. More success is to be expected from therapies such as amyloid breaker peptides or antibodies against amyloid. A better knowledge of the mechanisms leading to amyloid deposition is now necessary to determine how to block the pathological cascade of events. Potential approaches to prevent CAA progression include: inhibitors of Aβ cleavage from APP, potentiators of Aβ clearance, antagonists of vasoactive cytokines, and inhibitors of Aβ binding to APOE or the vascular extracellular matrix. The breakdown of amyloid-laden vessel walls might be prevented by inhibitors of Aβ toxicity, antioxidants, or anti-inflammatory agents (Greenberg, 1998). Appearance of small, clinically silent hemorrhagic lesions on gradient-echo MRI may be an efficient surrogate end point for pilot trials of promising therapeutic approaches to CAA (Greenberg and Rosand, 2001). The question of whether patients with CAA should be excluded from thrombolytic strategies (McCarron and Nicoll, 2004) for cerebral or myocardial ischemia is not answered, and the question has arisen as to how these patients can be identified in an emergency. Lowering blood pressure, irrespective of its level, is recommended, although there is no evidence that that reduces the risk of ICH in CAA patients.

Better knowledge of the mechanisms leading to amyloid deposition is now necessary to determine how to block the pathological cascade of events. Biochemical analysis of the amyloid vessels, genetic studies of so-called "sporadic cases," and determination of risk factors for amyloid deposition are the main research activities that will help to achieve this goal.

REFERENCES

Abrahamson, M., and Grubb, A. 1994. Increased body temperature accelerates aggregation of the Leu-68–>Gln mutant cystatin C, the amyloid-forming protein in hereditary cystatin C amyloid angiopathy. *Proc Natl Acad Sci U S A*, **91**, 1416–20.

Abrahamson, M., Jonsdottir, S., Olafsson, I., Jensson, O., and Grubb, A. 1992. Hereditary cystatin C amyloid angiopathy: identification of the disease-causing mutation and specific diagnosis by polymerase chain reaction based analysis. *Hum Genet*, **89**, 377–80.

Alonzo, N. C., Hyman, B. T., Rebeck, G. W., and Greenberg, S. M. 1998. Progression of cerebral amyloid angiopathy: accumulation of amyloid-beta40 in affected vessels. *J Neuropathol Exp Neurol*, **57**, 353–9.

Bakker, E., van Broeckhoven, C., Haan, J., *et al.* 1991. DNA diagnosis for hereditary cerebral hemorrhage with amyloidosis (Dutch type). *Am J Hum Genet*, **49**, 518–21.

Benedikz, E., Blondal, H., and Gudmundsson, G. 1990. Skin deposits in hereditary cystatin C amyloidosis. *Virchows Arch A Pathol Anat Histopathol*, **417**, 325–31.

Blondal, H., Guomundsson, G., Benedikz, E., and Johannesson, G. 1989. Dementia in hereditary cystatin C amyloidosis. *Prog Clin Biol Res*, **317**, 157–64.

Broderick, J., Brott, T., Tomsick, T., and Leach, A. 1993. Lobar hemorrhage in the elderly. The undiminishing importance of hypertension. *Stroke*, **24**, 49–51.

Buee, L., Hof, P. R., Bouras, C., *et al.* 1994. Pathological alterations of the cerebral microvasculature in Alzheimer's disease and related dementing disorders. *Acta Neuropathol (Berl)*, **87**, 469–80.

Castano, E. M., and Frangione, B. 1988. Human amyloidosis, Alzheimer disease and related disorders. *Lab Invest*, **58**, 122–32.

Cosgrove, G. R., Leblanc, R., Meagher-Villemure, K., and Ethier, R. 1985. Cerebral amyloid angiopathy. *Neurology*, **35**, 625–31.

De Jonghe, C., Zehr, C., Yager, D., *et al.* 1998. Flemish and Dutch mutations in amyloid beta precursor protein have different effects on amyloid beta secretion. *Neurobiol Dis*, **5**, 281–6.

de la Chapelle, A., Kere, J., Sack, G. H. Jr., Tolvanen, R., and Maury, C. P. 1992. Familial amyloidosis, Finnish type: G654—a mutation of the gelsolin gene in Finnish families and an unrelated American family. *Genomics*, **13**, 898–901.

Durlinger, E. T., Haan, J., and Roos, R. A. 1993. Hereditary cerebral hemorrhage with amyloidosis-Dutch type. *Neurology*, **43**, 1626–7.

Ellie, E., Camou, F., Vital, A., *et al.* 2001 Recurrent subarachnoid hemorrhage associated with a new transthyretin variant (Gly53Glu). *Neurology*, **57**, 135–7.

Finckh, U., von der Kammer, H., Velden, J., *et al.* 2000. Genetic association of a cystatin C gene polymorphism with late-onset Alzheimer disease. *Arch Neurol*, **57**, 1579–83.

Ghetti, B., Piccardo, P., Frangione, B., *et al.* 1996. Prion protein amyloidosis. *Brain Pathol*, **6**, 127–45.

Glenner, G. G. 1980a. Amyloid deposits and amyloidosis. The beta-fibrilloses (first of two parts). *N Engl J Med*, **302**, 1283–92.

Glenner, G. G. 1980b. Amyloid deposits and amyloidosis: the beta-fibrilloses (second of two parts). *N Engl J Med*, **302**, 1333–43.

Glenner, G. G., Henry, J. H., and Fujihara, S. 1981. Congophilic angiopathy in the pathogenesis of Alzheimer's degeneration. *Ann Pathol*, **1**, 120–9.

Glenner, G. G., and Wong, C. W. 1984. Alzheimer's disease: initial report of the purification and characterization of a novel cerebrovascular amyloid protein. *Biochem Biophys Res Commun*, **120**, 885–90.

Goren, H., Steinberg, M. C., and Farboody, G. H. 1980. Familial oculoleptomeningeal amyloidosis. *Brain*, **103**, 473–95.

Grabowski, T. J., Cho, H. S., Vonsattel, J. P., Rebeck, G. W., and Greenberg, S. M. 2001. Novel amyloid precursor protein mutation in an Iowa family with dementia and severe cerebral amyloid angiopathy. *Ann Neurol*, **49**, 697–705.

Graffagnino, C., Herbstreith, M. H., Schmechel, D. E., *et al.* 1995. Cystatin C mutation in an elderly man with sporadic amyloid angiopathy and intracerebral hemorrhage. *Stroke*, **26**, 2190–3.

Gray, F., Dubas, F., Roullet, E., and Escourolle, R. 1985. Leukoencephalopathy in diffuse hemorrhagic cerebral amyloid angiopathy. *Ann Neurol*, **18**, 54–9.

Greenberg, S. M. 1998. Cerebral amyloid angiopathy: prospects for clinical diagnosis and treatment. *Neurology*, **51**, 690–4.

Greenberg, S. M., Eng, J. A., Ning, M., Smith, E. E., and Rosand, J. 2004. Hemorrhage burden predicts recurrent intracerebral hemorrhage after lobar hemorrhage. *Stroke*, **35**, 1415–20.

Greenberg, S. M., Finklestein, S. P., and Schaefer, P. W. 1996. Petechial hemorrhages accompanying lobar hemorrhage: detection by gradient-echo MRI. *Neurology*, **46**, 1751–4.

Greenberg, S. M., and Hyman, B. T. 1997. Cerebral amyloid angiopathy and apolipoprotein E: bad news for the good allele? *Ann Neurol*, **41**, 701–2.

Greenberg, S. M., O'Donnell, H. C., Schaefer, P. W., and Kraft, E. 1999. MRI detection of new hemorrhages: potential marker of progression in cerebral amyloid angiopathy. *Neurology*, **53**, 1135–8.

Greenberg, S. M., and Rosand, J. 2001. Outcome markers for clinical trials in cerebral amyloid angiopathy. *Amyloid*, **8 Suppl 1**, 56–60.

Greenberg, S. M., Vonsattel, J. P., Stakes, J. W., Gruber, M., and Finklestein, S. P. 1993. The clinical spectrum of cerebral amyloid angiopathy: presentations without lobar hemorrhage. *Neurology*, **43**, 2073–9.

Griffiths, R. A., Mortimer, T. F., Oppenheimer, D. R., and Spalding, J. M. 1982. Congophilic angiopathy of the brain: a clinical and pathological report on two siblings. *J Neurol Neurosurg Psychiatry*, **45**, 396–408.

Gudmundsson, G., Hallgrimsson, J., Jonasson, T. A., and Bjarnason, O. 1972. Hereditary cerebral haemorrhage with amyloidosis. *Brain*, **95**, 387–404.

Gurol, M. E., Irizarry, M. C., Smith, E. E., *et al.* 2006. Plasma beta-amyloid and white matter lesions in AD, MCI, and cerebral amyloid angiopathy. *Neurology*, **66**, 23–9.

Haan, J., Algra, P. R., and Roos, R. A. 1990. Hereditary cerebral hemorrhage with amyloidosis-Dutch type. Clinical and computed tomographic analysis of 24 cases. *Arch Neurol*, **47**, 649–53.

Haan, J., Bakker, E., Bornebroek, M., and Roos, R. A. 2001. Van gen naar ziekte; het gen voor amyloid-beta-precursorproteine betrokken bij erfelijke cerebrale amyloidangiopathie. *Ned Tijdschr Geneeskd*, **145**, 1639–41.

Haan, J., Bakker, E., Jennekens-Schinkel, A., and Roos, R. A. 1992. Progressive dementia, without cerebral hemorrhage, in a patient with hereditary cerebral amyloid angiopathy. *Clin Neurol Neurosurg*, **94**, 317–8.

Haan, J., and Roos, R. A. 1990. Amyloid in central nervous system disease. *Clin Neurol Neurosurg*, **92**, 305–10.

Haan, J., Roos, R. A., and Bakker, E. 1995. No protective effect of apolipoprotein E epsilon 2 allele in Dutch hereditary cerebral amyloid angiopathy. *Ann Neurol*, **37**, 282.

Haan, J., Roos, R. A., Briet, P. E., *et al.* 1989. Hereditary cerebral hemorrhage with amyloidosis–Dutch type. Research-Group Hereditary Cerebral Amyloid-Angiopathy. *Clin Neurol Neurosurg*, **91**, 285–90.

Hamaguchi, T., Okino, S., Sodeyama, N., *et al.* 2005. Association of a polymorphism of the transforming growth factor-beta1 gene with cerebral amyloid angiopathy. *J Neurol Neurosurg Psychiatry*, **76**, 696–9.

Hendriks, L., van Duijn, C. M., Cras, P., *et al.* 1992. Presenile dementia and cerebral haemorrhage linked to a mutation at codon 692 of the beta-amyloid precursor protein gene. *Nat Genet*, **1**, 218–21.

Horita, Y., Imaizumi, T., Niwa, J., *et al.* 2003. [Analysis of dot-like hemosiderin spots using brain dock system]. *No Shinkei Geka – Neurol Surg*, **31**, 263–7.

Izumihara, A., Ishihara, T., Hoshii, Y., and Ito, H. 2001. Cerebral amyloid angiopathy associated with hemorrhage: immunohistochemical study of 41 biopsy cases. *Neurol Med Chir (Tokyo)*, **41**, 471–7; discussion 477–8.

Jeerakathil, T., Wolf, P. A., Beiser, A., *et al.* 2004. Cerebral microbleeds: prevalence and associations with cardiovascular risk factors in the Framingham Study. *Stroke*, **35**, 1831–5.

Jensson, O., Gudmundsson, G., Arnason, A., *et al.* 1987. Hereditary cystatin C (gamma-trace) amyloid angiopathy of the CNS causing cerebral hemorrhage. *Acta Neurol Scand*, **76**, 102–14.

Kang, J., Lemaire, H. G., Unterbeck, A., *et al.* 1987. The precursor of Alzheimer's disease amyloid A4 protein resembles a cell-surface receptor. *Nature*, **325**, 733–6.

Kim, S. H., Wang, R., Gordon, D. J., *et al.* 1999. Furin mediates enhanced production of fibrillogenic ABri peptides in familial British dementia. *Nat Neurosci*, **2**, 984–8.

Kim, Y., Wall, J. S., Meyer, J., et al. 2000. Thermodynamic modulation of light chain amyloid fibril formation. *J Biol Chem*, **275**, 1570–4.

Kiuru, S., Matikainen, E., Kupari, M., Haltia, M., and Palo, J. 1994. Autonomic nervous system and cardiac involvement in familial amyloidosis, Finnish type (FAF). *J Neurol Sci*, **126**, 40–8.

Knudsen, K. A., Rosand, J., Karluk, D., and Greenberg, S. M. 2001. Clinical diagnosis of cerebral amyloid angiopathy: validation of the Boston criteria. *Neurology*, **56**, 537–9.

Koennecke, H. C. 2006. Cerebral microbleeds on MRI: prevalence, associations, and potential clinical implications. *Neurology*, **66**, 165–71.

Larner, A. J., and Doran, M. 2006. Clinical phenotypic heterogeneity of Alzheimer's disease associated with mutations of the presenilin-1 gene. *J Neurol*, **253**, 139–58.

Lee, J. M., and Markus, H. S. 2006. Does the white matter matter in Alzheimer disease and cerebral amyloid angiopathy? *Neurology*, **66**, 6–7.

Levy, E., Carman, M. D., Fernandez-Madrid, I. J., et al. 1990. Mutation of the Alzheimer's disease amyloid gene in hereditary cerebral hemorrhage, Dutch type. *Science*, **248**, 1124–6.

Lofberg, H., Thysell, H., Westman, K., et al. 1987. Demonstration and classification of amyloidosis in needle biopsies of the kidneys, with special reference to amyloidosis of the AA-type. *Acta Pathol Microbiol Immunol Scand [A]*, **95**, 357–63.

Luyendijk, W., Bots, G. T., Vegter-van der Vlis, M., Went, L. N., and Frangione, B. 1988. Hereditary cerebral haemorrhage caused by cortical amyloid angiopathy. *J Neurol Sci*, **85**, 267–80.

Maat-Schieman, M. L., van Duinen, S. G., Haan, J., and Roos, R. A. 1992. Morphology of cerebral plaque-like lesions in hereditary cerebral hemorrhage with amyloidosis (Dutch). *Acta Neuropathol (Berl)*, **84**, 674–9.

Mandybur, T. I. 1986. Cerebral amyloid angiopathy: the vascular pathology and complications. *J Neuropathol Exp Neurol*, **45**, 79–90.

Masson, C., Henin, D., Colombani, J. M., and Dehen, H. 1998. [A case of cerebral giant-cell angiitis associated with cerebral amyloid angiopathy. Favorable evolution with corticosteroid therapy] *Rev Neurol (Paris)*, **154**, 695–8.

McCarron, M. O., and Nicoll, J. A. 2004. Cerebral amyloid angiopathy and thrombolysis-related intracerebral haemorrhage. *Lancet Neurol*, **3**, 484–92.

McCarron, M. O., Nicoll, J. A., Stewart, J., et al. 2000. Absence of cystatin C mutation in sporadic cerebral amyloid angiopathy-related hemorrhage. *Neurology*, **54**, 242–4.

Mead, S., James-Galton, M., Revesz, T., et al. 2000. Familial British dementia with amyloid angiopathy: early clinical, neuropsychological and imaging findings. *Brain*, **123(Pt 5)**, 975–91.

Nagai, A., Kobayashi, S., Shimode, K., et al. 1998. No mutations in cystatin C gene in cerebral amyloid angiopathy with cystatin C deposition. *Mol Chem Neuropathol*, **33**, 63–78.

Natte, R., Maat-Schieman, M. L., Haan, J., et al. 2001. Dementia in hereditary cerebral hemorrhage with amyloidosis-Dutch type is associated with cerebral amyloid angiopathy but is independent of plaques and neurofibrillary tangles. *Ann Neurol*, **50**, 765–72.

Nochlin, D., Bird, T. D., Nemens, E. J., Ball, M. J., and Sumi, S. M. 1998. Amyloid angiopathy in a Volga German family with Alzheimer's disease and a presenilin-2 mutation (N141I). *Ann Neurol*, **43**, 131–5.

Obici, L., Demarchi, A., de Rosa, G., et al. 2005. A novel AbetaPP mutation exclusively associated with cerebral amyloid angiopathy. *Ann Neurol*, **58**, 639–44.

Oh, U., Gupta, R., Krakauer, J. W., et al. 2004. Reversible leukoencephalopathy associated with cerebral amyloid angiopathy. *Neurology*, **62**, 494–7.

Palsdottir, A., Abrahamson, M., Thorsteinsson, L., et al. 1988. Mutation in cystatin C gene causes hereditary brain haemorrhage. *Lancet*, **2**, 603–4.

Panegyres, P. K., Kwok, J. B., Schofield, P. R., and Blumbergs, P. C. 2005. A Western Australian kindred with Dutch cerebral amyloid angiopathy. *J Neurol Sci*, **239**, 75–80.

Pasquier, F., and Leys, D. 1997. Why are stroke patients prone to develop dementia? *J Neurol*, **244**, 135–42.

Paunio, T., Kangas, H., Heinonen, O., et al. 1998. Cells of the neuronal lineage play a major role in the generation of amyloid precursor fragments in gelsolin-related amyloidosis. *J Biol Chem*, **273**, 16319–24.

Pfeifer, L. A., White, L. R., Ross, G. W., Petrovitch, H., and Launer, L. J. 2002. Cerebral amyloid angiopathy and cognitive function: the HAAS autopsy study. *Neurology*, **58**, 1629–34.

Plant, G. T., Revesz, T., Barnard, R. O., Harding, A. E., and Gautier-Smith, P. C. 1990. Familial cerebral amyloid angiopathy with nonneuritic amyloid plaque formation. *Brain*, **113(Pt 3)**, 721–47.

Probst, A., and Ulrich, J. 1985. Amyloid angiopathy combined with granulomatous angiitis of the central nervous system: report on two patients. *Clin Neuropathol*, **4**, 250–9.

Remes, A. M., Finnila, S., Mononen, H., et al. 2004. Hereditary dementia with intracerebral hemorrhages and cerebral amyloid angiopathy. *Neurology*, **63**, 234–40.

Ritter, M. A., Droste, D. W., Hegedus, K., et al. 2005. Role of cerebral amyloid angiopathy in intracerebral hemorrhage in hypertensive patients. *Neurology*, **64**, 1233–7.

Roob, G., Schmidt, R., Kapeller, P., et al. 1999. MRI evidence of past cerebral microbleeds in a healthy elderly population. *Neurology*, **52**, 991–4.

Rosand, J., Muzikansky, A., Kumar, A., et al. 2005. Spatial clustering of hemorrhages in probable cerebral amyloid angiopathy. *Ann Neurol*, **58**, 459–62.

Rovelet-Lecrux, A., Hannequin, D., Raux, G., et al. 2006. APP locus duplication causes autosomal dominant early-onset Alzheimer disease with cerebral amyloid angiopathy. *Nat Genet*, **38**, 24–6.

Salama, J., Gherardi, R., Amiel, H., et al. 1986. Post-anoxic delayed encephalopathy with leukoencephalopathy and non-hemorrhagic cerebral amyloid angiopathy. *Clin Neuropathol*, **5**, 153–6.

Sarazin, M., Amarenco, P., Mikol, J., et al. 2002. Reversible leukoencephalopathy in cerebral amyloid angiopathy presenting as subacute dementia. *Eur J Neurol*, **9**, 353–8.

Schmaier, A. H., Dahl, L. D., Rozemuller, A. J., et al. 1993. Protease nexin-2/amyloid beta protein precursor. A tight-binding inhibitor of coagulation factor IXa. *J Clin Invest*, **92**, 2540–5.

Schutz, H., Bodeker, R. H., Damian, M., Krack, P., and Dorndorf, W. 1990. Age-related spontaneous intracerebral hematoma in a German community. *Stroke*, **21**, 1412–8.

Scolding, N. J., Joseph, F., Kirby, P. A., et al. 2005. Abeta-related angiitis: primary angiitis of the central nervous system associated with cerebral amyloid angiopathy. *Brain*, **128**, 500–15.

Stokes, M. I., and Trickey, R. J. 1973. Screening for neurofibrillary tangles and argyrophilic plaques with Congo Red and polarized light. *J Clin Pathol*, **26**, 241–2.

Stone, M. J. 1990. Amyloidosis: a final common pathway for protein deposition in tissues. *Blood*, **75**, 531–45.

Strittmatter, W. J., Saunders, A. M., Schmechel, D., et al. 1993. Apolipoprotein E: high-avidity binding to beta-amyloid and increased frequency of type 4 allele in late-onset familial Alzheimer disease. *Proc Natl Acad Sci U S A*, **90**, 1977–81.

Suzuki, N., Iwatsubo, T., Odaka, A., et al. 1994. High tissue content of soluble beta 1–40 is linked to cerebral amyloid angiopathy. *Am J Pathol*, **145**, 452–60.

Takeda, S., Yamazaki, K., Miyakawa, T., et al. 2003. Subcortical hematoma caused by cerebral amyloid angiopathy: does the first evidence of hemorrhage occur in the subarachnoid space? *Neuropathology*, **23**, 254–61.

Tandon, A., Rogaeva, E., Mullan, M., and St George-Hyslop, P. H. 2000. Molecular genetics of Alzheimer's disease: the role of beta-amyloid and the presenilins. *Curr Opin Neurol*, **13**, 377–84.

Thomas, T., Thomas, G., McLendon, C., Sutton, T., and Mullan, M. 1996. beta-Amyloid-mediated vasoactivity and vascular endothelial damage. *Nature*, **380**, 168–71.

Timmers, W. F., Tagliavini, F., Haan, J., and Frangione, B. 1990. Parenchymal preamyloid and amyloid deposits in the brains of patients with hereditary cerebral hemorrhage with amyloidosis–Dutch type. *Neurosci Lett*, **118**, 223–6.

Tsushima, Y., Tanizaki, Y., Aoki, J., and Endo, K. 2002. MR detection of microhemorrhages in neurologically healthy adults. *Neuroradiology*, **44**, 31–6.

Uitti, R. J., Donat, J. R., Rozdilsky, B., Schneider, R. J., and Koeppen, A. H. 1988. Familial oculoleptomeningeal amyloidosis. Report of a new family with unusual features. *Arch Neurol*, **45**, 1118–22.

Van Broeckhoven, C., Haan, J., Bakker, E., *et al.* 1990. Amyloid beta protein precursor gene and hereditary cerebral hemorrhage with amyloidosis (Dutch). *Science*, **248**, 1120–2.

Van Den Boom, R., Bornebroek, M., Behloul, F., *et al.* 2005. Microbleeds in hereditary cerebral hemorrhage with amyloidosis-Dutch type. *Neurology*, **64**, 1288–9.

van Dijk, E. J., Prins, N. D., Vermeer, S. E., *et al.* 2004. Plasma amyloid beta, apolipoprotein E, lacunar infarcts, and white matter lesions. *Ann Neurol*, **55**, 570–5.

Van Nostrand, W. E., Wagner, S. L., Suzuki, M., *et al.* 1989. Protease nexin-II, a potent antichymotrypsin, shows identity to amyloid beta-protein precursor. *Nature*, **341**, 546–9.

Vidal, R., Revesz, T., Rostagno, A., *et al.* 2000. A decamer duplication in the 3' region of the BRI gene originates an amyloid peptide that is associated with dementia in a Danish kindred. *Proc Natl Acad Sci U S A*, **97**, 4920–5.

Vinters, H. V. 1992. Cerebral amyloid angiopathy and Alzheimer's disease: two entities or one? *J Neurol Sci*, **112**, 1–3.

Vinters, H. V., Secor, D. L., Read, S. L., *et al.* 1994. Microvasculature in brain biopsy specimens from patients with Alzheimer's disease: an immunohistochemical and ultrastructural study. *Ultrastruct Pathol*, **18**, 333–48.

Vonsattel, J. P., Myers, R. H., Hedley-Whyte, E. T., *et al.* 1991. Cerebral amyloid angiopathy without and with cerebral hemorrhages: a comparative histological study. *Ann Neurol*, **30**, 637–49.

Walker, D. A., Broderick, D. F., Kotsenas, A. L., and Rubino, F. A. 2004. Routine use of gradient-echo MRI to screen for cerebral amyloid angiopathy in elderly patients. *AJR Am J Roentgenol*, **182**, 1547–50.

Wang, Z. Z., Jensson, O., Thorsteinsson, L., and Vinters, H. V. 1997. Microvascular degeneration in hereditary cystatin C amyloid angiopathy of the brain. *Apmis*, **105**, 41–7.

Wattendorff, A. R., Bots, G. T., Went, L. N., and Endtz, L. J. 1982. Familial cerebral amyloid angiopathy presenting as recurrent cerebral haemorrhage. *J Neurol Sci*, **55**, 121–35.

Wildi, E., and Dago-Akribi, A. 1968. [Cerebral changes in the aged man]. *Bull Schweiz Akad Med Wiss*, **24**, 107–32.

Worster-Drought, C., Greenfield, J. G., and McMenemy, W. H. 1940. A form of familial presenile dementia with spastic paralysis, (including the pathological examination of a case). *Brain*, **63**, 237–54.

Yamada, M. 2004. Cerebral amyloid angiopathy and gene polymorphisms. *J Neurol Sci*, **226**, 41–4.

Yamada, M., Itoh, Y., Shintaku, M., *et al.* 1996. Immune reactions associated with cerebral amyloid angiopathy. *Stroke*, **27**, 1155–62.

Yamada, M., Tsukagoshi, H., Otomo, E., and Hayakawa, M. 1987. Cerebral amyloid angiopathy in the aged. *J Neurol*, **234**, 371–6.

Yasuda, M., Maeda, K., Ikejiri, Y., *et al.* 1997. A novel missense mutation in the presenilin-1 gene in a familial Alzheimer's disease pedigree with abundant amyloid angiopathy. *Neurosci Lett*, **232**, 29–32.

62

MOYA-MOYA SYNDROME

Harold P. Adams, Jr., Patricia Davis, and Michael Hennerici

Introduction

An uncommon cause of hemorrhagic or ischemic stroke in children and young adults, moya-moya was first described by Japanese investigators in 1955. Most of the initial reports about moya-moya were from Japan, but in the last 50 years, patients with moya-moya have been identified from around the world. Two subsets of patients with moya-moya have been identified; those with moya-moya disease, which probably is an inherited arteriopathy found primarily among persons of northeastern Asian ancestry, and those with moya-moya syndrome, which is diagnosed among persons of all ethnic groups and may be secondary to a large number of disorders.

The largely intracranial arteriopathy is associated with a progressive bilateral obliteration of the major arteries of the anterior circulation (distal segment of the internal carotid artery [ICA] and the proximal segments of the middle cerebral artery [MCA] and anterior cerebral artery [ACA]). As these arteries become occluded and disappear, they are replaced by a fine meshwork of small collateral vessels at the base of the brain that are the arteriographic and pathologic hallmark of moya-moya. The arteriographic appearance of these vessels, which resembles a "puff of smoke," is the source of the name of moya-moya. These same arteriographic findings may be found among patients with either moya-moya disease or moya-moya syndrome. The arteriographic findings in the absence of other conditions that may predispose to arterial occlusions in a child or young adult often lead to the diagnosis of moya-moya disease. In contrast, the arteriographic changes are associated with a large number of conditions, as described subsequently, and in these situations, the diagnosis of moya-moya syndrome is made. The latter scenario may be more common among young adults than among children. Differentiating moya-moya disease from moya-moya syndrome is important because the prognosis and treatment of the patient with the latter emphasizes management of the underlying disease.

The relentlessly progressive nature of the arteriographic changes is another key feature of moya-moya arteriopathy. Based on the arteriographic findings, six stages of the disease are defined (Suzuki, 1986) (Table 62.1). In general, a patient's clinical status corresponds to the stage of the arteriographic abnormalities. While approximately 10% of patients initially have changes of unilateral moya-moya, most of these patients eventually develop bilateral abnormalities. The angiographic findings of moya-moya syndrome are akin to those found with moya-moya disease (Natori et al., 1997). However, the presence of a unilateral process is more suggestive of moya-moya syndrome than of moya-moya disease. The diagnosis of moya-moya should be made with caution if the findings are strictly unilateral, particularly if the arterial changes do not worsen.

Epidemiology

Japan has the highest incidence and prevalence of moya-moya in the world. Wakai et al. (1997) estimated that 3900 Japanese patients with moya-moya are treated annually. Ikeda et al. (2006) recently concluded that the prevalence of moya-moya in the asymptomatic Japanese population is 50.7 per 100 000 people. The rate was considerably higher among Japanese women (94.3/100 000) than men (28.9/100 000.) Reports from Korea and Taiwan suggest that the incidence and prevalence of moya-moya are lower in these countries than in Japan but higher than elsewhere in the world (Hung et al., 1997; Ikezaki, Fukui, Inamura, et al., 1997; Ikezaki, Han, Kawano, et al., 1997). Presumably most of the cases in Northeast Asia represent true genetic moya-moya disease rather than moya-moya syndrome. In Japan, Wakai et al. (1997) found the incidence of moya-moya peaked in two age groups: children younger than 14 years and young adults between 25 and 49 years old. Approximately 50% of the patients had symptoms before the age of 10. The high frequency of disease in young children also suggests an inborn metabolic defect. Ikezaki, Fukui, Inamura, et al. (1997) found similar peaks among Korean patients, but the mean age could be higher. Another Korean study found two age peaks, 6–15 years and 31–40 years (Han et al., 2000). In Japan, the female-to-male ratio is approximately 1.6–1.8:1 (Fukui, 1997; Ikezaki, Han, Kawano, et al., 1997; Wakai et al., 1997). In Korea and Taiwan, the female-to-male ratio is approximately 1.3:1 (Hung et al., 1997; Ikezaki, Fukui, Inamura, et al., 1997; Ikezaki, Han, Kawano, et al., 1997).

Based on responses to a questionnaire mailed to institutions, Yonekawa et al. (1997) estimated that the incidence of moya-moya in Europe was approximately one-tenth of that found in Japan. Although most European patients were white, many of their clinical features were similar to those described in Japanese patients. Most European patients are children or young adults (Khan and Yonekawa, 2005). While moya-moya has been described in all ethnic groups in North America, surveys in Canada and the United States also show relatively low rates (Edwards-Brown and Quets, 1997; Numaguchi et al., 1997; Peerless, 1997). Uchino et al. (2005) looked at the frequency of moya-moya in Washington state and California and found an incidence of 0.086/100 000 persons. The incidence of moya-moya was considerably higher among

Uncommon Causes of Stroke, 2nd edition, ed. Louis R. Caplan. Published by Cambridge University Press. © Cambridge University Press 2008.

Table 62.1 Angiographic stages of moya-moya

Stage 1	There is narrowing of the distal segment of the ICA.
Stage 2	Basal moya-moya initially appears. There is dilation of the main cerebral arteries.
Stage 3	Basal moya-moya becomes more prominent. The proximal segments of the ACA and MCA are no longer visualized. Pial collaterals arise from branches of the posterior cerebral arteries (PCA).
Stage 4	The basal moya-moya begins to regress. Proximal segments of the PCA are involved.
Stage 5	The basal moya-moya decreases further. The major cerebral arteries are no longer visualized.
Stage 6	The basal moya-moya is no longer seen. The cerebral circulation is supplied only via meningeal-pial collaterals from branches of the external carotid arteries.

Table 62.2 Collateral vessels in moya-moya

External carotid artery
Middle meningeal artery
Facial artery
Temporal artery
Occipital artery
Superficial temporal artery
Ophthalmic artery
Ethmoidal arteries
Anterior falcine artery
PCA
Tectal plexus
Posterior choroidal artery
Thalamoperforating arteries
Dorsal callosal branches

Asian-Americans than among other ethnic groups. A higher rate of moya-moya in Hawaii than in the continental United States may be attributed to a higher concentration of persons of Japanese ancestry living in Hawaii (Graham and Matoba, 1997). Graham and Matoba (1997) found the prevalence and incidence of moya-moya among Japanese Americans to be similar to those found in Japan. The presentations of moya-moya in North America may differ from those found in Japan; for example, a relatively higher rate of hemorrhages is described (Peerless, 1997). This finding may support the hypothesis that most cases of moya-moya in North America are secondary to moya-moya syndrome instead of moya-moya disease. In the United States, a majority of cases are diagnosed in young adults (Cloft *et al.*, 1999; Edwards-Brown and Quets, 1997; Hallemeier *et al.*, 2006; Peerless, 1997). The differences in the age groups between Japan and North America also suggest a different underlying condition. A predominance of cases among young women also is reported in North America (Cloft *et al.*, 1999; Hallemeier *et al.*, 2006; Numaguchi *et al.*, 1997; Peerless, 1997).

Pathology of moya-moya

Pathological changes have been found in both intracranial and extracranial arteries, suggesting that moya-moya is not an isolated intracranial arteriopathy. Several reports have associated moya-moya disease with renal artery stenosis, a finding that implies that the disease is a multisystem vasculopathy in some patients (Halley *et al.*, 1988; Yamada *et al.*, 2000). Bilateral severe stenoses or occlusions of the terminal portions of the ICA and the proximal segments of the ACA and MCA are the hallmark of moya-moya. The disease also may affect the posterior circulation, most commonly the PCA, although the findings are less extensive and appear later than those found in the ICA and its major branches. Branches of the external carotid artery, especially the superficial temporal artery and middle meningeal artery also may be affected (Aoyagi *et al.*, 1996, 1997; Yang *et al.*, 1997).

Microscopic findings in the larger intracranial arteries included segmental narrowing, thickening of the intimal and medial layers, proliferation or degeneration of smooth muscle cells, and tortuosity or fragmentation of the internal elastic lamina (Fukui *et al.*, 2000; Hosoda *et al.*, 1997; Li *et al.*, 1991; Takebayashi *et al.*, 1984; Yamashita *et al.*, 1983). Inflammatory changes, calcification, and lipid deposits are not found in the arterial wall. These findings suggest that moya-moya is a vasculopathy that is distinct from either vasculitis or atherosclerosis (Haltia *et al.*, 1982).

The fine mesh of the basal collateral vessels, which is the clinical hallmark of moya-moya, usually involves the frontal basal regions (ethmoidal moya-moya). Less commonly, it can be generalized (vault moya-moya) (Suzuki, 1986). Collateral vessels contributing to the network of small-caliber vessels may arise from the middle meningeal artery, superficial temporal artery, facial artery, temporal artery, or occipital arteries. The ethmoidal arteries or the anterior falcine artery may serve as collaterals diverting blood from the ophthalmic artery to the hemisphere. In addition, pial or deep collateral vessels may develop from the tectal plexus, posterior choroidal artery, thalamoperforating arteries, or the dorsal callosal branches of the PCA (Table 62.2). Most of these vessels are leptomeningeal in location. Rather than being new arteries, these enlarged collateral channels appear to be normal arterioles and veins that are dilated. On microscopic examination, these vessels have fibrous intimal thickening and attenuation of the internal elastic lamina. Small penetrating arteries at the base of the brain also show fibrous thickening of the intima, thinning of the media, fragmentation of the internal elastic lamina, and microaneurysms (Yamashita *et al.*, 1983). Takebayashi *et al.* (1984) found moth-eaten changes in the walls of the lenticulostriate arteries and concluded that the changes mimicked severe hypertension or sustained arterial vasospasm.

The presumed etiology for the brain ischemia among patients with moya-moya is a gradually evolving hypoperfusion secondary to occlusion of the major arteries. The smaller caliber collateral channels are unable to maintain adequate blood supply to the brain, and infarctions (most commonly in a watershed pattern) develop. Multiple small infarctions most often develop in the basal ganglia and the deep white matter of the cerebral hemispheres. Larger infarctions, secondary to thromboembolic occlusions, usually are in the cortical distribution of the ACA or MCA. Infarctions in the posterior portions of the cerebral hemispheres, the brainstem, or the cerebellum are rare.

Microaneurysms or false aneurysms that may be the source of intracranial hemorrhage often are located on the small intracranial vessels. Most hemorrhages are located in the deep structures of the cerebral hemispheres. Small collateral vessels adjacent to the lateral ventricles may be the source of primary intraventricular hemorrhage. In addition, saccular aneurysms, most commonly located in the posterior circulation or on collateral vessels, also may be the source of subarachnoid hemorrhage (Kawaguchi et al., 1996b; Leblanc, 1992).

Genetic aspects of moya-moya disease

The familial occurrence of moya-moya disease and the much higher rates of the disease among persons of Japanese ancestry point towards a genetic factor (Graham and Matoba, 1997) Approximately 10% of affected Japanese patients have relatives with moya-moya disease. Cases of moya-moya disease in identical twins have been reported (Fukui, 1997). Familial aggregations of moya-moya disease are much less common in Europe and North America (Shetty-Alva and Alva, 2000). The two peaks of moya-moya disease in children and young adults suggest more than one genetic abnormality. Mineharu et al. (2006) concluded that most cases of familial moya-moya disease follow a pattern that is compatible with an autosomal dominant inheritance with incomplete penetrance. They also found a trend that affected mothers were more likely to have daughters with an adult onset of symptoms. A mother-to-child inheritance pattern in some families suggests that some cases of moya-moya disease might be because of a genetic mitochondrial disorder. In addition, the association of moya-moya with several genetic and inherited diseases (including Down syndrome, sickle cell disease, neurofibromatosis, and polycystic kidney disease) also suggests a possible genetic substrate (Cheong et al., 2005; Cramer et al., 1996; Hattori et al., 1998; Pracyk and Massey, 1989; Salih et al., 2006).

Inoue et al. (1997) reported that several alleles of the class II genes of the human leukocyte antigen (HLA) are associated with moya-moya disease. In a Korean population of patients with moya-moya disease, Han et al. (2003) found an association with the HLA-B35 allele, particularly among women and persons with adult-onset symptoms. Linkage studies among patients with moya-moya disease demonstrate several possible genetic loci. Cramer et al. (1996) postulated that a protein encoded on chromosome 21 might be related to the pathogenesis of moya-moya disease. Sakuri et al. (2004) found a location on gene 8q23. Ikeda et al. (1999) found a possible site on gene 3p24.2–p26. Other potential sites have been identified on chromosomes 6 and 17 (Fukui et al., 2000; Inoue et al., 2000; Yamauchi et al., 2000). Kang et al. (2006) reported that genes encoding tissue inhibitor of metalloproteinases 2 and 4 span previously identified sites on chromosomes 3 and 17 probably are related to moya-moya disease (Yamauchi et al., 2000). They also found a higher rate of changes in tissue inhibitor of metalloproteinase 2 among patients with moya-moya disease, and they speculated that these changes lead to changes in binding and transcription.

Presumably the inherited metabolic abnormality affects endothelial or arterial smooth muscle cells. The factor's primary actions must induce narrowing and occlusion of the large intracranial arteries. The development of the small collaterals (moya-moya phenomenon) may be a secondary reactive process in response to subacute ischemia. Abnormalities in levels of fibroblast growth factor, which is a mitogen for endothelial cells, may stimulate arterial growth. Increased immunoreactivity to fibroblast growth factor may be detected in specimens obtained from the dura or the superficial temporal artery (Hoshimaru et al., 1991; Malek et al., 1997; Suzui et al., 1994; Yamamoto et al., 1998). High fibroblast growth factor levels also are found in the smooth muscle and the intimal and medial layers in patients with moya-moya (Suzui et al., 1994). Elevated cerebrospinal fluid levels of fibroblast growth factor also may be found (Malek et al., 1997; Takahashi et al., 1993; Yoshimoto et al., 1996). Houkin et al. (1996) found that persons with unilateral moya-moya have lower levels of fibroblast growth factor than do patients with bilateral disease. Vascular endothelial growth factor, angiopoietins, platelet-derived growth factors, and integrins also may play a role in angiogenesis and cause arterial changes of moya-moya (Lim et al., 2006). Some of these factors may play a role in the evolution of moya-moya. Transforming growth factor β-1, which may lead to neovascularization of vessels and angiogenesis, also is implicated as a contributing factor in the pathogenesis of moya-moya (Yamamoto et al., 1997; Hojo et al., 1998). The smooth muscle cells obtained from the arteries of patients with moya-moya do not react to platelet-derived growth factor (Aoyagi et al., 1993, 1997). Masuda et al. (1993) detected increased generation of smooth muscle cells among patients with moya-moya disease by detecting the presence of proliferating cell nuclear antigen in cells. Although these findings are important and imply a nonatherosclerotic mechanism for the thickening of the arterial wall in moya-moya, additional research on the pathophysiology of the arteriopathy is needed.

Pathogenesis of moya-moya syndrome

The pathogenesis of moya-moya syndrome differs from that of moya-moya disease. Epidemiological variables and clinical presentations differ between the two groups of patients. Persons with moya-moya syndrome usually are young adults, who often have potential risk factors for stroke and a potential for intracranial hemorrhage. Moya-moya syndrome is associated with a large number of diseases (Table 62.3). Such relationships are not described among the Asian populations with moya-moya disease. Many diseases associated with moya-moya syndrome have a subacute or chronic course leading to brain ischemia, which serves as a potent stimulus for the growth and proliferation of small vessels at the base of the brain. Rather than a de novo arterial disease, many of the arterial changes may be secondary to the underlying illness, such as sickle cell disease, or may be a relatively nonspecific response to improve blood flow to deep brain structures that are ischemic.

Moya-moya syndrome may follow radiation therapy for treatment of an optic nerve glioma, particularly associated with neurofibromatosis, type 1 (Bitzer and Topka, 1995; Desai et al., 2006;

Table 62.3 Possible associations with moya-moya syndrome

Neurofibromatosis	Tuberous sclerosis
Turner syndrome	Retinitis pigmentosa
Down syndrome	Pseudoxanthoma elasticum
Glycogen storage disease – I	Sickle cell disease
Thalassemia	Protein C deficiency
Factor V Leiden	Protein S deficiency
Polycystic kidney disease	Eosinophilic granuloma
Noonan syndrome	Costello syndrome
Hypomelanosis of Ito	Livedo reticularis
Graves' disease – thyrotoxicosis	Rheumatoid arthritis
Arteriovenous malformation	Kawasaki disease
Oral contraceptive use	Smoking
Craniocerebral trauma	Cranial/basal irradiation
Parasellar tumors	Vasculitis
Polyarteritis nodosa	Fibromuscular dysplasia
Renal artery stenosis	Saccular aneurysm
Atherosclerosis	Tonsillitis/pharyngitis
Tuberculous meningitis	Leptospirosis
Anaerobic meningitis	*Propionibacterium acnes*

Table 62.4 Clinical presentations of moya-moya in children and adults

Children	Adults
Recurrent headaches	Subarachnoid hemorrhage
Seizures	Intracerebral hemorrhage
Ischemic stroke	Ischemic stroke
Focal motor signs	Focal motor signs
Sensory disturbances	Sensory disturbances
Speech disturbances	Speech disturbances
Impaired consciousness	Impaired consciousness
Movement disorders	Movement disorders
Mental retardation	Seizures
Cognitive decline	Headaches
Pituitary dysfunction	Vascular dementia

Kestle *et al.*, 1993). The interval from the radiation exposure until the appearance of the arterial changes has been 6–12 years (Bitzer and Topka, 1995; Desai *et al.*, 2006). Children receiving radiation therapy to the parasellar region before the age of 5 years seem to have the highest risk for secondary moya-moya (Desai *et al.*, 2006). Interactions between abnormalities in coagulation and recent infections and the development of moya-moya also are reported (Andeejani *et al.*, 1998; Bonduel *et al.*, 2001; Cheong *et al.*, 2005; Holz *et al.*, 1998; Tanigawara *et al.*, 1997; Tsuda *et al.*, 1997; Yamada *et al.*, 1997). The mesh of small vessels at the base of the brain (moya-moya phenomenon) also may be secondary to a gradual atherosclerotic occlusion of the major intracranial arteries. Reports correlate the development of moya-moya in young women with the use of oral contraceptives and smoking (Bruno, Adams, Biller, *et al.*, 1988; Levine *et al.*, 1991; Peerless, 1997). In contrast, Cloft *et al.* (1999) could find no relationship of moya-moya with common risk factors for stroke or use of oral contraceptives in a series of young American adults. An association between moya-moya and morning glory disc anomaly, thyrotoxicosis or Graves' disease also has been reported (Hsu *et al.*, 2006; Im *et al.*, 2005; Murphy *et al.*, 2005; Quah *et al.*, 2005; Squizzato *et al.*, 2005). The large number of conditions associated with moya-moya syndrome suggests that the arterial changes may be an epiphenomenon rather than a specific consequence of the primary illness.

Clinical presentations

Patients with either moya-moya disease or syndrome may have a number of presentations (Table 62.4). No one clinical presentation is specific for either form of moya-moya. Overall, the clinical findings in children differ slightly from those found among adults. In general, moya-moya disease is more likely in children and among persons of Northeastern Asian ancestry whereas moya-moya

syndrome is more likely in young adults and persons of other ethnic groups. Still, moya-moya (disease or syndrome) is included in the differential diagnosis of either ischemic or hemorrhagic stroke in children and young adults (Camilo and Goldstein, 2005; Chabrier *et al.*, 2000; deVeber, 2003; Wraige, Phol and Ganesan, 2005)

Affected children often present with headaches, motor impairments, or seizures (Namba et al 2006; Yamashiro *et al.*, 1984). Seol *et al.* (2005) reported that 44 of 204 children with moya-moya disease had severe headaches that interfered with daily activity and that occurred at least once a month. The headaches often have the clinical features of migraine. Seol *et al.* (2005) concluded that progressive recruitment of blood vessels and redistribution of blood flow could be potential causes of headaches in children. Because of the high risk for ischemia, treatment of headaches may be difficult. Seizures, which usually are generalized, may be an initial finding in approximately 5%–10% of children. Seizures also may occur at any time in the course of the illness. Ischemia is the most common clinical presentation (Han *et al.*, 2000). Recurrent ischemic strokes and transient ischemic attacks (TIA) provoked by hyperventilation also are reported (Battisella and Carollo, 1997; Hung *et al.*, 1997). The occurrence of a transient episode of focal neurological dysfunction following vigorous exercise or hyperventilation in a child should lead to consideration of moya-moya.

The signs of stroke or TIA usually reflect ischemia to a cerebral hemisphere. Children may have hemiparesis, dysarthria, sensory loss, movement disorders (Watanabe *et al.*, 1990), or focal cognitive impairments including aphasia. Infarctions may be located in either cortical or deep hemispheric structures. Many of the deep hemisphere infarctions are small, and on brain imaging their appearance may mimic the findings found among patients with lacunar infarctions secondary to chronic hypertension. Recurrent stroke may lead to progressive cognitive decline or mental slowing; this sequence of events is distressingly common among children with moya-moya disease (Kuroda *et al.*, 2004). Imaizumi *et al.* (1999) reported that intelligence begins to decrease after the onset of symptomatic moya-moya disease, but the decline usually stabilizes after approximately 10 years. Hogan *et al.* (2005)

found that intellectual decline among children with sickle cell disease was greater if they also had complicating moya-moya syndrome. Hypothalamic-pituitary dysfunction is a rare complication of moya-moya disease in children (Mootha et al., 1999). This complication should not be a surprising finding given the location of the vasculopathy.

Recurrent stroke or TIA also is a common presentation of moya-moya among young adults (Bruno, Adams, Biller, et al., 1988; Camilo and Goldstein, 2005; Chiu et al., 1998; Peerless, 1997). Ischemic lesions usually are in the border zone between the terminal perfusion beds of the ACA, MCA, and PCA. Infarctions may be located in the cortex, deep hemispheric white matter, or basal ganglia. Motor, sensory, or cognitive impairments often are prominent. A progressive ischemic syndrome affecting primarily the frontal lobes may lead to serious behavioral disturbances or disorders of executive function. Uncommonly, patients may present with movement disorders (Gonzalez-Alegre et al., 2003). A syndrome that mimics multi-infarction dementia may also occur. Brainstem ischemia is an atypical feature (Hirano et al., 1998). However, with involvement of the PCA, visual disturbances may occur (Miyamoto et al., 1986; Noda et al., 1987). Visual complaints include amaurosis fugax, visual field defects, decreased visual acuity, positive visual phenomena, and diplopia. Some of these complaints reflect disease in the carotid circulation, and others reflect posterior circulation ischemia. Seizures and headaches are much less common among adults than children. Adult patients with ischemic symptoms have a very high risk for recurrent stroke (Hallemeier et al., 2006).

Intracranial hemorrhage often is a presentation of moya-moya in adults. Han et al. (2000) reported that hemorrhage was the major clinical presentation in approximately 60% of the Korean adults with moya-moya disease. Asymptomatic microhemorrhages in the brain also may be detected by MRI (Ishikawa et al., 2005; Kikuta et al., 2005). Hemorrhages may be secondary to rupture of a collateral vessel, penetrating artery, small false aneurysm, an associated saccular aneurysm, or a vascular malformation (Iwama, Hashimoto, Tsukahara, et al., 1997; Iwama, Horimoto, Hashimoto, et al., 1997; Iwama, Todaka, Hashimoto, et al., 1997). Recurrent intracranial hemorrhages are frequent. Kawaguchi et al. (1996a) reported that recurrent bleeding occurs at a rate of approximately 2% per patient-year. In another study, Morioka et al. (2003) reported that rebleeding occurred in 22 of 36 patients with adult moya-moya. They found that rebleeding was most frequent among those patients 46–55 years old and that recurrent hemorrhage usually led to poor neurological outcomes. Approximately 60% of hemorrhages are intracerebral in location, approximately 30% are primarily intraventricular, and 5% are subarachnoid (Leblanc, 1992; Saeki et al., 1997). The common intraparenchymal sites for the hemorrhages are the basal ganglia and thalamus. Thalamic hemorrhages often are associated with an intraventricular extension (Irikura et al., 1996; Jayakumar et al., 1999). Hemorrhage arising from the caudate nucleus also can occur.

The location of the intracerebral hemorrhages in deep brain structures has led to the theory that bleeding is due to an overload of blood flow through penetrating arteries that supply these deep regions. These arteries become hypertrophied, are larger than usual, and show degenerative changes and microaneurysms when studied pathologically (Yamashita et al., 1983). They are not made to carry the extra load. This theory has led some clinicians to posit that surgical creation of bypasses might lessen the blood flow load of these penetrating arteries by providing alternative collateral pathways and so lessen the risk of brain hemorrhage. There are few data that test this hypothesis.

Small asymptomatic hemorrhages can be located in the paraventricular white matter, subcortex, or basal ganglia (Ishikawa et al., 2005). Although a potential association between cerebral arteriovenous malformation and moya-moya has been described, the number of cases is small (Lichtor and Mullan, 1987).

Subarachnoid hemorrhage is relatively rare among patients with moya-moya unless an intracranial saccular aneurysm also is present (Kawaguchi et al., 1996a). Although the number of patients with moya-moya and saccular aneurysms is relatively small, the disproportionately high rate of posterior circulation aneurysms raises the possibility of a cause-effect relationship. Presumably, augmented flow through the vertebrobasilar circulation, which is serving as a collateral channel for blood to reach the cerebral hemispheres, could lead to hemodynamic changes that stimulate growth of aneurysms (Iwama, Hashimoto, Tsukahara, et al., 1997; Iwama, Horimoto, Hashimoto, et al., 1997; Iwama, Todaka, Hashimoto, et al., 1997; Kodama et al., 1996; Muizelaar, 1988). Small false aneurysms found on the moya-moya collaterals at the base of the brain or along the ventricular surface also may produce subarachnoid hemorrhage (Konishi et al., 1985; Marushima et al., 2006).

Unilateral findings consistent with the diagnosis of moya-moya disease or syndrome can be detected in both children and young adults (Hirotsune et al., 1997; Houkin et al., 1996; Kawano et al., 1994). Most such patients subsequently develop bilateral disease, but some patients with unilateral moya-moya do not have the typical progressive course. However, some patients have persistent unilateral disease and they should be considered to have an atypical syndrome. The diagnosis of moya-moya disease should be made with considerable caution if the patient has clinical, brain, and vascular imaging findings of a unilateral process.

While oral contraceptive use may be associated with the development of moya-moya, there is no evidence that pregnancy worsens the arteriopathy. Isolated instances of successful outcomes of pregnancy among young women with moya-moya have been reported (Mehrkens et al., 2006). There is no evidence that pregnancy or delivery is associated with an increased risk of either ischemic or hemorrhagic stroke. Both Cesarean section and vaginal delivery have been performed, but special attention should be paid to avoid hypocapnia, hypotension, or hypertension.

Evaluation and diagnosis

Vascular imaging

The diagnosis of moya-moya requires visualization of the characteristic arterial findings. Thus, accurate imaging of the intracranial vasculature is a key for diagnosis, and this necessity usually means that the patient will need an arteriogram. Although arteriography

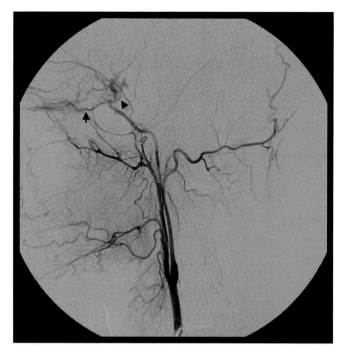

Figure 62.1 Woman (23-year-old) with moya-moya syndrome. A conventional angiogram with a right common carotid injection shows a large right ophthalmic artery (*arrow*) and occlusion of the terminal ICA with dilated lenticulostriate collaterals (*arrowhead*).

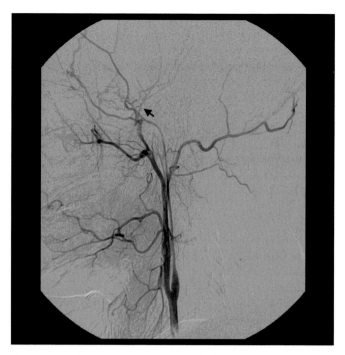

Figure 62.2 In the same patient, injection of the left common carotid shows a small collapsed left ICA with distal occlusion (*arrow*) and no filling of the left MCA and ACA.

is an invasive study that is associated with some risk, the likelihood of complications is quite low (Robertson *et al.*, 1998). The arterial changes are described in Tables 62.1 and 62.2 (Suzuki, 1986) (Figures 62.1 and 62.2). The presence of a terminal occlusion of one ICA with the finding of the typical basal network of fine-caliber vessels is not sufficient for the diagnosis. In this situation, a thromboembolic occlusion is common. Segmental stenoses of the proximal segments of the ACA and MCA secondary to vasospasm should not be misdiagnosed as moya-moya in a patient with a recent subarachnoid hemorrhage. Similarly, accelerated atherosclerosis in a young adult also may lead to stenosis or occlusion of the initial segment of an ACA or MCA. Several areas of segmental constrictions and dilations of cortical arteries are not consistent with moya-moya; these changes are more suggestive of a vasoconstrictive syndrome, vasculitis, or intracranial atherosclerosis, especially if the findings are most prominent in distal branches. Occlusions of the distal segments of the ACA or MCA are not typical for moya-moya even if pial or leptomeningeal collaterals are seen. Prominent fine-caliber collaterals arising from the ethmoidal arteries or other leptomeningeal vessels at the base of the brain are so typical of moya-moya that their absence should lead clinicians to question the diagnosis. During the early stages of moya-moya, prominent leptomeningeal collateral vessels arise from the PCA and its branches (Miyamoto *et al.*, 1984; Satoh *et al.*, 1988) (Figure 62.3). Although the finding of these collaterals on a posterior circulation arteriogram raises suspicion of moya-moya, these findings are not specific. Any obstruction of the proximal portions of the ACA or MCA may induce these changes. The PCA is affected as the moya-moya progresses (Yamada *et al.*, 1995; Yamada, Himeno, Suzuki, *et al.*, 1995). Thus, the absence of prominent collaterals arising from the

posterior circulation should not be surprising in advanced stages of the disease. Stenotic lesions similar to those found on major intracranial arteries also can be found on branches of the external carotid artery (Hoshimaru and Kikuchi, 1992). Intracranial saccular aneurysms, most commonly found on the posterior circulation, also may be visualized by arteriography. These aneurysms usually arise at arterial bifurcations. The false microaneurysms found on the penetrating collateral arterioles are not seen by arteriography.

Magnetic resonance angiography (MRA) or computed tomography angiography (CTA) usually detects the stenoses or occlusions of the distal ICA or the proximal anterior artery and MCA (Figure 62.4). However, these techniques have difficulty visualizing the basal moya-moya vessels. In comparison to conventional arteriography, MRA has a sensitivity and specificity for the diagnosis of moya-moya of 73% and 100%, respectively (Yamada *et al.*, 1995; Yamada, Himeno, Suzuki, *et al.*, 1995). Recently, Fushimi *et al.* (2006) reported that MRA performed using a 3-Tesla machine could detect the moya-moya vessels. CTA may be superior to MRA for visualization of the lesions of the major arteries of the Circle of Willis (Katz *et al.*, 1995). CTA also may detect the dilated basal collateral changes and the moya-moya vessels deep in the hemisphere (Tsuchiya *et al.*, 1994), and also has been used to monitor the progress of moya-moya (Kikuchi *et al.*, 1996).

Transcranial Doppler (TCD) ultrasonography has been used to measure changes in velocity and pulsatility, to search for the presence of major leptomeningeal collaterals, and to detect high-intensity transient signals in moya-moya (Horn *et al.*, 2005; Lee *et al.*, 2004; Perren *et al.*, 2005). Changes include diminished flow velocities in the MCA in comparison to the ICA and increased flow velocities in the ophthalmic arteries and PCA. These latter findings

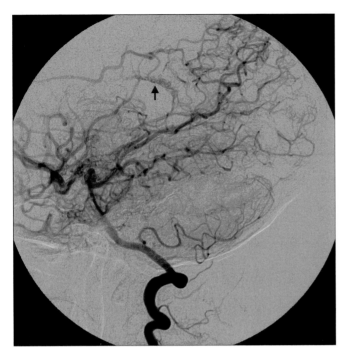

Figure 62.3 In the same patient, there is collateral flow from a right vertebral artery injection via the posterior communicating artery and pial collaterals from the PCA to the ACA (*arrow*).

reflect prominent collateral flow (Muttaqin *et al.*, 1993; Takase *et al.*, 1997). Overall the findings, which usually reflect hemodynamic changes rather than embolic events, correlate with the stage of moya-moya (Laborde *et al.*, 1993; Takase *et al.*, 1997). As the arteries become obliterated, the flow becomes very slow or stops. The findings also complement the changes detected by MRA. Sequential TCD studies may be performed to monitor the course of the disease. Because it is noninvasive, it is an ideal way to check for progression of the arteriopathy in children. The relative thinness of the skull in children makes the test easily performed. The shorter distances from the child's skull's surface to the Circle of Willis also make insonation technically clearer. TCD also can be used to monitor the patency of bypass operations (Perren *et al.*, 2005).

Duplex imaging of the carotid artery in the neck may provide clues for the presence of severe disease of the distal ICA or intracranial arteries by showing no flow at the neck or a very high resistance to flow (Muppala and Castaldo, 1994). The absence of a stenotic lesion at the carotid bifurcation and the finding of sluggish distal flow provide important clues about the location of the distal occlusion and the possible evidence of moya-moya. It is likely that these findings will lead to further investigation with MRA, CTA, or conventional arteriography. Thus, the results of the carotid duplex study could be helpful when screening a child or young adult with ischemic stroke.

Brain imaging

Both CT and MRI are used to assess the presence, extent, and location of hemorrhagic and ischemic brain lesions. Findings include multiple lesions (usually infarctions) located primarily in

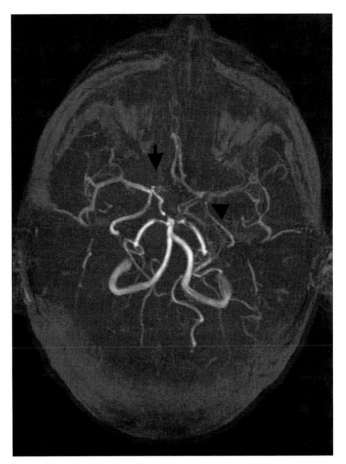

Figure 62.4 MRA of the same patient shows occlusion of the distal right ICA with dilated lenticulostriate collaterals (puff of smoke, *arrow*) with a small left ICA that is occluded in the cavernous portion (*arrowhead*). There is poor flow in the left MCA via collaterals.

deep hemispheric structures and the lobar white matter (Takeuchi *et al.*, 1982). Infarctions often take a border zone pattern between the terminal branches of the ACA and MCA. Takanashi *et al*, (1993) found that most ischemic lesions in children affect the cortex and immediate subcortical white matter whereas adults have more infarctions in the deep lobar white matter, basal ganglia, and centrum semiovale (Figure 62.5). Other findings include ventricular enlargement and cortical atrophy. Because many of the ischemic lesions are relatively small, MRI may be more sensitive than CT in detecting the deep infarctions (Bruno, Yuh, Biller, *et al.*, 1998; Takanashi *et al.*, 1993). MRI also provides information about the vasculature and the extent of the arterial disease. MRI may visualize the absence of normal flow voids in the ICA, MCA, or ACA in the suprasellar region and the collateral network in the basal ganglia. The arterial walls are seen as faint (Aoki *et al.*, 2002). MRI also may detect dilated leptomeningeal or transdural collateral arteries (Yamada *et al.*, 1995; Yamada, Himeno, Suzuki, *et al.*, 1995). Contrast enhancement increases the likelihood of detecting these arterial changes. Kassner *et al.* (2003) found that dynamic T2-weighted magnetic resonance perfusion imaging could be used to detect regional microvascular abnormalities that may represent angiogenic activity. Contrast-enhanced CT also may detect the

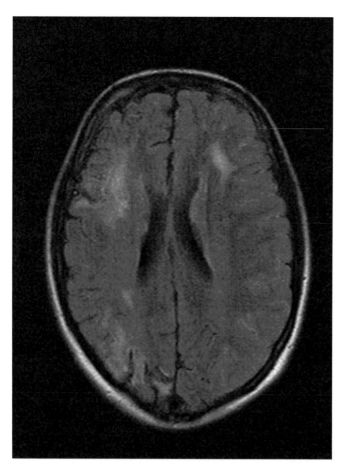

Figure 62.5 MRI fluid-attenuated inversion recovery (FLAIR) images (same patient as Figures 62.1–62.4) show bilateral subcortical and right parietal infarcts.

vascular changes deep in the cerebral hemispheres. Both CT and MRI will detect bleeding within the brain, ventricle, or subarachnoid space. Gradient-echo MRI may be used to detect small asymptomatic hemorrhages (Kikuta et al., 2005).

Electroencephalography and evoked potentials

Nonspecific abnormalities, most commonly diffuse slow activity, are commonly detected by electroencephalography performed among affected children. Hyperventilation may induce the "re-build-up phenomenon," which involves a gradual decrease in frequency but an increase in amplitude of electrical activity (Kurlemann et al., 1992; Kuroda et al., 1995). These changes probably relate to focal reduction in perfusion reserve provoked by vasoconstriction induced by the hyperventilation (Kuroda et al., 1995). Prolonged latencies, reduced amplitudes, and poor wave forms may be detected by brainstem auditory-evoked, visual-evoked, or somatosensory-evoked potentials (Chen et al., 1989). In general, changes in evoked potentials correlate with clinical, vascular imaging, and brain imaging findings. Abnormalities in visually evoked potentials correlate with involvement of the PCA, and the test could be used to monitor the progression of the arteriopathy (Tashima-Kurita et al., 1989).

Measurements of cerebral metabolism and blood flow

Changes in cerebral metabolism or blood flow may be assessed by positron emission tomography (PET), single photon emission computed tomography (SPECT), xenon-enhanced CT, and functional MRI (Horowitz et al., 1995; Obara et al., 1997; Piao et al., 2004; Sato et al., 1999; Shimizu et al., 1997; Tsuchiya et al., 1998; Khan and Yonekawa, 2005). Abnormalities include reduced cerebral blood flow, cerebral metabolic rate of oxygen, ratio of cerebral blood flow to cerebral blood volume, and cerebrovascular reserve (Piao et al., 2004). In contrast, cerebral blood volume and the oxygen extraction fraction are increased. These findings suggest that patients with moya-moya often have severe hemodynamic impairments. The changes may be enhanced by the administration of carbon dioxide or acetazolamide. Obara et al. (1997) reported different patterns of regional cerebral blood flow in reaction to hypercarbia among patients with moya-moya in comparison to patients with atherosclerotic occlusions of the ICA. They concluded that the relative preservation of regional cerebral blood flow with moya-moya may be secondary to the presence of abundant collaterals. Relative preservation of regional cerebral blood flow in the posterior portions of the cerebral hemispheres corresponds to the relative integrity of patency of the PCA. Detection of reduced blood flow in the occipital regions usually foretells development of stenotic or occlusive lesions in the vertebrobasilar territory (Yamada et al., 1996). The results of these studies provide data that outline the presence, location, and severity of perfusion defects in both children and adults with moya-moya. The changes in blood flow and metabolism may precede the arteriographic and brain imaging abnormalities. These tests may be used to help determine prognosis and develop treatment plans. For example, sequential deterioration of regional cerebral blood flow in a clinically stable patient might prompt consideration of a revascularization operation before the patient has a new stroke (Nakagawara et al., 1997). These tests also may be used to measure hemodynamic and metabolic responses after reconstructive operations.

Prognosis and treatment

In general, the prognosis of adults or children with moya-moya is guarded. Children with moya-moya disease have a very high risk for recurrent strokes that lead to cognitive decline and severe disability (Kim et al., 2004). Kim et al. (2004) noted that symptomatic children younger than 3 years had a particularly unfavorable prognosis. Young adults with moya-moya also have a high risk for recurrent strokes that lead to progressive motor, sensory, or cognitive impairments. The neurological sequelae often lead to dementia, disability, or long-term institutionalization.

Because of the very bleak natural history of moya-moya disease and the lack of effective therapies to treat the primary arteriopathy, medical or surgical measures to prevent both hemorrhagic and ischemic stroke are the focus of management. At present, no treatment is established as effective in limiting the neurological morbidity of moya-moya. Performing clinical trials to test the efficacy of any therapy is difficult because of the low incidence and prevalence of moya-moya, even in Japan. Most physicians also have limited experience with the disease. The diversity of clinical presentations and the variable course also makes a clinical trial complex and hard to perform. Despite these hurdles, a Japanese trial is planned to test the utility of extracranial-intracranial bypass surgery for treatment of adults with moya-moya who have had brain hemorrhage (Miyamoto *et al.*, 2004). The data supporting surgery for moya-moya syndrome are also retrospective and based on small sample sizes (Chiu *et al.*, 1998; Hallemeier *et al.*, 2006).

Management of patients with ischemic symptoms secondary to moya-moya is similar to that prescribed to patients with stroke secondary to other diseases. Treatment of acute ischemic stroke includes acute interventions aimed at limiting the neurological consequences of the ischemia, measures to forestall medical or neurological complications, rehabilitation, and interventions to prevent recurrent stroke. Although some young patients with acute ischemic stroke likely will be treated with thrombolysis, no data are available about either its safety or efficacy. Because of the potential for intracranial bleeding, emergency administration of anticoagulants or thrombolytic agents may be contraindicated. Hypoxia, hypercarbia, and hypotension should be avoided or treated in an effort to limit the ischemia. In contrast, markedly elevated blood pressures may need to be treated because of the associated risk of brain hemorrhage. Because affected patients are children and young adults who might live for several years, rehabilitation and other efforts to maximize recovery are crucial.

Patients with subarachnoid hemorrhage secondary to rupture of a complicating saccular aneurysm should have the aneurysm treated as soon as possible. Choices include surgical clipping or endovascular placement of coils (Arita *et al.*, 2003; Kodama *et al.*, 1996). Because aneurysms usually are in the posterior circulation, endovascular treatment probably is preferred. Measures to avoid dehydration or extremes of blood pressure are important because vasospasm secondary to subarachnoid hemorrhage might worsen the already borderline perfusion to the brain from the moya-moya. There are no data about the utility of nimodipine in preventing vasospasm among patients with subarachnoid hemorrhage and moya-moya. The utility of drug-induced hypertension or other measures to improve perfusion in the setting of vasospasm has not been tested. No surgical intervention is prescribed to treat the small aneurysms that arise on the penetrating collateral vessels. Treatment of intraventricular or intracerebral hemorrhage secondary to moya-moya is similar to that prescribed for hematomas secondary to other causes. Because the hematomas usually are deep in the cerebral hemispheres, surgical evacuation of the lesions is difficult.

Treatment of the underlying or associated condition is a fundamental component of care of patients with moya-moya syndrome. Hopefully, treatment of the concomitant disease slows the arterial process and it might lessen the likelihood of recurrent cerebrovascular events. For example, prevention of crises in children with sickle cell disease and early exchange transfusion may lessen the neurological consequences of moya-moya complicating the hemoglobinopathy. Children should be instructed to avoid activities that are associated with hyperventilation.

Factors associated with an increased risk of stroke should be addressed. Young women should halt use of oral contraceptives. Young adults should stop smoking. Hypercholesterolemia, diabetes mellitus, and arterial hypertension also should be treated. Lowering of the blood pressure should be performed slowly and cautiously because of the strong hemodynamic vulnerability of ischemia.

Because antiplatelet agents are effective in lowering the risk of stroke among patients with prior ischemic neurological symptoms, these medications often are prescribed. Still, no data demonstrating their usefulness are available. Data about the relative effectiveness of individual antiplatelet agents are absent. In general, low doses of aspirin are prescribed first. Other options include clopidogrel or the combination of aspirin and dipyridamole. Because of the lack of utility of the combination of clopidogrel and aspirin and the potential for bleeding, this regimen probably should be avoided. Because dipyridamole does have vasodilatory effects, it might affect flow among patients with moya-moya. Because headaches are frequent among patients with moya-moya and because of the potential side effect of headache, the role of dipyridamole may be limited. Because of the potential for intracranial hemorrhage, oral anticoagulants usually are not prescribed. Vasodilatory drugs and long-term volume expansion therapy are not effective.

Because of the limited success from medical interventions and because of the high probability of recurrent strokes, several surgical interventions are recommended for both children and adults with moya-moya. The operations include superficial temporal artery–MCA anastomosis, occipital artery-MCA anastomosis, encephaloduroarteriosynangiosis, encephalomyosynangiosis, encephalogaleosynagiosis, encephaloduroarteriomyosynangiosis, multiple cranial burr holes, and omental transposition. Some patients are treated with a combination of procedures that may be done unilaterally or bilaterally. In addition, cervical carotid sympathectomy and superior cervical ganglionectomy are proposed treatment options. The primary aim of the operations is to prevent recurrent ischemia by improving blood supply to the brain via surgical creation of new collaterals; areas of borderline perfusion would receive more blood flow. In addition, the operations might lower the risk of bleeding from the moya-moya vessels by reducing pressure in these small-caliber collaterals by providing new channels for blood to reach the brain (Houkin *et al.*, 1996). A multicenter trial testing surgery among adults with moya-moya is underway (Miyamoto *et al.*, 2004). In the interim, most currently available data are based on case series (Fung *et al.*, 2005; Goda *et al.*, 2004; Golby *et al.*, 1999; Han *et al.*, 2000; Kim *et al.*, 2004, 2007; Nussbaum and Erickson, 2000; Reis *et al.*, 2006; Smith and Scott, 2005; Yoshida *et al.*, 1999).

Patients are selected for surgery on the basis of their clinical status as well as the evidence of poor perfusion demonstrated by blood flow studies. Most studies suggest a positive response to surgery. The risk of recurrent brain ischemia appears to be reduced. Kuroda *et al.* (2004) reported that surgery also lessens the likelihood of intellectual decline. Responses to revascularization procedures among patients who have presented with intracranial hemorrhage have not been as promising as those among persons who primarily had ischemic symptoms (Okada *et al.*, 1998). Most studies report that perioperative morbidity is relatively low. However, Fung *et al.* (2005) reported that the risk of stroke was approximately 4%, and another 6% had reversible ischemic symptoms in the perioperative period. Unfortunately, the operations do not have success in halting the primary arterial occlusive process. Following surgery, some regression of the moya-moya collateral vessels has been reported (Okada *et al.*, 1998). No operative procedure has been shown to be effective in preventing rebleeding (Ikezaki, Han, Kawano, *et al.*, 1997).

Although direct arterial anastomosis is considered the best way to improve blood supply, the advanced state of the intracranial arterial disease may limit the availability of recipient vessels. Although direct arterial anastomoses can be used to treat children, the small caliber of both donor and recipient vessels make surgery a challenge. Thus, alternative operations to supply collaterals to the cerebral hemisphere have been developed. These synangiosis operations involve opening the dura and placing a piece of tissue with a vascular blood supply on the pial surface of the brain. The tissue can be placed on the lateral surface of the hemisphere or along the interhemispheric fissure. The goal is to indirectly improve blood supply via angiogenesis. There is evidence that both donor and recipient vessels dilate after the operation (Nariai *et al.*, 1994). Adjacent meningeal arteries, including the middle meningeal artery, also seem to participate in developing new collateral channels. Transposition or transplantation of a piece of omentum to the pial surface of the hemisphere also has been used (Ohtaki *et al.*, 1998; Touho *et al.*, 1996). Omental tissue is selected because of its potency in stimulating angiogenesis and improving vascularity of the brain. The omental tissue is placed on an extensive area of the surface of brain along with a branch of the superficial temporal artery or in combination with a direct anastomosis. Multiple calvarial burr holes could stimulate neovascularization of the dura surface via branches of the middle meningeal artery and superficial temporal artery (Kawaguchi *et al.*, 1996). Some patients will have staged operations with surgery performed on one side of the brain and then the other. Although angioplasty has been used to treat multiple areas of stenosis of intracranial arteries in other settings, its use in moya-moya is uncertain.

The experience to date suggests that either direct or indirect revascularization procedures offer the best promise in preventing recurrent ischemic stroke. The operations should be performed early in the course of the illness to lessen the likelihood of disabling sequelae of recurrent brain ischemia including cognitive impairments and mental decline. The superiority of either a direct approach using extracranial-intracranial arterial anastomoses or an indirect approach based on synangiosis is not established. Similarly, data have not established the superiority of one indirect revascularization operation over another.

Conclusions

The term moya-moya encompasses two clinical scenarios, moya-moya disease and moya-moya syndrome. The term moya-moya disease refers to an inherited disease that is most prevalent among persons from northeastern Asia. Although cases of moya-moya

disease likely do occur in other ethnic groups, the frequency appears to be much lower. Several genetic disorders likely produce the phenotype of moya-moya disease; this finding is reflected by the two age peaks of affected persons – children and young adults. Presumably the several genetic abnormalities induce metabolic changes in endothelial cells, smooth cells, or other vascular tissues that lead to the progressive occlusive arteriopathy. These disorders also may produce a factor that promotes angiogenesis of smaller vascular structures. These changes produce the characteristic findings detected by vascular imaging. The course of moya-moya disease that becomes symptomatic in younger children seems to be more fulminant than that reported among older children and adults. We have described in detail the clinical presentations, including both hemorrhagic and ischemic stroke. The hallmark of moya-moya disease is its relentlessly progressive nature with recurrent stroke leading to cognitive impairments, profound disability, institutionalization, or death.

Moya-moya syndrome remains a nonspecific diagnosis based primarily on the radiological findings that imitate those of moya-moya disease. In the future, a common thread may be identified that will denote a subset of patients with other intracranial arterial diseases who will also develop moya-moya syndrome. At present, the best approach is to assume that the radiological changes are an epiphenomenon induced by chronic ischemia secondary to a progressive arterial process of a wide variety of etiologies. The large number of associated conditions supports the concept that the development of the mesh of the fine collateral vessels deep in the cerebral hemispheres is in response to another vascular process. The finding of a unilateral process at the time of presentation probably should raise suspicion of moya-moya syndrome rather than moya-moya disease. Clinical presentations of moya-moya syndrome appear to be less stereotypical than those of moya-moya disease. Moya-moya syndrome appears to be relatively uncommon among children younger than 10 years but probably accounts for the majority of cases in young adults. Most patients outside of northeastern Asia who have the characteristic arteriographic findings of moya-moya probably have moya-moya syndrome. Although most patients with moya-moya syndrome have recurrent ischemic and hemorrhagic events, the prognosis may not be as grim as that for patients with moya-moya disease.

Although a number of vascular diseases can lead to ischemic or hemorrhagic stroke in children, moya-moya should be considered in the differential diagnosis of potential causes. Although moya-moya is a relatively uncommon cause of stroke in young adults, it should be included in the etiologic differential diagnosis of subarachnoid hemorrhage, intracerebral hemorrhage, and cerebral infarction – especially if one of the associated conditions is identified or if no other obvious explanation for the stroke is detected. Even if the moya-moya phenomenon is detected by vascular imaging in a young person with a stroke, the patient should be assessed for other contributing causes or explanation for the arterial changes.

While brain imaging, especially MRI, provides clues for the diagnosis of moya-moya, vascular imaging, especially conventional arteriography, remains the standard way to assess the presence, location, and extent of the arterial abnormalities. Noninvasive studies of blood flow and metabolism may be used to monitor the course of the disease and to aid in the selection of patients who might benefit from revascularization procedures.

Acute treatment of ischemic stroke secondary to moya-moya probably does not differ considerably from the management of patients with stroke secondary to other causes. Treatment of hemorrhagic stroke in a patient with moya-moya should parallel that prescribed to patients with intracranial bleeding from other sources.

Prevention of recurrent stroke is the focus of management of patients with moya-moya. Direct or indirect revascularization procedures should be offered early in the course of the illness in order to prevent recurrent ischemic stroke. Antiplatelet agents are prescribed. Because of the potential of bleeding complications, oral anticoagulants usually are avoided. The underlying disease associated with moya-moya syndrome also is treated. Control of risk factors, such as hypertension and smoking, also is recommended.

REFERENCES

Andeejani, A. M., Salih, M. A., Kolawole, T., *et al.* 1998. Moya-moya syndrome with unusual angiographic findings and protein C deficiency. *J Neurol Sci*, **159**, 11–6.

Aoki, S., Hayashi, N., Abe, O., *et al.* 2002. Radiation-induced arteritis: thickened wall with prominent enhancement on cranial MR images report of 5 cases and comparison with 18 cases with moya-moya disease. *Radiology*, **223**, 683–8.

Aoyagi, M., Fukai, N., Matsushima, Y., Yamamoto, M., and Yamamoto, K. 1993. Kinetics of 125I-PDGF binding and down-regulation of PDGF receptor in arterial smooth muscle cells derived from patients with moya-moya disease. *J Cell Physiol*, **154**, 281–8.

Aoyagi, M., Fukai, N., Yamamoto, M., Matsushima, Y., and Yamamoto, K. 1997. Development of intimal thickening in superficial temporal arteries in patients with moya-moya disease. *Clin Neurol Neurosurg*, **99(Suppl 2)**, S213–7.

Aoyagi, M., Fukai, N., Yamamoto, M., *et al.* 1996. Early development of intimal thickening in superficial temporal arteries in patients with moya-moya disease. *Stroke*, **27**, 1750–4.

Arita, K., Kurisu, K., Ohba, S., *et al.* 2003. Endovascular treatment of basilar tip aneurysms associated with moya-moya disease. *Neuroradiology*, **45**, 441–4.

Battistella, P. A., and Carollo, C. 1997. Clinical and neuroradiological findings of moyamoya disease in Italy. *Clin Neurol Neurosurg*, **99(suppl 2)**, S54–7

Bitzer, M., and Topka, H. 1995. Progressive cerebral occlusive disease after radiation therapy. *Stroke*, **26**, 131–6.

Bonduel, M., Hepner, M., Sciuccati, G., Torres, A. F., and Tenembaum, S. 2001. Prothrombotic disorders in children with moya-moya syndrome. *Stroke*, **32**, 1786–92.

Bruno, A., Adams, H. P. Jr., Biller, J., *et al.* 1988. Cerebral infarction due to moya-moya disease in young adults. *Stroke*, **19**, 826–33.

Bruno, A., Yuh, W. T., Biller, J., Adams, H. P. Jr., and Cornell, S. H. 1988. Magnetic resonance imaging in young adults with cerebral infarction due to moya-moya. *Arch Neurol*, **45**, 303–6.

Camilo, O., and Goldstein, L. B. 2005. Non-atherosclerotic vascular disease in the young. *J Thromb Thrombolysis*, **20**, 93–103.

Chabrier, S., Husson, B., Lasjaunias, P., Landrieu, P., and Tardieu, M. 2000. Stroke in childhood. Outcome and recurrence risk by mechanism in 59 patients. *J Child Neurol*, **15**, 290–4.

Chen, Y. J., Kurokawa, T., Kitamoto, I., and Ueda, K. 1989 Multimodality evoked potentials in children with moya-moya disease. *Neuropediatrics*, **20**, 20–4.

Cheong, P. L., Lee, W. T., Liu, H. M., and Lin, K. H. 2005 Moya-moya syndrome with inherited proteins C and S deficiency: report of one case. *Acta Paediatr Taiwan*, **46**, 31–4.

Chiu, D., Sheddon, P., Bratina, P., and Grotta, J. C. 1998. Clinical features of moya-moya disease in the United States. *Stroke*, **29**, 1347–51.

Cloft, H. J., Kalimes, D. F., Snider, R., and Jensen, M. E. 1999 Idiopathic supraclinoid and internal carotid bifurcation steno-occlusive disease in young American adults. *Neuroradiology*, **41**, 772–6.

Cramer, S. C., Robertson, R. L., Dooling, E. C., Scott, R. M. 1996. Moya-moya and Down syndrome. Clinical and radiological features. *Stroke*, **27**, 2131–5.

Desai, S. S., Paulino, A. C., Mai, W. Y., and Teh, B. S. 2006. Radiation-induced moya-moya syndrome. *Int J Radiat Oncol Biol Physics*, **64**, 1222–7.

deVeber, G. 2003. Arterial ischemic strokes in infants and children. An overview of current approaches. *Semin Thromb Hemost*, **29**, 567–73.

Edwards-Brown, M. E., and Quets, J. P. 1997. Midwest experience with moya-moya disease. *Clin Neurol Neurosurg*, **99(Suppl 2)**, S36–8.

Fukui, M. 1997. Current state of study on moya-moya disease in Japan. *Surg Neurol*, **47**, 138–43.

Fukui, M., Kono, S., Sueishi, K., and Ikezaki, K. 2000. Moya-moya disease. *Neuropathology*, **20(Suppl)**, S61–4.

Fung, L. W., Thompson, D., and Ganesan, V. 2005. Revascularization surgery for paediatric moya-moya: a review of the literature. *Childs Nerv Syst*, **21**, 358–64.

Fushimi, Y., Miki, Y., Kikuta, K., *et al.* 2006. Comparison of 3.0 and 1.5 T three-dimensional time-of-flight MR angiography in moya-moya disease: preliminary experience. *Radiology*, **239**, 232–7.

Goda, M., Isono, M., Ishii, K., *et al.* 2004. Long-term effects of indirect bypass surgery on collateral vessel formation in pediatric moya-moya disease. *J Neurosurg*, **100(2 Suppl)**, 156–62.

Golby, A. J., Marks, M. P., Thompson, R. C., and Steinberg, G. K. 1999. Direct and combined revascularization in pediatric moya-moya disease. *Neurosurgery*, **45**, 50–8.

Gonzalez-Alegre, P., Ammache, Z., Davis, P. H., and Rodnitzky, R. L. 2003. Moya-moya-induced paroxysmal dyskinesia. *Mov Disord*, **18**, 1051–6.

Graham, J. F., and Matoba, A. 1997. A survey of moya-moya disease in Hawaii. *Clin Neurol Neurosurg*, **99(Suppl 2)**, S31–5.

Hallemeier, C. L., Rich, K. M., Grubb, R. L. Jr., *et al.* 2006. Clinical features and outcome in North American adults with moya-moya phenomenon. *Stroke*, **37**, 1490–6.

Halley, S. E., White, W. B., Ramsby, G. R., and Voytovich, A. E. 1988. Renovascular hypertension in moya-moya syndrome. Therapeutic response to percutaneous transluminal angioplasty. *Am J Hypertens*, **114(Part 1)**, 348–52.

Haltia, M., Iivanaianen, M., Majuri, H., and Puranen, M. 1982. Spontaneous occlusion of the circle of Willis (moya-moya syndrome). *Clin Neuropathol*, **1**, 11–22.

Han, D. W., Kwon, O. K., Byun, B. J., *et al.* 2000. A co-operative study. Clinical characteristics of 334 Korean patients with moya-moya disease treated at neurosurgical institutes (1976–1994). The Korean Society for Cerebrovascular Disease. *Acta Neurochirguica (Wien)*, **142**, 1263–73.

Han, H., Pyo, C. W., Yoo, D. S., *et al.* 2003. Associations of moya-moya patients with HLA class I and class II alleles in the Korean population. *J Korean Med Soc*, **18**, 876–80.

Hattori, S., Kiguchi, H., Ishii, T., Nakajima, T., and Yatsuzuka, H. 1998. Moya-moya disease with concurrent von Recklinghausen's disease and cerebral arteriovenous malformation. *Pathol Res Pract*, **196**, 363–9.

Hirano, T., Uyama, E., Tashima, K., Mita, S., and Uchino, M. 1998. An atypical case of adult moya-moya disease with initial onset of brain stem ischemia. *J Neurol Sci*, **157**, 100–4.

Hirotsune, N., Meguro, T., Kawada, S., Nakashima, H., and Ohmoto, T. 1997. Long-term follow-up study of patients with unilateral moya-moya disease. *Clin Neurol Neurosurg*, **99(Suppl 2)**, S178–81.

Hogan, A. M., Kirkham, F. J., Isaacs, E. B., Wade, A. M., and Vargha-Khadem, F. 2005. Intellectual decline in children with moya-moya and sickle cell anaemia. *Dev Med Child Neurol*, **47**, 824–9.

Hojo, M., Hoshimaru, M., Miyamoto, S., *et al.* 1998. Role of transforming growth factor-beta 1 in the pathogenesis of moya-moya disease. *J Neurosurg*, **89**, 623–9.

Holz, A., Woldenberg, R., Miller, D., *et al.* 1998. Moya-moya disease in a patient with hereditary spherocytosis. *Pediatr Radiol*, **28**, 95–7.

Horn, P., Lanczik, O., Vajkoczy, P., *et al.* 2005. Hemodynamic reserve and high-intensity transient signals in moya-moya disease. *Cerebrovasc Dis*, **19**, 141–6.

Horowitz, M., Yonas, H., and Albright, A. L. 1995. Evaluation of cerebral blood flow and hemodynamic reserve in symptomatic moya-moya disease using stable Xenon-CT blood flow. *Surg Neurol*, **44**, 251–61.

Hoshimaru, M., and Kikuchi, H. 1992. Involvement of the external carotid arteries in moya-moya disease. Neuroradiological evaluation of 66 patients. *Neurosurgery*, **31**, 398–400.

Hoshimaru, M., Takahashi, J. A., Kikuchi, H., Nagata, I., and Hatanaka, M. 1991. Possible roles of basic fibroblast growth factor in the pathogenesis of moya-moya disease. An immunohistochemical study. *J Neurosurg*, **75**, 267–70.

Hosoda, Y., Ikeda, E., and Hirose, S. 1997. Histopathological studies of spontaneous occlusion of the circle of Willis (cerebrovascular moyamoya disease). *Clin Neurol Neurosurg*, **99(Suppl 2)**, S203–8

Houkin, K., Abe, H., Yoshimoto, T., and Takahashi, A. 1996. Is unilateral moya-moya disease from moya-moya disease? *J Neurosurg*, **85**, 772–6.

Hsu, S. W., Chaloupka, J. C., and Fattal, D. 2006. Rapidly progressive fatal bihemispheric infarction secondary to moya-moya syndrome in association with Graves thyrotoxicosis. *Am J Neuroradiol*, **27**, 643–7.

Hung, C. C., Tu, Y. K., Lin, L. S., Shih, C. J. 1997. Epidemiological study of moya-moya disease in Taiwan. *Clin Neurol Neurosurg*, **99(Suppl 2)**, S23–5.

Ikeda, H., Sasaki, T., Yoshimoto, T., Fukui, M., and Arinami, T. 1999. Mapping of a familial moya-moya disease gene to chromosome 3p24.2–p26. *Am J Hum Genet*, **64**, 533–7.

Ikeda, K., Iwasaki, Y., Kashihara, H., *et al.* 2006. Adult moya-moya disease in the asymptomatic Japanese population. *J Clin Neurosci*, **13**, 334–8.

Ikezaki, K., Fukui, M., Inamura, T., *et al.* 1997a. The current status of the treatment of hemorrhagic type of moya-moya disease based on a 1995 nationwide survey in Japan. *Clin Neurol Neurosurg*, **99(Suppl 2)**, S183–6.

Ikezaki, K., Han, D. M., Kawano, T., Inamura, T.. and Kukui, M. 1997b. Epidemiological survey of moya-moya disease in Korea. *Clin Neurol Neurosurg*, **99(Suppl 2)**, S6–10.

Im, S. M., Oh, C. W., Kwon, O. K., Kim, J. E., and Han, D. H. 2005. Moya-moya disease associated with Graves disease: special considerations regarding clinical significance and management. *J Neurosurg*, **103**, 1013–7.

Imaizumi, C., Imaizumi, T., Osawa, M., Fukuyama, Y., and Takeshita, M. 1999. Serial intelligence test scores in pediatric moya-moya disease. *Neuropediatrics*, **30**, 294–9.

Inoue, T. E., Ikezaki, K., Saszzuki, T., Matsushima, T., and Fukui, M. 1997 Analysis of class II genes of human leukocyte antigen in patients with moya-moya diseases. *Clin Neurol Neurosurg*, **99(Suppl 2)**, S234–7.

Inoue, T. K., Ikezaki, K., Sasazuki, T., Matsushima, T., and Fukui, M. 2000 Linkage analysis of moya-moya disease on chromosome 6. *J Child Neurol*, **15**, 179–82.

Irikura, K., Miyasaka, Y., Kurata, A., *et al.* 1996. A source of haemorrhage in adult patients with moyamoya disease. The significance of tributaries from the choroidal artery. *Acta Neurochir (Wien)*, **138**, 1282–6.

Ishikawa, T., Kuroda, S., Nakayama, N., *et al.* 2005. Prevalence of asymptomatic microbleeds in patients with moya-moya disease. *Neurol Med Chir (Tokyo)*, **45**, 495–500.

Iwama, T., Hashimoto, M., Tsukahara, T., and Miyake, H. 1997a. Superficial temporal artery to anterior cerebral artery direct anastomosis in patients with moya-moya disease. *Clin Neurol Neurosurg*, **99(Suppl 2)**, S134–6.

Iwama, T., Horimoto, M., Hashimoto, N., *et al.* 1997b. Mechanism in intracranial bleeding in moya-moya disease. *Clin Neurol Neurosurg*, **99(Suppl 2)**, S187–90.

Iwama, T., Todaka, T., and Hashimoto, N. 1997c. Direct surgery for major artery aneurysm associated with moya-moya disease. *Clin Neurol Neurosurg*, **99(Suppl 2)**, S191–3.

Jayakumar, P. N., Vasudev, M. K., and Srikanth, S. G. 1999. Posterior circulation abnormalities in moya-moya disease: a radiological study. *Neurol India*, **47**, 112–7.

Kang, H. S., Kim, S. K., Cho, B. K., *et al.* 2006. Single nucleotide polymorphisms of tissue inhibitor of metalloproteinase genes in familial moya-moya disease. *Neurosurgery*, **58**, 1074–80.

Kassner, A., Zhu, X. P., Li, K. L., and Jackson, A. 2003. Neoangiogenesis in association with moya-moya syndrome shown by estimation of relative recirculation based on dynamic contrast-enhanced MR images. *AJNR Am J Neuroradiol*, **24**, 810–8.

Katz, D. A., Marks, M. P., Napel, S. A., Bracci, P. M., and Roberts, S. L. 1995. Circle of Willis. Evaluation with spiral CT angiography, MR angiography and conventional angiography. *Radiology*, **195**, 445–9.

Kawaguchi, S., Sakaki, T., Kakizaki, T., *et al.* 1996a. Clinical features of the hemorrhage type moya-moya disease based on 31 cases. *Acta Neurochir*, **138**, 1200–10.

Kawaguchi, S., Sakaki, T., Morimoto, T., Kakizaki, T., and Kamada, K. 1996b. Characteristics of intracranial aneurysms associated with moya-moya disease. A review of 111 cases. *Acta Neurochir*, **138**, 1287–94.

Kawaguchi, T., Fujita, S., Hosoda, K. *et al.* 1996. Multiple burr-hole operation for adult moya-moya disease. *J Neurosurg*, **84**, 468–76.

Kawano, T., Fukui, M., Hashimoto, N., and Yonekawa, Y. 1994. Follow-up study of patients with 'unilateral' moya-moya disease. *Neurol Med Chir (Tokyo)*, **34**, 744–7.

Kestle, J. R., Hoffman, H. J., and Mock, A. R. 1993. Moya-moya phenomenon after radiation for optic nerve glioma. *J Neurosurg*, **79**, 32–5.

Khan, N.. and Yonekawa, Y. 2005. Moya-moya angiopathy in Europe. *Acta Neurochir*, **94(Suppl)**, 149–52.

Kikuchi, M., Asato, M., Sugahara, S., *et al.* 1996. Evaluation of surgically formed collateral circulation in moya-moya disease with 3D-CT angiography. Comparison with MR angiography and X-ray angiography. *Neuropediatrics*, **27**, 45–9.

Kikuta, K., Takagi, Y., Nozaki, K., *et al.* 2005. Asymptomatic microbleeds in moya-moya disease. T2-weighted gradient-echo magnetic resonance imaging study. *J Neurosurg*, **102**, 470–5.

Kim, D. S., Kang, S. G., Yoo, D. S., *et al.* 2007. Surgical results in pediatric moya-moya disease: angiographic revascularization and the clinical results. *Clin Neurol Neurosurg*, **109**, 125–31. Epub 2006 Jul 26.

Kim, S. K., Seol, H. J., Cho, B. K., *et al.* 2004. Moya-moya disease among young patients: its aggressive clinical course and the role of active surgical treatment. *Neurosurgery*, **54**, 840–4.

Kodama, N., Sato, M., and Sasaki, T. 1996. Treatment of ruptured cerebral aneurysm in moya-moya disease. *Surg Neurol*, **46**, 62–6.

Konishi, Y., Kadowaki, C., Hara, M., and Takeuchi, K. 1985. Aneurysm associated with moya-moya disease. *Neurosurgery*, **16**, 484–91.

Kurlemann, G., Fahrendorf, G., Krings, W., Sciuk, J., and Palm, D. 1992. Characteristic EEG findings in childhood moya-moya syndrome. *Neurosurg Rev*, **15**, 57–60.

Kuroda, S., Houkin, K., Ishikawa, T., *et al.* 2004. Determinants of intellectual outcome after surgical revascularization in pediatric moya-moya disease: a multivariate analysis. *Childs Nerv Syst*, **20**, 302–8.

Kuroda, S., Kamiyama, H., Isobe, M., *et al.* 1995. Cerebral hemodynamics and 'rebuild-up' phenomenon on electroencephalogram in children with moya-moya disease. *Childs Nerv Syst*, **11**, 214–9.

Laborde, G., Harders, A., Klimek, L., and Hardenack, M. 1993. Correlation between clinical, angiographic, and transcranial Doppler sonographic findings in patients with moya-moya disease. *Neurol Res*, **15**, 87–92.

Leblanc, R. 1992. Cerebral amyloid angiopathy and moya-moya disease. *Neurosurg Clin North Am*, **2**, 625–36.

Lee, Y. S., Jung, K. H., and Roh, J. K. 2004. Diagnosis of moya-moya disease with transcranial Doppler sonography: correlation study with magnetic resonance angiography. *J Neuroimaging*, **14**, 319–23.

Levine, S. R., Fagan, S. C., Pessin, M. S., *et al.* 1991. Accelerated intracranial occlusive disease, oral contraceptives, and cigarette use. *Neurology*, **41**, 1893–901.

Li, B., Wang, C. C., Zhao, Z. Z., *et al.* 1991. A histological, ultrastructural and immunohistochemical study of superficial temporal arteries and middle meningeal arteries in moya-moya disease. *Acta Pathol Jpn*, **41**, 521–30.

Lichtor, T., and Mullan, S. 1987. Arteriovenous malformation in moya-moya syndrome. Report of three cases. *J Neurosurg*, **67**, 603–8.

Lim, M., Cheshier, S., and Steinberg, G. K. 2006. New vessel formation in the central nervous system during tumor growth, vascular malformations, and Moyamoya. *Curr Neurovasc Res*, **3**, 237–45.

Malek, A. M., Connors, S., Robertson, R. L., Folkman, J., and Scott, R. M. 1997. Elevation of cerebrospinal fluid levels of basic fibroblast growth factor in moya-moya and central nervous system disorders. *Pediatr Neurosurg*, **27**, 182–9.

Marushima, A., Yanaka, K., Matuski, T., Kojima, H., and Nose, T. 2006. Subarachnoid hemorrhage not due to ruptured aneurysm in moya-moya disease. *J Clin Neurosci*, **13**, 146–9.

Masuda, J., Ogata, J., and Yutani, C. 1993. Smooth muscle cell proliferation and localization of macrophages and T cells in the occlusive intracranial arteries in moya-moya disease. *Stroke*, **24**, 1960–7.

Mehrkens, J. H., Steiger, H. J., Strauss, A., and Winkler, P. A. 2006. Management of haemorrhagic type moya-moya disease with intraventricular haemorrhage during pregnancy. *Acta Neurochir (Wien)*, **148**, 685–9.

Mehta, S. H., and Adams, R. J. 2006. Treatment and prevention of stroke in children with sickle cell disease. *Curr Treat Options Neurol*, **8**, 503–12.

Mineharu, Y., Takenaka, K., Yamakawa, H., *et al.* 2006. Inheritance pattern of familial moya-moya disease: autosomal dominant mode and genomic imprinting. *J Neurol Neurosurg Psychiatry*, **77**, 1025–9.

Miyamoto, S., and Japan Adult Moya-moya Trial Group. 2004. Study design for a prospective randomized trial of extracranial-intracranial bypass surgery for adults with moya-moya disease and hemorrhagic onset – the Japan Adult Moya-moya Trial Group. *Neurol Med Chir (Tokyo)*, **44**, 218–9.

Miyamoto, S., Kikuchi, H., Karasawa, J., *et al.* 1986. Study of the posterior circulation in moya-moya disease. Part 2. Visual disturbances and surgical treatment. *J Neurosurg*, **65**, 454–60.

Miyamoto, S., Kikuchi, H., Karasawa, J., *et al.* 1984. Study of the posterior circulation in moya-moya disease. Clinical and neuroradiological evaluation. *J Neurosurg*, **61**, 1032–7.

Mootha, S. L., Riley, W. J., and Brosnan, P. G. 1999. Hypothalamic-pituitary dysfunction associated with moya-moya disease in children. *J Pediatr Endocrinol Metab*, **12**, 449–53.

Morioka, M., Hameda, J., Todaka, T., *et al.* 2003. High-risk age for rebleeding in patients with hemorrhagic moya-moya disease: long-term follow-up study. *Neurosurgery*, **52**, 1049–54.

Muizelaar, J. P. 1988. Early operation of ruptured basilar artery aneurysm associated with bilateral carotid occlusion (moya-moya disease). *Clin Neurol Neurosurg*, **90**, 349–55.

Muppala, M., and Castaldo, J. E. 1994. Unilateral supraclinoid internal carotid artery stenosis with moya-moya-like vasculopathy. Noninvasive assessments. *J Neuroimaging*, **4**, 11–6.

Murphy, M. A., Perlman, E. M., Rogg, J. M., Easton, J. D., and Schuman, J. S. 2005. Reversible carotid artery narrowing in morning glory disc anomaly. *J Neuroophthalmol*, **25**, 198–201.

Muttaqin, Z., Ohba, S., Arita, K., *et al.* 1993. Cerebral circulation in moya-moya disease. A clinical study using transcranial Doppler sonography. *Surg Neurol*, **40**, 306–13.

Nakagawara, J., Takeda, R., Suematsu, K., and Nakamura, J. 1997. Quantification of regional cerebral blood flow and vascular reserve in childhood moya-moya disease using (123) IMP-ARG method. *Clin Neurol Neurosurg*, **99(Suppl 2)**, S96–9.

Nanba, R., Kuroda, S., Tada, M., *et al.* 2006. Clinical features of familial moya-moya disease. *Childs Nerv Syst*, **22**, 258–67.

Nariai, T., Suzuki, R., Matsushima, Y., *et al.* 1994. Surgically induced angiogenesis to compensate for hemodynamic cerebral ischemia. *Stroke*, **25**, 1014–21.

Natori, Y., Ikezaki, K., Matsushima, T., and Fukui, M. 1997. 'Angiographic moya-moya' its definition, classification and therapy. *Clin Neurol Neurosurg*, **99(Suppl 2)**, S162–78.

Noda, S., Hayasaka, S., Setogawa, T., and Matsumoto, S. 1987. Ocular symptoms in moya-moya disease. *Am J Ophthalmol*, **103**, 812–6.

Numaguchi, Y., Gonzalez, C. F., Davis, P. C., *et al.* 1997. Moya-moya disease in the United States. *Clin Neurol Neurosurg*, **99(Suppl 2)**, S26–30.

Nussbaum, E. S., and Erickson, D. L. 2000. Extracranial–intracranial bypass for ischemic cerebrovascular disease refractory to maximal medical therapy. *Neurosurgery*, **46**, 37–42.

Obara, K., Fukuuchi, Y., Kobari, M., Watanabe, S., and Dembo, T. 1997. Cerebral hemodynamics in patients with moya-moya disease and in patients with atherosclerotic occlusion of the major cerebral artery trunks. *Clin Neurol Neurosurg*, **99(Suppl 2)**, S86–9.

Ohtaki, Y., Ueda, T., Morimoto, S., *et al.* 1998. Intellectual functions and regional cerebral hemodynamics after extensive omental transplantation over both frontal lobes in childhood moya-moya disease. *Acta Neurochir*, **140**, 1043–53.

Okada, Y., Shima, T., Nishida, M., *et al.* 1998. Effectiveness of superficial temporal artery-middle cerebral artery anastomosis in adult moya-moya diseases. Cerebral hemodynamics and clinical course in ischemic and hemorrhagic varieties. *Stroke*, **29**, 625–30.

Peerless, S. J. 1997. Risk factors of moya-moya disease in Canada and the USA. *Clin Neurol Neurosurg*, **99(Suppl 2)**, S45–8.

Perren, F., Meiars, S., Schmiedek, P., Hennerici, M., and Horn, P. 2005. Power Doppler evaluation of revascularization in childhood moya-moya. *Neurology*, **64**, 558–60.

Piao, R., Oku, N., Kitagawa, K., *et al.* 2004. Cerebral hemodynamics and metabolism in adult moya-moya disease: comparison of angiographic collateral circulation. *Ann Nucl Med*, **18**, 115–21.

Pracyk, J. B., and Massey, J. M. 1989. Moya-moya disease associated with polycystic kidney disease and eosinophilic granuloma. *Stroke*, **20**, 1092–4.

Quah, B. L., Hamilton, J., Blaser, S., Heon, E., and Tehrani, N. N. 2005. Morning glory disc anomaly, midline cranial defects, and abnormal carotid circulation: an association worth looking for. *Pediatr Radiol*, **35**, 525–8.

Reis, C. V., Safavi-Abbasi, S., Zabramski, J., *et al.* 2006. The history of neurosurgical procedures for moya-moya disease. *Neurosurg Focus*, **20**, E7

Robertson, R. L., Chavali, R. V., Robson, C. D., *et al.* 1998. Neurologic complications of cerebral angiography in childhood moya-moya syndrome. *Pediatr Radiol*, **28**, 824–9.

Saeki, N., Nakazaki, S., Kubota, M., *et al.* 1997. Hemorrhagic type moya-moya disease. *Clin Neurol Neurosurg*, **99(Suppl 2)**, S196–201.

Sakuri, K., Horiuchi, Y., Ikeda, H., *et al.* 2004. A novel susceptibility locus for moya-moya disease on chromosome 8q23. *J Hum Genet*, **49**, 278–81.

Salih, M. A., Murshid, W. R., Al-Salman, M. M., *et al.* 2006. Moya-moya syndrome as a risk factor for stroke in Saudi children. Novel and unusual association. *Saudi Med J*, **27(Suppl 1)**, S69–80.

Sato, S., Shirane, R., Marouka, S., and Yoshimoto, T. 1999. Evaluation of neuronal loss in adult moya-moya disease by 123I-iomazenil SPECT. *Surg Neurol*, **51**, 158–63.

Satoh, S., Shibuya, H., Matzushima, Y., and Suzuki, S. 1988. Analysis of the angiographic findings in cases of childhood moya-moya disease. *Neuroradiology*, **30**, 111–9.

Seol, H. J., Wang, K. C., Kim, S. K., *et al.* 2005. Headache in pediatric moya-moya disease: review of 204 consecutive cases. *J Neurosurg*, **103(5 Suppl)**, 439–42.

Shetty-Alva, N., and Alva, S. 2000. Familial moya-moya disease in Caucasians. *Pediatr Neurol*, **23**, 445–7.

Shimizu, H., Shitame, B., Fujiwara, S., Takahashi, A., and Yoshimoto, T. 1997. Proton magnetic resonance spectroscopy in children with moya-moya disease. *Clin Neurol Neurosurg*, **99(Suppl 2)**, S64–7.

Smith, E. R., and Scott, R. M. 2005. Surgical management of moya-moya syndrome. *Skull Base*, **15**, 15–26.

Squizzato, A., Gerdes, V. E., Brandjes, D. P., Butler, H. R., and Stam, J. 2005. Thyroid diseases and cerebrovascular disease. *Stroke*, **36**, 2302–10.

Suzui, H., Hoshimaru, M., Takahashi, J. A., *et al.* 1994. Immunohistochemical reactions for fibroblast growth factor receptor in arteries of patients with moya-moya disease. *Neurosurgery*, **35**, 20–4.

Suzuki, J. 1986. *Moya-moya Disease*. Berlin: Springer-Verlag.

Takahashi, A., Sawamura, Y., Houkin, K., Kamiyama, H., and Abe, H. 1993. The cerebrospinal fluid in patients with moya-moya disease (spontaneous occlusion of the circle of Willis) contains high levels of basic fibroblast growth factor. *Neurosci Lett*, **160**, 214–6.

Takanashi, J., Sugita, K., Ishii, M., *et al.* 1993. Moya-moya syndrome in young children. MR comparison with adult onset. *AJN Am J Neuroradiol*, **145**, 1139–43.

Takase, K., Kashihara, M., and Hashimoto, T. 1997. Transcranial Doppler ultrasonography in patients with moya-moya disease. *Clin Neurol Neurosurg*, **99(Suppl 2)**, S101–5.

Takebayashi, S., Matsuo, K., and Kaneko, M. 1984. Ultrastructural studies of cerebral arteries and collateral vessels in moya-moya disease. *Stroke*, **15**, 728–32.

Takeuchi, S., Kobayashi, K., Tsuchida, T., *et al.* 1982. Computed tomography in moya-moya disease. *J Comput Assist Tomogr*, **6**, 24–32.

Tanigawara, T., Yamada, H., Sakai, N., *et al.* 1997. Studies of cytomegalovirus and Epstein-Barr virus infection in moya-moya disease. *Clin Neurol Neurosurg*, **99(Suppl 2)**, S225–8.

Tashima-Kurita, S., Matsushima, T., Kato, M., *et al.* 1989. Moya-moya disease. Posterior cerebral artery occlusion and pattern-reversal visual-evoked potential. *Arch Neurol*, **46**, 550–3.

Touho, H., Karasawa, J., Tenjin, H., and Ueda, S. 1996. Omental transplantation using a superficial temporal artery previously used or encephaloduroarteriosynangiosis. *Surg Neurol*, **45**, 550–8.

Tsuchiya, K., Inaoka, S., Mizutani, Y., and Hachiya, J. 1998. Echo-plane perfusion MR of moya-moya disease. *Am J Neuroradiol*, 19, 211–6.

Tsuchiya, K., Makita, K., and Furui, S. 1994. Moya-moya disease. Diagnosis with three-dimensional CT angiography. *Neuroradiology*, **36**, 432–4.

Tsuda, H., Hattori, S., Tanabe, S., *et al.* 1997. Thrombophilia found in patients with moya-moya disease. *Clin Neurol Neurosurg*, **99(Suppl 2)**, S229–33.

Uchino, K., Johnston, S. C., Becker, K. J., and Tirschwell, D. L. 2005. Moya-moya disease in Washington state and California, *Neurology*, **65**, 956–8.

Wakai, K., Tamakoshi, A., Ikezaki, K., *et al.* 1997. Epidemiological features of moya-moya disease in Japan. Findings of a nationwide study. *Clin Neurol Neurosurg*, **99(Suppl 2)**, S1–5.

Watanabe, K., Negoro, T., Maehara, M., *et al.* 1990. Moya-moya disease presenting with chorea. *Pediatr Neurol*, **6**, 40–2.

Wraige, E., Pohl, K. R., Ganesan, V. 2005. A proposed classification for subtypes of arterial ischaemic stroke in children. *Dev Med Child Neurol*, **47**, 252–6.

Yamada, H., Deguchi, K., Tanigawara, T., *et al.* 1997. The relationship between moya-moya disease and bacterial infection. *Clin Neurol Neurosurg*, **99(Suppl 2)**, S221–4.

Yamada, I., Himeon, Y., Matsushima, Y., and Shibuya, H. 2000. Renal artery lesions in patients with moya-moya disease: angiographic findings. *Stroke*, **32**, 733–7.

Yamada, I., Himeno, Y., Suzuki, S., and Matsushima, Y. 1995a. Posterior circulation in moya-moya disease. Angiographic study. *Radiology*, **197**, 239–46.

Yamada, I., Murata, Y., Umehara, I., Suzuki, S., and Matsushima, Y. 1996. SPECT and MRI evaluations of the posterior circulation in moya-moya disease. *J Nucl Med*, **37**, 1613–7.

Yamada, I., Suzuki, K., and Matsushima, Y. 1995b. Moya-moya disease. Comparison of assessment with MR angiography and MR imaging versus conventional angiography. *Radiology*, **196**, 211–8.

Yamamoto, M., Aoyagi, M., Fukui, N., Matsushima, Y., and Yamamoto, K. 1998. Differences in cellular responses to mitogens in arterial smooth muscle cells dervided from patients with moya-moya disease. *Stroke*, **29**, 1188–93.

Yamamoto, M., Aoyagi, M., Tajima, S., *et al.* 1997. Increase in elastin gene progression and protein synthesis in arterial smooth muscle cells derived from patients with moya-moya disease. *Stroke*, **28**, 1733–8.

Yamashiro, Y., Takahashi, H., and Takahashi, K. 1984. Cerebrovascular moya-moya disease. *Eur J Pediatr*, **1243**, 44–50.

Yamashita, M., Oka, K. I., and Tanaka, K. 1983. Histopathology of the brain vascular network in moya-moya disease. *Stroke*, **14**, 50–8.

Yamauchi, T., Houkin, K., Tada, M., and Abe, H. 1997. Familial occurrence of moya-moya disease. *Clin Neurol Neurosurg*, **99(Suppl 2)**, S162–7.

Yamauchi, T., Tada, M., Houkin, K., *et al.* 2000. Linkage of familial moya-moya disease (spontaneous occlusion of the circle of Willis) to chromosome 17q25 *Stroke*, **32**, 930–5.

Yang, S. H., Li, B., Wang, C. C., and Zhao, J. Z. 1997. Angiographic study of moya-moya disease and histological study of the external carotid artery system. *Clin Neurol Neurosurg*, **99(Suppl 2)**, S61–3.

Yonekawa, Y., Ogata, N., Kaku, Y., Taub, E., and Imhof, H. G. 1997. Moyamoya disease in Europe, past and present status. *Clin Neurol Neurosurg*, **99(Suppl 2)**, S58–60.

Yoshida, Y., Yoshimoto, T., Shirane, R., and Sakurai, Y. 1999. Clinical course, surgical management, and long-term outcome of moya-moya patients with rebleeding after an episode of intracerebral hemorrhage. An extensive follow-up study. *Stroke*, **30**, 2272–6.

Yoshimoto, T., Houkin, K., Takahashi, A., and Abe H. 1996. Angiographic factors in moyamoya disease. *Stroke*, **27**, 2160–5.

63 DILATATIVE ARTERIOPATHY (DOLICHOECTASIA)

Louis R. Caplan and Sean I. Savitz

Dolichoectasia describes enlarged, tortuous, and dilated arteries. Because dilatation seems to be the most important feature, the condition is now often referred to as *dilatative arteriopathy*. Dilatation can be so severe that portions of the artery become a fusiform aneurysm.

Location and pathogenesis of stroke

Dilatative arteriopathy involves preferentially the intracranial vertebral and basilar arteries. Figures 63.1 and 63.2 are examples of tortuous elongated vertebrobasilar arteries. Carotid and middle cerebral artery ectasia occurs but much less often. Elongation and angulation of the intracranial arteries can stretch and distort the orifices of arterial branches leading to decreased blood flow, especially in penetrating branches of the large arteries, causing, for example, basilar artery branch territory infarcts in the pons (Passero and Filosomi, 1998; Pessin *et al.*, 1989). Transcranial Doppler studies of dolichoectatic arteries show reduced mean blood flow velocities, with relatively preserved peak flow velocities (Hennerici *et al.*, 1987; Schwartz *et al.*, 1993). Blood flow is often to and fro within the dilated artery causing reduced antegrade flow (Hennerici *et al.*, 1987; Schwartz *et al.*, 1993).

Reduced flow can lead to stagnation of the blood column and thrombus formation within dilated arterial segments (De Georgia *et al.*, 1999; Pessin *et al.*, 1989). Extensive atherosclerotic plaques, often with calcification, encroachment on the lumen of penetrating arteries that branch from the parent artery, and thrombus formation, are often found at autopsy. On microscopic examination, there are often fibrotic changes in the vessel wall, with reduced muscularis and attenuated, fragmented, or absent elastica (Pico *et al.*, 2003; Shokunbi *et al.*, 1988). Thrombi often form due to reduced blood flow in portions of the dilated lumens. Luminal thrombi may obstruct arterial branches, and portions of the clot can embolize distally (De Georgia *et al.*, 1999; Pessin *et al.*, 1989). Brain ischemia, either transient or persistent, results. Occasionally the thin dilated arteries break, leading to subarachnoid and brain hemorrhage (De Georgia *et al.*, 1999; Kubis *et al.*, 2003; Pessin *et al.*, 1989).

Compression of brain structures

Tortuous elongated arteries can compress and distort brain structures especially in the medulla and pons. Stretching of cranial nerves exiting the brainstem can lead to irritative symptoms such as trigeminal pain, hemifacial spasm (Garibaldi and Miller, 2003),

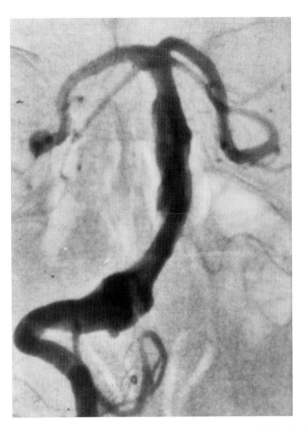

Figure 63.1 Vertebrobasilar angiogram (anteroposterior view), showing dilated tortuous left vertebral and basilar arteries.

vertigo, and tinnitus. Loss of cranial nerve function including numbness in the fifth nerve distribution, facial palsy, deafness, and so on, can develop. Lower cranial nerve neuropathies are also common (Castelnovo *et al.*, 2003). Rarely, the dilated arteries can compress the third ventricle, contributing to hydrocephalus. There are also reports that describe compression of the pons and the medulla (Savitz *et al.*, 2006) by dilated and tortuous vertebral and basilar arteries. Figure 63.3 shows an example of medullary compression by a very large curved vertebral artery. Patients with brainstem compression can present with transient symptoms or permanent deficits. Motor and vestibulocerebellar features are the most common clinical presentations (Savitz *et al.*, 2006). There is poor correlation, however, between radiographic features and symptoms (Savitz *et al.*, 2006).

In our experience, some patients have had recurrent episodes, mostly vestibulocerebellar, that can occur for years without the

Uncommon Causes of Stroke, 2nd edition, ed. Louis R. Caplan. Published by Cambridge University Press. © Cambridge University Press 2008.

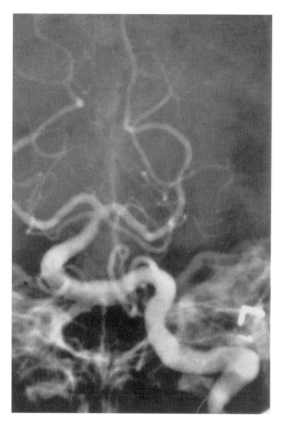

Figure 63.2 Vertebrobasilar angiogram (anteroposterior view and subtraction technique), showing very irregular dilated aneurysmal right vertebral and basilar arteries.

patient necessarily developing a stroke. Hemorrheologic and systemic vascular factors could explain these attacks, or they could be explained by reduced antegrade perfusion through dilated arteries that already show compromised fragile levels of brain perfusion.

Occurrence, pathology, and associations

Approximately one patient in eight who has brain imaging has some increase in the length and diameter of intracranial arteries (Pico *et al.*, 2004; Smoker *et al.*, 1986). Although most often recognized in adults, dilatative arteriopathy also occurs in children and adolescents. Hereditary factors probably play an important role, especially in young persons. In one family, three brothers all had large fusiform basilar artery aneurysms, and all had α-glucosidase deficiency (Makos *et al.*, 1987). Autopsy in an 11-year-old girl who died from a ruptured dolichoectatic basilar artery aneurysm showed that the artery had large gaps in the internal elastic lamina with only short segments of elastica remaining in some regions (Read and Esiri, 1979). The pathology in other young patients with dolichoectasia has shown deficiencies in the muscularis and internal elastic lamina with irregular thickness of the media, multiple gaps in the internal elastica, and regions of fibrosis. At times, the intima is thickened, and there is severe elastic tissue degeneration and an increase in the vasa vasorum (Hirsch and Roessmann, 1975). Dolichoectasia occurs in young

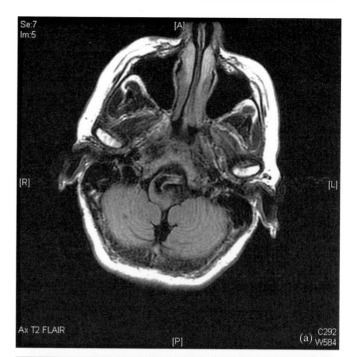

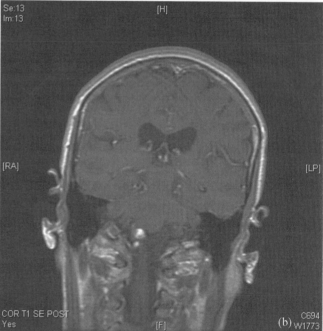

Figure 63.3 (a) Axial MRI using fluid-attenuated inversion recovery (FLAIR) techniques showing very large right vertebral artery compressing the medulla; (b) coronal view; (c) sagittal view showing the relationship of the dilated vertebral artery to the medulla oblongata.

patients with Marfan's syndrome (Silverman *et al.*, 2000; Zambrino *et al.*, 1999) and in Ehlers-Danlos syndrome. Children with AIDS and Fabry's disease (Mitsias and Levine, 1996) and children and adults with sickle cell disease also may develop dolichoectatic intracranial arteries and fusiform aneurysms. Genetic, infectious, inflammatory, immunological, and degenerative factors all may cause or contribute to the formation and progression of dolichoectasia.

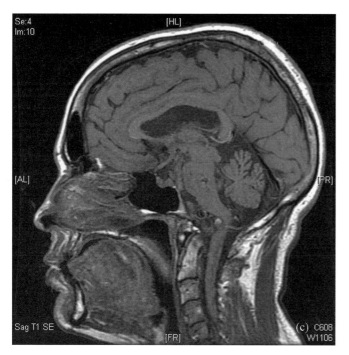

Figure 63.3 (*cont.*)

Association with vascular risk factors and penetrating artery territory brain infarcts

Amarenco and colleagues collected long-term epidemiological data on intracranial dolichoectasia, which they defined based on the consensus of subjective visual impression of two neurologists and an independent systematic reading in which the lateral position and height of bifurcation of the basilar artery was quantified and the diameters of the seven main intracranial arteries measured with a lens. Their GENIC (Etude du Profil Genetique de l'Infarctus Cerebral) studies found that dilatative arteriopathy is associated with older age, male sex, hypertension, a history of myocardial infarction, and an increased diameter of the thoracic aorta (Pico *et al.*, 2003).

Patients with dolichoectasia have also been found to have lacunar infarcts, severe leukoaraiosis, and severe etat crible (dilated Virchow-Robin spaces around penetrating arteries) (Pico *et al.*, 2005). White matter lesions and lacunar infarcts are generally attributed to disease of small penetrating intracranial arteries. Therefore, intracranial dolichoectasia is likely part of a systemic disorder involving large arteries, but is also associated with microscopic arterial disease.

The link between abnormal connective tissue in penetrating arteries and white matter abnormalities

The media and adventitia of large extracranial and intracranial arteries are composed of smooth muscle and elastic tissue in a connective tissue matrix. Small penetrating arteries have prominent medial coats. A common abnormality involving elastic fibers

or connective tissue matrix could affect both large brain-supplying and penetrating arteries.

Penetrating arterial pathology involves thickening of the arterial media that contains abnormal amounts of fibrinoid material and lipids. Dilatative arteriopathy and penetrating arterial disease are similar in that they are both diseases of the arterial wall rather than intimal-endothelialopathies. Much less research has been directed at the arterial media and adventitia than on the intima and endothelium. Abnormal connective tissue within the arterial wall affects biochemical constituents such as matrix metalloproteinases. Abnormal composition of matrix metalloproteinases can alter vascular permeability.

Rosenberg *et al.* (2001) and Pfefferkorn and Rosenberg, (2003) showed that disease of the arterial media is accompanied by up-regulation of matrix metalloproteinases (Pfefferkorn and Rosenberg, 2003; Rosenberg *et al.*, 2001). Increased activity of matrix metalloproteinases makes small arteries more permeable and loosens the blood–brain barrier. In patients with severe white matter disease, extracellular matrix macromolecules are found in increased concentrations around lacunar infarcts and within the abnormal white matter (Rosenberg *et al.*, 2001). Loosening of the blood–brain barrier can permit proteins and fluid to leak from the abnormal walls of the penetrating arteries and can lead to chronic demyelination, gliosis, and white matter damage – leukoariosis (Rosenberg *et al.*, 2001; Wardlaw *et al.*, 2003).

Many questions remain: How do the connective tissue abnormalities cause arterial dilatation? How does abnormal function of the arterial wall lead to dilatation and clinical disease? Further study of arterial dolichoectasia may yield important clues to many present cerebrovascular mysteries.

REFERENCES

Castelnovo, G., Jomir, L., Le Bayon, A., *et al.* 2003. Lingual atrophy and dolichoectatic artery. *Neurology*, **61**, 1121.

De Georgia, M., Belden, J., Pao, L., *et al.* 1999. Thrombus in vertebrobasilar dolichoectatic artery treated with intravenous urokinase. *Cerebrovasc Dis*, **9**, 28–33.

Garibaldi, D. C., and Miller, N. R. 2003. Tortuous basilar artery as cause of hemifacial spasm. *Arch Neurol*, **60**, 626–7.

Hennerici, M., Rautenberg, W., and Schwartz, A. 1987. Transcranial Doppler ultrasound for the assessment of intracranial arterial flow velocity–Part 2. Evaluation of intracranial arterial disease. *Surg Neurol*, **27**, 523–32.

Hirsch, C. S., and Roessmann, U. 1975. Arterial dysplasia with ruptured basilar artery aneurysm: report of a case. *Hum Pathol*, **6**, 749–58.

Kubis, N., Mikol, J., Von Langsdorff, D., *et al.* 2003. Dolichoectatic basilar artery: subarachnoid hemorrhage is not so rare. *Cerebrovasc Dis*, **16**, 292–5.

Makos, M. M., McComb, R. D., Hart, M. N., and Bennett, D. R. 1987. Alpha-glucosidase deficiency and basilar artery aneurysm: report of a sibship. *Ann Neurol*, **22**, 629–33.

Mitsias, P., and Levine, S. R. 1996. Cerebrovascular complications of Fabry's disease. *Ann Neurol*, **40**, 8–17.

Passero, S., and Filosomi, G. 1998. Posterior circulation infarcts in patients with vertebrobasilar dolichoectasia. *Stroke*, **29**, 653–9.

Pessin, M. S., Chimowitz, M. I., Levine, S. R., *et al.* 1989. Stroke in patients with fusiform vertebrobasilar aneurysms. *Neurology*, **39**, 16–21.

Pfefferkorn, T., and Rosenberg, G. A. 2003. Closure of the blood-brain barrier by matrix metalloproteinase inhibition reduces rtPA-mediated mortality in cerebral ischemia with delayed reperfusion. *Stroke*, **34**, 2025–30.

Pico, F., Labreuche, J., Cohen, A., Touboul, P. J., and Amarenco, P. 2004. Intracranial arterial dolichoectasia is associated with enlarged descending thoracic aorta. *Neurology*, **63**, 2016–21.

Pico, F., Labreuche, J., Touboul, P. J., and Amarenco, P. 2003. Intracranial arterial dolichoectasia and its relation with atherosclerosis and stroke subtype. *Neurology*, **61**, 1736–42.

Pico, F., Labreuche, J., Touboul, P. J., Leys, D., and Amarenco, P. 2005. Intracranial arterial dolichoectasia and small-vessel disease in stroke patients. *Ann Neurol*, **57**, 472–9.

Read, D., and Esiri, M. M. 1979. Fusiform basilar artery aneurysm in a child. *Neurology*, **29**, 1045–9.

Rosenberg, G. A., Sullivan, N., and Esiri, M. M. 2001. White matter damage is associated with matrix metalloproteinases in vascular dementia. *Stroke*, **32**, 1162–8.

Savitz, S. I., Ronthal, M., and Caplan, L. R. 2006. Vertebral artery compression of the medulla. *Arch Neurol*, **63**, 234–41.

Schwartz, A., Rautenberg, W., and Hennerici, M. 1993. Dolichoectatic intracranial arteries: review of selected aspects. *Cerebrovasc Dis*, **3**, 273–9.

Shokunbi, M. T., Vinters, H. V., and Kaufmann, J. C. 1988. Fusiform intracranial aneurysms. Clinicopathologic features. *Surg Neurol*, **29**, 263–70.

Silverman, I. E., Dike, G. L., *et al.* 2000. Vertebrobasilar dolichoectasia associated with Marfan syndrome. *J Stroke Cerebrovasc Dis*, **9**, 196–8.

Smoker, W. R., Price, M. J., Keyes, W. D., Corbett, J. J., and Gentry, L. R. 1986. High-resolution computed tomography of the basilar artery: 1. Normal size and position. *AJNR Am J Neuroradiol*, **7**, 55–60.

Wardlaw, J. M., Sandercock, P. A., Dennis, M. S., and Starr, J. 2003. Is breakdown of the blood-brain barrier responsible for lacunar stroke, leukoaraiosis, and dementia? *Stroke*, **34**, 806–12.

Zambrino, C. A., Berardinelli, A., Martelli, A., *et al.* 1999. Dolicho-vertebrobasilar abnormality and migraine-like attacks. *Eur Neurol*, **41**, 10–4.

64 PARADOXICAL EMBOLISM AND STROKE

Cyrus K. Dastur and Steven C. Cramer

Introduction

Paradoxical embolism can take many forms but generally refers to a venous clot that passes through an intracardiac shunt and produces an ischemic stroke. Convincing demonstration that a paradoxical embolism has unequivocally occurred is uncommonly present, so it is considered a rare cause of stroke. However, increasing attention to specific components of paradoxical embolism pathophysiology suggests that this might in fact be a common cause of stroke; for example, direct evidence comes from new methods for diagnosing venous thrombi, and indirect evidence comes from the increased study of patients with patent foramen ovale (PFO). Increased study is needed to clarify the precise frequency with which paradoxical embolism is the pathophysiological mechanism underlying ischemic stroke.

Paradoxical embolism refers to a circulatory event whereby material arising from the venous circulation passes paradoxically to the arterial circulation, as in the case of stroke, to the cerebral arterial circulation. The phenomenon was first described by Cohnheim (1877). Any material potentially found in venous blood can cause a paradoxical embolic stroke, including thrombus, fat, air, bone marrow, and amniotic fluid. There are important differences in pathogenesis among these different materials, for example, in the manner by which the substance accesses the arterial circulation (Horowitz, 2002; Koessler and Pitto, 2002; Parisi et al., 2002). However, the most frequently cited substances in this context are thrombi, and this chapter is restricted to this form.

The diagnosis of a paradoxical embolus can be confidently made only when four requirements are met (Chant and McCollum, 2001; Ward et al., 1995):

1. A venous thrombus as source. Note that in conditions such as stroke, where a potentially paradoxical embolism can result in new venous thrombi, the venous thrombus must be reasonably distinguished as being a cause rather than a consequence (Cramer et al., 2003), as discussed below
2. An anatomical conduit from venous to arterial circulation such as a PFO or atrial septal defect
3. A pressure gradient that promotes venous to arterial passage
4. A thrombus in the arterial circulation

The first two are the topic of increasing focus in medicine and are discussed below. The third is very common, albeit transiently, across the cardiac cycle (Adams, 2004). For example, a right-to-left cardiac pressure gradient is generated during coughing or the Valsalva maneuver (Dubourg et al., 1984), a fact that occasionally raises the question of paradoxical embolism when stroke arises during urination or defecation. The fourth, for stroke, is the cerebral arterial circulation although a paradoxical embolism can end up in any number of recipient arterial beds (Georgopoulos et al., 2001; Loscalzo, 1986; Thompson and Evans, 1930; Ward et al., 1995).

Cryptogenic stroke

Confirmation that a stroke is attributable to paradoxical embolism is uncommon; rarely are all four of the above criteria diagnosed with high certainty. Likely, a fraction of occurrences of paradoxical embolism are instead classified as cryptogenic stroke. Clues as to the cause and treatment of paradoxical embolic stroke might therefore come from literature pertaining to cryptogenic stroke.

Cryptogenic strokes are those in which an established pathophysiological mechanism is not found (Mohr, 1988). This is a common situation. Thus, across all patients with ischemic stroke, 30%–40% are cryptogenic (Albers et al., 2001; Mohr et al., 1978, 2001; Sacco et al., 1989; The National Institute of Neurological Disorders and Stroke rt-PA Stroke Study Group, 1995; The Publications Committee for the Trial of ORG 10172 in Acute Stroke Treatment [TOAST] Investigators, 1998).

Furthermore, the fraction of strokes that remains cryptogenic after careful evaluation is increased in younger stroke patients. For example, one study found that the fraction of ischemic strokes that are cryptogenic in patients age 20–45 is 31% higher than that in patients older than 45 years (Jacobs et al., 2002). In a study of patients <55 years old, no cause for stroke was apparent in 64% of them (Cabanes et al., 1993).

Cryptogenic stroke likely represents a number of different disease processes. However, some lines of evidence listed below suggest that a significant subset of cryptogenic strokes might actually be attributable to paradoxical embolism. Chief among these is the increased prevalence of a PFO in patients with cryptogenic stroke (Overell et al., 2000).

PFO

Anatomic closure of the foramen ovale normally follows functional closure after birth, but autopsy studies have found that a patent interatrial communication remains in a fraction of healthy

Uncommon Causes of Stroke, 2nd edition, ed. Louis R. Caplan. Published by Cambridge University Press. © Cambridge University Press 2008.

subjects. An early autopsy study (Thompson and Evans, 1930) found that 6% of subjects had a PFO that was pencil patent (>5 mm in diameter) and 29% of subjects had a PFO that was probe patent (2–5 mm). More recently, Hagen *et al.* (1984) found that, across all subjects at autopsy, 27.3% of subjects had a PFO with a mean diameter of 5 mm. This study also found that subjects younger than 30 years had a higher prevalence of PFO (34.3%), suggesting that the impact of any disease processes directly related to a PFO may be greater in younger patients.

Echocardiographic studies have varied in their estimates of PFO prevalence among healthy subjects, but the frequencies are generally lower than those found in autopsy studies. This finding suggests that echocardiography has reduced sensitivity for identifying PFO as compared to anatomical inspection. Note too that echocardiographic methods not only underestimate the prevalence, they also underestimate the size of PFOs. (Schuchlenz, Weihs, Beitzke, *et al.*, 2002) The prevalence of PFO found in most echocardiography studies of healthy subjects has been between 10% (Lechat *et al.*, 1988) and 22% (Hausmann *et al.*, 1992).

A PFO has been found to be present more often in patients with cryptogenic stroke than in patients with stroke of determined origin (Cabanes *et al.*, 1993; Di Tullio *et al.*, 1992; Hausmann *et al.*, 1992; Homma *et al.*, 1994, 2002; Jeanrenaud *et al.*, 1990; Job *et al.*, 1994; Klotzsch *et al.*, 1994; Lechat *et al.*, 1988; Petty *et al.*, 1997; Ranoux *et al.*, 1993; Steiner *et al.*, 1998) or in healthy controls (Cabanes *et al.*, 1993; de Belder *et al.*, 1992; De Castro *et al.*, 2000; Hausmann *et al.*, 1992; Job *et al.*, 1994; Lechat *et al.*, 1988; Webster *et al.*, 1988). This finding has been confirmed in both young and aged patient populations (de Belder *et al.*, 1992; Di Tullio *et al.*, 1992). However, not all studies support this association; for example, Meissner *et al.* (2006), in a prospective, population-based study of 585 randomly sampled subjects examined by a single echocardiographer, found that the presence of a PFO was not a predictor of stroke over a 5-year period.

Some of the uncertainty regarding the relationship between PFO and cryptogenic stroke might be, in part, because of methodological differences between studies (Petty *et al.*, 1997). For example, differences in methods of studying patients with cryptogenic stroke have resulted in a wide range of prevalence rates reported for PFO, from 20% (Jones *et al.*, 1994) to 78% (Klotzsch *et al.*, 1994), although the majority of studies report rates of 42%–57%. Variance from the latter range is largely related to two factors. First, the association appears to be weaker for transient ischemic attack (TIA) than for stroke. Thus most studies enrolling patients with TIA have the lowest rates (20%–26%) of PFO in cryptogenic stroke patients (de Belder *et al.*, 1992; Jones *et al.*, 1994). Second, the choice of contrast agent influences sensitivity for detecting PFO. Most studies using contrast agents besides saline agitated with air have the highest rates (66%–78%) of PFO in cryptogenic stroke patients (Job *et al.*, 1994; Klotzsch *et al.*, 1994).

Other factors can influence sensitivity for detecting PFO. Transesophageal echocardiography (TEE) has approximately twofold greater sensitivity for diagnosing PFO as compared to transthoracic echocardiography (TTE) (Hausmann *et al.*, 1992; Lethen *et al.*, 1997), although the addition of harmonic imaging using saline contrast can increase the sensitivity of TTE (Ha *et al.*, 2001).

Transcranial Doppler (TCD) has sensitivity that approaches that of TEE (Droste *et al.*, 2002; Klotzsch *et al.*, 1994; Stendel *et al.*, 2000), but decreased specificity. While TCD provides less information on cardiac structure than does echocardiography, it is more sensitive to extracardiac right-to-left shunts.

The choice of vein used to introduce echocardiographic contrast also influences the sensitivity for detecting a PFO. Blood entering the right atrium via the inferior vena cava (IVC) is more directed towards the interatrial septum region where a PFO is found, as compared to blood entering the right atrium via the superior vena cava. Studies have been consistent in finding a 2.5-fold increase in diagnostic sensitivity for a PFO when agitated saline contrast was injected via the femoral vein rather than the antecubital vein (Gin *et al.*, 1993; Hamann *et al.*, 1998).

The coexistence of other cardiac findings increases the strength of association between PFO and paradoxical embolism. For example, a PFO with concomitant atrial septal aneurysm (ASA) is also found more often in patients with cryptogenic stroke, particularly younger patients, and when both are present the risk of stroke recurrence increases sharply (Overell *et al.*, 2000). A dual diagnosis of PFO and ASA may have a particularly important association with stroke recurrence (Mas *et al.*, 2001; Messe *et al.*, 2004). Some authors have suggested that an ASA may in part be a reflection of a larger PFO size (Schuchlenz, Saurer, and Weihs, 2002). Others have speculated that this association is based on a flapping motion of the ASA that directs small thrombi coming from the IVC into a PFO (De Castro *et al.*, 2000). Persistence of a prominent eustachian valve and right atrial filamentous strands have also been associated with increased association of PFO with paradoxical embolism (Schneider *et al.*, 1995). The ASA also could promote local thrombosis at the site of dilatation of the atrial septal bulge.

A number of factors suggest that a significant fraction of cryptogenic strokes might be due to paradoxical embolism. The observation that cryptogenic stroke has in most studies been associated with an increased prevalence of PFO is one line of support for a model whereby a PFO is a conduit for a paradoxical thromboembolism to the brain. Clinical characteristics commonly found in patients with cryptogenic stroke provide further support for this model. Thus, a second link between cryptogenic stroke and paradoxical embolism is that the topography of cerebral infarct in patients with cryptogenic stroke and PFO is often suggestive of an embolic mechanism (Sacco *et al.*, 1989; Steiner *et al.*, 1998). Note that paradoxical emboli show a relatively high rate of involvement of the posterior circulation (Steiner *et al.*, 1998). Third, several studies suggest that PFO size is greater in patients with cryptogenic stroke than in normal subjects or patients with stroke of determined origin (Hausmann *et al.*, 1995; Homma *et al.*, 1994, 2002; Petty *et al.*, 1997; Schuchlenz *et al.*, 2000; Steiner *et al.*, 1998; Webster *et al.*, 1988). However, PFO size is not related to risk of stroke recurrence (Homma *et al.*, 2002; Kerut *et al.*, 2001). Fourth, the prevalence of PFO patency at rest, i.e. without induction of a Valsalva-related pressure gradient, may be greater in patients with stroke than in control subjects (De Castro *et al.*, 2000). Fifth, on rare occasion, a thrombus can be imaged as it traverses a PFO (Aggarwal *et al.*, 2002).

Deep venous thrombosis

A sixth line of evidence supporting a model whereby crypto-genic stroke arises on the basis of a paradoxical embolism passing through a PFO is that some studies show an increased prevalence of lower extremity deep venous thrombosis (DVT) in this sub-population. Gautier *et al.* (1991) performed venography 2 days to 7 months after cryptogenic TIA or stroke and found that 3 of 23 patients with PFO had leg DVT and three others had left common iliac vein compression. Ranoux *et al.* (1993) performed venogra-phy within 4 weeks of cryptogenic stroke and found that 1 of 13 patients with PFO had a leg DVT. Lethen *et al.* (1997) performed venography an average of 8 days after TIA or stroke of suspected cardiac origin, and found that 5 of 53 patients with PFO had iliac or calf DVT. Cramer *et al.* (2004) found that 9 of 46 patients with cryptogenic stroke and PFO studied with MRI venography (MRV) an average of 2 days after stroke had evidence for a pelvic DVT. Another study (Stollberger *et al.*, 1993) found a leg or pelvic DVT in 19 of 29 patients with PFO and a cryptogenic arterial, mostly cere-bral, embolus; however, five patients in this study had atrial fibril-lation as an alternative explanation for the embolic event, a rather high 13 of 29 patients had a history of prior venous thrombosis, and venograms were performed up to 90 days after the embolic event occurred, which might have captured the presence of poststroke DVTs that were a consequence, rather than a cause, of stroke. These concerns highlight some of the pitfalls in examining the relation-ship between PFO and cryptogenic stroke. We have defined a stan-dard for relating PFO and cryptogenic stroke on a "probable" basis (Cramer *et al.*, 2003), as reviewed below.

Note too that PFO and right-to-left intracardiac shunts have been linked with other brain disorders including migraine (Tobis and Azarbal, 2005) and cerebral complications of scuba divers, astronauts, and aviators (Foster *et al.*, 2003).

Of course, the presence of a PFO in association with crypto-genic stroke could also reflect pathophysiological events other than paradoxical embolism, such as direct embolization from a thrombus formed within a PFO or associated ASA, or an associ-ated atrial arrhythmia (Ay *et al.*, 1998; Berthet *et al.*, 2000; Lamy *et al.*, 2002; Overell *et al.*, 2000).

There are a number of limitations in interpreting data linking DVT with PFO-related stroke. Most studies addressing this point have evaluated only a subset, rather than a consecutive cohort, of stroke patients. Also, many studies have evaluated only part of the lower extremity venous system, or have used methods with lim-ited sensitivity in portions of the lower extremity venous system. Another frequent limitation has been the absence of an appro-priate control group, an important concern given the substantial increase in DVT prevalence that is found beginning approximately day 4 poststroke (Kelly *et al.*, 2001; Warlow *et al.*, 1976). These observations might explain why reported rates of DVT have varied so widely in prior studies of patients with PFO and cryptogenic stroke.

That venous thromboembolism occurs commonly in humans is not in doubt; indeed, estimates are that 600 000 incidents of pul-monary embolism occur each year in the United States (Fedullo and Tapson, 2003). That PFO is common in humans is also not in doubt. Whether the venous system has been consistently and sen-sitively interrogated in patients with PFO and cryptogenic stroke, however, is not clear. Thus it is possible that a thromboembolic source has rarely been found in patients with cryptogenic stroke because previously employed methods have lacked the sensitivity to consistently detect all relevant venous thrombi. Clinical diagno-sis of DVT is unreliable (Kearon and Hirsh, 1994). Contrast venog-raphy and ultrasonography are sensitive to DVT in the thigh but not in the pelvis (Bergqvist and Bergentz, 1990). The sensitivity of contrast venography for pelvic vein pathology can be improved by selectively cannulating these veins (Wheeler and Anderson, 1995), but this has infrequently been done because of the invasiveness of this procedure.

Data on prothrombotic states bolster the link between DVT and cryptogenic stroke. Bendixen *et al.* (2001), in a study of 1943 patients with stroke, concluded that prothrombotic states are a particularly important consideration in patients 15–35 years of age. Hypercoagulable disorders have been reported to be more common in younger patients with stroke (Chaturvedi, 1998; Dodge *et al.*, 2004; Tatlisumak and Fisher, 1996). Consistent with this, Pezzini *et al.* (2003) found that PFO played a pathogenic role in 36 of 125 young (mean age 35 years) patients with ischemic stroke. Among these 36 with PFO, the prevalence of a prothrombotic genetic variant, particularly the prothrombin G20210 A variant, was significantly increased as compared to patients in whom PFO was either absent or unrelated to stroke.

Venous thrombus sources with low impact on the lungs might have high impact on the brain

Diagnosis of a venous thrombus would influence the likelihood of diagnosing a cryptogenic stroke as due to paradoxical embolism, but venous evaluation is often incomplete. One issue that may be particularly important in this regard is evaluation of calf veins. Isolated calf vein DVT is more common than DVT in any other site following stroke (Landi *et al.*, 1992; Warlow *et al.*, 1976) and at autopsy (Havig, 1977a), and so also may be important before stroke. Proximal propagation may occur in 20%–28% of calf vein DVTs (Lohr *et al.*, 1995; Philbrick and Becker, 1988). Emboliza-tion can occur without propagation. For example, an isolated calf DVT was found at autopsy in 36%–46% of patients with pulmonary embolism (Havig, 1977b). Emboli from calf vein thrombi tend to be small and asymptomatic on reaching the lung (Hirsh and Hoak, 1996; Salzman, 1986), and in general medical practice, little emphasis is placed on treatment of calf vein DVT when extension to popliteal veins has not occurred (Kearon *et al.*, 1998).

A paradigmatic shift in thinking about calf vein thromboemboli may be needed when the final vascular bed is cerebral rather than pulmonary. That is, an embolus from a calf vein might be of little physiological significance upon reaching the pulmonary circula-tion, but of highly clinical significance upon reaching the cere-bral circulation (Mohr, 1988). DVT from calf veins may not be rare and, although of little significance to the lungs, can cause serious brain injury upon reaching the arterial circulation. A recent case series described several cryptogenic stroke patients with a calf vein DVT and PFO in whom the calf DVT was established as the cause of stroke on a probable basis (Cramer *et al.*, 2003). The high frequency of calf vein thromboemboli might be reasonably ignored when assessing embarrassment to pulmonary physiology, but in the setting of a right-to-left intracardiac shunt with cryptogenic brain embolism, this process requires more consideration.

Another issue of possible importance in the context of PFO and paradoxical stroke is evaluation of the pelvic veins. Autopsy studies have shown isolated pelvic vein or IVC thrombus in 16% of patients with pulmonary emboli (Modan *et al.*, 1972), and in autopsy studies of patients with a paradoxical embolism, the pelvic veins were the only source of thromboemboli in 22% of patients (Corrin, 1964; Johnson, 1951). A consecutive study of 769 MRI venograms (Spritzer *et al.*, 2001) found that 20% of the 167 DVTs identified were isolated to the pelvic veins. Pelvic DVTs have been described in patients with cryptogenic pulmonary embolism (Au *et al.*, 2001; Loud *et al.*, 2001; Stern *et al.*, 2002) and in patients with cryptogenic stroke with PFO (Cramer *et al.*, 1998, 2003; Greer and Buonanno, 2001; Noser *et al.*, 2001).

The Paradoxical Embolism from Large Veins in Ischemic Stroke (PELVIS) study (Cramer *et al.*, 2004) performed a pelvic MRV within 72 hours of stroke onset in young (18- to 60-year-old) consecutive stroke patients at five US academic centers. Testing to identify the cause of stroke was later performed during hospitalization. This study was designed to test the hypothesis that patients with cryptogenic stroke have an increased prevalence of pelvic DVTs as compared to patients with stroke of determined origin. This time cutoff of 72 hours was selected to minimize the influence of DVT arising after stroke onset. The age cutoff was selected to focus on young stroke patients given that the link between PFO and cryptogenic stroke is strongest in this group (Overell *et al.*, 2000). Enrolled patients had a mean age of 46 years. The PELVIS study found that patients with cryptogenic stroke (*n* = 46), compared to those with stroke of determined origin (*n* = 49), showed several significant differences, including younger age, higher prevalence of PFO (61% vs. 19%), and fewer atherosclerosis risk factors. Most importantly, cryptogenic patients had more MRV scans with a high probability for pelvic DVT (20%) than did patients with stroke of determined origin (4%, *p* <.03), with most of these having an appearance of a chronic DVT. The most commonly involved pelvic vein was the external iliac vein, followed by the common iliac vein, consistent with a prior report of pelvic DVT distribution in a more general population (Spritzer *et al.*, 2001). A limitation of this study was that inter-rater reliability for MRV interpretation was not high.

Superficial lower extremity veins have been associated with pulmonary embolism in a surprising proportion of cases, up to 33% (Leon *et al.*, 2005; Unno *et al.*, 2002; Verlato *et al.*, 1999). This result suggests that this venous system might be an important source of paradoxical thromboembolism. Any venous system that can give rise to pulmonary emboli, including the cerebral dural sinuses (Cakmak *et al.*, 2005), could potentially be a source of paradoxical emboli.

Further studies are needed to understand the significance of calf, pelvic, and other DVT in the pathogenesis of PFO-associated cryptogenic stroke. In some institutions, lower extremity venous duplex examinations do not include study of calf veins, but identification of such small DVTs might be necessary in the context of cryptogenic stroke. Imaging the pelvic veins traditionally has been limited. Bilateral contrast venography and other diagnostic methods have reduced diagnostic sensitivity for pelvic DVT (Bergqvist and Bergentz, 1990; Kelly *et al.*, 2001; Wheeler and Anderson, 1995). MRV was of diagnostic value in the PELVIS study (Cramer *et al.*, 2004), but inter-rater reliability was not high. A number of investigators are now examining improved methods to image lower extremity/pelvic veins, including gadolinium-enhanced MRV (Obernosterer *et al.*, 2002), MR direct thrombus imaging (Fraser *et al.*, 2002), venous enhanced subtracted peak arterial MRV (Fraser *et al.*, 2003), CT venography (Au *et al.*, 2001; Loud *et al.*, 2001), and signal-enhanced Doppler (Puls *et al.*, 1999).

Pulmonary embolism and paradoxical embolism

The incidence of paradoxical embolism in patients with acute pulmonary embolism has been estimated to be as high as 60% (Loscalzo, 1986). There is little controversy in the assertion that most pulmonary emboli occur due to venous thromboembolism, yet the proportion of pulmonary emboli that are classified as cryptogenic, i.e. in which no source of venous thrombus can be identified, might be as high as 23% (Loud *et al.*, 2001) to 50% (Fedullo and Tapson, 2003).

Right heart pressures often increase in parallel with pulmonary embolism, suggesting that a venous thromboembolic shower could increase the likelihood of paradoxical embolism. Data from one study support this hypothesis (Miller *et al.*, 1997). Also, patients with coexistent PFO and acute pulmonary embolism (whether the latter is hemodynamically significant or not) have elevated right-sided cardiac pressures. These cause an increase in right-to-left shunting through a PFO and a higher chance of further emboli migrating through the PFO to the cerebral arterial circulation (Maldjian *et al.*, 2006; Miller *et al.*, 1997). Consistent with this, among patients with pulmonary embolism, the rate of stroke is significantly higher when PFO is present (Konstantinides *et al.*, 1998).

Therapeutic considerations

When the presence of a paradoxical embolism is confirmed with high confidence, standard therapeutic responses to both the venous source of thrombus as well as the arterial embolus are invoked. However, in most cases, evidence for a paradoxical embolism is circumstantial and/or incomplete, and uncertainties in treatment exist at several levels.

The rate of stroke recurrence after a cryptogenic stroke is unclear, further complicating clinical decision making. In patients with cryptogenic stroke and/or TIA, reported annual rates of recurrence have included 16% (Comess *et al.*, 1994), 5.4% (De Castro *et al.*, 2000), 3.4% (Mas *et al.*, 1995), and 3.8% in one study where 84% of strokes were cryptogenic (Bogousslavsky *et al.*, 1996). Mas *et al.* (2001) found a stroke recurrence rate of 1% when both PFO and ASA were absent versus 3.8% when both were present. A recent large, prospective study found that the combined annual rate of death or recurrent ischemic stroke among patients with cryptogenic stroke was 7.8% (Mohr *et al.*, 2001), although a substudy found that the annual rate of death or recurrent stroke after a cryptogenic stroke was not significantly different when PFO was (7.2%) or was not (6.4%) present (Homma *et al.*, 2002). A recent meta-analysis concluded that "PFO is not associated with increased risk of subsequent stroke or death among medically treated patients with cryptogenic stroke. However, both PFO and ASA possibly increase the risk of subsequent stroke (but not death) in medically treated patients younger than 55 years" (Messe *et al.*, 2004). Future studies might examine the hypothesis that specific subgroups of patients with PFO and stroke can be identified in whom the risk of stroke recurrence is increased (Tong and Becker, 2004).

When concern for paradoxical embolism as the cause of stroke is high, several therapeutic options are available for secondary stroke prevention including antiplatelet agents, anticoagulation, and closure of the PFO via either a transcatheter or surgical approach. The risk-to-benefit ratio among these choices, however, remains unclear (McGaw and Harper, 2001; Wu *et al.*, 2004).

However, confidence that a cryptogenic stroke is because of paradoxical embolism is more often modest. Treatment of stroke in such a setting therefore remains controversial. Some experts recommend that secondary stroke prevention in a patient with a cryptogenic stroke, with or without PFO, is satisfactorily achieved with an antiplatelet agent (Albers *et al.*, 2004). Retrospective data suggest the possibility that warfarin could be superior to antiplatelet therapy (Orgera *et al.*, 2001). Consistent with this, one model suggests that, if the estimated risk of paradoxical stroke recurrence is >0.8% per year, secondary stroke prevention should be achieved with either anticoagulation or PFO closure (Nendaz *et al.*, 1998). PFO closure also has been advocated by some, and is under study in clinical trials (Furlan, 2004; Hara *et al.*, 2005).

Secondary stroke prevention in a patient with ischemic stroke and PFO remains unclear. Our approach to therapeutic decision making in the setting of ischemic stroke often involves prescription of an antiplatelet medication. The highest support for PFO closure is when a concomitant ASA is present. Warfarin is indicated only if a specific therapeutic target is present, such as a prothrombotic state, concomitant pulmonary embolism, or ischemic stroke arising from a DVT passing through a PFO as a paradoxical embolism on a probable basis. We have defined "probable basis" (Cramer *et al.*, 2003) as a diagnosis of a DVT less than 4 days (Warlow *et al.*, 1976) after stroke onset in the presence of a right-to-left intracardiac shunt such as PFO. Therefore, in this context, diagnostic evaluation should include imaging of the venous circulation including calf, popliteal, femoral, and pelvic veins. Hematological evaluation for both venous and arterial hypercoagulable states is included.

Conclusions

Cryptogenic stroke remains a common diagnosis, PFO is likely present with increased frequency in this setting, and several lines of evidence suggest a role of a PFO in stroke pathogenesis. These facts particularly pertain to younger stroke patients. Together, these data suggest that paradoxical embolism might account for an important fraction of ischemic strokes and be far from rare. However, further studies are needed in patients with cryptogenic stroke

and PFO, such as those related to prothrombic states, venous thrombosis, and thromboembolism recurrence, in order to clarify the frequency with which a paradoxical embolism has occurred. A paradigmatic shift in thinking about DVT in the small lower extremity veins, such as calf veins, may be needed, as emboli of no significance to the lung could, upon reaching the arterial circulation, cause substantial brain ischemia and disability. Preventing TIA, stroke, and death after a diagnosis of cryptogenic stroke may be best guided by a better understanding of the various pathophysiologies underlying PFO-associated cryptogenic stroke.

REFERENCES

Adams, H. P. Jr. 2004. Patent foramen ovale: paradoxical embolism and paradoxical data. *Mayo Clin Proc*, **79**, 15–20.

Aggarwal, K., Jayam, V. K., Meyer, M. A., Nayak, A. K., and Nathan, S. 2002. Thrombus-in-transit and paradoxical embolism. *J Am Soc Echocardiogr*, **15**, 1021–2.

Albers, G., Amarenco, P., Easton, J., Sacco, R., and Teal, P. 2001. Antithrombotic and thrombolytic therapy for ischemic stroke. *Chest*, **119**, 300S–320S.

Albers, G., Amarenco, P., Easton, J., Sacco, R., and Teal, P. 2004. Antithrombotic and thrombolytic therapy for ischemic stroke: the Seventh ACCP Conference on Antithrombotic and Thrombolytic Therapy. *Chest*, **126**, 483S–512S.

Au, V., Walsh, G., and Fon, G. 2001. Computed tomography pulmonary angiography with pelvic venography in the evaluation of thrombo-embolic disease. *Australas Radiol*, **45**, 141–5.

Ay, H., Buonanno, F., Abraham, S., Kistler, J., and Koroshetz, W. 1998. An electrocardiographic criterion for diagnosis of patent foramen ovale associated with ischemic stroke. *Stroke*, **29**, 1393–7.

Bendixen, B., Posner, J., and Lango, R. 2001. Stroke in young adults and children. *Curr Neurol Neurosci Rep*, **1**, 54–66.

Bergqvist, D., and Bergentz, S. E. 1990. Diagnosis of deep vein thrombosis. *World J Surg*, **14**, 679–87.

Berthet, K., Lavergne, T., Cohen, A., *et al.* 2000. Significant association of atrial vulnerability with atrial septal abnormalities in young patients with ischemic stroke of unknown cause. *Stroke*, **31**, 398–403.

Bogousslavsky, J., Garazi, S., Jeanrenaud, X., *et al.* 1996. Stroke recurrence in patients with patent foramen ovale: The Lausanne Study. *Neurology*, **46**, 1301–5.

Cabanes, L., Mas, J., Cohen, A., *et al.* 1993. Atrial septal aneurysm and patent foramen ovale as risk factors for cryptogenic stroke in patients less than 55 years of age. A study using transesophageal echocardiography. *Stroke*, **24**, 1865–73.

Cakmak, S., Nighoghossian, N., Desestret, V., *et al.* 2005. Pulmonary embolism: an unusual complication of cerebral venous thrombosis. *Neurology*, **65**, 1136–7.

Chant, H., and McCollum, C. 2001. Stroke in young adults: the role of paradoxical embolism. *Thromb Haemost*, **85**, 22–9.

Chaturvedi, S. 1998. Coagulation abnormalities in adults with cryptogenic stroke and patent foramen ovale. *J Neurol Sci*, **160**, 158–60.

Cohnheim, J. 1877. *Thrombose und Embolie, Vorlesungen Über Allgemeine Pathologie; ein Handbuch fur Aertze und Studierende*. Berlin: Hirschwald.

Comess, K., DeRook, F., Beach, K., *et al.* 1994. Transesophageal echocardiography and carotid ultrasound in patients with cerebral ischemia: prevalence of findings and recurrent stroke risk. *J Am Coll Cardiol*, **23**, 1598–603.

Corrin, B. 1964. Paradoxical embolism. *Br Heart J*, 26, 549–53.

Cramer, S., Maki, J., Waitches, G., *et al.* 2003. Paradoxical emboli from calf and pelvic veins in cryptogenic stroke. *J Neuroimaging*, **13**, 218–23.

Cramer, S., Rordorf, G., Kaufman, J., *et al.* 1998. Clinically occult pelvic-vein thrombosis in cryptogenic stroke. *Lancet*, **351**, 1927–8.

Cramer, S., Rordorf, G., Maki, J., *et al.* 2004. Increased pelvic vein thrombi in cryptogenic stroke: results of the Paradoxical Emboli from Large Veins in Ischemic Stroke (PELVIS) study. *Stroke*, **35**, 46–50.

de Belder, M., Tourikis, L., Leech, G., and Camm, A. 1992. Risk of patent foramen ovale for thromboembolic events in all age groups. *Am J Cardiol*, **69**, 1316–20.

De Castro, S., Cartoni, D., Fiorelli, M., *et al.* 2000. Morphological and functional characteristics of patent foramen ovale and their embolic implications. *Stroke*, **31**, 2407–13.

Di Tullio, M., Sacco, R., Gopal, A., Mohr, J., and Homma, S. 1992. Patent foramen ovale as a risk factor for cryptogenic stroke. *Ann Intern Med*, **117**, 461–5.

Dodge, S. M., Hassell, K., Anderson, *et al.* 2004. Antiphospholipid antibodies are common in patients referred for percutaneous patent foramen ovale closure. *Catheter Cardiovasc Interv*, **61**, 123–7.

Droste, D., Lakemeier, S., Wichter, T., *et al.* 2002. Optimizing the technique of contrast transcranial Doppler ultrasound in the detection of right-to-left shunts. *Stroke*, 33, 2211–6.

Dubourg, O., Rigaud, M., and Bardet, J. 1984. Contrast echocardiographic visualization of cough-induced right-to-left shunt through a patent foramen ovale. *J Am Coll Cardiol*, **4**, 587–94.

Fedullo, P. F., and Tapson, V. F. 2003. Clinical practice. The evaluation of suspected pulmonary embolism. *N Engl J Med*, **349**, 1247–56.

Foster, P. P., Boriek, A. M., Butler, B. D., Gernhardt, M. L., and Bove, A. A. 2003. Patent foramen ovale and paradoxical systemic embolism: a bibliographic review. *Aviat Space Environ Med*, **74**, B1–64.

Fraser, D., Moody, A., Davidson, I., Martel, A., and Morgan, P. 2003. Deep venous thrombosis: diagnosis by using venous enhanced subtracted peak arterial MR venography versus conventional venography. *Radiology*, **226**, 812–20.

Fraser, D., Moody, A., Morgan, P., Martel, A., and Davidson, I. 2002. Diagnosis of lower-limb deep venous thrombosis: a prospective blinded study of magnetic resonance direct thrombus imaging. *Ann Intern Med*, **136**, 89–98.

Furlan, A. 2004. Patent foramen ovale and recurrent stroke: closure is the best option: yes. *Stroke*, **35**, 803–4.

Gautier, J., Durr, A., Koussa, S., Lasault, G., and Grosgogeat, T. 1991. Paradoxical cerebral embolism with a patent foramen ovale. *Cerebrovasc Dis*, **1**, 193–202.

Georgopoulos, S., Chronopoulos, A., Dervisis, K., and Arvanitis, D. 2001. Paradoxical embolism. An old but, paradoxically, under-estimated problem. *J Cardiovasc Surg (Torino)*, **42**, 675–7.

Gin, K., Huckell, V., and Pollick, C. 1993. Femoral vein delivery of contrast medium enhances transthoracic echocardiographic detection of patent foramen ovale. *J Am Coll Cardiol*, **22**, 1994–2000.

Greer, D., and Buonanno, F. 2001. Cerebral infarction in conjunction with patent foramen ovale and May-Thurner syndrome. *J Neuroimaging*, **11**, 432–4.

Ha, J., Shin, M., Kang, S., *et al.* 2001. Enhanced detection of right-to-left shunt through patent foramen ovale by transthoracic contrast echocardiography using harmonic imaging. *Am J Cardiol*, **87**, 669–71, A11.

Hagen, P., Scholz, D., and Edwards, W. 1984. Incidence and size of patent foramen ovale during the first 10 decades of life: an autopsy study of 965 normal hearts. *Mayo Clin Proc*, **59**, 17–20.

Hamann, G., Schatzer-Klotz, D., Frohlig, G., *et al.* 1998. Femoral injection of echo contrast medium may increase the sensitivity of testing for a patent foramen ovale. *Neurology*, **50**, 1423–8.

Hara, H., Virmani, R., Ladich, E., *et al.* 2005. Patent foramen ovale: current pathology, pathophysiology, and clinical status. *J Am Coll Cardiol*, **46**, 1768–76.

Hausmann, D., Mugge, A., Becht, I., and Daniel, W. 1992. Diagnosis of patent foramen ovale by transesophageal echocardiography and association with cerebral and peripheral embolic events. *Am J Cardiol*, 70, 668–72.

Hausmann, D., Mugge, A., and Daniel, W. 1995. Identification of patent foramen ovale permitting paradoxic embolism. *J Am Coll Cardiol*, **26**, 1030–8.

Havig, O. 1977a. Deep vein thrombosis. *Acta Chir Scand*, **Suppl 478**, 4–11.

Havig, O. 1977b. Source of pulmonary emboli. *Acta Chir Scand*, **Suppl 478**, 42–7.

Hirsh, J., and Hoak, J. 1996. Management of deep vein thrombosis and pulmonary embolism. A statement for healthcare professionals. Council on Thrombosis (in consultation with the Council on Cardiovascular Radiology), American Heart Association. *Circulation*, **93**, 2212–45.

Homma, S., Di Tullio, M., Sacco, R., *et al.* 1994. Characteristics of patent foramen ovale associated with cryptogenic stroke. A biplane transesophageal echocardiographic study. *Stroke*, **25**, 582–6.

Homma, S., Sacco, R., Di Tullio, M., *et al.* 2002. Effect of medical treatment in stroke patients with patent foramen ovale: patent foramen ovale in the Cryptogenic Stroke Study. *Circulation*, **105**, 2625–31.

Horowitz, P. E. 2002. Fat embolism. *Anaesthesia*, **57**, 830–1; discussion 831.

Jacobs, B., Boden-Albala, B., Lin, I., and Sacco, R. 2002. Stroke in the young in the northern Manhattan stroke study. *Stroke*, **33**, 2789–93.

Jeanrenaud, X., Bogousslavsky, J., Payot, M., Regli, F., and Kappenberger, L. 1990. Patent foramen ovale and cerebral infarct in young patients. *Schweiz Med Wochenschr*, **120**, 823–9.

Job, F., Ringelstein, E., Grafen, Y., *et al.* 1994. Comparison of transcranial contrast Doppler sonography and transesophageal contrast echocardiography for the detection of patent foramen ovale in young stroke patients. *Am J Cardiol*, **74**, 381–4.

Johnson, B. 1951. Paradoxical emboli. *J Clin Pathol*, **4**, 316–32.

Jones, E., Calafiore, P., Donnan, G., and Tonkin, A. 1994. Evidence that patent foramen ovale is not a risk factor for cerebral ischemia in the elderly. *Am J Cardiol*, **74**, 596–9.

Kearon, C., Ginsberg, J., and Hirsh, J. 1998. The role of venous ultrasonography in the diagnosis of suspected deep venous thrombosis and pulmonary embolism. *Ann Intern Med*, **129**, 1044–9.

Kearon, C., and Hirsh, J. 1994. Factors influencing the reported sensitivity and specificity of impedance plethysmography for proximal deep vein thrombosis. *Thrombosis Haemost*, **72**, 652–8.

Kelly, J., Rudd, A., Lewis, R., and Hunt, B. 2001. Venous thromboembolism after acute stroke. *Stroke*, **32**, 262–7.

Kerut, E., Norfleet, W., Plotnick, G., and Giles, T. 2001. Patent foramen ovale: a review of associated conditions and the impact of physiological size. *J Am Coll Cardiol*, **38**, 613–23.

Klotzsch, C., Janssen, G., and Berlit, P. 1994. Transesophageal echocardiography and contrast-TCD in the detection of a patent foramen ovale. *Neurology*, **44**, 1603–6.

Koessler, M. J., and Pitto, R. P. 2002. Fat embolism and cerebral function in total hip arthroplasty. *Int Orthop*, **26**, 259–62.

Konstantinides, S., Geibel, A., Kasper, W., *et al.* 1998. Patent foramen ovale is an important predictor of adverse outcome in patients with major pulmonary embolism. *Circulation*, **97**, 1946–51.

Lamy, C., Giannesini, C., Zuber, M., *et al.* 2002. Clinical and imaging findings in cryptogenic stroke patients with and without patent foramen ovale: the PFO-ASA Study. Atrial Septal Aneurysm. *Stroke*, **33**, 706–11.

Landi, G., D'Angelo, A., Boccardi, E., *et al.* 1992. Venous thromboembolism in acute stroke: prognostic importance of hypercoagulability. *Arch Neurol*, **49**, 279–83.

Lechat, P., Mas, J., and Lascault, G. 1988. Prevalence of patent foramen ovale in patients with stroke. *N Engl J Med*, **318**, 1148–52.

Leon, L., Giannoukas, A. D., Dodd, D., Chan, P., and Labropoulos, N. 2005. Clinical significance of superficial vein thrombosis. *Eur J Vasc Endovasc Surg*, **29**, 10–7.

Lethen, H., Flachskampf, F., Schneider, R., *et al.* 1997. Frequency of deep vein thrombosis in patients with patent foramen ovale and ischemic stroke or transient ischemic attack. *Am J Cardiol*, **80**, 1066–9.

Lohr, J., James, K., Deshmukh, R., *et al.* 1995. Karmody Award. Calf vein thrombi are not a benign finding. *Am J Surg*, **170**, 86–90.

Loscalzo, J. 1986. Paradoxical embolism: clinical presentation, diagnostic strategies, and therapeutic options. *Am Heart J*, **112**, 141–5.

Loud, P., Katz, D., Bruce, D., Klippenstein, D., and Grossman, Z. 2001. Deep venous thrombosis with suspected pulmonary embolism: detection with combined CT venography and pulmonary angiography. *Radiology*, **219**, 498–502.

Maldjian, P. D., Anis, A., and Saric, M. 2006. Radiological reasoning: pulmonary embolism–thinking beyond the clots. *AJR Am J Roentgenol*, **186**, S219–23.

Mas, J.-L., Arquizan, C., Lamy, C., *et al.* 2001. Recurrent cerebrovascular events associated with patent foramen ovale, atrial septal aneurysm, or both. *N Engl J Med*, **345**, 1740–6.

Mas, J.-L., Zuber, M., the French Study Group on Patent Foramen Ovale and Atrial Septal Aneurysm. 1995. Recurrent cerebrovascular events in patients with patent foramen ovale, atrial septal aneurysm, or both and cryptogenic stroke or transient ischemic attack. *Am Heart J*, **130**, 1083–8.

McGaw, D., and Harper, R. 2001. Patent foramen ovale and cryptogenic cerebral infarction. *Intern Med J*, **31**, 42–7.

Meissner, I., Khandheria, B. K., Heit, J. A., *et al.* 2006. Patent foramen ovale: innocent or guilty? Evidence from a prospective population-based study. *J Am Coll Cardiol*, **47**, 440–5.

Messe, S., Silverman, I., Kizer, J., *et al.* 2004. Practice parameter: recurrent stroke with patent foramen ovale and atrial septal aneurysm. *Neurology*, **62**, 1042–50.

Miller, R. L., Das, S., Anandarangam, T., *et al.* 1997. Relation between patent foramen ovale and perfusion abnormalities in acute pulmonary embolism. *Am J Cardiol*, **80**, 377–8.

Modan, B., Sharon, E., and Jelin, N. 1972. Factors contributing to the incorrect diagnosis of pulmonary embolic disease. *Chest*, **62**, 388–93.

Mohr, J. 1988. Cryptogenic stroke. *N Engl J Med*, **318**, 1197–8.

Mohr, J., Caplan, L., Melski, J., *et al.* 1978. The Harvard Cooperative Stroke Registry: a prospective registry of patients hospitalized with stroke. *Neurology*, **28**, 754–62.

Mohr, J., Thompson, J., Lazar, R., *et al.* 2001. A comparison of warfarin and aspirin for the prevention of recurrent ischemic stroke. *N Engl J Med*, **345**, 1444–51.

Nendaz, M., Sarasin, F., Junod, A., and Bogousslavsky, J. 1998. Preventing stroke recurrence in patients with patent foramen ovale: antithrombotic therapy, foramen closure, or therapeutic abstention? A decision analytic perspective. *Am Heart J*, **135**, 532–41.

Noser, E., Felberg, R., and Alexandrov, A. 2001. Thrombolytic therapy in an adolescent ischemic stroke. *J Child Neurol*, **16**, 286–8.

Obernosterer, A., Aschauer, M., Schnedl, W., Lipp, R. 2002. Anomalies of the inferior vena cava in patients with iliac venous thrombosis. *Ann Intern Med*, **136**, 37–41.

Orgera, M., O'Malley, P., and Taylor, A. 2001. Secondary prevention of cerebral ischemia in patent foramen ovale: systematic review and meta-analysis. *South Med J*, **94**, 699–703.

Overell, J., Bone, I., and Lees, K. 2000. Interatrial septal abnormalities and stroke: a meta-analysis of case-control studies. *Neurology*, **55**, 1172–9.

Parisi, D. M., Koval, K., and Egol, K. 2002. Fat embolism syndrome. *Am J Orthop*, **31**, 507–12.

Petty, G., Khandheria, B., Chu, C.-P., Sicks, J., and Whisnant, J. 1997. Patent foramen ovale in patients with cerebral infarction. *Arch Neurol*, **54**, 819–22.

Pezzini, A., Del Zotto, E., Magoni, M., *et al.* 2003. Inherited thrombophilic disorders in young adults with ischemic stroke and patent foramen ovale. *Stroke*, **34**, 28–33.

Philbrick, J., and Becker, D. 1988. Calf deep venous thrombosis. A wolf in sheep's clothing? *Arch Intern Med*, **148**, 2131–8.

Puls, R., Hosten, N., Bock, J., *et al.* 1999. Signal-enhanced color Doppler sonography of deep venous thrombosis in the lower limbs and pelvis. *J Ultrasound Med*, **18**, 185–90.

Ranoux, D., Cohen, A., Cabanes, L., *et al.* 1993. Patent foramen ovale: is stroke due to paradoxical embolism? *Stroke*, 24, 31–4.

Sacco, R., Ellenberg, J., Mohr, J., *et al.* 1989. Infarcts of undetermined cause: the NINCDS Stroke Data Bank. *Ann Neurol*, **25**, 382–90.

Salzman, E. 1986. Venous thrombosis made easy. *N Engl J Med*, **314**, 847–8.

Schneider, B., Hofmann, T., Justen, M. H., and Meinertz, T. 1995. Chiari's network: normal anatomic variant or risk factor for arterial embolic events? *J Am Coll Cardiol*, 26, 203–10.

Schuchlenz, H., Saurer, G., and Weihs, W. 2002. Patent foramen ovale, atrial septal aneurysm, and recurrent stroke. *N Engl J Med*, **346**, 1331–2; author reply 1331–2.

Schuchlenz, H., Weihs, W., Beitzke, A., *et al.* 2002. Transesophageal echocardiography for quantifying size of patent foramen ovale in patients with cryptogenic cerebrovascular events. *Stroke*, **33**, 293–6.

Schuchlenz, H., Weihs, W., Horner, S., and Quehenberger, F. 2000. The association between the diameter of a patent foramen ovale and the risk of embolic cerebrovascular events. *Am J Med*, **109**, 456–62.

Spritzer, C., Arata, M., and Freed, K. 2001. Isolated pelvic deep venous thrombosis: relative frequency as detected with MR imaging. *Radiology*, **219**, 521–5.

Steiner, M., Di Tullio, M., Rundek, T., *et al.* 1998. Patent foramen ovale size and embolic brain imaging findings among patients with ischemic stroke. *Stroke*, **29**, 944–8.

Stendel, R., Gramm, H., Schroder, K., Lober, C., and Brock, M. 2000. Transcranial Doppler ultrasonography as a screening technique for detection of a patent foramen ovale before surgery in the sitting position. *Anesthesiology*, 93, 971–5.

Stern, J., Abehsera, M., Grenet, D., *et al.* 2002. Detection of pelvic vein thrombosis by magnetic resonance angiography in patients with acute pulmonary embolism and normal lower limb compression ultrasonography. *Chest*, **122**, 115–21.

Stollberger, C., Slany, J., Schuster, I., *et al.* 1993. The prevalence of deep vein thrombosis in patients with suspected paradoxical embolism. *Ann Intern Med*, **119**, 461–5.

Tatlisumak, T., and Fisher, M. 1996. Hematologic disorders associated with ischemic stroke. *J Neurol Sci*, **140**, 1–11.

The National Institute of Neurological Disorders and Stroke rt-PA Stroke Study Group. 1995. Tissue plasminogen activator for acute ischemic stroke. *N Engl J Med*, **333**, 1581–7.

The Publications Committee for the Trial of ORG 10172 in Acute Stroke Treatment (TOAST) Investigators. 1998. Low molecular weight heparinoid, ORG 10172 (Danaparoid), and outcome after acute ischemic stroke. *JAMA*, **279**, 1265–72.

Thompson, T., and Evans, W. 1930. Paradoxical embolism. *Q J Med*, **23**, 135–52.

Tobis, M. J., and Azarbal, B. 2005. Does patent foramen ovale promote cryptogenic stroke and migraine headache? *Tex Heart Inst J*, 32, 362–5.

Tong, D., and Becker, K. 2004. Patent foramen ovale and recurrent stroke: Closure is the best option: No. *Stroke*, **35**, 804–5.

Unno, N., Mitsuoka, H., Uchiyama, T., *et al.* 2002. Superficial thrombophlebitis of the lower limbs in patients with varicose veins. *Surg Today*, **32**, 397–401.

Verlato, F., Zucchetta, P., Prandoni, P., *et al.* 1999. An unexpectedly high rate of pulmonary embolism in patients with superficial thrombophlebitis of the thigh. *J Vasc Surg*, **30**, 1113–5.

Ward, R., Jones, D., and Haponik, E. 1995. Paradoxical embolism. *Chest*, **108**, 549–58.

Warlow, C., Ogston, D., and Douglas, A. 1976. Deep venous thrombosis of the legs after strokes. *Br Med J*, **1**, 1178–83.

Webster, M., Chancellor, A., Smith, H., *et al.* 1988. Patent foramen ovale in young stroke patients. *Lancet*, **2**, 11–2.

Wheeler, H., and Anderson, F. 1995. Diagnostic methods for deep vein thrombosis. *Haemostasis*, **25**, 6–26.

Wu, L., Malouf, J., Dearani, J., *et al.* 2004. Patent foramen ovale in cryptogenic stroke: current understanding and management options. *Arch Intern Med*, **164**, 950–6.

65 FIBROMUSCULAR DYSPLASIA

Louis R. Caplan

Fibromuscular dysplasia (FMD) was first described in 1938 in the renal arteries as a cause of arterial hypertension in a patient with unilateral kidney disease who had "an intraluminal mass of smooth muscle" (Leadbetter and Burkland, 1938; Sandok, 1989; Slovut and Olin, 2004). More than two decades later, McCormack et al. (1958, 1966) described the renal artery pathology of FMD. For many years, fibromuscular disease was assumed to be limited to the renal arteries. Palubinskas and Ripley (1964) were the first to report the angiographic appearance of FMD in extrarenal arteries. Their patient had involvement of the celiac artery and an angiographic lesion in an internal carotid artery (ICA). A year later, Javid (1965) first furnished histological proof of FMD in a carotid artery (Sandok, 1983). Connett and Lansche (1965) were the first to describe the radiological appearance of carotid artery FMD in a patient in whom the disease was confirmed pathologically.

FMD is probably not a single disease but may be a general term for a variety of different conditions that affect the arterial walls. FMD is a nonatheromatous multifocal condition now known to affect almost any systemic or brain-supplying artery, but this condition has special predilection for specific arterial sites. It tends to involve medium-sized muscular arteries, especially renal, splanchnic, and cervicocranial arteries. FMD is most often localized to the distal two-thirds of the renal arteries and the segments of the distal extracranial vertebral and carotid arteries adjacent to the second cervical vertebra (Josien, 1992; Watanabe et al., 1993). More rarely, FMD can involve the cavernous part of the carotid arteries and the arteries of the Circle of Willis.

Pathology

The arterial lesions consist of multiple, small saccular dilatations caused by areas of fragmentation of the arterial media with rings of fibrous and muscular hyperplasia (Corrin et al., 1981). Slavin and Gonzales-Vitale (1976) first described an arterial lesion found in splanchnic arteries characterized pathologically by lysis of the arterial media, gap formation in the arterial wall, aneurysms, and dissecting hematomas. Similar lesions, since then, have been extensively documented in other systemic and cervico-cranial arteries (Eskenasy-Cottier et al., 1994; Slavin et al., 1989, 1995). Although originally termed "segmental mediolytic arteritis," it later became clear that the lesion was not because of arterial inflammation and that it was a characteristic pathology in extracranial and intracranial lesions of FMD (Slavin et al., 1995).

FMD can involve any or all of the three layers of the arterial wall, but disease of the arterial media is the most common and important form. Three subtypes of the condition have been described. An adventitial form is characterized by narrowing of the vascular lumen by fibrous tissue hypertrophy surrounding an artery, and an intimal form is characterized by an increase in the fibrous components of the intima producing concentric narrowing of the arterial lumen. This form accounts for about 5% of cases and occurs mostly in children and adolescents, equally among boys and girls (Corrin et al., 1981). The most common form of FMD affects the media. Constricting bands composed of fibrous dysplastic tissue and proliferating smooth muscle cells in the media alternate with areas of luminal dilatation related to medial thinning and disruption of the elastic membrane (Luscher et al., 1987; Sandok, 1983, 1989). These abnormalities produce the characteristic "string-of-beads" appearance on arteriography. The medial form is by far the most common and occurs predominantly in women.

Frequency and angiographic appearance

FMD occurs predominantly in Caucasian women, mostly in the 4th to 6th decade of life. Children are also affected but less often (Lemahieu and Marchau, 1979; Sandok 1989). Infants have presented with fatal brain hemorrhages related to severe hypertension induced by aortic and renal artery FMD (Currie et al., 2001; Kaneko et al., 2004). Other children have had renal, splanchnic, and cervico-cranial fibromuscular lesions similar to those found in adults (DiFazio et al., 2000; Lemahieu and Marchau, 1979; Sandok, 1989).

In the cervico-cranial circulation, FMD is reported in <1% of nonselected consecutive cerebral arteriograms (Corrin et al., 1981; Sandok, 1989; So et al., 1981). The frequency of cephalic FMD in reported series ranges from 0.25% to 0.77% (Corrin et al., 1981; Harrington et al., 1970; Momose and New, 1973; Sandok, 1989; So et al., 1981). Among almost 14 000 angiograms performed at the Mayo Clinic and its affiliated hospitals, there were 82 instances of carotid FMD, a frequency of 0.6% (Corrin et al., 1981). There is no reliable information about its true frequency in patients evaluated for stroke. This blood vessel abnormality is most often reported in middle-aged women. Bilateral ICA involvement is common; abnormalities usually involve the pharyngeal portion of the artery and extend from the level of C1 proximally 7–8 cm, with sparing of the carotid bifurcation and the intracranial carotid artery. Twenty percent of patients have coexistent fibromuscular disease of the

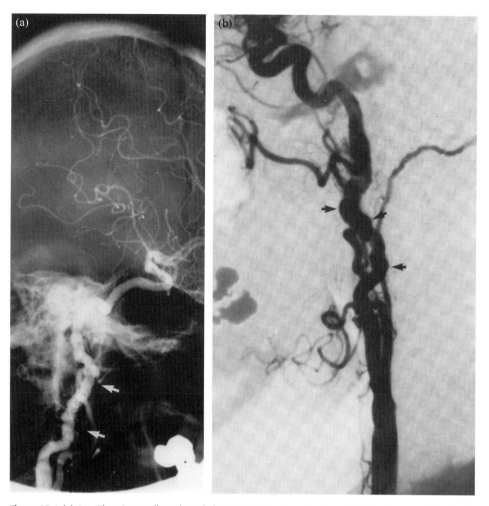

Figure 65.1 (a) Carotid angiogram (lateral view) showing prominent contractions of FMD (*white arrows*) in the pharyngeal carotid artery. (b) Subtraction cerebral carotid angiogram (anteroposterior view) showing string-of-beads appearance of FMD (*black arrows*) in the carotid artery above the bifurcation.

vertebral arteries in the neck (Corrin *et al.*, 1981). Intracranial FMD also occurs, but is much less common.

The most common finding is alternating zones of widening and narrowing of the arterial lumen on angiograms – the so-called string of beads appearance (Sandok, 1983; Slovut and Olin, 2004; Woldenberg *et al.*, 1997). Figures 65.1 and 65.2 show this typical appearance in lesions in the carotid and vertebral arteries in the neck. Dilatations in the artery are wider than the normal lumen and are separated from each other by sharply localized regions of vasoconstriction. Other types of appearances are also found. Some patients with typical string-of-beads lesions also have focal areas of tubular constriction and diverticulum-like aneurysmal dilatations. Hypertrophy of fibrous tissues in the adventitia or intima cause segmental areas of stenoses that can appear as shelves, ridges, or webs in the artery (Kubis *et al.*, 1999; Osborn and Anderson, 1977; So *et al.*, 1979; Watanabe *et al.*, 1993). Some patients with fibrous septa and webs have had typical string-of-beads abnormalities in the pharyngeal carotid arteries on angiography, but some have not had other obvious changes characteristic of FMD. Occasionally, patients have had band-like shelves or diaphragms within greatly enlarged carotid bulbs in the neck; superimposed

thrombi are sometimes present in these "megabulbs" (Kubis *et al.*, 1999).

Underlying conditions and associations

The most neurologically important associated conditions are intracranial aneurysms and arterial dissections. Intracerebral hemorrhages can develop because of the severe hypertension that sometimes accompanies renal artery FMD. FMD is often associated with aneurysms of the intracranial arteries. In one series among 37 patients with FMD, 19 patients had a total of 25 aneurysms (Mettinger and Ericson, 1982). In another series of 79 patients, 10 (12.6%) had intracranial aneurysms (Corrin *et al.*, 1981). Renal artery aneurysms are also well known in patients with renal artery FMD (Case records of the Massachusetts General Hospital, 1990). The frequency of detection of aneurysms will clearly depend on the indications for angiography; angiography for subarachnoid hemorrhage, brain ischemia, and conditions unrelated to stroke will result in very different frequencies of intracranial aneurysm detection.

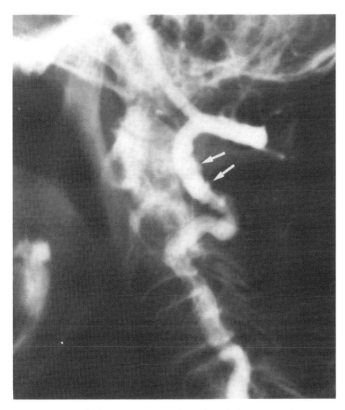

Figure 65.2 Vertebral artery angiogram (lateral view) showing FMD lesions (*white arrows*) in the distal portion of the extracranial vertebral artery.

Spontaneous cervical and intracranial artery dissection is an important complication of FMD (Ashleigh *et al.*, 1992; Baumgartner and Waespe, 1993; Bour *et al.*, 1992; Eskanasy-Cottier *et al.*, 1994; Gatalica *et al.*, 1992; Goldstein, 1982; Hugenholtz *et al.*, 1982; Nishiyama *et al.*, 1992; Shulze *et al.*, 1992; Watanabe *et al.*, 1993). Renal artery FMD is also sometimes complicated by dissections in the renal artery. Zardkoohi and Haupert (2007) suggest that the clinical syndrome of acute abdominal pain, systemic signs, and hypertension is a presentation of FMD that is more common in men than in women. Coronary artery FMD can also be complicated by coronary artery dissection and myocardial infarction (Huizar *et al.*, 2006; Lie and Berg, 1987).

The first descriptions of the relationship between FMD and arterial dissection appeared in the early 1980s. Goldstein (1982), in a single case report, described a 31-year-old woman who developed brainstem ischemia during a game of softball. The left cervical vertebral artery was irregularly narrowed beginning 2 cm beyond its origin until the level of C2. Goldstein commented on a "string of beads or wave-like appearance of the lumen." Hugenholtz *et al.* (1982) reported a 44-year-old woman who had cervical pain accentuated by turning the neck. Headache, vomiting, and transient bouts of hypertension (but no neurological symptoms or signs) were present. Angiography showed an irregular appearance of the cervical vertebral artery with a dissecting aneurysm at the C4–C6 level; analysis of the surgical specimen confirmed extensive fibromuscular degeneration with medial dysplasia and a dissection (Hugenholtz *et al.*, 1982). In many patients with dissection, foci of FMD are found angiographically in other regions or

proximate to the dissections. FMD has also been shown at autopsy in patients dying with cervico-cephalic arterial dissections.

Atherosclerotic-appearing lesions are also found in patients with FMD, but it is unclear how much the disorder of medial elastic and fibromuscular tissue promotes the development of atherosclerotic disease.

Clinical features

The diagnosis of FMD is occasionally made at the time of evaluation of patients who present with subarachnoid hemorrhage. FMD also predisposes patients to arterial dissections with related stroke syndromes. FMD is often discovered when patients present with a stroke related to arterial dissection. Although most FMD vascular lesions are asymptomatic, this vascular abnormality can cause brain ischemia.

In some patients who present with transient or persistent brain ischemia, FMD affecting an artery appropriate to explain the brain imaging and clinical findings is the only vascular abnormality found. The lumen may not appear severely compromised in these patients. The mechanism of the distal ischemia in this circumstance is unknown. Functional changes in vessel contraction (vasoconstriction) could lead to distal hypoperfusion. Altered blood flow with stasis could lead to thrombus formation and distal intra-arterial embolism. Either white platelet-fibrin thrombi or red erythrocyte-fibrin thrombi could form in regions of the artery affected by FMD. Alternatively, local dissections could precipitate thrombus formation.

A striking observation in series of patients with cervico-cranial FMD is the relative benignity of the condition. Even in patients who present with strokes, further vascular episodes are unusual and much less frequent than in patients with atherosclerotic vascular lesions (Patman *et al.*, 1980; Sandok 1989; Stewart *et al.*, 1986; Wells and Smith 1982; Wesen and Elliott 1986). In one large series, among 79 patients with carotid artery FMD, only three brain ischemia episodes developed during an average follow-up period of 5 years (Corrin *et al.*, 1981).

Imaging diagnosis of FD

Most diagnoses have been made using standard dye-contrast angiography. Zones of alternating vasoconstriction and vasodilatation are most typical – the so-called string of beads appearance. Localized tubular dilatations, focal constrictions, webs, shelves, and other focal regions of altered contractility are well-known manifestations seen on angiography. Tubular stenoses, diverticular appearance, and aneurysmal dilatation are sometimes found.

CT angiography (CTA) and MR angiography (MRA) also can identify FMD lesions (Ashleigh *et al.*, 1992; Heiserman *et al.*, 1992; Shulze *et al.*, 1992; Woldenberg *et al.*, 1997). For patients suspected of having FMD after duplex examination, MRA may avoid the need for conventional arteriography.

However, there are no large series that compare the diagnostic capability of these modalities versus standard catheter angiography. Because the lesions are usually well above the carotid artery bifurcation, ultrasound has been less effective in diagnosis than in patients with atherosclerotic lesions at the bifurcation. Occasional cervical FMD lesions have been diagnosed using Duplex ultrasound (Edell and Huang, 1981; Perren *et al.*, 2004). Duplex ultrasound is effective in showing and following the renal arterial FMD lesions (Slovut and Olin, 2004).

Treatment

Insufficient data are available to warrant rational therapeutic suggestions. Antiplatelet agents and anticoagulants have been prescribed to prevent recurrent episodes of brain ischemia, but the relatively benign natural history of FMD makes it difficult to know the effectiveness of these agents. Surgeons in the past have repaired the cervical lesions (Chiche *et al.*, 1997; Ehrenfeld and Wylie, 1974; Kelly and Morris, 1982; Moreau *et al.*, 1993). More recently, angioplasty with dilatation of the artery (Starr *et al.*, 1981) and stenting (Assadian *et al.*, 2005; Finsterer *et al.*, 2000; Meyers *et al.*, 2006) have been used to treat the fibromuscular lesions in the neck. The relative merits of medical, surgical, and endovascular treatment have not been formally studied.

A recent personal case has made me aware of the potential use of calcium-channel blockers. A patient of mine who had had angioplasty of a unilateral shelf-like stenosing lesion of the pharyngeal portion of one carotid artery developed, years later, a similar lesion in the contralateral carotid artery. An exploratory angiogram was performed prior to planned angioplasty-stenting of the lesion. After introducing the treating devices into the carotid artery, a second injection of dye showed that the lesion had temporarily disappeared. Clearly the shelf-like protrusion was because of hypercontractility. Because smooth muscle contraction is related to calcium entry, treatment with calcium-channel blockers such as verapamil, nimodipine, and nicardipine seems to me to be a logical approach. After this experience with my patient, I have routinely prescribed calcium-channel blockers and antiplatelets for patients who have FMD and related brain ischemia, but I have no data about the utility of this approach.

I usually prescribe antiplatelet aggregating agents but rarely use anticoagulants or recommend surgical repair or mechanical dilation of the arteries. I often prescribe calcium-channel blockers to prevent vasoconstriction. If the patient is hypertensive, the renal arteries should be studied. When FMD is found on angiography, CTA, or MRA, standard arteriography is warranted to exclude associated intracranial aneurysms.

Conclusion

Most research and clinical interest has been directed at atherosclerotic disease of the intima and subintima of arteries. Little is known about the other portions of the arterial wall. Clearly, disease of the artery walls can lead to altered contractility, dilatation with aneurysm formation, and tears with intramural hematomas. The disorder called FMD is pathologically heterogenous and may occur as a result of a variety of different etiologies that share abnormalities of connective tissue. The collagen, elastic tissue, and extracellular matrix can be involved. Knowledge of these disorders of vascular connective tissue is, at present, unfortunately rudimentary.

REFERENCES

Ashleigh, R. J., Weller, J. M., and Leggate, J. R. 1992. Fibromuscular hyperplasia of the internal carotid artery. A further cause of the 'Moya-moya' collateral circulation. *Br J Neurosurg*, **6**, 269–73.

Assadian, A., Senekowitsch, C., Assadian, O, *et al.* 2005. Combined open and endovascular stent grafting of internal carotid artery fibromuscular dysplasia: long term results. *Eur J Vasc Endovasc Surg*, **29**, 345–9.

Baumgartner, R. W., and Waespe, W. 1993. Behandelbare erkrankungen des nervensystems mit kataraktbildung. *Klin Monatsbl Augenheilkd*, **202**, 89–93.

Bour, P., Taghavi, I., Bracard, S., Frisch, N., and Fieve, G. 1992. Aneurysms of the extracranial internal carotid artery due to fibromuscular dysplasia: results of surgical management. *Ann Vasc Surg*, **6**, 205–8.

Case records of the Massachusetts General Hospital: Case 9–1990. 1990. *N Engl J Med*, **322**, 612–22.

Chiche, L., Bahnini, A., Koskas, F., *et al.* 1997, Occlusive fibromuscular disease of arteries supplying the brain: results of surgical treatment. *Ann Vasc Surg*, **11**, 496–504.

Connett, M. C., and Lansche, J. M. 1965. Fibromuscular hyperplasia of the internal carotid artery: report of a case. *Ann Surg*, **162**, 59–61.

Corrin, L. S., Sandok, B. A., and Houser, O. W. 1981. Cerebral ischemic events in patients with carotid artery fibromuscular dysplasia. *Arch Neurol*, **38**, 616–8.

Currie, A. D. M., Bentley, C. R., and Bloom, P. A. 2001. Retinal hemorrhage and fatal stroke in an infant with fibromuscular dysplasia. *Arch Dis Child*, **84**, 263–4.

DiFazio, M., Hinds, S. R. 2nd, Depper, M., Tom, B., and Davis, R. 2000. Intracranial fibromuscular dysplasia in a six-year old child: a rare cause of stroke. *J Child Neurol*, **15**, 559–62.

Edell, S. L., and Huang, P. 1981. Sonographic demonstration of fibromuscular hyperplasia of the cervical internal carotid artery. *Stroke*, **12**, 518–20.

Ehrenfeld, W. K., and Wylie, E. J. 1974. Fibromuscular dysplasia of the internal carotid artery: surgical management. *Arch Surg*, **109**, 161–6.

Eskenasy-Cottier, A. C., Leu, H. J., Bassetti, C., *et al.* 1994. A case of dissection of intracranial cerebral arteries with segmental mediolytic "arteritis." *Clin Neuropathol*, **13**, 329–37.

Finsterer, J., Strassegger, J., Haymerle, A., and Hagmuller, G. 2000. Bilateral stenting and asymptomatic internal carotid artery stenosis due to fibromuscular dysplasia. *J Neurol Neurosurg Psychiatry*, **69**, 683–6.

Gatalica, Z., Gibas, Z., and Martinez-Hernandez, A. 1992. Dissecting aneurysm as a complication of generalized fibromuscular dysplasia. *Hum Pathol*, **23**, 586–8.

Goldstein, S. J. 1982. Dissecting hematoma of the cervical vertebral artery: case report. *J Neurosurg*, **56**, 451–4.

Harrington, O. B., Crosby, V. G., and Nicholas, L. 1970. Fibromuscular hyperplasia of the internal carotid arteries. *Ann Thorac Surg*, **9**, 516–24.

Heiserman, J. E., Drayer, B. P., Fram, E. K., and Keller, P. J. 1992. MR angiography of cervical fibromuscular dysplasia. *AJNR Am J Neuroradiol*, **13**, 1454–7.

Hugenholtz, H., Pokrupa, R., Montpetit, V. J. A., *et al.* 1982. Spontaneous dissecting aneurym of the extracranial vertebral artery. *Neurosurgery*, **10**, 96–100.

Huizar, J. F., Awasthi, A., and Kozman, H. 2006. Fibromuscular dysplasia and acute myocardial infarction: evidence for a unique clinical and angiographic pattern. *J Invasive Cardiol*, **18**, E99–101.

Javid, H. 1965. Discussion of Hill LD, Antonius JL. Arterial dysplasia. *Arch Surg*, **90**, 595.

Josien, E. 1992. Extracranial vertebral artery dissection: nine cases. *J Neurol*, **239**, 327–30.

Kaneko, K., Someya, T., Ohtaki, R., *et al.* 2004. Congenital fibromuscular dysplasia involving multivessels in an infant with fatal outcome. *Eur J Pediatr*, **163**, 241–4.

Kelly, T. F. Jr., Morris, G. C. Jr. 1982. Arterial fibromuscular disease: observations on pathogenesis and surgical management. *Am J Surg*, **143**, 232–6.

Kubis, N., von Langsdorrff, D., Petitjean, C., *et al.* 1999. Thrombotic carotid megabulb: fibromuscular dysplasia, septae, and ischemic stroke. *Neurology*, **52**, 883–6.

Leadbetter, W. F., and Burkland, C. E. 1938. Hypertension in unilateral renal disease. *J Urol*, **39**, 611–26.

Lemahieu, S. F., and Marchau, M. M. B. 1979. Intracranial fibromuscular dysplasia and stroke in children. *Neuroradiology*, **18**, 99–102.

Lie, J. T., and Berg, K. K. 1987. Isolated fibromuscular dysplasia of the coronary arteries with spontaneous dissection and myocardial infarction. *Hu Pathol*, **18**, 654–6.

Luscher, T. F., Lie, J. T., Stanson, A. W., *et al.* 1987. Arterial fibromuscular dysplasia. *Mayo Clin Proc*, **62**, 931–52.

McCormack, L. J., Hazard, J. B., and Poutasse, E. F. 1958. Obstructive lesions of the renal artery associated with remediable hypertension. *Am J Pathol*, **34**, 582.

McCormack, L. J., Poutasse, E. F., Meaney, T. F., Noto, T. J. Jr., and Dunstan, H. P. 1966. A pathologic-arteriographic correlation of renal arterial disease. *Am Heart J*, **72**, 188–98.

Mettinger, K., and Ericson, K. 1982. Fibromuscular dysplasia and the brain. *Stroke*, **13**, 46–52.

Meyers, P. M., Schumacher, H. C., Higashida, R. T., Leary, M. C., Caplan, L. R. 2006. Use of stents to treat extracranial cerebrovascular disease. *Ann Rev Med*, **57**, 437–54.

Momose, K. J., and New, P. F. 1973. Non-atheromatous stenosis and occlusion of the internal carotid artery and its main branches. *Am J Roentgenol Radium Ther Nucl Med*, **118**, 550–66.

Moreau, P., Albat, B., and Thevenet, A. 1993. Fibromuscular dysplasia of the internal carotid artery: long term surgical results. *J Cardiovasc Surg*, **34**, 465–72.

Nishiyama, K., Fuse, S., Shimizu, J., Takeda, K., and Sakuta, M. 1992. A case of fibromuscular dysplasia presenting with Wallenberg syndrome, and developing a giant aneurysm of the internal carotid artery in the cavernous sinus. *Rhinsho Shinkeigaku*, **32**, 1117–20.

Osborn, A. G., and Anderson, R. E. 1977. Angiographic spectrum of cervical and intracranial fibromuscular dysplasia. *Stroke*, **8**, 617–26.

Palubinskas, A. J., Ripley, H. R. 1964. Fibromuscular hyperplasia in extrarenal arteries. *Radiology*, **82**, 451–5.

Patman, R. D., Thompson, J. E., Talkington, C. M., Garrett, W. V. 1980. *Natural history of fibromuscular dysplasia of the internal carotid artery. Stroke*, **11**, 135.

Perren, F., Urbano, L., Rossetti, A. O. *et al.* 2004. Ultrasound image of a single symptomatic carotid artery stenosis disclosed as fibromuscular dysplasia. *Neurology*, **62**, 1023–4.

Sandok, B. A. 1983. Fibromuscular dysplasia of the internal carotid artery. In *Neurologic Clinics*, Vol 1, H. J. M. Barnett (ed.), Philadelphia: Saunders, 17–26.

Sandok, B. A. 1989. Fibromuscular dysplasia of the cephalic arterial system. In *Handbook of Clinical Neurology*, Vol 11 (55). Vascular diseases, part 111. J. F. Toole (ed.), Amsterdam: Elsevier Science Publishers, 283–92.

Shulze, H. E., Ebner, A., and Besinger, U. A. 1992. Report of dissection of the internal carotid artery in three cases. *Neurosurg Rev*, **15**, 61–4.

Slavin, R. E., Cafferty, L., and Cartwright, J. 1989. Segmental mediolytic arteritis: a clinicopathologic and ultrastructural study of two cases. *Am J Surg Pathol*, **13**, 558–68.

Slavin, R. E., and Gonzalez-Vitale, J. C. 1976. Segmental mediolytic arteritis: a clinical pathologic study. *Lab Invest*, **35**, 23–9.

Slavin, R. E., Saeki, K., Bhagavan, B., and Maas, A. E. 1995. Segmental arterial mediolysis: a precursor to fibromuscular dysplasia. *Mod Pathol*, **8**, 287–94.

Slovut, D. P., and Olin, J. W. 2004. Fibromuscular dysplasia. *N Engl J Med*, **350**, 1862–71.

So, E. L., Toole, J. F., Dalal, P., *et al.* 1981. Cephalic fibromuscular dysplasia in 32 patients. *Arch Neurol*, **38**, 619–22.

So, E. L., Toole, J. F., Moody, D. M., and Challa, V. R. 1979. Cerebral embolism from septal fibromuscular dysplasia of the common carotid artery. *Ann Neurol*, **6**, 75–8.

Starr, D. S., Lawrie, G. M., and Morris, G. C. Jr. 1981. Fibromuscular disease of carotid arteries: long term results of graduated internal dilatation. *Stroke*, **12**, 196–9.

Stewart, M. T., Moritz, M. W., Smith, R. B. III, Fulenwider, J. T., and Perdue, G. D. 1986. The natural history of carotid fibromuscular dysplasia. *J Vasc Surg*, **3**, 305–10.

Watanabe, S., Tanaka, K., Nakayama, T., and Kazneko, M. 1993. Fibromuscular dysplasia at the internal carotid origin: a case of carotid web. *No Shinkei Geka*, **21**, 449–52.

Wells, R. P., and Smith, R. R. 1982. Fibromuscular dysplasia of the internal carotid artery: a long term follow-up. *Neurosurgery*, **10**, 39–43.

Wesen, C. A., and Elliott, B. M. 1986. Fibromuscular dysplasia of the carotid arteries. *Am J Surg*, **151**, 448–51.

Woldenberg, R., Holz, A., Black, K., *et al.* 1997. Fibromuscular dysplasia: a comparison of 2D time-of-flight magnetic resonance angiography, 3D time-of-flight magnetic resonance angiography and catheter angiography. *J Neurovasc Dis*, **2**, 74–8.

Zardkoohi, O., and Haupert, G. T. Jr. 2007 Scarce among men. *Am J Med*, **120**, 136–9.

PART VII: VENOUS OCCLUSIVE CONDITIONS

66 CEREBRAL VENOUS SINUS THROMBOSIS

Manu Mehdiratta, Sandeep Kumar, Magdy Selim, and Louis R. Caplan

Cerebral venous sinus thrombosis (CVST), although a relatively rare cause of stroke, is important to diagnose and treat early because of the significant morbidity and mortality associated with it. Diagnosis can be challenging as there are often a wide range of symptoms and signs, many of which are nonspecific in nature. In order to make the diagnosis of CVST, the physician must have enough clinical suspicion and thus order the appropriate investigations. Radiological studies are essential in making the diagnosis. If appropriate treatment is instituted soon after symptom onset, neurological outcomes are better than in arterial stroke.

Epidemiology

The annual incidence rate of CVST is approximately 3–4 cases per million. In children, the incidence can be as high as seven cases per million (Stam, 2005). It is likely that the true incidence is much higher, especially in developing countries where it may not be possible to definitively diagnose the condition. CVST causes 1%–9% of all deaths because of stroke and cerebrovascular disease, according to autopsy studies (Biousse and Bousser, 1999).

CVST tends to affect younger patients, who have fewer traditional risk factors, than do arterial infarcts. The mean age ranges from the mid 30s to 40s. Among young adults who develop CVST, 70%–80% of cases affect young women (de Bruijn, 1998; deVeber and Andrew, 2001; Ferro *et al.*, 2004). This is likely because of predisposing factors in this group such as oral contraceptive use and pregnancy and peripartum states, which are known to increase blood coagulability. Recent studies have shown that the risk of developing CVST is higher during the third trimester of pregnancy and postpartum. Peripartum and postpartum CVST occur at a frequency of about 12 cases per 100 000 deliveries (Lanska and Kryscio, 2000).

CVST also occurs in infants with dehydration and in the elderly who have concomitant disease causing a hypercoagulable state.

Predisposing factors

A hypercoagulable risk factor is found in approximately 85% of patients with CVST (Stam, 2005). In most cases, an environmental risk factor such as pregnancy, which is known to increase coagulability, contributes to CVST in a genetically susceptible individual. The risk factors for CVST (such as venous stasis, hypercoagulability, or damage to the vascular endothelium through extrinsic compression or invasion of venous sinuses) affect various aspect of Virchow's triad.

In women, common predisposing risk factors include pregnancy, postpartum states, and the use of oral contraceptives (Cantu and Barinagarrementeria, 1993; Lanska and Kryscio, 2000). Postpartum venous sinus thrombosis appears to be especially common in Mexico and India. Poverty, a vegetarian diet, and anemia are all posited to cause hyperhomocysteinemia and hypercoagulability, increasing the risk of venous occlusions. Studies have shown that the oral contraceptive pill can be prothrombotic and (especially in patients with a genetic susceptibility, such as Factor V Leiden or prothrombin gene mutation), can lead to CVST (Ludemann *et al.*, 1998; Martinelli *et al.*, 1998).

Infections such as mastoiditis and otitis can lead to occlusion of the transverse and sigmoid sinuses; this is seen especially in children (deVeber and Andrew, 2001). Meningitis can also lead to occlusion of adjacent sinuses.

Hematologic and inflammatory conditions contributing to hypercoagulability are also associated with CVST, especially in patients with Factor V Leiden mutation, protein C and S deficiency, prothrombin gene mutation, and anti-thrombin III deficiency. Other hematologic conditions associated are thrombocytosis, anti-phospholipid antibody syndrome, polycythemia vera, and paroxysmal nocturnal hemoglobinuria. Iron deficiency anemia can also promote venous and dural sinus thrombosis and may be a contributory factor to puerperal occurrences. Inflammatory conditions, such as ulcerative colitis and Crohn's disease, increase acute phase reactants promoting venous thrombosis. Patients with Behçet's disease also have an increased risk of developing CVST (Bousser *et al.*, 1985; Kumral, 2001; Wechsler *et al.*, 1992).

Neoplasms can invade the dura mater and cause occlusion of the adjacent dural sinuses. This occurs most often in patients with meningiomas. Tumors that invade the skull, for example, breast cancer and myeloma, can spread to the subjacent dura and dural sinuses. CVST can also follow traumatic injury to the venous sinuses or jugular veins after neurosurgical or other procedures. Patients with dural arteriovenous fistulas are sometimes shown to have accompanying thrombosis of dural venous sinuses and draining veins. The venous thrombosis can predispose to the development of a fistula, and fistulas can be the cause of subsequent venous thrombosis.

Occasionally CVST follows lumbar puncture or spontaneous cerebrospinal fluid (CSF) leaks. One posited mechanism explaining this occurrence is that low CSF pressure causes a downward shift of the brain with increased pressure on the cerebral veins and sinuses. This pressure may compress the venous walls

Uncommon Causes of Stroke, 2nd edition, ed. Louis R. Caplan. Published by Cambridge University Press. © Cambridge University Press 2008.

Table 66.1 Frequency of various clinical findings in patients with intracranial venous thromboses in some series

Clinical finding	C&B, 1993 puerper $n = 67$	C&B, 1993 nonpuer $n = 46$	Ameri and Bousser, 1992 $n = 110$	Einhaupl et al., 1990 $n = 71$	Tsai et al., 1995 $n = 29$	B&B, 1992 $n = 76$	Daif et al., 1995 $n = 40$	de Bruijn et al., 2001 $n = 59$	Ferro et al., 2004 $n = 624$
Headache	59 (88%)	32 (70%)	83 (75%)	63/69 (91%)	9 (31%)	61 (80%)	33 (82%)	56 (95%)	553 (88.1%)
Seizures	40 (60%)	29 (63%)	41 (37%)	34 (48%)	3 (10%)	22 (29%)	4 (10%)	28 (47%)	245 (39.3)
Focal findings	53 (79%)	35 (76%)	57 (52%)	47 (66%)	9 (31%)	34 (48%)	11 (27%)	27 (46%)	n/a
Altered conscious	42 (63%)	27 (59%)	33 (30%)	40 (56%)	27 (93%	18 (27%)	4 (10%)	32 (54%)	87 (13.9)
Papilledema	27 (40%)	24 (52%)	54 (49%)	19 (27%)	2 (7%)	38 (50%)	32 (80%)	23 (41%)	174 (28.3)

increasing the risk of thrombosis (Wilder-Smith et al., 1997). Low-CSF-pressure venous sinus thrombosis is especially difficult to diagnose, as these patients often present with a headache similar to that seen after lumbar puncture. The headache accompanying CVST continues to worsen early on in the disease course, whereas a post-lumbar-puncture headache usually improves.

Pathophysiology

CVST causes obstruction of both major veins and sinuses within the cerebrum. These usually occur in tandem, but each has its own secondary effect. The occlusion of cerebral veins leads to brain edema, venous infarction, and hemorrhage. Occlusion of larger cerebral venous sinuses results in increased intracranial pressure from impaired venous outflow and decreased absorption of CSF through the arachnoid villi. Under normal circumstances, CSF is eventually transported into the major draining dural sinuses, but in patients with CVST the pressure in the sinuses is increased, resulting in impaired absorption of CSF. The CSF retention further contributes to increased intracranial pressure and, in some patients, leads to a pseudotumor cerebri syndrome. The pseudotumor syndrome is most often found in patients with lateral sinus occlusions. When multiple dural sinuses are occluded, raised intracranial pressure becomes a very important clinical concern.

Raised venous pressure causes a failure of drainage and results in increased pressure in the arteries that supply the region drained by the occluded venous system. This pressure can be transmitted to the arterioles and veins leading to bleeding. Failure to adequately perfuse the region of increased pressure can lead to brain infarction. The increased venous pressure and inadequate drainage causes fluid to accumulate in the brain much like blocked street drains during a rainstorm leads to fluid piling up on the street. Brain edema in patients with CVST can be both cytotoxic and vasogenic. Often areas drained by blocked veins and dural sinuses contain an admixture of edema, infarction, and hemorrhage. At autopsy, patients who died with CVST usually have gross brain findings of dilated veins, brain edema, ischemic neurons, and evidence of hemorrhage.

Clinical features

Symptoms vary with cause and location of the venous occlusion. Table 66.1 shows the frequency of various findings in large series of patients reported by different authors. Headache is the most common presenting complaint in patients with CVST. Headache is seen in more than 90% of adult patients with CVST. Headache is explained by two major factors – the local process within the veins and dural sinuses, and increased intracranial pressure. The dura mater, overlying skull, and the venous sinuses are invested with pain-sensitive fibers unlike the brain itself. Distention of the sinuses (especially when because of inflammation) activates these pain-sensitive fibers. The headache can occur suddenly, as in subarachnoid hemorrhage, or gradually increase over the course of a few days (de Bruijn et al., 1996). Headache may precede neurological symptoms and signs by days or even weeks. Headache may be the only symptom or sign of CVST. In one large study, 17 (13.8%) of 123 consecutive patients with cerebral venous thrombosis and normal brain imaging, and CSF analysis had headache as the only symptom (Cumurciuc et al., 2005). The authors reviewed the clinical findings among these patients compared to those who had other findings. Fifteen had involvement of the lateral sinus. The onset of headache was progressive in 11, acute in three, and thunderclap in three. Once established, the headache continued unabated in 15. Headache was diffuse in four and unilateral in 13 (Cumurciuc et al., 2005).

Seizures are also common, occurring in up to 40% of patients with CVST (Stam, 2005). Seizures can be focal or generalized and rarely may result in status epilepticus. Although diminished level of consciousness is not a common presenting symptom at some time during the course, 191/439 patients (43.5%) in cumulative series had an alteration in the level of alertness (Table 66.1). Some patients may present even at onset with symptoms of increased intracranial pressure such as transient visual obscurations and vomiting.

Symptoms are often related to the location of the venous thrombosis. Table 66.2 shows the distribution of dural sinus occlusion in a number of series. If the thrombosis occurs in the superior sagittal sinus, the cerebral hemispheres are preferentially involved usually asymmetrically resulting in lateralizing symptoms such as aphasia, weakness, or neglect. The opposite cerebral hemisphere

Table 66.2 Distribution of venous structures involved in various studies

Vein	Cantu and Barinagarrementeria, 1993 puerp n = 67	Cantu and Barinagarrementeria, 1993 nonpuerp n = 46	Ameri and Bousser, 1992 n = 110	Southwick et al., 1986 septic n = 179	Tsai et al., 1995 n = 29	Bousser and Barnett, 1992 n = 76	Daif et al., 1995 n = 40	Ferro et al., 2004 n = 624
SSS	60 (22)	45 (11)	79 (14)	23 (7)*	19 (11)	53	34 (22)	313
LS	23 (1)	20 (1)	78 (10)	64 (4)*	15 (8)	55	13 (4)	536
SS	0	0	3 (1)		3	10	3	112
CS	0	0	3	92 (8)*	0	2	0	8
DV	17 (4)	10	9 (1)		1	3	4 (1)	68
CCV	13	14	30 (2)		0	29	0	110
>1	39	34	85		9	56	14	

Numbers in parenthesis represent cases in which structure was involved alone.

* Numbers in parenthesis represent personally studied cases – the rest are from literature review.

SSS = superior sagittal sinus; LS = lateral sinus; SS = straight sinus; CS = cavernous sinus; DV = deep venous system; CCV = cortical or cerebellar superficial veins.

>1 = more than one venous structure involved

also may become involved within a few days. Bilateral and midline cortical dysfunction may also occur due to superior sagittal sinus involvement.

Lateral sinus occlusion is as common as sagittal sinus thrombosis. In the past, thrombosis of the lateral sinus was almost entirely explained by spread of infection from acute or chronic ear and mastoid infections. The infective process within the ear structures often led to a local thrombophlebitis, and infections spread through emissary veins or directly through the thin sinus plate into the lateral sinus. The sigmoid portion of the lateral sinus lies adjacent to the mastoid air cells from its origin to the jugular bulb. Infection can spread from the lateral sinus into the jugular vein. Lateral sinus occlusions involve dysfunction of the temporal lobes and occasionally the cerebellum. Aphasia, agitation, and visual field abnormalities predominate. Lateral sinus occlusions are also most often associated with a pseudotumor syndrome. The left transverse (lateral) sinus is often hypoplastic. When the right transverse sinus and jugular vein become occluded, increased intracranial pressure becomes a very important problem.

Cavernous sinus thrombosis causes proptosis, an injected red eye, and impaired eye movements. This is usually associated with ethmoid, sphenoid, orbital, or facial infections.

With involvement of the deep venous structures such as the straight sinus and basal vein of Rosenthal, basal ganglionic and thalamic lesions may ensue resulting in nonspecific behavioral symptoms such as delirium, memory loss, or mutism (Kothare et al., 1998). Bilateral basal ganglionic and thalamic infarcts or hemorrhages are pathognomic of deep venous involvement. Stiffness of the limbs with decerebrate postures, coma, and vertical gaze palsy are the most common clinical findings in patients with extensive basal ganglionic and thalamic hemorrhagic infarcts and edema. Some patients present with apathy and are found on examination to be abulic and to have poor memory as the predominant signs. When patients who present with stupor or coma recover,

they often show residual signs of lack of initiative and spontaneity and may also have poor memory.

Occasional patients have occlusion of veins that drain the cerebellum (Caplan, 1996; Eng et al., 1990; Rousseaux et al., 1987). The findings are similar to those found in patients with infarcts caused by arterial occlusions – ataxia, veering, dizziness, diplopia. Headache is often occipital or nuchal.

The decreased CSF absorption in patients with CVST and the mass effect of brain edema and hemorrhage often lead to signs of increased intracranial pressure. If there is sufficient generalized increased intracranial pressure, displacement of the diencephalon and brainstem and herniation with subsequent coma or death may result. Coma may also be related to ongoing seizures, such as in nonconvulsive status epilepticus.

Because of the myriad of clinical symptoms, the diagnosis is often challenging. A high clinical suspicion needs to be maintained in patients who are young or middle-aged with new-onset headache, especially if headache is accompanied by seizures or focal neurological symptoms. This is especially true for younger patients who do not have a history of traditional vascular risk factors. Examination findings that can be helpful in making the diagnosis include papilledema, 6th nerve palsies, and focal neurological signs.

Brain and vascular imaging

MRI and CT scanning are essential in confirming the diagnosis of CVST. There can be indirect signs on imaging that raise suspicion for CVST such as hydrocephalus and mastoiditis. Direct signs indicating thrombosis can also be observed when examination of the cerebral veins and sinuses is undertaken.

Findings on CT scan in patients with CVST are often very subtle. As a result, the CT scan is read as normal in 25%–40% of patients who are later found to have CVST (Provenzale et al., 1998;

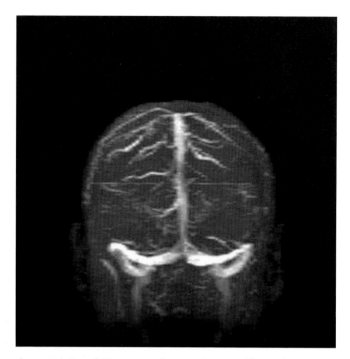

Figure 66.1 Normal MR venogram demonstrating normal flow in the superior sagittal sinus and transverse sinuses.

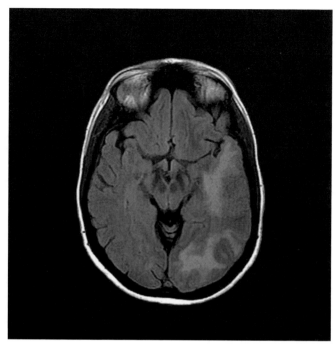

Figure 66.2 T2 fluid-attenuated inversion recovery (FLAIR) image demonstrating venous infarcts in the left temporo-occipital areas in a patient with left transverse sinus thrombosis.

Rao *et al.*, 1981). When intracranial venous occlusions are suspected, CT scanning should always be done with contrast to increase reliability, unless there is a contraindication. Even with the use of contrast, CT scanning is not optimal for diagnosing CVST unless a CT venogram is also performed.

Indirect signs found on CT include edema and venous infarcts in the parenchyma. Venous infarcts are hemorrhagic in up to 40% of CVST patients (Provenzale *et al.*, 1998; Rao *et al.*, 1981). It is difficult to differentiate hemorrhages due to venous infarcts from other secondary causes of brain hemorrhage. However, certain red flags should increase suspicion for a venous etiology, including: multiple hemorrhages, hemorrhage in a nonarterial distribution, subcortical hemorrhages, hemorrhages that are located bilaterally in the thalamus and/or basal ganglia, irregular appearance, and hemorrhages with an area of hypodensity at the periphery, indicating that the bleeding began in an area of brain edema (Rao *et al.*, 1981; Stam, 2005).

Direct signs of venous sinus thrombosis on CT are usually seen in patients given contrast or who have undergone a CT venogram. These include the "empty delta or empty triangle sign" which is seen on contrast CT as a bright triangle surrounding a hypodense core. The bright triangle corresponds with contrast enhancement of the dilated veins surrounding the thrombus, and the hypodense core is the area of decreased contrast flow due to thrombus (Virapongse *et al.*, 1987). MRI is superior to CT in confirming CVST because it is more sensitive in showing both the direct and indirect signs of intracranial venous occlusions such as subtle parenchymal abnormalities, petechial hemorrhages, and thrombi (Selim *et al.*, 2002). Also, MRI is less susceptible to bone artifacts than is CT and is capable of multiplanar imaging to aid in diagnosis (Bianchi

et al., 1998; Connor and Jarosz, 2002). A normal MR venogram is shown in Figure 66.1.

Direct and indirect changes suggestive of CVST are shown using a number of different MRI sequences including T1- and T2-weighted MRI, echo-planar T2* (susceptibility), and diffusion-weighted MRI. On standard T1- and T2-weighted MRI with CVST, there is a loss of the normal signal flow void that is usually seen. In addition, there are signal changes produced by the venous thrombosis and associated changes in blood flow and hemoglobin degradation. The actual thrombus within the vein or sinus is prone to the same degradation process as hemorrhage and therefore initially appears isointense on T1 and hypointense on T2 during the first 1–5 days because of the presence of oxyhemoglobin within the red blood cells (Bianchi *et al.*, 1998; Connor and Jarosz, 2002; Provenzale *et al.*, 1998). Venous infarcts may also be seen as shown in Figure 66.2.

On T2*-weighted images, intravenous thrombus appears hypointense (loss of signal) because of the formation of deoxyhemoglobin. T2* can be especially useful in visualizing small areas of hemorrhage, such as petechial bleeding, within venous infarcts (Idbaih *et al.*, 2006; Selim *et al.*, 2002).

Diffusion-weighted imaging produces a wide variety of changes in patients with CVST and is therefore not very sensitive or specific for the diagnosis of intracranial venous occlusive disease. It is helpful, however, in the detection of early venous congestion and edema that may not be evident on standard T1, T2, and FLAIR images at an early stage (Chu *et al.*, 2001; Lovblad *et al.*, 2001; Wasay *et al.*, 2002).

In order to definitively diagnose CVST, direct imaging of the veins and sinuses is necessary. MR venography (MRV), CT

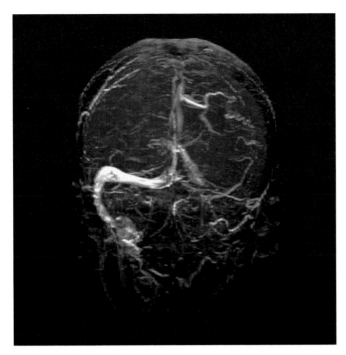

Figure 66.3 MR venogram of a 58-year-old woman with protein C deficiency with superior sagittal sinus and left transverse and sigmoid sinus thromboses.

venography (CTV), and conventional angiography are all accepted modalities, although MRV is the most commonly used of the three. The key finding on MRV is lack of flow signal within a venous sinus with nonopacification of the sinus (Figure 66.3). MRV has many limitations, the most significant being lack of flow signal because of artifact. This is often seen in a hypoplastic transverse sinus and is due to slow blood flow within the sinus (Ayanzen *et al.*, 2000; Bianchi *et al.*, 1998).

CTV has evolved recently due to the advent of newer generation spiral CT scanners. Like MRV, the key finding is lack of flow in the venous sinus. In addition, contrast enhancement of the sinuses and venous collaterals that have developed may also be seen on CTV. CTV is more readily accessible than MRV for most centers, and is less costly and may better visualize smaller sinuses and veins (Casey *et al.*, 1996).

The use of four-vessel cerebral angiography for the diagnosis of CVST has decreased significantly during the past decade, largely due to the advent of newer techniques such as MR and CT angiography and venography, which are noninvasive and pose little or no risk to the patient. Now, four-vessel angiography is mainly used in CVST patients who have had an inconclusive MRI/MR venogram or CT venogram, such as in isolated cortical vein thrombosis, or in those who are being considered for intrasinus use of thrombolytics or other recanalization therapies.

Transcranial Doppler (TCD) has also been applied in the diagnosis and follow-up of patients with dural sinus thrombosis (Caplan, 1996; Stolz *et al.*, 2002; Valdueza *et al.*, 1995, 1999; Wardlaw *et al.*, 1994). Venous signals can be detected and displayed from the region of the basal vein of Galen, which lies adjacent to the P2 portion of the posterior cerebral artery. In patients with dural sinus occlusions, the veins of Labbe and Rosenthal often serve as collateral channels. Increased blood flow in these veins increases the blood flow velocities as measured by TCD. The mean blood flow velocities in the region of the basal vein of Rosenthal have been quite elevated acutely in some patients and then have returned to normal after treatment and presumed recanalization of the original dural sinus occlusion (Valdueza *et al.*, 1995, 1999; Wardlaw *et al.*, 1994). TCD may be most useful in monitoring changes in venous flow and so documenting the effect of treatment. Too few patients have been studied and reported to know the effect of the location of the dural sinus occlusion on the frequency and reliability of the TCD results.

Management

General measures

The clinical course of CVST is highly variable. Some patients present with minor symptoms such as headaches, whereas others are comatose at presentation. The initial assessment is therefore directed towards identifying patients at higher risk of further deterioration and ensuring their immediate hemodynamic stability. Those with intracerebral hemorrhage, substantial brain edema, diminished level of responsiveness, or involvement of deep or a combination of deep and superficial venous systems should be monitored in intensive care units. Correction of dehydration with intravenous fluids is important, as intravascular depletion may promote further thrombosis. Any source of infection – especially involving the ear, mastoid, or sinuses – should be searched for and treated with appropriate antibiotics.

Seizures often complicate the picture in patients with CVST (Stam, 2005). Most seizures are partial in nature and respond well to antiepileptic medication, although some patients may develop status epilepticus. The long-term management with antiseizure medicines must be individualized as the existing data remain inconclusive in these patients (Nagpal, 1983; Preter *et al.*, 1996). Concurrently, a search for any predisposing conditions should be initiated promptly as their subsequent identification will influence the long-term treatment of these individuals. Many patients with intracranial venous occlusions have more than one predisposing condition (Stefini *et al.*, 1999).

Intracranial hypertension

The major pathology in CVST is thrombosis of cerebral veins or dural sinuses leading to impaired drainage, venous hypertension with subsequent edema formation, venous infarction, and hemorrhage. Patients with significant brain edema or hemorrhage often have elevated intracranial pressures. Application of general measures to reduce the elevated intracranial pressure, such as head elevation, is helpful in augmenting venous return. Short-term hyperventilation, often reserved for patients with severe brain edema, may also provide temporary benefit by inducing respiratory alkalosis and vasoconstriction, thereby reducing the total cerebral blood volume.

Hyperosmolar treatment with mannitol, glycerol, and hypertonic saline are usually helpful in reducing brain edema and

Table 66.3 Retrospective nonrandomized studies of the effects of anticoagulation in patients with intracranial venous thrombosis

	Anticoagulated		Not anticoagulated	
	Survived Improved	Died	Survived Improved	Died
Krayenbuhl, 1954	16	1	32	24
Bousser et al., 1985	23	0	11	4
*Case reports 1942–1987	25	3 bled	25	44
*Walker (unpublished)	6	0	7	1
Jacewicz and Plum, 1990	4	1 (veg)	4	5
Totals	74 (94%)	5 (6%)	79 (50%)	78 (50%)

* These cases are tabulated in Jacewicz and Plum, 1990.

lowering intracranial pressure. However, care should be exercised to avoid intravascular volume depletion with judicious supplementation of intravenous fluids, as dehydration may be counterproductive. Surgical options should be explored under special circumstances. Large hematomas exerting mass effect in patients with severe intracranial hypertension may be amenable to surgical evacuation. In patients with life-threatening brain edema, decompression with hemicraniectomy has also been attempted (Nagpal, 1983; Stefini et al., 1999).

Anticoagulation

Anticoagulation plays a central role in management of intracranial venous occlusive disease. Anticoagulants likely prevent further thrombus growth and propagation, helping to arrest the thrombotic process. Martin and Sheehan (1941) were first to advocate heparin treatment for CVST. Beginning in the 1960s, a number of single case reports and retrospective reviews began to support the safety and utility of heparin and other anticoagulants in the treatment of patients with intracranial venous thrombosis (Bousser and Barnett, 1992; Caplan, 1996; Jacewicz and Plum, 1990). In some patients, a dramatic improvement was noted a day or so after the starting of heparin in patients who had previously been steadily worsening. Table 66.3 tabulates retrospective nonrandomized results from case reports and series of patients with intracranial venous thromboses treated or not treated with anticoagulants. Among 79 patients given anticoagulants, 94% improved and survived, whereas only about one-half of the 157 patients not given anticoagulants survived (Jacewicz and Plum, 1990). Although these studies cannot prove effectiveness, they show that anticoagulants are probably seldom harmful.

Heparin therapy is now endorsed by most experts as the first line of treatment for patients with CVST (Bousser, 1999; Einhaupl et al., 2006). The effect of heparin has been studied in three, randomized controlled trials (de Bruijn and Stam, 1999; Einhaupl et al., 1991; Nagaraja et al., 1995). The first trial compared dose-adjusted intravenous heparin to placebo but was stopped after only 20 patients were enrolled because of the dramatic differences observed between the two groups; there were three deaths in the placebo group and none in the heparin-treated patients, whereas only one patient in the placebo group recovered completely compared to 8 of the 10 patients in the heparin group (Einhaupl et al., 1991). However, lingering doubts about the study methodology and concerns about risks of bleeding prompted another trial using low-molecular-weight heparin (de Bruijn and Stam, 1999). In this trial, 60 patients were randomized to receive nadroparin versus placebo, followed by an open arm of 10 weeks of warfarin treatment in those subjects who received heparin. There were no significant differences in outcomes between the two groups. However, there was a trend for all predefined outcomes in favor of anticoagulation. The third study performed on women with puerperal sinus thrombosis found a nonsignificant benefit of intravenous heparin treatment (Nagaraja et al., 1995). Though the results of these trials did not provide unequivocal evidence of efficacy of heparin treatment, heparin treatment appeared to be safe even in the presence of hemorrhagic lesions.

Another very important reason to use anticoagulants is to prevent pulmonary embolism from venous thrombi that often extend into the jugular vein and could, like any other peripheral venous occlusion, extend to the heart. Diaz et al. (1992) reported a patient with superior sagittal sinus thrombosis who died of a fatal pulmonary embolus. They also reviewed the available literature on patients with dural sinus occlusion studied between 1942 and 1990, and found that in 23/203 (11%) patients the dural sinus occlusion was complicated by pulmonary embolism, and all but 1 of these 23 patients died (Diaz et al., 1992).

The total duration of oral anticoagulation in patients with intracranial venous occlusive disease is not known. Some clinicians anticoagulate patients with transient risk factors with warfarin treatment for 3 months. Those patients with idiopathic CVST and those with mild thrombophilia are often treated for 6–12 months, whereas indefinite anticoagulation is considered in those with recurrent episodes of CVST (two or more) and in those with severe hereditary thrombophilia (Einhaupl et al., 2006).

Thrombolytic treatment

Endovascular thrombolysis with urokinase and tissue plasminogen activator, as well as mechanical thrombolysis, has been attempted in some patients with CVST (Canhao et al., 2003; Chow et al., 2000; Frey et al., 1999; Kim and Suh, 1997). However, the existing published data are limited to case reports and uncontrolled studies. Based on these reports, it is not possible to infer whether thrombolytic therapy is superior to heparin. Thrombolysis may help in restoring blood flow more promptly, but it is unclear whether this leads to a better clinical recovery (Frey et al., 1999; Kim and Suh, 1997). Thrombolysis might be most useful in patients with extensive venous occlusions who have limited egress of blood from the cranium. Hemorrhage risk is probably greater in patients who receive thrombolysis, especially in those with pre-existing hemorrhage (Frey et al., 1999; Kim and Suh, 1997). Thrombolytic treatment should therefore be reserved for those patients with a poor prognosis or in those who continue to worsen despite adequate anticoagulation and possibly have no associated hemorrhage. The role of mechanical treatment of dural sinus stenosis is also not clear at the present time.

Prognosis

Prospective studies that have examined the long-term outcome after CVST have reported a mortality rate ranging from 0% to 39% (Cakmak *et al.*, 2003; Rondepierre *et al.*, 1995). The death/dependence rate ranged from 9% to 44% (Ferro *et al.*, 2002; Rondepierre *et al.*, 1995). However, more recent data from a multicenter study (the Cerebral Venous Thrombosis Portuguese Collaborative Study Group; VENOPORT), which followed 624 patients with CVST for a median of 16 months, showed a better prognosis with a total mortality rate of 8% in this cohort (Ferro *et al.*, 2004). Patients presenting with isolated intracranial hypertension fared better (7% dead/dependent) than the remaining patients (13.6% dead/dependent). The study also analyzed risk factors for an unfavorable outcome that included male sex (hazard ratio [HR] = 1.6), age > 37 years (HR = 2.0), coma (HR = 2.7), mental status disorder (HR = 2.0), intracerebral hemorrhage on admission (HR = 1.9), thrombosis of the deep cerebral venous system (HR = 2.9), central nervous system infection (HR = 3.3), and cancer (HR = 2.9). Seizures (10%) and new thrombotic events (4%) were the most frequent complications during follow-up. The rate of recurrent sinus thrombosis was low at 2.2%.

The outcome of patients with early intracerebral hemorrhage after CVST was reported from this cohort (Girot *et al.*, 2007). A mortality rate of 6% within 30 days was observed in this subset of patients, and a 21% rate of death or dependency. Analysis of risk factors indicated that older age, male sex, thrombosis of the deep venous system, and motor deficits were associated with a worse outcome than was heparin use. Heparin treatment, in contrast, did not influence the risk of subsequent hemorrhage.

REFERENCES

Ameri, A., and Bousser, M.-G. 1992. Cerebral venous thrombosis. *Neurol Clin*, **10**, 87–111.

Ayanzen, R. H., Bird, C. R., Keller, P. J., *et al.* 2000. Cerebral MR venography: normal anatomy and diagnostic pitfalls. *AJNR Am J Neuroradiol*, **21**, 74–8.

Bianchi, D., Maeder, P. H., Bogousslavsky, J., Schnyder, P., and Meuli, R. A. 1998. Diagnosis of cerebral venous thrombosis with routine magnetic resonance: an update. *Eur Neurol*, **40**, 179–90.

Biousse, V., and Bousser, M. G. 1999. Cerebral venous thrombosis. *Neurologist*, **5**, 326–49.

Bousser, M. G. 1999. Cerebral venous thrombosis. Nothing, heparin, or local thrombolysis. *Stroke*, **30**, 481–3.

Bousser, M.-G., and Barnett, H. J. M. 1992. *Stroke. Pathophysiology, Diagnosis, and Management*, 2nd edn. H. Barnett, J. P. Mohr, B, M. Stein, F. M. Yatsu (eds.), New York: Churchill Livingstone, pp. 517–37.

Bousser, M.-G., Chiras, J., Bories, J., and Castaigne, P. 1985. Cerebral venous thrombosis: a review of 38 cases. *Stroke*, **16**, 199–213.

Cakmak, S., Derex, L., Berruyer, M., *et al.* 2003. Cerebral venous thrombosis: clinical outcome and systematic screening of prothrombotic factors. *Neurology*, **60**, 1175–8.

Canhao, P., Falcao, F., and Ferro, J. M. 2003. Thrombolysis for cerebral sinus thrombosis: a systematic review. *Cerebrovasc Dis*, **15**, 159–66.

Cantu, C., and Barinagarrementeria, F. 1993. Cerebral venous thrombosis associated with pregnancy and puerperium: review of 67 cases. *Stroke*, **24**, 1880–4.

Caplan, L. R. 1996. Venous and dural sinus occlusions in Posterior Circulation Disease. Clinical findings, diagnosis, and management. Boston: Blackwell Science, pp. 569–92.

Casey, S., Alberico, R. A., and Patel, M. 1996. Cerebral CT venography. *Radiology*, **198**, 163–70.

Chow, K., Gobin, P., Saver, J., *et al.* 2000. Endovascular treatment of dural sinus thrombosis with rheolytic thrombectomy and intra-arterial thrombolysis. *Stroke*, **31**, 1420–5.

Chu, K., Kang, D. W., Yoon, B. W., and Roh, J. K. 2001. Diffusion weighted magnetic resonance imaging in cerebral venous thrombosis. *Arch Neurol*, **58**, 1569–76.

Connor, S. E., and Jarosz, J. M. 2002. Magnetic resonance imaging of cerebral venous thrombosis. *Clin Radiol*, **57**, 449–61.

Cumurciuc, R., Crassard, I., Sarov, M., Valade, D., and Bousser, M. G. 2005. Headache as the only neurological sign of cerebral venous thrombosis: a series of 17 cases. *J Neurol Neurosurg Psychiatry*, **76**, 1084–7.

Daif, A., Awada, A., Al-Rajeh, S., *et al.* 1995. Cerebral venous thrombosis in adults. A study of 40 cases from Saudi Arabia. *Stroke*, **26**, 1193–5.

de Bruijn, S. F. T. M. (ed.) 1998. Cerebral Venous Sinus Thombosis: Clinical and Epidemiological Studies. Amsterdam: Thesis.

de Bruijn, S. F., and Stam, J. 1999. Randomized, placebo-controlled trial of anticoagulant treatment with low-molecular-weight heparin for cerebral sinus thrombosis. *Stroke*, **30**, 484–8.

de Bruijn, S. F., Stam, J., and Kappelle, L. J. 1996. Thunderclap headache as a first symptom of cerebral venous sinus thrombosis. *Lancet*, **348**, 1623–5.

deVeber, G., and Andrew, M. 2001. Cerebral sinovenous thrombosis in children. *N Engl J Med*, **345**, 417–23.

Diaz, J. M., Schiffman, J. S., and Urban, E. S. 1992. Superior sagittal sinus thrombosis and pulmonary embolism: a syndrome rediscovered. *Acta Neurol Scand*, **86**, 390–6.

Einhaupl, K., Bousser, M. G., de Bruijn, S. F., *et al.* 2006. EFNS guideline on the treatment of cerebral venous and sinus thrombosis. *Eur J Neurol*, **13**, 553–9.

Einhaupl, K., Villringer, A., Haberl, R. L., *et al.* 1990. Clinical spectrum of sinus venous thrombosis. In *Cerebral Sinus Thrombosis, Experimental and Clinical Aspects*, K. Einhaupl, O. Kemski, and A. Baethmann (eds.), New York: Plenum Press, pp. 149–55.

Einhaupl, K., Villringer, A., Meister, W., *et al.* 1991. Heparin treatment in sinus venous thrombosis. *Lancet*, **338**, 597–600.

Eng, L. J., Longstreth, W. T., Shaw, C. M., *et al.* 1990. Cerebellar venous infarction: case report with clinicopathologic correlation. *Neurology*, **40**, 837–8.

Ferro, J. M., Canhao, P., Stam, J., Bousser, M. G., and Barinagarrementeria, F. 2004. Prognosis of cerebral vein and dural sinus thrombosis: results of the International Study on Cerebral Vein and Dural Sinus Thrombosis (ISCVT). *Stroke*, **35**, 664–70.

Ferro, J. M., Lopes, M. G., Rosas, M. J., Ferro, M. A., and Fontes, J., for the Cerebral Venous Thrombosis Portuguese Collaborative Study Group (VENOPORT). 2002. Long-term prognosis of cerebral vein and dural sinus thrombosis: results of the VENOPORT Study. *Cerebrovasc Dis*, **13**, 272–8.

Frey, J. L., Muro, G. J., McDougall, C. G., Dean, B. L., and Jahnke, H. K. 1999. Cerebral venous thrombosis: combined intrathrombus rtPA and i.v. heparin. *Stroke*, **30**, 489–94.

Girot, M., Ferro, J. M., Canhao, P., *et al.* 2007. Predictors of outcome in patients with cerebral venous thrombosis and intracerebral hemorrhage. *Stroke*, **38**, 337–42.

Idbaih, A., Boukobza, M., Crassard, I., *et al.* 2006. MRI of clot in cerebral venous thrombosis: high diagnostic value of susceptibility-weighted images. *Stroke*, **37**, 991–5.

Jacewicz, M., and Plum, F. 1990. Aseptic cerebral venous thrombosis in cerebral sinus thrombosis. In *Experimental and Clinical Aspects*. New York: Plenum Press, pp. 157–70.

Kim, S. Y., and Suh, J. H. 1997. Direct endovascular thrombolytic therapy for dural sinus thrombosis: infusion of alteplase. *AJNR Am J Neuroradiol*, **18**, 639–45.

Kothare, S. V., Ebb, D. H., Rosenberger, P. B., *et al.* 1998. Acute confusion and mutism as a presentation of thalamic strokes secondary to deep cerebral venous thrombosis. *J Child Neurol*, **13**, 300–3.

Krayenbuhl, H. 1954. Cerebral venous thrombosis. The diagnostic value of cerebral angiography. *Schweiz Archiv Neurol Neurochir Psychiatr*, **74**, 261–87.

Kumral, E. 2001. Behcet's disease. In *Uncommon Causes of Stroke*, J. Bogous-slavsky, and L. R. Caplan (eds.). Cambridge: Cambridge University Press, pp. 150–6.

Lanska, D. J., and Kryscio, R. J. 2000. Risk factors for peripartum and postpartum stroke and intracranial venous thrombosis. *Stroke*, **31**, 1274–82.

Lovblad, K. O., Bassetti, C., Schneider, J., *et al.* 2001. Diffusion-weighted MR in cerebral venous thrombosis. *Cerebrovasc Dis*, **11**, 169–76.

Ludemann, P., Nabavi, G. D., Junker, R., *et al.* 1998. Factor V Leiden mutation is a risk factor for cerebral venous thrombosis: a case-control study of 55 patients. *Stroke*, **28**, 2507–10.

Martin, J., and Sheehan, H. 1941, Primary thrombosis of cerebral veins. *Br Med J*, **1**, 349–53.

Martinelli, I., Sacchi, E., Landi, G., *et al.* 1998. High risk of cerebral-vein thrombosis in carriers of prothombin-gene mutation and in users of oral contraceptives. *N Engl J Med*, **338**, 1793–7.

Nagaraja, D., Rao, B. S. S., Taly, A. B., and Subhash, M. N. 1995. Randomized controlled trial of heparin in puerperal cerebral venous/sinus thrombosis. *Nimhans J*, **13**, 111–15.

Nagpal, R. D. 1983. Dural sinus and cerebral venous thrombosis. *Neurosurg Rev*, **6**, 155–60.

Preter, M., Tzourio, C., Ameri, A., and Bousser, M. G. 1996. Long-term prognosis in cerebral venous thrombosis. Follow-up of 77 patients. *Stroke*, **27**, 243–6.

Provenzale, J. M., Joseph, G. J., and Barboriak, D. P. 1998. Dural sinus thrombosis: findings on CT and MR imaging and diagnostic pitfalls. *AJNR Am J Radiol*, **170**, 777–83.

Rao, K. C., Knipp, H. C., and Wajner, E. J. 1981. CT findings in cerebral and venous sinus thrombosis. *Radiology*, **140**, 391–8.

Rondepierre, P., Hamon, M., Leys, D., *et al.* 1995. Thromboses veineuses cerebrales: etude de l'evolution. *Rev Neurol (Paris)*, **151**, 100–4.

Rousseaux, P., Lesoin, F., Barbaste, P., and Jomin, M. 1987, Infarctus cerebelleux pseudotumoral d'origine veineuse. *Rev Neurol (Paris)*, **144**, 209–11.

Selim, M., Fink, J., Linfante, I., *et al.* 2002. Diagnosis of cerebral venous thrombosis with echo-planar T2*-weighted magnetic resonance imaging. *Arch Neurol*, **59**, 1021–6.

Southwick, F. S., Richardson, E. P., and Swartz, M. N. 1986. Septic thrombosis of the dural venous sinuses. *Medicine*, **65**, 82–106.

Stam, J. 2005. Thrombosis of cerebral veins and sinuses. *N Engl J Med*, **352**, 1791–8.

Stefini, R., Latronico, N., Cornali, C., Rasulo, F., and Bollati, A. 1999. Emergent decompressive craniectomy in patients with fixed dilated pupils due to cerebral venous and dural sinus thrombosis: report of three cases. *Neurosurgery*, **45**, 626.

Stolz, E., Gerriets, T., Bodeker, R. H., Hugens-Penzel, M., and Kaps, M. 2002. Intracranial venous hemodynamics is a factor related to a favorable outcome in cerebral venous thrombosis. *Stroke*, **33**, 1645–50.

Tsai, F., Wang, A.-M., Matovich, V. B., *et al.* 1995. MR staging of acute dural sinus thrombosis: correlation with venous pressure measurements and implications for treatment and prognosis. *AJNR Am J Neuroradiol*, **16**, 1021–9.

Valdueza, J. M., Hoffmann, O., Weih, M., Mehraein, S., and Einhaupl, K. M. 1999. Monitoring of venous hemodynamics in patients with cerebral venous thrombosis by transcranial Doppler ultrasound. *Arch Neurol*, **56**, 229–34.

Valdueza, J. M., Schultz, M., Harms, L., and Einhaupl, K. M. 1995. Venous transcranial Doppler ultrasound monitoring in acute dural sinus thrombosis. Report of two cases. *Stroke*, **26**, 1196–9.

Virapongse, C., Cazenave, C., Quisling, R., Sarwar, M., and Hunter, S. 1987. The empty delta sign. *Radiology*, **162**, 779–85.

Wardlaw, J. M., Vaughan, G. T., Steers, A. J. W., and Sellar, R. J. 1994. Transcranial Doppler ultrasound findings in venous sinus thrombosis. *J Neurosurg*, **80**, 332–5.

Wasay, M., Bakshi, R., Bobustuc, G., *et al.* 2002. Diffusion-weighted magnetic resonance imaging in superior sagittal sinus thrombosis. *J Neuroimaging*, **12**, 267–9.

Wechsler, B., Vidailhet, M., Piette, J. C., *et al.* 1992. Cerebral venous thrombosis in Behcet's disease: clinical study and long-term follow-up of 25 cases. *Neurology*, **42**, 614–8.

Wilder-Smith, E., Kothbauer-Margretier, I., Lammle, B., *et al.* 1997. Dural puncture and activated protein C resistance: risk factors for cerebral venous sinus thrombosis. *J Neurol Neurosurg Psychiatry*, **63**, 351–6.

PART VIII: VASOSPASTIC CONDITIONS AND OTHER MISCELLANEOUS VASCULOPATHIES

67 REVERSIBLE CEREBRAL VASOCONSTRICTION SYNDROMES

Aneesh B. Singhal, Walter J. Koroshetz, and Louis R. Caplan

Introduction

Segmental narrowing or "beading" of intracranial arteries on contrast cerebral angiograms is often associated with pathological conditions such as atherosclerosis, infectious arteritis, vasculitis, and fibromuscular dysplasia. In these conditions the arteries are histologically abnormal and the luminal narrowing is progressive unless the underlying condition can be treated. Several other conditions, however, are associated with reversible segmental narrowing of arteries that appear normal on routine histological examination. This phenomenon of reversible segmental arterial vasoconstriction is poorly understood and can affect cerebral as well as systemic arteries (Table 67.1).

Cerebral vasoconstriction has been associated with several diverse conditions (Table 67.1), including pregnancy (postpartum angiopathy), vasoconstrictive drugs (drug-induced "arteritis"), and headache disorders. While there may be differences in the etiopathogenesis of cerebral vasoconstriction with each associated condition, the clinical, laboratory, imaging, and angiographic features of these patients are remarkably similar, justifying the use of the inclusive term "reversible cerebral vasoconstriction syndromes" (RCVS). Most patients are young adults who present with acute-onset, severe, recurrent headaches. The vasoconstriction can persist for days to weeks and can progress to precipitate cerebral ischemia and stroke. Nevertheless, most patients have a benign outcome. Some are left with neurological deficits resulting from brain infarcts or hemorrhages. A minority develop a fulminant course with poor outcome including death. Although RCVS are considered rare, they are probably under-recognized and frequently misdiagnosed as primary cerebral vasculitis because the latter condition has overlapping angiographic and, to some degree, clinical features. With the advent of newer, relatively noninvasive angiographic techniques such as CT angiography (CTA) and MR angiography (MRA), and with the escalating use of vasoconstrictive drugs like "ecstacy" and cocaine, it is likely that physicians will encounter more patients with RCVS.

Historical background

Stroke and brain ischemia were associated with intracranial arterial "spasm" for decades; however, after the recognition of carotid artery stenosis, embolic stroke, and lacunar disease in the 1960s, subarachnoid hemorrhage and migraine emerged as the only two conditions associated with stroke from cerebral vasospasm. In the 1970s, several unusual cases were reported of women who, during

pregnancy or the early puerperium, developed sudden headaches, nausea, vomiting, seizures, and focal neurological deficits, and recovered spontaneously within a few weeks (Fisher, 1971; Millikan, 1975). The cerebrospinal fluid (CSF) was normal, and known thromboembolic etiologies were ruled out. Cerebral angiogram showed slow arterial filling or arterial irregularities that proved to be reversible on serial angiograms. At the Second Conference on Cerebrovascular Diseases at the Salpêtrière Hospital in Paris, Rascol et al. (1979) presented four such cases, and the entity came to be recognized as "postpartum angiopathy." Similar cases continued to be reported in association with pregnancy (Dupuy et al., 1979; Henry et al., 1984; Rousseaux et al., 1983), migraine (Fisher, 1986; Geraud and Fabre, 1984; Laurent et al., 1984; Michel et al., 1985; Serdaru et al., 1984), and even unruptured saccular aneurysms (Bloomfield and Sonntag, 1985; Day and Raskin, 1986; Friedman et al., 1983; Raynor and Messer, 1980). Because the ergot derivatives were frequently used in pregnancy and migraine, increased sympathomimetic tone was implicated in the pathophysiology (Henry et al., 1984; Raroque et al., 1993).

In 1987, Dr. Marie Fleming presented two patients with RCVS at the Boston Society of Neurology and Psychiatry meeting at Massachusetts General Hospital. Dr. C. Miller Fisher recognized the similarity between these and the other previously published cases of reversible cerebral vasoconstriction, including the patients with postpartum angiopathy (Rascol et al., 1979) presented at the Salpêtrière conference. In a collaborative effort Drs. Call, Fleming, Fisher, and others reported 19 patients in whom the vasoconstriction was either idiopathic or associated with the use of ergot derivatives, unruptured saccular aneurysms, carotid endarterectomy, and Guillain-Barré syndrome (Call et al., 1988). Although the precise pathophysiology was unknown, "migrainous vasospasm" was considered likely. Thereafter some authors reported patients with RCVS as having Call's syndrome or Call-Fleming syndrome (Martin-Araguz et al., 1997; Modi and Modi, 2000; Noskin et al., 2006; Nowak et al., 2003; Singhal et al., 2002).

In the rheumatology literature, patients with reversible changes on cerebral angiography were interpreted to have a benign form of cerebral vasculitis (Bettoni et al., 1984; Snyder and McClelland, 1978; van Calenbergh et al., 1986) because they responded promptly and completely to a short course of steroids, unlike other biopsy-proven cases of cerebral vasculitis. In 1993, Calabrese et al. reviewed these cases and proposed the term "benign angiopathy of the central nervous system" to characterize this subset of patients. Their group recently analyzed clinical characteristics and

Table 67.1 Conditions associated with reversible arterial vasoconstriction

Cerebral arteries

1. Pregnancy and puerperium

Early puerperium, late pregnancy, eclampsia*, pre-eclampsia*, delayed postpartum eclampsia*

2. Exposure to drugs and blood products

Phenylpropanolamine, pseudoephedrine, ergotamine tartrate, methergine, bromocriptine, lisuride, selective serotonin reuptake inhibitors (SSRIs)*, sumatriptan*, isometheptene, cocaine, ecstacy, amphetamine derivatives*, marijuana*, lysergic acid diethylamide (LSD), tacrolimus (FK-506), cyclophosphamide*, erythropoietin*, intravenous immune globulin (IVIG)*, red blood cell transfusions*

3. Miscellaneous

Hypercalcemia, porphyria*, pheochromocytoma, bronchial carcinoid tumor, unruptured saccular cerebral aneurysm, head trauma, spinal subdural hematoma, postcarotid endarterectomy*, neurosurgical procedures

4. Idiopathic

No identifiable precipitating factor

Associated with headache disorders such as migraine, primary thunderclap headache*, benign exertional headache, benign sexual headache, primary cough headache

Systemic arteries

1. Extremities: Raynaud's phenomenon, digit ischemia from vasoconstrictive drugs

2. Coronary: Prinzmetal's angina, cocaine-induced coronary vasospasm

3. Renal: possible small-vessel vasoconstriction due to tacrolimus, cyclosporine

4. Mesenteric: associated with carcinoid tumor, sumatriptan

5. Uterine: eclampsia

* These conditions are also associated with the Reversible Posterior Leukoencephalopathy Syndrome (RPLS)

long-term outcomes of this entity and concluded that it is probably a cerebral vasoconstriction syndrome (Hajj-Ali et al., 2002).

Stroke and angiographic "beading" associated with the use of nasal decongestants, diet pills, and other sympathomimetic drugs such as cocaine, amphetamines, ephedrine, ergot derivatives, pseudoephedrine, and phenylpropanolamine have been reported as drug-induced cerebral "arteritis" (Bostwick, 1981; Forman et al., 1989; Margolis and Newton, 1971; Merkel et al., 1995; Mourand et al., 1999; Ryu and Lin, 1995; Stoessl et al., 1985; Yu et al., 1983). However, this diagnosis was based almost exclusively on angiography alone, without other evidence for vasculitis (Aggarwal et al., 1996; Buxton and McConachie, 2000; Kaye and Fainstat, 1987; Nolte et al., 1996), although at times there was indication of vascular inflammation more consistent with nonspecific injury or vascular necrosis (Merkel et al., 1995; Rumbaugh et al., 1971) or a "reactive" inflammation (Calado et al., 2004b). Similar abnormalities have been associated with exposure to serotonergic agents such as ecstasy, sumatriptan, and the selective serotonin reuptake inhibitors (Conde Lopez et al., 1998; Meschia et al., 1998;

Nighoghossian et al., 1998; Noskin et al., 2006; Singhal et al., 2002). It is likely that these clinical angiographic abnormalities result from vasoconstrictive effects of the drugs and not from an underlying inflammatory vasculitis.

Patients with cerebral vasoconstriction have been reported by stroke neurologists, headache specialists, obstetricians, and rheumatologists under different eponymic labels based on the associated conditions and theories of pathogenesis. Patients with identical clinical, imaging, and laboratory features have been reported as having "postpartum angiopathy," "migraine angiitis," "thunderclap headache associated vasospasm," "drug induced angiopathy," "Call-Fleming syndrome," "benign cerebral angiopathy," benign angiopathy of the central nervous system," and "reversible cerebral angiitis." The confusing nomenclature has probably hampered the recognition of RCVS and limited research concerning its causes and pathogenesis. Only recently have some authors started defining the unifying clinical and imaging features of patients with cerebral vasoconstriction (Singhal, 2002a, 2004a; Singhal and Bernstein, 2005; Singhal et al., 2003), and have proposed that cerebral vasoconstriction in the setting of any associated condition be uniformly referred to as a reversible cerebral vasoconstriction syndrome or RCVS (Calabrese et al., 2007). These efforts have already started improving the recognition and diagnosis of patients with cerebral vasoconstriction. For example, Ducros et al. (2007) recently published their series of 67 patients with RCVS accumulated over a 3-year period. This large prospective series confirms many of the clinical-imaging features identified in prior reviews and smaller case series. In this series, RCVS was spontaneous in 37% and secondary to one or more risk factors in 63% of patients. Identifying the precipitating secondary cofactor or disease is important, because it may guide management (e.g. stopping the vasoactive drug) and eventually lead toward a better understanding of the pathogenesis. Finally, recent publications have drawn attention to the overlapping clinical and imaging features of reversible cerebral vasoconstriction syndromes, recurrent primary thunderclap headache, and the reversible posterior leukoencephalopathy syndrome, raising the possibility of a shared pathophysiology between these entities (Calabrese et al., 2007; Chen et al., 2006; Singhal, 2004b).

Clinical features

The RCVS affects women more often than men. Most reported patients are between 20 and 50 years of age, although children can be affected (Kirton et al., 2006). The typical patient presents with a sudden, "worst-ever" headache that reaches its peak intensity within seconds, often referred to as a "thunderclap headache" (Day and Raskin, 1986; Dodick, 2002). Thunderclap headache is most characteristic of aneurysmal subarachnoid hemorrhage and can be the presenting symptom of conditions such as primary brain hemorrhage, carotid artery dissection, and cerebral venous sinus thrombosis. As a result, patients are often (and appropriately) subjected to a battery of tests to evaluate for ruptured saccular aneurysms or other intracranial causes of sudden, severe headache. The onset headache may be occipital or diffuse, severe and throbbing, and accompanied by nausea, emesis, and photosensitivity. Sudden-onset headaches can recur for days to weeks (Ducros et al., 2007); however, their intensity and frequency diminish over time. Headache recurrence can be spontaneous while the patient is at rest, or precipitated by exertion or Valsalva maneuver.

A past medical history or a family history of migraine and depression is often present, and some patients can later develop chronic migraine-like headaches or depression. Precipitating conditions include pregnancy or puerperium, vasoconstrictive drug exposure, head trauma, neurosurgical manipulation, and others (Table 67.1). Emotional disturbances (e.g. sudden fear, orgasm, excitement) are frequently reported at the onset (Kapoor et al., 1990; Silbert et al., 1989; Valenca et al., 2004). We have encountered a young man whose syndrome was precipitated by an intense burning sensation of the palate after ingestion of a spicy red jalapeno pepper! Blood pressure may be normal or elevated, although usually not elevated to the levels seen in hypertensive encephalopathy.

Severe neurological symptoms and signs can develop from ischemia in brain regions that are perfused by an artery that is severely constricted. Brain hemorrhage can occur and explain neurological dysfunction (Singhal, 2007). Generalized motor seizures may occur at the onset, but epilepsy does not ensue; the seizures are attributable to brain edema or ischemia from severe vasoconstriction. Neurological deficits, if present, occur in the first few days after onset of the headache and often localize to the parieto-occipital lobes and "borderzone" arterial territories. Visual dysfunction (cortical blindness, Balint's syndrome, flashing lights, and scotomas) is frequent (Calabrese et al., 2007; Singhal, 2002a). Most patients have exaggerated muscle reflexes and tremor. Confusion, apraxia, dysarthria, aphasia, numbness, hemiparesis, and ataxia have been reported. Clinical deficits usually recover within days to weeks, and headaches usually improve within a few weeks, either spontaneously or after treatment with vasodilators or steroids. There are rare instances of a devastating course and even death (Buckle et al., 1964; Geraghty et al., 1991; Singhal, 2002b).

Brain and vascular imaging

Up to one-third of patients with RCVS show no abnormality on parenchymal brain imaging (Singhal et al., 2003) despite having multifocal cerebral arterial narrowing on angiograms. Normal brain scans are virtually unknown in patients with primary cerebral vasculitis, a mimic of RCVS, and this feature helps to separate the two conditions.

The most frequent head CT or brain MRI abnormality is bihemispheric, symmetric infarcts in arterial borderzone regions (Figures 67.1 and 67.2). Ischemic lesions are often crescentic or horseshoe-shaped; however, with severe ischemia the cortex becomes affected and lesions appear more wedge-shaped. Perfusion imaging may show areas of hypoperfusion distal to the affected artery. Some patients have shown infarct progression within these hypoperfused regions (Figure 67.1), supporting the hypothesis that ischemic stroke results from severe cerebral hypoperfusion (Rosenbloom and Singhal, 2007; Singhal et al., 2002). On MRI, fluid-attenuated inversion recovery (FLAIR) sequences often show dot-shaped or linear hyperintensities along

the cortical surfaces, which may reflect slow flow within dilated vessels (Doss-Esper et al., 2005; Iancu-Gontard et al., 2003; Rosenbloom and Singhal, 2007; Singhal, 2004b). Up to one-third of patients develop brain hemorrhage, including parenchymal hemorrhages (Campos and Yamamoto, 2006; Fallis and Fisher, 1985; Maertens et al., 1987; Roh and Park, 1998; Singhal, 2007; Ursell et al., 1998; Yu et al., 1983) and small "non-aneurysmal" subarachnoid hemorrhages overlying the cortical surface (Doss-Esper et al., 2005; Rosenbloom and Singhal, 2007; Singhal, 2007). The timing of brain hemorrhages and ischemic strokes appears to be different, with hemorrhages occurring early and infarcts occurring later, mainly in the second week after onset (Ducros et al., 2007). The mechanism of hemorrhage is unclear, but may be related to ischemia-reperfusion injury and leakage or rupture of cortical surface vessels in the setting of abrupt hypertension and impaired autoregulation. Recent drug exposure appears to be more common in patients with brain hemorrhage. Brain edema, in a topographical pattern resembling the reversible posterior reversible leukoencephalopathy syndrome, has been reported (Dodick et al., 2003; Doss-Esper et al., 2005; Singhal, 2004b).

The diagnosis of RCVS rests on showing reversible vasoconstriction in the cerebral vasculature (Figures 67.1 and 67.2). Transfemoral angiography, CTA, MRA, and TCD ultrasound have all been used for this purpose. Indirect tests such as CTA may be preferable because of their lower risks. The medium-sized cerebral arteries (the middle and anterior cerebral arteries and the intracranial vertebral, basilar, posterior cerebral, superior cerebellar, anterior inferior cerebellar, and posterior inferior cerebellar arteries) are most frequently involved, and show multifocal areas of segmental narrowing as well as vasodilatation ("beading"). It is possible that the angiographic changes start distally and progress proximally towards the larger arteries (Ducros et al., 2007). Rarely, the extracranial internal carotid artery can become involved and even occlude from severe vasoconstriction (Janzarik et al., 2006). Small, unruptured, cerebral aneurysms have been shown in some patients (Day and Raskin, 1986; Friedman et al., 1983; Raynor and Messer, 1980; Singhal, 2002b; Wijdicks et al., 1988). The prevailing view is that these unruptured aneurysms are incidental (Wijdicks et al., 1988). TCD studies show diffusely elevated intracranial blood flow velocities (Bogousslavsky et al., 1989; Gomez et al., 1991; Ihara et al., 2000; Nowak et al., 2003; Zunker et al., 2002) and are most useful as follow-up tests to establish reversal of vasoconstriction (Figure 67.1).

The most specific evidence for the diagnosis of an RCVS is complete or near-complete reversibility of vasoconstriction in a timely manner, invariably within 3 months. It cannot be overemphasized that the angiographic findings, although highly characteristic, are not specific for RCVS and cannot be differentiated from the angiographic abnormalities seen with cerebral vasculitis (Calabrese et al., 1997). The diagnosis of RCVS is heavily influenced by the pretest probability derived from the clinical findings, the presence of associated conditions (Table 67.1), and the results of adjunctive studies such as CSF examination. Clearing of clinical symptoms and vascular imaging abnormalities over time without immunosuppressant treatment are other important diagnostic findings that support characterization of the condition as an RCVS.

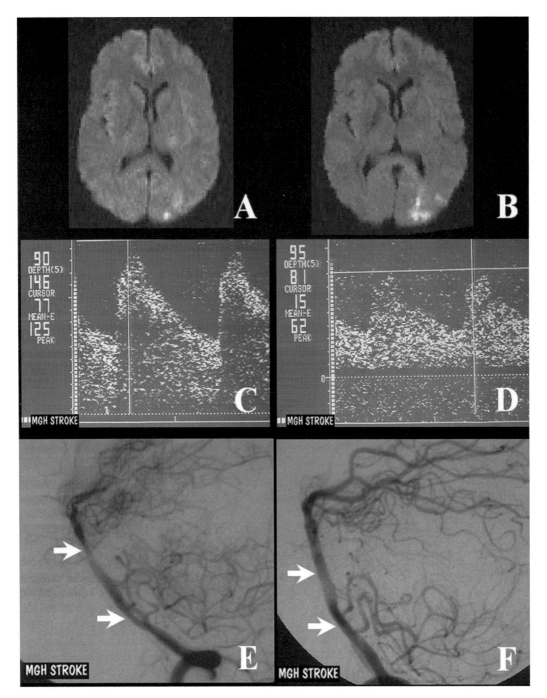

Figure 67.1 Brain imaging in a woman with RCVS. (**A**) Initial diffusion-weighted MRI (DWI) shows small occipital infarctions. Surrounding areas of hypoperfusion, suggesting vasoconstriction, were present on perfusion MRI (not shown). (**B**) Follow-up DWI after 1 week shows progressive infarction within the hypoperfused areas. (**C**) Initial transcranial Doppler (TCD) ultrasound shows marked elevation of blood flow velocities in the right middle cerebral artery. (**D**) Follow-up TCD ultrasound after 3 months shows normal blood flow velocities. (**E**) Initial cerebral angiogram shows vasoconstriction of the basilar and posterior cerebral arteries (*arrows*). (**F**) Follow-up angiogram after 4 months shows reversal of the vasoconstriction.

Etiology and pathophysiology

The etiology of the sudden, prolonged, and spontaneously reversible vasoconstriction is not known. A disturbance in the control of cerebral vascular tone appears to be a critical element. Many authors have implicated "migrainous vasospasm" in view of the frequent prior history of migraine and the severe headache, nau-

sea, vomiting, and visual symptoms that characterize the onset. Migraine is a common condition, and as discussed below the relationship between migraine and RCVS is unclear. However, a migraine association may imply that there is a pre-existing genetic susceptibility to vasoconstriction in migraineurs, which makes them vulnerable to develop severe persistent vasoconstriction after an appropriate vasoactive stimulus. The association with

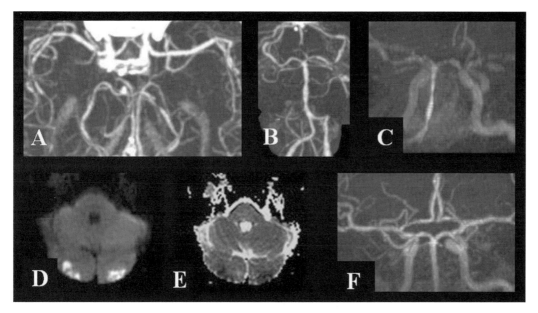

Figure 67.2 Brain imaging in a 46-year-old male with RCVS. The patient, who had a past medical history of migraine without aura, hypertension, hyperlipidemia, and cannabis abuse, developed a severe postcoital thunderclap headache. Severe headaches recurred, and on day 3 he developed cortical blindness and mild left hemiparesis. Admission CTA showed multifocal segmental stenosis ('beading') of the bilateral middle cerebral arteries (**A**) and the basilar, posterior cerebral and superior cerebellar arteries (**B**). These abnormalities were also present on brain MRA (**C**). Diffusion-weighted MRI (**D**) and apparent diffusion coefficient maps (**E**) showed symmetric lesions in the bilateral occipital lobes, consistent with ischemic strokes. In addition, brain MRI showed small infarcts in the bilateral cerebellar hemispheres and in the right frontal lobe (not shown). Serological tests and the results of two CSF examinations showed no evidence for vasculitis or subarachnoid hemorrhage. The patient was treated with analgesics and verapamil. His deficits resolved completely over a period of 3 weeks, and a follow-up MRA (**F**) showed resolution of the cerebral arterial vasoconstriction. Reproduced with permission from Calabrese, L. H., Dodick, D. W., Schwedt, T. J., and Singhal, A. B. 2007. Narrative review: reversible cerebral vasoconstriction syndromes. *Ann Intern Med*, **146**, 34–44.

sympathomimetic or serotonergic drugs and tumors (Armstrong and Hayes, 1961; Henry *et al.*, 1984; Le Coz *et al.*, 1988; Nighoghossian *et al.*, 1994, 1998; Noskin *et al.*, 2006; Raroque *et al.*, 1993; Razavi *et al.*, 1999; Singhal *et al.*, 2002), acute porphyria (Black *et al.*, 1995; Kupferschmidt *et al.*, 1995), hypercalcemia (Kaplan, 1998; Walker *et al.*, 1980; Yamamoto *et al.*, 1999; Yarnell and Caplan, 1986), IVIG (Doss-Esper *et al.*, 2005; Sztajzel *et al.*, 1999; Voltz *et al.*, 1996), carotid endarterectomy (Brick *et al.*, 1990; Dagher *et al.*, 2005; Lopez-Valdes *et al.*, 1997; Rosenbloom and Singhal, 2007), neurosurgical trauma (Chang *et al.*, 1999; Hyde-Rowan *et al.*, 1983; LeRoux *et al.*, 1991; Lopez-Valdes *et al.*, 1997; Schaafsma *et al.*, 2002; Suwanwela and Suwanwela, 1972) and uncontrolled hypertension (Goldstein *et al.*, 1991; Kontos *et al.*, 1978) have led to speculation that chemical factors (e.g. circulating catecholamines, serotonin, endothelin-1, calcium, nitric oxide, prostaglandins) as well as mechanical factors (e.g. shear stress) may be involved in the pathophysiology. The frequent occurrence in women, particularly around the time of delivery, menarche, and menopause, suggests a role for hormonal influences. Some authors speculate that the vasoconstriction is related to transient inflammation, although the results of pathological, serological, and CSF tests have not shown evidence for inflammation. Sudden alterations in blood flow and blood volume as occur during pregnancy and puerperium and after carotid artery surgery could also stress cranial blood vessels that are predisposed to vasoactivity.

Approach to diagnosis

For the experienced clinician familiar with the syndrome, RCVS is not difficult to recognize and diagnose: most patients report acute-onset, severe headaches at onset, have benign CSF findings, characteristic brain-imaging features, and vascular abnormalities that are fully reversible. Ideally the patient should have all of the features outlined in Table 67.2.

Sudden-onset (thunderclap) headaches may herald conditions such as subarachnoid hemorrhage, embolic occlusion of the posterior or middle cerebral arteries, intracerebral hemorrhage, arterial dissection, viral meningitis, spontaneous intracranial hypotension, pituitary apoplexy, and cerebral venous sinus thrombosis (Headache Classification Subcommittee, 2004; Dodick, 2002). The initial evaluation should uniformly include a head CT scan to exclude these more common and ominous conditions. If the CT scan does not reveal any etiology for thunderclap headache, neurovascular imaging should be performed to investigate for vascular causes of headache such as arterial dissection, cerebral venous sinus thrombosis, and reversible cerebral vasoconstriction. Indirect tests such as CTA and MRA are appropriate first-line imaging techniques to evaluate for reversible cerebral vasoconstriction; however, conventional catheter-based angiography still remains the gold standard. Once arterial vasoconstriction is shown, further tests should be directed towards excluding alternate causes of angiographic narrowing. CSF examination

Table 67.2 Summary of critical elements for the diagnosis of RCVS

1. Transfemoral angiography or indirect CTA or MRA documenting segmental cerebral artery vasoconstriction
2. No evidence for aneurysmal subarachnoid hemorrhage
3. Normal or near-normal CSF analysis (proteins < 80 mg/dL, white blood cells < 10/mm³, normal glucose)
4. Severe, acute headache, with or without additional neurologic signs or symptoms

The diagnosis cannot be confirmed until reversibility of the angiographic abnormalities is documented within 12 weeks after onset or (if death occurs before the follow-up studies are completed) autopsy rules out conditions such as vasculitis, intracranial atherosclerosis, and aneurysmal subarachnoid hemorrhage, which can also manifest with headache and stroke.

Source: Calabrese, L. H., Dodick, D. W., Schwedt, T. J., and Singhal, A. B. 2007. Narrative review: reversible cerebral vasoconstriction syndromes. *Ann Intern Med*, **146**, 34–44, with permission]

should be performed to exclude "CT negative" subarachnoid hemorrhage and inflammatory conditions such as infection and cerebral vasculitis. In a systematic review (Singhal, 2002a) of 152 patients with the RCVS, CSF results were entirely normal in 80% of patients, and 95% of patients had CSF cell counts < 10 per mm³ and protein levels < 80 mg/dL. Blood tests such as erythrocyte sedimentation rate, rheumatoid factor, anti-nuclear and anti-neutrophil cytoplasmic antibody titers, and urine vanillylmandelic acid and 5-hydroxy indoleacetic acid levels are useful to evaluate for systemic vasculitis and pheochromocytoma. Serum calcium, and in some instances parathyroid hormone, levels should be drawn because hypercalcemia is a known cause of cerebral vasoconstriction and can cause strokes. Some patients with an RCVS may not have a classic thunderclap headache, and the CSF might show minor elevations of protein and cell counts such that a diagnosis of cerebral vasculitis should still be seriously considered. In this circumstance, particularly if there are neurological deficits and/or diffuse parenchymal abnormalities or multifocal strokes on MRI, a brain biopsy to exclude cerebral vasculitis may be indicated.

Blood flow velocities in intracranial arteries measured by TCD are helpful in following patients with RCVS. Velocities are invariably elevated at onset and decrease when the condition remits either spontaneously or after treatment.

Differential diagnosis

The differential diagnosis primarily includes disorders that present with acute, severe thunderclap headache (Dodick, 2002), which can be excluded with appropriate brain and vascular imaging as discussed above. If imaging is negative and the patient does not prove to have vasoconstriction, primary headache disorders such as primary thunderclap headache, primary exertional headache or orgasmic headache should be considered (Headache Classification Subcommittee, 2004; Silbert *et al.*, 1989). In a prospective study of recurrent thunderclap headaches, Chen

et al. found evidence for cerebral vasoconstriction in 39% of patients. The clinical features of patients with and without vasoconstriction was remarkable similar. These observations suggest that recurrent primary thunderclap headache and cerebral vasoconstriction syndrome constitute different spectra of the same disorder (Chen *et al.*, 2006). Migraine is an important differential diagnosis because many patients have a past history of migraine, the topography of brain infarcts can be similar, serotonergic mechanisms are implicated in both conditions (Singhal *et al.*, 2002), and because migraine headache has been associated with cerebral angiographic abnormalities (Fisher, 1983; Garnic and Schellinger, 1983; Gomez *et al.*, 1991; Lieberman *et al.*, 1984; Masuzawa *et al.*, 1983; Monteiro *et al.*, 1985; Sanin and Mathew, 1993; Schluter and Kissig, 2002; Schon and Harrison, 1987; Serdaru *et al.*, 1984; Solomon *et al.*, 1990). Some authors have questioned whether RCVS is simply a severe prolonged migraine attack ("status migrainosis") with the fortuitous documentation of angiographic vasoconstriction (Gilbert, 2002). However, there are important differences. The angiographic abnormalities in RCVS, although reversible, usually persist for days to weeks, whereas most patients with migraine have normal arteriograms. The presenting headache in RCVS is invariably hyperacute, is not preceded by the premonitory or aura symptoms often seen with migraine, and does not resemble the patient's prior attacks of migraine. Unlike RCVS, migraine is a recurrent disorder, and has a primarily neuronal basis.

Intracranial atherosclerosis, fibromuscular dysplasia, inflammatory vasculitis, and infectious arteritis are conditions that can cause stroke, are associated with headache, and have similar angiographic features but carry a significantly worse prognosis. A careful medical history usually helps to distinguish these conditions from RCVS. For example, atherosclerosis tends to affect older individuals with risk factors such as chronic hypertension or diabetes and results in chronic strokes. Intracranial atherosclerosis of branch arteries is especially common among blacks and individuals of Asian origin and is more common in women than men. The demonstration of prompt resolution of vasoconstriction decreases the likelihood of misdiagnosis. Patients with aneurysmal subarachnoid hemorrhage typically present with thunderclap headache and can develop cerebral vasospasm; however, the vasospasm usually develops later (day 4–11) and is restricted to the artery surrounded by blood rather than affecting multiple arteries as in the RCVS.

The condition that is often difficult to distinguish from RCVS is primary angiitis of the central nervous system (CNS), an inflammatory condition affecting brain arteries that often requires brain biopsy for definitive diagnosis and that warrants urgent treatment with immunosuppressive agents. Features such as headache, focal deficits, stroke, seizures, and angiographic irregularities are common to both conditions. It is important to distinguish RCVS from primary angiitis of the CNS because consideration of vasculitis can unnecessarily expose patients with an RCVS to the risks of brain biopsy and to the adverse effects of long-term immunosuppressive therapy.

While angiograms can be identical in both conditions, the diagnosis is secured within the context of clinical presentation, CSF analysis, and the presence of associated conditions such as pregnancy. Patients with primary angiitis of the CNS tend to have insidious, dull headaches, a stepwise clinical progression, abnormal CSF results, and multifocal infarctions widely distributed in the gray and white matter, with or without diffuse white matter hyperintensities, on brain MRI (Singhal *et al.*, 2003). Conversely, patients with RCVS have dramatic clinical presentations with explosive headaches and normal CSF findings, and one-third show no abnormality on brain MRI. Though rare exceptions exist (Calado *et al.*, 2004a), the reversibility over days to weeks is the feature that best distinguishes this disorder from CNS vasculitis.

The reversible posterior leukoencephalopathy syndrome (RPLS) is a reversible brain edema syndrome characterized by onset headaches, visual symptoms, and reversible gray and white matter lesions on brain MRI. Associated conditions include eclampsia, hypertensive encephalopathy, porphyria, and exposure to chemotherapeutic immunosuppressant agents, and its etiology is related to endothelial dysfunction and a disturbance in cerebral autoregulation (Hinchey *et al.*, 1996). Similar clinical features and edematous MRI lesions are found in patients with cerebral vasoconstriction (Boughammoura *et al.*, 2003; Dodick *et al.*, 2003; Doss-Esper *et al.*, 2005; Henderson *et al.*, 2003; Lin *et al.*, 2003; Rosenbloom and Singhal, 2007; Singhal, 2004b; Singhal and Bernstein, 2005; Zunker *et al.*, 2000). These features, and the similar associated conditions, suggest that RCVS and RPLS are overlapping disorders sharing a pathophysiologic disturbance in cerebral arterial tone.

Management

The treatment of RCVS is guided by personal experience and observational data. There is no "standard of care," and no clinical trials have been conducted to prove that any treatment can alter the natural history of this syndrome. RCVS is often self-limited, with spontaneous clinical improvement and resolution of headaches and angiographic abnormalities occurring during a few weeks. Successful outcomes including alleviation of symptoms and rapid reversibility of vascular abnormalities have been reported with a variety of modalities including calcium-channel blockers (Dodick, 2003; Lu *et al.*, 2004; Nowak *et al.*, 2003), brief courses of glucocorticoids (Hajj-Ali *et al.*, 2002), and magnesium sulfate (Singhal, 2004b). Calcium-channel blockers such as verapamil, nimodipine, and nicardipine show more effects on cervico-cranial arteries, and these agents may be preferred. It is difficult to ascertain the true effectiveness of these treatments because the headache and angiographic abnormalities are known to fluctuate and to resolve spontaneously even with simple observation (Ducros *et al.*, 2007; Hajj-Ali *et al.*, 2002; Singhal, 2004b; Singhal *et al.*, 2002).

All potentially vasoconstrictive drugs should be discontinued whenever this diagnosis is suspected. Headaches should be treated with analgesic medications, and drugs like sumatriptan, which have vasoconstrictive effects, should be avoided (Meschia *et al.*, 1998; Singhal *et al.*, 2002). Because the Valsalva maneuver can precipitate headache exacerbations, precautionary measures such as the use of stool softeners and avoidance of heavy physical exertion are probably beneficial. Seizures, if present, usually do not recur after the initial few days, and prolonged use of antiepileptics is unnecessary in the absence of brain hemorrhage or chronic stroke-induced seizures. Because distinction between RCVS and primary angiitis of the CNS can be difficult in the initial stages, a short course of steroids to treat possible vasculitis is sometimes justified. Long-term steroid therapy is fraught with complications, and steroids should be discontinued if serial angiography shows resolution. A brief course of steroids does not cure true vasculitis, so reversible cerebral vasoconstriction is a more likely diagnosis if complete remission follows a short steroid course.

Most patients remain stable despite severe angiographic abnormalities and do not require admission to the neurological critical care unit. Patients who deteriorate usually do so within the first week, and should be promptly transferred to the intensive care unit for careful hydration and blood pressure and TCD monitoring. Blood pressure management in this syndrome can be challenging. Acute hypertension can precipitate further vasoconstriction, and pharmacologically induced hypertension should be avoided (Rosenbloom and Singhal, 2007). In contrast, hypotension can theoretically reduce cerebral perfusion pressure and result in stroke. Some patients can develop progressive vasoconstriction and stroke, and in this circumstance emergent intervention with balloon angioplasty (Ringer *et al.*, 2001) or intra-arterial nicardipine (Badjatia *et al.*, 2004) may be considered, although some patients deteriorate despite these aggressive measures (Song *et al.*, 2004).

Prognosis

Most patients with RCVS recover completely or near-completely within days to weeks. Fulminant vasoconstriction resulting in progressive symptoms (Ringer *et al.*, 2001) or death (Buckle *et al.*, 1964; Geraghty *et al.*, 1991; Singhal, 2002b) can occur in rare cases. There may be a lag in the resolution of the clinical or angiographic features after either has resolved. It should be noted that "reversibility" in the term RCVS refers to reversibility of vasoconstriction, and that some patients may be left with permanent neurological deficits from infarcts or hemorrhages. Recurrence of an RCVS episode (i.e. after headaches stop recurring and after vasoconstriction reversal has been documented) is virtually unknown and has been reported in only one patient with postpartum angiopathy (Ursell *et al.*, 1998). There is no evidence that the risk for complications such as eclampsia or pre-eclampsia in subsequent pregnancies is increased following an episode of postpartum angiopathy.

REFERENCES

Aggarwal, S. K., Williams, V., Levine, S. R., Cassin, B. J., and Garcia, J. H. 1996. Cocaine-associated intracranial hemorrhage: absence of vasculitis in 14 cases. *Neurology*, **46**, 1741–3.

Armstrong, F. S., and Hayes, G. J. 1961. Segmental cerebral arterial constriction associated with pheochromocytoma. *J Neurosurg*, **18**, 843–6.

Badjatia, N., Topcuoglu, M, A., Pryor, J. C., *et al.* 2004. Preliminary experience with intra-arterial nicardipine as a treatment for cerebral vasospasm. *AJNR Am J Neuroradiol*, **25**, 819–26.

Bettoni, L., Juvarra, G., Bortone, E., and Lechi, A. 1984. Isolated benign cerebral vasculitis. Case report and review. *Acta Neurol Belg*, **84**, 161–73.

Black, K. S., Mirsky, P., Kalina, P., *et al.* 1995. Angiographic demonstration of reversible cerebral vasospasm in porphyric encephalopathy. *AJNR Am J Neuroradiol*, **16**, 1650–2.

Bloomfield, S. M., and Sonntag, V. K. 1985. Delayed cerebral vasospasm after uncomplicated operation on an unruptured aneurysm: case report. *Neurosurgery*, **17**, 792–6.

Bogousslavsky, J., Despland, P. A., Regli, F., and Dubuis, P. Y. 1989. Postpartum cerebral angiopathy: reversible vasoconstriction assessed by transcranial Doppler ultrasounds. *Eur Neurol*, **29**, 102–5.

Bostwick, D. G. 1981. Amphetamine induced cerebral vasculitis. *Hum Pathol*, **12**, 1031–3.

Boughammoura, A., Touze, E., Oppenheim, C., Trystram, D., and Mas, J. L. 2003. Reversible angiopathy and encephalopathy after blood transfusion. *J Neurol*, **250**, 116–8.

Brick, J. F., Dunker, R. O., and Gutierrez, A. R. 1990. Cerebral vasoconstriction as a complication of carotid endarterectomy. Case report. *J Neurosurg*, **73**, 151–3.

Buckle, R. M., Du Boulay, G., and Smith, B. 1964. Death due to cerebral vasospasm. *J Neurol Neurosurg Psychiatry*, **27**, 440–4.

Buxton, N., and McConachie, N. S. 2000. Amphetamine abuse and intracranial haemorrhage. *J Roy Soc Med*, **93**, 472–7.

Calabrese, L. H., Dodick, D. W., Schwedt, T. J., and Singhal, A. B. 2007. Narrative review: reversible cerebral vasoconstriction syndromes. *Ann Intern Med*, **146**, 34–44.

Calabrese, L. H., Duna, G. F., and Lie, J. T. 1997. Vasculitis in the central nervous system. *Arthritis Rheum*, **40**, 1189–201.

Calabrese, L. H., Gragg, L. A., and Furlan, A. J. 1993. Benign angiopathy: a distinct subset of angiographically defined primary angiitis of the central nervous system. *J Rheumatol*, **20**, 2046–50.

Calado, S., Vale-Santos, J., Lima, C., and Viana-Baptista, M. 2004. Postpartum cerebral angiopathy: vasospasm, vasculitis or both? *Cerebrovasc Dis*, **18**, 340–1.

Call, G. K., Fleming, M. C., Sealfon, S., *et al.* 1988. Reversible cerebral segmental vasoconstriction. *Stroke*, **19**, 1159–70.

Campos, C. R., and Yamamoto, F. I. 2006. Intracerebral hemorrhage in postpartum cerebral angiopathy associated with the use of isometheptene. *Int J Gynaecol Obstet*, **95**, 151–2.

Case records of the Massachusetts General Hospital. 1985. Weekly clinicopathological exercises. Case 35–1985. Abrupt onset of headache followed by rapidly progressive encephalopathy in a 30-year-old woman. *N Engl J Med*, **313**, 566–75.

Chang, S. D., Yap, O. W., and Adler, J. R. Jr. 1999. Symptomatic vasospasm after resection of a suprasellar pilocytic astrocytoma: case report and possible pathogenesis. *Surg Neurol*, **51**, 521–6; discussion 526–7.

Conde Lopez, V. J., Ballesteros Alcalde, M. C., Blanco Garrote, J. A., and Marco Llorente, J. 1998. [Cerebral infarction in an adolescent girl following an overdose of paroxetine and caffedrine combined with theodrenaline]. *Actas Luso Esp Neurol Psiquiatr Cienc Afines*, **26**, 333–8.

Dagher, H. N., Shum, M. K., and Campellone, J. V. 2005. Delayed intracranial vasospasm following carotid endarterectomy. *Cerebrovasc Dis*, **20**, 205–6.

Day, J. W., and Raskin, N. H. 1986. Thunderclap headache: symptom of unruptured cerebral aneurysm. *Lancet*, **2**, 1247–8.

Dodick, D. W. 2002. Thunderclap headache. *J Neurol Neurosurg Psychiatry*, **72**, 6–11.

Dodick, D. W. 2003. Reversible segmental cerebral vasoconstriction (Call-Fleming syndrome): the role of calcium antagonists [comment]. *Cephalalgia*, **23**, 163–5.

Dodick, D. W., Eross, E. J., Drazkowski, J. F., and Ingall, T. J. 2003. Thunderclap headache associated with reversible vasospasm and posterior leukoencephalopathy syndrome. *Cephalalgia*, **23**, 994–7.

Doss-Esper, C. E., Singhal, A. B., Smith, M. S., and Henderson, G. V. 2005. Reversible posterior leukoencephalopathy, cerebral vasoconstriction, and strokes after intravenous immune globulin therapy in Guillain-Barré syndrome. *J Neuroimaging*, **15**, 188–92.

Dupuy, B., Lechevalier, B., Chevalier, D., Theron, J., and Dijkstra, R. 1979. [Recurrent cerebral vascular complications connected with methergine in obstetrics]. *Rev Otoneuroophtalmol*, **51**, 293–9.

Fallis, R. J., and Fisher, M. 1985. Cerebral vasculitis and hemorrhage associated with phenylpropanolamine. *Neurology*, **35**, 405–7.

Fisher, C. M. 1971. Cerebral ischemia – less familiar types (review). *Clin Neurosurg*, **18**, 267–336.

Fisher, C. M. 1983. Honored guest presentation: painful states: a neurological commentary. *Clin Neurosurg*, **31**, 32–53.

Fisher, C. M. 1986. Late-life migraine accompaniments–further experience. *Stroke*, **17**, 1033–42.

Forman, H. P., Levin, S., Stewart, B., Patel, M., and Feinstein, S. 1989. Cerebral vasculitis and hemorrhage in an adolescent taking diet pills containing phenylpropanolamine: case report and review of literature. *Pediatrics*, **83**, 737–41.

Friedman, P., Gass, H. H., and Magidson, M. 1983. Vasospasm with an unruptured and unoperated aneurysm. *Surg Neurol*, **19**, 21–5.

Garnic, J. D., and Schellinger, D. 1983. Arterial spasm as a finding intimately associated with the onset of vascular headache. A case report. *Neuroradiology*, **24**, 273–6.

Geraghty, J. J., Hoch, D. B., Robert, M. E., and Vinters, H. V. 1991. Fatal puerperal cerebral vasospasm and stroke in a young woman. *Neurology*, **41**, 1145–7.

Geraud, G., and Fabre, N. 1984. [Benign acute cerebral angiopathy]. *Presse Med*, **13**, 1095.

Gilbert, G. J. 2002. Cerebral vasoconstriction and stroke after use of serotonergic drugs. *Neurology*, **59**, 651–2; author reply 652.

Goldstein, M., Wright, J., and Churg, J. 1991. *Vasculitis and Hypertension*. New York, Tokyo: Ikagu-Schoin.

Gomez, C. R., Gomez, S. M., Puricelli, M. S., and Malik, M. M. 1991. Transcranial doppler in reversible migrainous vasospasm causing cerebellar infarction: report of a case. *Angiology*, **42**, 152–6.

Hajj-Ali, R. A., Furlan, A., Abou-Chebel, A., and Calabrese, L. H. 2002. Benign angiopathy of the central nervous system: cohort of 16 patients with clinical course and long-term followup. *Arthritis Rheum*, **47**, 662–9.

Headache Classification Subcommittee of the International Headache Society. 2004. The International Classification of Headache Disorders: 2nd edition. *Cephalalgia*, 24(Suppl1), 9–160.

Henderson, R. D., Rajah, T., Nicol, A. J., and Read, S. J. 2003. Posterior leukoencephalopathy following intrathecal chemotherapy with MRA-documented vasospasm. *Neurology*, **60**, 326–8.

Henry, P. Y., Larre, P., Aupy, M., Lafforgue, J. L., and Orgogozo, J. M. 1984. Reversible cerebral arteriopathy associated with the administration of ergot derivatives. *Cephalalgia*, **4**, 171–8.

Hinchey, J., Chaves, C., Appignani, B., *et al.* 1996. A reversible posterior leukoencephalopathy syndrome. *N Engl J Med*, **334**, 494–500.

Hyde-Rowan, M. D., Roessmann, U., and Brodkey, J. S. 1983. Vasospasm following transsphenoidal tumor removal associated with the arterial changes of oral contraception. *Surg Neurol*, **20**, 120–4.

Iancu-Gontard, D., Oppenheim, C., Touze, E., *et al.* 2003. Evaluation of hyperintense vessels on FLAIR MRI for the diagnosis of multiple intracerebral arterial stenoses. *Stroke*, **34**, 1886–91.

Ihara, M., Yanagihara, C., and Nishimura, Y. 2000. Serial transcranial color-coded sonography in postpartum cerebral angiopathy. *J Neuroimaging*, **10**, 230–3.

Janzarik, W. G., Ringleb, P. A., Reinhard, M., and Rauer S. 2006. Recurrent extracranial carotid artery vasospasms: report of 2 cases. *Stroke*, **37**, 2170–3.

Kaplan, P. W. 1998. Reversible hypercalcemic cerebral vasoconstriction with seizures and blindness: a paradigm for eclampsia? *Clin Electroencephalogr*, **29**, 120–3.

Kapoor, R., Kendall, B. E., and Harrison, M. J. 1990. Persistent segmental cerebral artery constrictions in coital cephalgia. *J Neurol Neurosurg Psychiatry*, **53**, 266–7.

Kaye, B. R., and Fainstat, M. 1987. Cerebral vasculitis associated with cocaine abuse. *JAMA*, **258**, 2104–6.

Kirton, A., Diggle, J., Hu, W., and Wirrell, E. 2006. A pediatric case of reversible segmental cerebral vasoconstriction. *Can J Neurol Sci*, **33**, 250–3.

Kontos, H. A., Wei, E. P., Navari, R. M., *et al.* 1978. Responses of cerebral arteries and arterioles to acute hypotension and hypertension. *Am J Physiol*, **234**, H371–383.

Kupferschmidt, H., Bont, A., Schnorf, H., *et al.* 1995. Transient cortical blindness and bioccipital brain lesions in two patients with acute intermittent porphyria. *Ann Intern Med*, **123**, 598–600.

Laurent, B., Michel, D., Antoine, J. C., and Montagnon, D. 1984. [Basilar migraine with alexia but not agraphia: arterial spasm on arteriography and the effect of naloxone]. *Rev Neurol (Paris)*, **140**, 663–5.

Le Coz, P., Woimant, F., Rougemont, D., *et al.* 1988. [Benign cerebral angiopathies and phenylpropanolamine]. *Rev Neurol (Paris)*, **144**, 295–300.

LeRoux, P. D., Haglund, M. M., Mayberg, M. R., and Winn, H. R. 1991. Symptomatic cerebral vasospasm following tumor resection: report of two cases. *Surg Neurol*, **36**, 25–31.

Lieberman, A. N., Jonas, S., Hass, W. K., *et al.* 1984. Bilateral cervical carotid and intracranial vasospasm causing cerebral ischemia in a migrainous patient: a case of "diplegic migraine." *Headache*, **24**, 245–8.

Lin, J. T., Wang, S. J., Fuh, J. L., *et al.* 2003. Prolonged reversible vasospasm in cyclosporin A-induced encephalopathy. *AJNR Am J Neuroradiol*, **24**, 102–4.

Lopez-Valdes, E., Chang, H. M., Pessin, M. S., and Caplan, L. R. 1997. Cerebral vasoconstriction after carotid surgery. *Neurology*, **49**, 303–4.

Lu, S. R., Liao, Y. C., Fuh, J. L., Lirng, J. F., and Wang, S. J. 2004. Nimodipine for treatment of primary thunderclap headache. *Neurology*, **62**, 1414–6.

Maertens, P., Lum, G., Williams, J. P., and White, J. 1987. Intracranial hemorrhage and cerebral angiopathic changes in a suicidal phenylpropanolamine poisoning. *South Med J*, **80**, 1584–6.

Margolis, M. T., and Newton, T. H. 1971. Methamphetamine ("speed") arteritis. *Neuroradiology*, **2**, 179–82.

Martin-Araguz, A., Fernandez-Armayor, V., Moreno-Martinez, J. M., *et al.* 1997. [Segmental arteriographic anomalies in migranous cerebral infarct]. *Rev Neurol*, **25**, 225–9.

Masuzawa, T., Shinoda, S., Furuse, M., *et al.* 1983. Cerebral angiographic changes on serial examination of a patient with migraine. *Neuroradiology*, **24**, 277–81.

Merkel, P. A., Koroshetz, W. J., Irizarry, M. C., and Cudkowicz, M. E. 1995. Cocaine-associated cerebral vasculitis. *Semin Arthritis Rheum*, **25**, 172–83.

Meschia, J. F., Malkoff, M. D., and Biller, J. 1998. Reversible segmental cerebral arterial vasospasm and cerebral infarction: possible association with excessive use of sumatriptan and Midrin. *Arch Neurol*, **55**, 712–4.

Michel, D., Vial, C., Antoine, J. C., *et al.* 1985. [Benign acute cerebral angiopathy. 4 cases]. *Rev Neurol (Paris)*, **141**, 786–92.

Millikan, C. 1975. Accidents vasculaires cerebraux chez les femmes agees de 15 a 45 ans. In *Maladies Vasculaires Cerebrales. I Conference de la Salpêtrière*, Hospital de la Salpetriere, Paris. P. L. F. Castaigne, and J.-C. Gautier (eds.), Paris: J.-B. Balliere, 77–84.

Modi, M., and Modi, G. 2000. Case reports: postpartum cerebral angiopathy in a patient with chronic migraine with aura. *Headache*, **40**, 677–81.

Monteiro, P., Carneiro, L., Lima, B., and Lopes, C. 1985. Migraine and cerebral infarction: three case studies. *Headache*, **25**, 429–33.

Mourand, I., Ducrocq, X., Lacour, J. C., *et al.* 1999. Acute reversible cerebral arteritis associated with parenteral ephedrine use. *Cerebrovasc Dis*, **9**, 355–7.

Nighoghossian, N., Derex, L., and Trouillas, P. 1998. Multiple intracerebral hemorrhages and vasospasm following antimigrainous drug abuse. *Headache*, **38**, 478–80.

Nighoghossian, N., Trouillas, P., Loire, R., *et al.* 1994. Catecholamine syndrome, carcinoid lung tumor and stroke. *Eur Neurol*, **34**, 288–9.

Nolte, K. B., Brass, L. M., and Fletterick, C. F. 1996. Intracranial hemorrhage associated with cocaine abuse: a prospective autopsy study [see comment]. *Neurology*, **46**, 1291–6.

Noskin, O., Jafarimojarrad, E., Libman, R. B., and Nelson, J. L. 2006. Diffuse cerebral vasoconstriction (Call-Fleming syndrome) and stroke associated with antidepressants. *Neurology*, **67**, 159–60.

Nowak, D. A., Rodiek, S. O., Henneken, S., *et al.* 2003. Reversible segmental cerebral vasoconstriction (Call-Fleming syndrome): are calcium channel inhibitors a potential treatment option? *Cephalalgia*, **23**, 218–22.

Raroque, H. G. Jr., Tesfa, G., and Purdy, P. 1993. Postpartum cerebral angiopathy. Is there a role for sympathomimetic drugs? *Stroke*, **24**, 2108–10.

Rascol, A., Guiraud, B., Manelfe, C., and Clanet, M. 1979. Accidents vasculaires cerebraux de la grossesse et du post partum, In *Maladies Vasculaires Cere-* *brales*. II. Conference de la Salpêtrière sue les maladies vasculaires cerebrales, Hospital de la Salpêtrière, Paris. P. L. F. Castaigne, and J.-C. Gautier (eds.), Paris: J.-B. Balliere, 84–127.

Raynor, R. B., and Messer, H. D. 1980. Severe vasospasm with an unruptured aneurysm: case report. *Neurosurgery*, **6**, 92–5.

Razavi, M., Bendixen, B., Maley, J. E., *et al.* 1999. CNS pseudovasculitis in a patient with pheochromocytoma. *Neurology*, **52**, 1088–90.

Ringer, A. J., Qureshi, A. I., Kim, S. H., *et al.* 2001. Angioplasty for cerebral vasospasm from eclampsia. *Surg Neurol*, **56**, 373–8; discussion 378–9.

Roh, J. K., and Park, K. S. 1998. Postpartum cerebral angiopathy with intracerebral hemorrhage in a patient receiving lisuride. *Neurology*, **50**, 1152–4.

Rosenbloom, M. H., and Singhal, A. B. 2007. CT angiography and diffusion-perfusion MR imaging in a patient with ipsilateral reversible cerebral vasoconstriction after carotid endarterectomy. *AJNR Am J Neuroradiol*, **28**, 920–2.

Rousseaux, P., Scherpereel, B., Bernard, M. H., and Guyot, J. F. 1983. [Acute benign cerebral angiopathy. 6 cases]. *Presse Med*, **12**, 2163–8.

Rumbaugh, C. L., Bergeron, R. T., Scanlan, R. L., *et al.* 1971. Cerebral vascular changes secondary to amphetamine abuse in the experimental animal. *Radiology*, **101**, 345–51.

Ryu, S. J., and Lin, S. K. 1995. Cerebral arteritis associated with oral use of phenylpropanolamine: report of a case. *J Formos Med Assoc*, **94**, 53–5.

Sanin, L. C., and Mathew, N. T. 1993. Severe diffuse intracranial vasospasm as a cause of extensive migrainous cerebral infarction [see comment]. *Cephalalgia*, **13**, 289–92.

Schaafsma, A., Veen, L., and Vos, J. P. 2002. Three cases of hyperperfusion syndrome identified by daily transcranial Doppler investigation after carotid surgery. *Eur J Vasc Endovasc Surg*, **23**, 17–22.

Schluter, A., and Gissig, B. 2002. MR angiography in migrainous vasospasm. *Neurology*, **59**, 1772.

Schon, F., and Harrison, M. J. 1987. Can migraine cause multiple segmental cerebral artery constrictions? *J Neurol Neurosurg Psychiatry*, **50**, 492–4.

Serdaru, M., Chiras, J., Cujas, M., and Lhermitte, F. 1984. Isolated benign cerebral vasculitis or migrainous vasospasm? *J Neurol Neurosurg Psychiatry*, **47**, 73–6.

Silbert, P. L., Hankey, G. J., Prentice, D. A., and Apsimon, H. T. 1989. Angiographically demonstrated arterial spasm in a case of benign sexual headache and benign exertional headache. *Aust N Z J Med*, **19**, 466–8.

Singhal, A. B. 2002a. Cerebral vasoconstriction without subarachnoid blood: associated conditions, clinical and neuroimaging characteristics. *Ann Neurol*, S59–60.

Singhal, A. B. 2002b. Thunderclap headache, reversible cerebral arterial vasoconstriction, and unruptured aneurysms. *J Neurol Neurosurg Psychiatry*, **73**, **96**; author reply 96–7.

Singhal, A. B. 2004a. Cerebral vasoconstriction syndromes. *Top Stroke Rehabil*, **11**, 1–6.

Singhal, A. B. 2004b. Postpartum angiopathy with reversible posterior leukoencephalopathy. *Arch Neurol*, **61**, 411–6.

Singhal, A. B. 2007. Brain hemorrhages in RCVS. *Neurology*, (abstract, in press).

Singhal, A. B, and Bernstein, R. A. 2005. Postpartum angiopathy and other cerebral vasoconstriction syndromes. *Neurocrit Care*, **3**, 91–7.

Singhal, A. B., Caviness, V. S., Begleiter, A. F., *et al.* 2002. Cerebral vasoconstriction and stroke after use of serotonergic drugs. *Neurology*, **58**, 130–3.

Singhal, A. B., Topcuoglu, M. A., Caviness, V. S., and Koroshetz, W. J. 2003. Call-Fleming Syndrome versus isolated cerebral vasculitis: MRI lesion patterns. *Stroke*, **34**, 264.

Snyder, B. D., and McClelland, R. R. 1978. Isolated benign cerebral vasculitis. *Arch Neurol*, **35**, 612–4.

Solomon, S., Lipton, R. B., and Harris, P. Y. 1990. Arterial stenosis in migraine: spasm or arteriopathy? *Headache*, **30**, 52–61.

Song, J. K., Fisher, S., Seifert, T. D., *et al.* 2004. Postpartum cerebral angiopathy: atypical features and treatment with intracranial balloon angioplasty. *Neuroradiology*, **46**, 1022–6.

Stoessl, A. J., Young, G. B., and Feasby, T. E. 1985. Intracerebral haemorrhage and angiographic beading following ingestion of catecholaminergics. *Stroke*, **16**, 734–6.

Suwanwela, C., and Suwanwela, N. 1972. Intracranial arterial narrowing and spasm in acute head injury. *J Neurosurg*, **36**, 314–23.

Sztajzel, R., Le Floch-Rohr, J., and Eggimann, P. 1999. High-dose intravenous immunoglobulin treatment and cerebral vasospasm: a possible mechanism of ischemic encephalopathy? *Eur Neurol*, **41**, 153–8.

Ursell, M. R., Marras, C. L., Farb, R., *et al.* 1998. Recurrent intracranial hemorrhage due to postpartum cerebral angiopathy: implications for management. *Stroke*, **29**, 1995–8.

Valenca, M. M., Valenca, L. P., Bordini, C. A., *et al.* 2004. Cerebral vasospasm and headache during sexual intercourse and masturbatory orgasms. *Headache*, **44**, 244–8.

van Calenbergh, F., van den Bergh, V., and Wilms, G. 1986. Benign isolated arteritis of the central nervous system. *Clin Neurol Neurosurg*, **88**, 267–73.

Voltz, R., Rosen, F. V., Yousry, T., Beck, J., and Hohlfeld, R. 1996. Reversible encephalopathy with cerebral vasospasm in a Guillain-Barré syndrome patient treated with intravenous immunoglobulin. *Neurology*, **46**, 250–1.

Walker, G. L., Williamson, P. M., Ravich, R. B., and Roche, J. 1980. Hypercalcaemia associated with cerebral vasospasm causing infarction. *J Neurol Neurosurg Psychiatry*, **43**, 464–7.

Wijdicks, E. F., Kerkhoff, H., and van Gijn, J. 1988. Cerebral vasospasm and unruptured aneurysm in thunderclap headache. *Lancet*, **2**, 1020.

Yamamoto, Y., Georgiadis, A. L., Chang, H. M., and Caplan, L. R. 1999. Posterior cerebral artery territory infarcts in the New England Medical Center Posterior Circulation Registry. *Arch Neurol*, **56**, 824–32.

Yarnell, P. R., and Caplan, L. R. 1986. Basilar artery narrowing and hyperparathyroidism: illustrative case. *Stroke*, **17**, 1022–4.

Yu, Y. J., Cooper, D. R., Wellenstein, D. E., and Block, B. 1983. Cerebral angiitis and intracerebral hemorrhage associated with methamphetamine abuse. Case report. *J Neurosurg*, **58**, 109–11.

Zunker, P., Golombeck, K., Brossmann, J., Georgiadis, D., and Deuschl, G. 2002. Post-partum cerebral angiopathy: repetitive TCD, MRI, MRA, and EEG examinations. *Neurol Res*, **24**, 570–2.

Zunker, P., Steffens, J., Zeller, J. A., and Deuschl, G. 2000. Eclampsia and postpartal cerebral angiopathy. *J Neurol Sci*, **178**, 75–8.

68 ECLAMPSIA AND STROKE DURING PREGNANCY AND THE PUERPERIUM

Kathleen B. Digre, Michael Varner, and Louis R. Caplan

Introduction

Eclampsia derives from an ancient Greek word that means "to shine forth." The term was originally used to describe epileptic convulsions or seizures. In the twentieth century the term became synonymous with the pregnancy-specific condition pre-eclampsia or toxemia of pregnancy. Toxemia of pregnancy (toxemia gravidarum) is an old term that suggested a spectrum of findings related to the acute or subacute development of hypertension during pregnancy. The term literally means a "toxin in the blood," reflecting the idea that some toxic substance released from the uterus, placenta, or fetus was responsible for the disorder. The terms eclampsia and pre-eclampsia are now preferred.

Pre-eclampsia is a syndrome unique to human pregnancy characterized by the new onset of hypertension (>140/90 mmHg) and proteinuria after 20 weeks of gestation in previously normotensive, nonproteinuric women (American College of Obstetricians and Gynecologists [ACOG], 2002). In its "purest" form, it is described in previously healthy young (age < 25 years) women in their first pregnancy with no antecedent history of hypertension or proteinuria (Chesley, 1985). Severe pre-eclampsia is characterized by even higher elevation of blood pressure, and/or more than 5 grams of protein in the urine.

Eclampsia is a life-threatening complication and is characterized by the same findings as pre-eclampsia but, in addition, includes generalized seizure, altered consciousness, or blindness in a pre-eclamptic woman with no other obvious explanation for her seizures. Criteria for the diagnosis of pre-eclampsia, severe pre-eclampsia, and eclampsia have been developed (Tables 68.1, 68.2, 68.3).

Severe pre-eclampsia and eclampsia (SPE/E) may be complicated by the syndrome of HELLP – hemolysis, elevated liver function tests, and low platelets. HELLP occurs in about 1 in 5 women with severe pre-eclampsia (Sibai, 1992). HELLP syndrome is associated with poor outcome to pregnancy and even maternal and fetal death (Sibai, 1992). The term was coined by Weinstein (1982) to aid the clinician in the recognition of a complication of severe pre-eclampsia that was associated with significant liver dysfunction. The importance of recognizing HELLP syndrome is that women who meet criteria for this syndrome are at high risk for serious maternal complications such as disseminated intravascular coagulation (DIC), abruptio placenta, acute renal failure, hepatic failure, pulmonary edema, cerebral edema, stroke, and death and require immediate hospitalization and treatment (O'Brien and Barton, 2005).

SPE/E usually develop in the third trimester or within 48 hours after delivery. Delayed postpartum eclampsia (or delayed-onset eclampsia) is the same condition but occurring more than 48 hours after delivery. While most women develop SPE/E while pregnant, up to 48% (Sibai, 1992) can have the occurrence postpartum. Delayed or late-onset postpartum SPE/E can occur up to 4 weeks after delivery, but most occur within 1 week (Douglas and Redman, 1994; Hirshfeld-Cytron et al., 2006). The symptoms and signs may develop in a woman who has delivered uneventfully and within days has a headache, generalized seizure, or alteration of consciousness. The imaging features are similar to typical eclampsia.

Sometimes there is difficulty in recognition of the syndrome postpartum, and patients don't always exhibit pre-eclampsia before delivery. The origin of late postpartum eclampsia remains unclear. On occasion, retained placental fragments are found (Hirshfeld-Cytron et al., 2006).

The incidence of pre-eclampsia in the United States ranges between 5% and 10% of pregnancies (Cunningham et al., 2005; Kaunitz et al., 1985; Schobel et al., 1996). Severe pre-eclampsia occurs in 5.6/1000 deliveries; eclampsia is less common, occurring in 1/1000 deliveries (Samadi et al., 1996). A recent study in Scandinavia noted an incidence of eclampsia to be in 5.0/10 000 maternities (confidence interval [CI], 4.3–5.7/10 000) (Andersgaard et al., 2006). In the developing world, however, the incidence of SPE/E is much higher and the mortality rate is up to 10 times higher (Lopez-Jaramillo et al., 2005). Although the frequency of eclampsia has declined in the United States, pre-eclampsia and eclampsia are still major causes of maternal and perinatal mortality. Pre-eclampsia and eclampsia make up 20% of all maternal mortality (MacKay et al., 2001), and mortality is 2–5/100 cases (Cunningham et al., 2005).

The pre-eclampsia-eclampsia syndrome commonly occurs in women with underlying microvascular diseases, particularly chronic hypertension, diabetes, renal disease, or autoimmune disease (Fisher et al., 1981). A systematic review of >1000 controlled studies published from 1966 to 2002 found that a previous history of pre-eclampsia, multiple pregnancy, nulliparity, pre-existing diabetes, high body mass index (BMI) before pregnancy, maternal age ≥40 years, renal disease, hypertension, >10 years since previous pregnancy, and presence of anti-phospholipid antibodies all increased a woman's risk of developing pre-eclampsia (Duckitt, 2005). These latter observations are germane to the discussion of pathophysiology because the prospect of underlying conditions, be they previously recognized or not, being identified in the clinical scenario of pre-eclampsia-eclampsia must always be considered.

Uncommon Causes of Stroke, 2nd edition, ed. Louis R. Caplan. Published by Cambridge University Press. © Cambridge University Press 2008.

Table 68.1 Criteria for pre-eclampsia

Blood pressure of 140 mmHg systolic or higher OR 90 mmHg diastolic or higher after 20 weeks gestation in a woman with previously normal blood pressure

Proteinuria, 0.3 grams of protein or higher in a 24-hour urine specimen

Source: Diagnosis and Management of Pre-Eclampsia and Eclampsia ACOG Technical Bulletin 33. Washington, DC: ACOG, 2002. Reprinted with permission from ACOG.

Table 68.2 Criteria for severe pre-eclampsia

Diagnosis of severe pre-eclampsia

- Pre-eclampsia is considered severe if one or more of the following criteria are present:
- Blood pressure > 160 mmHg systolic or > 110 mmHg diastolic
- Proteinuria > 5 g/24 h (normal < 300 mg/24 h) or > 3+ on two random urine samples
- Oliguria < 500 cc in 24 hours
- Cerebral or visual disturbances
- Pulmonary edema or cyanosis
- Epigastric or right upper quadrant pain
- Impaired liver function
- Thrombocytopenia
- Fetal growth restriction

Source: Diagnosis and Management of Pre-Eclampsia and Eclampsia ACOG Technical Bulletin 33. Washington, DC: ACOG, 2002. Reprinted with permission from ACOG.

Table 68.3 Criteria for eclampsia

Eclampsia is the presence of a new onset of seizure in a pre-eclamptic woman without other obvious underlying etiology.

Elevated BMI as well as elevated inflammatory markers such as C-reactive protein and elevated triglycerides seem to be risk factors for the development of SPE/E (Bodnar *et al.*, 2005). Table 68.4 lists risk factors for the development of SPE/E.

African-American women face a higher frequency of SPE/E and a higher mortality rate (MacKay *et al.*, 2001). Many reasons have been given for this, ranging from higher levels of homocysteine in African-American women to increased rates of premorbid hypertension. A recent large population-based study by the Centers for Disease Control and Prevention (CDC) found that African-American women did not have that much higher a prevalence of SPE/E as Caucasian women did, but they died from SPE/E three times more frequently (Tucker *et al.*, 2007).

There is no single test that can predict who is going to get pre-eclampsia. Although uric acid is used as a screening tool, its predictive value is only about 33% (Lim, 1998), and a meta-analysis of several trials found uric acid levels to be a very poor predictor of

Table 68.4 Risk factors for the development of SPE/E

Women during their first pregnancy
Pre-eclampsia in past pregnancies
History of chronic hypertension, diabetes, or other vascular and connective tissue disease
Family history of pre-eclampsia, cardiovascular disease, heart disease, stroke, or renal disorders
History of anti-phospholipid antibody syndrome and other thrombophilias
Poorly nourished women
Women older than 35 years
Low plasma volume
BMI over 35
Elevated C-reactive protein
Elevated triglycerides
Elevated homocysteine
Multiple pregnancies
African-American race

Sources: Aardenburg, *et al.*, 2006; Sibai, 1989; ACOG, 2002; Duckitt, Harrington, 2005

SPE/E (Thangaratinam *et al.*, 2006). Fortunately, the fundamental tenets of perinatal care (serial determinations of blood pressure, proteinuria, and weight gain at increasingly frequent intervals) are designed to detect pre-eclampsia before it progresses to SPE/E.

Most women with pre-eclampsia have no neurologic symptoms. However as the disease progresses, the most common initial symptoms are headache and scotomas. Any pre-eclamptic woman with symptoms has advanced to severe pre-eclampsia (Table 68.2). As the disease progresses, the symptoms increase to include headache (present in the vast majority), photophobia, difficulty concentrating, and lethargy. If the patient develops seizures, coma, cortical blindness, or stroke, the patient has eclampsia.

The diagnoses of pre-eclampsia and eclampsia are based on clinical symptoms and signs and on laboratory abnormalities. Elevation of uric acid, thrombocytopenia, decreased level of antithrombin III, DIC, and HELLP syndrome all establish the diagnosis.

Complications of SPE/E include pulmonary edema, respiratory failure, kidney and liver failure, the HELLP syndrome, abruption of the placenta with or without DIC, seizures, status epilepticus, hypoxia from recurrent seizures, aspiration pneumonia, and stroke (including the posterior reversible encephalopathy syndrome [PRES]) (Ringelstein and Knecht, 2006). The outcome for the neonate in SPE/E should also be considered. Pre-eclampsia is an independent risk factor for stroke in neonates (Wu *et al.*, 2004).

Having pre-eclampsia may be a risk factor for future cerebrovascular disease (Brown *et al.*, 2006; Irgens *et al.*, 2001; Sattar and Greer, 2002; Wilson, Watson *et al.*, 2003). A family history of pre-eclampsia increases a woman's odds of having pre-eclampsia by almost 3 (Relative Risk 2.9) (Duckitt and Harrington, 2005). Furthermore, if two or more first-degree relatives have cardiovascular disease, the risk for pre-eclampsia is doubled, and if there is heart disease or stroke in two or more first-degree relatives, the risk is tripled (Ness *et al.*, 2003). Sattar and Greer (2002) suggest that a history of pre-eclampsia should increase surveillance for other vascular disorders.

The only cure for pre-eclampsia is delivery. In general, this should be recommended whenever the woman has reached the diagnosis of SPE/E or the fetus is either mature or developing in utero compromise (see discussion on treatment).

Strokes and posterior encephalopathy associated with pre-eclampsia and eclampsia

The three pregnancy-specific causes of stroke are: eclampsia, amniotic fluid embolism, and choriocarcinoma. The rest of the causes of stroke, although they may be increased in pregnancy, are generally ischemic, venous, or embolic. While pre-eclampsia and eclampsia are often thought to be the most common causes of stroke in pregnancy, other causes (particularly cardiac embolism) should be considered (Liang, *et al.*, 2006). Eclampsia is the most common pregnancy-specific cause of stroke.

Recognition of stroke with SPE/E includes the development of sudden onset of focal neurological deficits in patients who have the neurologic features of headache, confusion, and seizures that accompany SPE/E.

In two population-based studies, pre-eclampsia and eclampsia accounted for 24%–47% of ischemic strokes during pregnancy or the puerperium (Kittner *et al.*, 1996; Sharshar *et al.*, 1995), and also accounted for 14%–44% of intracerebral hemorrhages during this same time period (Kittner *et al.*, 1996; Sharshar *et al.*, 1995). Intraparenchymal hemorrhages are a common finding in fatal cases; they are found in >40% of patients studied at autopsy (Mas and Lamy, 1998a,b; Sheehan and Lynch, 1973). While eclampsia is a common cause of hemorrhagic stroke, consideration of other causes such as an underlying arteriovenous malformation, bleeding diathesis, and aneurysmal hemorrhage should also be considered when hemorrhage is detected (Liang *et al.*, 2006; Witlin *et al.*, 1997).

In a large study of 4024 maternal deaths monitored at the CDC, 20% of the deaths (790) were equally split between pre-eclampsia and eclampsia. Cerebrovascular ischemia made up the majority of deaths in SPE/E in this study (39%). Thirty-five percent of the deaths were from cerebral hemorrhage, 3% from cerebral edema, and only 1% from embolism. HELLP syndrome accounted for 7% of the deaths in patients with SPE/E (MacKay *et al.*, 2001).

Almost all studies show that brain hemorrhages cause the major morbidity and mortality from stroke in patients with SPE/E. Sheehan and Lynch who published the classic monograph of "The Pathology of Toxemia in Pregnancy" in 1973 noted that those who died within 24 hours of a brain hemorrhage bled into the basal ganglia or pons (Sheehan and Lynch, 1973). At autopsy, intracerebral hemorrhages range from multiple scattered cortical and subcortical petechiae, to small hemorrhages most often located at cortical-subcortical junctions, to massive hematomas (Mas and Lamy, 1998a,b; Richards *et al.*, 1988; Sheehan and Lynch, 1973). However, subarachnoid hemorrhage has been reported in

association with eclampsia in individuals without underlying aneurysm or arteriovenous malformation (Shah, 2003).

Patients with intracerebral hemorrhage have a poorer outcome compared to patients with ischemic stroke: A study by Martin *et al.* (2005) showed that 25 of 28 women who had a stroke during SPE/E had brain hemorrhages. Fifty-three percent of these women died, and only three women had good outcomes.

The "Ile de France" study showed similar findings. Seven patients had hemorrhagic strokes. Of these, eclampsia was associated with the HELLP syndrome in two patients, and DIC in another two patients. Most intracerebral hemorrhages were lobar (4/7), with hemorrhages in the brainstem (2/7) and lenticulostriate territory (1/7) accounting for the rest (Sharshar *et al.*, 1995).

Most of the strokes and hemorrhages in SPE/E occur in the late third trimester and in the immediate postpartum period. Martin *et al.* (2005) found that more than half of his patients had their strokes postpartum. See Table 68.5 for a review of published series on strokes associated with SPE/E.

More common than strokes in SPE/E is an encephalopathic disorder that is reversible if hypertension is effectively and rapidly controlled. The initial symptom is usually headache followed by agitation and reduced alertness. Visual aberrations are common and range from severe cortical blindness, to vivid visual hallucinations, to visual agnosias of the Balint type. Difficulties making new memories, impaired concentration, and loss of precision in language are often found when sought. Gerstmann syndrome has also been reported (alexia, agraphia, acalculia, right-left confusion, and finger agnosia) (Kasmann and Ruprecht, 1995). Hemianopia can occur but is less common. Minor motor weakness and ataxia occur, but frank paralysis is rare. If untreated, stupor and coma may intervene. The encephalopathy is identical to that found in patients with hypertensive encephalopathy and/or acute glomerulonephritis with uremia and in some patients who are given immunosuppressant therapy after organ transplantation (Hinchey *et al.*, 1996). Although the encephalopathy is reversible in most people, some may have brain infarction and persistent neurological signs including death associated with the encephalopathy. In the Witlin *et al.* (1997) series of cerebrovascular disorders in pregnancy, 3 of 24 women had hypertensive encephalopathy, and all three women died. When stroke does occur, consideration for underlying hypercoagulable factors may be helpful. One patient with pre-eclampsia had a postpartum stroke complicated not only by HELLP but also by a prothrombin gene mutation (Altamura *et al.*, 2005).

Cortical blindness is a frequent presenting sign of SPE/E encephalopathy. Patients present with complaints of blindness along with other variable features of SPE/E including headache, nausea, and seizures. Various visual syndromes such as alexia, simultanagnosia, homonymous hemianopia, and Balint syndrome are also reported. Why cortical blindness should be relatively common (estimated as up to 15% of cases of eclampsia) should not be surprising, because the posterior circulation vasculature is most often involved. The reason for the posterior circulation involvement is thought to be less sympathetic innervation of the posterior circulation (Manfredi *et al.*, 1997; Schwartz *et al.*, 2000). The diagnosis of cortical blindness is made when the patient

Table 68.5 Strokes in SPE/E

Study: Stroke in SPE/E	N	No. strokes w SPE/E	Timing	Hemorrhagic	Ischemic	Outcome
Simolke et al., 1991	15 preg	3	Third	3	0	1 death; 1 left hemiparesis
Awada et al., 1995	12 preg	1	Third	0	1	0 deaths because of E
Sharshar et al., 1995	31 preg	14 (45%)	1 pp 6 third	7	7	3 deaths of ICH group
Kittner et al., 1996	31 preg	6 (19%)	4 third 2 pp	2	4	?
Witlin et al., 1997	23 Preg	4 (17%)	?	2	2	2 deaths
Jaigobin and Silver, 2000	34 preg	7 (21%)		1	3 (+3 venous sinus thrombosis)	0 deaths
Lanska, 2000	183 preg	98 (54%)	57 peri 30 pp	?	? + 11 with venous sinus thrombosis	0 deaths
Jeng et al., 2004	49 preg	8 (16%)	?	7	1	?
Liang et al., 2006	32 preg	7 (22%)	?	5	2	?
Douglas and Redman, 1994	382 E	8 (2%)	?	1 ended in persistent vegetative state	7	Only 7 deaths total in the E group
Loureiro et al., 2003	17 SPE/E	4		0	4	0 deaths
Zeeman et al., 2004	24 E	6		0	6	0 deaths; 5 with gliotic changes on MRI
Martin et al., 2005	28 PE/E	28 all strokes in SPE/E	12 third 16 pp	25	2	15/28 (53%) mortality; only 3 without major disability
Andersgaard et al., 2006	211 PE/E	3 (1.4%)	?	?	?	Severe deficits

Preg = series of pregnant women with stroke; PE/E: series of women with pre-eclampsia/eclampsia; E = series with eclampsia. Timing: pp = postpartum; peri = peripartum; third = third trimester; ICH = intracranial hemorrhage.

exhibits no visual behavior (e.g. does not have eye movement to an optokinetic drum) and has intact pupillary light reflexes. One of the best tests for diagnosing simultanagnosia (not being able to see the whole visual field at once) is the Cookie Theft Picture from the Boston Naming test. In one study, 97% (29/30) women with eclampsia could not describe the picture. This finding correlated completely with abnormalities seen on the MRI (Hoffmann et al., 2002). Fortunately, most cases of cortical blindness associated with SPE/E resolve with few neurological deficits (Cunningham et al., 1995). Although most authors report that the visual symptoms are reversible and most patients have a return to normal vision, if there is hemorrhagic infarction, particularly with the HELLP syndrome, permanent defects can result (Murphy and Ayazifar, 2005).

Visual loss in SPE/E can also occur from retinal, choroidal, and optic nerve ischemia and infarction. Chorioretinal infarcts have been reported to cause serous retinal detachments and visual loss with SPE/E. While the incidence may be even higher, choroidal infarcts with serous retinal detachments are thought to occur in about 1% of pre-eclampsia cases (Iida and Kishi, 2002; Sathish and Arnold, 2000). Because retinal changes and optic disc swelling may also cause visual loss, a funduscopic examination is also recommended (Digre and Corbett, 2003). Although most of the changes in the fundus are reversible, permanent retinal changes and visual loss can occur (Moseman and Shelton, 2002; Murphy and Ayazifar, 2005). An Amsler Grid is helpful in making the diagnosis of focal chorioretinal lesions. See Figure 68.1 for an example of a woman with visual aberrations that showed defects on the Amsler Grid. Amsler Grid abnormalities actually correlated with finding MRI abnormalities (Digre et al., 1995).

Rarely, cerebral brain herniation has been described with SPE/E-associated PRES. The outcome can vary (Belogolovkin et al., 2006; Cunningham and Twickler, 2000).

Brain and vascular imaging

Brain imaging has become essential in properly diagnosing acute neurological changes in pregnant women. Imaging assists in the diagnosis of tumor, aneurysm, arteriovenous malformations, and dural venous sinus thrombosis that may have clinical presentations similar to SPE/E. Imaging characteristics of SPE/E are essential in differentiating this condition from other complications that may mimic it; imaging also can show the complication of stroke. In one study, imaging diagnosed a different condition than the suspected eclampsia (Witlin et al., 1997).

CT is most useful in separating hemorrhage from ischemia from encephalopathy in patients with typical eclampsia.

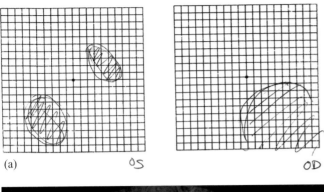

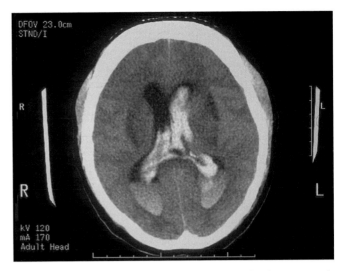

Figure 68.2 An acute intraventricular hemorrhage occurred in this woman with eclampsia.

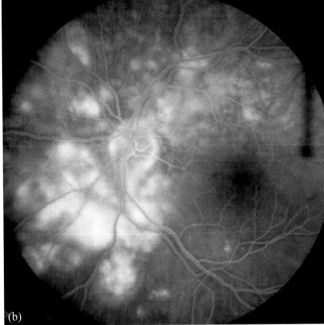

Figure 68.1 (**a**) Amsler Grid findings in a woman with severe pre-eclampsia who had choroidal infarctions. OD = right eye, OS = left eye. (**b**) A fluorescein angiogram of a woman with severe-pre-eclampsia showing choroidal infarctions. These resolved postpartum. From Digre and Corbett, 2003 (with permission from authors).

Hemorrhage may be lobar, intraventricular, or subarachnoid. In the encephalopathy syndrome of eclampsia, CT scans show white matter hypodensities that are usually symmetric, in the cerebral cortex, subcortical white matter, and the supratentorial deep gray matter. (See Figure 68.2, typical intraventricular hemorrhage). These abnormalities are predominantly located within the occipital and parietal areas, but they spare the paramedian, calcarine, and peristriate regions and are seen in women with SPE/E who have the acute encephalopathy syndrome that usually includes acute development of seizures and occasionally cortical blindness (Colosimo *et al.*, 1985; Dahmus *et al.*, 1992; Duncan *et al.*, 1989; Kirby and Jaindl, 1984; Lau *et al.*, 1987).

Whereas CT scans have been abnormal in 33% of eclamptic patients (Dahmus *et al.*, 1992), MRI scans are abnormal in 48–100% of patients with eclampsia (Dahmus *et al.*, 1992; Demirtas *et al.*, 2005; Digre *et al.*, 1993; Raps *et al.*, 1993; Sengar *et al.*, 1997). The changes found on MRI include punctate or confluent areas of increased foci on T2-weighted images in the centrum semiovale and the deep white matter, predominantly in the posterior parietal and occipital lobes (Dahmus *et al.*, 1992; Hinchey *et al.*, 1996; Schwartz *et al.*, 2000), at the gray-white junction, and in the external capsule, the basal ganglia, and occasionally in the cerebellum (Sengar *et al.*, 1997). In one study, all patients with abnormal MRI showed changes in the occipital lobe, followed by parietal, frontal, and temporal lobes (Demirtas *et al.*, 2005). In this study, patients with abnormal MRI were more likely to have seizures, visual disturbances, and alteration in consciousness than were those who had no lesions. However, the occipital lobe is not always the predominate site. There are reports of basal ganglia and frontal lobe involvement alone, but these are thought to be atypical manifestations (Ahn *et al.*, 2004).

The MRI findings in pre-eclamptic patients are somewhat different from those found in eclampsia. In one study, the abnormalities in pre-eclampsia were present in the white matter only, and predominantly in the frontal and parietal areas, and not at the gray-white junction (Digre *et al.*, 1993). Patients with eclampsia have a characteristic curvilinear abnormality at the gray-white matter junction that was not seen in patients with pre-eclampsia; this finding was used to help differentiate various causes of neurological symptoms in pregnant women (Digre *et al.*, 1993; Schwartz *et al.*, 2000; Sengar *et al.*, 1997). Most often, there is no evidence of microhemorrhages or microinfarcts, but this may be secondary to the microscopic size of the lesions and to the limits of the MRI resolution, or the absence of microhemorrhages and microinfarcts may be more in keeping with the findings being mainly vasogenic edema (Figures 68.3, a–d).

The MRI abnormalities of hyperintense signal on T2-weighted and hypointense signal on T2-weighted images, respectively, located in the posterior parietal and occipital lobes, are usually reversible in most of the patients studied (Duncan *et al.*, 1989; Hinchey *et al.*, 1996; Raps *et al.*, 1993; Raroque *et al.*, 1990; Sanders *et al.*, 1991; Schwartz *et al.*, 1992; Sengar *et al.*, 1997; Singhal, 2004). These types of changes have been termed reversible posterior

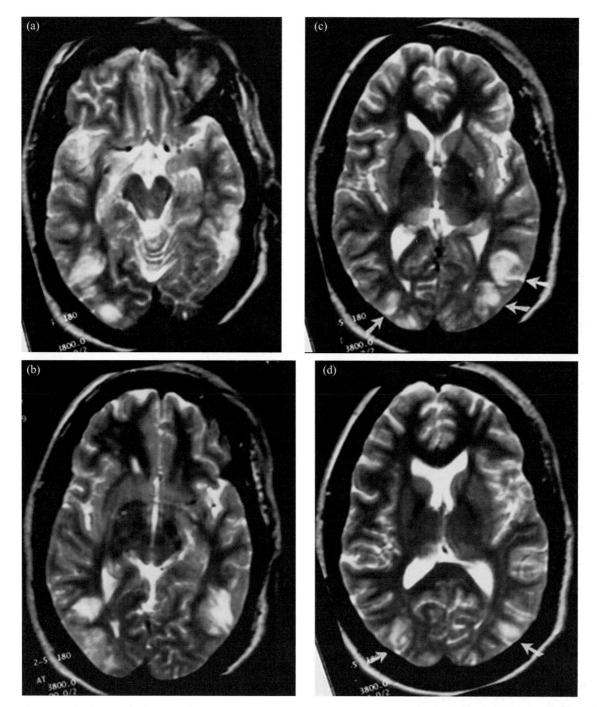

Figure 68.3 (**a–c**) T2-weighted images of a woman with severe pre-eclampsia. Notice the predominance of signals in the posterior parietal and occipital regions (*arrows*). (**d**) Compare with (**c**), where the lesions have almost totally resolved within 1 month.

leukoencephalopathy or PRES and are thought to represent a peripartum angiopathy (Singhal, 2004). See Figure 68.4, a and b, for a typical case of cortical blindness on MRI.

Newer techniques such as diffusion-weighted imaging (DWI) and apparent diffusion coefficient (ADC) are very helpful in understanding the relationship of edema and infarction. DWI detects water molecule changes in tissues. If there is vasogenic edema with increased extracellular fluid, the characteristic signal is either normal or reduced brightness. If there is cytotoxic edema, a hyperintense or very bright signal is produced. Bright signal on DWI can also be "T2 shine though"; therefore, it is not entirely clear using only the DWI whether infarction has occurred. The ADC map is independent of T2 effects. Therefore, decreased attenuation or darkness on an ADC map shows restricted flow of water, and therefore signifies ischemic stroke in that area. If the ADC is elevated or bright, then what is seen on DWI represents vasogenic edema (Hoffmann *et al.*, 2002; Koch *et al.*, 2001; Schaefer *et al.*, 1997; Schwartz *et al.*, 2000; Zeeman *et al.*, 2004).

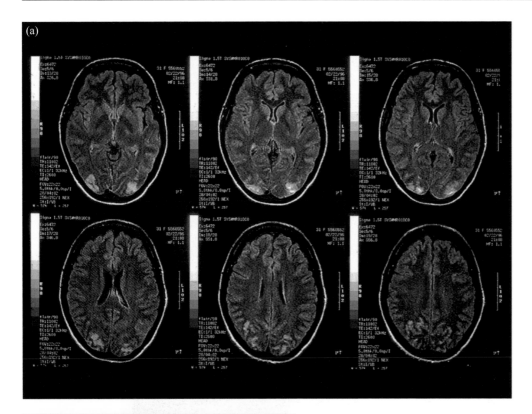

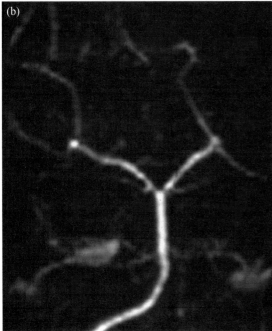

Figure 68.4 (**a**) Woman with postpartum cortical blindness and eclampsia (hypertension, seizure) showed typical abnormalities on MRI. She completely recovered within 24 hours. (**b**) Her magnetic resonance angiography (MRA) showed vasoconstriction of the posterior cerebral arteries and basilar artery. From Digre *et al.*, 2005 with permission.

Factors that bode well for reversibility include cortical lesions and subcortical lesions. Brain stem and deep white matter change did less well (Pande *et al.*, 2006). Eclampsia as a cause of PRES is more likely to be reversible and have fewer permanent residues than other PRES syndromes (Pande *et al.*, 2006). Although hemorrhages are occasionally found, these are much less common than areas of vasogenic edema. Some have used MRI to correlate with other findings in eclampsia. Schwartz *et al.* (2000) found that MRI vasogenic edema correlated best with aberrant red cell morphology and lactate dehydrogenase levels rather than with the height of the blood pressure.

Not all PRES is reversible, however. In a prospective study, Zeeman *et al.* (2004) found that, of 25 of 27 women with eclampsia, two had MRI abnormalities that have been described in PRES. Fifteen of the 27 had hyperintense lesions on DWI (meaning that at least vasogenic edema was present in 55%). Six had infarction on ADC mapping (low-intensity lesions), and gliosis was seen in five of the six patients who had repeat imaging postpartum. The authors posited that the sixth patient probably had gliosis below the limit of detection of the MRI scan (Zeeman *et al.*, 2004). Others have had similar experience (Loureiro *et al.*, 2003). See Figure 68.5, a and b, showing vasogenic edema on both the DWI and ADC map.

Angiography is characteristic in patients with eclampsia (Call *et al.*, 1988; Raps *et al.*, 1993; Tommer *et al.*, 1988). The vasoconstriction usually involves large arteries along the Circle of Willis as well as small circumferential branch arteries. The constriction is most often multifocal, but it can also be diffuse. Some areas of vasoconstriction alternate with regions of vasodilatation, giving the vessels a sausage-shaped appearance. MRA has shown similar vascular abnormalities (Ito *et al.*, 1995; Sengar *et al.*, 1997) (see Figure 68.4b). The angiographic abnormalities are usually reversible when follow-up studies are performed (Sengar *et al.*, 1997). The severity of vasoconstriction does not correlate with the severity of the hypertension (Easton *et al.*, 1998). Transcranial Doppler (TCD) ultrasound is a good noninvasive way to monitor the vasoconstriction. Qureshi *et al.* (1996) studied 11 women with eclampsia using TCD, and found elevated blood flow velocities and lower average pulsatility indexes compared to those in pre-eclamptic women and those in women with normal pregnancies. In one study TCD correlated with narrowing found in MRA, and as the vasculature normalized by MRA, TCD measurements did as well (Ikeda *et al.*, 2002) TCD has also been used effectively to study patients with postpartum cerebral angiopathy (Bogousslavsky *et al.*, 1989). Patients whose angiography shows vasoconstriction have usually had multifocal white matter abnormalities on brain-imaging scans.

Fluorodeoxyglucose-positron emission tomography (FDG-PET) imaging has shown altered glucose metabolism in areas of the T2 signal abnormalities that normalize after resolution of the eclampsia (Zunker *et al.*, 2003).

Electroencephalography (EEG) has been reported to correlate with abnormal MRI scans, and in one patient with an intracerebral hemorrhage, the EEG abnormalities persisted for more than 6 months (Osmanagaoglu *et al.*, 2005).

Differential diagnosis

The differential diagnosis of SPE/E includes dural sinus thrombosis and a reversible cerebral vasoconstriction syndrome. Cerebral dural sinus thrombosis is more common during the puerperium than during pregnancy (Cantu and Barinagarrementeria, 1993; Chopra and Banerjee, 1989; Srinivasan, 1983,1988). Headache and seizures are prominent features of both dural sinus occlusion and eclampsia, but patients with dural sinus occlusions are usually not hypertensive, and the clinical and CT abnormalities in patients with dural sinus occlusions are usually focal and not as multifocal

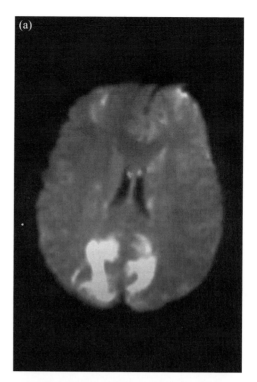

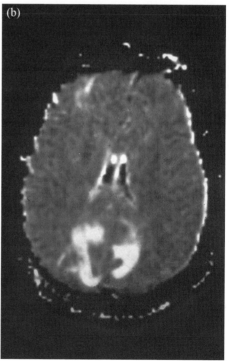

Figure 68.5 (a) DWI is bright and the correlating (b) ADC map is also bright, indicating vasogenic edema in this woman with eclampsia.

as in eclampsia. The majority of cerebral venous thromboses occur postpartum and are more common in women with complicated deliveries.

The reversible cerebral vasoconstriction syndrome (sometimes called the Call-Fleming syndrome) is a clinical and angiographic syndrome characterized by onset of a severe headache (sometimes

Table 68.6 Differential diagnosis of SPE/E
Venous thrombosis: especially cortical vein thrombosis
Embolic stroke
Reversible angiopathy (often postpartum)
Drug abuse: cocaine, amphetamines, sympathomimetics
Seizure disorder: epilepsy
Intracranial hemorrhage
Thrombotic thrombocytopenia purpura
Hypertension: chronic, renal disease, primary aldosteronism, Cushing's syndrome, pheochromocytoma, coarctation of the Aorta, glomerulonephritis, and other renal disease
Vasculitis
Behavioral disturbances
Acute fatty metamorphosis of pregnancy
Long-chain 3-hydroxyacyl-coenzyme A dehydrogenase deficiency (LCHAD deficiency)
Systemic lupus erythematosis
Budd-Chiari
Watershed infarction

Source: Adapted from Varner, 2002.

called a "thunderclap" headache), seizures, focal neurological findings, and angiographic evidence of multiple arterial constrictions. This disorder is most common in women and often develops in the postpartum period (Call *et al.*, 1988; Neudecker *et al.*, 2006). When reversible cerebral vasoconstriction syndrome occurs in the puerperium, it is called postpartum cerebral angiopathy (Barinagarrementeria *et al.*, 1992; Bogousslavsky *et al.*, 1989; Comabella *et al.*, 1996; Raroque *et al.*, 1993; Roh and Park, 1998; Singhal 2004; Ursell *et al.*, 1998). While the headache, seizures, and neurological deficits mimic SPE/E, the angiopathy on the scan involves white matter less frequently and less extensively than SPE/E does. Furthermore, many (but not all) of the patients do not have hypertension. Small cortical hemorrhages can accompany and complicate the angiopathy (Roh and Park, 1998; Singhal, 2004; Ursell *et al.*, 1998). The angiopathy and angiographic findings are difficult to separate from reversible posterior leukoencephalopathy (Singhal, 2004). In fact, this condition really overlaps with SPE/E enough that some have proposed that the two conditions suggest a similar underlying process (Singhal, 2004). Certain pharmacological agents have been associated with the syndrome, including bromocriptine (Comabella *et al.*, 1996), ergonovine (Barinagarrementeria *et al.*, 1992), ergotamines (Modi and Modi, 2000), lisuride (Roh and Park, 1998), and even serotonin reuptake inhibitors such as fluoxetine (Singhal, 2004). The imaging findings are usually reversible. Reversible cerebral vasoconstriction syndrome is further discussed in Chapter 67.

The differential diagnosis of SPE/E of pregnancy should also include other conditions that occur unrelated to pregnancy, e.g. brain embolism from cardiac disease, watershed infarction, bleeding diathesis, arterial dissection, and so forth. See Table 68.6 for a list of conditions in the differential diagnosis of SPE/E.

Pathology and pathophysiology of pre-eclampsia–eclampsia

Although the precise etiology of eclampsia and pre-eclampsia remains unknown, the consensus opinion remains focused on abnormalities of placental implantation. Placental implantation site biopsies in pre-eclamptic women show characteristic inadequate secondary trophoblast invasion (Granger *et al.*, 2001; Khong *et al.*, 1986). Hypoxia to the placenta leads to release of vascular mediators such as vascular endothelial growth factor (VEGF), which leads to endothelial cell injury through unknown mediators. This leads to widespread vasospasm, and this vasospasm is considered to be central to the condition. Vasoconstriction leads to increased resistance to blood flow with resultant hypertension and generalized endothelial disruption. These underlying pathophysiologies are central to the findings in all organ systems.

How stroke occurs in this setting is not completely understood, but there are plausible theories. First, because the pathological change is in the endothelium of blood vessels, any genetic tendency toward thrombophilia along with the pathologic endothelial change could be responsible for an ischemic event. Second, the endotheliopathy may be partially responsible for the lack of autoregulation when there is hypertension, and this could lead to ischemia and hemorrhagic stroke (Bushnell *et al.*, 2006).

Wilson, Goodwin *et al.* (2003) suggest that behind pre-eclampsia lies a genetic predisposition to the condition. Multiple genes that regulate blood pressure, especially in the renin-angiotensin system, and placental development factors are most attractive. However, there are three other abnormalities that lead to the development of pre-eclampsia according to them. The first is abnormal maternal immune adaptation, which may be in response to paternally derived antigens. Further complicating the immune maladaption are antibodies to endothelial cells. The second is placenta ischemia, which occurs when the spiral arteries do not adequately widen to the demands of an increasing size of the placenta. The third is oxidative stress, which leads to damage of the endothelial cell in the placenta but also in the entire systemic circulation (Wilson, Goodwin *et al.*, 2003).

Easton *et al.* (1998) reviewed many theories of brain involvement in eclampsia. Hypertensive encephalopathy is frequently cited as the underlying syndrome of eclampsia in the brain that causes edema and hemorrhages. The brain pathology is similar to that seen in hypertensive encephalopathy caused by other factors. Cerebral blood flow is constant over a wide range of blood pressures and is independent of systemic blood pressure until the blood pressure rises above the level of autoregulation. At that point, vasodilation can occur, tight junctions are loosened, and plasma proteins can be extravasated. This process leads to microhemorrhages and edema formation. Easton, Mas, *et al.*, 1998, believe that eclampsia represents an endotheliopathy. Additional evidence for systemic endothelial injury is the frequent biochemical abnormalities that are found in eclamptic persons. High circulating levels of von Willebrand factor, endothelin, and the cellular epitope of fibronectin have been reported (Easton *et al.*, 1998). These substances are all known to be released by damaged endothelial cells.

Endothelial changes in the brain lead to a breakdown in the normal blood-brain barrier and a capillary leak syndrome. The vasoconstriction and vasodilatation could also represent a vascular reaction to the endothelial abnormality that affects the brain's blood vessels. The sympathetic nervous system must also play a role in the brain findings in eclampsia because Schobel et al. (1996) showed that the rate of sympathetic nerve activity in patients with pre-eclampsia was more than three times higher than that found in normotensive pregnant women and more than twice as high as that found in hypertensive women who were not pregnant. Heightened sympathetic nerve activity could contribute to hypertension and vasoconstriction.

Other theories that have been used to explain the pathologic findings include immunological dysfunction, coagulation abnormalities, endocrine dysfunction, vasospasm, and even dietary factors (Sibai, 1992).

The neurologic signs and symptoms of pre-eclampsia-eclampsia are essentially the same as those seen in hypertensive encephalopathy (Barton and Sibai, 1991). These findings are most often caused by vasogenic edema that arises from the escape of fluid from the intravascular compartment into the interstitium because of breakthrough of autoregulation. Because the vertebrobasilar system and posterior cerebral arteries are sparsely innervated by sympathetic nerves, the occipital lobes and other posterior brain regions may be particularly susceptible to breakthrough of autoregulation with elevated systemic pressures. Investigators in recent Doppler ultrasonographic studies have demonstrated elevated cerebral perfusion pressures and reduced cerebrovascular resistance (Belfort et al., 1999) in patients with eclampsia, and increased regional cerebral blood flow to the occipital lobes has been found in those patients who undergo single photon emission computed tomography (SPECT) (Belfort et al., 2005) and xenon CT (Ohno et al., 1999).

Older autopsy series have reported findings consistent with the aforementioned pathophysiology. Small hemorrhages and microinfarctions (0.3–1.0 mm) are found scattered in the cerebral cortex, usually in an asymmetric distribution, and frequently in arterial border-zone regions. These lesions are most commonly seen in the occipital lobe, followed by the parietal lobe, frontal lobe, and then the temporal lobe, but are rarely found in the cerebellum (Sheehan and Lynch, 1973). The cortical lesions are only 0.3–1.0 mm in size, compared to the subcortical hemorrhages that are 2–6 mm in size. Small hemorrhages (3–5 mm) may also be located in the deep white matter and in the caudate and brainstem. Large intracerebral hemorrhages may occur in the basal ganglia, pons, or cerebral hemispheres, and depending on the location may extend to the ventricular system. In all hemorrhagic lesions, the pathology shows congested capillaries with surrounding hemorrhage.

The small cerebral blood vessels often show fibrinoid necrosis of the vascular walls. Fibrin thrombi also occlude some small arteries and arterioles. Perivascular small hemorrhages are also common (Easton et al., 1998).

Richards et al. (1988) correlated the neuroradiologic findings and clinical status with neuropathologic findings in seven patients, and identified seven major neuropathological abnormalities including vasculopathy with acute vessel wall damage, perivascular microhemorrhages and/or microinfarcts as listed above, and intracerebral hemorrhages including subarachnoid and intraventricular hemorrhages. They also described edema located throughout the brain and not limited to regions of microinfarctions, and hypoxic brain damage distributed diffusely and in border-zone regions; in one patient, there was evidence of transtentorial herniation.

SPE/E shows vascular pathology in almost all of the organs examined in postmortem studies (Sheehan and Lynch, 1973). The kidneys show "glomerular endotheliosis" (Lindheimer and Katz, 1991a). Glomeruli are swollen because of swelling of the endothelial and mesangial cells; the swelling results in capillary lumen narrowing. Fibrin and thrombi are found in the capillaries (Cunningham et al., 2005) and lead to changes to the glomeruli and reduction of glomerular filtration; proteinuria results. VEGF was found to be elevated in patients with pre-eclampsia undergoing renal biopsy, and this may account for some of the endothelial proliferation (Tang et al., 2005). The liver is also the seat of frequent pathological changes. Periportal hemorrhagic necrosis develops in the peripheral portion of liver lobules. Frank hemorrhages can occur and can lead to enlargement of the liver and even rupture of the liver capsule. Liver function tests are often abnormal (Cunningham et al., 2005). See Figure 68.6, a and b, for a summary of the pathological changes seen in eclampsia.

Treatment

The goal of treatment in eclampsia is to medically stabilize the woman, stop seizures, lower the blood pressure, decrease cerebral edema, and deliver a healthy baby. Magnesium sulfate has been proven superior to other treatments in the prevention of further seizures. Termination of pregnancy has long been recognized as the only permanent effective treatment. Delivery is associated with resolution of the eclamptic syndrome (Donaldson, 1989). The fetus should be delivered expeditiously, although immediate cesarean delivery is not mandatory, and in many cases induction of labor and vaginal delivery are both possible and preferred. The ACOG suggests using magnesium sulfate with a 6 gram loading dose diluted in fluid, and delivered intravenously (IV) for 15–20 minutes followed by a 2 g/h infusion (ACOG, 2002; Cunningham et al., 2005).

Magnesium does not effectively treat the associated hypertension, and control of hypertension is essential. At times, the blood pressure elevation is in the moderate range of hypertension (150–170 mmHg systolic), but for that patient this level represents a significant and relatively acute rise from her previous blood pressures during pregnancy. It is very important in these patients to lower the blood pressure. Treatment of the hypertension is usually achieved by using hydralazine 5–10 mg IV every 15–20 minutes until the target pressure is reached (Cunningham et al., 2005). Labetalol also has been suggested to be given in a 20-mg IV bolus; if not effective, 40 mg; if still not effective, 80 mg every 10 minutes to a maximum dose of 220 mg total (ACOG, 2002; Cunningham et al., 2005). Hydralazine and labetalol were compared in one large randomized trial, and there was no difference in the efficacy between the two drugs (Vigil-De Gracia et al., 2006). In a recent

(a)

REPORTED CNS LESIONS IN ECLAMPSIA (PATHOLOGY)

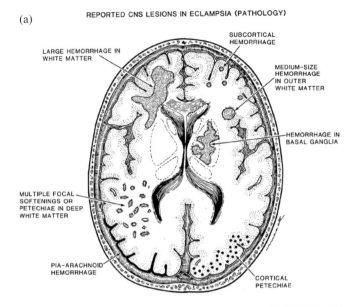

SUBCORTICAL HEMORRHAGE

LARGE HEMORRHAGE IN WHITE MATTER

MEDIUM-SIZE HEMORRHAGE IN OUTER WHITE MATTER

HEMORRHAGE IN BASAL GANGLIA

MULTIPLE FOCAL SOFTENINGS OR PETECHIAE IN DEEP WHITE MATTER

PIA-ARACHNOID HEMORRHAGE

CORTICAL PETECHIAE

GROSS SPECIMEN ECLAMPSIA

(b)

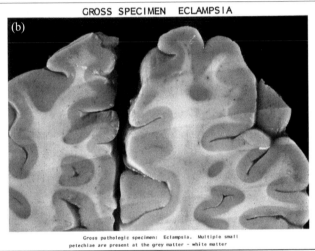

Gross pathologic specimen: Eclampsia. Multiple small petechiae are present at the grey matter - white matter

Figure 68.6 (**a**) A composite diagram of the pathological specimens reported by Sheehan and Lynch (1973). (**b**) Actual postmortem of woman who died of eclampsia. Note the small petechial hemorrhages at the gray-white junction. See color plate. From Digre *et al.*, 1993 with permission. Copyright © 1993, American Medical Association. All rights reserved.

Cochrane review, no drug was superior to another, but based on the evidence reviewed, Duley *et al.* (2006) recommended avoiding diazoxide, ketanserin, nimodipine, and magnesium sulfate for the treatment of hypertension. They recognized that magnesium may be used to prevent eclampsia, but as an antihypertensive agent, there was no evidence for its effectiveness (Duley *et al.*, 2006). The goal of therapy should be to reduce the blood pressure below levels associated with maternal vascular risks (generally <160/110) but to maintain sufficient pressure to adequately perfuse both mother and fetus.

Magnesium has been the key treatment of eclampsia for many years. A randomized trial showed that magnesium sulfate was superior to phenytoin in preventing eclamptic seizures in hypertensive women admitted to the hospital for delivery (Lucas *et al.*, 1995). Magnesium sulfate has also been shown to be superior to

both phenytoin and diazepam in preventing recurrent seizures in women with eclampsia who have already had a seizure (Eclampsia Trial Collaborative Group, 1995). Another randomized trial showed that magnesium was superior to nimodipine in preventing seizures in pre-eclampsia (Belfort *et al.*, 2003). The largest study of magnesium sulfate (the Magpie Study) once again affirmed the effectiveness of magnesium in preventing eclamptic seizures. Not only was the frequency of eclamptic seizures reduced by half, but maternal mortality was reduced, and there were no adverse effects on the infant (Altman *et al.*, 2002).

Treatment of HELLP syndrome, which complicates severe pre-eclampsia with glucocorticoids, has been shown to improve laboratory values such as liver function tests, renal function, and platelet numbers, but no improvement is made in maternal mortality (Sibai, 2004). Women whose pregnancies are complicated by HELLP are at higher risk for development of pre-eclampsia in subsequent pregnancies (O'Brien and Barton, 2005). Although some centers have seen improved outcomes for women with postpartum HELLP syndrome using high-dose semisynthetic corticosteroids (Rose *et al.*, 2004), this finding has not been universally reproduced (Barton and Sibai, 2004).

Reports of successful angioplasty for vasospasm associated with eclampsia have been reported in unusually refractory cases (Ringer *et al.*, 2001). While treatment of strokes with thrombolytics has been reported in pregnancy (Murugappan *et al.*, 2006), tissue plasminogen activator (t-PA) has not been used for the treatment of stroke in eclampsia.

Prevention of eclampsia-related strokes and hemorrhages seems to be directed toward aggressive treatment of pre-eclampsia and severe pre-eclampsia with control of hypertension. Martin *et al.* (2005) found that, besides careful attention to the diastolic pressures, attention to systolic pressure may be important in preventing hemorrhagic strokes.

Prevention of pre-eclampsia in women with high-risk profiles seems to be best with low-dose aspirin (Ruano *et al.*, 2005).

SPE/E remains an important cause of stroke for young women. While many controversies exist, treatment is geared at preventing and/or stopping seizures, lowering blood pressure, and treating with magnesium for the best outcome for mother and infant.

Acknowledgments

This work was supported in part by an unrestricted grant from Research to Prevent Blindness, to the Moran Eye Center, University of Utah.

REFERENCES

American College of Obstetricians and Gynecologists (ACOG) Committee on Practice Bulletins – Obstetrics. 2002. ACOG practice bulletin. Diagnosis and management of preeclampsia and eclampsia. Number 33, January 2002. *Obstet Gynecol*, **99**, 159–67.

Ahn, K. J., You, W. J., Jeong, S. L., *et al.* 2004. Atypical manifestations of reversible posterior leukoencephalopathy syndrome: findings on diffusion imaging and ADC mapping. *Neuroradiology*, **46**, 978–83.

Altamura, C., Vasapollo, B., Tibuzzi, F, Novelli, G. P., Valensise, H., Rossini, P. M., Vernieri, F. Postpartum cerebellar infarction and haemolysis, elevated liver enzymes, low platelet (HELLP) syndrome. *Neurol Sci*. 2005 Apr;26(1):40–2

Altman, D., Carroli, G., Duley, L., *et al.* Magpie Trial Collaboration Group. 2002. Do women with pre-eclampsia, and their babies, benefit from magnesium sulphate? The Magpie Trial: a randomised placebo-controlled trial. *Lancet*, **359**, 1877–90.

Andersgaard, A. B., Herbst, A., Johansen, M., *et al.* 2006. Eclampsia in Scandinavia: incidence, substandard care, and potentially preventable cases. *Acta Obstet Gynecol Scand*, **85**, 929–36.

Aardenburg, R., Spaanderman, M. E., van Eijndhoven, H. W., de Leeuw, P. W., and Peeters, L. L. 2006. A low plasma volume in formerly preeclamptic women predisposes to the recurrence of hypertensive complications in the next pregnancy. *J Soc Gynecol Investig*, **13**(8), 598–603.

Awada, A., al Rajeh, S., Duarte, R., and Russell, N. 1995. Stroke and pregnancy. *Int J Gynecol and Obstet*, **48**, 157–61.

Barinagarrementeria, F., Cantu, C., and Balderrama, J. 1992. Postpartum cerebral angiopathy with cerebral infarction due to ergonovine use. *Stroke*, **23**, 1364–6.

Barton, J. R., and Sibai, B. M. 1991. Cerebral pathology in eclampsia. *Clin Perinatol*, **18**, 891–910.

Barton, J. R., and Sibai, B. M. 2004. Diagnosis and management of hemolysis, elevated liver enzymes, and low platelets syndrome. *Clin Perinatol*, **31**, 807–33, vii.

Belfort, M. A., Anthony, J., Saade, G. R., Allen, J. C. Jr., and the Nimodipine Study Group. 2003. A comparison of magnesium sulfate and nimodipine for the prevention of eclampsia. *N Engl J Med*, **348**, 304–11.

Belfort, M. A., Grunewald, C., Saade, G. R., Varner, M., and Nissell, H. 1999. Preeclampsia may cause both overperfusion and underperfusion of the brain. *Acta Obstet Gynecol Scand*, **78**, 586–591.

Belfort, M. A., Kennedy, A., and Rassner, U. A. 2005. Novel techniques for cerebral evaluation in preeclampsia and eclampsia. *Clin Obstet Gynecol*, **48**, 387–405.

Belogolovkin, V., Levine, S. R., Fields, M. C., and Stone, J. L. 2006. Postpartum eclampsia complicated by reversible cerebral herniation. *Obstet Gynecol*, **107**(2 Pt 2), 442–5.

Bodnar, L. M., Ness, R. B., Harger, G. F., and Roberts, J. M. 2005. Inflammation and triglycerides partially mediate the effect of prepregnancy body mass index on the risk of preeclampsia. *Am J Epidemiol*, **162**, 1198–206.

Bogousslavsky, J., Despland, P. A., Regli, F., and Dubuis, P. Y. 1989. Postpartum cerebral angiopathy: reversible vasoconstriction assessed by transcranial Doppler ultrasound. *Eur Neurol*, **29**, 102–5.

Brown, D. W., Dueker, N., Jamieson, D. J., *et al.* 2006. Preeclampsia and the risk of ischemic stroke among young women: results from the Stroke Prevention in Young Women Study. *Stroke*, **37**, 1055–9.

Bushnell, C. D., Hurn, P., Colton, C., *et al.* 2006. Advancing the study of stroke in women: summary and recommendations for future research from an NINDS-Sponsored Multidisciplinary Working Group. *Stroke*, **37**, 2387–99.

Call, G. K., Fleming, M. C., Sealfon, S., *et al.* 1988. Reversible cerebral segmental vasoconstriction. *Stroke*, **19**, 1159–70.

Cantu, C., and Barinagarrementeria, F. 1993. Cerebral venous thrombosis associated with pregnancy and puerperium. Review of 67 cases. *Stroke*, **24**, 1880–4.

Chesley, L. C. 1985. Diagnosis of preeclampsia. *Obstet Gynecol*, **65**, 423–5.

Chopra, J. S., and Banerjee, A. K. 1989. Primary intracranial sinovenous occlusions in youth and pregnancy. In *Handbook of Clinical Neurology*, Vol 10: *Vascular Diseases, part II*, P. J. Vinken, G. W. Bruyn, and H. L. Klawans (eds.), Amsterdam: Elsevier Science Publishers, pp. 425–52.

Colosimo, C., Fileni, A., Moschini, M., and Guerrini, P. 1985. CT findings in eclampsia. *Neuroradiology*, **27**, 313–7.

Comabella, M., Alvarez-Sabin, J., Rovira, A., and Codina, A. 1996. Bromocriptine and postpartum cerebral angiopathy: a causal relationship? *Neurology*, **46**, 1754–6.

Cunningham, F. G., Fernandez, C. O., and Hernandez, C. 1995. Blindness associated with preeclampsia and eclampsia. *Am J Obstet Gynecol*, **172**(4 Pt 1), 1291–8.

Cunningham, F. G., Gant, N. F., Leveno, K. J., *et al.* 2001. Hypertensive disorders in pregnancy. In *Williams' Obstetrics*, 21th ed., F. G. Cunningham, J. W. N. F. Gant, K. J. Leveno, L. C. Gilstrap, J. C. Hauth, K. D. Wenstrom (eds.), New York: McGraw Hill 2001, pp. 567–618

Cunningham, F. G., and Twickler, D. 2000. Cerebral edema complicating eclampsia. *Am J Obstet Gynecol*, **182**(1 Pt 1), 94–100.

Dahmus, M. A., Barton, J. R., and Sibai, B. M. 1992. Cerebral imaging in eclampsia: magnetic resonance imaging versus computed tomography. *Am J Obstet Gynecol*, **167**, 935–41.

Demirtas, O., Gelal, F., Vidinli, B. D., *et al.* 2005. Cranial MR imaging with clinical correlation in preeclampsia and eclampsia. *Diagn Interv Radiol*, **11**, 189–94.

Digre, K. B., and Corbett, J. J. 2003. Practical viewing of the optic disc. Boston: Butterworth, 605–25.

Digre, K. B., Varner, M. W., Osborn, A. G., and Crawford, S. 1993. Cranial magnetic resonance imaging in severe preeclampsia vs. eclampsia. *Arch Neurol*, **50**, 399–406.

Digre, K. B., Varner, M. W., Skalabrin, E., and Belfort, M. 2005. Diagnosis and treatment of cerebrovascular disorders in pregnancy. In *Handbook of Cerebrovascular Diseases*, H. P. Adams (ed.), New York: Marcel-Dekker, 805–50.

Donaldson, J. O. 1989. Eclampsia. In *Neurology of Pregnancy*, Philadelphia: WB Saunders, pp. 269–310.

Douglas, K. A., and Redman, C. W. 1994. Eclampsia in the United Kingdom. *BMJ*, **309**, 1395–400.

Duckitt, K., and Harrington, D. 2005. Risk factors for pre-eclampsia at antenatal booking: systematic review of controlled studies. *BMJ*, **330**, 565.

Duley, L., Henderson-Smart, D. J., and Meher, S. 2006. Drugs for treatment of very high blood pressure during pregnancy. *Cochrane Database Syst Rev.* 2006 Jul 19;3:CD001449.

Duncan, R., Hadley, D., Bone, I., *et al.* 1989. Blindness in eclampsia: CT and MR imaging. *J Neurol Neurosurg Psychiatry*, **52**, 899–902.

Easton, J. D., Mas, J.-L., Lamy, C., *et al.* 1998. Severe preeclampsia/eclampsia: hypertensive encephalopathy of pregnancy? *Cerebrovasc Dis*, **8**, 53–8.

Eclampsia Trial Collaborative Group. 1995. Which anticonvulsant for women with eclampsia? Evidence from the collaborative Eclampsia Trial. *Lancet*, **345**, 1455–63.

Fisher, K. A., Luger, A., Spargo, B. H., and Lindheimer, M. D. 1981. Hypertension in pregnancy: clinical-pathological correlations and remote prognosis. *Medicine (Baltimore)*, **60**, 267–76.

Granger, J. P., Alexander, B. T., Llinas, M. T., Bennett, W. A., and Khalil, R. A. 2001. Pathophysiology of hypertension during preeclampsia linking placental ischemia with endothelial dysfunction. *Hypertension*, **38**(3 Pt 2), 718–22.

Hinchey, J., Chaves, C., Appignani, B., *et al.* 1996. A reversible posterior leukoencephalopathy syndrome. *N Engl J Med*, **334**, 494–500.

Hirshfeld-Cytron, J., Lam, C., Karumanchi, S. A., and Lindheimer, M. 2006. Late postpartum eclampsia: examples and review. *Obstet Gynecol Surv*, **61**, 471–80.

Hoffmann, M., Keiseb, J., Moodley, J., and Corr, P. 2002. Appropriate neurological evaluation and multimodality magnetic resonance imaging in eclampsia. *Acta Neurol Scand*, **106**, 159–67.

Iida, T., and Kishi, S. 2002. Choroidal vascular abnormalities in preeclampsia. *Arch Ophthalmol*, **120**, 1406–7.

Ikeda, T., Urabe, H., Matsukage, S., Sameshima, H., and Ikenoue, T. 2002. Serial assessment in eclampsia of cerebrohemodynamics by combined transcranial Doppler and magnetic resonance angiography. *Gynecol Obstet Invest*, **53**, 65–7.

Irgens, H. U., Reisaeter, L., Irgens, L. M., and Lie, R. T. 2001. Long term mortality of mothers and fathers after pre-eclampsia: population based cohort study. *BMJ*, **323**, 1213–7.

Ito, T., Sakai, T., Inagawa, S., Utsu, M., and Bun, T. 1995. MR angiography of cerebral vasospasm in preeclampsia. *AJNR Am J Neuroradiol*, **16**, 1344–6.

Jaigobin, C., and Silver, F. L. 2000. Stroke and pregnancy. *Stroke*, **31**, 2948–51.

Jeng, J. S., Tang, S. C., and Yip, P. K. 2004. Incidence and etiologies of stroke during pregnancy and puerperium as evidenced in Taiwanese women. *Cerebrovasc Dis*, **18**, 290–5.

Kasmann, B., and Ruprecht, K. W. 1995. Eclamptogenic Gerstmann's syndrome in combination with cortical agnosia and cortical diplopia. *Ger J Ophthalmol*, **4**, 234–8.

Kaunitz, A. M., Hughes, J. M., Grimes, D. A., *et al.* 1985. Causes of maternal mortality in the United States. *Obstet Gynecol*, **65**, 605–12.

Khong, T. Y., De Wolf, F., Robertson, W. B., and Brosens, I. 1986. Inadequate maternal vascular response to placentation in pregnancies complicated by preeclampsia and by small-for-gestational age infants. *Br J Obstet Gynaecol*, **93**, 1049–59.

Kirby, J. C., and Jaindl, J. J. 1984. Cerebral CT findings in toxemia of pregnancy. *Radiology*, **151**, 114.

Kittner, S. J., Stern, B. J., Feeser, B. R., *et al.* 1996. Pregnancy and the risk of stroke. *N Engl J Med*, **335**, 768–74.

Koch, S., Rabinstein, A., Falcone, S., and Forteza, A. 2001. Diffusion-weighted imaging shows cytotoxic and vasogenic edema in eclampsia. *AJNR Am J Neuroradiol*, **22**, 1068–70.

Lanska, D. J., and Kryscio, R. J. 2000. Risk factors for peripartum and postpartum stroke and intracranial venous thrombosis. *Stroke*, Jun;31(6):1274–82.

Lau, S. P., Chan, F. L., Yu, Y. L., Woo, E., and Huang, C. Y. 1987. Cortical blindness in toxemia of pregnancy: findings on computed tomography. *Br J Radiol*, **60**, 347–9.

Liang, C. C., Chang, S. D., Lai, S. L., *et al.* 2006. Stroke complicating pregnancy and the puerperium. *Eur J Neurol*, **13**, 1256–60.

Lim, K. H., Friedman, S. A., Ecker, J. L., Kao, L., and Kilpatrick, S. J. 1998. The clinical utility of serum uric acid measurements in hypertensive diseases of pregnancy. *Am J Obstet Gynecol*, **178**(5), 1067–71.

Lindheimer, M. D., and Katz, A. I. 1991a. The kidney and hypertension in pregnancy. In *The Kidney*, 4th edn., B. M. Brenner, and F. C. Rector (eds.), Philadelphia: W. B. Saunders, pp. 1551–95.

Lindheimer, M. D., and Katz, A. I. 1991b. Hypertension in pregnancy: advances and controversies. *Clin Nephrol*, **36**, 166–73.

Lopez-Jaramillo, P., Garcia, R. G., and Lopez, M. 2005. Preventing pregnancy-induced hypertension: are there regional differences for this global problem? *J Hypertens*, **23**, 1121–9.

Loureiro, R., Leite, C. C., Kahhale, S., *et al.* 2003. Diffusion imaging may predict reversible brain lesions in eclampsia and severe preeclampsia: initial experience. *Am J Obstet Gynecol*, **189**, 1350–5.

Lucas, M. J., Leveno, K. J., and Cunningham, F. G. 1995. A comparison of magnesium sulfate with phenytoin for the prevention of eclampsia. *N Engl J Med*, **333**, 201–5.

MacKay, A. P., Berg, C. J., and Atrash, H. K. 2001. Pregnancy-related mortality from preeclampsia and eclampsia. *Obstet Gynecol*, **97**, 533–8.

Manfredi, M., Beltramello, A., Bongiovanni, L. G., *et al.* 1997. Eclamptic encephalopathy: imaging and pathogenetic considerations. *Acta Neurol Scand*, **96**, 277–82.

Martin, J. N. Jr., Thigpen, B. D., Moore, R. C., *et al.* 2005. Stroke and severe preeclampsia and eclampsia: a paradigm shift focusing on systolic blood pressure. *Obstet Gynecol*, **105**, 246–54.

Mas, J.-L., and Lamy, C. 1998a. Stroke in pregnancy and the puerperium. *J Neurol*, **245**, 305–13.

Mas, J.-L., and Lamy, C. 1998b. Stroke in pregnancy and the postpartum period, In *Cerebrovascular Disease. Pathophysiology, Diagnosis, and Management*, M. D. Ginsberg, and J. Bogousslavsky (eds.), Malden, MA: Blackwell Science, pp. 1684–97.

Modi, M., and Modi, G. 2000. Case reports: postpartum cerebral angiopathy in a patient with chronic migraine with aura. *Headache*, **40**, 677–81.

Moseman, C. P., and Shelton, S. 2002. Permanent blindness as a complication of pregnancy induced hypertension. *Obstet Gynecol*, **100**(5 Pt 1), 943–5.

Murphy, M. A., and Ayazifar, M. 2005. Permanent visual deficits secondary to the HELLP syndrome. *J Neuroophthalmol*, **25**, 122–7.

Murugappan, A., Coplin, W. M., Al-Sadat, A. N., *et al.* 2006. Thrombolytic therapy of acute ischemic stroke during pregnancy. *Neurology*, **66**, 768–70.

Ness, R. B., Markovic, N., Bass, D., Harger, G., and Roberts, J. M. 2003. Family history of hypertension, heart disease, and stroke among women who develop hypertension in pregnancy. *Obstet Gynecol*, **102**, 1366–71.

Neudecker, S., Stock, K., and Krasnianski, M. 2006. Call-Fleming postpartum angiopathy in the puerperium: a reversible cerebral vasoconstriction syndrome. *Obstet Gynecol*, **107**(2 Pt 2), 446–9.

O'Brien, J. M., and Barton, J. R. 2005. Controversies with the diagnosis and management of HELLP syndrome. *Clin Obstet Gynecol*, **48**, 460–77.

Ohno, Y., Wakahara, Y., Kawai, M., and Arii, Y. 1999. Cerebral hyperperfusion in patient with eclampsia. *Acta Obstet Gynecol Scand*, **78**, 555–6.

Osmanagaoglu, M. A., Dinc, G., Osmanagaoglu, S., Dinc, H., and Bozkaya, H. 2005. Comparison of cerebral magnetic resonance and electroencephalo-gram findings in pre-eclamptic and eclamptic women. *Aust NZJ Obstet Gynaecol*, **45**, 384–90.

Pande, A. R., Ando, K., Ishikura, R., *et al.* 2006. Clinicoradiological factors influencing the reversibility of posterior reversible encephalopathy syndrome: a multicenter study. *Radiat Med*, **24**, 659–68.

Qureshi, A. I., Frankel, M. R., Ottenlips, J. R., and Stern, B. J. 1996. Cerebral hemodynamics in preeclampsia and eclampsia. *Arch Neurol*, **53**, 1226–31.

Raps, E. C., Galetta, S. L., Broderick, M., and Atlas, S. W. 1993. Delayed peripartum vasculopathy: cerebral eclampsia revisited. *Ann Neurol*, **33**, 222–5.

Raroque, H. G., Orrison, W. W. & Rosenberg, G. A. (1990). Neurologic involvement in toxemia of pregnancy: reversible MRI lesions. *Neurology*, **40**, 167–9.

Raroque, H. G., Tesfa, G., and Purdy, P. 1993. Postpartum cerebral angiopathy. Is there a role for sympathomimetic drugs? *Stroke*, **24**, 2108–10.

Richards, A., Graham, D., and Bullock, R. 1988. Clinicopathological study of neurological complications due to hypertensive disorders of pregnancy. *J Neurol Neurosurg Psychiatry*, **51**, 416–21.

Ringelstein, E. B., and Knecht, S. 2006. Complications of SPE/E from cerebral small vessel diseases: manifestations in young women. *Curr Opin Neurol*, **19**, 55–62.

Ringer, A. J., Qureshi, A. I., Kim, S. H., *et al.* 2001. Angioplasty for cerebral vasospasm from eclampsia. *Surg Neurol*, **56**, 373–8; discussion 378–9.

Roh, J. K., and Park, K. S. 1998. Postpartum cerebral angiopathy with intracerebral hemorrhage in a patient receiving lisuride. *Neurology*, **50**, 1152–4.

Rose, C. H., Thigpen, B. D., Bofill, J. A., *et al.* 2004. Obstetric implications of antepartum corticosteroid therapy for HELLP syndrome. *Obstet Gynecol*, **104**(5 Pt 1), 1011–4.

Ruano, R., Fontes, R. S., and Zugaib, M. 2005. Prevention of preeclampsia with low-dose aspirin – a systematic review and meta-analysis of the main randomized controlled trials. *Clinics*, **60**, 407–14.

Samadi, A. R., Mayberry, R. M., Zaidi, A. A., *et al.* 1996. Maternal hypertension and associated pregnancy complications among African-American and other women in the United States. *Obstet Gynecol*, **87**, 557–63.

Sanders, T. G., Clayman, D. A., Sanchez-Ramos, L., Vines, F. S., and Russo, L. 1991. Brain in eclampsia: MR imaging with clinical correlation. *Radiology*, **180**, 475–8.

Sathish, S., and Arnold, J. J. 2000. Bilateral choroidal ischaemia and serous retinal detachment in pre-eclampsia. *Clin Experiment Ophthalmol*, **28**, 387–90.

Sattar, N., and Greer, I. A. 2002. Pregnancy complications and maternal cardiovascular risk: opportunities for intervention and screening? *BMJ*, **325**, 157–60.

Schaefer, P. W., Buonanno, F. S., Gonzalez, R. G., and Schwamm, L. H. 1997. Diffusion-weighted imaging discriminates between cytotoxic and vasogenic edema in a patient with eclampsia. *Stroke*, **28**, 1082–5.

Schobel, H. P., Fischer, T., Heuszer, K., Geiger, H., and Schmieder, R. E. 1996. Preeclampsia – a state of sympathetic overactivity. *N Engl J Med*, **335**, 1480–5.

Schwartz, R. B., Feske, S. K., Polak, J. F., *et al.* 2000. Preeclampsia-eclampsia: clinical and neuroradiographic correlates and insights into the pathogenesis of hypertensive encephalopathy. *Radiology*, **217**, 371–6.

Schwartz, R. B., Jones, K. M., Kalina, P., *et al.* 1992. Hypertensive encephalopathy: findings on CT, MR imaging, and SPECT imaging in 14 cases. *Am J Roentgenol*, **159**, 379–83.

Sengar, A. R., Gupta, R. K., Dhanuka, A. K., Roy, R., and Das, K. 1997. MR imaging, MR angiography, and MR spectroscopy of the brain in eclampsia. *Am J Neuroradiol*, **18**, 1485–90.

Shah, A. K. 2003. Non-aneurysmal primary subarachnoid hemorrhage in pregnancy-induced hypertension and eclampsia. *Neurology*, **61**, 117–20.

Sharshar, T., Lamy, C., and Mas, J. L. 1995. Incidence and causes of strokes associated with pregnancy and puerperium: a study in public hospitals of Ile de France. *Stroke*, **26**, 930–6.

Sheehan, H. L., and Lynch, J. B. 1973. Cerebral lesions. In *Pathology of Toxaemia of Pregnancy*, H. L. Sheehan, and J. B. Lynch (eds.), London: Churchill Livingstone, pp. 525–54.

Sibai, B. M. 1989. Preeclampsia–eclampsia. In *Gynecology and Obstetrics*, Vol 2, J. J. Sciarra (ed.), Philadelphia: J. B. Lippincott, pp. 1–12.

Sibai, B. M. 1992. Eclampsia. In *Neurological Disorders of Pregnancy*, 2nd edn., P. J. Goldstein, and B. J. Stern (eds.), Mount Kisco, NY: Futura Publishing.

Sibai, B. M. 2004. Diagnosis, controversies, and management of the syndrome of hemolysis, elevated liver enzymes, and low platelet count. *Obstet Gynecol*, **103**, 981–91.

Simolke, G. A., Cox, S. M., and Cunningham, F. G. 1991. Cerebrovascular accidents complicating pregnancy and the puerperium. *Obstet Gynecol*, **78**, 37–42.

Singhal, A. B. 2004. The key to the diagnosis of reversible cerebral angiopathy is that there is no associated hypertension or other features of SPE/E. Postpartum angiopathy with reversible posterior leukoencephalopathy. *Arch Neurol*, **61**, 411–6.

Srinivasan, K. 1983. Cerebral venous and arterial thrombosis in pregnancy and puerperium, a study of 135 patients. *Angiology*, **34**, 733–46.

Srinivasan, K. 1988. Puerperal cerebral venous and arterial thrombosis. *Semin Neurol*, **8**, 222–5.

Tang, Z., Ren, H., Yang, G., *et al.* 2005. Significance of vascular endothelial growth factor expression in renal tissue of patients with preeclamptic nephropathy. *Am J Nephrol*, **25**, 579–85.

Thangaratinam, S., Ismail, K. M., Sharp, S., *et al.* 2006. Accuracy of serum uric acid in predicting complications of pre-eclampsia: a systematic review. *BJOG*, **113**, 369–78.

Tommer, B. L., Homer, D., and Mikhael, M. A. 1988. Cerebral vasospasm and eclampsia. *Stroke*, **19**, 326–9.

Tucker, M. J., Berg, C. J., Callaghan, W. M., and Hsia, J. 2007. The Black-White disparity in pregnancy-related mortality from 5 conditions: differences in prevalence and case-fatality rates. *Am J Public Health*, 97, 247–51.

Ursell, M. R., Marras, C. L., Farb, R., *et al.* 1998. Recurrent intracranial hemorrhage due to postpartum cerebral angiopathy. Implications for management. *Stroke*, **29**, 1995–8.

Varner, M. W. 2002. The differential diagnosis of preeclampsia and eclampsia. In Hypertension and Pregnancy, M. A. Belfort, M. Thornton, and G. R. Saade (eds.), New York: Marcel Dekker, 57–83.

Vigil-De Gracia, P., Lasso, M., Ruiz, E., *et al.* 2006. Severe hypertension in pregnancy: hydralazine or labetalol. A randomized clinical trial. *Eur J Obstet Gynecol Reprod Biol*, **128**, 157–62.

Weinstein, L. 1982. Syndrome of hemolysis, elevated liver enzymes, and low platelet count: a severe consequence of hypertension in pregnancy. *Am J Obstet Gynecol*, **142**, 159–67.

Wilson, B. J., Watson, M. S., Prescott, G. J., *et al.* 2003. Hypertensive diseases of pregnancy and risk of hypertension and stroke in later life: results from cohort study. *BMJ*, **326**, 845.

Wilson, M. L., Goodwin, T. M., Pan, V. L., and Ingles, S. A. 2003. Molecular epidemiology of preeclampsia. *Obstet Gynecol Surv*, **58**, 39–66.

Witlin, A. G., Friedman, S. A., Egerman, R. S., Frangieh, A. Y., and Sibai, B. M. 1997. Cerebrovascular disorders complicating pregnancy–beyond eclampsia. *Am J Obstet Gynecol*, **176**, 1139–45; discussion 1145–8.

Wu, Y. W., March, W. M., Croen, L. A., *et al.* 2004. Perinatal stroke in children with motor impairment: a population-based study. *Pediatrics*, **114**, 612–9.

Zeeman, G. G., Fleckenstein, J. L., Twickler, D. M., and Cunningham, F. G. 2004. Cerebral infarction in eclampsia. *Am J Obstet Gynecol*, **190**, 714–20.

Zunker, P., Georgiadis, A. L., Czech, N., *et al.* 2003. Impaired cerebral glucose metabolism in eclampsia: a new finding in two cases. *Fetal Diagn Ther*, **18**, 41–6.

MIGRAINE AND MIGRAINE-LIKE CONDITIONS

Sean I. Savitz and Louis R. Caplan

Various migraine disorders have been associated with stroke. This chapter focuses on the complex relationship of migraine with stroke and the different mechanisms by which migraine can predispose to stroke. Poorly understood migraine-like disorders that can lead to ischemic infarction are also discussed.

Migrainous stroke

There is a higher than expected prevalence of migraine among individuals with stroke. Retrospective and prospective studies have found an increased risk of ischemic stroke especially among migraineurs with aura (Henrich and Horwitz, 1989; Stang *et al.*, 2005). A meta-analysis of several observational studies showed a twofold risk of ischemic stroke in patients with migraine and a threefold risk if migraine was accompanied with aura (Etminan *et al.*, 2005). The association between migraine and brain infarction in young women is even stronger (Chang *et al.*, 1999; Tzourio *et al.*, 1993, 1995). It is also important to point out that, in men, prospective data from the Physician's Health Study showed a twofold risk for ischemic stroke among male doctors with migraine (Buring *et al.*, 1995).

Symptoms that occur during migraine auras closely resemble symptoms that result from brain ischemia. One set of symptoms so closely resembles vertebrobasilar artery disease that it has been dubbed "basilar artery migraine." Such intermittent symptoms of brainstem and cerebellar dysfunction attributable to migraine are not limited to the young but occur even in older patients, the same population that has arteriosclerotic disease of arteries that supply the posterior circulation.

Various mechanisms have been posited to explain how migraine can predispose to stroke. First, ischemic infarction can occur during a migraine, a phenomenon that has been termed "migrainous stroke." According to the International Headache Society (Olesen, 2006), a migrainous stroke is one that occurs in a patient who has migraine with aura, and the typical symptoms of the aura in a migraine attack persist for more than 1 hour. In addition, imaging shows that (i) infarction occurs in a relevant brain area that subserves the neurological function appropriate to the aura, (ii) neurological symptoms and signs are prolonged, and (iii) no other cause is identified.

During the aura phase of a migraine, spreading depression causes vasoconstriction leading to a decline in cerebral blood flow to a level that may cause ischemic injury. Vasoconstriction can persist and severely compromise blood flow in regions supplied by that artery. Vasoconstriction can cause changes in the vascular endothelium that lead to activation of platelets and the coagulation cascade promoting thrombosis within the constricted artery. In addition, if a patient had vascular risk factors predisposing to local thrombosis, the threshold for ischemic injury in the face of blood flow reduction may be even lower. However, strokes can occur in migraineurs at times when there is no preceding typical aura (Caplan 1991, 1996; Heinrich, 1986). Bilateral hypoperfusion has even been observed in patients during a migraine attack without aura (Woods *et al.*, 1994).

Migraine and silent infarcts

There is an increased prevalence of silent infarcts in migraineurs. A population-based MRI study found a higher prevalence of cerebellar infarcts in patients with migraine compared to those without migraine (Kruit *et al.*, 2004). The odds ratio for posterior circulation infarcts varied according to migraine subtype and attack frequency (Kruit *et al.*, 2004). Spreading depression has been implicated as an important mechanism that may reduce blood flow to the cerebellum and cause asymptomatic infarcts. Similarly, Kruit *et al.* (2004) also found that women with migraine have a higher prevalence of silent high deep white matter lesions, which may represent infarcts, but their clinical significance is unknown (Kruit *et al.*, 2004).

Other mechanisms and associated medical conditions predisposing to stroke

In addition to cortical spreading depression and vasoconstriction, migraine may predispose to ischemia by several other mechanisms listed in Table 69.1. Persistent vomiting can lead to intravascular volume depletion and result in cerebral blood flow reduction. There is a strong association between patent foramen ovale and migraine (Beda and Gill, 2005). A patent foramen ovale permits the passage of paradoxical emboli and may allow for chemical mediators from the systemic circulation to enter the intracranial vasculature and trigger mechanisms within the central nervous system that lead to migraines.

Migraine is also associated with a number of different medical conditions that pose risks for stroke. For example, migraine is thought to predispose to edema of vascular walls and an increased susceptibility to arterial dissection. Systemic lupus erythematosis (SLE), the antiphospholipid antibody syndrome, MELAS (mitochondrial encephalomyopathy, lactic acidosis, and stroke-like episodes), CADASIL (cerebral autosomal dominant arteriopathy

Uncommon Causes of Stroke, 2nd edition, ed. Louis R. Caplan. Published by Cambridge University Press. © Cambridge University Press 2008.

Table 69.1 Posited relationships between migraine and strokes in migraineurs

1. Migraine is incidental, and the stroke has another well-recognized cause.
2. Systemic disorders cause both migraine headaches and strokes (MELAS, CADASIL, cocaine use, SLE, MVP, etc.).
3. Structural occlusive and other arterial diseases (AVMs, dissections, SLE) cause symptoms that mimic migraine. An inherited tendency for migraine such as a channelopathy may magnify the likelihood that migraine-like phenomena might occur during the course of other vascular conditions.
3. Migraine causes an arterial dissection which, in turn, causes a brain infarct.
4. Migraine accentuates the development of vascular lesions that predispose to stroke (aneurysms, fibromuscular dysplasia, dissections, etc.).
5. Migraines are associated with severe vasoconstriction. Prolonged and intense vasoconstriction can cause ischemia in the territory supplied by the constricted artery.
6. Migraine and vascular constriction activate platelets that then potentiate white thrombus formation.
7. Migraine and vasoconstriction cause irritation or damage to the vascular endothelium with release of substances that activate the coagulation cascade and predispose to red clot formation. Red clots and white clots are more apt to form in the lumen of the constricted arteries and may cause an occlusive thrombosis of the artery with subsequent brain infarction.
8. Migraineurs have a high prevalence of patent foramen ovale, which could permit the passage of paradoxical emboli to the brain.
9. Dehydration and vomiting during migraine cause hypovolemia and increase the tendency to thrombosis.
10. Reperfusion of brain regions and arterioles and capillaries rendered ischemic during a migraine attack can cause ICH.

MELAS = mitochondrial encephalomyopathy, lactic acidosis, and stroke-like episodes; CADASIL = cerebral autosomal dominant arteriopathy with subcortical infarcts and leukoencephalopathy; SLE = systemic lupus erythematosus; MVP = mitral valve prolapse; AVM = arteriovenous malformation; ICH = intracerebral hemorrhage.

with subcortical infarcts and leukoencephalopathy), and mitral valve prolapse (MVP) are all associated with migraine or migraine-like episodes and strokes or stroke-like episodes. Finally, migraine-like events have been reported to occur in patients with prosthetic heart valves (Caplan *et al.*, 1976) and Hodgkin's disease (Feldmann and Posner, 1986).

Migraine and transient global amnesia

There is a higher prevalence of migraine in patients with transient global amnesia. Patients may actually have a migraine attack associated with the amnestic event. There is an extensive literature supporting the possibility that the mechanism for some types of transient global amnesia is because of a migrainous etiology involving spreading depression (Teive *et al.*, 2005). Some studies have even documented abnormalities on diffusion and perfusion imaging during or days after amnesia (Sedlaczek *et al.*, 2004), suggesting an ischemic mechanism.

Pseudomigraine with pleocytosis (Bartleson syndrome)

Bartleson syndrome is another disorder associated with focal neurological signs and prominent headache. This disorder occurs mostly in young men and is characterized by attacks resembling migrainous auras that occur in a flurry and are accompanied by prominent headache and cerebrospinal fluid pleocytosis (Bartleson *et al.*, 1981). Sometimes, a fever occurs. The pleocytosis has a lymphocytic predominance (>100 cells) with an elevated protein, and is not accompanied by other spinal fluid abnormalities such as elevated glucose or oligoclonal bands. Although some studies suggest that MRI shows no specific structural lesions (Gomez-Aranda *et al.*, 1997), we have seen patients with this syndrome who have ischemic infarctions. No evidence has been found for lyme disease, neurosyphilis, Herpes simplex virus (HSV), neurobrucellosis, mycoplasma, HIV meningitis, or granulomatous or neoplastic arachnoiditis (Gomez-Aranda *et al.*, 1997). This disorder may represent a primary migraine disorder with an inflammatory etiology, but other possibilities include a viral meningovascular infection or some other undefined aseptic meningitis. The clinical course of this syndrome is typically self-limited, lasting usually from 6 to 12 weeks.

Stroke-like migraine attacks after radiation therapy

Stroke-like migraine attacks after radiation therapy (SMART) is a relatively new syndrome in which stroke-like migraine attacks occur as a late consequence of brain irradiation (Black *et al.*, 2006; Pruitt *et al.*, 2006). Patients begin to have episodes years after radiation. The migraine-like events consist of prolonged, but reversible, neurological dysfunction that can last for several weeks. Headaches are often (but not always) preceded by aura. MRI shows diffuse cortical enhancement that self-resolves. No pattern to date has been found that associates the dose of radiation, tumor type, or specific chemotherapeutic agents with the occurrence of this syndrome.

Cerebral reversible vasoconstriction syndrome (Call-Fleming Syndrome)

Call *et al.* (1988) called attention to a syndrome that they dubbed reversible cerebral segmental vasoconstriction. This condition is extensively reviewed in Chapter 67. Many of the patients have had or will develop typical migraine. Many of the transient episodes resemble migrainous attacks. The onset is often with a thunderclap headache (Chen *et al.*, 2006). This condition most often affects young women, especially during the puerperium, but also develops at menopause and is found at all ages. Some patients have developed this syndrome after carotid surgery (Lopez-Valdes *et al.*,

1997). Vasoconstriction involves many large, medium, and small cerebral arteries. The clinical findings include severe headache, decreased alertness, seizures, and changing multifocal neurological signs. Focal abnormal areas of ischemia are sometimes found on MRI scans. Angiography shows sausage-shaped focal regions of vasodilatation and multifocal regions of vascular narrowing.

Brain hemorrhage after migraine attacks

Cerebral hemorrhages occasionally are reported after a severe migraine attack (Caplan 1988; Cole and Aube 1990; Gautier *et al.*, 1993). The posited explanation is that initially intense vasoconstriction during the migraine headache leads to ischemia of a local brain region with edema and ischemia of the small vessels perfused by the constricted artery. When the headache improves vasoconstriction abates, blood flow to the region is augmented, and the reperfusion can cause hemorrhage from the damaged arteries and arterioles (Caplan, 1988). The mechanism is the same as that found in hemorrhage after carotid endarterectomy and in reperfusion after brain embolization.

REFERENCES

Bartleson, J. D., Swanson, J. W., and Whisnant, J. P. 1981. A migrainous syndrome with cerebrospinal fluid pleocytosis. *Neurology*, **31**, 1257–62.

Beda, R. D., and Gill, E. A. Jr. 2005 Patent foramen ovale: does it play a role in the pathophysiology of migraine headache? *Cardiol Clin*, **23**, 91–6.

Black, D. F., Bartleson, J. D., Bell, M. L., and Lachance, D. H. 2006 SMART: stroke-like migraine attacks after radiation therapy. *Cephalalgia*, **26**, 1137–42.

Buring, J. E., Hebert, P., Romero, J., *et al.* 1995. Migraine and subsequent risk of stroke in the Physicians' Health Study. *Arch Neurol*, **52**, 129–34.

Call, G. K., Fleming, M. C., Sealfon, S., *et al.* 1988. Reversible cerebral segmental vasoconstriction. *Stroke*, **19**, 1159–70.

Caplan, L. R. 1988. Intracerebral hemorrhage revisited. *Neurology*, **38**, 624–7.

Caplan, L. R. 1991. Migraine and vertebrobasilar ischemia. *Neurology*, **41**, 55–61.

Caplan, L. R. 1996. Migraine and posterior circulation ischemia. In Posterior Circulation Disease. *Clinical Findings, Diagnosis, and Management*, L. R. Caplan (ed.), Boston: Blackwell Science, 544–68.

Caplan, L. R., Weiner, H., Weintraub, R. M., and Austen, W. G. 1976. "Migrainous" neurologic dysfunction in patients with prosthetic cardiac valves. *Headache*, **16**, 218–21.

Chang, C. L., Donaghy, M., and Poulter, N. 1999. Migraine and stroke in young women: case-control study. The World Health Organization Collaborative Study of Cardiovascular Disease and Steroid Hormone Contraception. *Br Med J*, **318**, 13–8.

Chen, S. P., Fuh, J. L., Lirng, J. F., Chang, F. C., and Wang, S. J. 2006. Recurrent primary thunderclap headache and benign CNS angiopathy. *Neurology*, **67**, 2164–9.

Cole, A. J., and Aube, M. 1990 Migraine with vasospasm and delayed intracerebral hemorrhage. *Arch Neurol*, **47**, 53–6.

Etminan, M., Takkouche, B., Isorna, F. C., and Samii, A. 2005. Risk of ischaemic stroke in people with migraine: systematic review and meta-analysis of observational studies. *Br Med J*, **330**, 63.

Feldmann, E., and Posner, J. B. 1986. Episodic neurologic dysfunction in patients with Hodgkin's disease. *Arch Neurol*, **43**, 1227–33.

Gautier, J. C., Majdalani, A., Juillard, J. B., *et al.* 1993. Hemorragies cerebrales au cours de la migraine. *Rev Neurol (Paris)*, **149**, 407–10.

Gomez-Aranda, F., Canadillas, F., Marti-Masso, J. F., *et al.* 1997. Pseudomigraine with temporary neurological symptoms and lymphocytic pleocytosis. A report of 50 cases. *Brain*, **120**, 1105–13.

Henrich, J. B., and Horwitz, R. I. 1989. A controlled study of ischemic stroke risk in migraine patients. *J Clin Epidemiol*, **42**, 773–80.

Kruit, M. C., van Buchem, M. A., Hofman, P. A., *et al.* 2004. Migraine as a risk factor for subclinical brain lesions. *JAMA*, **291**, 427–34.

Lopez-Valdes, E., Chang, H. M., Pessin, M. S., and Caplan, L. R. 1997. Cerebral vasoconstriction after carotid surgery. *Neurology*, **49**, 303–4.

Olesen, J. 2006 International Classification of Headache Disorders, Second Edition (ICHD-2): current status and future revisions. *Cephalalgia*, **26**, 1409–10.

Pruitt, A., Dalmau, J., Detre, J., Alavi, A., and Rosenfeld, M. R. 2006. Episodic neurologic dysfunction with migraine and reversible imaging findings after radiation. *Neurology*, **67**, 676–8.

Sedlaczek, O., Hirsch, J. G., Grips, E., *et al.* 2004. Detection of delayed focal MR changes in the lateral hippocampus in transient global amnesia. *Neurology*, **62**, 2165–70.

Stang, P. E., Carson, A. P., Rose, K. M., *et al.* 2005. Headache, cerebrovascular symptoms, and stroke: the Atherosclerosis Risk in Communities Study. *Neurology*, **64**, 1573–7.

Teive, H. A., Kowacs, P. A., Maranhao Filho, P., Piovesan, E. J., and Werneck, L. C. 2005. Leao's cortical spreading depression: from experimental "artifact" to physiological principle. *Neurology*, **65**, 1455–9.

Tzourio, C., Iglesias, S., Hubert, J. B., *et al.* 1993. Migraine and risk of ischaemic stroke: a case-control study. *Br Med J*, **307**, 289–92.

Tzourio, C., Tehindrazanarivelo, A., Iglesias, S., *et al.* 1995. Case-control study of migraine and risk of ischaemic stroke in young women. *Br Med J*, **310**, 830–3.

Woods, R. P., Iacoboni, M., and Mazziotta, J. C. 1994. Brief report: bilateral spreading cerebral hypoperfusion during spontaneous migraine headache. *N Engl J Med*, **331**, 1689–92.

70 INTRAVASCULAR LYMPHOMA

Elayna O. Rubens

Introduction

Intravascular lymphoma is a rare, extranodal, large B-cell lymphoma in which neoplastic, lymphoid cells proliferate within the lumina of small to medium-sized vessels. The disease was first described in 1959 by Pfleger and Tappeiner and called angioendotheliomatosis proliferans systemisata (Pfleger and Tappeiner, 1959). Subsequently, the disease was referred to as "neoplastic angioendotheliomatosis", "malignant angioendotheliomatosis" or "angiotropic lymphoma" (Case records of the Massachusetts General Hospital, 1986; Petito et al., 1978). The current nomenclature – intravascular lymphoma or intravascular lymphomatosis – is based on the knowledge that the neoplastic cells are of lymphoid rather than endothelial origin (Bhawan et al., 1985).

The proliferating lymphoid cells occlude the involved blood vessels thereby compromising tissue blood flow. The result is ischemic damage affecting a variety of organ systems, including the brain and spinal cord. The variable sites and extent of the ischemia lead to diverse clinical presentations. This clinical heterogeneity combined with the rarity of the disease itself makes diagnosis challenging. The pathologic process is often not identified until autopsy (Devlin et al., 1998). Without treatment, the disease is nearly universally fatal. With the use of aggressive, combined chemotherapy, however, some patients may achieve complete remission and even long-term, disease-free survival (DiGiuseppe et al., 1994). Diagnosis requires knowledge of the disease process, its diagnostic features, and a high index of suspicion.

Epidemiology

Intravascular lymphoma is a rare disease with an estimated incidence of less than one case per million people. It usually occurs in the sixth or seventh decade of life, although it has been reported in patients ranging from 34 to 90 years old (Zuckerman et al., 2006). Men and women are equally affected. An ethnic or racial propensity for the disease has not been reported, although there are regional differences in clinical presentation. A cutaneous variant of intravascular lymphoma that has been reported in women in western countries seems to have a more favorable prognosis than does typical intravascular lymphoma (Ferreri, et al., 2004). Additionally, a Japanese study may have identified an "Asian variant" of the disease that is typically associated with a hemophagocytic syndrome, less neurological impairment, and no cutaneous involvement (Murase et al., 2007).

Clinical features

Our knowledge of the disease manifestations and prognosis is confined to a number of small case series and individual case reports. Prognosis of the disease is dismal overall with a median survival of untreated patients of 4–7 months. With chemotherapy, prognosis is improved, although reported follow-up is usually short. Anghel et al. (2003) reviewed the outcomes of 33 reported patients treated with chemotherapy. After a median follow-up of 8 months, 67% of patients had died. Of those alive, 23% had no evidence of disease, including some patients with follow-up of more than 4 years (Anghel et al., 2003). Poor prognostic factors include age > 60 years, thrombocytopenia, and lack of anthracycline-based chemotherapy treatment (Murase et al., 2007).

The most common findings occur in the skin and central nervous system (CNS), although renal, pulmonary, hepatic, splenic, adrenal, and cardiac manifestations also occur. Non-neurologic presentations include fever of unknown origin, rash, night sweats, weight loss, renal failure, and shortness of breath (DiGiuseppe et al., 1994; Anghel et al., 2003; Kanda et al., 1999). Neurological findings develop in about two-thirds of patients and usually present as multifocal cerebrovascular events, subacute encephalopathy, spinal cord or nerve root vascular syndromes, or peripheral and cranial neuropathies (Beristain and Azzarelli, 2002; Debiais et al., 2004; Glass et al., 1993).

Brain infarction

In the brain, intravascular lymphoma manifests primarily as multiple infarcts. Among patients with neurological symptoms, 76% have multifocal infarcts (Glass et al., 1993). Reported symptoms include confusion, rapidly progressive dementia, dysarthria, aphasia, diplopia, focal motor or sensory complaints, ataxia, paraparesis, vertigo, seizures, myoclonus, and incontinence (Baehring et al., 2003; Beristain and Azzarelli, 2002; DiGiuseppe et al., 1994; Ferreri et al., 2004; Gaul et al., 2006; Glass et al., 1993; Heinrich et al., 2005; Murase et al., 2007). Recurrent, focal neurological signs are often accompanied by a progressive encephalopathy (Imamura et al., 2006). The strokes may involve any area of the brain, although supratentorial infarcts are more prevalent than cerebellar or brainstem infarction (Baehring et al., 2005). The differential diagnosis often includes CNS angiitis, acute disseminated encephalomyelitis, progressive multifocal leukoencephalopathy, paraneoplastic encephalomyelitis, and Creutzfeld-Jakob disease (Gaul et al., 2006; Lozsadi et al., 2005).

Uncommon Causes of Stroke, 2nd edition, ed. Louis R. Caplan. Published by Cambridge University Press. © Cambridge University Press 2008.

Imamura *et al*. (2006) described a 75-year-old woman who presented with multiple stroke-like episodes that initially responded to conventional stroke therapy. She first had a pseudobulbar palsy and was found to have a left frontal lobe infarct. Her deficits resolved. One month later, she developed acute onset sensory aphasia and had a new, left temporal lesion. The aphasia improved with antiplatelet therapy. The next month, she presented with confusion and was found to have diffuse, subcortical white matter T2 lesions with gyriform enhancement. Biopsy revealed intravascular lymphoma. The stroke episodes and confusional state were associated with fever. She eventually died of pulmonary complications 10 months later (Imamura *et al.*, 2006).

At our hospital, a 71-year-old, previously healthy woman presented with headache and transient speech difficulty. Imaging, electroencephalogram (EEG), cerebrospinal fluid (CSF) profile, laboratory studies including erythrocyte sedimentation rate (ESR), and cardiac evaluation were all normal. One month later, she developed a fluent aphasia, balance difficulties, episodic confusion, and memory problems. She was found to have multiple acute infarcts in the bilateral cerebellar hemispheres and left thalamus. During the next weeks, she became increasingly confused and agitated and had incomprehensible speech. Repeat MRI showed a new, right parieto-occipital infarct. A brain biopsy showed intravascular lymphoma. Unfortunately, she was unable to receive chemotherapy because of poor performance status, and she died several weeks later.

Encephalopathy and rapidly progressive dementia

Other patients with cerebral pathology present with a gradual cognitive decline, subacute encephalopathy, or fluctuating level of consciousness. Encephalopathy is observed in 27% of intravascular lymphoma patients and may be accompanied by focal neurological signs or seizures (Glass *et al.*, 1993). These findings are attributed to multiple infarctions or are caused by other metabolic or infectious processes associated with the systemic disease process.

Martin-Duverneuil *et al* . (2002) reported one such case of a 44-year-old woman who complained of memory difficulties, mental slowing, hypersomnia, and headaches for 9 months. An MRI showed multiple, hyperintense areas in the white matter on T2-weighted images involving periventricular white matter, posterior portion of the corpus callosum, and cerebellar white matter. Brain biopsy revealed proliferation of atypical lymphoid cells in the lumen of small vessels. Despite chemotherapy and radiotherapy, her dementia progressed and she eventually became paraplegic. The patient died 1 year after presentation (Martin-Duverneuil *et al.*, 2002).

A German group reported another 80-year-old woman with no vascular risk factors who presented with cognitive slowing and impairment of concentration, short-term memory problems, and hallucinations (visual and auditory). Examination revealed temporal disorientation, naming difficulty, paraphasic errors, ideomotor apraxia, psychomotor agitation, and mild left-leg monoparesis. Imaging showed several small periventricular, T2-bright lesions, a cortical-subcortical left temporal lesion, and a left cerebellar white matter lesion. She died suddenly of a pulmonary embolism prior to further diagnostic work-up. At autopsy, there was accumulation of lymphoid cells within the small and medium leptomeningeal and intracerebral blood vessels which occasionally invaded the vascular wall. Where vessels were completely occluded, there were associated infarcts of the adjacent brain tissue (Heinrich *et al.*, 2005).

Spinal cord and radicular syndromes

Glass *et al* . (1993) reported that 38% of patients with neurological symptoms had spinal cord involvement manifesting as paraparesis (either spastic or flaccid), pain, and incontinence. Similarly, in a case series from Brigham and Women's Hospital, those patients with spinal cord involvement had rapidly progressive paraparesis, spasticity, allodynia, and bladder dysfunction (Baehring *et al.*, 2003). Occasionally spinal cord presentation is associated with good outcome (Debiais *et al.*, 2004). Any spinal cord or root level can be involved, and pathology reveals involvement of associated blood vessels and infarction of the cord or affected roots.

A 63-year-old man with progressive numbness and weakness in his legs followed by urinary retention and, later, language difficulty was found at postmortem examination to have intravascular lymphoma involving the spinal cord and brain. At presentation, he had a flaccid paraplegia, a T5 sensory level, and sphincter dysfunction. MRI of the spinal cord showed T2-hyperintense lesions and gadolinium enhancement in the thoracic cord and conus. He was initially thought to have autoimmune encephalomyelitis and was treated with immunosuppressive therapy. He died 18 months after symptom onset of nosocomial pneumonia. At autopsy, he was found to have intravascular lymphoma involving the vessels of the brain, spinal cord, and skeletal muscle.

Neuropathy

Because of involvement of the vasa nervorum, intravascular lymphoma may also affect the peripheral and cranial nerves. The most commonly reported cranial nerve findings are facial, abducens, vestibulocochlear, oculomotor, trigeminal, and optic neuropathies (Glass *et al.*, 1993). The peripheral neuropathy observed in intravascular lymphoma is a predominantly axonal neuropathy. As the peripheral nerves are commonly involved, these may serve as a potential site for diagnostic biopsy in symptomatic patients (Devlin *et al.*, 1998).

Intracranial hemorrhage

Intracranial hemorrhage is an exceedingly rare complication of intravascular lymphoma. Lui *et al* . (2003) reported a 41-year-old woman who presented with eye pain, blurred vision from the left eye, left lateral gaze palsy, and mental status changes. She later developed disseminated intravascular coagulopathy and multiorgan failure. A CT scan revealed diffuse, subcortical hemorrhages.

The diagnosis of intravascular lymphoma was subsequently made at autopsy (Lui *et al.*, 2003).

Venous infarction

The proliferation of lymphomatous cells within the venules and dural venous sinuses may lead to venous occlusion, infarction, and hemorrhagic transformation. Kenez *et al*. (2000) reported a case of a 43-year-old woman who presented with repeated episodes of seizure and aphasia followed by right hemiparesis and mental status changes. During her course, she was found to have multiple, T2-bright cortical and subcortical white matter lesions that fluctuated in their appearance. In addition, there was moderate hemorrhagic transformation. MR venogram showed a small lesion in the superior sagittal sinus and vein of Galen, whereas the internal cerebral vein and the venous angle were not visualized. She died 9 months after the onset of the illness. Autopsy findings revealed neoplastic invasion of the walls of the superior sagittal sinus, meningeal veins, and small and medium-sized cerebral arteries. Areas of adjacent infarcted tissue were also identified. The authors surmise that the fluctuating MRI appearance reflected disturbed venous outflow and opening of collaterals due to lymphomatous venous occlusion (Kenez *et al.*, 2000).

Diagnostic studies

Pathology

Ultimately, the diagnosis of intravascular lymphoma must be made by pathologic examination of affected tissue. When neurological symptoms are present, a search for other sites more amenable to biopsy should be undertaken. In the absence of systemic involvement, a brain biopsy can be performed. In some series, brain biopsy was nondiagnostic in up to 60% of patients (Baehring *et al.*, 2003). In order to decrease such false-negative results, it is imperative that the tissue obtained from the brain be from a clinically involved region of the nervous system.

Biopsy or postmortem examination of the brain in intravascular lymphoma shows distention and occlusion of small cerebral and meningeal capillaries, arterioles, and venules by malignant lymphocytes (Figure 70.1). These lymphocytes usually have a B-cell phenotype (Figure 70.2), although they may rarely be of T-cell or natural killer (NK)-cell origin (Zuckerman *et al.*, 2006). Vessel occlusion often coexists with brain infarction, sometimes hemorrhagic, distributed throughout the brain and spinal cord (Martin-Duverneuil *et al.*, 2002). Occasionally, malignant cells extend beyond the vessel walls, but extravasation is exceptional (Beristain and Azzarelli, 2002). Other commonly involved organs include the skin, liver, spleen, bone marrow, kidney, lung, and prostate (Ferreri *et al.*, 2004). Adrenal glands, thyroid, gallbladder, nasal mucosa, and muscle are also sites of disease, whereas lymph nodes are usually spared (Glass *et al.*, 1993).

The explanation for the intravascular accumulation of lymphoid cells has not yet been elucidated. The neoplastic lymphocytes in some cases have been found to lack normal adhesion and homing molecules (specifically CDIIa/CD18) required for endothelial cell

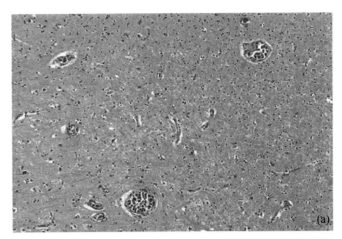

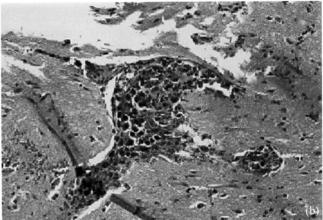

Figure 70.1 (a) Hematoxylin and eosin staining showing lymphocyte accumulation in small to medium-sized vessels in the brain. (b) Higher power hematoxylin and eosin staining showing lymphocyte accumulation in small to medium-sized vessels in the brain. See color plate.

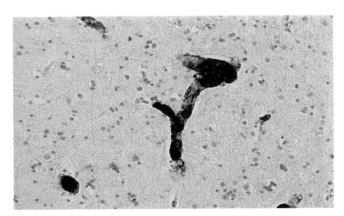

Figure 70.2 The tumor cells within the vessels stain with B-cell marker CD20. See color plate.

binding and extravasation (Jalkanen *et al.*, 1989). Other studies, however, have not replicated these findings and suggest that cell adhesion molecules may play a role in the intravascular replication of the neoplastic cells (Kanda *et al.*, 1999).

Imaging

Like its clinical features, the diagnostic imaging results in patients with intravascular lymphoma are variable. CT and cerebral angiography may show characteristics of stroke and vessel occlusion, but findings are often nonspecific and, in many instances, these studies are normal. MRI seems to be more sensitive, though in one case series, brain MRI had a false-negative rate of nearly 50% (Ferreri et al., 2004). Similarly, MRI of the spine may be normal even in cases where extensive cord involvement is evident on pathologic examination (Devlin et al., 1998). Nevertheless, asymptomatic brain lesions may be detected in some cases, and MRI should be included in the staging and work-up of patients with suspected intravascular lymphoma, even in the absence of neurological symptoms (Ferreri et al., 2004).

In a report of the imaging findings of four intravascular lymphoma patients and review of the literature, Williams et al. (1998) found that all patients with intravascular lymphoma had multifocal abnormalities. These abnormalities included nonspecific white matter changes (45%), infarct-like lesions (36%), focal mass lesion (36%), and meningeal or parenchymal enhancement (64%). Common infarct patterns include multifocal lesions on diffusion-weighted imaging (DWI) in association with corresponding T2 signal abnormalities, resolution of some DWI or T2 lesions along with the appearance of new lesions during the course of the disease, and gadolinium enhancement in proximity to T2 or DWI changes (Baehring et al., 2003). In some patients treated with chemotherapy, DWI and fluid-attenuated inversion recovery (FLAIR) abnormalities were partially reversible relative to the response to treatment (Baehring et al., 2005). Intravascular lymphomatosis has also been reported to mimic posterior leukoencephalopathy on MRI in a woman who presented with complete visual loss and confusion. The T2 hyperintensity involved the subcortical white matter of the parietal and occipital lobes including the U fibers, but sparing overlying cortex (Moussouttas, 2002).

Other studies

Supportive diagnostic findings include an elevated ESR, anemia, and elevated lactate dehydrogenase. Bone marrow biopsy is often unrevealing. CSF analysis can be normal in intravascular lymphoma, even in the presence of neurological signs (Lozsadi et al., 2005). More often, elevated CSF protein is found. About half of patients have a mild to moderate CSF pleocytosis (Beristain and Azzarelli, 2002). CSF cytology is usually negative for malignant cells, although rare exceptions of malignant lymphoid cells in the CSF do occur (Baehring et al., 2003; Ossege et al., 2000). Immunoglobulin G index may also be elevated (Moussouttas, 2002).

EEG can reveal background slowing indicative of diffuse cerebral dysfunction, focal slowing in the areas of localized vascular infiltration, or paroxysmal activity in the setting of seizures. Occasionally, focal EEG abnormalities are seen prior to changes on MRI (Baumann et al., 2000).

Treatment

Various treatment options have been shown to improve symptoms and outcome. Given the widespread nature of intravascular lymphoma, systemic chemotherapy with anthracycline-based regimens has been the most commonly pursued treatment in the literature (cyclophosphamide, doxorubicin, vincristine, and prednisone [CHOP] or rituximab [R]-CHOP). In one case series of 22 patients treated with chemotherapy, ten (45%) achieved a complete remission, three (14%) achieved partial remission, seven (32%) progressed, and two (9%) died of toxicity (Ferreri et al., 2004). Only five of these treated patients had CNS involvement, and four of them died within 4 months of diagnosis despite treatment. One patient with neurological symptoms who was treated with high-dose chemotherapy and autologous stem cell transplantation was alive and disease free at 19 months. The poor outcome among patients with neurological manifestations highlights the importance of using chemotherapy regimens with adequate CNS penetration (Ferreri et al., 2004). High-dose methotrexate alone or in combination with CHOP has also been used in six patients with neurological findings; half of these patients had complete remission (Baehring et al., 2003).

In another series, 48% of ten patients treated with combination chemotherapy achieved complete remission and were free of disease after ≥ 3 years of follow-up (DiGiuseppe et al., 1994). High-dose chemotherapy with autologous stem cell transplantation was performed on two women with intravascular lymphoma. Both of these patients achieved complete remission and were relapse free up to 71 months from diagnosis (Ferreri et al., 2004). Systemic chemotherapy and intrathecal methotrexate in combination with the anti-CD20 monoclonal antibody rituximab was shown to produce complete remission in three patients with systemic intravascular lymphoma, all of whom remained disease free at 24–45 months of follow-up (Bouzani et al., 2006). Steroids and plasmapheresis have also been used with temporary alleviation of symptoms (Harris et al., 1994).

Conclusion

Intravascular lymphoma is an extremely rare malignancy that evades diagnosis because of its rarity, variable clinical presentation, and lack of definitive diagnostic findings other than biopsy. Inclusion of intravascular lymphoma in the differential diagnosis of multifocal brain infarctions may improve yield of antemortem diagnosis and therefore increase access to available treatments.

REFERENCES

Anghel, G., Pettinato, G., Severino, A., et al. 2003. Intravascular B-cell lymphoma: report of two cases with different clinical presentation but rapid central nervous system involvement. Leuk Lymphoma, **44**, 1353–9.

Baehring, J. M., Henchcliffe, C., Ledezma, C. J., Fulbright, R., and Hochberg, F. H. 2005. Intravascular lymphoma: magnetic resonance imaging correlates of disease dynamics within the central nervous system. J Neurol Neurosurg Psychiatry, **76**, 540–4.

Baehring, J. M., Longtine, J., and Hochberg, F. H. 2003. A new approach to the diagnosis and treatment of intravascular lymphoma. J Neurooncol, **61**, 237–48.

Baumann, T. P., Hurwitz, N., Karamitopolou-Diamantis, E., *et al*. 2000. Diagnosis and treatment of intravascular lymphomatosis. *Arch Neurol*, **57**, 374–7.

Beristain, X., and Azzarelli, B. 2002. The neurological masquerade of intravascular lymphomatosis. *Arch Neurol*, **59**, 439–43.

Bhawan, J., Wolff, S. M., and Ucci, A. A. 1985. Malignant lymphoma and malignant angioendotheliomatosis: one disease. *Cancer*, **55**, 570–6.

Bouzani, M., Karmiris, T., Rontogianni, D., *et al*. 2006. Disseminated intravascular B-cell lymphoma: clinicopathological features and outcome of three cases treated with anthracycline based immunochemotherapy. *Oncologist*, **11**, 923–8.

Case records of the Massachusetts General Hospital. Weekly clinicopathological exercises. Case 39–1986. A 66-year-old woman with fever, fluctuating neurologic signs, and negative blood cultures. 1986. *N Engl J Med*, **315**, 874–5.

Debiais, S., Bonnaud, I., Cottier, J. P., *et al*. 2004. A spinal cord intravascular lymphomatosis with exceptional good outcome. *Neurology*, **63**, 1329–30.

Devlin, T., Moll, S., Hulette, C., and Morgenlander, J. C. 1998. Intravascular malignant lymphomatosis with neurologic presentation: factors facilitating antemortem diagnosis. *South Med J*, **91**, 672–6.

DiGiuseppe, J. A., Nelson, W. G., Seifter, E. J., Boitnott, J. K., and Mann, R. B. 1994. Intravascular lymphomatosis: a clinicopathologic study of 10 cases and assessment of response to chemotherapy. *J Clin Oncol*, **12**, 2573–9.

Ferreri, A. J. M., Campo, E., Ambrosetti, A., *et al*. 2004. Anthracycline-based chemotherapy as primary treatment for intravascular lymphoma. *Ann Oncol*, **15**, 1215–21.

Ferreri, A. J. M., Campo, E., Seymour, J. F., *et al*. 2004. Intravascular lymphoma: clinical presentation, natural history, management and prognostic factors in a series of 38 cases, with special emphasis on the 'cutaneous variant'. *Br J Haematol*, **127**, 173–83.

Ferry, J. A., Harris, N. L., Picker, L. J., *et al*. 1988. Intravascular lymphomatosis (malignant angioendotheliomatosis). A B-cell neoplasm expressing surface homing receptors. *Mod Pathol*, **1**, 444–52.

Gaul, C., Hanisch, F., Neureiter, D., *et al*. 2006. Intravascular lymphomatosis mimicking disseminated encephalomyelitis and encephalomyelopathy. *Clin Neurol Neurosurg*, **108**, 486–9.

Glass, J., Hochberg, F. H., and Miller, D. C. 1993. Intravascular lymphomatosis – a systemic disease with neurologic manifestations. *Cancer*, **71**, 3156–64.

Harris, C. P., Sigman, J. D., and Jaeckle, K. A. 1994. Intravascular malignant lymphomatosis: amelioration of neurological symptoms with plasmapheresis. *Ann Neurol*, **35**, 357–9.

Heinrich, A., Vogelgesang, S., Kirsch, M., and Khaw, A. V. 2005 Intravascular lymphomatosis presenting as rapidly progressive dementia. *Eur Neurol*, **54**, 55–8.

Imamura, K., Awaki, E., Aoyama, Y., *et al*. 2006. Intravascular large B-cell lymphoma following a relapsing stroke with temporary fever: a brain biopsy case. *Intern Med*, **45**, 693–5.

Jalkanen, S., Aho, R., Kallajoki, M., *et al*. 1989. Lymphocyte homing receptors and adhesion molecules in intravascular malignant lymphomatosis. *Int J Cancer*, **44**, 777–82.

Kanda, M., Suzumiya, J., Ohshima, K., Tamura, K., and Kikuchi, M. 1999. Intravascular large cell lymphoma: clinicopathological, immuno-histochemical and molecular genetic studies. *Leuk Lymphoma*, **34**, 569–80.

Kenez, J., Barsi, P., Majtenyi, K., *et al*. 2000. Can intravascular lymphomatosis mimic sinus thrombosis? A case report with 8 months' follow up and fatal outcome. *Neuroradiology*, **42**, 436–40.

Lozsadi, D. A., Wieshmann, U., and Enevoldson, T. P. 2005. Neurological presentation of intravascular lymphoma: report of two cases and discussion of diagnostic challenges. *Eur J Neurol*, **12**, 710–4.

Lui, P. C. W., Wong, G. K. C., Poon, W. S., and Tse, G. M. K. 2003. Intravascular lymphomatosis. *J Clin Pathol*, **56**, 468–70.

Martin-Duverneuil, N., Mokhrari, K., Behin, A., *et al*. 2002. Intravascular malignant lymphomatosis. *Neuroradiology*, **44**, 749–54.

Moussouttas, M. 2002. Intravascular lymphomatosis presenting as posterior leukoencephalopathy. *Arch Neurol*, **59**, 640–1.

Murase, T., Yamaguchi, M., Suzuki, R., *et al*. 2007. Intravascular large B-cell lymphoma (IVLBCL): a clinicopathologic study of 96 patients with special reference to the immunophenotypic heterogeneity of CD-5. *Blood*, **109**, 478–85.

Ossege, L. M., Postler, E., Pleger, B., Muller, K. M., and Malin, J. P. 2000. Neoplastic cells in the cerebrospinal fluid in intravascular lymphomatosis. *J Neurol*, **247**, 656–8.

Petito, C. K., Gottlieb, G., Dougherty, J. H., and Petito, F. A. 1978. Neoplastic angioendotheliosis: ultrastructural study and review of the literature. *Ann Neurol*, **3**, 393–9.

Pfleger, L., and Tappeiner, J. 1959. Zur Kenntnis der systemisierten endotheliomatose der cutanen blutgefasse. *Hautarzt*, **10**, 359–63.

Williams, R. L., Meltzer, C. C., Smirniotopoulos, J. G., Fukui, M. B., and Inman, M. 1998. Cerebral MR imaging in intravascular lymphomatosis. *AJNR Am J Neuroradiol*, **19**, 427–31.

Zuckerman, D., Seliem, R., and Hochberg, E. 2006. Intravascular lymphoma: the oncologist's "great imitator." *Oncologist*, **11**, 496–502.

71 OTHER CONDITIONS

Louis R. Caplan

A number of unrelated vascular conditions that are potential causes of stroke have not been included as complete chapters in this edition of Uncommon Causes. Some of these conditions, which I summarize briefly in this final chapter, are rare whereas others are more common, but stroke is an unusual or minor feature of the condition.

Aortic dissections

Aortic dissections have been recognized since the time of Morgagni more than 200 years ago. Moersch and Sayre (1950) were the first to emphasize the importance of neurological complications of aortic dissection. The first analysis of a large number of cases of aortic dissection was by Hirst *et al.* (1958). They reported the findings among 505 cases of documented dissection of the aorta and emphasized the difficulty in diagnosis. Others have defined the various types and locations of the dissections, the frequency of various symptoms and signs, diagnostic testing results, outcomes, and treatment (DeSanctis *et al.*, 1987; Hagan *et al.*, 2000; Spittell *et al.*, 1993). Some reports analyze the neurological features of aortic dissection (Chase *et al.*, 1968; Gaul *et al.*, 2007; Gerber *et al.*, 1986).

Aortic dissections are often classified into two large groups: type A that involves the ascending aorta and type B that begins beyond the aortic arch. The dissection originates in the ascending aorta in about two-thirds of patients, and the transverse portion of the aortic arch in 10% (Crawford, 1990). In another one-fifth of patients, the dissection begins in the proximal descending aorta beyond the origin of the left subclavian artery and in the distal descending aorta in only about 5% of cases (Crawford, 1990). Dissections can be short, extending only a few centimeters, or be quite long, extending almost from the ascending aorta to the iliac arteries. The cleavage plane in the media of the aorta usually occupies about half and sometimes the entire circumference of the aorta (Crawford, 1990; Roberts, 1981). The plane of dissection (false lumen) characteristically follows the curvature of the ascending aorta and arch. The false lumen containing the hematoma almost always communicates with the true lumen through an intimal tear located near the proximal end of the dissection (Crawford, 1990; Roberts, 1981).

When the dissection begins in the ascending aorta, the large brain and arm supplying branches of the aorta are often obstructed by the intramural hematoma. Partial obstructions can become complete by promoting local thrombus formation or by an intimal tear forming a flap that blocks the lumen (Hirst *et al.*, 1958). Occasionally the aortic dissection extends into the cervical portions of the arteries (Stecker *et al.*, 1997). Table 71.1 contains data about the location of dissections and the aortic branch arteries compromised among 505 cases reviewed. Dissections can also extend into the aortic valve causing acute aortic insufficiency and can block the orifices of the coronary ostia above the aortic valve causing myocardial ischemia. The dissections can also rupture into the chest causing shock and into the pericardium causing cardiac tamponade. Chronic dissecting aneurysms can also cause obstruction of the superior vena cava.

Aortic dissections are 2–3 times more common in men than in women (Hirst *et al.* 1958). In nearly all patients, histological analysis of the aorta reveals some degree of medial degeneration. The most common presentation of aortic dissection is pain (DeSanctis *et al.*, 1987; Hagan *et al.*, 2000; Hirst *et al.*, 1958; Spittell *et al.*, 1993). The location of pain varies considerable and can be in the chest, back, abdomen, or head and neck. Occasional patients have painless dissections (Gerber *et al.*, 1986). The blood pressure is usually normal or high, but in about one-quarter of patients hypotension is found on presentation to the hospital, and about one in eight patients presents in shock (Hagan *et al.*, 2000). Examination may show a loss of the pulse, especially of the common carotid, left subclavian, and femoral arteries. Bruits are often heard over the neck arteries. About 30% of patients have neurological symptoms, but a smaller percentage (about 6% of those with a proximal aortic dissection) present with an obvious stroke (Hagan *et al.*, 2000). Among 7000 autopsies performed at the Massachusetts General Hospital between 1959 and 1965, there were 54 persons with nontraumatic dissections of the ascending aorta, among whom 16 (30%) had systems, signs, and pathological evidence of brain ischemia (Chase *et al.*, 1968).

Neurological presentations are divided into four major types:

1. Stupor and coma due to systemic hypoperfusion or caused by blockage of multiple aortic brain-supplying branches
2. Focal or multifocal brain infarcts caused by obstruction of one or more branches or because of extension of the dissection into one or more of the brachiocephalic arteries
3. Spinal cord ischemia and infarction
4. Ischemic peripheral neuropathy caused by blockage of arteries supplying a limb.

In the large compilation of cases of Hirst *et al.* (1958), 95/505 (19%) patients had prominent neurological findings; two thirds of the patients with neurological signs had unilateral motor and/or sensory signs indicating a focal brain deficit, and 27 (28%) were paraplegic due to spinal cord infarction. In another series, among 236 patients, only 13 (5.5%) had prominent neurological findings – six paraparesis, two coma, three focal cerebral signs, and two

Uncommon Causes of Stroke, 2nd edition, ed. Louis R. Caplan. Published by Cambridge University Press. © Cambridge University Press 2008.

Table 71.1 Location and arteries compromised among 505 cases

Location within the aorta (among 398 patients)

Ascending aorta, 244 (61%)

Aortic arch, 37 (9.2%)

Arterial origins obstructed

   Iliac, 132 (26%)

   Innominate, 67 (13%)

   Right common carotid, 27 (5%)

   Right subclavian, 15 (3%)

   Left common carotid, 59 (12%)

   Left subclavian, 48 (9.5%)

Source: Hirst *et al.*, 1958, with permission.

Table 71.2 Patterns of radiation-induced brain and vascular presentations

1. Acute radionecrosis presenting as a focal brain mass
2. Chronic dementing brain disease
3. Moyamoya obliteration of basal arteries, especially in children and young adults
4. Focal brain infarcts and strokes in patients with stenosis of intracranial arteries
5. Stenosis of extracranial arteries found in patients who have no brain symptoms or have transient ischemic attacks or strokes

ischemic neuropathy (Spittell *et al.*, 1993). Comatose presentations are most common in patients who are hypotensive on admission. Hypotension or frank shock is usually associated with rupture of the aorta into the pleural or pericardial spaces (DeSanctis *et al.*, 1987). Some have had cardiac tamponade related to the large amount of blood discharged under arterial pressure rapidly into the pericardium. Coexistence of blockage of the aortic cervicocranial arteries often leads to concurrent important brain infarcts in these comatose patients. Occasionally coma is related to interruption of multiple brain-supplying arteries without concurrent hypotension. Paraparesis or paraplegia is a complication of dissection of the descending aorta blocking the artery of Adamkiewicz and other aortic branches that supply the spinal cord.

In some patients the dissection in the aorta extends into the brachiocephalic branches of the aorta. Zurbrugg *et al.* (1988) used duplex ultrasonography to study the carotid arteries in 39 patients years after aortic dissections and found that 13 had carotid artery dissections. Stecker *et al.* (1997) imaged the brachiocephalic arteries in 24 patients within 1 month of acute aortic dissections using duplex ultrasound and enhanced MRI and CT studies. They found that half of the 20 innominate arteries studied contained dissections whereas two-fifths of the left common carotid and left subclavian arteries were dissected. Dissections were much less common in arteries located at a distance from the arch (Stecker *et al.*, 1997).

Rapid diagnosis using modern imaging techniques and treatment is essential in this highly morbid and mortal condition.

Radiation-induced vascular disease and strokes

Radiation-related damage to tissues and blood vessels has long been recognized, but the realization was markedly increased after the atom bomb explosions in Hiroshima and Nagasaki. Herein I will comment only on blood vessel-related damage after iatrogenic therapeutic radiation for malignant diseases.

The frequency of delayed radiation-related strokes has been studied most thoroughly in children. In reports from the Childhood Cancer Survival Study, strokes were most common after radiation therapy for leukemia, brain tumors, and Hodgkin's disease (Bowers *et al.*, 2005, 2006). The relative risk of stroke in leukemia survivors was 6.4 (95% confidence interval, 3–13.8) and 29 for brain tumor survivors (95% confidence interval, 13.8–60.6) (Bowers *et al.* (2006). The mean cranial radiation therapy dose was associated in a dose-dependent manner with the frequency of later stroke (Bowers *et al.*, 2006). Hodgkin's disease survivors also had a very high rate of late strokes (83.6 per 100 000 person-years), especially after mantle radiation therapy (Bowers *et al.*, 2005).

The pathology of radiation-induced brain damage emphasizes vascular injury. Vascular lesions are time, location, and dose dependent (Fajardo and Berthrong, 1988). Capillaries and sinusoids are most vulnerable, followed by arterioles and small, medium-sized, and large arteries (Dion *et al.*, 1990; Fajardo and Berthrong, 1988). Endothelial cells are most vulnerable (Fajardo and Berthrong, 1988; Haymaker *et al.*, 1968; St Louis *et al.*, 1974). The pathology includes denudation of the endothelial layer; infiltration of foam cells, histiocytes, fibrin, fibroblasts, and collagen in the subendothelium and intima; myointimal proliferation and fibrosis and sometimes calcification; narrowing of arterial lumens; thinning and fragmentation of the elastic membranes; and adventitial fibrosis (Burger *et al.*, 1979; Conomy and Kellermeyer, 1975; Fajardo and Berthrong, 1988; Haymaker *et al.*, 1968). Often vessels are surrounded by perivascular chronic inflammatory cells (Burger *et al.*, 1979; Haymaker *et al.*, 1968; Rizzoli and Pagnanelli, 1984). Thrombi are often present within damaged vessels.

Some authors have emphasized worsening of atherosclerosis as a major complication of therapeutic radiation.(Cheng *et al.*,1999, Murros and Toole, 1989) The endothelial and intimal abnormalities induced by irradiation could increase permeability to lipids (Atkinson *et al.*, 1989; Silverberg *et al.*, 1978). Inflammation is also known to accelerate atherosclerosis and is prominent in histological sections of vessels and brain tissue. Vascular imaging in patients with therapeutic radiation often shows lesions in areas that are often involved in atherosclerosis, in unusual areas, and also invariably within the field of irradiated tissue.

Clinically, there are several patterns of presentation in patients with radiation-related brain and vascular injury. These are listed in Table 71.2. Patients may present acutely with brain focal mass lesions, transient brain ischemia, or strokes.(Kang *et al.* (2002) Others develop a chronic syndrome related to brain atrophy and multiple small, presumably vascular lesions. Vascular occlusive lesions are often found intracranially and extracranially, some in usual loci for atherosclerosis and some in unusual areas for atherosclerosis.

Patients treated with radiation to the nervous system often present months and years later with focal mass lesions. These lesions can involve the brain or spinal cord. Biopsy of these lesions shows fibrinoid degeneration of blood vessels, coagulative necrosis, and gliosis (Glantz *et al.*, 1994). In some patients, multifocal enhancing lesions are found that represent radiation necrosis (Peterson *et al.*, 1995). In other patients, the brain damage is more diffuse, and a clinical picture of dementia with other neurological signs develops insidiously years after brain radiation (DeAngelis *et al.*, 1989). These patients have brain atrophy and a leukoencephalopathy characterized by hyperintensity of the white matter and loss of white matter substance. Enhancement of focal lesions is also found in some patients with this diffuse dementing syndrome (DeAngelis *et al.*, 1989).

Children who have been irradiated for brain tumors may develop a moyamoya pattern of intracranial arterial occlusion (Bitzer and Topka (1995). Ullrich *et al.*, 2007). Among 345 children (average age at start of therapy 101 = 54 months) who were irradiated for brain tumors, 33 (10%) had prominent vascular abnormalities during follow-up that averaged 4 1/2 years. Among those with vascular lesions, 12 had a moyamoya pattern. Vascular ectasia and focal regions of narrowing were also common, and many had brain infarcts. The presence of neurofibromatosis type 1 and higher radiation doses were associated with the development of moyamoya (Ullrich *et al.*, 2007).

Positing that some or much of the brain damage might be because of brain ischemia related to the radiation-induced small-vessel vasculopathy, anticoagulants (Glantz *et al.*, 1994; Rizzoli and Pagnanelli, 1984) and pentoxifylline (Dion *et al.*, 1990), an agent with hemorrheological properties, have been considered to be possibly useful in ameliorating the nervous system damage, but there are few convincing studies.

Hypereosinophilic syndrome

A markedly increased number of eosinophils in the peripheral blood can be caused by a neoplastic process (eosinophilic leukemia), represent a reactive process to a systemic condition, or reflect an idiopathic condition usually referred to as a hypereosinophilic syndrome. Hypereosinophilia is most often a secondary process in response to drugs, allergies, and/or parasitic diseases (Durack *et al.*, 1979; Fauci, 1982; Fletcher and Bain, 2007). In these reactive conditions, the eosinophils are not clonal and are produced in response to eosinophilopoietic cytokines (Fletcher and Bain, 2007).

Recently, four partner genes that fuse to platelet-derived growth factor receptor, alpha polypeptide (PDGFRA) to encode an active tyrosine kinase that drives clonal eosinophil production have been described (Bain, 2004; Fletcher and Bain, 2007; Robyn *et al.*, 2005; Tanaka *et al.*, 2006). The most common abnormality is a microdeletion on chromosome 4q12 resulting in (FIPILI)-PDGFRA fusion (Bain, 2004; Fletcher and Bain, 2007). Patients with this genetic abnormality are now considered to have (or to develop) eosinophilic leukemia or systemic mastocytosis (Bain, 2004; Fletcher and Bain, 2007; Robyn *et al.*, 2005; Tanaka *et al.*, 2006). Patients with the hypereosinophilic syndrome do not have this genetic finding.

Table 71.3 Mechanisms of eosinophil-induced neurotoxicity

Direct neural tissue infiltration

Damage related to eosinophil function by direct cytotoxicity or by antibody-dependent cellular cytotoxicity

Damage related to eosinophil products, by secretion into neurons, or by secretion of intracytoplasmic granules contained in the circulation, with subsequent damage to neural tissue

Embolic cerebral infarction related to local development of thrombi or a generalized hypercoagulable state

Nervous system damage secondary to eosinophil-mediated action in remote organ systems

The idiopathic hypereosinophilic syndrome is a leukoproliferative disorder characterized by cytokine-induced overproduction of eosinophils with resultant multiorgan infiltration and damage. The diagnostic criteria include evidence of end organ damage, exclusion of all other causes of eosinophilia, and a sustained absolute eosinophil count of 1500 cells/μl that has been present for at least 6 months (Osowo *et al.*, 2006).

Eosinophils have several toxic effects that can damage brain and other tissues. Both the central and peripheral nervous system can be affected by these undesirable toxic effects (Dorfman *et al.*, 1983; Durack *et al.*, 1979; Fauci, 1982).

The potential mechanisms of eosinophil-induced neuronal damage are multiple and are noted in Table 71.3 (Weaver *et al.*, 1988). Proteins derived from eosinophils can potentially injure cells and tissues. Three basic proteins have been isolated: medial-basic protein, eosinophil-cationic protein, and eosinophil-derived neurotoxin (Durack *et al.*, 1979). Release of medial-basic protein can damage endothelial cells and can promote thrombosis and artery-to-artery emboli (Durack *et al.*, 1979; Fauci, 1982). Eosinophil-cationic protein can contribute to a thrombotic tendency. Eosinophil-derived neurotoxin has a direct toxic action on neuronal tissue and on myelinated axons. In patients with eosinophilic leukemia, a high leukocrit can pack small blood vessels and contribute to thrombosis and small hemorrhages (Kawanami *et al.*, 2002), and accompanying thrombocytopenia can promote bleeding in the brain and other organs.

Loeffler's endomyocardiopathy (Corssmit *et al.*, 1999) is at times complicated by cardiac thrombi (Kocaturk and Yilmaz, 2005) and peripheral venous (Terrier *et al.*, 2006) and peripheral limb small and large arterial occlusive thrombosis (Chusid et al, 1975; Funahashi *et al.*, 2006; Ponsky *et al.*, 2005). Endothelial injury and hypercoagulability are often manifest in systemic vessels. The three most common clinical neurological syndromes that represent eosinophil-induced neurotoxicity are axonal peripheral neuropathy, dementia, and stroke (Dorfman *et al.*, 1983; Weaver *et al.*, 1988).

Brain infarction is most likely attributable to medial-basic protein-mediated endothelial damage, eosinophil-cationic protein-mediated hypercoagulability, and eosinophil-mediated cardiopathy. The patient reported by Weaver *et al.* (1988) first had a left occipital cerebral infarction followed 3 months later by a right parietal cerebral infarction. Dementia developed 1 year later, and neurophysiological study showed a polyneuropathy (Weaver *et al.*, 1988).

Management consists of the treatment of hypereosinophilia and includes prednisone and hydroxyurea. Interferon-α (Yoon *et al.*, 2000) and monoclonal antibodies (Fletcher and Bain, 2007) have also been used effectively. Concerning embolic cerebral infarctions, Weaver *et al.* (1988) recommended anticoagulation in preference to antiplatelet therapy.

Lymphomatoid granulomatosis

Lymphomatoid granulomatosis is an angiocentric lymphoproliferative condition predominantly affecting the lungs that was first described by the pathologist Dr. Averill Liebow (Katzenstein *et al.*, 1979; Liebow *et al.*, 1972). The pathology of this condition is rather distinct. Lesions consist of focal regions of polymorphic lymphoid infiltrates composed of lymphocytes, plasma cells, and large atypical mononuclear cells with frequent necrosis within the lymphoid nodules. The term granulomatosis was used by Liebow to describe the focal regions of necrosis, not to denote granulomatous inflammation (as would be found in tuberculosis and sarcoidosis) (Myers, 1990; Pisani and DeRemee, 1990). The abnormal lymphoid collections are centered around arteries and veins with transmural infiltration of the walls of the vessels by the lymphoid cells.

Series of cases show that men are affected more than women in a range of 2:1 or 3:; most often symptoms and signs develop in the fifth or sixth decade of life (Fauci *et al.*, 1982; Katzenstein *et al.*, 1979; Koss *et al.*, 1986; Myers, 1990; Pisani and DeRemee, 1990), although occasional patients develop the condition in their teens (Mizuno *et al.*, 2003). The clinical course varies considerably with some reports of prolonged courses and even spontaneous remissions (Schmidley, 2008). Pulmonary symptoms and signs predominate (Calfee *et al.*, 2007; Hochberg *et al.*, 2006; Katzenstein *et al.*, 1979). Lymphomatoid granulomatosis has recently been found to be caused by an Epstein-Barr viral infection of B lymphocytes and is classified as an Epstein-Barr virus-associated form of lymphoproliferative disease (Hochberg *et al.*, 2006; Wilson *et al.*, 1996). Lower grades of lymphomatoid granulomatosis may represent B-cell proliferation of as yet uncertain malignant potential, whereas severe lymphomatoid granulomatosis is considered a mature, diffuse B-cell form of lymphoma accompanied by an extensive but benign T-cell reaction (Schmidley, 2008).

The lung and brain regions of necrosis are presumably related to infarction caused by the cellular vascular infiltrate ("angiitis"). This condition differs from neoplastic angioendotheliosis (intravascular lymphoma described in Chapter 70) in which the lymphomatous cells pack the blood vessels, whereas in lymphomatoid granulomatosis the abnormal cells invade the vessel walls causing vessel-related damage to the tissue supplied. Some patients have responded to immunosuppressant treatment, interferon-α2b, and rituximab (Calfee *et al.*, 2007; Hochberg *et al.*, 2006; Mizuno *et al.*, 2003; Wilson *et al.*, 1996).

The most common extrapulmonary findings are in the skin and nervous system – each accounting for about one-third of patients. The skin lesions usually consist of a raised erythematous rash and occasionally skin nodules, especially on the trunk. Central nervous system (CNS) lesions are more common than are cranial or peripheral neuropathies, and usually consist of focal and multifocal brain mass lesions (Fauci *et al.*, 1982; Katzenstein *et al.*, 1979; Koss *et al.*, 1986).

The neurological symptoms usually have a gradual onset and consist of multifocal abnormalities – loss of cognition, amnesia, hemiparesis, ataxia, and so forth. Sudden-onset deficits compatible with strokes are not described. The symptoms and signs usually accumulate during months to years.

Reviews of the MRI findings in patients with lymphomatoid granulomatosis emphasize multifocal small and large mass-type lesions that involve the cerebral hemispheres and sometimes the brainstem and cerebellum (Bhagavatula and Scott, 1997; Carone *et al.*, 2006; Patsalides *et al.*, 2005; Tateishi *et al.*, 2001). The lesions usually enhance with gadolinium either in a punctate or linear fashion, but sometimes ring enhancement is noted. Brain atrophy may develop during months to years. Enhancement of the leptomeninges and dura mater sometimes occurs as does cranial nerve enhancement. The lesions can involve the orbit and cavernous sinuses (Patsalides *et al.*, 2005). The spinal fluid sometimes reveals a slight pleocytosis.

Divry-van Bogaert syndrome

Diffuse meningocerebral angiomatosis and leukoencephalopathy is a congenital recessively transmitted condition that involves both adults and children (van Bogaert, 1967; Vonsattel and Hedley-Whyte, 1989). This syndrome was first described in 1946 by Divry and van Bogaert, who had examined three brothers who had livedo reticularis and who gradually developed dementia, seizures, and pyramidal signs that developed in all three brothers about 15 years after the diagnosis (van Bogaert, 1967). Autopsy showed leptomeningeal "angiopathies" and brain infarcts. Demyelination was also present (van Bogaert, 1967).

Two forms have been traditionally separated. The adult-onset form includes skin lesions and neurological findings. The skin findings consist of the presence of a diffuse symmetrical livedo reticularis, which can increase at the onset of neurological problems. Skin biopsies show increased dermal capillaries with focal loss of "zonulae occludens" between endothelial cells (Alarcón-Segovia and Sanchez-Guerrero (1989); van Bogaert, 1967). The neurological findings include seizures, dementia, and motor disturbances. Among these symptoms, cognitive and behavioral abnormalities predominate (van Bogaert, 1967; Vonsattel and Hedley-Whyte, 1989). Motor signs are related to the presence of brain infarcts. Generally, death occurs between 10 and 15 years after the onset of neurological symptoms (van Bogaert, 1967; Vonsattel and Hedley-Whyte, 1989).

In the infantile form, the onset of symptoms occurs after the age of 3 years (van Bogaert, 1967). In one patient, a poliomyelitis vaccination was the presumptive cause (Vonsattel and Hedley-Whyte, 1989). This form includes skin anomalies and neurological disorders. In contrast to the adult form, skin lesions can be absent in children but do not differ from those found in the adult form, when present (van Bogaert, 1967; Vonsattel and Hedley-Whyte, 1989).

The neurological signs include seizures, motor involvement, and cognitive decline. The duration of the disease is shorter in adults, and death occurs generally within 24 months after onset of neurological signs (van Bogaert, 1967).

Neuropathologic abnormalities are brain infarcts, demyelination of white matter, and cerebromeningeal angiomatosis, which is the most constant and pathognomonic finding of this disease (Bussone *et al.*, 1984; Julien *et al.*, 1971; van Bogaert, 1967; Vonsattel and Hedley-Whyte, 1989). It is a large corticomeningeal network with vascular congestion and multiple vessel occlusions. Microscopic examination shows fibrotic changes of the vascular walls with fatty degeneration and amyloid deposits. These abnormalities lead to multifocal cerebral infarctions in the gray and white matters. In addition, demyelination of the central white matter is observed in nearly all the patients, and consists of axonal and oligodendrocytic loss with astrogliosis (van Bogaert, 1967). These abnormalities occur mostly predominantly around blood vessels.

Distinction of the syndrome described by Divry and van Bogaert from Snedden's syndrome (Chapter 56) is difficult and arbitrary (Ellie *et al.*, 1987). At the time of the original description, neither brain nor vascular imaging was available and anti-phospholipid antibody testing was unknown. The only distinction between the two designated conditions is the meningeal neovascularization described in the Divry-van Bogaert syndrome. However, there are few autopsies in patients with Snedden's syndrome, so the extent of meningeal vascular changes is unclear. The two conditions should be thought of as a continuum of conditions that cause livedo reticularis and small-artery CNS strokes, some of which are genetically determined and familial, and some are associated with high titers of anti-phospholipid antibodies.

Blue rubber bleb nevus syndrome

The Blue rubber bleb nevus syndrome is a very uncommon systemic disorder characterized by cutaneous and visceral cavernous hemangiomas. The name comes from the nature of the skin lesions, which are characteristically rubbery textured and easily compressible. The skin lesions are usually bluish purple, are present in childhood, and occur mostly over the trunk and extremities (Bedocs and Gould, 2003). Gastrointestinal angiomas appear most often in the small bowel, a site that appears to dominate visceral involvement. Brain angiomas have been described early in life (Kim, 2000). Angiomas may also involve the orbit, occasionally bilaterally (Chang and Rubin, 2002). Developmental venous anomalies are also sometimes found (Gabikian *et al.*, 2003).

Patients with the blue rubber bleb nevus syndrome may present with anemia from chronic gastrointestinal bleeding, and require lifelong treatment with iron and blood transfusions. Often there are many angiomatous lesions that are located throughout the gastrointestinal tract. Some have treated these lesions surgically with success (Fishman *et al.*, 2005). Children and young adults may present with seizures (Bedocs and Gould, 2003) or progressive focal neurological deficits (Satya-Murti *et al.*, 1986).

Brain imaging usually reveals multiple angiomatous lesions, some large.

REFERENCES

Alarcón-Segovia D, Sanchez-Guerrero J. (1989) Primary antiphospholipid syndrome. *Journal of Rheumatol* 16, 482–488.

Atkinson, J. L. D., Sundt, T. M. Jr., Dale, A. J. D., Cascino, T. L., and Nichols, D. A. 1989. Radiation-associated atheromatous disease of the cervical carotid artery: report of seven cases and review of the literature. *Neurosurgery*, 24, 171–8.

Bain, B. J. 2004. Relationship between idiopathic hypereosinophilic syndrome, eosinophilic leukemia, and systemic mastocytosis. *Am J Hematol*, 77, 82–5.

Bedocs, P. M., and Gould, J. W. 2003. Blue rubber-bleb nevus syndrome: a case report. *Cutis*, 71, 315–8.

Bhagavatula, K., and Scott, T. F. 1997. Magnetic resonance appearance of cerebral lymphomatoid granulomatosis. *J Neuroimaging*, 7, 120–1.

Bitzer, M., and Topka, H. 1995. Progressive cerebral occlusive disease after radiation therapy. *Stroke*, 26, 131–6.

Bowers, D. C., Liu, Y., Leisenring, W., *et al.* 2006. Late-occurring stroke among long-term survivors of childhood leukemia and brain tumors: a report from the Childhood Cancer Survivor Study. *J Clin Oncol*, 24, 5277–82.

Bowers, D. C., McNeil, D. E., Liu, Y., *et al.* 2005. Stroke as a late treatment effect of Hodgkin's disease: a report from the Childhood Cancer Survivor Study. *J Clin Oncol*, 23, 6508–15.

Burger, P. C., Mahaley, M. S. Jr., Dudka, L., *et al.* 1979. The morphological effects of radiation administered therapeutically for intracranial gliomas: a postmortem study of 25 cases. *Cancer*, 44, 1256–72.

Bussone, G., Parati, E. A., Boiardi, A., *et al.* 1984. Divry-van Bogaert syndrome. Clinical and ultrastructural findings. *Arch Neurol*, 41, 560–2.

Calfee, C. S., Shah, S. J., Wolooters, P. J., Saint, S., and King, T. E. Jr. 2007. Anchors away. *N Engl J Med*, 356, 504–9.

Carone, D. A., Benedict, R. H., Zivadinov, R., Singh, B., and Ambrus, J. L. 2006. Progressive cerebral disease in lymphomatoid granulomatosis causes anterograde amnesia and neuropsychiatric disorder. *J Neuroimaging*, 16, 163–6.

Chang, E. L., and Rubin, P. A. 2002. Bilateral multifocal hemangiomas of the orbit in the blue rubber bleb nevus syndrome. *Ophthalmology*, 109, 537–41.

Chase, T. N., Rosman, N. P., and Price, D. L. 1968. The cerebral syndromes associated with dissecting aneurysm of the aorta. A clinicopathological study. *Brain*, 91, 173–90.

Cheng, S. W. K., Ting, A. C. W., Lau, H., Lam, L. K., and Wei, W. I. 1999. Irradiation-induced extracranial carotid stenosis in patients with head and neck malignancies. *Am J Surg*, 178, 323–8.

Chusid, M. J., Dale, D. C., West, B. C., and Wolff, S. M. 1975. The hypereosinophilic syndrome. Analysis of 14 cases with review of the literature. *Medicine*, 54, 1–27.

Conomy, J. P., and Kellermeyer, R. W. 1975. Delayed cerebrovascular consequences of therapeutic radiation. A clinicopathologic study of a stroke associated with radiation-related carotid arteriopathy. *Cancer*, 36, 1702–8.

Corssmit, E. P., Trip, M. D., and Durrer, J. D. 1999. Loffler's endomyocarditis in the idiopathic hypereosinophilic syndrome. *Cardiology*, 91, 272–6.

Crawford, E. S. 1990. The diagnosis and management of aortic dissection. *JAMA*, 264, 2537–41.

DeAngelis, L. M., Delattre, J.-Y., and Posner, J. B. 1989. Radiation-induced dementia in patients cured of brain metastases. *Neurology*, 39, 789–96.

DeSanctis, R. W., Doroghazi, R. M., Austen, W. G., and Buckley, M. J. 1987. Aortic dissection. *N Engl J Med*, 317, 1060–7.

Dion, M. W., Hussey, D. H., Doornbos, J. F., *et al.* 1990. Preliminary results of a pilot study of pentoxifylline in the treatment of late radiation soft tissue necrosis. *J Radiat Oncol Biol Phys*, 19, 401–7.

Dorfman, L. J., Ransom, B. R., Formo, L. S., and Klets, A. 1983. Neuropathy in the hypereosinophilic syndrome. *Muscle Nerve*, 6, 291–8.

Durack, D. T., Sumi, S. M., and Klebanoff, S. J. 1979. Neurotoxicity of human eosinophils. *Proc Natl Acad Sci U S A*, 76, 1443–7.

Ellie, E., Julien, J., Henry, P., Vital, C., and Ferrer, X. 1987. Divry-van Bogaert cortico-meningeal angiomatosis and Sneddon's syndrome. Nosological study. *Rev Neurol (Paris)*, **143**, 798–805.

Fajardo, L. F., and Berthrong, M. 1988. Vascular lesions following irradiation. *Pathol Ann*, **23**, 297–330.

Fauci, A. S. 1982. NIH conference: the idiopathic hypereosinophilic syndrome. *Ann Intern Med*, **97**, 78–92.

Fauci, A. S., Haynes, B. F., Costa, J., Katz, P., and Wolff, S. M. 1982. Lymphomatoid granulomatosis: prospective clinical and therapeutic experience over 10 years. *N Engl J Med*, **306**, 68–74.

Fishman, S. J., Smithers, C. J., Folkman, J., *et al.* 2005. Blue rubber bleb nevus syndrome: surgical eradication of gastrointestinal bleeding. *Ann Surg*, **241**, 523–8.

Fletcher, S., and Bain, B. 2007. Diagnosis and treatment of hypereosinophilic syndromes. *Curr Opin Hematol*, **14**, 37–42.

Funahashi, S., Masaki, I., and Furuyama, T. 2006. Hypereosinophilic syndrome accompanying gangrene of the toes with peripheral arterial occlusion–a case report. *Angiology*, **57**, 231–4.

Gabikian, P., Clatterbuck, R. E., Gailloud, P., and Rigamonti, D. 2003. Developmental venous anomalies and sinus pericranii in the blue rubber-bleb nevus syndrome. Case report. *J Neurosurg*, **99**, 409–11.

Gaul, C., Dietrich, W., Friedrich, I., Sirch, J., and Erbguth, F. J. 2007. Neurological symptoms in Type A aortic dissections. *Stroke*, **38**, 292–7.

Gerber, O., Heyer, E. J., and Vieux, U. 1986. Painless dissections of the aorta presenting as acute neurologic syndromes. *Stroke*, **17**, 644–7.

Glantz, M. J., Burger, P. C., Friedman, A. H., *et al.* 1994. Treatment of radiation-induced nervous system injury with heparin and warfarin. *Neurology*, **44**, 2020–7.

Hagan, P. G., Nienaber, C. A., Isselbacher, E. M. *et al.* 2000. The International Registry of Acute Aortic Dissection (IRAD). New insights into an old disease (2000). *JAMA*, **283**, 897–903.

Haymaker, W., Ibrahim, M. Z. M., Miquel, J., *et al.* 1968. Delayed radiation effects in the brains of monkeys exposed to x and gamma rays. *J Neuropathol Exp Neurol*, **27**, 50–79.

Hirst, A. E. Jr., Johns, V. J., and Kime, S. W. 1958. Dissecting aneurysm of the aorta: a review of 505 cases. *Medicine*, **37**, 217–79.

Hochberg, E. P., Gilman, M. D., and Hasserjian, R. P. 2006. Case records of the Massachusetts General Hospital. Case 17–2006–a 34-year-old man with cavitary lung lesions. *N Engl J Med*, **354**, 2485–93.

Julien, J., Vital, C., Henry, P., Barrat, M., and Coquet, M. 1971. Corticomeningeal angiomatosis of Divry and van Bogaert. *Rev Neurol (Paris)*, **125**, 39–52.

Kang, J. H., Kwon, S. U., and Kim, J. S. 2002. Radiation-induced angiopathy in acute stroke patients. *J Stroke Cerebrovasc Dis*, **11**, 315–9.

Katzenstein, A.-L. A., Carrington, C. B., and Liebow, A. 1979. Lymphomatoid granulomatosis. A clinicopathologic study of 152 cases. *Cancer*, **43**, 360–73.

Kawanami, T., Kurita, K., Yamakawa, M., Omoto, E., and Kato, T. 2002. Cerebrovascular disease in acute leukemia: a clinicopathological study of 14 patients. *Intern Med*, **41**, 1130–4.

Kim, S. I. 2000. Blue rubber bleb nevus syndrome with central nervous system involvement. *Pediatr Neurol*, **22**, 410–2.

Kocaturk, H., and Yilmaz, M. 2005. Idiopathic hypereosinophilic syndrome associated with multiple intracardiac thrombi. *Echocardiography*, **22**, 675–6.

Koss, M. N., Hochholzer, I., Langloss, J. M., *et al.* 1986. Lymphomatoid granulomatosis: a clinicopathologic study of 42 patients. *Pathology*, **18**, 283–8.

Liebow, A. A., Carrington, C. R. B., and Friedman, P. J. 1972. Lymphomatoid granulomatosis. *Hum Pathol*, **3**, 457–558.

Mizuno, T., Takanashi, Y., Onodera, H., *et al.* 2003. A case of lymphomatoid granulomatosis/angiocentric immunoproliferative lesion with long clinical course and diffuse brain involvement. *J Neurol Sci*, **213**, 67–76.

Moersch, F. P., and Sayre, G. P. 1950. Neurologic manifestations associated with dissecting aneurysm of the aorta. *JAMA*, **144**, 1141–8.

Murros, K. E., and Toole, J. F. 1989. The effect of radiation on carotid arteries. *Arch Neurol*, 46, 449–55.

Myers, J. L. 1990. Lymphomatoid granulomatosis: past, present, & future. *Mayo Clin Proc*, **65**, 274–8.

Osowo, A., Fetten, J., and Navaneethan, S. 2006. Idiopathic hypereosinophilic syndrome: a rare but fatal condition presenting with common symptoms. *South Med J*, **99**, 188–9.

Patsalides, A. D., Atac, G., Hedge, U., *et al.* 2005. Lymphomatoid granulomatosis: abnormalities of the brain at MR imaging. *Radiology*, **237**, 265–73.

Peterson, K., Clark, H. B., Hall, W. A., and Truwit, C. L. 1995. Multifocal enhancing magnetic resonance imaging lesions following cranial irradiation. *Ann Neurol*, **38**, 237–44.

Pisani, R. J., DeRemee, R. A. 1990. Clinical implications of the histopathologic diagnosis of pulmonary lymphomatoid granulomatosis. *Mayo Clin Proc*, **65**, 151–63.

Ponsky, T. A., Brody, F., Giordano, J., *et al.* 2005. Brachial artery occlusion secondary to hypereosinophilic syndrome. *J Vasc Surg*, **42**, 796–9.

Rizzoli, H. V., and Pagnanelli, D. M. 1984. Treatment of delayed radiation necrosis of the brain. *J Neurosurg*, **60**, 589–94.

Roberts, W. C. 1981. Aortic dissection: anatomy, consequences, and causes. *Am Heart J*, **101**, 195–214.

Robyn, J., Lemery, S., McCoy, J. P., *et al.* 2005. Multilineage involvement of the fusion gene in patients with FILIPI/PDGFRA positive hypereosinophilic syndrome. *Br J Haematol*, **132**, 286–92.

Satya-Murti, S., Navada, S., and Eames, F. 1986. Central nervous system involvement in blue-rubber-bleb-nevus syndrome. *Arch Neurol*, **43**, 1184–6.

Schmidley, JW. 2008. An unusual case of multiple discrete brain lesions. *Reviews in Neurological Diseases*. **5**, 27–28, 38–41.

Silverberg, G. D., Britt, R. H., and Goffinet, D. R. 1978. Radiation-induced carotid artery disease. *Cancer*, **41**, 130–7.

Spittell, P. C., Spittell, J. A., Joyce, J. W. *et al.* 1993. Clinical features and differential diagnosis of aortic dissection: experience with 236 cases (1980 through 1990). *Mayo Clin Proc*, 68, 642–51.

St Louis, E. L., McLoughlin, M. J., and Wortzman, G. 1974. Chronic damage to medium and large arteries following irradiation. *J Can Assoc Radiol*, 25, 94–104.

Stecker, M. M., Bavaria, J. E., Barclay, D. K., *et al.* 1997. Carotid dissection with acute aortic dissection. *J Neurovasc Dis*, **2**, 166–71.

Tanaka, Y., Kurata, M., Togami, K., *et al.* 2006. Chronic eosinophilic leukaemia with the FIPILI-PDGFR alpha fusion gene in a patient with a history of combination chemotherapy. *Int J Hematol*, **83**, 152–5.

Tateishi, U., Terae, S., Ogata, A., *et al.* 2001. MR imaging of the brain in lymphomatoid granulomatosis. *AJNR Am J Neuroradiol*, **22**, 1283–90.

Terrier, B., Piette, A. M., Kerob, D., *et al.* 2006. Superficial venous thrombophlebitis as the initial manifestation of hypereosinophilic syndrome: study of the first 3 cases. *Arch Dermatol*, **142**, 1606–10.

Ullrich, N. J., Robertson, R., Kinamon, D. D. *et al.* 2007. Moyamoya following cranial irradiation for primary brain tumors in children. *Neurology*, **68**, 932–8.

van Bogaert, L. 1967. [On meningeal angiomatosis with leukodystrophy]. *Wien Z Nervenheilkd Grenzgeb*, **25**, 131–6.

Vonsattel, J.-P. G., and Hedley-Whyte, T. 1989. Diffuse meningocerebral angiomatosis and leucoencephalopathy. In *Handbook of Clinical Neurology. Vascular Diseases*, P. J. Vinken, G. W. Bruyn, and H. L. Klawans (eds.), Part III, J. F. Toole (ed.), vol. 55, The Netherlands: Elsevier Science Publishers, pp. 317–24.

Weaver, D. F., Heffernan, L. P., Purdy, R. A., Ing, V. W. 1988. Eosinophil-induced neurotoxicity: axonal neuropathy cerebral infarction, and dementia. *Neurology*, **38**, 144–146.

Wilson, W. H., Kingma, D. W., Raffeld, M., Wittes, R. E., and Jaffe, E. S. 1996. Association of lymphomatoid granulomatosis with Epstein-Barr viral infection of B lymphocytes and response to interferon-alpha 2b. *Blood*, **87**, 4531–7.

Yoon, T. Y., Ahn, G. B., and Chang, S. H. 2000. Complete remission of hypereosinophilic syndrome after interferon-alpha therapy: report of a case and literature review. *J Dermatol*, **27**, 110–5.

Zurbrugg, H. R., Leupi, F., Schupbach, P., and Althaus, U. 1988. Duplex scanner study of carotid artery dissection following surgical treatment of aortic dissection type A. *Stroke*, **19**, 970–6.

INDEX